Laboratory Applications in Clinical Pediatrics

Laboratory Applications
in Clinical Pediatrics

IRVING J. WOLMAN, M.D.

*Director of Laboratories and Hematologist,
The Children's Hospital of Philadelphia;
Associate Professor of Pediatrics, Undergraduate
and Graduate Schools of Medicine, University
of Pennsylvania; Editor, Quarterly Review
of Pediatrics; Diplomate in Pediatrics,
Pathology and Clinical Pathology*

The Blakiston Division

McGraw-Hill Book Company, Inc.
New York   Toronto   London   1957

To ROSLYN, CAROL, and JAMES

Preface

Every physician who deals with children refers constantly to the clinical laboratory. This holds true whether the immediate problem is diagnosis and treatment of an acute or chronic illness, or evaluation of an apparently well child for subclinical signs of malnutrition or disease. Even the simple "health examination" is not complete without a urine analysis and blood count.

From the standpoint of practice, the laboratory aspects of pediatrics are as distinct from those of internal medicine as are the clinical aspects of these two specialties. Normal values and the interpretations to be applied to abnormal findings often change significantly during the successive phases of growth from birth through adolescence. Furthermore, determinations on infants and young children frequently require specialized techniques because of the peculiarities of the illnesses and the much smaller volumes of the specimens.

Every pediatrician should be familiar with the scientific meaning and clinical applicability of the many available test procedures, the differences in physiologic limits at different ages, and the pathogenesis of the derangements which may develop in disease states. He should have some insight into the biochemical, cytologic, and microbiologic processes which can be assayed by laboratory analyses, and be able to interpret any disturbances which are revealed by these approaches. And for both psychologic and economic reasons he should learn to be selective rather than indiscriminate when soliciting help from the laboratory.

This book has been prepared as an aid in these directions. Intended for students and residents, for laboratory directors in general hospitals, and particularly for practitioners who are not in close contact with pediatrics teaching centers, it endeavors to condense and discuss those major laboratory phenomena which seem pertinent to the clinical care of infants and children.

Usefulness for diagnosis has been the primary touchstone. Information not immediately pertinent to practice is omitted or given but brief mention. Encyclopedic expositions are avoided, and key references only are cited. Comments concerning treatment are restricted to situations in which laboratory controls play a major role. Instructions on how to perform individual tests are left out purposely, save for those new ones not yet in the standard manuals whose performance is within the capacity of the office laboratory.

Most of the diseases are presented under the specific approaches most likely to uncover abnormal findings. This arrangement, though perhaps inconsistent with formal logic, is in accord with what happens in office and hospital. Patients usually come for medical care because of symptoms or complaints—not because of the known existence of a specific ailment.

The author assumes sole responsibility for the countless decisions concerning the choice and extent of the presentations. The validity of much of the basic material has been verified by firsthand experience gained in the study of pathology in several leading hospitals for children in this country, as a laboratory director in the United States Public Health Service during World War II, and especially during years of observation and graduate and undergraduate teaching on the wards and in the laboratories of The Children's Hospital of Philadelphia. In so far as possible, the information contained has been checked by reference to authoritative articles, monographs, and related references in the aggressively expanding fields of clinical pathology, pediatrics, and related disciplines.

Profound thanks are due my many professional friends and colleagues who were kind enough to comment constructively on preliminary drafts of the chapters. Acknowledgments are due also to various medical journals, notably the *American Journal of Medical Sciences* and the *Quarterly Review of Pediatrics*, for permission to reproduce small portions from numerous original reviews and editorials which have already appeared in print.

IRVING J. WOLMAN

Contents

CHAPTER 1

Hemoglobin Level, Erythrocyte Count, and Related Variables

Within the body economy the prime function of the circulating hemoglobin is to carry oxygen. The immature red cells or rubricytes of the bone marrow synthesize the hemoglobin, and the mature red cells transport the hemoglobin through the circulation.

The average infant or child daily produces 1 to 4 gm of hemoglobin and 3 to 12 billion new red cells to meet the needs of replacement and growth. An acceleration in the normal rate of production is accompanied usually by a peripheral reticulocytosis.

HEMOGLOBIN

Iron is essential to the formation of the heme component of the hemoglobin molecule. Amino acids and related proteinogenic substances are needed for the globin and protoporphyrin fractions. Copper, cobalt, pyridoxine, niacin, vitamin B_{12}, the citrovorum factor, and other trace nutrients are indispensable also. An inadequate intake of any of these may be reflected in a depressed blood hemoglobin level. The most common form of malnutritional anemia in all countries is that which results from a shortage of iron.

Since the life span of the average erythrocyte is approximately 110 to 120 days, a little less than 1 per cent of the total mass of circulating red cells is broken down every 24 hours. The effete erythrocytes either disintegrate in the circulation or are destroyed by the spleen or other elements of the reticuloendothelial system. The protoporphyrin ring within the hemoglobin, made up of iron, globin, and bilirubin, is first oxidatively opened. The iron is removed and combined in ferric form with the iron-binding protein of serum, to be transported to the bone marrow for formation of new hemoglobin or to the liver or spleen or elsewhere for storage. The globin-bilirubin complex, which gives the "indirect" or delayed van den Bergh reaction, is also released into the circulation. Within the liver the globin in this complex is released to the body protein pool,

1

and the bilirubin when not wholly excreted into the bile appears in the plasma to give a "direct" van den Bergh reaction.

When red cells are being destroyed with extreme rapidity, as in severe hemolytic disorders, free hemoglobin and heme pigments such as methemalbumin may make their appearance in the plasma. Overflow of free hemoglobin into the urine takes place when the plasma level reaches 100 mg per 100 ml.

Hemoglobinometry

A movement is under way in the United States for the general acceptance of a national Standard of Reference for hemoglobin. This will be in the form of a preparation of crystalline human hemoglobin which conforms with rigid chemical and physical criteria. From this a Standard for Distribution will be prepared in the form of a certified solution of cyanmethemoglobin to be distributed to clinical laboratories for calibration of hemoglobinometers. The iron content of hemoglobin is accepted as 0.335 per cent; this corresponds with an equivalent weight for hemoglobin of 16,700 per atom of iron and with an oxygen capacity of 1.34 ml per gm of hemoglobin.

Many possibilities for error will still attend the collecting of the blood samples and the manipulation of the instruments. The eye's capacity to judge color value is a variable in many procedures. There are, in addition, a few situations such as the shock syndrome and the newborn period in which the ooze from a skin puncture does not truly represent the central circulation.

DIRECT CHEMICAL ANALYSIS. Direct chemical measurement of hemoglobin is used mostly in research, in the establishment of standards, and in calibrating visual and photoelectric hemoglobinometers. Though the most accurate, this approach requires fairly large samples of venous blood and more skill, time, and equipment than are available to the average individual who does blood counts.

Hemoglobin concentration when determined by the oxygen- or carbon monoxide–combining capacities of whole blood regularly proves to be 2 to 3 per cent lower than when determined by iron analysis. The small amounts of methemoglobin and sulfhemoglobin and other inert pigments in the blood which contain iron but fail to carry blood gases account for this slight discrepancy. The results obtained by photoelectric or colorimetric methods are in close accordance with those of iron analysis.

In methemoglobinemia or sulfhemoglobinemia a patient may have pronounced air hunger and other signs of oxygen lack, yet the hemoglobin readings by methods not based on gas-carrying capacity may fall within the normal range.

COLORIMETRIC METHODS. A number of such methods are in common use. The trend is more and more toward using photoelectric devices in order to minimize subjective errors.

Photoelectric Colorimetry. This is perhaps the most accurate of the simpler approaches, in that the instruments are highly sensitive and the personal equation reduced to a minimum. In duplicate determinations on venous blood specimens from 200 subjects examined in a survey, Wiehl found the standard error of single determinations to be only ± 0.145 gm per 100 ml. Once the apparatus has been calibrated, which requires some skill, the only sources of inaccuracy lie in the measurement of the diluent and the filling of the pipet with blood. Readings are performed quickly and conveniently.

Direct Colorimetric Comparison. The methods of Dare, Gowers, and Tallqvist and the Tintometer and related methods, all based on direct visual comparison of color, are no longer widely used. They have been found subject to numerous sources of error such as dirt on the glass, cloudiness of the serum, air bubbles, improper size of the drop, and subjective difficulties in the precise matching of color. Serial readings from the same blood specimen are often not closely reproducible.

"Gray" Photometers. Green light of a properly chosen wave length appears gray when passed through oxyhemoglobin solution. This principle has been applied to the construction of highly reliable hemoglobinometers, in which the intensity of the gray light is compared visually with that of an accurately calibrated wedge of neutral gray glass.

Carbon Monoxide Hemoglobin. The Haldane method, more popular in England than in the United States, measures the carbon monoxide hemoglobin after coal gas has been passed for at least 2 minutes through blood diluted with slightly alkaline fluid. This method is satisfactory in experienced hands. One needs a source of carbon monoxide, a standard undeteriorated solution for comparison, a jaundice-free specimen since bilirubin alters the color, and a good eye for color matching. The carbon monoxide method has proven highly accurate when adapted to photoelectric colorimetry.

Cyanmethemoglobin and Alkaline Hemoglobin. These two derivatives can be measured in dilute solutions with visual standards or a calibrated electric photometer. The use of the cyanide reagent is dangerous outside of research departments.

Acid Hematin. The Sahli, Newcomer, Hellige, Haden-Hauser, Autenrieth, and similar methods measure the intensity of the brown color of acid hematin produced by acidification of the blood, usually in dilute solution.

SOURCES OF VARIATION IN CLINICAL HEMOGLOBINOMETRY. *Physiologic Factors.* Blood samples from the ear lobes of children often give slightly higher readings than those secured by venipuncture. Blood flowing freely from any finger tip, except in the neonatal period, gives readings identical with venous blood. Moderate squeezing of the finger tip to hasten the flow has an unimportant influence (though the results of tests for coagulability may be much distorted thereby). Should extremely representative readings be desired, several independent estimations can be made and the average taken.

Differences amounting up to 2 gm hemoglobin per 100 ml of circulating blood may be encountered in the same child tested on consecutive days or on the morning and afternoon of the same day. Generally these variations are less than 1 gm per 100 ml. They are due to fluctuations in plasma volume and to stagnation changes at the site of puncture. Exercise or excitement may cause a minor transitory hemoconcentration, mediated apparently through splenic contraction which introduces additional red cells into the circulation.

Infants under 1 month of age almost invariably show significantly higher hemoglobin levels and red cell counts in blood from a toe, heel, or finger puncture than in blood drawn from a vein. Here, local stagnation and greater permeability of the immature capillaries produce a mild local hemoconcentration. Oettinger and Mills found, in 24 infants, an average difference of 3.6 gm per 100 ml between venous and capillary (toe) blood in the first hour of life. At 5 days of age the average difference was 2.2 gm and at 3 weeks 1.1 gm. A similar phenomenon of even greater magnitude may take place at any age during the shock reaction.

Personal Error in Color Matching. Individuals vary considerably in their ability to match colors exactly. Experiments with physicians and technicians have shown that those whose readings deviate appreciably from the normal tend always to do so in the same direction, too high or too low. The extent of this visual deviation from the actual value for hemoglobin as determined chemically or photometrically may amount to as much as ±4.0 gm per 100 ml. It is important, therefore, for everyone who uses a visual method to ascertain both the extent of his subjective bias (if any) as well as the reliability of his instrument. This can be done by comparing a series of personal readings made on one's own instrument with others obtained on the same specimens with a standardized photoelectric device. The average deviation thus determined may then be utilized with all future readings. If this correction is large, a less deviant instrument should be procured.

Variations in Colored Standards. Another difficulty with visual readings is that the color of the standard does not always match that of the hemoglobin solution. This holds especially for the tinted-glass standards incorporated in most portable instruments. Sometimes already inaccurate when newly purchased, the hue of glass may fade with age. Every instrument which contains a colored-glass standard should be subjected to recalibration every few months.

Conversion of Acid Hematin. The conversion of adult hemoglobin to acid hematin at room temperature tends to be approximately 75 per cent complete at 1 minute, 95 per cent at 5 minutes, 99 per cent at 15 to 30 minutes, and 100 per cent in 1 to 2 hours. Fetal hemoglobin (p. 108), present in significant amounts during the first months in all infants and throughout life in some of the severe hereditary red cell dyscrasias, is converted more slowly. Hence when instruments employing the acid hematin reaction such as the Sahli and Haden-Hauser are being used with such patients, reading should be deferred until at least 30 minutes have passed.

Reporting in Per Cent. The expressing of childhood hemoglobin levels in terms of per cent is to be condemned. The reference standard for 100 per cent is supposed to represent the mean or optimum value for healthy adult men; and there is little sense in comparing young children with adults. More importantly, unanimity is lacking as to what hemoglobin level constitutes 100 per cent. Some laboratory apparatuses take 13.5 gm as 100 per cent, others 14.5 gm, and still others 17.2 gm. Logically, if the 100 per cent concept is to be used, separate sets of standards must be provided for each year of childhood and for the first few postnatal months, inasmuch as mean and optimal values alter significantly with growth.

Normal Childhood Levels

There is no precise uniformity as to the "normal" ranges of variation in childhood population groups for either the hemoglobin level or the red cell count. Presumably healthy children of the same age have readings which give a wide scatter. These divergences have been ascribed to dietary differences, physiologic or hereditary or constitutional deviations, recent intercurrent infections, proximity to meals or exercise, time of day, birth weight, emotional factors, home conditions, and nutritional and endocrine status. Altitude is of significance; children being reared in cities like Denver (altitude 5,000 ft), Mexico City (7,500 ft), and La Paz (20,000 ft) have more circulating red cells and hemoglobin per unit volume of blood than those residing near sea level, as in Philadelphia or San Diego. Averages for economically depressed groups tend to be lower than for those economically privileged. Levels usually drop a little during the winter months when growth is slower and respiratory tract infections more common. Widespread administration of liberal amounts of iron-containing foods or of medicinal iron tends to raise the mean hemoglobin levels of population groups. Data on ambulatory childhood populations have been published by Washburn, Mack, Kaucher, Wintrobe, Osgood, Hawkins, and many others.

More studies are needed of groups of healthy children who have had an ample intake of iron and other pertinent food substances—studies so designed that with these nutritive variables at their optimum one can elucidate more adequately the importance of race, body weight, barometric pressure, speed of body growth, endocrinal function, and other suspected influences. The accumulation of "standards" by these approaches will then make it feasible to truly contrast an individual child under certain circumstances with other essentially healthy children in the same circumstances.

If "normal" is thought of as being synonymous with "optimal," then perhaps a good working definition of a normal hemoglobin level for any single child would be that level which can not be pushed higher by the giving of iron or other nutritional hematinic agents, excluding of course those situations in which factors other than dietary are causing an unphysiologic depression.

Data gathered from random population groups are not satisfactory for reference purposes, inasmuch as children with anemia have not necessarily been excluded. The optimal figures listed in Table 1-1 are based on selected published surveys from the United States, Canada, and Great Britain and the author's own observations on healthy Philadelphia children who were in good nutrition and free from obvious disease.

Table 1-1. Red Cells and Hemoglobin and Related Variables

(Approximate optimal mean values for healthy well-nourished full-term infants and children *)

Age	Hemoglobin (gm per 100 ml)	Red blood cells (millions per cu mm)	Hematocrit (per cent)	Mean cellular volume (cu μ)	Mean cellular hemoglobin (μμgm)
6–48 hours	16–22	4.8–6.6	53–63	95–110	35
3–7 days	13–20	4.6–6.4	50–60	95–110	35
2 weeks	18	5.5	57	104	34
3 weeks	17	5.2	52	102	33
4 weeks	16	4.8	47	98	32
5 weeks	15	4.6	43	94	31
6 weeks	14	4.4	39	90	30
7 weeks	13	4.2	36	85	29
8 weeks	12	4.0	34	85	28
3 months	11.5	4.1	34	84	28
4 months	11.8	4.4	35	80	28
5 months	11.8	4.5	35	79	26
6 months	12	4.7	36	77	25
9–12 months	12	4.8	36	76	25
18 months	12.5	5.0	37	75	25
2–6 years	13	5.0	38	76	26
7–12 years	14	5.2	41	79	27
13–17 years (girls)	14	5.2	41	79	29
13–17 years (boys)	15	5.7	44	78	28

Hemoglobin concentration in packed red cells: 33 to 34 per cent at all ages

* Based on published and original data from the United States, Canada, and Great Britain.

With preschool children beyond infancy a hemoglobin level of 12 or 13 gm per 100 ml may be deemed optimal. This rises slowly in later childhood and becomes 13 or 14 gm at the onset of puberty. A further rise ensues during adolescence, more prominent in boys than in girls. Upper normal limits are 16 to 18 gm for adolescent boys, depending on age and maturity, and 14 to 16 gm for adolescent girls. There are no appreciable sex differences before puberty.

NEWBORN PERIOD. The ranges of normal variation for hemoglobin level as well as for all other blood constituents are considerably wider in the first few weeks than in any other period of life. Diverse variable influences play a role here—body weight, gestational age, management of the cord, postuterine age of the infant in hours or days, neonatal lability of the blood volume, and site of the sample taken for test.

Clement Smith has calculated from published data that on the first day of life the hemoglobin level has a mean of 19.85 gm per 100 ml in peripheral blood and 17.0 gm in venous blood. With 133 normal newborn English infants Mollison and Cutbush found a mean concentration in cord blood of 16.55 gm per 100 ml, with a standard deviation of ±1.5 gm. Of the readings, 95 per cent fell between 13.6 and 19.6 gm. The above figures are derived chiefly from studies of cord specimens. Blood collected from a vein after the first hour or two of life gives somewhat higher.values.

From the first to the eighth day the hemoglobin level tends to remain constant. The postnatal fall then becomes apparent. It is probable that this decline actually begins on the first day, but is obscured by shrinkage of blood volume in association with the physiologic decrease of body weight that takes place in the first week. Chuinard, Osgood, and Ellis give mean values for the first week of 16.3 gm per 100 ml, with 95 per cent of the readings falling between 12.3 and 20.3 gm. In newborn infants the individual red cells have a higher content of hemoglobin than in older children and adults.

Time of Clamping the Cord. The hemoglobin and red count levels of the newborn period are influenced by the time interval before the umbilical cord is clamped or cut. In two groups of 25 infants studied by DeMarsh, Alt, and Windle, the peripheral blood during the first week when the cords were clamped instantly averaged 5.45 million red cells per cu mm and 19.5 gm of hemoglobin, whereas when the cords were clamped after an appreciable number of minutes the averages were 6.01 million and 22.1 gm. The group with immediate clamping of the cord maintained a reticulocytosis of 6 to 8 per cent for the first 5 days, whereas those in whom tying was delayed had a mean peak of 5.8 per cent recticulocytes at 24 hours and a mean of 4 per cent at 48 hours.

From 75 to 135 ml of blood is contained in the umbilical veins. Most of this will be forced into the infant circulation if time is allowed for the emptied uterus to contract around the blood-filled placenta. Failure to receive such placental blood may predispose to later anemia, especially in premature infants.

In a series of cesarean section infants studied by Stevenson and Erhard, the mean red cell count on the first day was 4.84 million and the hemoglobin 16.1 gm; in a control series of infants delivered vaginally, 5.42 million and 17.3 gm. In both groups the umbilical cords were clamped immediately.

POSTNEONATAL INFANCY. A slow but steady decline in the blood hemoglobin level becomes apparent after the first week. This is due to diminution in the rate of hemopoiesis in the presence of growing body size and blood volume. The rate of hemodestruction is increased very little if at all (p. 13). For example, Guest found a fall in Cincinnati, Ohio, infants from a mean level of 19 gm per 100 ml in the first 10 days of life to 12 gm at 2 months.

In Horan's series of 249 normal infants in Birmingham, England, the mean peripheral hemoglobin level was 20.7 gm per 100 ml at age 0 to 48 hours and 19.8 gm at 3 to 7 days. This fell to 11.7 gm at 9 to 12 weeks, rose slowly to 12.4 gm at 5 to 6 months of age, and was 11.6 gm at 1 year.

With healthy Minnesota infants Leichsenring and associates found a mean hemoglobin level of approximately 12.5 gm at 1 month of age. This receded to 11.4 gm at 2 months, rose to 12.4 gm in the succeeding 3 months, fell slightly again, and returned to about 12.2 gm at 1 year.

The mean level of white infants between the ages of 4 and 12 months has been said to be higher by 0.5 to 1.0 gm per 100 ml than that of Negro infants of corresponding age. This difference may be of nutritional rather than of racial origin.

Woodruff and Bridgeforth conducted a study in Nashville, Tenn., to determine whether a moderate maternal anemia during late pregnancy would result in lowered hemoglobin levels in the infant. No significant differences were found during the first year between the offspring of 89 mothers with a mean hemoglobin level of 9.91 per 100 ml and of 93 mothers with a mean hemoglobin level of 13.09 gm. The mean hemoglobin curve was almost identical with that of Leichsenring's normal infants. This is in contrast with the earlier observation of Strauss that severe maternal iron-deficiency anemia (e.g., with hemoglobin levels of about 5 gm) is often followed by the development of infantile nutritional anemia. An important variable is the age at which the feeding of iron-containing foods is begun. When the congenital reserve of iron is meager, the starting of these foods soon after the second month helps to protect against later nutritional anemia (Chap. 51).

PREMATURELY BORN INFANTS. In the fetus aged 18 weeks the hemoglobin level is approximately 10 gm per 100 ml. This average increases slowly, being about 12 gm at 24 weeks, 13 gm at 32 weeks, and 14 gm shortly before term. These values have been determined by study of the cord blood of premature infants. With these the same postnatal rise and the same relations to early and late clamping of the cord take place as with full-term infants. It would seem more important to delay tying the cords of premature infants than of full-term ones because (1) prematurely born infants are more prone to develop anemia in later infancy, and (2) a larger proportion of their total blood and therefore of their iron reserve lies in the placenta.

Much of the hemoglobin in the fetus and the premature infant at birth is more resistant to denaturation by alkali, has a greater avidity for oxygen, and will reach a higher degree of saturation under a diminished oxygen tension than the adult type of hemoglobin.

The hemoglobin level in capillary blood of prematurely born infants tends to remain more or less constant from the first to tenth day of age, once the postpartum adjustments have been made. The encountered readings may range from 12 to 20 gm per 100 ml, with most falling between 14 and 18 gm. Birth weight is of negligible influence here; an infant weighing but 1,000 gm may have a higher concentration of hemoglobin in his blood than another weighing 2,500 gm. Greater peripheral stasis or dehydrative shrinkage of blood volume can balance out any inherent difference referable to smaller body weight.

The extent of postneonatal hemoglobin and red cell changes in prematurely born infants depends in part on birth weight and prenatal factors and in part on the management during the first year of life. Those who do not receive transfusions or supplemental iron suffer a progressive fall in hemoglobin which is more pronounced and much more prolonged than that of full-term infants.

Whether given antianemic treatment or not, the mean hemoglobin for premature infants of birth weight below 1,500 gm at 3 months averages 8 to 9 gm per 100 ml; for those of birth weight between 1,500 and 2,000 gm, 9.5 gm; for those of birth weight between 2,000 and 2,500 gm, 10 gm. The ones with the greatest weight gains are likely to have the lowest hemoglobin values at 3 months, perhaps because the more rapid increase in blood volume serves as a dilution factor. If dietary supplements of iron are given after the first few weeks, the hemoglobin levels begin to rise after the third month and reach the range for full-term infants at 6 to 15 months of age. The levels in infants below 1,500 gm often rise faster and reach normal limits sooner than in those of heavier birth weight. If not given iron, infants of birth weight under 1,500 gm reach a low point of 6 to 8 gm of hemoglobin sometime between 6 and 12 months of age and may not experience an appreciable rise for 6 months or more thereafter. With higher birth weights the fall is not so pronounced. The lowest point is more likely to be 8 or 9 gm reached at 4 to 6 months of age, and recovery is more rapid.

Factors influencing the extent and duration of this "physiologic anemia of prematurity," in addition to birth weight, are diet, infections, maternal iron stores, twinning, and transfusions. Transfusion therapy is not needed unless the hemoglobin level falls below a determined threshold. Judgments differ as to whether this threshold should be set as high as 8 gm or as low as 5 gm per 100 ml, at or after the third month of life. Pertinent objections to transfusions seem to be (1) the inadvisability of subjecting infants to a procedure which may be unnecessary, and (2) the fear of reactions in the broad sense, including late complications such as serum hepatitis. These are counterbalanced by the general clinical impression that transfusion when given to subthreshold infants does improve nutritional status, rate of weight gain, and perhaps resistance to infection. Any major operative procedure should be preceded or accompanied by a transfusion if the hemoglobin level is below 10 gm per 100 ml.

Premature infants who are given transfusions frequently, commencing at about the third week of life, will have hemoglobin curves which run

Table 1-2. Ranges in Hemoglobin Values with Age and Sex among Selected Healthy 7- to 14-year-old Saskatoon Children *

	Age (years)	No. of Children	Range (gm Hb per 100 ml)	Average	Standard deviation
Boys	7	91	11.2–14.9	13.1	0.91
	8	114	11.8–15.4	13.4	0.83
	9	74	11.6–15.8	13.6	0.95
	10	87	11.5–15.2	13.6	0.85
	11	91	11.9–16.7	13.6	0.84
	12	84	12.0–16.1	13.8	1.01
	13	92	12.3–16.2	14.1	0.88
	14	103	12.0–16.4	14.4	1.11
Girls	7	99	10.9–15.0	13.0	0.84
	8	98	11.5–15.6	13.2	0.84
	9	99	11.5–15.4	13.4	0.83
	10	100	10.0–16.1	13.6	0.92
	11	92	12.1–16.1	13.6	0.82
	12	82	11.5–16.1	13.9	0.90
	13	101	11.8–16.2	14.0	0.97
	14	77	12.2–16.3	13.9	0.97
Boys	7–14	736	11.2–16.7	13.7	0.89
Girls	7–14	748	10.0–16.3	13.6	0.87
Entire group	7–14	1,484	10.0–16.7	13.6	0.77

SOURCE: Reprinted by permission, Hawkins and Kline, *Blood* 5:278–285, 1950.

* The determinations were made carefully with capillary blood taken from the finger tip and measured by the cyanmethemoglobin method of Collier, utilizing 0.340 as the percentage of iron in hemoglobin.

approximately parallel to those of full-term infants, with a minimum at about the eighth week.

CHILDHOOD. The hemoglobin levels in 392 Detroit children 2 to 18 years old studied by Kaucher and associates ranged from 10.5 to 18 gm per 100 ml and averaged 13.5 gm. No great differences were found between determinations in the fall and spring or in boys and girls. The only trend in this series was a rise from 12.5 gm per 100 ml at 3 years to 13.5 gm at 10 years.

The distribution and averages for hemoglobin levels in a selected population of healthy school children are well illustrated in the report of

Hawkins and Kline. In order to prepare a table of normal values these authors in 1948 surveyed 1,669 school children in Saskatoon, Saskatchewan, Canada. Preliminary medical examination excluded 11 per cent of the children from the tabulations because they had had more than the usual degree of illness. The general level of health and body weight in the remaining 89 per cent was extremely good (Table 1-2). Saskatoon is only about 1,600 ft above sea level, an altitude hardly sufficient to elevate the average hemoglobin level appreciably.

ADOLESCENCE. Wiehl found the mean hemoglobin level for well-nourished white New York City girls aged 12 to 17 years to remain at approximately 13.8 gm per 100 ml of blood. For adolescent boys of comparable status the mean hemoglobin at 12 years was about 13.6 gm. This rose to 14.9 gm at 14 years and more slowly to 15.2 gm at 17 years. Interestingly, the hemoglobin level in the boys was correlated more closely with physical maturity than with chronologic age. The mean for all boys with no pubic hair was 13.5 gm (about the same as that for age 12 years); for those with sparse pubic hair, 14.1 gm; for those with a moderate amount, 14.9 gm; and for those with an abundance, 15.2 gm (approximately the mean for ages 16 and over).

ERYTHROCYTE COUNT

Enumeration of the number of erythrocytes per cubic millimeter of circulating blood by the hemocytometer method is far from precise. Successive counts made accurately with the standard methods have an inherent error up to ±8 per cent, which is ±0.4 million when the true red cell count is 5.0 million per cu mm. This potentially wide range of variation is the summation of the random deviations inherent in each of the successive steps in the procedure. The greatest variable is the uneven distribution of the cells in the counting chamber.

Photoelectric methods have been proposed to determine the red cell count by measuring the light scattering of erythrocytes in a standardized suspension. Since the property measured is influenced not only by the number but also by the shape and size of the suspended particles, the reliability of this approach in pediatrics, where normal cells vary in size with age and where different diseases give rise to various morphologic abnormalities, is subject to question.

Normal Values

The red cell count displays a trend somewhat similar to that of hemoglobin concentration (Table 1-1). It is above adult level at birth and in the first few days of life and falls gradually to a low point at 2 to 4 months of age. It rises more rapidly than the hemoglobin value and reaches the prepuberty level before the end of the first or second year.

Significant sex differences are not noted prior to the onset of adolescence. At this time a slight rise occurs, more prominent in boys than in girls.

NEWBORN PERIOD. From reports published by others, Clement Smith calculated the mean red cell count for full-term newborns at the time of birth to be 5.64 million for peripheral blood and 4.80 for venous blood, chiefly cord specimens. Normal variability is wide. Incompatibilities between mother and infant with respect to ABO, Rh, or related blood factors affect the red cell and hemoglobin levels only exceptionally (Chap. 13).

Evidences of the fetal blood picture still remain in the newborn period. Reticulocyte levels up to 5 per cent of all red cells are not uncommon in cord blood. These fall to less than 2 per cent within a few days, and to less than 1 per cent after the second week. Nucleated red cells may also be free in the circulation at birth, in numbers up to 10 per 100 leukocytes; these rarely persist beyond the third or fourth day.

Higher counts of nucleated red cells, or their undue persistence, may be found in association with certain abnormal states: prematurity, erythroblastosis fetalis, congenital syphilis, prolonged asphyxia or anoxemia, maternal diabetes, bacterial infections, severe congenital heart disease, cytomegalic inclusion disease, and pronounced damage to the liver.

The red cell count rises significantly in the first 2 or 3 hours after birth. Thus Findlay's studies of 11 newborn infants of varying degrees of maturity showed augmentations of hemoglobin, red cells, and hematocrit ranging from 13 to 70 per cent. The average rises in Windle's infants amounted to 1 million cells at 1 hour in 25 whose cords were clamped at the instant of birth, and to 1.5 million in 25 whose cords were not clamped until enough time had elapsed to permit much placental blood to flow into the infant.

With 293 newborn infants, Wegelius found a mean red cell rise in the first 2 hours of about 450,000 cells, or 9 per cent. Higher increases were noted in the presence of asphyxia. Since the magnitude of the rise is the same in venous as in capillary blood, peripheral stasis cannot explain the phenomenon. There was a corresponding adjustment of the hemoglobin level, an absolute rise in reticulocytes, an increase in mean diameter of the red cells from 7.6 to 7.8 μ, and in the packed red cell volume (hematocrit) from 57.2 to 64.1 per cent. The leukocyte pattern showed negligible changes.

Because of these physiologic variations and shifts, all descriptions of the blood pattern in groups of infants "at birth" should note how many in the group were prematurely born, the exact ages of the infants in hours at the time of the test, whether the samples were taken from the peripheral skin or the veins, and whether or not the infants had received placental blood by late clamping of the cord.

POSTNEONATAL INFANCY. With 615 white Cincinnati infants and children from birth to 5¼ years who had never received medicinal iron, Guest, Brown, and Wing found the mean count in cord blood to be 4.8 million, with a range from 3.8 to 6 million. During the first 10 days of life the mean count was 5.2 million, with a range from 3.8 to 7 million. It then declined rapidly to 3.8 million at 30 to 90 days with a range of 2.4 to 5.4 million (the many lower values in this series were probably due in part to inclusion of some cases of iron-deficiency anemia). The red cell counts in Horan's British breast-fed infants gave considerably higher values, presumably because all were maturely full-term and healthy. At birth the mean red cell count was 6.54 million per cu mm; at 9 to 12 weeks, 4.14; at 25 to 28 weeks, 5.14; at 33 to 36 weeks, 4.72; and then rose steadily to 5.41 million at 53 to 56 weeks.

Physiologic Anemia of the Newborn. Once normal respiration has been established in the newborn infant, prenatal oxygen-carrying mechanisms prove to be in physiologic excess, and fetal hemoglobin (p. 108) begins to disappear. The high red cell and hemoglobin concentrations an infant is born with constitute an ample reserve in the direction of satisfying the oxygen needs of the body for the next 2 months. During this interval, while physical exertions are at a minimum, the production of new red cells appears to come almost to a standstill, to wait until the normal processes of attrition and aging and the body growth of the infant have reduced the oxygen supply in the blood to where the bone marrow becomes stimulated once more. Evidences of sluggish red cell formation during the first 2 months include a subnormal reticulocyte count and an unduly high ratio of granulocytes to rubricytes within the bone marrow. There is little evidence that red cell destruction is much accelerated during this period of hemopoietic adjustment. Should some special situation impose an unusual demand for new red cells, however, such as a hemolytic episode, a sudden hemorrhage, or a cyanotic heart lesion, the bone marrow will be found able to resume red cell proliferation immediately. The responsiveness of the bone marrow to red cell need nevertheless appears to be less sensitive in the early months than later.

The extent of this neonatal drop is highly variable, as indicated in the foregoing data from Guest's studies. With prematurely born infants the numerical value of the drop is more pronounced and even more variable, as discussed on page 9.

Reexcitation of red cell and hemoglobin formation usually begins between the sixth and tenth weeks when iron deficiency is not present and may be heralded by a 1 to 4 per cent reticulocytosis lasting for a few weeks. This reticulocytosis is governed in sharpness and duration by the rapidity of weight gain, the extent of the previous decline of the red cell count, and the availability of iron in the diet or the body reserves. After enough new cells have been produced to reach a level efficient for the infant economy, the reticulocytosis subsides to a maintenance level slightly under 1 per cent, the exact value varying with the individual.

From the standpoints of volumetric measurements and appearances in the stained film, the red cells are normochromic or slightly macrocytic through the first 2 months of life. Size variations are a little more pronounced than in later life. The average size of the red cells then becomes somewhat smaller (Table 1-1). The extent of this microcytic tendency depends upon the management of the infant. If no iron supplement is in the diet, the microcytosis and hypochromia become clearly evident. When supplemental iron is fed, these changes are minimal. Conversely, infections and prematurity may promote their development. Exceptionally the usual postneonatal fall in blood values occurs belatedly, or may even fail to appear.

If after the first 3 months the count should fail to rise properly, the possibility of iron-deficiency anemia or of a hereditary dysfunction must be looked into. Anemia is more likely to develop if the infant was born prematurely, or came from a multiple pregnancy, or had bleeding in the neonatal period, or if the maternal diet during pregnancy had been severely deficient in iron.

Exceptionally one sees infants often prematurely born whose postneonatal status is that of a pronounced normochromic anemia which cannot be explained in terms of hemorrhage, excessive hemodestruction, blood group incompatibility, or other recognized causes. They may have a peripheral reticulocytosis. The spleen and liver are not enlarged, and neonatal icterus has not been pronounced or prolonged. In some of these there may have been an intrauterine communication between infant and maternal circulations, as shown by the compatibility of the blood groups and the demonstration of declining amounts of fetal hemoglobin in the maternal blood stream for some weeks after birth.

PREMATURELY BORN INFANTS. The red cell pattern of prematurely born infants at the moment of birth depends to some extent upon gestational age. Red cell formation begins in the yolk sac, but shifts to the body mesenchyme and blood vessels at about the fifth week. The liver is the most active hemopoietic organ from the second month until midfetal life. The spleen starts to produce red cells at the end of the second month, and the bone marrow during the third month. The first red cells to appear are like primitive marrow cells, with large nuclei and only recognizable traces of hemoglobin in their cytoplasm. At 3 months the circulating red cells are approximately 90 per cent reticulocytes; at 6 months, 15 to 30 per cent; and just before birth, 4 to 6 per cent. Nucleated red cells circulate in the fetus, diminishing with maturation until they number only about 0.1 per cent at the end of full gestation.

The fetal red cell count rises from less than 400,000 per cu mm at 5 weeks gestational age to 3.5 million at 6 months and 4 to 5 million at 8 months. Infants of 800 to 1,500 gm birth weight have 3.5 to 5.5 million red cells in the first few days after delivery, usually about 4.5 million. Infants of 1,500 to 2,500 gm birth weight have from 4 to 7 million red cells after delivery, usually about 5.5 million.

In the fetus and smaller premature the red cells are large, less uniform, and have a high hemoglobin content. In dry smears their average diameter has been reported as 9.2 μ at 3 months and 8.1 μ at 6 months.

Prematurely born infants usually display nucleated red cells in their circulation at birth. These may be as many as 20 per cent of all the red cells when the weight is very low and are believed to reflect the existence of extramedullary foci of hemopoiesis. They disappear during the first week regardless of the birth weight. Reticulocytosis is prominent also in prematurely born infants and may take as long as 3 months to subside.

Just as with full-term infants, the red cell count of prematurely or immaturely born infants falls to a low point at the eighth to twelfth week, and then slowly rises again. Wide scatter of readings occurs in all weight ranges. Regardless of birth weight the red cell counts in such infants average about 3.4 million at 12 weeks and 3.8 to 2.2 million at 6 months. Supplements of dietary iron or medication with liver or vitamins seem to have only a minimal influence in counteracting the extent of this "physiologic" decline or in promoting a more rapid rise to levels normal for full-term infants. If small weekly transfusions are given during the first few months, the red cell curve will be less depressed, according to Rossier and Potiron.

CHILDHOOD. The mean red cell count in Osgood and Baker's 21 Oregon children aged 4 to 13 years was almost exactly 5 million. The lowest figure was 4.06 and the highest 6.16 million; the 95 per cent range was 4.2 to 5.8 million. Studies in other geographic areas have revealed essentially identical value ranges, with a slight rise above 5 million beginning after age 6 years.

ADOLESCENCE. In several hundred well-nourished boys aged 12 to 18 years studied by Wiehl in New York City the average red cell count at each year was approximately 5.7 million, except for an elevation to 6.0 million at 13 years. The 80 percentile range was approximately 5.3 to 6.2 million, and slightly higher at age 13. The mean red cell count for girls exhibited a downward trend from an average of 5.4 million at 12 years to 5.1 million at 17 years, with no rise at 13 years. The 80 percentile range was 4.7 to 5.6 million.

MEAN ERYTHROCYTE MEASUREMENTS

Packed Cell Volume (PCV, Hematocrit)

MEASUREMENT. That fraction of a unit volume of whole blood constituted by the red cells and their contained hemoglobin can be measured by centrifuging a sample of blood containing an anticoagulant in a hematocrit tube and noting the comparative volume of the mass of packed cells:

$$\frac{\text{Red cell volume} \times 100}{\text{whole blood volume}} = \text{PCV (expressed as \%)}$$

The necessary anticoagulant must be chosen with care. Either powdered heparin or a dry mixture of 4 mg potassium oxalate monohydrate and 6 mg ammonium oxalate monohydrate per ml of blood will not change the size or shape of the red cells. Sufficient centrifugal force must be exerted to pack the cells to where further centrifugation will produce no further packing. Actually, this is a state in which somewhat less than 5 per cent of the measured volume is still serum. To compress the cells beyond this limit requires enormous forces inexpedient for routine determinations. Packing will be adequate if the centrifuging of venipuncture blood is done at 2,500 rpm for 15 to 20 minutes in a large laboratory centrifuge in which the radius from the center axis to the midpoint of the mass of cells when packed is at least 15 cm. In smaller centrifuges the speed should be considerably higher.

For infants and young children there are available "micro" hematocrit devices designed for use with drops of blood from peripheral sources. The hematocrit tubes of the Van Allen type have proved in our hands to have a wider margin of error than the "macro" methods; they are nevertheless satisfactory if the test is carried out in duplicate and the pair of observations do not deviate from each other. New high-speed centrifuges are available which permit accurate determinations of the hematocrit in narrow glass capillary tubes. When accurately measured, 1 hematocrit unit is equal approximately to 0.34 gm of hemoglobin per 100 mm or 107,000 red cells per cu mm, provided the cells are normochromic and normocytic.

NORMAL VALUES. (Table 1-1). *Newborn Period.* Clement Smith cites the mean values for cord blood as from 51.3 to 57.2 per cent, with readings in most infants falling between 46 and 60 per cent. A slight rise occurs for the first few days, followed by a steady drop to a low value of around 35 per cent at about the third month. An illustration of the scatter which may be encountered is given in Chuinard, Osgood, and Ellis' series of 195 infants in the first 10 days of life: the mean was 43.4 per cent, with a range from 25.5 to 61 per cent.

Infancy and Childhood. In Horan's series the mean PCV was 60 per cent at 3 to 7 days, 44 per cent at 3 to 5 weeks, 37 per cent at 6 to 8 weeks, and 34 per cent at 9 to 12 weeks. It then rose steadily to between 36 and 37 per cent at 17 to 20 weeks and remained at that level for the remainder of the first year.

The mean PCV for adolescent boys in Wiehl's series rose steadily from 43.4 per cent at 12 years to 49.3 at 17 to 18 years. Since the mean red cell counts were constant over this period, this hematocrit rise must be attributable to expanding size of the red cells. For adolescent girls aged 12 to 17 years the mean hematocrit oscillated between 43.6 and 45.5 per cent. For both sexes the 80 percentile spread was approximately 3 per cent above and below the medians.

ABNORMAL STATES. The PCV becomes abnormal whenever there are disturbances in either red cell count or mean red cell size. It is low in anemia of all kinds and rises as recovery occurs. In congenital heart disease and other disorders accompanied by chronic cyanosis it may become elevated if erythrocytosis (polycythemia) develops.

Acute decreases in blood volume as a consequence of shock, dehydration, or burns may result in readings as high as 60 to 70 per cent. The values may be higher in finger tip than in venous blood, although elevated in both, because of peripheral vascular stagnation and local fluid loss.

Mean Erythrocyte Measurements

MEAN CELLULAR VOLUME (MCV). The size or volume of the average single erythrocyte corpuscle can be calculated from the relationship between PCV and erythrocyte count:

$$\frac{\text{Hematocrit (volume of packed cells, in ml per 100 ml blood)} \times 10}{\text{erythrocyte count (millions per cu mm)}}$$
$$= \text{MCV (expressed in cu } \mu)$$

A blood picture in which the MCV is normal is *normocytic;* larger than normal, *macrocytic;* smaller than normal, *microcytic.* Deviations from normocytic are not deemed significant unless they exceed twice the standard deviation from the mean for healthy children of the same age.

NORMAL VALUES. *Infancy and Childhood.* The red cells are unusually large at birth (Table 1-1). In Guest, Brown, and Wing's series the MCV in cord blood was 113 cu μ, with individual values distributed from 90 to 124 cu μ. Immediately after birth the mean volume began to diminish, reaching 73 cu μ at 8 months and 72 cu μ at 12 to 18 months. At 2 years of age it was 74 cu μ; at 3 years, 78 cu μ; at 4½ years, 80 cu μ. In optimally nourished children over 1½ years of age nearly all of the readings fell between 75 and 90 cu μ. In Horan's infants the curve for mean volume declined from approximately 96 cu μ at birth to 73 cu μ at 17 to 20 weeks, and more slowly to 69 cu μ at 1 year of age.

In premature infants at birth the red cells are larger than those of full-term infants, especially in those of very low birth weights, and continue so for the first 8 or 10 weeks of life. Study of the direct smears shows anisocytosis and anisochromia over this period.

Adolescence. Wiehl found mean values of 76.5 cu μ in boys of 12 and 13 years of age. Progressive enlargement occurred from 80.8 at 14 years to 87.7 at 17 to 18 years. Girls of 12 years of age had a mean of 82.0, which rose slowly to 87.8 at 17 years. The normal range for adults is approximately 78 to 94, with a mean of 87.

ABNORMAL STATES. Microcytosis, i.e., MCV below 60 cu μ, is confined almost exclusively to iron-deficiency anemia and to individuals who carry the Mediterranean anemia trait. Macrocytosis, i.e., mean volumes above 100 or 105 cu μ, is not uncommon in the other varieties of nutritional anemia, in pernicious anemia, and in chronic cyanotic disturbances with erythrocytosis.

The anemias secondary to chronic infections, nephritis, hypothyroidism, leukemia, malignancy, and other acquired disorders of childhood as a rule have erythrocytes which are of normal volume and diameter unless an iron-deficiency state is superimposed. Every child with a normocytic anemia who presents no other recognizable hematologic disturbance should have a survey of the organ systems for evidences of some underlying disease. In acidosis, whether induced by drugs or metabolic derangements, the red cells temporarily increase in size while retaining normal shape. In alkalosis the opposite occurs.

Mean Cellular Hemoglobin (MCH)

The average quantity of hemoglobin per individual cell is calculated from the ratio between hemoglobin level and erythrocyte count:

$$\frac{\text{Gm hemoglobin per 100 ml blood} \times 10}{\text{erythrocyte count (in millions per cu mm)}} = \text{MCH (expressed in } \mu\mu\text{gm)}$$

Red cells of normal hemoglobin content are termed *normochromic;* above normal, *hyperchromic;* below normal, *hypochromic.*

NORMAL VALUES. *Infancy and Childhood.* In Guest, Brown, and Wing's series the MCH in cord blood was 37.5 $\mu\mu$gm and 36.7 in the first 10 days. From 1 to 3 months of age this averaged 32.0; from 3 to 7 months, 27.1; in the first year, 23.0; at 2 years, 24.2; at 3 years, 26.5; and at 4½ years, 27.4. Horan found a mean of 31 at birth and for the first 3 weeks. This fell steadily to 22 to 23 at 8 months of age and remained there for the rest of the year. Mean values for children beyond 4 years of age are usually between 25 and 29 $\mu\mu$gm, near the adult value (Table 1-1).

Adolescence. The mean hemoglobin content per cell in Wiehl's series of adolescent boys increased from 24.0 $\mu\mu$gm at 12 years to 27.4 $\mu\mu$gm at 17 to 18 years. In girls this value remained at about 26.0 during the ages 12 to 15 years, and then increased to 27.2 at 16 and 17 years. Above age 13 years the means for the two sexes were approximately equal.

Hemoglobin Content of Packed Red Cells
(Mean Cellular Hemoglobin Concentration, MCHC)

The percentage of hemoglobin contained in a unit mass of circulating erythrocytes is calculated from the hemoglobin level and the PCV:

$$\frac{\text{Gm hemoglobin per 100 ml blood} \times 100}{\text{vol. packed erythrocytes per 100 ml blood}} = \text{MCHC (expressed as \%)}$$

This ratio describes the content of hemoglobin in a unit volume of red cells. The number of red cells does not enter the calculation. The percentage reading is the numerical equivalent of the number of grams of hemoglobin per 100 ml of packed red cells.

NORMAL VALUES. This ratio normally shows little age variation (Table 1-1). Guest, Brown, and Wing found the mean in cord blood to be 33.3 per cent, with a range from 29 to 36 per cent. In infants aged 30 to 90 days the mean rose slightly to 34.8 per cent, with a range from 31 to 37.9 per cent. From then on, in infants and children from upper economic levels, most of the values fell consistently between 34 to 35 per cent, the adult value. The means in Horan's series showed little variation throughout the first year, fluctuating between 33 and 35 per cent.

The means fluctuated between 30.0 and 31.8 per cent in the adolescent boys and girls of ages 12 to 17 years studied by Wiehl. These slightly lower figures than those of other workers were attributed to differences in techniques.

Electrophysical considerations suggest that a concentration of hemoglobin in the mass of packed red cells of about 34 per cent is the highest compatible with an orderly molecular lattice of hemoglobin which permits rapid diffusion and acceptance of oxygen.

Mean Cellular Diameter (MCD)

The diameter of erythrocytes when fixed and stained on glass slides can be ascertained either with a microscope having an ocular micrometer or with any of several optical diffraction methods. In normal subjects nearly all the red cells are of about the same diameter.

NORMAL VALUES. Price-Jones found the diameters of red cells of normal adults to fall in a narrow bell-shaped distribution between 6.718 and 7.718 μ, with a mean of 7.2 μ. Wintrobe gives the normal for both male and female adults as 7.5±0.3 μ. In the neonatal period the mean cellular diameter narrows gradually from 8.6 μ in cord blood to 7.4 μ at 6 to 12 months of age, where it remains throughout childhood.

The presence of generalized macrocytosis or microcytosis within a red cell population can be estimated from the other blood constants with much greater ease than by this method of direct measurement.

Anisocytosis, the extent of the scatter of the cell diameters, is easily recognized in the blood smear. It can be measured quantitatively only by the Price-Jones type of curves, which show spreading at the base and broadening of the peak.

Comments on Mean Erythrocyte Measurements in Childhood

The high values for mean cellular volume and mean cellular hemoglobin in the newborn period confirm that the individual red cells in the fetus and at birth are larger and contain more hemoglobin than those of older persons. After the first 2 months the red cells tend to be slightly microcytic in comparison with those of adults. This proportionately lower hemoglobin level continues from late infancy until adolescence.

The ratios of mean corpuscular volume, mean cellular hemoglobin, and mean corpuscular hemoglobin content are utilized more often in adult than in pediatric hematology. The swing in the normal levels for red cells and hemoglobin in growing infants and children makes the application of these ratios somewhat involved. Another difficulty is that the ratios fail to portray the scatter of the measurements about the mean. Anisocytosis, poikilocytosis, and related cytologic alterations as seen in the stained blood smears (p. 19) are much more helpful clinically than computed statistical averages.

Many of the indexes used in the past to portray the blood status have been found unsatisfactory for pediatrics, largely because the so-called "standards" incorporated into the calculations gave little or no attention to age variations. Among the relationships thus being abandoned are the expressing of hemoglobin readings in percentages, the hemoglobin coefficient, the volume coefficient, the color index, the volume index, and the saturation index.

BIBLIOGRAPHY

TECHNIQUES OF MEASUREMENT

Berkson, J., T. B. Magath, and *M. Hurn,* Laboratory Standards in Relation to Chance Fluctuations of the Erythrocyte Count as Estimated with the Hemocytometer, *J. Am. Statist. A.* 30:414, 1935.

——, ——, and ——, Error of Estimate of Blood Cell Count as Made with Hemocytometer, *Am. J. Physiol.* 128:309, 1940.

Biggs, R., and *R. L. Macmillan,* The Error of the Red Cell Count, *J. Clin. Path.* 1:288, 1948.

—— and ——, The Errors of Some Hematological Methods as They Are Used in a Routine Laboratory, *J. Clin. Path.* 1:269, 1948.

Cannan, R. K., Proposal for the Distribution of a Certified Standard for Use in Hemoglobinometry, *Am. J. Clin. Path.* 25:376, 1955.

Guest, G. M., and *V. E. Siler,* A Centrifuge Method for the Determination of Cells in Blood, *J. Lab. & Clin. Med.* 19:757, 1934.

Hamilton, L. H., Errors in Blood Cell Counting. I. Technical Errors, *Canad. J. Med. Tech.* 17:137, 1955.

——, Errors in Blood Cell Counting. II. Statistical Errors, *Canad. J. Med. Tech.* 18:8, 1956.

Karr, W. G., and *J. H. Clark,* Comparison of Various Hemoglobin Methods as Performed in Hospital and Physicians' Laboratories, *Am. J. Clin. Path.* 11:127, 1941.

King, E. J., M. Gilchrist, and G. E. Delory, Accuracy of Haemoglobin Methods, Lancet 1:239, 1944.

Lange, H. F., and H. Palmer, Studies of Erythrocyte Counting. I. Technical Errors, Acta med. scandinav. 131:555, 1948. II. Technical-physiological Errors, ibid. 131:555, 1948. III. Physiological Variations, ibid. 132:2, 1948.

Oettinger, L., Jr., and W. B. Mills, Simultaneous Capillary and Venous Hemoglobin Determinations in the Newborn Infant, J. Pediat. 35:362, 1949.

Orona, M. M., and R. Stenkamp, Hematologic Variations in Capillary Blood, Northwest Med. 48:472, 1949.

Schlenker, F. S., and J. Noll, On the Determination of Packed Cell Volume, J. Lab. & Clin. Med. 39:582, 1952.

Strumia, M. M., A. B. Sample, and E. D. Hart, An Improved Micro Hematocrit Method, Am. J. Clin. Path. 24:1016, 1954.

Sunderman, F. W., R. P. MacFate, D. A. MacFadyen, G. F. Stevenson, and B. E. Copeland, Symposium on Clinical Hemoglobinometry, Am. J. Clin. Path. 23:519, 1953.

Thorell, B., "Studies on the Formation of Cellular Substances during Blood Cell Production," Kimpton, London, 1947.

NORMAL VALUES IN INFANCY AND CHILDHOOD

Dickstein, B., and I. J. Wolman, The Normal Red Cell in Infancy and Childhood: Some Recent Advances, Am. J. M. Sc. 215:694, 1948.

Faxén, N., Red Blood Picture in Healthy Infants, Acta paediat. (suppl. 1) 19:1, 1937.

Gil, J. R., and C. G. Terán, Determination of the Number of Erythrocytes, Volume of Packed Red Cells, Hemoglobin and Other Hematologic Standards in Mexico City (Altitude: 7,457 feet): Study Made on Two Hundred Healthy Persons, Blood 3:660, 1948.

Guest, G. M., and E. W. Brown, Erythrocytes and Hemoglobin of the Blood in Infancy and Childhood. I. Size and Hemoglobin Content of the Erythrocytes in Nutrition Anemia, Am. J. Dis. Child. 52:616, 1936.

———, ———, and M. Wing, Erythrocytes and Hemoglobin of the Blood in Infancy and in Childhood. II. Variability in Number, Size and Hemoglobin Content of the Erythrocytes during the First Five Years of Life, Am. J. Dis. Child. 56:529, 1938.

Hawkins, W. W., and D. K. Kline, Hemoglobin Levels among Seven to Fourteen Year Old Children in Saskatoon, Canada, Blood 5:278, 1950.

———, E. Speck, and V. G. Leonard, Variation of the Hemoglobin Level with Age and Sex, Blood 9:999, 1954.

Horan, M., Studies in Anaemia of Infancy and Childhood: The Haemoglobin, Red Cell Count, and Packed Cell Volume of Normal English Infants during the First Year of Life, Arch. Dis. Childhood 25:110, 1950.

Kaucher, M., E. Z. Moyer, A. P. Harrison, R. U. Thomas, M. M. Rutledge, W. Lameck, and E. F. Beach, Nutritional Status of Children. VII. Hemoglobin, J. Am. Dietet. A. 24:496, 1948.

Leichsenring, J. M., L. M. Norris, and M. L. Halbert, Hemoglobin, Red Cell Count and Mean Corpuscular Hemoglobin of Healthy Infants, A.M.A. Am. J. Dis. Child. 84:27, 1952.

Mack, P. B., J. M. Smith, C. H. Logan, A. T. O'Brien, J. J. Shaw, and P. Dodd, Hemoglobin Values in Pennsylvania: Studies in Human Nutrition, Milbank Mem. Fund Quart. 19:282, 1941.

Mackay, H. M. M., L. Wills, and K. Bingham, Economic Status and the Haemoglobin Level of Children of Men in the Fighting Service and of Civilians, Brit. M. J. 1:711, 1946.

Merritt, K. K., and *L. T. Davidson,* The Blood during the First Year of Life. I. Normal Values for Erythrocytes, Hemoglobin, Reticulocytes, and Platelets and Their Relationship to Neonatal Bleeding and Coagulation Time, *Am. J. Dis. Child.* 46:990, 1933.

Mugrage, E. R., and *M. I. Andresen,* Values for Red Blood Cells of Average Infants and Children, *Am. J. Dis. Child.* 51:775, 1936.

Munday, B., M. L. Shepherd, L. Emerson, B. M. Hamil, M. W. Poole, I. G. Macy, and *T. E. Raiford,* Hemoglobin Differences in Healthy White and Negro Infants, *Am. J. Dis. Child.* 55:776, 1938.

Osgood, E. E., and *R. L. Baker,* Erythrocyte, Hemoglobin, Cell Volume and Color, Volume and Saturation Index: Standards for Normal Children of School Age, *Am. J. Dis. Child.* 50:343, 1935.

Pett, L. B., and *G. E. Ogilvie,* Hemoglobin Levels at Different Ages, *Canad. M. A. J.* 58:353, 1948.

Post, R. L., and *C. R. Spealman,* Variation of Total Circulating Hemoglobin and Reticulocyte Count of Man with Season and Following Hemorrhage, *J. Appl. Physiol.* 1:227, 1948.

Reedy, M. E., S. O. Schwartz, and *E. B. Plattner,* Anemia of the Premature Infant: A Two-year Study of the Response to Iron Medication, *J. Pediat.* 41:25, 1952.

Wiehl, D. G., Medical Evaluation of Nutritional Status: III. Hemoglobin and Erythrocyte Values for Adolescents in High-income Families, *Milbank Mem. Fund Quart.* 19:45, 1941.

———, Accuracy of Hemoglobin Determinations on Finger-tip Blood, *Milbank Mem. Fund Quart.* 24:5, 1946.

Wolman, I. J., The Peripheral Blood Count of Children, *J. Nat. M. A.* 47:1, 1955.

Wolstein, M., The Normal Blood in Infants and Children, in Hal Downey (ed.), "Handbook of Hematology," vol. II, Paul B. Hoeber, Inc., New York, 1938.

NORMAL RED CELL AND HEMOGLOBIN LEVELS IN THE NEWBORN PERIOD AND IN PREMATURITY

Chuinard, E. G., E. E. Osgood, and *D. M. Ellis,* Hematologic Standards for Healthy Newborn Infants: Erythrocyte Count, Hemoglobin Content, Cell Volume, Color Index, Volume Index and Saturation Index, *Am. J. Dis. Child.* 62:1188, 1941.

DeMarsh, Q. B., H. L. Alt, and *W. F. Windle,* Effect of Depriving Infant of Its Placental Blood on Blood Picture during First Week of Life, *J.A.M.A.* 116:2568, 1941.

———, ———, and ———, Factors Influencing the Blood Picture of the Newborn: Studies on Sinus Blood on the First and Third Days, *Am. J. Dis. Child.* 75:860, 1948.

———, *W. F. Windle,* and *H. L. Alt,* Blood Volume of Newborn Infant in Relation to Early and Late Clamping of Umbilical Cord, *Am. J. Dis. Child.* 63:1123, 1942.

Findlay, L., The Blood in Infancy, *Arch. Dis. Childhood* 21:195, 1946.

Gilmour, J. R., Normal Haemopoiesis in Intra-uterine and Neonatal Life, *J. Path. & Bact.* 52:25, 1941.

Langley, F. A., Haemopoiesis and Siderosis in the Foetus and Newborn, *Arch. Dis. Childhood* 26:64, 1951.

Mackay, H. M. M., The Early Anaemia of Premature Infants: The Haemoglobin Level of Immature Babies in the First Half-year of Life and the Effect during the First Three Months of Blood Injections and Iron Therapy, *Arch. Dis. Childhood* 10:195, 1935.

McCausland, A. M., F. Holmes, and *W. R. Schumann,* Management of Cord and Placental Blood and Its Effect upon the Newborn, *California Med.* 71:190, 1949.

Mollison, P. L., and *M. Cutbush,* Haemolytic Disease of the Newborn: Criteria of Severity, *Brit. M. J.* 1:123, 1949.

Parsons, L. G., Studies in the Anaemias of Infancy and Early Childhood, *Arch. Dis. Childhood* 8:85, 1933.

Rossier, A., and *L. Potiron,* The Anemia of Prematurity: Prophylactic Treatment by Early Repeated Blood Transfusion (L'Anémie des prematures: son traitement preventif par les transfusions de sang, précoces et repetées), *Arch. franç. pédiat.* 9:113, 1952.

Smith, Clement A., "The Physiology of the Newborn Infant," Charles C Thomas, Springfield, Ill., 1951.

Stevenson, S. S., and *L. H. Erhard,* Early Clamping of the Umbilical Cord during Cesarean Section, *J. Pediat.* 40:64, 1952.

Strauss, M. B., Anemia of Infancy from Maternal Iron Deficiency in Pregnancy, *J. Clin. Invest.* 12:345, 1933.

Washburn, A. H., Blood Cells in Healthy Young Infants: Postnatal Readjustments of Red Blood Cells in Individual Babies, *Am. J. Dis. Child.* 62:530, 1941.

Wegelius, R., On the Changes in the Peripheral Blood Picture of the Newborn Infant Immediately after Birth, *Acta paediat.,* vol. 35, suppl. 4, 1948.

Windle, W. F., Development of the Blood and Changes in the Blood Picture at Birth, *J. Pediat.* 18:538, 1941.

Woodruff, C. W., and *E. B. Bridgeforth,* Relationship between the Hemogram of the Infant and That of the Mother during Pregnancy, *Pediatrics* 12:681, 1953.

CHAPTER 2

Anemia and Its Manifestations

Anemia may be defined as a condition in which the hemoglobin level or the erythrocyte count, singly or in combination, are significantly below the physiologic normal range. It will be noted that there are two components in this definition and that a decrease in only one is needed for the term *anemia* to be applicable. The packed cell volume (hematocrit) will be subnormal whenever either the red cell count or hemoglobin level is reduced.

Since there are almost no childhood disturbances in which the red cell count and hematocrit become depressed while the hemoglobin level remains undisturbed, the term anemia for pediatric purposes is synonymous with a reduced hemoglobin level, or *hemoglobinopenia*. It has been proposed that the line of demarcation be set statistically as two standard deviations below the mean of the readings obtained by the same laboratory method with healthy persons of the same age and sex as the patient, but full sets of data which give the normal scatter of hemoglobin and related blood measurements in healthy infants and children are not yet available.

In the erythrocytosis of cyanotic congenital heart disease, the hemoglobin level may be proportionately lower than the red cell count as the consequence of a masked hypochromic iron-deficiency anemia, even while both are increased above the "normal."

So many counterbalancing mechanisms, chiefly cardiovascular, compensate for mild degrees of oxygen-carrying deficiency that the gap is broad between the level of hemoglobin which customarily obtains in the blood stream during health and the level low enough to produce anoxemic difficulties.

Fully hemoglobinized arterial blood is 95 to 97 per cent saturated with oxygen and contains about 20 ml of oxygen per 100 ml. An average of 5 ml of oxygen per 100 ml is released to the tissues as the blood traverses the capillary bed. This leaves a content of 15 ml per 100 ml, or 70 per cent saturation, in the mixed venous blood returning to the right auricle. With mildly anemic states the absolute oxygen-carrying capacity per volume of arterial blood is reduced parallel to the diminished hemoglobin level, reducing the oxygen tension within the tissues. Tissue uptake of oxygen, however, remains at about 5 ml per 100 ml of blood, so that the per cent saturation of the returning venous blood is disproportionately lowered. With more severe anemia the exaggerated arteriovenous oxygen difference reaches a critical level and the cardiac output rises. Other homeostatic mechanisms are then stimulated also—dilatation of the peripheral arterioles, a reduced basal metabolic rate, and a reduced total blood volume.

Erythrocytopenia—diminished erythrocyte count—is found in most childhood anemias. The count may not be reduced significantly in children with milder iron deficiency and in some carriers of Mediterranean anemia.

For practical purposes in office or clinic, the threshold values in Table 2-1 will be found dependable for the recognition of anemia on the basis of single tests. The criteria have been derived from reported and personal data, with approximately 10 per cent added to twice the approximate standard deviations to allow for technical errors in performance. When

Table 2-1. Threshold Values for Diagnosis of Anemia in Childhood *

	1–9 months	9 months–6 years	6–12 years, girls; 6–15 years, boys	12–18 years, girls; 15–18 years, boys
Hemoglobin (gm per 100 ml)	9 or less	10 or less	11 or less	12 or less
Erythrocyte count (millions)	4.0 or less	4.2 or less	4.5 or less	4.5 or less (girls) 5.0 or less (boys)
Packed cell volume (per cent)	30 or less	32 or less	36 or less	40 or less

* In the absence of congenital heart disease or other disease which evokes erythrocytosis.

two or three red cell characteristics are measured, slightly higher threshold values may be taken. In borderline situations it is important to confirm the existence of anemia by clinical studies, repetition of the determinations, and scrutiny of peripheral blood films.

To recognize anemia, especially of mild degree, laboratory studies are needed. Pallor of the skin and mucous membranes, those traditional clinical features, are often highly misleading. One child with pink gums and flushed cheeks may have a hemoglobin level startlingly lower than another whose skin appears sallow or pale.

MORPHOLOGIC CLASSIFICATION

From the morphologic viewpoint, the anemias may be classified according to the size of the unit vehicle, the red cell. This gives three primary divisions: (1) normocytic, (2) microcytic, (3) macrocytic. Normocytic has been defined by the Committee on Nomenclature as "a blood picture in which the erythrocytes have a mean corpuscular volume or volume index within plus or minus two standard deviations of the mean normal determined by the same method on the bloods of healthy person of the patient's age and sex group." Microcytic refers to cell populations in which the mean corpuscular volume is less than the normal range as thus defined; whereas macrocytic signifies the opposite. A hemoglobin level within similar normal limits is called *normochromic;* below this, *hypochromic.* There are no known "hyperchromic" states.

Though purely descriptive, this approach to cataloguing can be of great assistance in narrowing the list of diagnostic possibilities when an obscure case of anemia is first seen. Hemoglobin production and red cell formation are so intertwined that anemic disturbances rarely affect one without involving the other.

DYNAMIC CLASSIFICATION

From the broad physiologic viewpoint, anemia is often discussed as the result of an altered balance between two opposing metabolic equilibria:

1. Erythropoiesis—rate of production of red cells and hemoglobin
2. Hemodestruction or hemolysis—rate of destruction of red cells and hemoglobin

When this balance becomes distorted, many of the ensuing hematologic derangements can be described in terms of direction and degree, i.e., whether hyper- or hypo- and to what extent.

Convenient laboratory methods for estimating the status of erythropoiesis in an anemic child include (1) study of the morphologic aspects of the peripheral blood as seen in direct smears, (2) reticulocyte count, and (3) cellularity and quality of the rubricytic pattern within the bone marrow. Convenient methods for detecting accelerated blood destruction are (1) total serum bilirubin level and its fractional components, and (2) quantitive output of urobilinogen and related pigments in urine and stools.

The more abrupt and severe the development of an anemia, the more pronounced the dyspnea and tachycardia and other signs of anoxic strain. In acutely developing hemorrhagic or hemolytic disorders the patient may be made desperately ill by a red cell count no lower than 2.5 million, whereas with gradual onset the adjustment to much lower levels can be made without conspicuous difficulty. Red cell counts below 800,000, though highly exceptional and barely compatible with life, may be seen at times in slowly developing and long-standing disturbances and especially those which date back to early infancy. When erythrocytopenia of this degree develops suddenly in a previously well infant or

Table 2-2. Etiologic Classification of the Childhood Anemias

I. The malnutritional anemias
    Hypochromic microcytic anemia (iron-deficiency anemia)
    The macrocytic anemias
        Deficiency in the folic acid–vitamin B_{12}–ascorbic acid complex
        Deficiency in amino acids or other essential nutrients
    The normocytic anemias
        Von Jaksch's anemia
        Malignant malnutrition (kwashiorkor)
        Malnutritional anemia associated with intestinal parasitism
II. Familial dystrophies of the red cells
    Hereditary spherocytosis (congenital hemolytic icterus)
    Mediterranean or Cooley's anemia
    Sickle cell anemia and variant forms
    Hereditary elliptocytosis
    Familial erythroid multinuclearity
    Acanthrocytosis
    The nonspherocytic congenital hemolytic anemias
    Congenital methemoglobinemia
III. Anemias secondary to toxic and systemic disturbances
    Aplastic anemia
    Bacterial and viral infections
    Burns
    Drugs and poisons
        Lead poisoning
        Naphthalene poisoning
    Erythroblastosis fetalis and related maternal–fetal blood group incompatibilities
    Favism
    Hypothyroidism
    Chronic kidney disease
    Leukemia and other malignant diseases
    Leukoerythroblastotic reaction
    Malaria
    Marrow infiltration
    Posthemorrhagic anemia
    Essential pulmonary hemosiderosis
IV. Constitutional aplastic and hypoplastic anemias
    Chronic congenital aregenerative anemia (pure red cell anemia)
    Constitutional pancytopenia associated with multiple developmental defects
    Familial hypoplastic anemia
    Congenital photosensitive porphyria
V. Hemolytic anemias caused by autogenous mechanisms
    Acquired hemolytic anemia of autogenous origin
    Hypersplenism (Banti's syndrome, Gaucher's disease, etc.)
    Paroxysmal hemoglobinemia due to cold autohemagglutinins
    Paroxysmal hemoglobinuria due to cold autohemolysins
    Paroxysmal nocturnal hemoglobinuria

child, as in acute favism or naphthalene poisoning, the outcome almost certainly will be fatal unless corrective transfusions are given quickly. Children with congenital red cell dystrophies of pronounced severity tend to stabilize their erythrocyte and hemoglobin values at subnormal levels and destroy transfused red cells if in excess of what they have become physiologically adjusted to.

ETIOLOGIC CLASSIFICATION

For the best management of a patient, the results of morphologic and physiologic studies must be coordinated with additional information relating to all the fundamental pathogenetic mechanisms responsible for the development of the anemia. It is from this viewpoint that the specific varieties of anemia are discussed in the ensuing chapters (Table 2-2).

With every child with anemia a thorough inquiry should be made as to bleeding episodes in the past; familial blood disorders; adequacy of protein, vitamins, and iron-containing foods in the diet; recent infections and their character; and possible exposure to drugs or medications. The child should be disrobed and examined for icterus, lymph node enlargement, hepatomegaly, splenomegaly, hemorrhages, infections, skeletal aberrations, and constitutional diseases. The choice of laboratory tests depends upon the judgment of the physician as guided by the history and physical examination. The red cells should be studied as discussed in the ensuing pages, and pertinent tests performed on urine, stool, and blood. Roentgenography of the bones and other special procedures are performed as needed.

Whenever the findings indicate the possibility of a hereditary red cell dystrophy the effort should be made to test all other siblings, both parents, and as many grandparents and close relatives as will cooperate. Disclosing a pattern of inheritance will not only substantiate the diagnosis in a child but almost invariably will discover other affected members within the family.

LABORATORY ABNORMALITIES IN ANEMIA

Depression of Red Cell and Hemoglobin Levels

As stated, there is almost no condition in infancy or childhood which can depress the red cell count or the packed cell volume without simultaneously decreasing the hemoglobin level. In the so-called normochromic anemias such as occur in nephritis, persistent infections, and related chronic disorders, one finds the red cells, the hemoglobin, and the hematocrit all reduced about equally. In microcytic iron-deficiency anemia, the most prevalent of the childhood anemias, the hemoglobin level has to sink to the neighborhood of 8 gm per 100 ml before the red cell count shows any appreciable drop. In the milder forms of the hereditary anemias the hemoglobin level is often depressed whereas the red cell count may or may not show a significant change. In the macrocytic anemias the rule is for both the red cells and the hemoglobin to be reduced, with the red cells being the more affected. With any anemia the red cell count or hemoglobin level or both may be brought temporarily to the normal zone if the patient is made acutely dehydrated by a sudden illness, but restoration of the fluid shortage will uncover the true state of affairs.

Estimation of hemoglobin alone, therefore, when accurately done, is better for detecting the presence of anemia in infants and children than is the red cell count. When assayed by a photometer or photoelectric colorimeter the hemoglobin estimation has the added advantage of being technically more reliable. A discrepancy between red cell count and hemoglobin level when the latter is in the normal range is practically always due to an error in red cell counting. Only when the hemoglobin reading falls in the anemic zone or when other findings are abnormal need a red cell count be performed. The appearance of the red cells in the stained film of the peripheral blood serves as a check on the hemoglobin estimation. An adequate hematocrit procedure is another reliable screening approach for the detection of the possible presence of anemia.

Morphology of the Red Cells in Blood Films

Direct inspection by microscopy is the simplest approach to detecting abnormalities of the red cells with respect to shape, size distribution, hemoglobinization, deposits, parasites, and various other intracellular changes. Fresh wet preparations studied by direct or darkfield or polarized illumination may be employed for special purposes such as search for Heinz bodies, but the nonprofessional hematologist relies almost exclusively on scrutiny of the dried and stained blood smear. Wright's stain or similar derivatives of the Romanowsky formula are employed most widely in this country. Other stains are useful for special purposes, such as brilliant cresyl blue for reticulocytes, Giemsa for malaria, Prussian blue for iron-containing bodies, Feulgen for desoxyribonucleoprotein, etc.

PREPARATION OF THE BLOOD SMEAR. The physician should include the study of a blood smear in the examination of every patient who is ill. Prerequisite are facilities for staining, a good batch of stain, microscopic familiarity with deviating cell forms, and the judgment needed to relate the normal or abnormal observations to the clinical history and physical and other findings. In only a few minutes the red cells, white cells, and platelets can be inspected and their character and comparative numbers noted. Should any of the morphologic appearances be suggestive of disease, further studies are made as indicated or the slide saved for submission to the nearest pathologist or hematologist for consultation.

The best site for the procuring of blood samples for direct smears is the finger tip in infants and children or the heel or great toe in newborn and premature infants. Venipuncture specimens containing citrate or oxalate are satisfactory for inspection of the red cells if smears are prepared within a few minutes after collection. Exposure of the leukocytes to anticoagulants other than heparin results almost immediately in distorted shapes, artefactual vacuoles, and irregular staining.

The glass slides used should be scrupulously clean and free from grease or finger marks. The smear should be thin enough for the red cells to lie singly and the cytoplasm of the leukocytes to be spread out. The buffer solution employed in dilution of Wright's stain should be tested frequently and kept at a pH close to 6.7 to 6.8. Too acid a reaction gives a pink tone; too alkaline, a blue tone. For good preparations one should permit the blood to dry for at least 10 minutes before proceding with the staining. Unsatisfactory preparations should be discarded. A well-stained slide will be free from precipitate and be uniformly tinted throughout, the red cells will not be distorted or vacuolated, and any polychromatophilic or other intracellular changes will stand out clearly. The leukocytes and platelets will show distinctly all cytoplasmic granules and nuclear irregularities.

DEVIATIONS. Red cells from normal subjects show little variability in size, shape, or staining qualities. Their mean diameter when dried on a slide may fall between 7.0 and 8.0 μ, and is usually between 7.3 and 7.5. Some 35 to 45 per cent of the water content is lost during drying; fresh cells in plasma have a mean diameter closer to 8.5 μ. The frequency distribution of the cell diameters within a red cell population ordinarily gives a bell-shaped curve.

The method of Price-Jones calls for measuring the diameters of 1,000 individual cells and plotting the readings on graph paper. With this approach, the curves for Mediterranean anemia show a depressed peak and a spread wider than normal. With hereditary spherocytosis or iron-deficiency anemia the means are in the direction of a smaller diameter (*microcytosis*) and the curve is skewed. With vitamin B$_{12}$ deficiency and related anemias the shift is in the opposite direction (*macrocytosis*). Because the determination of osmotic fragility and the calculation of the red cell measurements yield data of equivalent or superior clinical utility with less expenditure of time, Price-Jones measurements of curves of diameter distribution are no longer widely used.

Pronounced differences in diameter (*anisocytosis*) may be seen in iron-deficiency anemia, the macrocytic anemias, chronic aregenerative anemia, the severe forms of the hereditary anemias, and in hyperactive blood regeneration after a sudden hemorrhage or hemolytic episode. In a few disorders, such as severe burns, elliptocytosis, and Mediterranean anemia, some red cells seem to be disintegrating in the blood stream into smaller units—a process known as *fragmentation*.

The intensity of red cell staining reflects the hemoglobin content. In the anemia of iron deficiency the red cells, whether of normal or small diameter, tend to have little or no hemoglobin at their centers (*hypochromia*). In hereditary spherocytosis and in hemolytic anemia caused by circulating antibodies they have a normal content of hemoglobin, or may even stain unusually deeply at the center. In wet preparations these cells tend to be biconvex and thicker (*spherocytes*), rather than the normal biconcaval with a central depression more pronounced on one side. When normal red cells are transfused into a patient with a hemolytic anemia due to circulating antibodies, they may undergo a spherocytic change in shape. Spherocytes have normal cell volumes.

In the condition known as *anisochromia* the hemoglobin is distributed unevenly through the cytoplasm. This is a not uncommon finding in the blood of prematurely born infants.

Poikilocytes are red cells of distorted shape which occur in inconstant numbers in diverse severe anemias and represent a defect in cellular architecture. During childhood they are most frequent in Mediterranean anemia and severe iron deficiency. In intensity this change parallels the severity of the disturbance.

Ovalocytes are oval or elliptic cells which appear in the circulation, usually in small numbers, in pronounced cases of sickle cell anemia, Mediterranean anemia, and other severe anemias. Ovalocytosis is a customary companion of poikilocytosis and anisocytosis. A distinction can be made, on etiologic grounds mainly, between those ovalocytes and the similar-appearing cells found in hereditary elliptocytosis (p. 69).

Leptocytes are unusually thin and have an increased diameter. Their typical structure is that of a narrow peripheral rim of hemoglobin and a large central achromic area. Sometimes the scanty content of hemoglobin is distributed irregularly.

Target cells are leptocytes which when stained exhibit a central dotlike mass and a peripheral ring of hemoglobin, separated by a clear zone.

In fresh wet preparations leptocytes are bowl- or hat-shaped and their edges fold over. Such cells may be encountered in hemoglobin C disease, Mediterranean anemia, sickle cell anemia, liver disease, and posthemorrhagic and postsplenectomy states. Severe dehydration during life, or osmotically hypertonic solutions in the test tube, may produce reversibly a similar change in normal red cells. The leptocytes which appear in the circulation after splenectomy are of unexplained origin. Leptocytes may have a normal hemoglobin content and cell volume even though their diameter and surface area are greater than normal.

Burr cells are irregular red cells found in small numbers in the peripheral blood of patients with uremia, malignancy, and bleeding peptic ulcer. One or more coarse spiny projections extend from the periphery in both wet preparations and stained blood films. They differ from *crenated* red cells, such as those found in the cerebrospinal fluid after bleeding, in that the projections of the latter are more numerous and are arranged symmetrically.

RETICULOCYTES. A reticulocyte is an immature red cell in which enough of the formative early cytoplasm remains to take a basophilic cresyl blue dye. It is important that a laboratory always use the same counting method in order to maintain constant limits for normality. Reticulocytes with a high content of reticulum can be recognized in routine films stained with Wright's stain by their *polychromatophilic* or *basophilic* tint. Reticulocytes have a somewhat greater diameter than mature erythrocytes and when present in abundance can simulate the appearance of macrocytosis. They are believed to mature into erythrocytes within a day or so after entering the circulation.

The peripheral count of reticulocytes goes up whenever erythropoiesis is accelerated. This is believed to be an expression of an accelerated normal process, along with an actual lowering of the unknown threshold mechanism which releases red cells from the marrow spaces. Normal reticulocyte counts in children usually range between 0.5 and 1.0 per cent. Values between 1.2 and 15 per cent may be termed a "mild" or "moderate" reticulocytosis; above 15 per cent, "marked." During and soon after an acute hemolytic episode the reticulocytes may temporarily become so numerous as to form a majority of the circulating erythrocytes.

In anemias of iron deficiency or those consequent to hemorrhage, a rise in reticulocytes is a sign of regeneration or proliferation on the part of the marrow rubricytes. The same interpretation explains the reticulocytosis which may be brought about by the chemotherapy of leukemia or the administration of corticotropin or cortisone for any systemic or hematologic disease associated with anemia. The reticulocytosis in Mediterranean anemia and the sickle cell group of disorders is of more complex origin and not well understood.

Only a few days may be needed for a reticulocytosis to become manifest after a hemorrhage or after corrective therapy for an anemia is begun. When a hemolytic injury has been unusually severe, as in drug sensitivity, the erythropoietic resurgence as evidenced by reticulocytosis, marrow rubricytosis, and rise of the red cell count may be delayed for weeks or even months.

Thus from changes in the reticulocyte levels of anemic patients it is possible to draw important deductions with reference to the red cell productivity of the bone marrow and the efficacy of therapy. With many anemias, once an initial bone marrow examination has been made for diagnostic information, serial reticulocyte counts can give adequate insight into red cell production without further marrow aspirations being required.

Reticulocytes when abundant will give rise to an opaque irregular upper zone at the top of the red cell layer in sedimentation tests done in long narrow tubes such as those of Westergren. Reticulocytes resist rouleaux formation and settle downward more slowly.

In hereditary spherocytosis the reticulocytes resemble those of normal subjects in being disk-shaped and of large size but differ in being thicker and of smaller diameter. This indicates that the abnormality of the red cells is already present before the cells are delivered into the blood stream.

When erythropoiesis is depressed, as in infiltration or aplasia of the bone marrow, the reticulocyte count subsides to less than 0.5 per cent and may be so low as to be uncountable. Sometimes in these conditions, however, a slight increase to 1.0 or 2.0 per cent may be noted. This apparent paradox results from hyperplastic activity of the uninjured hemopoietic foci still in the marrow.

NUCLEATED RED CELLS. These are normal constituents of the circulating blood of the fetus and of the infant at birth. The absolute count in the normal full-term infant rarely exceeds 1,200 per cu mm, but may be higher in the premature infant. They disappear rapidly during the first few days and are almost never found after the fourth day. Their presence in the blood stream of the newborn in great numbers or for a longer period is indicative of some disorder.

Mild stimulation of red cell production as the result of a sudden hemorrhage or acute hemolytic disorder brings out the reticulocytes; a more violent demand for red cells brings out normoblasts, or even the highly immature megaloblasts in extreme stimulation. The threshold for the appearance of nucleated forms corresponds ordinarily to a reticulocyte count of about 20 per cent, though this may be lower after splenectomy.

The release of nucleated red cells in Mediterranean anemia and to a lesser extent in the sickle cell and other hereditary anemias seems to reflect a disturbance in red cell production and marrow oxygen content as well as an abnormal peripheral demand. Nucleated red cells are not uncommon in small numbers in leukemia, especially the chronic granulocytic variety and erythroleukemia; in assorted poisonings; in severe heart failure and other disorders which are attended by tissue anoxia; in overwhelming septic infections; in malignancies and related disorders accompanied by marrow infiltrations; and in all abnormal conditions attended by extramedullary hemopoiesis. Circulating normoblasts are a regular phenomenon after splenectomy for any cause.

INCLUSION BODIES. Single or multiple dark-staining inclusion bodies are found within the red cells in many hematologic disturbances. These are most often rounded, with diameters ranging from punctate dots up to 2 μ, though usually under 0.5 μ. Rod-shaped forms or club-shaped or irregular masses 1 to 6 μ in length may be seem. Stippled basophilic granules often appear in lead poisoning (p. 83).

Heinz bodies are refractile round red cell inclusions which are best seen in fresh wet preparations rather than in stained smears. They may appear in patients receiving medications or exposed to chemicals which are potentially hemolytic; many of these substances possess a benzene-ring nucleus. Some degree of methemoglobinemia is often associated. Whenever they are detected it is advisable to question thoroughly regarding possible exposure to toxic drugs or chemicals.

Heinz bodies are typically found in congenital agenesis of the spleen. This anomaly occasionally accompanies major abnormalities of the heart and great vessels along with partial situs inversus of the abdominal viscera. Other pertinent blood findings resemble those observed after splenectomy—circulating target cells and nucleated red cells, leukocytosis, and thrombocytosis. Gasser has reported 14 premature or underweight full-term infants who showed a constitutional hemolytic disturbance in association with these erythrocyte inclusions.

SIDEROCYTES AND SIDEROBLASTS. Small particles of nonhemoglobin iron, stainable with potassium ferrocyanide–hydrochloric acid technique, appear in certain circumstances within the mature erythrocytes (siderocytes) and marrow normoblasts (sideroblasts). As a rule these particles are not apparent in blood films stained with Wright's or similar Romanowsky dyes; when seen, they are sometimes called *Pappenheimer bodies*. They vary in size from just within the limit of visibility up to 2 μ in diameter. Only rarely does a single cell contain more than a dozen granules. Red cells in any stage of normal or distorted development may be siderocytic.

Siderocytes appear in the peripheral blood in erythroblastosis fetalis, hereditary spherocytosis, hemolytic anemia due to autogenous mechanisms, lead poisoning, uremia, myelosclerosis, and other disturbances. They frequently become abundant in the peripheral blood after splenectomy for any cause.

Sideroblasts are present in normal marrow in appreciable numbers. Presumably these granules are utilized in hemoglobin formation, since they disappear at the reticulocyte stage or earlier. Sideroblasts are greatly diminished in iron deficiency states, usually being less than 1 per cent of all normoblasts. Conversely, they are exceptionally abundant in lead poisoning, thalassemia major, megaloblastic anemia, and diverse hemolytic disorders.

Hemodestructive Processes

Not much is known of the physiologic mechanisms which normally terminate the life span of individual red cells within the circulation. It is believed that each red cell ages continuously and that the aging process uses up enzymes and other substances essential to the cell's integrity. The terminal event may be intravascular fragmentation or disintegration (hemolysis), reticuloendothelial phagocytosis, or dissolution within the recesses of the spleen.

Some of the drugs and poisons which cause abnormal hemodestruction appear to attack the interior of the cells, altering their metabolism and particularly that of the hemoglobin-methemoglobin-choleglobin system.

Among these substances are the benzol derivatives, phenylhydrazine, aromatic amino and nitro compounds, silver and lead salts, carbon tetrachloride and bisulfide, and the sulfonamides. Saponin, lecithin, and lysolecithin also cause intracellular breakdown.

Hemolytic antibodies induce surface injuries which lead either to hemolysis directly or to agglutination followed by hemolysis. Among these are the isohemagglutinins and isohemolysins related to transfusion reactions and hemolytic disturbances of the newborn and the autogenous antibodies of the so-called "acquired" hemolytic anemias. Most of the isohemolysins alter the surface membranes, but do not actually destroy the red cells unless complement is present. Disruption of the intricate molecular architecture then liberates the hemoglobin, and a colorless "ghost" remains.

Curiously, lower concentrations of antibodies are needed for hemagglutination and hemolysis in vivo than in vitro. It has been suggested that red cells whose surface has been altered by an isoantibody tend to stagnate in the capillaries of various organs, where substances liberated by the tissues ("tissue lysins") bring about increases in fragility. The enhanced fragility, in turn, accelerates the susceptibility of the cells to disintegration by mechanical stress and strain or by the normal hemodestructive processes of the body.

Erythrophagocytosis

Leukocytes containing one or two engulfed red cells—so-called erythrophagocytes—are seen occasionally in peripheral blood films in disorders in which hemolysis is extremely rapid. Among these disorders are severe bacterial and protozoan infections, acquired hemolytic anemia, leukemia, erythroblastosis fetalis, paroxysmal cold hemoglobinuria, transfusion reactions, and acute poisoning by potassium chlorate or naphthalene. Erythrophagocytes occur usually in such small numbers that the smears have to be thoroughly surveyed for their detection.

Zinkham and Diamond have proposed an in vitro test to uncover a latent propensity to erythrophagocytosis: 5 ml of venous blood are placed in a dry centrifuge tube containing 0.6 ml of 0.1 M sodium oxalate or 1 mg of heparin. After standing at room temperature for 30 minutes the sample is centrifuged. The buffy coat is then drawn off with a capillary pipet and incubated in test tubes at 37°C for 1 to 2 hours. When the peripheral leukocyte count is over 10,000 per ml, whole blood may be taken instead of the buffy coat. Stained smears are then made. The percentage of leukocytes which contain ingested red cells is called the *erythrophagocytic index*. The authors found indexes of less than 0.1 per cent in blood specimens from healthy children and those with most other hematologic conditions, and 5 to 83 per cent in 3 of 4 children with "acquired" hemolytic anemia.

In the process of erythrophagocytosis the red cells first adhere to the neutrophils and monocytes and are then engulfed by them. This initial adherence may be so marked that the red cells appear agglutinated in the Coombs and other hemagglutinin tests unless the white cells have been removed previously.

Red Cell Survival Time

The life span of an individual normal erythrocyte within the blood stream may range from as little as 40 days to as much as 200 days or more. The average survival time appears to be somewhere between 110 and 130 days. Thus approximately 0.9 per cent of the circulating red cells wear out daily, and an equivalent number of new cells are formed. In the child, slightly more are produced than are destroyed to keep pace with growth. When abnormal factors destroy the circulating red cells with unusual rapidity (*hyperhemolysis*) the average survival time ranges from under 100 days in mild disturbances to but a few days in extreme situations. The abnormal destruction becomes superimposed on those of normal senescence.

The so-called Ashby method of differential agglutination follows the rate of disappearance of transfused compatible red cells of a different ABO or MN group. As the transfused red cells become obsolescent and are eliminated, the steadily diminishing ratio of nonagglutinable to agglutinable cells within the circulation of the recipient is estimated with the aid of potent grouping serums.

Red cells may be withdrawn from a patient, exposed to or "tagged" with radioactive isotopes such as Fe^{55}, Fe^{59}, C^{14}, N^{15} or Cr^{51}, and then reintroduced into the circulation. This approach permits one to follow the survival rate of a patient's red cells within his own internal environment.

Such studies can be helpful, for example, in determining whether a recently developing anemic process is due to inhibition of erythropoiesis or acceleration of erythrodestruction. Decisions with respect to such procedures as splenectomy may then be made on a sounder basis.

When an intracellular structural defect is the cause of the anemia, as in most hereditary red cell dyscrasias, such imperfect cells disappear unusually rapidly on being transfused into a normal person, whereas normal red cells survive their normal length of time when the patient is the recipient. Conversely, when the accelerated destruction is due to circulating antibodies or hypersplenic activity, normal red cells will disappear at an exceptional rate when transfused into the patient. Erythrocytes from individuals with iron-deficiency anemia, or from asymptomatic carriers of sicklemia or Mediterranean anemia, usually exhibit normal or nearly normal survival times when transfused into normal recipients.

Disturbances in Metabolism of Bile (Blood) Pigments

In many forms of anemia the metabolic cycles of hemoglobin, bilirubin, and urobilinogen are disturbed. Changes can be detected in the blood levels or fecal output, and the urine may contain urobilinogen, hemosiderin, coproporphyrin, bilirubin, or even hemoglobin. Prolonged excessive excretion of bile pigments by the liver is conducive to the formation of pigment gallstones.

When hemoglobin is being liberated into the blood stream at an excessive rate, much of it is converted promptly into hematin and other heme pigments. Combinations of these with the plasma albumin may form a brown pigment known as methemalbumin, which often circulates for some days after the hemolytic process has ceased. This may be searched for when intravascular hemolysis is suspected, as after transfusion reactions. It appears to be a constant finding in the serum of individuals with paroxysmal nocturnal hemoglobinuria. Like methemoglobin and sulfhemoglobin, methemalbumin reacts with benzidine and gives rise to specific spectroscopic absorption bands.

HEMOGLOBINEMIA. The normal range for free extracorpuscular hemoglobin is 1 to 4 mg per 100 ml of plasma. A higher reading can be taken as evidence of intravascular hemolysis due to hemolytic disease. With levels above 40 mg per 100 ml the plasma appears reddish. With levels above the renal threshold of approximately 100 mg per 100 ml, hemoglobinuria appears; this occurs only when the red cell destruction is extremely rapid and severe. With any degree of hemoglobinemia the urine usually contains hemosiderin, in quantities roughly proportional to the level of free hemoglobin.

Crosby and Dameshek found hemoglobinemia in acquired hemolytic anemia, erythroblastosis fetalis, acute disseminated lupus erythematosus, and severe Mediterranean anemia and sickle cell anemia. Patients with moderately severe Mediterranean anemia may have no elevation in plasma hemoglobin until after splenectomy, suggesting that abnormal red cells previously being destroyed in the spleen without raising the plasma hemoglobin are now being hemolyzed intravascularly. The level is normal in the usual case of hereditary spherocytosis. In single patients the hemoglobinemia tends to follow the fluctuating severity of the hemolytic process and to cease as the activity subsides.

Osmotic Fragility

Human plasma is isotonic osmotically with an 0.85 per cent solution of sodium chloride. When red cells are transferred from plasma to proper artificial environments such as hypotonic salt solutions, the cells imbide water by osmosis, grow progressively larger, and ultimately liberate their hemoglobin. With normal red cells this lysis occurs at about 175 per cent of the initial volume. Red cells which are already rounded to begin with tend to become lysed at 150 per cent of the initial volume or less. Such increased osmotic fragility occurs regularly in hereditary spherocytosis and with considerable frequency in acquired hemolytic anemia, erythroblastosis fetalis, some drug intoxications, and after extensive third-degree burns. Reversely, red cells which are unusually thin can resist rupture until distended to 200 to 220 per cent above normal size. This is the finding in the sickle cell anemias, Mediterranean anemia, and occasionally in severe degrees of iron-deficiency anemia.

SALINE FRAGILITY TEST. Osmotic resistance may be measured by placing small numbers of red cells in solutions having a progressively diminishing content of pure (silver-free; Merck) sodium chloride. After these have stood for a standard time the limits of minimal and complete hemolysis are noted. A blood specimen from a known normal subject serves as a control. Hemolysis normally begins in 0.46 to 0.42 per cent solution and is complete in 0.34 to 0.30 per cent.

In hereditary spherocytosis with the red cells already rounded, liberation of hemoglobin may begin in 0.60 to 0.50 per cent saline and be complete at or around 0.40 per cent. In sickle cell and Mediterranean anemia, in which the capacity of the flattened cells to swell before rupture is exceptional, hemolysis may begin in the usual saline dilution but may not be complete until below 0.30 or 0.20 per cent or even less. The extent of hemoglobin liberation in each tube may be estimated visually or measured by a photoelectric device.

The alterations in osmotic resistance run roughly parallel to the morphologic changes in the red cells. Abnormalities are sometimes indicated by this test when anemia and splenomegaly are lacking and inspection of the cells fails to uncover cell forms which are decisively abnormal.

The fragility test is of little assistance in differentiating between the carrier and active states of a hereditary anemia. Changes in osmotic resistance may take place at all levels of severity. In clinically latent individuals with any of the hereditary disturbances, normal or only slightly altered readings may be encountered. Most children with active Mediterranean anemia exhibit curves of less resistance than those of their carrier parents, because they receive transfusions frequently and hence go about with a mixture of normal and abnormal red cells.

Rigid control of all details is essential for reliable test results. A difference of 10°C in temperature gives changes equivalent to about an 0.01 per cent alteration in saline concentration. The more acid the environment, the smaller and more resistant the cells; a change of as little as 0.01 pH unit will produce measurable osmotic effects. Red cells saturated with carbon dioxide have a greater cell volume than when saturated with oxygen. Significant amounts of bile pigment in the plasma or toxins derived from hemolytic organisms may also influence the results. It is most important that each laboratory standardize the performance of its osmotic tests into a rigid pattern with control of all the sources of variation cited above.

All normal curve patterns are not exactly alike. Each normal person tends to retain essentially the same individual curve throughout his lifetime. In the hereditary red cell dyscrasias the patterns display wider variability but tend to remain constant for any one patient except after splenectomy or transfusion. In the acquired hemolytic anemias due to autoantibodies the pattern is labile, with shifts that parallel the severity of the process.

The Screening Saline Fragility Test. This survey approach indicates whether the osmotic reactions of the red cells are normal or abnormal and, if the latter, in which direction. Finger tip blood is introduced into two test tubes, containing saline mixtures of 0.42 per cent and 0.32 per cent, respectively. After an hour's standing a normal blood will show only a trace or absent hemolysis in the 0.42 per cent mixture but complete or nearly complete hemolysis in the 0.32 per cent mixture. In hereditary and other forms of spherocytosis the 0.42 per cent tube will display striking hemolysis. In disorders characterized by increased osmotic resistance an unhemolyzed residue will be prominent in the 0.32 per cent tube. When this screening test uncovers osmotic abnormalities the more detailed procedure should be applied.

The Incubation Test. In blood stored at 37°C, whether clotted or mixed with anticoagulant, fresh red cells from patients with hereditary spherocytosis tend to hemolyze considerably in 24 hours, whereas control red cells from normal subjects have but traces of hemolysis after that period and only moderate destruction after 48 hours.

Mechanical Fragility

In vitro procedures can be set up for study purposes in which freshly drawn blood is subjected to friction and agitation, simulating exaggeratedly the mechanical wear and tear which red cells are exposed to in the circulation. By standardizing such agitation it is possible to compare one blood specimen with another. Most of the methods employ rotating glass flasks containing glass beads and a small volume of blood which has been defibrinated or otherwise made incoagulable. After a given period, aliquot samples of the rotated blood and an unrotated control are placed in slightly hypertonic saline solutions and centrifuged. The excess of hemoglobin in the supernatant of the rotated specimen as compared with the control is taken as a measure of the mechanical hemolysis. Increased values are obtained usually with red cells from hereditary spherocytosis and hemolytic anemia due to antibodies and with cells which are sickled or agglutinated. Abnormal readings in mechanical fragility and osmotic fragility procedures do not always run parallel.

BIBLIOGRAPHY

ANEMIA AND ITS MANIFESTATIONS

Baar, H. A., and *T. W. Lloyd*, Studies in the Anaemias of Infancy and Early Childhood. XII. The Regeneration Rate of Haemoglobin and the Life Span of

Erythrocytes in Normal and Pathological Conditions, *Arch. Dis. Childhood* 18:1, 1943.

——— and ———, Studies in the Anaemias of Infancy and Early Childhood. XIV. The Fate of Transfused Erythrocytes, *Arch. Dis. Childhood* 18:124, 1943.

Bush, J. A., and **L. E. Ainger,** Congenital Absence of the Spleen with Congenital Heart Disease: Report of a Case with Ante Mortem Diagnosis on the Basis of Hematologic Morphology, *Pediatrics* 15:93, 1955.

Cartwright, G. E., C. M. Huguley, Jr., H. Ashenbrucker, J. Fay, and **M. M. Wintrobe,** Studies on Free Erythrocyte Protoporphyrin, Plasma Iron and Plasma Copper in Normal and Anemic Subjects, *Blood* 3:501, 1948.

Chernoff, A. I., and **A. M. Josephson,** Acute Erythroblastopenia in Sickle-cell Anemia and Infectious Mononucleosis, *A.M.A. Am. J. Dis. Child.* 82:310, 1951.

Cooper, M. B., Erythrophagocytosis in Hemolytic Disease of the Newborn: A Report of Twenty-five Cases, *Blood* 5:678, 1950.

Clark, B. B., and **R. W. Morrissey,** Relation of Methemoglobin to Hemolysis, *Blood* 6:532, 1951.

Crosby, W. H., The Pathogenesis of Spherocytes and Leptocytes (Target Cells), *Blood* 7:261, 1952.

——— and **W. Dameshek,** The Significance of Hemoglobinemia and Associated Hemosiderinuria, with Particular Reference to Various Types of Hemolytic Anemia, *J. Lab. & Clin. Med.* 38:829, 1951.

Dickstein, B., W. E. Landmesser, Jr., W. E. Love, T. H. Wilson, and **I. J. Wolman,** The Osmotic Resistance of Human Erythrocytes in Normal, Carrier and Anemic States: With Special Reference to Changes Due to Age, Race, Sickle-cell Anemia, Mediterranean (Cooley's) Anemia and Congenital Hemolytic Icterus, *Am. J. M. Sc.* 217:53, 1949.

Dornhorst, A. C., Analytical Review: The Interpretation of Red Cell Survival Curves, *Blood* 6:1284, 1951.

Douglas, A. S., and **J. V. Dacie,** The Incidence and Significance of Iron-containing Granules in Human Erythrocytes and Their Precursors, *J. Clin. Path.* 6:307, 1953.

Fairley, N. H., Methaemalbumin: Clinical Aspects, *Quart. J. Med.* 10:95, 1941.

Gasser, C., Die hämolytische Frühgeburtenämie mit spontaner Innenkörper-bildung, *Helvet. paediat. acta* 8:491, 1953.

Goldbloom, R. B., E. Fischer, J. Reinhold, and **D. Yi-Yung Hsia,** Studies on the Mechanical Fragility of Erythrocytes. I. Normal Values for Infants and Children, *Blood* 8:165, 1953.

Granick, S., The Chemistry and Functioning of the Mammalian Erythrocyte, *Blood* 4:404, 1949.

Ham, T. H., W. B. Castle, F. H. Gardner, and **G. A. Daland,** Laboratory Diagnosis of Polycythemia and Anemia, *New England J. Med.* 243:815, 860, 1950.

Jacobs, M. H., and **D. R. Stewart,** A Simple Method for the Quantitative Measurement of Cell Permeability, *J. Cell. & Comp. Physiol.* 1:71, 1932.

Jacobsen, E., Reticulocytes and Their Humoral Regulation, *J. Clin. Path.* 1:19, 1947.

McFadzean, A. J. S., and **L. J. Davis,** Iron-staining Erythrocytic Inclusions with Especial Reference to Acquired Haemolytic Anaemia, *Glasgow M. J.* 28:237, 1947.

Metcalf, W. K., Study of Intracellular Hemoglobin, *Blood* 6:1114, 1951.

Mills, H., and **S. P. Lucia,** Familial Hypochromic Anemia Associated with Post-splenectomy Erythrocyte Inclusion Bodies, *Blood* 4:891, 1949.

Ponder, E., "Hemolysis and Related Phenomena," Grune & Stratton, Inc., New York, 1948.

Price-Jones, C., "Red Blood Cell Diameters," Oxford University Press, London, 1933.

Rozsa, G., and *S. S. Spicer,* Nature of Heinz Bodies, *Nature* 171:84, 1953.

Schwartz, S. O., Significance of Nucleated Red Blood Cells in Peripheral Blood, *J.A.M.A.* 154:1339, 1954.

——— and *S. A. Motto,* The Diagnostic Significance of "Burr" Red Blood Cells, *Am. J. M. Sc.* 218:563, 1949.

Sutherland, D. A., M. S. McCall, M. T. Groves, and *E. E. Muirhead,* The Survival of Normal Erythrocytes Estimated by Means of Cells Tagged with Radioactive Chromium: A Study of the Normal State, *J. Lab. & Clin. Med.* 43:717, 1954.

Zinkham, W. H., and *L. K. Diamond,* In Vitro Erythrophagocytosis in Acquired Hemolytic Anemia, *Blood* 7:592, 1952.

CHAPTER 3

Malnutritional Anemias

The fact that the hemoglobin, hematocrit, and red cell levels tend to be low when there is a major deficiency in the intake or utilization of one or more essential hemopoietic nutrients has led to the clinical application of these measurements in appraising nutritional status. When iron deficiency is the sole cause of the anemia, the hemoglobin level becomes depressed much more than the erythrocyte count, resulting in a hypochromic and often microcytic type of anemia. Conversely, when iron stores are adequate but the hemopoietic vitamins are lacking, as in folic acid or vitamin B_{12} deficiency, the erythrocyte count may become more depressed than the hemoglobin level and macrocytosis follows. When the dietary intake is defective primarily in calories and protein, any mild anemia which develops is typically normochromic and normocytic. The total blood volume may or may not be diminished in any of these forms of anemia; unfortunately there is no simple method for measuring this important variable.

A low hemoglobin level per se does not enhance susceptibility to infections, but infection when once established is often more severe and speed of recovery in the absence of antibiotics is often retarded. The pathogenesis of this difficulty is not clear, but is related presumably to other disturbed mechanisms which are produced by or are coincident with the anemia. In Great Britain during World War II Mackay and associates noted that improving the diet, including the addition of iron, was followed by a rise in the mean hemoglobin level of children up to 6 years of age by about 6 per cent and also by a 25 per cent reduction in their illnesses.

HYPOCHROMIC MICROCYTIC ANEMIA (HYPOCHROMIC OR ACHROMIC ANEMIA, HYPOFERRIC ANEMIA, IRON-DEFICIENCY ANEMIA, CHLOROTIC ANEMIA OF CHILDHOOD)

Iron deficiency leads to poor hemoglobin formation, the erythrocytic stroma being involved secondarily. Hypochromic microcytosis is so characteristic as to be essentially diagnostic. No other hematologic disturbances in childhood produce changes in this direction except the carrier state of Mediterranean anemia.

Causes

Known influences which predispose to iron deficiency during infancy and childhood are: (1) Not enough iron in the diet or its poor absorption through the intestinal mucosa (Chap. 51). Since milk itself is almost devoid of iron, the infant must be given a liberal intake from other sources, such as vegetables, meats, and fortified cereals. The comparatively limited range of food taken in infancy makes it easy for milk to become the principal or sole food item when iron-containing foods are rejected or not offered. (2) Body growth. The rapid growth of cellular tissues and blood volume during infancy, and the concomitant increase in absolute mass of circulating hemoglobin, tend to deplete the iron reserves of the body. This physiologic need lies behind the aphorism that the growing infant tends to bleed into his own increasing blood volume. (3) Infectious diseases. The poor iron absorption and inhibition of erythrocyte formation which infections may bring about can continue for some time after the clinical subsidence of the infection. (4) Blood loss, as from a gastrointestinal ulcer. This can be persistent or intermittent. Loss of blood from obvious or occult hemorrhage is not common in infancy and is usually evident when it occurs. (5) Gestational and obstetric factors which reduce the reserve iron stores of the newborn infant. Among these are prematurity, maternal anemia, multiple births, early clamping of the umbilical cord, and neonatal hemorrhage.

Iron-deficiency anemia in the early years is usually wholly of nutritional origin. Enhancing the quantity of iron being taken, or restoring it by injection or transfusion, will usually correct the disturbance promptly.

With older children, in contrast, hemorrhages, menstruation, infections, faulty assimilation, or depressive chronic diseases are more likely to complicate the pathogenesis. Even though the absolute demand for iron is greater than in infancy, the variety of foods taken makes it difficult to escape ingesting this element. Once in a great while, however, an older child may be seen who through some quirk of mind has limited himself almost exclusively to milk. When hypochromic microcytosis is found in a child of school age, the physician should make a careful diagnostic survey for some lesion which can lead to occult bleeding, and also for the carrier state of Mediterranean anemia. Stools and urine should be examined for blood frequently, because the loss may be intermittent rather than continuous. If these prove negative, complete gastrointestinal roentgenography is called for. The anemia which develops in a child with chronic blood loss who has been receiving a well-balanced diet rich in iron tends to be normochromic and normocytic.

Symptoms and Blood Findings

Pallor, fatigability, and poor appetite are the predominant symptoms, with minor retardation of growth if the disorder is long-continued. In a series of Philadelphia cases personally studied, 90 per cent fell within the age range of 6 to 30 months. The gastric hypochlorhydria or achlorhydria, frequently found when searched for, is secondary rather than primary; nevertheless, once developed it contributes to perpetuation of the disturbance.

Iron-deficiency anemia can complicate anemia from other causes. In such cases the institution of iron therapy usually produces a transitory reticulocytosis followed by a moderate rise in hemoglobin level and leaves the blood changes of the underlying constitutional disease more clearly evident.

In the anemia of iron deficiency the red cell count does not become much diminished until after the hemoglobin level has fallen to approximately 8 gm per 100 ml. The hemoglobin content of the packed red cells may range from 25 to 35 per cent (normal for children, 33 to 35 per cent). The red cells show central pallor and irregular diminution in size. The reticulocytes are almost always below normal so long as the diet remains devoid of iron, but one may find a reticulocytosis of 1 to 2 per cent or higher if some food which contains iron has been ingested recently. A few nucleated red cells may appear in the peripheral blood. Price-Jones curves show not only a mean microcytosis but an abnormal range of spread in cell diameters (anisocytosis). The more severe the anemia, the more pronounced are all blood changes. In most untreated cases the values for mean cellular hemoglobin are less than 20 and may be as low as 12 $\mu\mu$gm (normal, 26 to 28). The mean cellular volume, calculated from the hematocrit and erythrocyte count, is usually between 50 and 65 cu μ, but may be as small as 40 cu μ (normal range for infants, 74 to 78 cu μ). The osmotic fragility of the red cells remains unaltered. The granulocytes and platelets may be diminished in advanced cases associated with malnutrition. The plasma iron level is subnormal (Chap. 51).

Therapy

Iron is the specific remedy for hypochromic microcytic anemia of nutritional origin, as shown by the prompt response which follows its use. When iron is supplied the active synthesis of hemoglobin is reassumed quickly and the red cells mature once more in normal fashion, giving a transient reticulocytosis. Trace amounts of copper or cobalt sometimes are given as supplementary therapy, but are not indispensable. Vitamins, a high-protein diet, and a good supply of other important nutrients help to relieve a concomitant poor nutritional state if present.

Ferrous salts are more satisfactory than ferric salts as oral medication for iron-deficiency anemia. Nearly every child will respond satisfactorily. Excellent results are secured usually by a daily intake of 0.1 to 0.5 gm of ferrous sulfate per day, the size of the dose depending on the age of the patient. Supplementary ascorbic acid may enhance absorption. The therapy should be continued for several months after the peripheral hemoglobin level has been restored and the cause of the anemia corrected, since reaccumulation of storage iron in tissue depots is always a slow process.

Colloidal suspensions of iron are available for parenteral injection. These can be recommended when oral iron fails to produce results or is not satisfactory because of gastrointestinal symptoms or lack of cooperation on the part of patient or parents. Reactions to injections are exceptional, provided they are given in accordance with the instructions which accompany each package.

When apparently adequate amounts of iron fail to elicit a satisfactory hematologic response, an occult infection, a chronic bleeding focus, or the presence of some other anemia-producing disease should be suspected. We have seen such refractoriness in several patients with cyanotic congenital heart disease.

Results of Iron Therapy

Clinical evidences of improvement become evident early. Appetite may improve within 24 hours. Pallor disappears as the hemoglobin rises, and vigor and sense of well-being become restored. Complete recovery takes 15 to 45 days, as a rule. The recovery time is longer in the more severe cases. It is also longer for patients who receive the medication by the oral route.

A rise in hemoglobin level can be detected as early as the second day after an intravenous injection, or on the fourth or fifth day after initiation of oral therapy. With regular treatment the restoration of the hemoglobin continues steadily until recovery from the anemia is complete. The rate of increase varies from 0.1 to 0.3 gm of hemoglobin per 100 ml per day. The return of the red cell count when depressed is almost as rapid.

Reticulocyte counts, if taken serially, will reveal a begining rise by the second to fifth day and a peak between the fifth and tenth day. The reticulocytosis may fade away as swiftly as it appeared or continue at low grade until the anemia has been fully corrected. The extent of the rise is inversely proportional to the initial hemoglobin level. The average peak may be 15 to 30 per cent with initial hemoglobin levels less than 5 gm per 100 ml, but only about 4 to 10 per cent when the levels are between 6 and 9 gm.

The hematocrit depression tends to be directly proportional to the hemoglobin level. Readings are nearly always below 30 per cent and may even fall below 20 per cent. Return to normal during treatment parallels the hemoglobin rise or may be more rapid. The mean cellular hemoglobin, mean cellular volume, and hemoglobin content of the mass of packed red cells recover at approximately the same rate, and the structural irregularities of the red cells fade away. As mentioned, when improvement after prolonged iron therapy is only partial, the patient should be restudied for some other underlying disturbance.

THE MACROCYTIC ANEMIAS

In this group of anemias (1) the red cells are significantly greater in volumetric size than normal, (2) the bone marrow shows the patterns of red cell dysplasia and maturation arrest at the prorubricyte or megaloblast level (*megaloblastic anemia*), and (3) administration of agents of the folic acid–vitamin B_{12} system or related nutrients induces a specific therapeutic response. In mild cases only one of these features may be prominent enough to be recognized. Sometimes enough microcytes are present coincidentally to result in a normal value for calculated mean red cell volume; in these circumstances it is probable that a superimposed iron deficiency or other handicap obscures the full development of macrocytosis. Macrocytic blood changes in association with a more normal bone marrow have been described in hypothyroidism, some hemolytic syndromes, and occasional refractory anemias of uncertain origin.

Etiology

The macrocytic enlargement of the red cells is best understood as resulting from intracellular deficiencies of vitamin-like nutrients other than iron—folic (pteroylglutamic) acid, the citrovorum factor (folinic acid), or vitamin B_{12}. Folic acid appears to be the precursor of citrovorum factor.

Vitamin B_{12} and folic acid seem to complement each other in nucleic acid synthesis; when one is absent the other becomes less effective. In vitamin-C deficiency, the intermediary metabolism of folic acid is hampered. Subclinical scurvy can aggravate the severity of the anemia or precipitate the development of overt symptoms.

The majority of instances of macrocytic anemia encountered in the childhood years result from a deficient intake of folic acid, often associated with an ascorbic acid deficiency. Macrocytic anemia due to failure of synthesis of intrinsic factor within the gastric mucosa is almost never seen. Defective absorption of vitamin B_{12} or folic acid may be responsible in sprue, the celiac syndrome, enterocolic fistulas, and other steatorrheic states. Defective intrahepatic storage occurs in cirrhosis and related severe liver diseases. Rarely a macrocytic anemia will develop in a child with leukemia who receives folic acid antagonists for a long time.

General Features

The laboratory findings in a typical childhood case of any macrocytic anemia are similar to those of pernicious anemia in adults. There is a low blood hemoglobin content (3 to 8 gm per 100 ml) and even greater lowering of the red cell count (1 to 2.5 million), a comparatively high packed cell volume (15 to 25 per cent), an augmented corpuscular volume (90 to 130 cu μ), and a normal or nearly normal hemoglobin content in the packed mass of red cells (30 to 35 per cent) and in the individual red cells (28 to 40 $\mu\mu$gm). The peripheral blood smear may show anisocytosis and Howell-Jolly bodies, Cabot rings, punctate or diffuse basophilia, or highly immature nucleated forms. Neutrophilopenia and thrombocytopenia are not uncommon, with hypersegmented and giant neutrophils in the peripheral blood. All changes are most pronounced in advanced cases.

Mild urobilinogenuria and bilirubinemia are usually demonstrable. Hypoproteinemia is usually present. The serum iron level is elevated, and the urobilinogen content of feces increased. The bone marrow findings are those of erythropoietic proliferation and dysgenesis with a piling up of immature and atypical megaloblasts in early stages of development and distortions in the appearance of the granulocyte precursors (p. 325).

The macrocytic anemias of infancy and childhood differ from pernicious anemia of adults in not being accompanied by neurologic disturbances or glossitis. Achlorhydria is usually, but not invariably, present. Therapeutic responses to folic acid, citrovorum factor, or vitamin B_{12} individually are far from uniform, but folic acid is usually the most effective.

Acute macrocytic disturbances of dietary origin in childhood do not recur after corrective therapy unless the deficient food intake is returned to. Recovery sometimes is initiated by transfusion alone.

The nursing infant of a mother receiving a poor diet who has had macrocytic anemia during pregnancy is likely to exhibit megaloblastic blood changes unless the antianemic vitamins are given. Correction of the deficiency in the mother will also heal the baby, showing that the protective vitamins are transmitted through the breast milk.

Megaloblastic Anemia

This name is applied to a form of macrocytic anemia which occurs typically in infants 3 months to 2 years of age. The fundamental lesion appears to be a deficient or suboptimal intake of hemopoietic vitamins. There are usually contributory influences in the form of a comparatively low intake of protein or vitamin C or both, premature or immature birth, or recent gastroenteritis or other intercurrent infection. As a rule the feeding regime has consisted principally of goat's milk, breast milk, or a powdered modified cow's-milk preparation not fortified with ascorbic acid in liberal amounts. The disorder is characterized by pallor, weakness, irritability, undernutrition, persistent upper respiratory infection, anorexia, and macrocytic anemia. Scurvy, overt or subclinical, is often concomitant. There may be transitory gastric achlorhydria, even after histamine. Proof of the diagnosis rests upon the demonstration of characteristic distortions in the immature red cells and granulocytes of the bone marrow.

This disturbance always clears quickly when crude liver extract is given. Large doses of folic acid, and vitamin B_{12} less regularly, are nearly as effective. If vitamin B_{12} fails to produce appreciable improvement within a few days, folic acid should be given, and vice versa. A high protein diet and large doses of vitamin C are valuable adjuvants. The marrow megaloblasts begin to mature immediately. A peripheral reticulocytosis is usually evident within a week. The erythrocyte count and hemoglobin rise more gradually and may take 1 to 2 months to return to normal.

Pernicious Anemia

A few instances of true Addisonian anemia have been observed in childhood, and some of these have been familial. Their features are identical with those of adult cases, save that the gastric mucosa has been sometimes capable of elaborating a little hydrochloride acid when stimulated by histamine. Central nervous system lesions may develop, simulating dorsolateral sclerosis of the cord. These are alleviated by vitamin B_{12} therapy, but are refractory to or may even be aggravated when folic acid is given.

Before treatment the red cells present marked anisocytosis and poikilocytosis. Many are round or oval macrocytes. Circulating rubriblasts and bosophilic stippling may also be evident. Reticulocytes are few. Leukopenia and neutropenia tend to occur, with overlarge neutrophils having five- to eight-lobed nuclei. Platelets are normal or diminished. The bone marrow is hypercellular and shows a preponderance of primitive large nucleated red cells. Fecal urobilinogen and serum bilirubin level may be in moderate excess of normal. The red cells have a shortened survival period. Papillary atrophy of the tongue may develop during relapses and subside during remissions.

Specific antipernicious anemia therapy with liver-extract injections or vitamin B_{12}, or at times with folic acid, is followed by an immediate clinical and hematologic remission. In the early phases the increase in hemoglobin may lag behind the recovery of the red cell count. This transient hypochromia represents a depletion of the iron stores and can be corrected by administration of ferrous sulfate. Unlike what occurs with other forms of macrocytic anemia, withdrawal of specific therapy is followed by a relapse, usually within a few months. Relapses are often preceded by acute infections.

Transfused blood may contain sufficient quantities of the absent substances to induce more normal maturation in a rubriblastic marrow and bring about a reticulocytosis. Since several weeks may then be needed for the marrow to resume a hyperplastic appearance, suspected cases should undergo a marrow examination prior to transfusion.

THE NORMOCYTIC ANEMIAS

Von Jaksch's Anemia

This disturbance is a rare and extreme chronic anemia of nutritional origin. Splenomegaly, hepatomegaly, and general malnutrition are usually associated, often with rickets and recurrent infections. The red cells, low in absolute numbers, may be normocytic or macrocytic or microcytic. The total leukocyte count may be eleveted, and the platelets diminished. The peripheral blood contains reticulocytes, nucleated red cells, and immature granulocytes. The bone marrow is hypocellular, with many reticulum cells. There are no evidences of excessive blood destruction in the form of bilirubinemia or urobilinogenuria. The blood calcium and phosphorus levels tend to be low along with the rickets, and the plasma alkaline phosphatase elevated. The vitamin and prothrombin levels of the blood are usually low.

The disturbance is reversible. After a normal diet has been given for some months the immature cells disappear from the blood, the enlargement of liver and spleen subsides, and the bone marrow reverts to normal. A high intake of vitamins and iron accelerates the recovery.

Minimal and mild forms of this syndrome are more prevalent than the extreme pattern outlined above. Many children in nutritionally poor state as the result of multiple dietary deficiencies exhibit a red cell and marrow picture which seems to be a combination of iron-deficiency and megaloblastic anemia and have along with it a mild leukocytosis, a depressed platelet count, small numbers of circulating immature cells, and slight enlargement of the liver and spleen.

Kwashiorkor

This is a severe nutritional disorder seen in young children in Africa, Central America, and other areas where the food intake of the population is grossly defective. Known also as the "malignant-malnutrition" or "plurideficiency" syndrome, the disorder is characterized clinically by edema, stunted growth, mental apathy, rawness of the skin, weakness, enlarged liver, and depigmentation of the hair. Anemia is often mild; when moderate or advanced it is usually hypochromic and microcytic. Occasional cases have a macrocytic picture. There are no characteristic deviations in the leukocyte or thrombocyte counts or in differential leukocyte distribution. The bone marrow is usually of normal cellularity, with no consistent irregularities in the forming rubricytes or granulocytes.

Serum albumin and globulin are customarily reduced, and liver function tests often give abnormal results. Intestinal parasites are frequent in the stools.

Malnutritional Anemia Associated with Intestinal Parasitism

The anemia shown by undernourished children in tropical climates is largely hypochromic and microcytic in its early or mild phases. The poor intake or absorption of iron-containing food and the blood loss from the intestine with infestations such as those of hookworm combine to produce an anemia which fundamentally is one of iron deficiency. As the disturbance progresses and becomes severe a macrocytic change becomes superimposed. This is attributed pathogenetically to a superimposed faulty intake and absorption of protein and vitamin nutrients, and losses from diarrhea. Poor dietary and living conditions contribute to the tendency of these children to develop later a malnutritional form of celiac syndrome or liver disease, or even kwashiorkor.

STARVATION

During acute starvation the erythrocytes and the hemoglobin levels may fall a little, though the loss may be masked by the concomitant dehydration. The leukocyte count tends to drop also, leading to a relative lymphocytosis. The bone marrow sometimes becomes moderately hypoplastic, with plasma cells comparatively numerous. Anemia is unusual in chronic starvation of adults; when it appears it tends to be normocytic and normochromic. With growing children, on the other hand, anemia of the hypochromic microcytic character of iron deficiency is more prone to develop, often with associated megaloblastic components.

BIBLIOGRAPHY

HYPOCHROMIC MICROCYTIC ANEMIA

Davidson, W. M., and *R. F. Jennison,* The Relationship between Iron Storage and Anaemia, *J. Clin. Path.* 5:281, 1952.

Darby, W. J., Iron and Copper, *J.A.M.A.* 142:1288, 1950.

Dickstein, B., I. J. Wolman, C. Tan, B. Slaughter, H. Butson, and *R. Cohen,* Intravenous Iron Therapy in the Iron-deficiency Anemia of Infancy and Childhood, *A.M.A. Am. J. Dis. Child.* 84:52, 1952.

Finch, C. A., M. Hegsted, T. D. Kinney, E. D. Thomas, C. E. Rath, D. Haskins, S. Finch, and *R. G. Fluharty,* Iron Metabolism: The Pathophysiology of Iron Storage, *Blood* 5:983, 1950.

Fullerton, H. W., The Iron-deficiency Anaemia of Late Infancy, *Arch. Dis. Childhood* 12:91, 1937.

Granick, S., Iron Metabolism and Hemochromatosis, *Bull. New York Acad. Med.* 25:403, 1949.

Guest, G. M., and *E. W. Brown,* Erythrocytes and Hemoglobin of the Blood in Infancy and in Childhood. I. Size and Hemoglobin Content of the Erythrocytes in Nutritional Anemia, *Am. J. Dis. Child.* 52:616, 1936.

Heath, C. W., and *A. J. Patek,* The Anemia of Iron Deficiency, *Medicine* 16:267, 1937.

Josephs, H. W., Hypochromic Microcytic Anemia of Infancy: Iron Depletion as a Factor, *Pediatrics* 18:959, 1956.

Mackay, H., R. H. Dobbs, and *K. Bingham,* The Effect of National Bread, of Iron Medicated Bread, and of Iron Cooking Utensils on the Haemoglobin Level of Children in Wartime Day Nurseries, *Arch. Dis. Childhood* 20:56, 1945.

————, ————, ————, and *W. J. Martin,* The Etiology and the Effects of Minor Grades of Anaemia in Young Children: Studies at a Group of War-time Day Nurseries, *Arch. Dis. Childhood* 21:145, 1946.

———— and *L. Goodfellow,* Nutritional Anemia in Infancy, *Med. Res. Council Spec. Rep.* 157, 1931.

Niccum, W. L., R. L. Jackson, and *G. Stearns,* Use of Ferric and Ferrous Iron in the Prevention of Hypochromic Anemia in Infants, *A.M.A. Am. J. Dis. Child.* 86:553, 1953.

Parsons, L. G., Studies in the Anemias of Infancy and Early Childhood. I. Introduction, *Arch. Dis. Childhood* 8:85, 1933.

Smith, C. A., W. L. Caton, C. C. Roby, D. E. Reid, R. S. Caswell, and *J. G. Gibson,* Transplacental Iron: Its Persistence during Infancy as Studied Isotopically, II, *Am. J. Dis. Child.* 80:856, 1950.

Strauss, M. B., Hypochromic Anemia, *Am. Pract.* 3:65, 1948.

THE MACROCYTIC ANEMIAS

Bethell, F. H., Treatment of Macrocytic Anemias with Vitamin B_{12}, *J. Am. Dietet. A.* 26:89, 1950.

Delbèke, M. J., Anémie pernicieuse de l'enfant constatée chez deux frères, *Arch. franç. pédiat.* 9:837, 1952.

Girdwood, R. H., The Interrelationships of Factors That Influence the Megaloblastic Anemias, *Blood* 7:77, 1952.

Heck, F. J., Proper Use of Iron, Liver Extract, Vitamin B_{12}, and Folic Acid in Anemias, *J.A.M.A.* 148:783, 1952.

Imerslund, O., Red Blood Cell Diameters in Megaloblastic Anemia in Children Needing Continuous Treatment, *Acta paediat.* 40:82, suppl. 83, 1951.

Lindgren, G., Macrocytosis in Acute Hepatitis and Pernicious Anemia: A Comparison Based on 830 Price-Jones' Curves, *Acta med. scandinav.* 136:39, 1949.

May, C. D., C. T. Stewart, A. Hamilton, and *R. J. Salmon,* Infection as Cause of Folic Acid Deficiency and Megaloblastic Anemia, *A.M.A. Am. J. Dis. Child.* 84:718, 1952.

Reisner, E. H., Jr., J. A. Wolff, R. J. McKay, Jr., and *E. F. Doyle,* Juvenile Pernicious Anemia, *Pediatrics* 8:88, 1951.

Sturgis, C. C., Pernicious Anemia and Other Macrocytic Anemias, chap. 6 in "Hematology," 2d ed., Charles C Thomas, Springfield, Ill., 1955.

Unglaub, W. G., and *G. A. Goldsmith,* Folic Acid and Vitamin B_{12} in Medical Practice, *J.A.M.A.* 161:623, 1956.

THE NORMOCYTIC ANEMIAS AND STARVATION

Altmann, A., and *J. F. Murray,* The Anaemia of Malignant Malnutrition (Infantile Pellagra Kwashiorkor): Protein Deficiency as a Possible Aetiological Factor, *South African J. M. Sc.* 13:91, 1948.

Davidson, C. S., H. L. Wilcke, and *P. J. Reiner,* A Nutritional Survey of Starvation in a Group of Young Men, *J. Lab. & Clin. Med.* 31:721, 1946.

Gomez, F., R. R. Galván, J. Cravioto, and *S. Frenk,* Malnutrition in Infancy and Childhood, with Special Reference to Kwashiorkor, *Advances Pediat.* 7:131, 1955.

Spies, T. D., S. Dreizen, G. S. Parker, D. J. Silberman, Detection and Treatment of Nutritive Failure in Children, *J.A.M.A.* 148:1376, 1952.

Tovar-Excobar, C., and *B. L. DeMajo,* Multiple Deficiency Syndromes in Infants and Children (Venezuelan Kwashiorkor), *Docum. med. geog. et trop.* 7:116, 1955.

Veneklaas, G. M. H., Aplasia of the Bone Marrow: A New Cause of the von Jaksch Syndrome, *Arch. Dis. Childhood* 27:134, 1952.

CHAPTER 4

Hereditary Dystrophies of the Red Cells

HEREDITARY SPHEROCYTOSIS

This has been known also as congenital hemolytic icterus and Minkowski-Chauffard disease. The fundamental defect appears to be in the red cell stroma, producing fragile "spherocytic" cells which have a shortened life span in symptomatic patients.

The disease is inherited as a dominant mendelian character and is more common in whites than in Negroes. Its severity is variable, with symptoms ranging from extremely marked to completely absent. Once the florid picture has been established it remains so, with little likelihood of appreciable spontaneous regression.

Statistically, when a parent has this red cell defect, 50 per cent of his children will be affected. Clinical expressions of the disorder, however, are unpredictably variable.

The onset is usually insidious. Symptoms when present indicate a chronic fluctuating hemolytic process—pallor, weakness, splenomegaly, and slight jaundice. The hematologic changes are those of hemolytic anemia—reticulocytosis, elevated serum bilirubin, rubricytic hyperplasia in the bone marrow, and increased urobilinogen in stool and urine. Some patients have marked anemia and negligible jaundice; in others the reverse is true. The liver and spleen are often palpable. A family history is usually obtainable, or by a laboratory survey the pediatrician may be the first to recognize the subclinical existence of the disorder in other members.

Spherocytosis

The characteristic red cell in this disease is somewhat rounded with unusually small diameter and abnormal thickness. In blood films these cells appear smaller than normal and more deeply staining. In some patients only a few such cells may be seen, whereas in others nearly all the cells will seem affected. Since overstaining makes normal red cells stain like spherocytes it is important when making this evaluation to find unaffected cells with normal pallor at their centers. If there has been protracted excessive hemodestruction there may be associated hypochromia, polychromasia, or anisocytosis. Unusually large red cells may be scattered among those with decreased diameter.

The apparent smallness can be demonstrated by preparing a smear of the patient's blood on one half of a glass slide and of normal blood on the other half. Both preparations are then stained simultaneously, and their microscopic appearances compared. Deviations in cell size are recognized easily.

Direct microscopy of red cells in a fresh cover-slip preparation reveals that some of the cells which lie edgewise are biconvex. Others may appear cup-shaped or spheroidal with a dimple at one end. Rouleaux when present are curved and short because rounded red cells do not become closely stacked.

Quantitative measurements have shown the mean red cell diameter to be between 6 and 7 μ (normal 7.7 μ) and the cross-sectional thickness 2.2 to 4.7 μ (normal 1.7 to 2.5 μ). The mean corpuscular volume remains approximately unaltered, but may rise above normal when blood destruction and erythropoiesis have been unusually active. No significant correlation can be established between the mean diameter of the red cells and the presence or severity of the clinical symptoms, the onset of hemolytic crises, or the rapidity of red cell regeneration after a crisis.

When transfused into healthy recipients the affected cells have a shorter survival time than normal. Contrariwise, normal cells when transfused into patients with congenital spherocytosis exhibit a normal survival time. Circulating or absorbed hemolysins are not found, and cold isoagglutinins are exceptional. In uncomplicated cases the red cells are not agglutinated by Coombs' antiglobulin serum.

Red Cell Fragility

Related to the spheroid shape of the red cells is their diminished resistance to osmotic and mechanical strains (p. 37). Prior incubation of the blood for 24 hours at 37°C under sterile conditions will enhance the fragility (p. 39).

Other Laboratory Findings

The distinction between "active" and "latent" cases is entirely one of degree. Sensitive methods have shown that both hemopoiesis and hemodestruction proceed at an accelerated rate even when no signs of anemia are elicitable. No abnormalities have been found in the hemoglobin. Asymptomatic parents are as likely to transmit this genetically dominant trait to their offspring.

Anemia when present tends to be normochromic and normocytic. The red cell count may become stabilized anywhere between 2.5 and 5.5 million (Table 4-1). Reticulocytes range from 2 to 50 per cent, but are usually between 5 and 20 per cent. Polychromatophilic and nucleated red cell forms are not uncommon. The bone marrow exhibits hyperplasia

Table 4-1. Typical Abnormalities in the Hereditary Red Cell Dystrophies

	Hereditary spherocytosis		Thalassemia		Sicklemia		Hb C disturbances		Hb C— sickle cell disease	Thalassemia— sickle cell disease †
	Latent	Active	Trait	Disease	Trait	Disease	Trait	Disease		
Hemoglobins	AA	AA	AA	AAF	AS	SSF	AC	CC	SC	AS (F) †
RBC osmotic behavior *	Frag. ±	Frag.	Res.	Res.	Res.	Res.	Res. ±	Res.	Res.	Res.
Hb level (gm/100 ml)	12–15	8–12	10–12	<9	12–15	6–9	11–15	11–15	7–11	7–11
RBC (meters/cu mm)	5.0	2.5–4.5	3.5–5.5	4.0	5.0	4.5	4.0–5.0	4.0–5.0	3.0–4.5	3.0–4.5
Reticulocytes (%)	1–5	5–20	1–5	5–20	0.5	1–20	0.5–1.5	0.5–2.5	3–6	3–6
Urobilinogenuria	+	+++	+	+++	0	++	0	+	++	++
Splenomegaly	0	+	0	+++	0	±	0	±	+	++
Sickling:										
Holly leaf	0	0	0	0	+++	0	0	0	0	0
Filamentous	0	0	0	0	0	++++	0	0	++++	+++
Stained blood smears:										
Anisocytosis	+	++	+	++++	0	++	0	+	++	+
Microcytosis	++	+++	0	±	0	±	0	0	±	±
Macrocytosis	+	++	++	++	0	++	0	0	+	+
Leptocytosis	0	0	±	+	+	+	+	++++	++++	+
Ovalocytosis	0	0	+	++	0	0	0	0	0	0
Hypochromia	0	0	+	++	0	++	+	++	++	++
Sickle cells	0	0	0	0	0	++	0	0	±	±
Siderocytes	0	0	0	+	0	0	0	0	0	0
Nucleated RBC:										
Before splenectomy	0	0	0	+	0	0	0	0	0	0
After splenectomy	0	+	0	++	0	+	0	+	+	+
WBC (thousands)	5–10	5–10	5–10	5–10	5–10	10–20	5–10	5–10	5–15	5–10
Bone marrow										
RBC hypercellularity	+	+++	+	++++	0	+++	0	++	+++	+++

* Frag. = more fragile than normal; Res. = more resistant than normal.
† Heterozygous combinations of thalassemia with the abnormal hemoglobin C or E give a somewhat similar hematologic pattern but without sickling. The presence of fetal hemoglobin is inconstant.

of the red cell series even when the disease is clinically latent. The mean volume and mean hemoglobin content of the red cells may be normal, increased, or decreased. The serum bilirubin tends to be between 1 and 5 mg per 100 ml, with no increase in the 1-minute component. Sometimes the granulocyte and platelet counts remain unusually low; when this occurs a superimposed hypersplenic activity seems the likely explanation. The urine almost always contains urobilinogen in excess. The fecal urobilinogen output is greatly augmented; it tends to be between 300 and 800 mg per day, depending on the severity of the disturbance and the age of the child. The hemolytic index becomes 50 to 150 instead of the normal 10 to 20 (p. 704). Supportive transfusions as a rule are not needed, except when the equilibrium between red cell production and destruction is disturbed by episodes of hemolytic destruction.

Crises

These are acute explosions of acute hemolysis and prostration in which the rate of red cell destruction goes up rapidly and the spleen enlarges. All symptoms including jaundice and anemia become transiently aggravated. The episodes may be initiated by febrile illnesses, though more often no precipitating cause can be detected. Probably because of the spread of a subclinical virus infection, crises sometimes occur within a few days of each other among all affected members of a family. The bone marrow may temporarily take on a hypoplastic or even aplastic appearance (p. 328).

In some cases the predominant symptoms seem to be more hepatic than hemolytic. The patient has nausea, vomiting, fever, jaundice, and upper right quadrant pain. The serum bilirubin rises rapidly with change in reaction from slow-acting to immediate, and the liver becomes enlarged and tender. Hemoglobinuria may occur. The fecal urobilinogen output often rises further, as much as 1,000 mg per day.

After a crisis which has been treated with transfusion the urobilinogen output may temporarily subside to as low as 100 mg per day. This reflects a normal rate of destruction of the donor's red cells and the previous wiping out of many of the patient's own cells. Within a few weeks the output rises again as the patient's shorter-lived cells once more become preponderant.

Transfusions are usually advisable during crises if the drop in hemoglobin is severe. Occasionally, however, a transfusion is followed by increased hemodestruction and a further fall in hemoglobin level.

Spleen

In hereditary spherocytosis the parenchyma of the spleen is jammed with red cells. Erythrophagocytosis is inconspicuous, indicating that some humoral rather than cellular mechanism is destroying the red cells or rendering them more susceptible to other influences. Affected cells tend to be trapped within the spleen, whereas normal transfused cells have less difficulty in traversing the parenchyma.

SPLENECTOMY. The only satisfactory treatment for the persistent ictero-anemic symptoms and the recurrent crises lies in splenectomy. After splenectomy the excessive blood destruction and blood formation are arrested immediately, and red cell and reticulocyte counts begin to return to normal, and crises no longer occur. Emergency splenectomy can be lifesaving in a severe crisis.

After splenectomy, Howell-Jolly bodies become evident and may persist for years. The spherocytosis and increased red cell fragility recede only partially. The red cells and hemoglobin attain normal levels in about a month. Reticulocytosis is usually not prominent after the second week. Leukocyte counts between 30,000 and 60,000 per cu mm are not unusual for some weeks after the operation. This increase is chiefly in the neutrophils, but the absolute number of monocytes may rise also. The platelets mount similarly to between 500,000 and 800,000 per cu mm, as a rule, but may exceed 1 million; their return to normal may take many weeks in some cases.

Symptoms due to increased hemolysis have recurred in rare patients after several symptom-free months or years following splenectomy. Since recurrences have been often associated with accessory spleens, these should be searched for and removed during the primary operation. Accessory spleens occur in about 10 per cent of normal adults; they may be more frequent in childhood and infancy. Their location may be hilar, gonadal, or gastrointestinal. Hypertrophy of the hemolymph tissues has been observed in a few autopsied cases in which symptoms had returned following splenectomy.

Splenectomy is advisable for every infant or child who has active symptoms of the disorder, even if hemolytic crises have not yet occurred. One reason is that the operation may ultimately have to be done at some future time anyway; another is that an appreciable physiologic burden will be removed early; a third is that a prophylactic splenectomy in childhood may forestall a cholecystectomy in adult life. Parents frequently comment that they had not appreciated the physical handicap their child had been under until they saw how more energetic and well nourished he became subsequent to the operation.

It is advantageous to study the blood of every infant born into a family in which other members, and especially a parent, are known to be affected with this hereditary dyscrasia. If the infant has the red cell defect, any clinical signs which may develop such as weakness, splenomegaly, anemia, or intermittent icterus can be evaluated in the light of this knowledge. Splenectomy occasionally becomes necessary as early as the first month of life.

MEDITERRANEAN (COOLEY'S) ANEMIA

The severe and readily recognizable form of Mediterranean anemia, when first separated as an entity by Cooley from the miscellaneous group then known as von Jaksch's anemia, was named "erythroblastic anemia" because of the large numbers of immature red cells in the peripheral blood. This term was soon abandoned because of the confusion in nomenclature with erythroblastosis fetalis due to blood group incompatibility and because of the discovery of mild or "trait" forms which typically had neither anemia nor nucleated red cells in the circulation. The early recognition of the disease in children of Italian, Greek, Syrian, or Armenian parents then led to the introduction of *Mediterranean anemia* or *thalassemia,* from the Greek word for "great sea." For the grades of severity the modifying adjectives "severe," "mild," and "intermediate," or "thalassemia major" and "thalassemia minor" have been suggested.

Gradations in Severity

Individuals affected by the mild or minor form are ordinarily free from symptoms, and the existence of a hematologic disturbance is not suspected until specific blood studies are made. Patients with the severe or major form exhibit the well-known features of stunted growth, hypertrophy of the bones, marked distortion of the red cells, cardiac enlargement, and failure to survive beyond early childhood without supportive transfusions. Gallstones and orthopedic deformities are common late complications. Myocardial failure sometimes develops.

Genetic studies have explained these differences in severity. When one gene carries the determining factor the disease is minimal. When both genes are affected the major disturbance appears. In other words, the mild case is heterozygous and the florid severe case homozygous. Every time a patient is encountered it is important to survey the parents and all siblings, to assist in determining whether the patient is homozygous or heterozygous, and to detect other cases that may be in need of medical observation or eugenic advice.

Intermediate cases are sometimes seen in which the manifestations fall between the severe florid disturbance which goes with homozygosity and the almost negligible symptoms of the usual heterozygote carrier. These patients exhibit clinically evident anemia, bizarre red cells, reticulocytosis, hyperplasia of the bone marrow, and other related features which indicate moderate activity of the disorder. Splenomegaly may be detectable. The bones may show moderate thinness of the cortex and decrease in density. The fetal hemoglobin content in these patients may vary from a negligible level to over 90 per cent of all the hemoglobin.

Family surveys do not always uncover the same background of genetic possibilities. Sometimes both parents have the Mediterranean anemia trait; sometimes only one. Numerous cases are on record in which the "intermediate" syndrome has been associated with the interaction of Mediterranean anemia trait from one parent and of hemoglobin S, C, or E from the other. Elliptocytosis may enter the inheritance pattern.

Red Cell Changes

Florid cases have a progressive erythrocytopenia which, if not corrected by supportive transfusions, may fall to excessively low levels. The red cells in blood smears show pallor, leptocytosis, target forms, anisocytosis, poikilocytosis, oval and sausage-shaped cells, basophilic stippling, nucleated forms, Howell-Jolly bodies, Cabot rings, nuclear or reticular markings, and fragmenting forms. There is a marked reticulocytosis (5 to 20 per cent) and increased osmotic resistance of the red cells. All these changes tend to be proportional to the severity of the symptoms.

The typical child with the severe disease requires transfusions of red cells every few weeks or months to be comfortably sustained. Consequently the hematologic studies of such a patient usually reflect a mixture of donor and abnormal blood, except when there are long intervals between transfusions.

The child or adult with the mild form of the disease is not sufficiently affected to require transfusions or other treatment. He shows typically an absent to mild anemia (hemoglobin 14 to 10 gm per 100 ml), a red cell count which may be normal, slightly subnormal, or slightly increased (4 to 7 million), a hematocrit which is usually at the lower limit of normal (34 to 44 per cent), and a mild reticulocytosis (0.8 to 2 per cent). The morphologic appearances of the red cells are of the same character as in patients with the florid disturbance but much less prominent; careful search is sometimes needed for their detection. The osmotic resistance of the red cells is nearly always increased.

In all affected individuals the average cell diameter in dried smears tends to be about 7 μ (normal 7.2 to 7.4). The packed masses of red cells have a hemoglobin content of 22 to 30 per cent in the active disease and 22 to 34 per cent in the carrier state (normal 32 to 34 per cent). The calculated values for mean hemoglobin per cell in both kinds of cases have ranged from 16 to 30 $\mu\mu$gm. The mean red cell volume in both forms similarly varies widely, from 60 to 90 cu μ (normal range for children, 75 to 90 cu μ).

Other Laboratory Abnormalities

In florid cases the total serum bilirubin tends to be mildly or moderately elevated with the 1-minute fraction not disturbed. Readings range from 1 to 6 mg per 100 ml, as a rule. The bone marrow is extremely hypercellular (p. 327). The urine may or may not exhibit a slight increase of urobilinogen; occasionally it contains other pigments not readily identifiable.

Studies have thus far failed to detect any abnormal hemoglobin in this disease except that 2 to over 90 per cent of the hemoglobin in patients with florid symptoms may be of the fetal or F form (p. 101). In the carrier state the above changes are not seen and the fetal hemoglobin is in the normal range.

Pathogenesis

The hematologic changes seem best explainable in terms of an inability of the red cells within the bone marrow to mature properly, apparently as a result of an anomaly within the hemoglobinizing red cell stroma. In the more primitive red cells the nuclear chromatin seems identical with that of the normal rubriblast. In older cells the nuclear structure shrinks gradually to become small, compact, pyknotic, and uniformly stained. The hemoglobin in the cytoplasm, on the other hand, seems to be formed in diminished amounts, and often in punctate fashion.

Iron metabolism is disturbed. In children with the severe disease the iron-binding component of the serum, though quantitatively at or near normal, is fully saturated with iron, instead of being only about one-third saturated as occurs normally. The same phenomenon is seen also in the mild or trait stage of the disorder, but with less consistency. Iron-containing and iron-free pigment granules accumulate in great numbers throughout the body, especially in the cells of the liver, stomach, pancreas, salivary glands, adrenals, thyroid, parathyroids, and pituitary. Their presence can be explained as being due in part to hemosiderosis from the transfusions so interminably needed, and in part to an aberrant metabolism of iron or hemoglobin. Ellis, Schulman, and Smith have presented evidence of excessive absorption of iron from the intestinal tract.

Red cells from healthy subjects when transfused into patients with Mediterranean anemia usually persist for the normal length of time. Red cells from active patients have a curtailed survival time when transfused into healthy subjects. Survival time is only a little shortened when the donor has the trait.

None of the known antianemia remedies (iron, crude liver extract, vitamin B_{12}, folic acid, citrovorum factor, cortisone) have proven of benefit. Transfusions, repeated regularly, are the best supportive measure.

Splenectomy

In florid cases the spleen tends to become large and hard and may grow to occupy the left flank. Most patients ultimately have to be subjected to operation, to remove a large heavy spleen which mechanically crowds the other viscera and may throw the gait off balance. The operation also reduces the need for transfusions when hypersplenic activity has become superimposed.

After splenic removal the proportion of nucleated red cells in the peripheral blood goes up markedly. But unlike the transient postsplenectomy rises in most other dyscrasias which subside partially, the nucleated red cells in Mediterranean anemia permanently persist in great numbers after the operation.

Mediterranean Hemopathic Syndromes

These are as yet unclassified hereditary red cell disturbances which are occasionally seen in individuals of Italian and Greek descent. Oval cells, microcytes, macrocytes, elliptocytes, or other abnormal varieties of erythrocytes may be seen in varying numbers in the peripheral blood. Some of the patients exhibit jaundice or splenomegaly or may have hemolytic crises. Splenectomy may reduce the blood destruction but is without effect on the morphologic changes which may become accentuated afterward.

SICKLE CELL ANEMIA AND RELATED HEMOGLOBIN DISORDERS

The prevalence of individuals in the Negro population of the United States whose red cells exhibit sickling appears to vary in different cities. The best studies suggest that the over-all average is 8 to 9 per cent and that between 2.5 and 20 per cent of these are affected with the active disease. In Africa the sickle cell phenomenon varies from less than 1 per cent in the South African Bantu to about 20 per cent in the West African Negro. It has been found also among certain population groups in Greece and the Dravidian-speaking inhabitants of southern India.

Hemoglobin S

Electrophoretic studies with the Tiselius apparatus and paper strips have shown the hemoglobin in sickle cells to be quantitatively distinguishable from normal hemoglobin. This special form, known as hemoglobin S, moves more slowly in the electrophoretic field (p. 116).

The occurrence of S hemoglobin is a hereditary anomaly, transmitted genetically as a simple mendelian factor. Homozygous individuals have red cells which sickle readily and give rise to a pronounced set of resulting symptoms. Heterozygous individuals have red cells which sickle only when the oxygen in the environment is markedly reduced, and characteristically have no symptoms.

Alkali-resistant hemoglobin of the fetal type (hemoglobin F) is found also in patients with the active disease, in concentrations varying from 2 to 24 per cent of the total pigment. By deducting the fetal hemoglobin from the total hemoglobin one will have an approximate estimate of the hemoglobin S content, since normal or A hemoglobin occurs in these patients in only 1 or 2 per cent concentration, as a rule.

The severity of the anemia, the reticulocyte output, and the varying quantities of F pigment in different patients have thus far not exhibited any striking correlations. It has been suggested that F hemoglobin may not be equally distributed in all erythrocytes and that the cells containing it may survive longer.

In households where only one parent is affected, approximately 50 per cent of the offspring will be *carriers* of the trait, or *sicklemics,* and none will have sickle cell disease. When both parents are carriers, 25 per cent of all offspring will have the active disease, 50 per cent will be carriers, and only 25 per cent will have no S hemoglobin.

The solubility of oxy-S-hemoglobin appears to approximate that of normal A hemoglobin, whereas that of reduced S hemoglobin is very much less. In the nondissolved state, reduced S hemoglobin forms thin rodlike solidified particles in parallel arrangement which are known as tactoids. These can be visualized with phase microscopy of highly concentrated solutions. It is presumed that sickling is caused by tactoid-like crystallization of reduced S hemoglobin within the erythrocytes. Reduced A and F hemoglobin do not form tactoids; the high content of F hemoglobin in the neonatal period seems to explain why only a minority, if any, of the cells exhibit sickling in apparently normal newborn infants in whom florid sickle cell disease later becomes manifest.

In the presence of a high or saturated oxygen tension most or all intracellular S hemoglobin exists in the combined form as oxy-S-hemoglobin, which permits the red cells to remain normal in shape and behavior. If experimentally the oxygen tension of a suspension of affected red cells is lowered gradually, one by one they begin to assume an abnormal shape as the contained oxyhemoglobin becomes correspondingly reduced, until finally no rounded cell forms are left. Each red cell appears to possess its own specific threshold for sickling, determined in part if not predominantly by a far from uniform percentage of contained S hemoglobin. The phenomenon is reversible; sickled cells revert to the biconcave form as the surrounding oxygen tension is increased.

With active sickle cell anemia the phenomenon of sickling can be seen in wet or stained smears of venous blood in a fair percentage of the cells, whereas with the trait this does not occur.

Tests for Sickling

The various procedures for detecting the propensity to sickling are based upon removal of oxygen from the environment. Most of the methods require only one or two drops of free-flowing blood from the finger tip. Best results are obtainable when a rubber band is allowed to remain for several minutes around the finger before the puncture is made.

COVER-SLIP TESTS. A drop of blood taken from a vein or finger tip is placed on a glass slide under a cover slip. A drop of normal saline solution may be added to facilitate the observing of individual cell changes, if desired. The preparations should be set up rapidly to minimize reoxygenation from the air. The edges are sealed with a rim of oil or petroleum jelly. The preparation is then set aside at room temperature or in an incubator at 37°C and inspected microscopically over a period of 3 or even 4 days.

Various solutions containing reducing agents have been devised to accelerate the loss of oxygen in cover-slip preparations. Some supravital stain or a droplet from a broth culture of aerobic bacteria or normal feces may be added. Sodium metabisulfite is the reducing substance most widely used, but others which are effective include ascorbic acid, sodium hydrosulfite, and cysteine. Such preparations need not be sealed since with these adjuvants potential sickling becomes manifest in 15 to 30 minutes as a rule.

In trait cases the A hemoglobin contained in the cells permits the sickling process to go only part way. The sickled shapes which develop when the oxygen is diminished are predominantly irregular and "holly leaf" in character, with short jagged protrusions along the surface. All cells may not sickle until the oxygen seems nearly absent, which may take several days in the absence of added reducing agents.

In the active disease all the cells will assume sickle shapes much more rapidly; the majority will be long, slender, and curved, with a delicate tapering filament at one or both ends.

BECK AND HERTZ METHOD. A drop of blood is introduced into a corked test tube containing 1 ml of equal parts of physiologic saline and 3 per cent sodium citrate brought to a pH of 6.9 by 1 per cent acetic acid. This is incubated for 24 hours at 32°C. An equal amount of a physiologic saline–10 per cent neutral formalin mixture is next added, without agitation, to fix the red cells irreversibly in whatever shape they have assumed. A few drops are then examined microscopically.

The Sicklemic Trait (Sickle Cell Trait)

Heterozygously affected individuals have an essentially normal clinical story and physical findings. The hemoglobin, red cell, and hematocrit levels and erythrocyte constants are normal or nearly normal, and there is no reticulocytosis, leukocytosis, hyperbilirubinemia, or signs of excessive hemodestruction. The erythrocytes show few if any morphologic changes in direct smears. Crises do not occur.

Sickle Cell Disease (Active Sickle Cell Anemia)

The child with the active disease tends to appear slender and undernourished, with comparatively elongated extremities. He frequently has recurrent episodes of weakness, pains in the abdomen, extremities or joints (sometimes with local swelling), or other symptoms. Moderate splenomegaly is sometimes detectable. Cardiac murmurs and cardiomegaly are common and may simulate rheumatic fever. Leg ulcers occur mostly after adolescence. The sclerae and mucous membranes are pale or icteric.

The distinction between the active disease and the simple trait can be difficult clinically with infants and young children who for other reasons are anemic or in a state of active blood regeneration after an anemia.

The response to hemopoietic stumulants will usually clarify the differentiation. One encounters, however, occasional sicklemics at all ages with mild anemia and mild hemolytic symptoms in whom the intensity of the disturbance seems intermediate between the trait and the active disease.

Children with the anemia of active sickle cell disease are prone to exhibit cyanosis or laryngospasm during anesthesia, presumably secondary to the assumption of sickled shape by the red cells as a consequence of the anoxemia. They also have a greater tendency to bleed from incised areas than do normal children. For this reason, when an operation is needed, it is wise to (1) temporarily raise the hemoglobin level to 10 gm per 100 ml or higher by preoperation transfusions, (2) employ an anesthetic which does not lower the blood oxygen tension, (3) keep matched blood in readiness in the operating room for emergency transfusion if hemorrhage becomes extreme, and (4) observe the child carefully during the postoperative period to detect beginning complications.

HEMATOLOGIC ASPECTS. The typical manifestation of the active disturbance is a chronic hemolytic anemia (Table 4-1). The erythrocyte count is generally below 3 million per cu mm, and occasionally below 2 million. The hemoglobin level is reduced in normocytic proportions, usually becoming stabilized at between 8 and 6 gm per 100 ml. The hematocrit is lowered also, ranging from 28 to 20 per cent. Sickled forms are often seen in direct smears of the blood and marrow and in red cell suspensions being counted in a hemocytometer. The circulating reticulocytes are regularly increased, usually between 3 and 20 per cent. There is usually a leukocytosis with a total white cell count between 10,000 and 20,000 per cu mm; both neutrophils and lymphocytes are increased. The bone marrow shows red cell hyperplasia. The serum bilirubin is usually in the range between 0.5 and 4 mg per 100 ml and predominantly slow or indirectly reacting.

The red cells when not in the sickled phase may display poikilocytosis, anisocytosis, anisochromia, basophilia, target forms, and other irregularities. Nucleated cells and Howell-Jolly bodies are common, especially after splenectomy.

The character of the red cells is usually normochromic with a tendency toward macrocytosis. The mean cell volumes range from 85 to 100 cu μ, the mean cell hemoglobin between 28 and 34 $\mu\mu$gm, and the hemoglobin concentration in the packed red cells between 32 and 35 per cent. The osmotic resistance of the red cells to hypotonic saline solutions and related test media in active cases is so increased that some of the cells may fail to disintegrate even in distilled water. In heterozygous asymptomatic individuals the osmotic resistance is less altered and even may give normal readings with the customary tests.

Cross-transfusion experiments have shown that red cells from subjects with the sickle cell trait, when transfused into normal children or those with the active disturbance, have a normal life span averaging 120 days. Contrariwise, red cells from patients with active sickle cell anemia, when transfused into normal children or those with the sickle cell trait, have markedly reduced survival times. This briefer survival time lies behind the excessive erythrodestruction and compensatory regeneration in the active disease.

By immediately introducing blood from patients with the active disease into a saline-formalin solution without exposure to air, Sherman found that 10 to 20 per cent of the red cells in the arteries and 30 to 60 per cent of those in the veins were in the sickled phase. Subjects with the trait had almost no circulating sickled forms. Sherman noted also that oxygen pressures reduced to approximately 50 mm Hg regularly produced sickling in cells from active cases but not in those from individuals with the trait. Hence, as mentioned, when patients with the active disease are to be operated on, it is important to use an anesthetic which does not induce anoxemia.

Red cells in the sickled phase usually fail to form rouleaux or to settle appreciably with the standard sedimentation tests. This retardation becomes greater when the environmental oxygen is reduced. Applying this observation, Winsor and Burch have devised an ingenious test called the *diagnostic parameter*. A tourniquet or blood-pressure cuff is applied to an arm for a few minutes to induce venous stasis. A sample of 5 ml of venous blood is withdrawn into a small stoppered vial containing an anticoagulant. A portion is then set up for a Westergren sedimentation measurement without mixing the blood with air. The remaining blood is then aerated by being rotated in air in a small beaker or Erlenmeyer flask, and another sedimentation test set up. If the patient has active sickle cell anemia, the difference between the sedimentation rates of the aerated and nonaerated samples should be greater than 20 mm per hour.

PATHOGENESIS OF SYMPTOMS. The symptoms are attributed to local intravascular sickling. In its discoid form, the red cell may be flexible and elastic, but, as Murphy and Shapiro express it, the moment it sickles it becomes "fixed and rigid as a crystal of ice as it moves about and abuts against cells and fixed objects." The end-to-end length becomes two to five or more times as great as the diameter of the intact red cell, exclusive of the long processes which taper from the ends. These distorted and rigid cell forms tend to jam within the small blood vessels if in sufficient numbers. As the local circulation slows, the ensuing local anoxemia induces sickling of other cells. Thrombosis or local necrosis may develop in areas where the collateral circulation is poor.

Practically every organ of the body may be affected by this phenomenon. Transitory obstructions in the abdominal viscera can mimic ruptured peptic ulcer, ruptured gall bladder, or acute appendicitis, giving rise to the so-called "abdominal crises." Pulmonary occlusions may resemble pneumonia. Lesions of the nervous system have produced paralytic phenomena resembling poliomyelitis. Death is usually due to some complication related to circulatory stasis.

The spleen is usually palpable in childhood, small and fibrotic in adult life. The splenic parenchyma tends to retain the sickled forms. Persistent compact packing with these cells leads ultimately to recurrent thrombosis, hemorrhage, scarring, and calcium and iron deposition. Interestingly, trait cases may exhibit the same splenic lesions as do active cases, though to a much lesser degree.

HEMOLYTIC CRISES. In many patients with the active disease the disturbance, after having been stable for months or even years, may exhibit sudden exacerbations. The severity may vary from a minor exaggeration of symptoms to sudden jaundice, rapidly progressive anemia, and other signs of acutely augmented blood destruction. The pathogenesis of such hemolytic crises is not understood. They are often induced by acute bacterial or viral infections.

When hemolytic crises become frequent or prolonged, or when the hemoglobin level and red cell count fail to remain stabilized and repeated transfusions are called for, it is important to give serious consideration to splenectomy, if this organ is enlarged. The operation will usually be followed by a cessation or reduction of crises and the need for transfusions. Splenectomy arrests the symptoms of hypersplenism but has no effect on the other manifestations of the disease.

APLASTIC CRISES. Singer had directed attention to this unusual complication, which depends on the occasional tendency for acute virus infections to inhibit the production of red cells in the marrow for as long as 10 days (p. 328). Such cessation of the output of red cells in a normal individual is of little consequence, being easily compensated for later. In active sickle cell disease or other chronic hemolytic disturbances, however, the failure of delivery of new red cells when there is a markedly shortened red cell survival time can result in a pronounced aggravation of anemic symptoms within a very few days.

URINE. Through some mechanism not well understood as yet, patients with active sickle cell anemia are not able to excrete a concentrated urine. Urine specimens, even during periods of fluid deprivation, rarely attain a specific gravity much above the 1.016 range. The other components of the urine analysis are not disturbed. This phenomenon is not encountered in Mediterranean anemia or aregenerative anemia in which the red cell and hemoglobin levels are often lower.

Hemoglobin C

This form of hemoglobin is even slower in electrophoretic mobility than the abnormal sickle cell hemoglobin S (p. 116). It appears to be transmitted by a mendelian gene similar to that of hemoglobin S. It has been found in a frequency of 10 per cent in one group of natives of the northern Gold Coast of West Africa, and in lower frequency in other parts of the world where West African slaves were brought in the past. In American Negroes the incidence of this gene has varied from 1 to 3 per cent in different cities; the subjects are nearly always heterozygous, and have the gene in AC or SC combinations.

Individuals who are homozygous for the hemoglobin C gene (CC) exhibit splenomegaly and minor clinical symptoms. They have a mild anemia with a usual hemoglobin level of 10 to 12 gm per 100 ml (Table 4-1). The majority (50 to 100 per cent) of the red cells in the peripheral smear are target forms. Sickling does not occur. The red cells display increased osmotic resistance in hypotonic saline solutions, and have a shortened life span in the circulation.

Heterozygotes with hemoglobin C combined with structurally normal hemoglobin are asymptomatic, and their red cells do not sickle (Table 4-1). Their hemoglobin levels, red cell and erythrocyte counts, and serum bilirubin levels fall within normal limits. The red cells appear normal in ordinary smears apart from numerous target cells (3 to 30 per cent). The rates of red cell survival and destruction seem to be unaltered in most cases. The osmotic fragility of the red cells may be normal or decreased.

Variants of Sickle Cell Disease

The recent discoveries of the genetically transmissible variants of hemoglobin have made it possible to distinguish clinically and hematologically several different forms of sickle cell and related anemias. All combinations of the variant genes for hemoglobin with each other or with those for thalassemia, spherocytosis, and other inherited red cell disorders are theoretically possible, and a moderate number have already been identified and reported (Table 4-1).

THALASSEMIA MINOR–SICKLE CELL DISEASE. This highly uncommon form results from the marriage of a subject having thalassemia with one having the sickle cell trait (Table 4-1). Siblings with simultaneous heterozygosity for both S hemoglobin and the thalassemia gene exhibit a syndrome similar either to mild sickle cell anemia or to "intermediate" thalassemia (p. 59). The term *microdrepanocytic disease* has been applied to the hemoglobin S–thalassemia combination.

HEMOGLOBIN C–SICKLE CELL DISEASE (SICKLE CELL–C DISEASE). The genetic combination of hemoglobin C and sickle cell hemoglobin S results in a hemolytic disturbance similar to but less severe than active sickle cell anemia. The syndrome is characterized by a mild persistent anemia, with hemoglobin levels stabilized at 9 to 10 gm per 100 ml and red cell counts at 3.5 to 4.5 million. Reticulocytes range from 2 to 8 per cent of all red cells. The bone marrow exhibits rubricytic hyperplasia, though less than in active sickle cell disease. Leukocytosis is ordinarily absent. In stained smears the individual red cells tend to be leptocytic in appearance; they are uniform in size and contour, and sickle cell forms are infrequent. Target forms are numerous and conspicuous and range in frequency from 40 to 85 per cent of all cells. This is a most distinctive feature. Corpuscular measurements reveal only minimal diminution in diameter but considerable reduction in volume and hemoglobin content. Cells containing iron-staining cytoplasmic granules (siderocytes) are unusual, in comparison with their prevalence in sickle cell anemia. The exhibition of sickling in an anaerobic environment is rapid and complete, producing filamentous sickle forms. The osmotic fragility is decreased, just as in sickle cell anemia. The serum bilirubin level is normal or may be very slightly augmented (0.1 to 1.3 mg per 100 ml). Icterus is not apparent. The excretion of fecal urobilinogen is moderately increased. The red cells have a moderately shortened survival time when transfused into normal recipients.

Nutrition, bone growth, and physical activity are not hampered as a rule. Episodes of acute hemolysis, abdominal or musculosketal pain, or cardiac murmurs or enlargement are highly unusual. There may be moderate enlargement of the liver and spleen in the childhood years, which later subsides.

Other Abnormal Hemoglobins

The forms of hemoglobin encountered most often in the United States and about which most is known are adult hemoglobin (A), fetal hemoglobin (F), sickle cell hemoglobin (S), and C hemoglobin. Hemoglobin A appears to exert a dominant influence when in heterozygous combination with any of the other hemoglobins—most such individuals appear well and exhibit only subclinical changes in their red cells. Hemoglobin F is present in the blood of the fetus and newborn in appreciable amounts (Chap. 9); it normally disappears during the first year but often fails to do so in patients with a hereditary form of anemia. The full character of this hemoglobin has not been fully explored; there may be several subvarieties. Genetic factors may influence its appearance. Other variants of hemoglobin which have been described at the time of this writing include D, E, G, H, I, J, and K. Hemoglobins S and C have been discussed on the preceding pages.

HEMOGLOBIN D. With paper electrophoresis (p. 116) this hemoglobin has the same motility as S. Sickling does not occur, however, presumably because in its reduced state it is more soluble and does not crystallize into tactoids. It has been found in 0.4 per cent of American Negroes, occasional Caucasians, and 1 per cent of Sikhs living in the Punjab area of India.

HEMOGLOBIN E. With paper electrophoresis this migrates to a position intermediate between C and S. Approximately 10 per cent of some native groups in Thailand and Burma are said to carry the gene. A somewhat lower incidence has been found in Indonesia, Ceylon, and Bengal. Heterozygous carriers are asymptomatic, and their blood smears may show occasional target cells. Homozygous individuals exhibit symptoms resembling a mild form of thalassemia major.

HEMOGLOBIN G, H, I, J, AND K. These have been recognized thus far in only a few individuals, and little is known as yet concerning their clinical or anthropologic significance.

OTHER FAMILIAL ANEMIAS

Hereditary Elliptocytosis

In this malformational group of disorders many of the red cells appear oval or elliptic or rod-shaped in the blood smear and may be microcytic or hypochromic (*microelliptocytes*). There may be transient periods of erythrocytosis with red cell counts above 6 million. The anomaly is congenital, non-sex-linked, persists through life, and is seen only in the mature red cell. The erythroblasts and even the reticulocytes have a normal shape. The elliptocytes remain unaltered when suspended in plasma of normal individuals of the same blood group or in hypotonic solutions and do not exhibit the property of sickling.

Elliptocytosis can occur with or without signs of increased blood destruction and anemia. It has been described in many members of a number of families, chiefly with Dutch, German, or Italian parentage. No abnormality of the hemoglobin has been detected thus far, and alkali-resistant hemoglobin is not increased. As in sickle cell anemia, the percentage of elliptic cells is almost negligible at birth and the condition may not be apparent until after the first few months.

The familial condition is to be distinguished from assorted other forms of anemia in which oval-shaped red cells may make their appearance, apparently as secondary changes.

True elliptocytosis seems to occur in three stages of intensity. The *asymptomatic elliptocytic carrier* is free from evidences of increased red cell production or destruction. There are normal levels for red cells and hemoglobin, and no reticulocytosis, with only a minority of the cells (usually 10 to 30 per cent) appearing elliptocytic. Genetically these individuals are presumed to be heterozygous for a mendelian gene.

Elliptocytosis with compensated hemolysis refers to those patients with a reduced red cell survival time and other phenomena of excessive hemodestruction but no overt symptoms of anemia.

Elliptocytosis with hemolytic anemia is an exceptional condition characterized by excessive erythrodestruction, marked ovalocytosis, poikilocytosis, and microcytosis, usually with some splenic enlargement. Symptoms may be relieved in part by splenectomy. These individuals may be hemozygotes; parents and siblings should be studied also.

Familial Erythroid Multinuclearity

This unusual red cell anomaly, of familial origin, is characterized by giant-sized and nucleated red cells having coarse cytoplasmic stippling and karyorrhexis within the circulation and of giant multinucleated red cell precursors within the marrow. The patients, although asymptomatic, tend to have a mild anemia which is refractory to oral iron therapy. The red cell count is proportionately lower than the hemoglobin, the latter usually being normal or low normal. Anisocytosis and poikilocytosis are constant. Reticulocyte counts are normal. The multinucleated red cells in the marrow seem to result from normal nuclear fission with suppression of cytoplasmic division. Somewhat similar changes in red cell formation may be observed secondarily in other blood disorders of severe degree.

Acanthrocytosis

A rare erythrocytic anomaly in which the surfaces of the red cells show irregularly spaced large and coarse projections has been described by Singer and associates. Many cells resemble spherocytes with pseudopods. The term *acanthrocyte* (thorny red cell) is proposed for this particular type of misshapen erythrocyte. The osmotic fragility of these cells is slightly decreased in hypotonic saline, markedly increased with lysolecithin or mechanical strain. Affected individuals may have the celiac syndrome in early childhood, a progressive ataxic neuropathy, and, less regularly, retinitis pigmentosa. They have not exhibited evidences of an exaggerated hemolytic process in vivo.

Hereditary Nonspherocytic Hemolytic Anemias

Numerous families with unusual forms of hereditary anemia have been described. In these the red cells may or may not be distorted in size or shape. As a rule the same atypical forms prevail within a family. Affected individuals exhibit hemolytic phenomena of varying severity or may be asymptomatic carriers. The osmotic resistance of the red cells is usually normal, but the survival time of erythrocytes transfused into normal recipients tends to be abnormally short. Normocytic or macrocytic anemia, hyperhemolysis, enlargement of liver and spleen, and sometimes even osseous changes, may be found. Circulating antibodies are not demonstrable by the Coombs test, but episodes of aggravated hemolysis, presumably of hypersplenic origin, may occur. Splenectomy when done is usually of scant value. Transmission is typically as a mendelian dominant, non-sex-linked.

In some of these families many of the red cells have shown marked punctate basophilia. A familial hypochromic microcytic anemia associated with postsplenectomy inclusion bodies has been described by Mills and Lucia, and somewhat similar, probably sex-linked, anemias by Rundles and Falls and by Cooley. In the family studied by Kaplan and Zuelzer the erythrocytes showed a moderate degree of elliptocytosis.

An unusual form of familial hemolytic anemia, superficially similar to Mediterranean anemia, has been observed by Stransky in the Philippine Islands. Symptoms begin in early childhood or later, with stunting growth, severe anemia, splenomegaly, and marked jaundice. Hemoglobin of the fetal type has been found in moderate amounts in a few cases. Splenectomy is of little benefit.

BIBLIOGRAPHY

HEREDITARY SPHEROCYTOSIS

Battle, J. D., Jr., Hereditary Spherocytosis: Pathogenesis of the "Acute Crisis," *J. Lab. & Clin. Med.* 38:784, 1951.

———, Hereditary Spherocytosis (Congenital Hemolytic Jaundice): Pathogenesis of the "Hemolytic" Crisis, *Am. J. M. Sc.* 224:82, 1952.

Clinical Conference: Two Cases of Hereditary Spherocytosis Manifest in the Newborn Period, *J. Pediat.* 44:213, 1954.

Dacie, J. V., P. L. Mollison, N. Richardson, J. G. Selwyn, and *L. Shapiro,* Atypical Congenital Haemolytic Anaemia, *Quart. J. Med.* 22:79, 1953.

Macaulay, D., Achloruric Jaundice in a Newborn Infant, *Arch. Dis. Childhood* 26:241, Anemia, *Blood* 9:414, 1954.
1951.

Selwyn, J. C., and *J. V. Dacie,* Autohemolysis and Other Changes Resulting from the Incubation in Vitro of Red Cells from Patients with Congenital Hemolytic

Young, L. E., M. J. Izzo, and *R. F. Platzer,* Hereditary Spherocytosis. I. Clinical, Hematologic and Genetic Features in Twenty-eight Cases, with Particular Reference to the Osmotic and Mechanical Fragility of Incubated Erythrocytes, *Blood* 6:1073, 1951.

——— and *G. Miller,* Differentiation between Congenital and Acquired Forms of Hemolytic Anemia: Observations on 47 Cases of Hereditary Spherocytosis and 24 Cases of Autoimmune Disease, *Am. J. M. Sc.* 226:664, 1953.

———, *R. F. Platzer, D. M. Ervin,* and *M. J. Izzo,* Hereditary Spherocytosis. II. Observations on the Role of the Spleen, *Blood* 6:1099, 1951.

MEDITERRANEAN ANEMIA

Astaldi, G., and *P. Tolentino,* Studies on the Pathogenesis of Thalassaemia, *J. Clin. Path.* 5:140, 1952.

Banks, L. O., and *R. B. Scott,* Thalassemia in Negroes, *Pediatrics* 11:622, 1953.

Banton, A. H., A Genetic Study of Mediterranean Anemia in Cyprus, *Am. J. Human Genet.* 3:47, 1951.

Ellis, J. T., Generalized Siderosis with Fibrosis of Liver and Pancreas in Cooley's (Mediterranean) Anemia with Observation on the Pathogenesis of the Siderosis and Fibrosis, *Am. J. Path.* 30:287, 1954.

Gatto, I., and L. Valentino, Thalassemia (Microcarterocitosis) Minima, Pediatria 61:313, 1953.

Hanlon, D. G., J. B. Selby, and E. D. Bayrd, Hereditary Leptocytosis (Thalassemia Minor), J.A.M.A. 161:1132, 1956.

Horemis, K., and L. Zanos, Hereditary Hemolytic Anemias in Greece, World M. A. Bull. 5:28, 1953.

Rich, A., Studies on the Hemoglobin of Cooley's Anemia and Cooley's Trait, Proc. Nat. Acad. Sc. 38:187, 1952.

Smith, C. H., and J. E. Morgenthau, Case Report: Cholelithiasis in Severe Mediterranean (Cooley's) Anemia, Blood 6:1147, 1951.

———, I. Schulman, R. E. Ando, and G. Stern, Studies in Mediterranean (Cooley's) Anemia. I. Clinical and Hematologic Aspects of Splenectomy, with Special Reference to Fetal Hemoglobin Synthesis, Blood 10:582, 1955.

———, T. R. C. Sison, W. H. Floyd, Jr., and S. Siegal, Serum Iron and Iron-binding Capacity of the Serum in Children with Severe Mediterranean (Cooley's) Anemia, Pediatrics 5:799, 1950.

Sturgeon, P., H. A. Itano, and W. R. Bergren, Genetic and Biochemical Studies of 'Intermediate' Types of Cooley's Anemia, Brit. J. Haemat. 1:264, 1955.

SICKLE CELL ANEMIA

Banks, L. O., R. B. Scott, and J. Simmons, Studies in Sickle Cell Anemia: Inheritance Factor, Including Effect of Interaction of Genes for Sicklemia and Thalassemia, A.M.A. Am. J. Dis. Child. 84:601, 1952.

Beck, J. S. P., and C. S. Hertz, Standardizing Sickle Cell Method and Evidence of Sickle Cell Trait, Am. J. Clin. Path. 5:325, 1935.

Daland, G. A., and W. B. Castle, A Simple and Rapid Method for Demonstrating Sickling of the Red Blood Cells: The Use of Reducing Agents, J. Lab. & Clin. Med. 33:1082, 1948.

Dickstein, B., and I. J. Wolman, Sickle Cell Anemia: Recent Progress of Pediatric Interest, Am. J. M. Sc. 213:728, 1947.

Diggs, L. W., The Crisis in Sickle Cell Anemia: Hematologic Studies, Am. J. Clin. Path. 26:1109, 1956.

Erlandson, M., C. H. Smith, and I. Schulman, Thalassemia-Hemoglobin C Disease in White Siblings, Pediatrics 17:740, 1956.

Frazier, C. A., and C. E. Rice, Neonatal Sickle Cell Anemia, J.A.M.A. 143:1065, 1950.

Kaplan, E., W. W. Zuelzer, and J. V. Neel, Further Studies on Hemoglobin C. II. The Hematologic Effects of Hemoglobin C Alone and in Combination with Sickle Cell Hemoglobin, Blood 8:735, 1953.

Margolies, M. P., Sickle Cell Anemia: A Composite Study and Survey, Medicine 30:351, 1951.

Murphy, R. C., and S. Shapiro, Sickle Cell Disease, Arch. Int. Med. 74:28, 1944.

Neel, J. V., Data Pertaining to the Population Dynamics of Sickle Cell Disease, Am. J. Human Genet. 5:154, 1953.

Neel, J. V., H. A. Itano, and J. S. Lawrence, Two Cases of Sickle Cell Disease Presumably Due to the Combination of the Genes for Thalassemia and Sickle Hemoglobin, Blood 8:434, 1953.

Scott, R. B., A. D. Ferguson, M. E. Jenkins, and H. M. Clark, Studies in Sickle-cell Anemia. VIII. Further Observations on the Clinical Manifestations of Sickle-cell Anemia in Children, A.M.A. Am. J. Dis. Child. 90:682, 1955.

Sherman, I. J., Sickling Phenomenon, with Special Reference to Differentiation of Sickle Cell Anemia from Sickle Cell Trait, Bull. Johns Hopkins Hosp. 67:309, 1940.

Shotton, D., C. L. Crockett, Jr., and *B. S. Leavell,* Splenectomy in Sickle Cell Anemia: Report of a Case and Review of the Literature, *Blood* 6:365, 1951.

Silvestroni, E., and *I. Bianco,* Genetic Aspects of Sickle Cell Anemia and Micro-drepanocytic Disease, *Blood* 7:429, 1952.

Singer, K., Review: The Pathogenesis of Sickle Cell Anemia, *Am. J. Clin. Path.* 21:858, 1951.

—— and *A. I. Chernoff,* Studies on Abnormal Hemoglobins. III. The Interrelationship of Type S (Sickle Cell) Hemoglobin and Type F (Alkali Resistant) Hemoglobin in Sickle Cell Anemia, *Blood* 7:47, 1952.

—— and *B. Fisher,* Studies on Abnormal Hemoglobins. V. The Distribution of Type S (Sickle Cell) Hemoglobin and Type F (Alkali Resistant) Hemoglobin within the Red Cell Population in Sickle Cell Anemia, *Blood* 7:1216, 1952.

—— and ——, Studies on Abnormal Hemoglobins. VII. The Composition of the Non-S Hemoglobin Fraction in Sickle-cell Anemia Bloods: A Comparative Quantitative Study by the Methods of Electrophoresis and Alkali Denaturation, *J. Lab. & Clin. Med.* 42:193, 1953.

——, *S. Robin, J. C. King,* and *R. N. Jefferson,* The Life Span of the Sickle Cell and the Pathogenesis of Sickle Cell Anemia, *J. Lab. & Clin. Med.* 33:975, 1948.

Wasserman, C. F., V. R. Phelps, and *A. J. Hertzog,* Chronic Hemolytic Anemia in a White Child Due to Thalassemia and Sicklemia, *Pediatrics* 9:286, 1952.

Wells, I. C., and *H. A. Itano,* Ratio of Sickle-cell Anemia Hemoglobin to Normal Hemoglobin in Sicklemics, *J. Biol. Chem.* 188:65, 1951.

Williams, A. W., and *J. P. Mackay,* Rapid Determination of the Sickle Cell Trait by the Use of a Reducing Agent, *J. Clin. Path.* 2:141, 1949.

HEMOGLOBIN E

Chernoff, A. I., V. Minnich, S. Chongcharoensuk, S. Na-Nakorn, and *R. Chernoff,* Clinical, Hematological and Genetic Studies of Hemoglobin E, *J. Lab. & Clin. Med.* 44:780, 1954.

Itano, H. A., Clinical States Associated with Alterations of the Hemoglobin Molecule, *A.M.A. Arch. Int. Med.* 96:287, 1955.

Minnich, V., S. Na-Nakorn, S. Chongcharoensuk, and *S. Kochaseni,* Mediterranean Anemia: A Study of Thirty-two Cases in Thailand, *Blood* 9:1, 1954.

Singer, K., Hereditary Hemolytic Disorders Associated with Abnormal Hemoglobins, *Am. J. Med.* 18:633, 1955.

ABNORMAL HEMOGLOBINS—MISCELLANEOUS

Chernoff, A. I., On the Prevalence of Hemoglobin D in the American Negro, *Blood* 11:907, 1956.

Neel, J. V., J. Hiernaux, J. Linhard, A. Robinson, W. W. Zuelzer, and *F. B. Livingstone,* Data on the Occurrence of Hemoglobin C and Other Abnormal Hemoglobins in Some African Populations, *Am. J. Human Genet.* 8:138, 1956.

Zuelzer, W. W., J. V. Neel, and *A. R. Robinson,* Abnormal Hemoglobins. Progress in Hematology, vol. I, L. M. Tocantins (ed.), Grune & Stratton, Inc., New York, 1956.

ELLIPTOCYTOSIS

Berlin, R., and *S. Hedenstedt,* The Life Span of Elliptocytes, *Acta med. scandinav.* 143:273, 1952.

Heilmeyer, L., and *H. Begemann,* Blut und Blutkrankheiten, in "Handbuch der Inneren Medizin," vol. 2, p. 334, Springer-Verlag OHG, Berlin, 1951.

Kirkegaard, A., and *K. Larsen,* Elliptische Erythrocyten in einer daenischen Familie und einige Untersuchungen ueber die Natur der Elliptocytose, *Acta med. scandinav.* 110:521, 1942.

Lipton, E. L., Elliptocytosis with Hemolytic Anemia: The Effects of Splenectomy, *Pediatrics* 15:67, 1955.

Motulsky, A. G., K. Singer, W. H. Crosby, and *V. Smith,* The Life Span of the Elliptocyte: Hereditary Elliptocytosis and Its Relationship to Other Familial Hemolytic Diseases, *Blood* 9:57, 1954.

Vecchio, F., and *L. Tropeano:* Anemic-hemolytic Syndrome with Macrocytic Elliptocytosis in a Breastfed Child (Su una particolare sindrome anemico-emolitica con ellittocitosi macrocitica in un lattante), *Pediatria* 55:240, 1947.

Wyandt, H., P. M. Bancroft, and *T. O. Winship,* Elliptic Erythrocytes in Man, *Arch. Int. Med.* 68:1043, 1941.

HEREDITARY NONSPHEROCYTIC HEMOLYTIC ANEMIAS

Bruton, O. C., W. H. Crosby, and *A. G. Motulsky,* Hereditary Nonspherocytic Hemolytic Anemia Presenting as Hemolytic Disease of the Newborn Infant, *Pediatrics* 13:41, 1954.

Crigler, J. F., Jr., and *V. A. Najjar,* Congenital Familial Nonhemolytic Jaundice with Kernicterus, *Pediatrics* 10:169, 1952.

Crosby, W. H., Hereditary Nonspherocytic Hemolytic Anemia, *Blood* 5:233, 1950.

Feinberg, A. W., and *J. Watson,* Nonspherocytic Chronic Hemolytic Anemia with Basophilic Stippling: Report of a Case in a Negro, *Blood* 6:357, 1951.

Haden, R. L., A New Type of Hereditary Hemolytic Jaundice without Spherocytosis, *Am. J. M. Sc.* 214:255, 1947.

Holliday, T. D. S., Familial Non-spherocytic Hemolytic Anemia, *J. Clin. Path.* 6:219, 1953.

Kaplan, E., and *W. W. Zuelzer,* Familial Nonspherocytic Hemolytic Anemia, *Blood* 5:811, 1950.

Krivit, W., R. T. Smith, J. F. Martin, R. Read, and *R. A. Good,* Congenital Nonspherocytic Hemolytic Anemia: Two Nonfamilial Cases with Red Cell Survival Studies, *J. Pediat.* 49:245, 1956.

Lipton, E. L., H. J. Grossman, and *J. B. Richmond,* Chronic Familial Nonspherocytic Hemolytic Anemia, *Pediatrics* 12:384, 1953.

Mills, H., and *S. P. Lucia,* Familial Hypochromic Anemia Associated with Postsplenectomy Erythrocyte Inclusion Bodies, *Blood* 4:891, 1949.

Motulsky, A. G., W. H. Crosby, and *H. Rappaport,* Hereditary Nonspherocytic Hemolytic Disease: A Study of a Singular Familial Hemolytic Syndrome, *Blood* 9:749, 1954.

Singer, K., B. Fisher, and *M. A. Perlstein,* Acanthrocytosis: A Genetic Erythrocytic Malformation, *Blood* 7:577, 1952.

Wolff, J. A., and *F. H. von Hofe,* Familial Erythroid Multinuclearity, *Blood* 6:274, 1951.

CHAPTER 5

Anemias Secondary to Toxic
and Systemic Disturbances

The possibility of a childhood anemia being caused by some acquired systemic disturbance must always be explored when preliminary hematologic survey indicates the presence of a normochromic normocytic type of anemia, and ancillary evidence seems to exclude anemia of hereditary or malnutritional origin.

ACUTE INFECTIONS

Red cells are often destroyed at an enhanced rate during severe acute infections such as septicemia, pneumonia, and fulminating osteomyelitis. Red cell and hemoglobin levels may fall markedly within a few days. The responsible bacterium in such an illness is usually a strain of streptococci, pneumococci, staphylococci, coliform bacilli, or bacilli of the *Clostridium welchii* type with hemolytic activity in vitro. Very occasionally the hemolysis is so rapid that hemoglobinuria occurs; in newborn infants this process is termed Winckel's disease.

Supplementing direct red cell destruction is a not infrequent transitory cessation of erythropoiesis induced by acute infections caused by either viruses or bacteria (p. 328). With bacterial pneumonia before modern chemotherapeutic agents were available, about 25 per cent of infants and younger children would become sufficiently anemic to require transfusion before the illness had run its course. It was not uncommon, in such patients who died, to encounter siderosis of the spleen with or without hypocellularity of the bone marrow as pathologic changes.

CHRONIC INFECTIONS AND RELATED DISEASES

Protracted infections are likely to be accompanied by stabilization of the red cells and hemoglobin at levels lower than normal for the age. The list of such diseases includes tuberculosis, rheumatic fever, osteomyelitis, lung abscess, bronchiectasis, pyelonephritis, brucellosis, histoplasmosis, wound infections, subacute bacterial endocarditis, congenital

75

syphilis, and intestinal parasitism. Somewhat similar forms of anemia may be seen with ulcerative colitis, malignant tumors, chronic arthritis, chronic kidney disease, and after traumatic injuries.

Pathogenesis

Not much is known concerning the disturbed metabolism responsible for this form of anemia. Depression of erythropoiesis from action of toxins on bone marrow cells seems more responsible than acceleration of erythrodestruction. Contributory influences may be impaired gastrointestinal absorption, unusual affinity of reacting tissues for iron, direct blood loss into the inflamed area, anorexia followed by an inadequate intake of hemopoietic substances during the illness, or other abnormal conditions.

In general, the more severe or protracted the disorder the greater the likelihood of anemia. Since the pathogenesis is largely through depression of hemopoiesis, it may take several weeks after the onset of the disturbance for sufficient effete red cells to become obsolescent and unreplaced to make the anemia demonstrable. The severity of the anemia does not reflect necessarily either the duration or the intensity of the disease process. The latter is usually more prominent than the anemia. The anemia subsides as the patient improves.

Anemia in chronic infection tends to be normochromic and normocytic unless a deficiency of iron or other hemopoietics is superimposed. The reticulocyte count is not elevated, and the urine urobilinogen and the serum bilirubin are not increased. When the infection subsides hemopoiesis begins to become unusually active, a reticulocytosis appears, and the peripheral blood picture returns to normal.

Therapy

Tonics or injections of iron and vitamins or liver extract give but little benefit unless a malnutritional status is superimposed. Nevertheless, every effort should be exerted to see that the food intake is adequate in calories and protein and rich in vitamins.

Transfusions may temporarily restore depressed hemoglobin and red cell levels to normal, but these may regress to their former levels within a few weeks if the infection remains active.

Malaria

In this disease the invaded red cells rupture, coincidentally with the maturation of each crop or brood of plasmodia. The anemia is normochromic and normocytic as a rule, though some macrocytosis or microcytosis may be associated. Contributory to the anemia may be some of the indirect mechanisms which are operative in other chronic infections. Paroxysms of acute hemolysis and hemoglobinuria, known as blackwater fever, are rare in the childhood years.

Oroya Fever

This is a severe febrile infection with prominent hemolytic symptoms encountered in Peru. It is caused by *Bartonella bacilliformis*. The insect vector is the sand fly Phlebotomus.

Kidney Diseases

In acute glomerulonephritis and the nephrotic syndrome, which are the most common parenchymal kidney diseases of childhood, the red cell count and hemoglobin normally show only minor deviations. There may be a mild anemia when edema is present, which fades away after diuresis. Superimposed infections may depress the red cell count and hemoglobin levels, which return to normal after the infection has subsided.

In chronic nephritis with nitrogen retention, on the other hand, pronounced anemia of normochromic normocytic character is a fairly constant feature. In the subacute stages the red cell counts typically range from 2 to 4 million and there may be a mild reticulocytosis or leukocytosis. In the late stages with chronic uremia the anemia may become more pronounced, the reticulocyte count subnormal, and the bone marrow hypocellular, often extremely so. In chronic pyelonephritis the depressant action of the infection is superimposed on the intoxication from the excretory disturbance. Hemopoietic stimulants are as ineffective as in the anemia associated with chronic infections. Repeated supportive transfusions are sometimes necessary to keep the red cells and hemoglobin at comfortable levels. Exceptionally the chronic kidney disease develops so insidiously that its presence is not recognized until after the cause of the anemia has been elucidated. Improvement in the blood follows subsidence of the uremic symptoms.

HYPOTHYROIDISM

A mild to moderate normocytic or macrocytic normochromic anemia occurs in most cases of untreated juvenile hypothyroidism, whether of congenital or postneonatal origin. The hemoglobin level typically remains between 8 and 11 gm per 100 ml, and the red cell count between 3.5 and 4.5 million. The reticulocyte count is subnormal. The bone marrow shows general hypocellularity, with all myeloid series being depressed. Carotenemia may be present coincidentally and simulate jaundice (p. 657). If the hemoglobin level is disproportionately lower than the red cell count and the red cells appear microcytic in the blood smears, an iron-deficiency anemia is probably superimposed.

Replacement therapy with thyroid substance corrects this anemia. The first sign of activation of the bone marrow is the appearance of reticulocytosis. The red cell and hemoglobin levels may decline slightly in the first few weeks of treatment, during restoration of the plasma volume.

LATE STAGE OF ERYTHROBLASTOSIS FETALIS

In the first few days of life, while hemolysis is most active (p. 166), the infant with erythroblastosis fetalis nearly always has a bone marrow picture of increased cellularity. Nevertheless, an interval of protracted aregenerative anemia may follow and last for several months. Within the marrow only primitive rubriblasts may be seen, with few red cells more mature. Granulocyte and thrombocyte production are not impaired. One or more supportive transfusions may be required until red cell regeneration begins.

MARROW INFILTRATION

Massive infiltration of the bone marrow and other organs by leukemia, metastatic sarcoma, the reticuloendothelioses, or other space-filling disorders may hamper the formation of red cells, granulocytes, and thrombocytes within the bone marrow—a true depressive panhemocytopenia. Similar changes can occur in generalized bone diseases. The resulting anemia, usually progressive, tends to be normochromic and normocytic, but macrocytosis is seen occasionally. The reticulocyte count tends to be reduced. When thrombocytopenia is marked there may be hemorrhagic phenomena. Whether the productive elements of the marrow in uninvolved areas are hyperplastic or aplastic seems to depend upon the reaction of the normal marrow cells to the foreign tissue. The impaired blood production is sometimes complicated by excessive hemodestruction, as shown by poor or negligible benefit after transfusion and liberal deposits of hemosiderin in the organs at autopsy.

GAUCHER'S DISEASE

In this disease the changes in the bones advance so slowly that blood changes do not present themselves until after infancy, as a rule, and may not be prominent till late childhood or adult life. The cell pattern in the peripheral blood is influenced by the severity of the foreign-cell infiltration in the bone marrow and by the presence or absence of superimposed hypersplenism (p. 295). Focal hemorrhages, necrosis, or atrophy of some of the hemopoietic tissue and ultimate fibrosis have all been described.

LEUKOERYTHROBLASTOTIC REACTION (EXTRAMEDULLARY HEMOPOIESIS)

When blood cell formation becomes restricted or distorted as the result of space-occupying or depressant disturbances within the bone marrow, hemopoiesis sometimes begins again in the liver, spleen, and elsewhere, simulating the conditions which exist normally in the fetus. The peripheral blood will then exhibit the so-called leukoerythroblastotic reaction.

This is characterized by many myelocytes and progranulocytes in the peripheral blood, accompanied by intermittent showers of nucleated red cells. The red cell and hemoglobin levels may or may not be decreased, and the total leukocyte count may range from pronounced leukopenia to leukocytosis. Reticulocytosis or thrombocytopenia or both may be noted. The circulation may contain giant platelets and megakaryocytic fragments, and excessive numbers of megakaryocytes may be demonstrable later in the marrow, spleen, or lymph nodes at autopsy. Difficulty in obtaining specimens of marrow upon repeated aspirations—so-called "dry taps"—often call for marrow biopsy in order to determine the provocative cause. A somewhat similar blood cell picture may be seen in erythroleukemia (p. 219), but here the circulating erythrocytes and leukocytes usually show structural abnormalities.

The epinephrine stimulatory test has been suggested by Doan and Wright as a confirmatory test for the leukoerythroblastotic reaction:
Two complete blood counts including platelet and reticulocyte counts are taken during a 15- to 30-minute preliminary period, and the splenic outline traced (if palpable). With a child a dose of about 0.5 ml of 1:1,000 epinephrine chloride is then injected subcutaneously. All studies are then repeated every 10 to 15 minutes for 2 hours or longer. A pronounced rise in immature cells or even of mature forms, which reaches its peak soon after the greatest contraction of the spleen, is believed to be a sign of extramedullary blood formation and a contraindication to splenectomy. More recent evidence suggests that such cellular reserves mobilized by epinephrine may come from the lungs as well.

APLASTIC ANEMIA (APLASTIC PANCYTOPENIA, REFRACTORY ANEMIA, PANMYELOPHTHISIS)

In this syndrome, less common in children than in adults, pancytopenia of all cellular elements of the peripheral blood develops from progressive inadequacy of the bone marrow *after previously normal hemopoietic functioning.* When a cause can be demonstrated the diagnosis is often qualified as "symptomatic" or "secondary"; when unknown it may be called "primary" or "idiopathic." Among the etiologic situations presumably responsible in observed cases have been (1) septic infections, due most often to staphylococci, diphtheria bacilli, brucella, or *Salmonella choleraesuis;* (2) drugs and poisons such as benzol, phenol, toluol, and their derivatives, arsenicals, chloramphenicol, cinchophen, gold salts, insecticides, mustard gas and the nitrogen mustard derivatives, nirvanol, quinine, sulfonamides, tridione, and trinitrotoluene; (3) physical agents such as radium, roentgen rays, radioactive phosphorus, and products of atomic fission or atomic bomb explosions; and (4) chronic constitutional diseases resulting in severe malnutrition or cachexia, such as chronic nephritis, generalized tuberculosis, pituitary insufficiency, parasitic infestations, and malignant disease. Individual susceptibility is important, as in the rare chloramphenicol reactions. Other cases have been interpreted as exhaustion of a constitutionally or nutritionally inferior bone marrow under extreme stress. The disturbance, as a rule, is irreversible.

Manifestations

The onset may be abrupt or gradual; the clinical course insidious or fulminating. Much depends on whether the bone marrow has been completely depressed or whether hemopoietic activity still remains. The principal symptoms are those of anemia: pallor, weakness, anorexia, fatigability, and breathlessness on exertion. Complicating hemorrhages are common, especially into the skin and from the nose and gastrointestinal tract. Prophylactic chemotherapy is advisable to avoid infections.

In cases of moderate severity the red cell count may fluctuate between 2 and 3 million. In most patients, however, the red cell count tends to fall steadily, with death soon ensuing unless transfusions are given. The individual erythrocytes tend to be normal and normochromic, but immature or bizarre forms sometimes appear in quantity. Calculation from the hematocrit often shows a macrocytosis, with mean red cell volume over 90 cu μ. There are no signs of excessive hemolysis, as a rule, and no disturbances in osmotic fragility. Reticulocytes are scanty or absent, though some patients have intermittent reticulocytosis of mild degree, between 1 and 3 per cent or a little higher. The leukocyte count tends to be between 2,000 and 4,000 per cu mm as a consequence of a drop in the absolute count of granulocytes; abnormal granulocytes are not common. Sometimes the lymphocytes are quantitatively diminished also. A relative eosinophilia is suggestive of some sensitivity cause and may presage a more favorable prognosis. The platelets are depressed also, usually below 50,000 per cu mm, and later become too few to count. The bleeding and clotting times tend to be prolonged, and clot retraction becomes imperfect. The sedimentation rate is extremely rapid, and the serum protein level may fall in the terminal stages.

In atypical cases, such as those caused by chronic exposure to poisons, the hematologic reactions may be bizarre and baffling. Erythrocytosis, leukemoid reactions, leukocytosis, thrombocytopenia or thrombocytosis, or granulocytopenia with only immature cells circulating may be seen. In a minority of patients the marrow injury is restricted to only one or two of the hemopoietic cell series or is partial rather than complete. The patient may then be left with hypoplastic anemia, thrombocytopenia, or granulocytopenia in any combination.

The bone marrow may appear hypocellular, completely aplastic, or even hypercellular (p. 329). There is no close correlation between the cellularity of the marrow and the clinical course of the patient. Compensatory extramedullary hemopoiesis as evidenced by splenomegaly and immaturity of circulating leukocytes and red cells is infrequent.

Death is due usually to exhaustion or hemorrhage. Terminal infections are not as frequent as before antibiotics were available. At necropsy, in addition to the bone marrow changes, one finds scattered hemorrhages, hemosiderosis of the organs if many transfusions have been given, and hypertrophy of the heart in long-standing disturbances.

Differential Diagnosis

In the early stages the hematologic picture in this aplastic disturbance may simulate other blood dyscrasias such as agranulocytosis, leukemia, thrombocytopenic purpura, chronic aregenerative anemia, or the reactions induced by hypersplenism or myelofibrotic or neoplastic infiltration of the bone marrow. For this reason, and in order to check on the progress of the patient, it is advisable to take at least two bone marrow aspirations or even biopsies from different sites and separated by a time interval. The appearance of the circulating granulocytes and lymphocytes should be studied carefully in order not to overlook leukemic cells.

Therapy

Therapy is difficult and as a rule unsatisfactory. Every effort should be made to find a probable cause in order to remove it from the environment. Hemopoietic stimulants of all kinds should be given, though as a rule they are not of much benefit. British anti-Lewisite (BAL) may be administered if heavy metal poisoning seems responsible. Corticotropin or cortisone may provide some regenerative bone marrow stimulation, but only rarely is this permanent. Marrow transplantation has proved unsuccessful. Nursing supervision and emotional support of the patient are most important. An intractable hemorrhagic episode may be brought under temporary control by slow intravenous infusions of corticotropin along with transfusions of fresh blood.

Supportive blood transfusions should be given as often as needed. Freshly collected blood may help combat bleeding. Transfusions of packed red cells are less likely to produce cardiac failure, allergic manifestations, or transfusion reactions. All cross matchings should be done with extreme care, employing the indirect globulin procedure (p. 135).

A few instances are on record in which splenectomy was followed by an alleviation of symptoms, sometimes permanent. Splenectomy should not be considered unless (1) there are indications of undue hemolysis such as hyperbilirubinemia and urobilinogenuria (ordinarily not present), and (2) the peripheral blood picture and perhaps the epinephrine test have made it clear that the spleen is not serving as a source of extramedullary blood cell formation.

Prognosis

Enough patients have exhibited recovery after having been kept alive for many months or even several years by successive transfusions to justify tireless repetition of this procedure as frequently as needed. This may become difficult technically as the available veins become thrombosed after repeated venipunctures and local extravasations.

Repeated bone marrow examinations are not essential to follow progress. Some granulocytes, reticulocytes, and thrombocytes in the blood stream, albeit in small numbers, are indications that these normal cellular elements are still being produced. Subsidence of the injurious process and the beginning of recovery are heralded by a rise in the levels of these cells.

DRUGS AND POISONS

Acute toxic inhibition or hemolytic destruction of the red cells can be brought about by many chemical agents. Some drugs, such as phenylhydrazine, naphthalene, potassium chlorate, snake venom, and mushroom poison directly lyse the red cells of all individuals, with the severity of symptoms being proportional to the amount ingested. Other drugs, among them promin, quinine, and the sulfonamides, seem to cause hemolysis or hemodepression only if there is unusual susceptibility on the part of the host. Immediate symptoms may be those of sudden hemolysis. Various abnormal autohemagglutinins or autohemolysins may appear transitorily in the circulation (p. 94). With idiosyncratic sensitivities the manifestations recur when the drug is administered again, even in small dosage.

Some drugs and poisons such as the derivatives of benzol, phenol, toluol, and aniline may produce methemoglobinemia or sulfhemoglobinemia as well as affecting red cell production or destruction. Still others, such as lead, act primarily by depressing the bone marrow, and accelerate destruction only minimally if at all. With profound bone marrow depression the pattern of aplastic anemia may be produced in the peripheral blood.

Lead Poisoning

HEMOGLOBIN AND RED CELLS. Children with acute or chronic lead poisoning almost invariably exhibit some degree of anemia. The hemoglobin level as a rule is depressed somwhat more than the red cell count. Most patients exhibit between 6 and 12 gm of hemoglobin per 100 ml, and a red cell count between 2.5 and 4.5 million. The relative *rate of production* of hemoglobin is retarded as the result of injury to many of the maturing rubricytes of the marrow, but the *quality* of the hemoglobin that forms, so far as is known, remains unaltered. A mild reticulocytosis of 1 to 2 per cent is typically present; the reticulocyte count may be 5 per cent or higher.

Morphologically the red cells in the stained peripheral smear exhibit, in addition to mild hypochromia, numerous distortions in the form of anisocytosis (variation in size) and poikilocytosis (bizarre shapes).

Another prominent though less constant feature is that of stippling. In about two-thirds of the cases, from 0.10 to 2.0 per cent of the circulating erythrocytes contain basophilic rounded granules of variable diameter. These are believed to be cytoplasmic remnants derived from incomplete hemoglobin production. They contain ribonucleic acid. Iron stainable by the ferrocyanide reaction may be demonstrable in granules of substantial size. The largest granules are found in small distorted achromic cells whose stroma clearly has been poorly formed.

The anemia of lead poisoning is the consequence of both defective production of hemoglobin and accelerated destruction of abnormal red cells by the spleen and presumably also by the reticuloendothelial system. The red cells when tested for osmotic fragility in a graded series of hypotonic saline solutions may display a diminution in fragility (increase in resistance).

BONE MARROW. This may seem moderately hypoplastic, comparatively normal, or even at times slightly hyperactive. Basophilic stippling may be found in some of the developing normoblasts and polychrome erythrocytes whose staining qualities indicate that hemoglobin has already formed in their substance. The marrow aspirate may also exhibit large reticuloendothelial cells containing hemosiderin, phagocytized red cells, and basophilic granular masses. Such observations suggest that stippling is the result of faulty erythrogenesis rather than the direct effect of lead upon the released mature red cells. Small particles of nonhemoglobin iron demonstrable by special staining are abundant in both normoblasts and mature erythrocytes (p. 34).

Some normoblasts may contain so much excess of protoporphyrin as to fluoresce when viewed microscopically under ultraviolet light (*fluorescytes*). This microfluorescence may appear also but less prominently in the other cells and bony trabeculae of the marrow.

OTHER LABORATORY FINDINGS. A leukocytosis up to 25,000 or more cells per cu mm in total count may be evident during a period of acute symptoms. Most of the increased cells are neutrophils, which sometimes contain toxic granules. Eosinophilia is uncommon. Monocytes or lymphocytes or both may be increased. Platelets are usually unaltered in numbers but may be diminished.

That blood destruction may be accelerated is suggested in some cases by a mild hyperbilirubinemia with an increased output of bilirubin in bile and urine. Many patients have hemosiderosis of the body tissues. Coproporphyrin III is usually detectable in the urine (p. 353). The urine may contain protein, glucose, or ketone bodies. If cerebral symptoms are present there will be changes in the cerebrospinal fluid (p. 469). Coagulation difficulties are almost never seen.

Naphthalene Poisoning

Ingestion of naphthalene and related substances may bring about an episode of acute hemolysis severe enough to be fatal. These accidents are seen most often in children about 2 years of age who suck moth balls which consist of naphthalene. An episode in a newborn infant 6 days old has been ascribed to oiling of the skin followed by contact with diapers which had been stored previously with naphthalene crystals.

Symptoms consisting of diarrhea, vomiting, abdominal pain, fever, prostration, pallor, and passage of dark hemoglobin-containing urine begin 2 to 5 days after the exposure. The red cell and hemoglobin levels drop abruptly, sometimes to as low as one-fifth normal value. Studies of the blood show leukocytosis, anisocytosis, microspherocytosis, reticulocytosis, and increased saline fragility. Some red cells usually exhibit partial fragmentation or other distortions in shape. There may be clear colorless areas near the cell borders with the hemoglobin concentrated in other regions. Heinz bodies may be apparent in fresh wet preparations. The urine may have the odor of naphthalene. Chemical examination reveals it to contain alpha and beta naphthol and alpha and beta naphthoquinone in large amounts. The nature of the disturbance is often not recognized until after the parents have been questioned specifically as to contact of the child with moth balls or naphthalene flakes. Treatment consists of whole-blood transfusions and a liberal fluid intake, either parenterally or by mouth.

BURNS

Patients with severe third-degree burns often experience a rapidly developing anemia. Part of the explanation may lie in toxic depression of the bone marrow, but a major component is actual injury to many of the red cells by the physical effects of heat.

FAVISM (BROAD BEAN INTOXICATION)

This is a sensitization disease to *Vicia faba* (broad bean, horse bean, fava bean), which expresses itself acutely as a paroxysm of red cell hemolysis. Favism is seen most often in Sicily, Calabria, and Sardinia, where the bean is an important dietary staple, but more and more cases are being described in the United States.

Attacks are induced by inhalation of the pollen or eating of the bean. For reasons not well understood, sensitization is exhibited by only a small minority of those who are exposed. Various parts of the plant are antigenic, but the principal allergen is in the bean protein. The initial sensitization is induced by massive inhalation of pollen. It has been suggested that denaturization may have been incomplete when symptoms follow ingestion of cooked beans. Patients who have had one episode may have recurrences on further contact with the bean.

An attack of favism consists of an acute hemolytic episode accompanied by fever, malaise, gastrointestinal symptoms, anemia, and jaundice and may be fatal. It begins in a few hours to a few days after exposure to the bean and continues for several days. The severity may vary. In less than a day the red cell count can be reduced to 1 million or less, and the hemoglobin level to as low as 2 gm per 100 ml. There is leukocytopenia at first, followed in a few hours by leukocytosis and later by eosinophilia. Anisocytosis, poikilocytosis, basophilia, and erythroblastosis are found in the smear. Hemoglobinemia and hemoglobinuria appear. Jaundice, hepatomegaly, and splenomegaly soon follow. Recovery begins within a day or two, heralded by subsidence of the symptoms and a rise in reticulocytes. The best immediate therapy is liberal transfusions, along with other measures. Iron and other hematinics are advisable afterward.

The possibility of favism or of accidental ingestion of naphthalene moth balls or other hemolytic poison should always be considered whenever a child exhibits acute jaundice and anemia without a cause being evident. Many of the cases of so-called Lederer's acute hemolytic anemia are probably due to some such mechanism.

POSTHEMORRHAGIC ANEMIA

The degree of anemia which follows the loss of large amounts of blood depends upon several factors: (1) the total quantity lost, (2) the time period over which this has occurred, (3) the individual's regenerative capacity, (4) the presence or absence of associated red cell difficulties, and (5) persistence and duration of the bleeding. A sudden hemorrhage throws much more strain on the adjustment mechanisms than does a gradual one. One child with a massive traumatic hemorrhage may have serious air hunger and shock when one-third of his blood volume is gone, whereas another with slower bleeding continuing over several days may lose nearly 50 per cent of his red cells and yet have few symptoms. Slow bleeding permits compensatory fluid to pass from tissue spaces into the vascular channels, and shock is much less. The hemoglobin, hematocrit, and red cell levels are not reliable measures of the total amount of blood lost, since they do not take into account the extent of either vasoconstriction or hemodilution.

Studies of children with chronic anemia from hemorrhage indicate that they are as likely to have an excessively large as an abnormally small blood volume. An iron deficiency may be superimposed as a consequence of the unusual rate of loss of this element from the body economy.

The immediate hematologic signs of sudden hemorrhage, other than lowered red cell hemoglobin and hematocrit values, are (1) a thrombocytosis which may reach a level of as high as 1 million per cu mm within an hour or two, (2) a coincident shortening of the blood coagulation time, (3) a neutrophilic leukocytosis of 10,000 to 25,000, with many immature granulocytes and even metamyelocytes developing within a few hours. These associated reactions subside within a day or two, but the red cell count may continue to fall for a little longer as the blood volume is restored. If the hemorrhage has been in the upper intestinal tract the concentration of nitrogenous elements of the blood may go up a little and fever may appear. A rise in blood urea nitrogen above 50 mg per 100 ml signifies an excessive loss of blood.

Whether acute, subacute, or chronic, every hemorrhage evokes compensatory regenerative action on the part of the erythropoietic system. A reticulocytosis begins on the second or third day, and marrow aspirates show rubricytic hyperactivity. Nucleated red cells may appear in the peripheral blood if the loss has been very great. The red cell count rises steadily; the anemia following a single acute hemorrhage can be expected to be completely corrected in 4 to 6 weeks. The newly forming red cells are identical with those previously present, except that in the presence of inadequate iron the new cells will be hypochromic and microcytic. If full recovery does not occur, a recurrence of the bleeding, a dietary deficiency, or some other kind of systemic disturbance must be searched for.

When bleeding is external it is apparent at once. With internal bleeding, however, the disturbance may not be recognized until air hunger supervenes. When the signs and symptoms point to internal bleeding but the exact location is obscure, suspected body cavities may be aspirated diagnostically if a gastrointestinal source can be excluded. An underlying disturbance of coagulation should be considered whenever a child exhibits spontaneous bleeding without obvious cause.

ESSENTIAL PULMONARY HEMOSIDEROSIS

This is a chronic and usually progressive disturbance characterized by attacks of dyspnea and hemoptysis secondary to recurrent hemorrhages into the lungs. There is no abnormal general bleeding tendency and no eosinophilia. During the attacks bilirubinuria and urobilinogenuria may occur. Anemia appears, often of the hypochromic type, and may be refractory to iron therapy. The peripheral blood shows anisocytosis, poikilocytosis, and pallor of the red cells. Erythrocytosis may develop if lung insufficiency becomes chronic. A reticulocytosis is usually present. The bone marrow is normal except that immature red cells may be a little diminished. At autopsy the lung alveolae are filled with hemosiderin-containing phagocytes and the elastic tissue of the small pulmonary arterioles may appear altered.

SUDDEN SEVERE HEMORRHAGE AT BIRTH

Such accidents can give rise to a distinctive picture which superficially resembles erythroblastosis fetalis. The loss of blood may take place from the placental surface during abruptio placentae or placenta praevia, or later through the umbilical vessels if improperly tied. Bleeding which takes place before the infant leaves the uterine cavity may be masked by the mixing of fetal with maternal blood. An unintentional incision of the placenta during cesarian section can lead to pronounced fetal blood loss before delivery is accomplished. After any such accidents of delivery the blood count of the infant should be followed carefully.

Newborn infants with hemorrhagic complications tend to be pale and feeble. Edema, shock, or respiratory distress may supervene. Blood studies after the first few hours may show low red cell and hemoglobin levels and a marked leukocytosis. There are peripheral signs of bone marrow hyperactivity in the form of a reticulocytosis and an increase in the basophilic and nucleated red cells. Differentiation is made from erythroblastosis fetalis by the history, the absence of severe jaundice and splenomegaly, and the negative serologic tests of both mother and child for sensitization to the red cell antigens. It is possible, of course, for a severe posthemorrhagic anemia to be superimposed on erythroblastosis fetalis or some other blood dyscrasia.

Therapy consists primarily in giving prompt and large transfusions along with oxygen and other supportive measures until the blood picture and blood volume are restored to normal.

A similar reaction pattern of anemia with extremely active red cell regeneration may follow an acute episode of red cell destruction or of massive sudden hemorrhage in a previously well infant or child of any age.

ANEMIA ASSOCIATED WITH CHRONIC OBSTRUCTIVE SPLENOMEGALY

A normochromic normocytic form of chronic anemia is occasionally seen in splenomegaly with hypersplenism (p. 295).

BIBLIOGRAPHY

BACTERIAL AND VIRAL INFECTIONS

Chernoff, A. I., and *A. M. Josephson,* Acute Erythroblastopenia in Sickle-cell Anemia and Infectious Mononucleosis, *A.M.A. Am. J. Dis. Child.* 82:310, 1951.

Gasser, C., Acute Erythroblastopenia: 10 Cases of Aplastic Erythroblastic Crises with Giant Erythroblasts in Allergic-Toxic Conditions, *Helvet. paediat. acta* 4:107, 1949.

Hemmeler, G., Les anémies toxiques et hemolytiques, *Ann. paediat.* 169:13, 1947.

Parsons, W. B., Jr., T. Cooper, and *C. H. Scheifley,* Anemia in Bacterial Endocarditis, *J.A.M.A.* 153:14, 1953.

Smith, C. H., Anemias in Infancy and Childhood, *Bull. New York Acad. Med.* 30:155, 1954.

Vaughan, J., Anaemia Associated with Trauma and Sepsis, *Brit. M. J.* 1:35, 1948.

Wintrobe, M. M., Principles in the Management of Anemias, *Bull. New York Acad. Med.* 30:6, 1954.

APLASTIC ANEMIA

Abt, A. F., Aplastic Anemias in Childhood: Report of a Primary Idiopathic Refractory Type, with Splenectomy, in an Eleven Year Old Girl, *Am. J. Dis. Child.* 78:516, 1949.

Boon, T. H., and *J. N. Walton,* Aplastic Anaemia, *Quart. J. Med.* 20:75, 1951.

Ersley, A. J., C. K. Iverson, and *F. D. Lawrason,* Cortisone and ACTH in Hypoplastic Anemia, *Yale J. Biol. & Med.* 25:44, 1952.

Frumin, A. M., A. S. Conston, and *D. R. Meranze,* Aplastic Anemia with Platelet Thrombi, *Blood* 7:942, 1952.

Loeb, V., Jr., Studies on the Anemia of Chronic Primary Bone Marrow Failure (Refractory Anemia), *J. Lab. & Clin. Med.* 38:923, 1951.

Smith, C. H., Hypoplastic and Aplastic Anemias of Infancy and Childhood: With A Consideration of the Syndrome of Nonhemolytic Anemia of the Newborn, *J. Pediat.* 43:457, 1953.

Sturgeon, P., Idiopathic Aplastic Anemia in Children: Its Early Differentiation from Aleukemic Leukemia by Bone Marrow Aspiration, *Pediatrics* 8:216, 1951.

DRUGS AND POISONS

Fink, H. W., and *C. A. Smith,* Incidence of Reactions to Sulfonamide Drugs in Infants and Children, *J. Pediat.* 28:40, 1946.

Hodgkinson, R. Blood Dyscrasias Associated with Chloramphenicol: An Investigation into the Cases in the British Isles, *Lancet* 1:285, 1954.

Lewis, C. N., L. E. Putnam, F. D. Hendricks, I. Kerlan, and *H. Welch,* Chloramphenicol (Chloromycetin) in Relation to Blood Dyscrasias with Observations on Other Drugs: A Special Survey, *Antibiotics & Chemother.* 2:601, 1952.

Loyd, E. L., Aplastic Anemia Due to Chloramphenicol, *Antibiotics & Chemother.* 2:1, 1952.

Mackell, J. V., F. Rieders, H. Brieger, and *E. L. Bauer,* Acute Hemolytic Anemia Due to Ingestion of Naphthalene Moth Balls, *Pediatrics* 7:722, 1951.

Osgood, E. E., Hypoplastic Anemias and Related Syndromes Caused by Drug Idiosyncrasy, *J.A.M.A.* 152:816, 1953.

Steele, J. M., Aplastic Anemia Subsequent to Sulfonamide Administration: A Case Report, *New York J. Med.* 50:2963, 1950.

Sturgeon, P., Fatal Aplastic Anemia in Children Following Chloramphenicol (Chloromycetin) Therapy, *J.A.M.A.* 149:918, 1952.

Welch, H., C. N. Lewis, and *I. Kerlan,* Blood Dyscrasias: A Nationwide Survey, *Antibiotics & Chemother.* 4:607, 1954.

Zuelzer, W. W., and *L. Apt,* Acute Hemolytic Anemia Due to Naphthalene Poisoning: A Clinical and Experimental Study, *J.A.M.A.* 141:185, 1949.

FAVISM

Jacobs, A. H., Favism in Two Children in California, *Pediatrics* 6:51, 1950.

Lecks, H. I., Favism: Report of a Case in a Child, *J. Pediat.* 34:309, 1949.

Luisada, A., Favism: A Singular Disease Chiefly Affecting the Red Blood Cells, *Medicine* 20:229, 1941.

MISCELLANEOUS

Braid, F., Hypothyroidism in Childhood, *Brit. M. J.* 1:1169, 1951.

Camacho Camba, J., La Anemia carencial del tropico in el nino (necatoriasis—uncinariasis—anemia tropical) *Rev. colombiana pediatria y puericultura* 12:90, 1952.

Jonsson, B., B. Vahlquist, and *K. Agner,* Case Report: Essential Pulmonary Hemosiderosis, *Blood* 6:665, 1951.

Kahn, J. B., Jr., and *J. Furth,* The Pathogenesis of Postirradiation Anemia, *Blood* 7:404, 1952.

MacArthur, P., Anaemia in Nephritis, *Arch. Dis. Childhood* 17:1, 1942.

CHAPTER 6

Constitutional Aplastic Anemias

PURE RED CELL ANEMIA (CHRONIC CONGENITAL AREGENERATIVE ANEMIA, CONGENITAL HYPOPLASTIC ANEMIA, ESSENTIAL ERYTHROCYTOPENIA)

This disturbance is characterized by a congenital impairment of red cell production within the bone marrow with only minor, if any, impairment of granulocyte or thrombocyte production. Pallor, weakness, and anemia become evident in the first weeks or months of life, though exceptionally not until after the first year. Red cells produced by the patient are normocytic in size, and either normochromic or hypochromic. When transfusions are frequent, most of the red cells are normal in appearance, being derived in large measure from the successive donors. The bone marrow has a decreased proportion of immature red cells, whose formation may appear distorted (p. 327).

There is no sickling or altered red cell fragility, and circulating hemolysins and agglutinins are not found. Familial prevalence has been observed, suggesting that this is a recessively transmitted anomaly. Liver, spleen, and lymph nodes are not enlarged, except occasionally in infancy. Serum bilirubin is not increased. Serum iron may be slightly elevated. The urine is free from coproporphyrin and excess urobilinogen or urobilin. Leukocytosis attends bacterial infections, and lymphocytosis appears in pertussis. There are no evidences of extramedullary hemopoiesis in the peripheral blood or at necropsy examination.

As a rule, reticulocytes are absent from the peripheral blood or number 0.3 per cent or less of all red cells. Occasional patients, however, show a reticulocytosis up to 1.5 per cent and sporadic circulating normoblasts.

Nutritionally these children often appear thin. When the condition is recognized early in life and proper supportive therapy given, their growth in height is not retarded, their intelligence is unimpaired, and they have no undue susceptibility to infection.

The failure of red cell production seems to express itself either partially or completely. The transfusion requirement is related to the rate of spontaneous capacity to form red cells. Patients become active and have

90

good appetites immediately after adequate supportive transfusions, and then grow listless and anorexic as the donor red cells wear out. The fresher the blood the longer the benefit.

Mild cases need transfusions only every few months or may be able without transfusions to maintain levels of 6 to 8 gm of hemoglobin and 2 to 2.5 million red cells per 100 ml without any transfusions except during severe infections. Severe cases may need to be transfused as often as every 3 to 6 weeks.

Spontaneous remissions may occur, lasting for several months to several years. In the more severe cases, the skin tends to take on a slightly dusky hue, probably because of hemosiderosis consequent on the repeated transfusions. A mild granulocytopenia or thrombocytopenia may persist. With the progress of the years an apical systolic heart murmur may appear and the heart or liver may enlarge. Two of our patients developed generalized bony demineralization, and one of these had neurologic signs of tetany despite a blood calcium level in the normal range.

Restorative therapy with hemopoietic vitamins, liver extracts, and attempts at bone marrow implants have induced no improvement. A single instance has been reported of transitory marrow regeneration following short-wave diathermy to the long bones. With the partial cases the use of corticotropin or cortisone or related hormones will often stimulate the bone marrow and improve the over-all nutritional status. Maintenance dosages must be worked out by long-range observation of the individual patients. When such benefit is achieved, discontinuance of the hormone tends to be followed by recession of the blood cell levels.

CONSTITUTIONAL PANCYTOPENIA ASSOCIATED WITH MULTIPLE DEVELOPMENTAL DEFECTS (FANCONI'S ANEMIA, "FAMILIAL PERNICIOUSLIKE ANEMIA IN CHILDREN")

This is a form of progressive generalized hypoplasia of the bone marrow associated with a decrease in circulating erythrocytes, leukocytes, and platelets, in which the patients exhibit skin pigmentation or other congenital abnormalities such as skeletal or mental underdevelopment, deafness, anomalies of the heart, kidneys, or ears, or hypoplasia of the gonads. Both familial and sporadic cases have been described.

The existence of anemia in these children typically does not become apparent until late infancy or the early years of childhood. Pallor, hemorrhages due to thrombocytopenia, or resistant infections are frequent first indications of bone marrow inadequacy.

As a rule the anemia, thrombocytopenia, and granulocytopenia are equally advanced. Macrocytosis is common, though not present consistently. Occasional immature red or white cells may be found in the peripheral blood. Reticulocytes may be increased, up to 15 per cent. Blood coagulation is sometimes altered. The red cell fragility is normal. The marrow shows hypocellularity, with arrest of maturation of the red and white cell series at the early rubricyte and promyelocyte levels and megakaryocytes reduced or virtually absent. Terminally it may become wholly aplastic and appear fatty. Hemosiderosis of the internal organs is often found at necropsy. The nature of the metabolic fault is not known. The disturbance is refractory to all therapy other than supportive transfusions. Several cases are on record in which splenectomy seemed to have been followed by some improvement, but this operation is usually of no benefit.

FAMILIAL HYPOPLASTIC PANCYTOPENIA

This term may be applied to a disorder exhibited by multiple members of a family in which the affected individuals exhibit pallor, weakness, bleeding tendency, and a chronic diminution of otherwise normal-appearing red cells, granulocytes, and platelets. The bone marrow is morphologically hypoplastic, with all the blood-forming elements quantitatively diminished but qualitatively normal. A mild reticulocytosis is usually seen. The spleen is not enlarged. Minor anomalies of the skeleton or other organs may be present. Periodic transfusions are needed.

PORPHYRIA ERYTHROPOÏETICA (CONGENITAL PHOTOSENSITIVE PORPHYRIA)

This rare metabolic anomaly is characterized clinically by fluorescent deep-red urine and sensitivity of the skin to sunlight. Splenomegaly and normochromic anemia due to an increased rate of blood destruction are not uncommon. The urine contains uroporphyrin and coproporphyrin in large amounts, and there is an abundance of urobilinogen and coproporphyrin in the stools. There is usually a reticulocytosis. The red cells in the peripheral blood may show anisocytosis, poikilocytosis, and basophilia. The bone marrow aspirate exhibits active red cell hyperplasia, and some of the rubriblastic nuclei may show degenerative changes. The marrow reticuloendothelium may show phagocytosed erythrocytes or hemosiderin. After splenectomy the fecal and urinary porphyrin and fecal urobilinogen excretion decrease, and the other evidences of accelerated red cell production and destruction become less pronounced.

BIBLIOGRAPHY

CONSTITUTIONAL APLASTIC AND HYPOPLASTIC ANEMIAS

Aldrich, R. A., V. Hawkinson, M. Grinstein, and *C. J. Watson,* Photosensitive or Congenital Porphyria with Hemolytic Anemia. I. Clinical and Fundamental Studies before and after Splenectomy, *Blood* 6:685, 1951.

Beautyman, W., A Case of Fanconi's Anemia, *Arch. Dis. Childhood* 26:238, 1951.

Burgert, E. O., Jr., R. L. J. Kennedy, and *G. L. Pease,* Congenital Hypoplastic Anemia, *Pediatrics* 13:218, 1954.

Cathie, I. A. B., Erythrogenesis Imperfecta, *Arch. Dis. Childhood* 25:313, 1950.

Estren, S., and *W. Dameshek,* Familial Hypoplastic Anemia of Childhood: Report of Eight Cases in Two Families with Beneficial Effects of Splenectomy in One Case, *Am. J. Dis. Child.* 73:671, 1947.

———, *J. F. Suess,* and *W. Dameshek,* Congenital Hypoplastic Anemia Associated with Multiple Developmental Defects (Fanconi Syndrome), *Blood* 2:85, 1947.

Fisher, O. D., and *F. M. B. Allen,* Erythrogenesis Imperfecta or Congenital Hypoplastic Anemia (Diamond-Blackfan Type), *Arch. Dis. Childhood* 28:363, 1953.

Fitzgerald, J. H., Jr., and *A. H. London, Jr.,* Chronic Hypoplastic Anemia of the Newborn: Report of a Case with Apparent Recovery, *North Carolina M. J.* 7:215, 1946.

Lelong, M. R., C. Joseph, C. Polonowski, G. Desmonts, and *J. Colin,* L'Anémie chronique avec arrêt de la maturation normoblastique (type Blackfan-Diamond), *Arch. franç. pediat.* 8:473, 1951.

Levy, A., Aplastic Anemia in Siblings with Multiple Congenital Anomalies (the Fanconi Type), *J. Pediat.* 40:24, 1952.

Palmen, K., and *B. Vahlquist,* Stationary Hypoplastic Anemia, *Acta haematol.* 4:273, 1949.

Reinhold, J. S. L., E. Neumark, R. Lightwood, and *C. O. Carter,* Familial Hypoplastic Anemia with Congenital Abnormalities (Fanconi's Syndrome), *Blood* 7:915, 1952.

Rohr, K., Familial Panmyelophthisis: Fanconi Syndrome in Adults, *Blood* 4:130, 1949.

Rosenthal, I. M., E. L. Lipton, and *G. Asrow,* Effect of Splenectomy on Porphyria Erythropoietica, *Pediatrics* 15:663, 1955.

Silver, H. K., W. C. Blair, and *C. H. Kempe,* Fanconi Syndrome: Multiple Congenital Anomalies with Hypoplastic Anemia, *A.M.A. Am. J. Dis. Child.* 83:14, 1952.

Smith, C. H., Hypoplastic and Aplastic Anemias of Infancy and Childhood: With a Consideration of the Syndrome of Nonhemolytic Anemia of the Newborn, *J. Pediat.* 43:457, 1953.

Sunderman, F. W., Jr., and *F. W. Sunderman,* Practical Considerations of Diseases of Porphyrin Metabolism: Porphyria and Porphyrinuria, *Am. J. Clin. Path.* 25:1231, 1955.

CHAPTER 7

Hemolytic Anemias of Autogenous Origin

ACQUIRED HEMOLYTIC ANEMIA

This designation comprises a group of uncommon anemic disorders in which an individual's red cells, previously normal, begin to be destroyed at an accelerated rate as the result of the autogenous evolvement of abnormal isoantibodies, or occasionally through other immune processes. The presence of the autoantibodies is usually demonstrable by the Coombs and related tests, and sometimes they occur free in the plasma; occasionally, however, their existence must be inferred from the phenomena exhibited or the symptoms attributed to the pathologic development of other autoimmune mechanisms. It has been hypothesized that certain drugs, viruses, or bacteria at times may initiate the hemodestruction by causing minor chemical alterations in red cells. The altered cells then act as antigens to stimulate the immunity mechanisms of the body. These mechanisms then attack and injure other red cells, which in turn become antigenic, and so the cycle goes on. A related theory is that rare environmental antigens have affinity for the surfaces of red cells. As exposure to the antigen continues the endogenous reactive processes attack the red cells as well as the surface antigens.

When the hemolytic phenomena develop as a complication of some generalized disease the deranged cell system may be the source of the antibody. Thus infectious mononucleosis when severe may be accompanied by sudden anemia or other forms of cytopenia, often with the temporary exhibition of antibodies such as autohemagglutinins or hemolysins, or even a positive Donath-Landsteiner test. In chronic leukemia or lymphosarcoma the proliferating abnormal cells may release some abnormal globulin which acts as an antibody against red cells and leads to their early destruction. In a few cases of severe pyogenic infections an abnormal autoagglutinability of the red cells has been observed.

Current evidence indicates that anti–red cell autoantibodies may be formed by the reticuloendothelial system, the lymphoid system, the plasma cells, or the cells of the spleen. The spleen is a common offender, in that it is both the largest lymphoid organ of the body and the largest

94

compact unit of reticuloendothelial cells. The autoantibodies are somewhat nonspecific inasmuch as they will affix themselves to normal red cells as well.

When the disease arises slowly and is of moderate severity the patient exhibits a normochromic anemia usually with intermittent weakness, pallor, icterus, or splenomegaly. When it has an acute explosive onset there may be chills, malaise, or even hemoglobinuria, shock, air hunger, and anuria.

Laboratory Findings

The red cells tend to vary in size, with microcytic-appearing spherocytes, large basophilic forms, and perhaps occasional normoblasts. After the disease becomes long-standing the red cells may show central pallor. The stools and urine contain an excess of urobilinogen.

The blood plasma may contain traces of methemalbumin or of free hemoglobin which will spill over into the urine if the hemoglobinemia is marked. The serum bilirubin tends to be elevated with all except minimal degress of hemolysis, the major rise being in the slow-reacting fraction (indirect van den Bergh test). Cold isohemagglutinins make their appearance not infrequently.

The bone marrow is usually hypercellular and hyperactive with respect to the red cell series and gives rise to a peripheral reticulocytosis. Should the antibodies be extremely potent or of long duration, however, the bone marrow may become depressed and hypocellular; in this event no reticulocytosis takes place and the disorder may be confused with some form of hypoplastic anemia. The cells of the thrombocyte or granulocyte series may share in the stimulation or depression.

The osmotic and mechanical fragility of the red cells may be increased slightly in mild disturbances, and markedly so in the more severe. Normal red cells transfused into these patients undergo sphering and exhibit increased fragility, and their survival is diminished also.

Demonstration of Autoantibodies

Immunologic mechanisms capable of damaging the integrity of the red cells are as a rule demonstrable by one or more laboratory approaches:

DIRECT COOMBS TEST. The red cells from most patients will be agglutinated by Coombs testing serum, indicating that they are coated abnormally with antibody globulin. (This serum is prepared by injecting rabbits with human serum globulin until antibodies develop against the human globulin.) Positive-reacting sensitized cells will often agglutinate spontaneously when suspended in normal serum or in purified albumin solutions.

In performing the Coombs test it is important that the patient's red cells be given at least three preliminary washings with saline solution, or else an outer shell of normal plasma globulin may prevent the union of the rabbit serum with the autoantibody coating. A positive reaction may not appear until after the serum has been diluted (the prozone phenomenon). It is possible to titrate roughly the amount of antibody on the cells by using progressive dilutions of antiglobulin serum. The activity of the disease and the amount of absorbed antibody tend to run parallel.

INDIRECT COOMBS TEST. When the above test gives negative results it may be possible to demonstrate the existence of anti–red cell antibodies in the patient's plasma by first exposing normal red cells of compatible blood type or from a group O Rh-negative subject to the patient's plasma, and then noting agglutination of these red cells when rabbit antihuman globulin serum is added subsequently.

SERUM ISOHEMAGGLUTININS AND ISOHEMOLYSINS. A wide battery of procedures are available. The patient's red cells may be suspended in progressive dilutions of his own serum, normal serum, and an albumin solution, each at refrigerator, room, and body temperature. Sets of tubes containing the red cells and progressive dilutions of the serum are incubated at 37, 20, and 4°C, because the various red cell agglutinins and hemolysins may have different effective thermal ranges. Each of these tests may be set up in quadruplicate, using saline and 20 to 30 per cent bovine albumin as diluents, with and without the addition of complement. Variations in pH may also be introduced.

Agglutination or hemolysis may appear in one or more of these preparations if an antibody coating is present. Similar procedures are available for surveying the patient's serum, utilizing either his own cells or compatible red cells from a normal subject. The tests for free antibodies in the patient's serum are positive with less consistency than those for antibodies absorbed on the red cells.

It is sometimes possible to separate the antibody from the patient's red cells by washing the cells with normal saline at various temperatures. The eluate may then sensitize normal red cells for the antiglobulin reaction (indirect Coombs test) or agglutinate or hemolyze normal red cells or the patient's red cells after trypsinization or when suspended in albumin solution or normal human serum.

Included in any serologic work-up should be the search for unusual antibodies against other blood group antigens, particularly if the patient had received blood or plasma transfusions in the recent or remote past.

Preliminary exposure of the red cells used in all the above tests to a solution of trypsin or some other proteolytic enzyme for a brief period (usually a few minutes) may render them more susceptible to any abnormal antibodies. Trypsin enhances the agglutinability with cold isohemagglutinins, so that less significance can be placed on a high titer of cold agglutinins obtained with this technic. Red cells from patients with paroxysmal nocturnal hemoglobinuria have also been used with satisfactory results for the study of abnormal antibodies.

Judgment and experience are needed for the proper interpretation of results with all such highly sensitive methods of testing. Many of the reactions are weak and hard to read. Some of the positive responses may appear to be nonspecific; others will seem more clearly related to clinical phenomena. Positive reactions in a given patient do not necessarily mean that the hemolytic disturbances are caused by these immune substances.

ERYTHROPHAGOCYTOSIS. In vitro phagocytosis of red cells by leukocytes may take place if a tube of freshly drawn blood with an added anticoagulant is left to incubate for an hour or more at 37°C (p. 35). Erythrophagocytosis by the tissue reticuloendothelial cells is not uncommon in this disease, as shown by histologic studies at autopsy. In outstandingly severe cases the phenomenon may be recognized in direct smears of the circulating blood.

Treatment

With conservative therapy some patients undergo spontaneous re-missions; others do not. Transfusions of red cells or whole blood may relieve the anemia, but the respite tends to be shorter than with other diseases. Repeated transfusions often seem to aggravate the erythro-destruction and should be kept to an absolute minimum. Reliable cross matching can become extremely difficult if the circulating antibody is comparatively broad in specificity and reacts with the red cells of most prospective donors. In this situation the patient is best transfused with washed red cells of the O Rh-negative variety. Local irradiation of the spleen may be of benefit in chronic lymphomatosis or leukemic enlarge-ment, but is deemed useless or even dangerous in most other forms of acquired hemolytic anemia.

Administration of corticotropin or cortisone may arrest the hemolytic process for some weeks or months or even result in a permanent recession. Such therapy is advisable. Corticotropin is sometimes more effective than cortisone. Some or all of the laboratory tests for autoantibodies may become negative during the period of therapy.

Results of splenectomy are unpredictable. One merit of hormone therapy is that it may improve the status of an acutely ill patient long enough for splenectomy to be done without great risk. After the opera-tion the signs of anemia and hemolysis may subside completely and permanently, or only partially and for a brief period, or an exacerbation may follow. When the disease process recurs after an interval of im-provement, a second operation sometimes reveals a tiny hyperplastic accessory spleen whose excision may lead to another partial if not com-plete cessation of symptoms. If the disease becomes severe once more, the internal lymph nodes may be suspected of having taken on hypersplenic-like behavior and may be treated with nitrogen mustard or with x-ray irradiation of the chest and upper abdomen. The ultimate outcome in such progressive cases is usually fatal. At no time, however, should the aggressive therapeutic program with transfusions, steroid hormones, splenectomy, and other measures be relaxed.

When splenectomy is followed by disappearance of the autoantibodies and complete clinical arrest of the disturbance, it may be presumed that the spleen was the site of abnormal antibody formation and perhaps active also in the removal of antibody coated cells. When abnormal hemodestruction ceases after splenectomy but the autoantibodies are still demonstrable, it would seem that the extrasplenic tissues have been participating in the production of the injurious substances but that most, if not all, of the undue elimination of coated cells was being carried out by the spleen. If splenectomy does not alter the patient's course significantly, all or the greater part of the hemodestruction must be attributed to nonsplenic mechanisms.

When the differential count of the peripheral blood contains more than 1 or 2 per cent of myelocytes, metamyelocytes, and nucleated red cells and the bone marrow is hypoplastic, the possibility of extramedullary hemopoiesis within the enlarged spleen must be seriously considered. In that event, splenectomy may aggravate rather than relieve the anemia by removing an important compensatory blood-forming organ.

HEMOLYTIC EPISODES DUE TO COLD AUTOHEMAGGLUTININS

Circulating autohemagglutinins with maximum potency against red cells at 0 to 5°C but inactive at 37°C (cold hemagglutinins, cold isohemagglutinins) often appear in primary atypical pneumonia and hemolytic anemia caused by autoimmune mechanisms, and sporadically also in other acute infections, blood dyscrasias, and cirrhosis of the liver. They arise less commonly in children than in adults. Cold isohemolysins are sometimes demonstrable also, but in lower concentration.

Cold autohemagglutinins can bring about acute hemolytic episodes if the surface of the body is chilled. During or immediately after such an exposure the patient may exhibit chills, hemoglobinuria, normochromic anemia, splenomegaly, reticulocytosis, bilirubinemia, leukocytosis, and urobilinogenuria. The differential count may show a predominance of neutrophils, with some myelocytes and metamyelocytes. The fragility determinations and Coombs tests give normal results. Acrocyanosis or Raynaud's phenomenon or even local gangrene may ensue if exposure to cold is prolonged. In atypical pneumonia the respiratory complaints and physical signs may be minimal, so that chest roentgenography is needed to establish the diagnosis.

These hemolytic episodes must be differentiated from those of syphilitic paroxysmal cold hemoglobinuria; in the latter, cold autohemagglutinins are absent and complement is needed for the confirmatory serologic tests.

The relationship of cold autohemagglutinins to primary atypical pneumonia is of especial importance diagnostically, inasmuch as these antibodies do not develop in other infections of the respiratory tract. About three-fourths of all patients with this disease exhibit titers between 1:80 and 1:640 at 4°C, lasting usually only a few weeks. This rise may not begin until the third week after the onset of the illness or even later or may occur immediately and subside by 2 to 4 weeks.

Because low temperatures excite cold hemagglutinins to activity, it is important to avoid cold oxygen tents, alcohol sponging, cold drinks, and antipyretics in the medical management of all individuals who possess them. Patients must also protect themselves against outdoor cold in winter.

When a patient with cold isohemagglutinins needs a transfusion, the donor blood should be warmed before being introduced into the venous system. All typing and cross matching should be done in glassware warmed to 37°C, or the blood may clump in all preparations and appear as group AB Rh-positive. Accordingly, every blood specimen which seems to be of this group and which gives unsatisfactory cross matches should be retested at 37°C to rule out any possibility of cold isohemagglutination.

Laboratory Procedures

When serum is desired for cold autohemagglutinin studies the blood should be collected from the patient in a warm syringe and left at room temperature. If it is stored in a refrigerator the red cells in the clot will remove from the serum any cold hemagglutinins which may be present. If the serum is then separated before thorough warming, it will give a negative response.

In normal subjects the titer for cold autohemagglutinins with homologous red cells by standard laboratory methods is typically 1:4 or less, though it may be as high as 1:16. With trypsinized red blood cells the normal range is extended to 1:64, the most frequent titer being 1:32. With the albumin technic the usual level is 1:2. Customarily the test is made in saline dilutions; titers of 1:20 or higher are deemed positive. These agglutinins are somewhat heterospecific; they will act on red cells of other blood groups, and even on the red cells of some animals.

All agglutinations due to cold are reversed when the specimens are rewarmed at 37°C for 1 or 2 hours. Chilling the blood restores the phenomenon.

The first clue as to the existence of cold isohemagglutinins in high potency may be the recognition of agglutination in the glass chamber when a red cell count is made in cool equipment or the noting of granular clumping of blood in a cold syringe during a venipuncture or in a tube of blood stored in a refrigerator. A simple test which can be made at the bedside is to draw blood into a syringe or tube containing an anticoagulant, and then place the container under running cold water. Granular clumps which form under this circumstance and then dissociate when the tube is warmed denote a positive reaction. Chilling and rewarming a hanging drop or cover-slip preparation of fresh blood will also demonstrate these changes.

PAROXYSMAL HEMOGLOBINURIA DUE TO COLD AUTOHEMOLYSINS

This uncommon disease is becoming a rarity with the fading away of syphilis, congenital or acquired, which is nearly always a prerequisite for its emergence in childhood. Exposing the whole body or even part of one extremity to a low temperature is followed promptly by intravascular hemolysis with chills, fever, jaundice, and urticaria, accompanied by hemoglobinemia with or without hemoglobinuria.

The cause of the symptoms is the constant presence in the blood of an autohemolysin. At low temperatures the red cells absorb the hemolysin, but the cells do not rupture until warmed in the presence of complement.

Laboratory Procedures

In the Rosenbach test a typical systemic attack is precipitated by immersing both hands or feet in ice-cold water for 10 to 20 minutes. In the Ehrlich test, which is safer and less taxing, a finger or hand is immersed in ice water for 10 to 20 minutes while a tourniquet remains loosely in place around the digit or forearm. A venipuncture from the tested extremity will then show free hemoglobin in the blood.

The Donath-Landsteiner test is done in vitro. A test tube containing freshly drawn blood, after being left in the refrigerator for several hours, will on being rewarmed show a pink color in the supernatant serum as an expression of hemolysis. In the modified Mackenzie test, washed red cells from the patient and a normal subject of the same blood group are suspended individually, with added complement, in tubes of serum from each of these individuals. The mixtures are chilled for 10 to 30 minutes and then warmed again. The patient's serum will hemolyze both sets of red cells if a cold hemolysin is present, whereas the control serum will not.

Serologic study of these individuals with the tests for syphilis gives a positive reaction. The autohemolysin, which can fluctuate in titer with the passage of time, is believed to be evoked by the same immunologic mechanism which gives rise to the positive syphilis test. Long after the patient ceases to have paroxysms on exposure to cold, either as the result of spontaneous recovery or of specific treatment, the presence of the cold hemolysin remains demonstrable. The titers of the two do not run parallel, except that both usually decrease following antisyphilitic therapy.

In many patients with paroxysmal cold hemoglobinuria induced by syphilis, exposure to cold results in urticaria as well as chills and passage of dark-red urine. These patients appear to have a circulating "dermolysin" which is either the same substance as the hemolysin or closely allied to it. This antibody can be transferred passively. If the patient's serum is injected intradermally into a nonsensitive test subject and the injection site is chilled and warmed, an erythematous pruritic wheal appears. It is possible to adsorb away the dermolysin along with the hemolysin by exposing a tube of whole clotted blood to cold, followed by quick centrifugation in the cold.

PAROXYSMAL NOCTURNAL HEMOGLOBINURIA (MARCHIAFAVA-MICHELI SYNDROME)

This entity, rare in childhood, is a form of chronic hemolytic anemia which tends to produce episodes of hemoglobinuria on arising in the morning. The subject's red cells seem anomalously susceptible to some normal thermolabile component of human serum and become hemolyzed by it when carbon dioxide accumulates in the tissues during sleep and lowers the hydrogen-ion concentration of the blood below a critical level. Large doses of aspirin can produce the same effect. Febrile illnesses tend to aggravate the symptoms. Transfusions are the best remedial measures.

Unless sufficient hemoglobin is liberated to produce a serum level greater than the renal threshold, the patient may have hemoglobinemia without hemoglobinuria. Patients with atypical hemolytic anemia without demonstrable antibodies should be subjected to the diagnostic tests for paroxysmal nocturnal hemoglobinuria.

Laboratory Procedures

The heat-resistance test is positive in this disease. About 5 ml of clotted blood in a test tube is placed in an incubator at 37°C with control tubes set up at room and refrigerator temperatures. Hemolytic discoloration of the supernatant serum takes place after 4 to 24 hours in the incubator, but not at the lower temperatures. This spontaneous hemolysis occurs frequently at the normal pH of blood, but is decreased or eliminated at an alkaline pH of 7.6 to 8.0 or above. The patient's serum will not hemolyze compatible red cells from a normal subject. Since electrophoretic analysis indicates that the patient's hemoglobin has a normal structure, the erythrocyte stroma appears to be at fault.

The acid hemolysis test of Ham approaches more closely what takes place in the body. To acidified serum (pH 6.5 to 6.8) from normal defibrinated blood is added a 50 per cent suspension of washed red cells from the patient. Hemolysis represents a positive reaction, provided controls remain negative.

BIBLIOGRAPHY

AUTOIMMUNE MECHANISMS IN ACQUIRED HEMOLYTIC ANEMIA

Dacie, J. V., Haemolytic Anaemia, with Particular Reference to Cause and Mechanism, *Postgrad. M. J.* 24:70, 1948.

Dacie, J. V., Hemolysins in Acquired Hemolytic Anemia: Effect of pH on the Activity in Vitro of a Serum Hemolysin, *Blood* 4:928, 1949.

————, The Presence of Cold Haemolysins in Sera Containing Cold Haemagglutinins, *J. Path. & Bact.* 62:241, 1950.

———— and *G. C. Gruchy*, Auto-antibodies in Acquired Hemolytic Anemia, *J. Clin. Path.* 4:253, 1951.

Engleson, G., and *R. Grubb*, Abnormal Agglutinability of Red Cells in Pyogenic Infections: Report of Two Cases, *Am. J. Clin. Path.* 19:782, 1949.

Gardner, F. H., A. E. McElfresh, J. W. Harris, and *L. K. Diamond*, The Effect of Adrenocorticotrophic Hormone (ACTH) in Idiopathic Acquired Hemolytic Anemia as Related to the Hemolytic Mechanisms, *J. Lab. & Clin. Med.* 37:444, 1951.

Gasser, C., Acute Hemolytic Crises Following Plasma Transfusions in Dystrophic-toxic Infants (Akute hämolytische Krisen nach Plasma-transfusionen in dystrophisch-toxischen Säuglingen), *Helvet. paediat. acta* 1:38, 1945.

Liu, S. H., Chronic Hemolytic Anemia with Erythrocyte Fragility to Cold and Acid. I. Clinical and Laboratory Data of Two Cases, with Special Reference to the Cell Abnormality, *Blood* 6:101, 1951.

Meyer, L. M., and *N. D. Ritz*, Use of Corticotropin Therapy for Idiopathic Acquired Hemolytic Anemia, *J.A.M.A.* 155:742, 1954.

O'Connor, W. J., J. M. Vakiener, and *R. J. Watson*, Idiopathic Acquired Hemolytic Anemia in Young Children, *Pediatrics* 17:732, 1956.

Ponder, E., Certain Hemolytic Mechanisms in Hemolytic Anemia, *Blood* 6:559, 1951.

Sennott, J. S., Erythrophagocytosis in Acute Hemolytic Anemia of the Newborn: A Report of Three Cases, *Am. J. Dis. Child.* 71:269, 1946.

Zuelzer, W. W., Hemolytic Anemias: Mechanisms and Diagnostic Aspects, *J. Pediat.* 41:479, 1952.

COLD ISOHEMAGGLUTININS

Ames, R. G., Report of an Epidemic of Atypical Pneumonia in Children with Observations on Cold Agglutination Titers, *Cincinnati J. Med.* 28:791, 1947.

Bateman, J. C., Symptoms Attributable to Cold Hemagglutination. Report of Two Cases. *Arch. Int. Med.* 84:523, 1949.

Finland, M., and *M. W. Barnes*, Cold Agglutinins. VII. Tests of Cold Isohemagglutinins in Pneumonia and Other Acute Respiratory Infections over a Four Year Period, *Am. J. M. Sc.* 221:152, 1951.

Moffatt, G. M., Cold Auto-haemagglutination, *Canad. M. A. J.* 60:612, 1949.

Neely, F. L., W. H. Baria, C. Smith, and *C. F. Stone, Jr.*, Primary Atypical Pneumonia with High Titer of Cold Hemagglutinins, Hemolytic Anemia, and False Positive Donath-Landsteiner Test, *J. Lab. & Clin. Med.* 37:382, 1951.

PAROXYSMAL COLD HEMOGLOBINURIA

Becker, R. M., Paroxysmal Cold Hemoglobinurias, *Arch. Int. Med.* 81:630, 1948.

Jordan, W. S., Jr., L. Pillemer, and *J. H. Dingle*, The Mechanism of Hemolysis in Paroxysmal Cold Hemoglobinuria, *J. Clin. Invest.* 30:11, 22, 1951.

Malley, L. K., and *M. D. Hickey*, Paroxysmal Cold Haemoglobinuria of Non-syphilitic Type, *Lancet* 1:387, 1949.

Sweetman, W. P., E. F. Murphy, and *R. C. Woodcock*, Acute Idiopathic Paroxysmal Cold Haemoglobinuria of Non-syphilitic Type in a Child, *Brit. M. J.* 1:465, 1952.

PAROXYSMAL NOCTURNAL HEMOGLOBINURIA

Crosby, W. H., and *W. Dameshek*, Paroxysmal Nocturnal Hemoglobinuria: The Mechanism of Hemolysis and Its Relation to the Coagulation System, *Blood* 5:822, 1950.

Ham, T. H., Chronic Hemolytic Anemia with Paroxysmal Nocturnal Hemoglobinuria: Study of Mechanisms of Hemolysis in Relation to Acid Base Equilibrium, *New England J. Med.* 217:915, 1937.

Marks, J., The Marchiafava-Micheli Syndrome (Paroxysmal Nocturnal Hemoglobinuria), *Quart. J. Med.* 18:105, 1949.

McIlvanie, S. K., and *M. F. Beard*, Paroxysmal Nocturnal Hemoglobinuria: With Two New Case Reports, *Blood* 6:936, 1951.

CHAPTER 8

Erythrocytosis

Erythrocytosis (polycythemia, erythremia) refers to an abnormal increase in the red cell count, with the upper limit of normal ideally defined as more than two standard deviations above the mean for healthy persons of the same age and sex as the patient. Unfortunately, adequate data for the precise delimitation of the upper limits as related to age are still unavailable, so that one must rely on clinical experience and judgment when deciding when a red cell count is abnormally elevated.

As a rule, the hemoglobin level, hematocrit, and total blood volume are augmented as well as the red cell count. An exception occurs when iron-deficiency anemia is superimposed on the erythrocytosis of congenital cyanotic heart disease; here the red cell count may be elevated but the red cells themselves are unduly small and low in hemoglobin.

Erythrocytosis is an uncommon finding in the pediatric age period. It occurs most frequently in patients with congenital heart disease with pronounced arterial unsaturation of the peripheral blood. Pulmonary arteriovenous fistulas, chronic constricting bronchiolitis, and any other chronic lung or vascular lesion which can cause persistent arterial anoxemia may also elicit a persistent erythrocytosis. Prolonged existence at unusually high altitudes and congenital methemoglobinemia may have the same result.

A transitory erythrocytosis often accompanies states of sudden plasma loss or extreme dehydration, as in burns, crush injuries, diarrhea, excess vomiting, water deprivation, and after extreme diuresis or sweating. In any of these conditions the red cell counts may go as high as 8 to 10 million per cu mm. With extreme increases the combination of augmented blood volume, higher viscosity of the blood, and broadened capillary bed may retard the blood flow through the vessels sufficiently to favor spontaneous intravascular thrombosis with or without resultant infarctions. Essential polycythemia (polycythemia vera) is practically unheard of in the childhood years. Cobalt poisoning may induce a moderate increase in hemoglobin and red cell levels.

CYANOTIC CONGENITAL HEART DISEASE

Erythrocytosis develops with a fair degree of constancy in children with those forms of congenital heart anomalies having permanent venous-arterial shunts or extreme retardation of blood flow and resultant chronic oxygen unsaturation of the blood. With erythrocytosis the hemoglobin level is usually between 15 and 25 gm per 100 ml but may go to 30 gm in severe cases. The red cell count changes are more or less parallel and tend to be between 5.5 and 9 million. Exceptional values as high as 11 million have been recorded. Sometimes the erythrocytosis seems disproportionately higher than the hemoglobin increase, and vice versa. The hematocrit is likewise elevated; it may be between 65 and 85 per cent, paralleling the red cell count. The mean red cell volume is nearly always higher than in normal children of corresponding age and weight and tends to be between 80 and 110 cu μ. The highest mean volumes occur when the red cell counts are not much elevated. The mean content of hemoglobin in each red cell, as calculated from the blood hemoglobin level and the red cell count, is usually within normal limits but may range from 20 to 36 $\mu\mu$; in general this measurement is proportional to the mean cellular volume. The mean hemoglobin concentration in the packed mass of red cells is not infrequently decreased, ranging from 20 to 32 per cent. The mean osmotic resistance is sometimes a little altered: hemolysis in hypotonic saline dilutions may begin in concentration of 0.48 or 0.46 and not be complete until 0.30 or 0.28 (normal; approximately 0.44 to 0.32). There is often a mild reticulocytosis, between 1.0 and 2.0 per cent. The more severe the blood changes, the more marked tend to be the cyanosis and clubbing of the fingers, but the correlation is not close.

The total leukocyte count is usually between 4,000 and 8,000 per cu ml, with lymphocytes reduced perhaps more than the other white cell constituents. The bone marrow exhibits unusual prominence of red cell formation in some patients. The serum bilirubin is usually in the range between 0.9 and 2.0 mg per 100 ml, the slight increase being in the indirect portion. The serum iron is likewise increased, usually being between 130 and 300 mg per 100 ml. The platelet count is usually between 60,000 and 200,000 per cu mm despite a normal marrow content of megakaryocytes. There is no persistence of fetal (alkali-resistant) hemoglobin.

Prader, Rossi, and Wodenegg, using a dye technique, found the total blood volume in 20 children with congenital cyanotic heart disease averaged 65 per cent greater than the mean for 23 control healthy children, this rise being due to the circulating erythrocytes. The total erythrocyte volume was relatively enormously augmented (+189 per cent), whereas plasma volume was actually slightly diminished (−17 per cent).

The stimulus for the erythrocytosis and related changes seems to lie in the degree of oxygen unsaturation of the arterial blood, though this is not the complete explanation. The oxygen saturation in patients with congenital cyanotic heart disease can range from 15 to 90 per cent. It has been claimed that erythrocytosis does not occur unless the oxygen saturation is below 66 per cent, but exceptions to this rule in both directions have been encountered.

In infancy and early childhood the erythrocytosis may precede the development of recognizable cyanosis, or vice versa. Sometimes the erythrocytosis does not begin until after a few years of age. An acute anemia induced by an infection or nutritional inadequacy may transitorily efface an antecedent erythrocytosis and cause the cyanosis to disappear.

The oxygen saturation of the arterial blood becomes much higher immediately after a corrective operation. The hemoglobin level, however, may take 1 to 3 weeks to settle to 1 to 6 gm per 100 ml lower than the preoperative level. The hematocrit readings likewise become less. Diminution in the red cell count, on the other hand, may take 1 to 3 months. These variables do not go all the way back to normal unless the operation corrects the defect completely.

Newborn infants with congenital cyanotic heart disease may fail to experience the decrease in red cell and hemoglobin levels which normally takes place in the first 3 months of life. After this period, however, such infants are prone to develop a "relative" anemia, with a maintained or even rising red cell count but with a fall in hemoglobin level. Irritability, poor weight gain, and poor appetite may attend this development.

Masked Anemia

A concomitant iron-deficienccy anemia should be suspected whenever the hemoglobin level and hematocrit are not elevated in proportion to the red cell count. In fact, in many patients with congenital cyanotic heart disease the corpuscular measurements indicate that the red cells are not fully replete with hemoglobin.

The giving of iron therapy to such patients is usually followed by a rise in hemoglobin, hematocrit, and red cell levels. Iron medication given parenterally may produce these changes after iron given by the oral route has been ineffective. Just as in the iron-deficiency anemia of noncardiac cases, these children may show improvement in appetite and begin to gain weight before the red cell count or hemoglobin levels rise appreciably. In a group of such children studied by Rudolph, Nadas, and Borges, the administration of iron was followed by a gradual decrease in the number of cyanotic spells, improvement of exercise tolerance, rapid increase in weight, and general improvement in behavior over the next 2 to 6 months. In some instances this clinical improvement, still associated with severe cyanosis, continued for several weeks or months. Deterioration of the clinical condition began when the hematocrit reached 70 to 75 per cent. At and above this level the blood viscosity began to mount rapidly and was thought to be responsible for the unfavorable anoxic symptoms.

BIBLIOGRAPHY

ERYTHROCYTOSIS

Adams, F. H., and *S. C. Cunningham,* Further Studies on the Blood of Children with Cyanotic Heart Disease with Special Reference to the Hemoglobin, *J. Pediat.* 41:424, 1952.

Birkhill, F. R., M. A. Maloney, and *S. M. Levenson,* Effect of Transfusion Polycythemia upon Bone Marrow Activity and Erythrocyte Survival in Man, *Blood* 6:1021, 1951.

Josephs, H. W., The Mechanism of Reduction of Red Cells and Hemoglobin Following Operation for Tetralogy of Fallot, *Bull. Johns Hopkins Hosp.* 86:1, 1950.

Prader, A., E. Rossi, and *M. Wodenegg,* Blutuntersuchungen beim Morbus coeruleus, *Helvet. paediat. acta* 4:267, 1949; 5:159, 172, 185, 1950.

Rodes, C. B., Cavernous Hemangiomas of the Lung with Secondary Polycythemia, *J.A.M.A.* 110:1914, 1938.

Rudolph, A. M., A. S. Nadas, and *W. H. Borges,* Hematologic Adjustments to Cyanotic Congenital Heart Disease, *Pediatrics* 11:454, 1953.

Yater, W. M., J. Finnegan, and *H. M. Giffin,* Pulmonary Arteriovenous Fistula (Varix), *J.A.M.A.* 141:581, 1949.

CHAPTER 9

Derivatives of Hemoglobin

FETAL (ALKALI-RESISTANT) HEMOGLOBIN

The hemoglobin of the human fetus is strongly resistant to the denaturizing acting of alkali, in contrast to human adult hemoglobin which becomes converted rapidly into alkaline hematin at pH 13. Fetal hemoglobin on exposure to 1 per cent sodium or ammonium hydroxide solution requires 1 to 3 or more hours for complete denaturation, whereas adult hemoglobin changes completely into alkaline hematin within 5 minutes. These differences in resistance to strong alkali can be followed with any simple hand spectroscope. Rabbit antiserums have been prepared which are specific for fetal and adult hemoglobin, respectively. The two forms are unlike in crystalline structure, amino acid composition, spectrophotometric patterns, and motility in electrophoretic fields. More precise studies may reveal that there are several varieties of human alkali-resistant hemoglobin, but for the time being it is more convenient to view all abnormally denaturing hemoglobin as being fetal hemoglobin.

Fetal blood can absorb oxygen and release carbon dioxide more readily than can adult blood in environments corresponding to those which obtain in the uterus. This property has been traced, at least in part, to the fetal hemoglobin component.

In fetuses of 20 weeks gestation the blood contains 95 per cent of fetal oxyhemoglobin and 5 per cent of the adult type. At birth the fetal hemoglobin is 50 to 90 per cent of the total; at 2 months of age, 10 to 75 per cent; from 2 to 12 months, 2 to 30 per cent; from 12 to 24 months, usually under 5 per cent but sometimes up to 20 per cent; and in children and adults, less than 2 per cent. Fetal hemoglobin seems to fade away more rapidly in full-term babies after birth than in those born prematurely.

Schulman and Smith found a lowered fetal hemoglobin in infants with erythroblastosis fetalis. In cord blood of 96 normal infants the mean was 11.6 ± 1.2 gm per 100 ml of blood, whereas in cord blood of 33 erythroblastotic infants the mean was 8.4 ± 2.5 gm. Interestingly, the mean quantity of adult hemoglobin was higher than normal in the erythro-

108

blastotic infants who were not anemic, 15.9 gm compared with 14.7 gm in the controls, but not significantly different (14.1 gm) in those who were anemic.

The cherry-red color given by blood containing fetal hemoglobin when treated with sodium hydroxide makes it possible for medicolegal experts to identify fetal hemoglobin in old blood stains. When extracted material is treated with sodium hydroxide, a denaturation time of more than ½ hour means that the blood stain in question—once its human origin has been established—comes from a fetus or infant less than 6 months of age or from an active case of some red cell dyscrasia. Similarly, when a newborn infant vomits blood or has blood in the stools, one can establish whether the blood is of maternal or fetal origin by demonstrating the absence or presence of fetal hemoglobin within it (p. 707). On the other hand, when searching for evidences of carbon monoxide poisoning in a young infant, one cannot utilize the familiar Hoppe-Seyler alkali test which hinges upon a delay in the prompt change of normal blood to brown on addition of sodium hydroxide.

The resistance of fetal hemoglobin to alkali renders the alkaline hematin approach unreliable for quantitating the blood hemoglobin level with infants under 8 months of age, unless the specimen is left for at least 3 hours before the readings are taken. With this exception, the differences in molecular structure do not alter the readings, as determined by standard methods based on measurements of oxyhemoglobin or acid hematin.

The presence of fetal hemoglobin presumably helps to inhibit the sickling phenomenon in infants under 4 months of age who ultimately will display this trait. Only a small percentage of their erythrocytes will sickle, if any, and the time for the change to attain its maximum seems unusually long. This hemoglobin is perhaps the factor which inhibits intravascular sickling in the fetus despite the low oxygen tension which exists in intrauterine life.

Recognition of Fetal Hemoglobin

A simple office procedure is the following: 5 ml of a 1 per cent distilled water solution of hemoglobin is prepared in a test tube. Examination with the hand spectroscope by transmitted light shows the two absorption bands of the oxyhemoglobin spectrum between lines D and E (578 and 540 mμ). One milliliter of a 1 per cent sodium hydroxide solution is then added. This denatures the hemoglobin, changing its pinkish-red color to the brown of alkaline hematin. The time required for the oxyhemoglobin bands to fade away is followed with the spectroscope. In individuals above 4 to 6 months of age this is usually about a minute, though 5 minutes may be taken as maximum normal. If the blood contains much fetal hemoglobin, however, the disappearance time of the bands will be 1 to 3 hours.

A good quantitative method is that of Chernoff and Singer. After a measured quantity of hemoglobin has been exposed to an alkaline reagent for exactly 1 minute, the denaturation process is stopped by addition of a solution which simultaneously lowers the pH and precipitates the nonhemoglobin chromogens. After filtration, the unaltered (fetal) hemoglobin which remains is measured in a Beckman spectrophotometer at 540 mμ and expressed as a percentage of the initial total amount of hemoglobin.

Fetal Hemoglobin in the Anemias

In 100 hematologically normal individuals older than 3 years Singer, Chernoff, and Singer noted spectrophotometric readings for alkali-resistant hemoglobin of from 0.5 to 1.7 per cent of the total hemoglobin concentration. The mean was 1.0 per cent. These authors suggest a threshold of 2.0 per cent as just above the range of normal, inasmuch as this finding occurred only once in 370 determinations of healthy older subjects. Since 5 per cent of fetal hemoglobin may remain in the blood stream until the third year of life, evaluation of the abnormal persistence of fetal hemoglobin in patients under this age must include the consideration that the physiologically occurring form may not have disappeared completely.

In carriers of the sickle cell trait over 2 years of age the range of 1-minute denaturation values is identical with that of normals. In active sickle cell anemia the fetal type of hemoglobin usually falls between 2 and 25 per cent of the total with no marked relations to the severity of the anemia or other symptoms or the reticulocyte count. Transfusions lower the percentages temporarily in proportion to the amount of normal blood given. In Mediterranean anemia the patients with moderate or severe anemia tend to have unusually high denaturation values up to 90 per cent, whereas those with minimal blood changes have values which are normal or elevated only slightly. In hereditary spherocytosis and chronic aregenerative anemia a minority of the patients may have elevated fetal hemoglobin readings up to 5 per cent.

METHEMOGLOBIN

This normal derivative of oxyhemoglobin, present in minimal quantities in normal blood, may increase during life under the stimulation of certain chemical agents and result in cyanotic disturbances. Sulfhemoglobin is usually produced coincidentally under these circumstances, but methemoglobin is far more important clinically. The molecular structure of methemoglobin is almost identical with that of regular oxyhemoglobin, except that the iron in the heme portion is in the oxidized ferric rather than the ferrous form. This oxidation is readily reversible and does not injure the red cell stroma.

Hemoglobin has a natural tendency to become oxidized to methemoglobin, and in aqueous solution outside of the body will do so. Methemoglobin forms continuously within the red cells, and as continously is reconverted to hemoglobin by the intracellular enzyme systems, so that the intracorpuscular content is always maintained at about 1 per cent of the total hemoglobin. The most significant physiologic difference between methemoglobin and oxyhemoglobin is that methemoglobin is inert and cannot transport oxygen.

Methemoglobin may accumulate in the red cells either when the intracellular reduction mechanisms are functionally inadequate or when oxidant changes activate the production to a degree beyond the enzymatic capacity of the cell to reduce it. Methylene blue accelerates the enzymic reduction mechanism. Ascorbic acid, glutathione, cysteine, and BAL (2,3-dimercaptopropanol) act directly and can reduce methemoglobin in the absence of enzymes.

Methemoglobinemia becomes recognizable clinically when the quantity of methemoglobin is enough to produce noticeable cyanosis. It is often said that the thresholds for recognition of cyanosis are for methemoglobin 1.5 gm per 100 ml of blood, for reduced hemoglobin 5 gm, and for sulfhemoglobin less than 0.5 gm. Several very young infants have been described, however, whose skin had a grayish-blue color with a blood methemoglobin content below 1 gm per 100 ml. A high level of methemoglobin in the blood can produce serious hypoxia of the tissues, particularly when it develops quickly. This should be managed as an emergency and a reducing agent given at once.

The percentage of total hemoglobin in normal blood which is methemoglobin was found by Kravitz and associates to be slightly higher in infancy than later:

	Mean, %	Range, %
Prematures (birth–72 days)	2.2	0.02–4.7
Newborns (1–10 days)	1.5	0.00–2.8
Infants (1 month–1 year)	1.2	0.17–2.4
Children (1–14 years)	0.8	0.00–2.4
Adults (14–78 years)	0.8	0.00–1.9

Most methemoglobinemia is intracellular, in the sense that methemoglobin is confined to the interior of the red cells. Plasma methemoglobinemia, in which methemoglobin forms in the plasma after hemoglobin has been liberated from the red cells by intravascular hemolysis, has been described as occurring in acute hemolytic disorders, sepsis due to anaerobic organisms, Winckel's disease of the newborn, blackwater fever, and paroxysmal hemoglobinuria.

Congenital Methemoglobinemia

This is a rare anomalous disorder characterized by a persistently high level of methemoglobin and cyanosis. The condition because apparent in early babyhood and may be familial. There appears to be a deficiency in the major intracellular enzyme which normally reduces methemo-globin. The evidence suggests that the missing substance is coenzyme I or a cytochrome derivative.

In the cases reported the content of methemoglobin has ranged from 0.7 gm per 100 ml (5 per cent of the total hemoglobin) to 7.5 gm (60 per cent of the total). The oxygen dissociation curve of the blood is usually normal. Symptoms of headaches, fatigability, and breathlessness may develop as a consequence of the decreased oxygen-carrying capacity of the blood. Physiologic disturbances are surprisingly mild in these chronic cases, and may be nonexistent. In older children the total blood hemo-globin level and red cell count may be somewhat elevated, and subtract-ing the methemoglobin content from the total may reveal the functioning oxyhemoglobin to be approximately normal. In cyanotic infants with con-genital methemoglobinemia a systolic cardiac murmur and electrocardio-graphic disturbances may lead to the erroneous diagnosis of some con-genital heart disease such as tricuspid atresia. Therapy with daily inges-tion of ascorbic acid may reduce the cyanosis and erythrocytosis, but only slowly, taking several weeks or months. An intravenous injection of methylene blue in a dosage of 1.5 mg per kg body weight reduces the methemoglobin level and raises the oxygen-carrying capacity to normal within 60 minutes. With daily oral doses of methylene blue in a dosage of 3 to 5 mg per kg, the cyanosis may disappear. Maintenance therapy must be individualized and may consist of ascorbic acid or enteric-coated methylene blue, given orally as indicated.

Methemoglobinemia Due to Drugs

Any drug or poison which can activate the oxidation of intraheme iron from the ferrous to the ferric state may accelerate the production of methemoglobin. The list of such chemical agents includes phenacetin, acetanilid, plasmochin, some sulfonamides and especially sulfanilamide, nitrobenzene, toluene derivatives, pyridium, sodium and other nitrites, bismuth subnitrate, and potassium chlorate. Other unknown variables enter into this biologic reaction, else the rarity of this complication with some of the organic drugs is impossible to explain. The simpler inorganic salts such as nitrites and chlorates are more consistent in their action. These penetrate the red cell membranes readily and produce methemo-globin with regularity and rapidity at low concentrations.

Many of the causative substances are medicinals kept in the house for adult use and swallowed accidentally by children in the course of their play. Occasional instances of childhood methemoglobinemia have re-sulted from accidental ingestion or exposure to common household sub-stances—furniture polish or insect-exterminator sprays (nitrobenzene), shoe dyes or marking ink (aniline), colored wax crayons (paranitrani-line), or perfumes and essences (aromatic compounds). We have seen several infants affected by the feeding of infusions of so-called "medicinal herbs." Methemoglobinemia in newborn and premature infants has been produced by contact with aniline-containing inks used to mark the diapers, the aniline being absorbed through the skin. Concentrations of methemoglobin in acquired methemoglobinemia may amount to as much as 6 gm per 100 ml, or up to 60 per cent of the total hemoglobin.

The most prominent clinical feature is the intense gray cyanosis which comes on soon after ingestion of the toxic agent. The possibility should always be suspected whenever a child is found with acute cyanosis in the absence of any other possible cause. Inquiry with respect to possible contact with drugs, poison, or dyes must be made at once. Should the hemoglobin become progressively inactivated the child will develop signs of dangerous anoxemia in the form of coma, dyspnea, and circulatory failure. Associated symptoms of poisoning depend on the nature of the offending substance. These may include acidosis, acute red cell destruction, or impaired functioning of the liver, kidneys, or other viscera. Fluoroscopic demonstration of bismuth in the gastrointestinal tract is helpful in corroborating the possibility of nitrite poisoning from ingestion of bismuth subnitrate.

Methemoglobinemia Due to Well Water

Infant feeding mixtures prepared with well water which contains nitrates have often caused methemoglobinemia. The phenomenon ceases when the well water is discontinued and reappears when it is resumed. Continued exposure to such water may end fatally. Cases of this type seem more numerous in the North Central United States and the central provinces of Canada, though both private and public water supplies over a much wider geographic area have a high content of nitrates. The principal source of the offending nitrate appears to be animal or human excreta which after bacterial decomposition has seeped into the interior of the wells.

Epidemiologic surveys have demonstrated that the condition occurs typically in infants under 2 months of age and is almost never seen after 5 months. Because the added water is greater, feeding mixtures made from evaporated or powdered milk are incriminated more often than those made from whole cow's milk. The toxicity of well water seems to be contingent upon its nitrate nitrogen content, the total amount ingested per day, the number of days of exposure, the duration of the boiling (boiling for 30 minutes can triple the concentration of nitrates), and other unknown external considerations. Concentrations of nitrate nitrogen in excess of 40 parts per million (ppm) have been found in the majority of situations investigated, and concentrations in excess of 1,300 ppm have been reported. For public health control the critical level above which well water may be deemed unsafe for infant feeding appears to

be 10 ppm of nitrate nitrogen, because of the possibility of more dangerous levels being reached through boiling.

Escherichia coli and related coliform organisms in the upper gastrointestinal tract of the infants seem to be essential for the development of
this form of methemoglobinemia. Nitrates from water do not themselves
act upon hemoglobin—they are first converted to nitrites by the nitrate-
reducing bacteria in the upper alimentary tract. A favorable environment
for this reaction obtains only when the gastric juice is weak, as in early
infancy. Adding lactic acid to formulas of susceptible infants in concentrations of 0.5 to 1 per cent has been shown to prevent the development
of methemoglobinemia.

Recognition of Methemoglobinemia

A strong clue is the appearance of the venous blood on venipuncture. Blood
which contains methemoglobin has a distinctive chocolate-brown color which
fades in a few hours as the methemoglobin becomes converted to hemoglobin
on exposure to air. If this is at all marked and it is not feasible to make an
immediate chemical or spectroscopic examination, the blood specimen should
be oxalated or citrated and stored in a refrigerator under a layer of oil.

If blood from a suspected case is mixed with an anticoagulant and centrifuged, the absence of distinctive color in the plasma indicates that the cause
of the cyanosis lies in the cells. On next shaking the entire specimen vigorously
in air, normal blood will be converted completely to bright-red oxyhemoglobin
within 15 minutes, whereas in methemoglobinemia the color will remain dark.

Methemoglobinemia can be detected with a hand spectroscope. A blood
sample is diluted 10 to 100 times with tap or distilled water. This hemolyzes
the red cells and makes the preparation transparent enough for spectroscopy.
When the solution is examined by transmitted light, methemoglobin, if present,
will give rise to a dark band at 630 mμ. If a few drops of 5 per cent potassium
cyanide are next added, the methemoglobin will be reduced to hemoglobin
almost at once, whereas any accompanying sulfhemoglobin, whose absorption
band lies at 618, will remain unaltered. More precise spectrophometric and
other quantitative approaches are available in which the methemoglobin level
can be ascertained on a quantitative basis.

Therapy

In acquired methemoglobinemia, regardless of cause, any excess of
methemoglobin will become spontaneously reconverted to hemoglobin in
8 to 24 hours unless the inciting factor continues to operate. Hence when
treating a case it is essential to separate the patient from the cause if at
all possible. A laxative should be given if the offending substance has
been taken by mouth. Adjuvant therapy consists of oral or intravenous
glucose solution and oxygen inhalations.

With severe cases it is important to speed up the reconversion of methemoglobin to hemoglobin. Methylene blue and thionin act very rapidly
in this direction but are of short-lived benefit. The customary dose of

methylene blue is about 1.5 mg for each kilogram of body weight, given intravenously and slowly as a 1 per cent saline or glucose solution. The injection may have to be repeated, especially when the offending substance cannot be removed immediately. For less severe cases the methylene blue may be given orally as 10 to 20 mg per kg body weight; vomiting or diarrhea may follow unless the medication is enteric-coated. The cyanosis will disappear in 1 to 2 hours with intravenous therapy if effective, more slowly when given by mouth. The methylene blue powder employed for laboratory staining purposes can be employed intravenously or orally if of high pharmaceutic quality.

Ascorbic acid will also reconvert methemoglobin, but at a slower rate. An adequate intake is 300 mg a day, given orally in divided doses for as long as needed. Niacin and glutathione are said to have similar actions.

Relation to Cyanide Poisoning

Because methemoglobin has an unusual affinity for cyanides, the deliberate induction of methemoglobinemia has been proposed for the therapy of cyanide poisoning. Speed is important, but the prognosis is not hopeless so long as the heart is beating. One gives 0.3 to 0.5 gm of sodium nitrite intravenously in a 3 per cent solution over 5 to 10 minutes, followed by 50 ml of a 25 per cent solution of sodium thiosulfate intravenously over another 10 minutes. The latter combines with the cyanide to form thiocyanate, which is relatively nontoxic and is excreted. Inhalation of amyl nitrite is even more rapid in antidotal action and may be used first. If the poison has been taken by mouth, gastric lavage is important. Artificial respiration is indicated if the respiration has ceased but heart sounds are still audible. The intravenous therapy may have to be repeated in some hours if the symptoms recur.

SULFHEMOGLOBIN

This abnormal derivative of hemoglobin, of undetermined chemical structure, may appear in the red cells after ingestion of or exposure to the same oxidizing drugs which give rise to methemoglobinemia. Constipation or concomitant use of a sulfur-containing medication seem to be important adjuvants to its production. Both sulfhemoglobin and methemoglobin usually coexist in most cases of cyanosis due to drugs, in inconstant ratio.

Sulfhemoglobin does not carry oxygen. Unlike methemoglobin, it cannot be reversibly transmuted into hemoglobin. Once formed it persists for 3 to 4 months, according to the survival time of the red cells which carry it. Even in severe intoxications its concentration does not seem to rise above 15 to 20 per cent of all hemoglobin. Hence in the absence of concomitant methemoglobinemia it may induce prominent cyanosis but is not likely to be a cause of anoxemic symptoms. Sulfhemoglobinemia has been said to be responsible for the so-called enterogenous cyanosis associated with chronic constipation. No corrective therapy is known other than removal of the offending substance. Methylene blue and ascorbic acid are of no benefit.

The diagnosis is made by spectroscopy or spectrophotometry, as discussed under methemoglobin. When the blood is first withdrawn its color may be lavender or mauve if sulfhemoglobin is predominant. The reagents such as oxygen, ammonium sulfide, or potassium cyanide which reduce methemoglobin will leave sulfhemoglobin unaltered. Sulfhemoglobin does not appear in the plasma except when blood destruction is associated.

GENETIC ALLELES OF HEMOGLOBIN

As discussed in Chapter 4, there occur numerous variants of human adult (A) hemoglobin which are under genetic control and which, singly or in combination, can be responsible for significant clinical, hematologic, and anthropologic phenomena. Differences among these variants can be demonstrated by the approaches of moving boundary electrophoresis in the Tiselius apparatus, zone electrophoresis on filter paper, and solubility determinations. Of these, the so-called filter paper electrophoresis is by far the simplest and most practical. Apparatus for its performance can be found in many routine laboratories.

Filter Paper Electrophoresis

This procedure employs a broad sheet of filter paper moistened with alkaline barbital buffer and stretched between two electrodes which transmit a direct electric current. Details of technique can be found in the latest textbooks of hematology and clinical pathology. In our laboratory, satisfactory separations of the principal abnormal hemoglobins are attained with Whatman No. 3 filter paper, barbital buffer at pH 8.6 and ionic strength 0.06, 350 volts of power, and 8 to 12 hours running time. The hemoglobin solutions from patients under study move along the paper toward the anode for variable distances, contingent upon their character.

C hemoglobin is the least mobile. Relative mobilities may be schematized as follows:

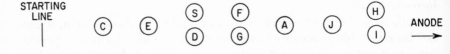

BIBLIOGRAPHY

FETAL HEMOGLOBIN

Beaven, G. H., H. Hoch, and E. R. Holiday, The Hemoglobins of the Human Fetus and Infant: Electrophoretic and Spectroscopic Differentiation of Adult and Fetal Types, Biochem. J. 49:374, 1951.

Chernoff, A. I., Immunologic Studies of Fetal Hemoglobin, J. Lab. & Clin. Med. 40:787, 1952.

———, Immunologic Studies of Hemoglobins. I. The Production of Antihemoglobin Sera and Their Immunologic Characteristics, Blood 8:399, 1953.

———, The Human Hemoglobins in Health and Disease, New England J. Med. 253:365, 1955.

——— and K. Singer, Studies on Abnormal Hemoglobins. IV. Persistence of Fetal Hemoglobin in the Erythrocytes of Normal Children, Pediatrics 9:469, 1952.

Gardikas, C., D. G. Scott, and J. F. Wilkinson, Observations on Foetal Haemoglobin, Arch. Dis. Childhood 28:38, 1953.

Helpern, M., and G. Strassmann, Differentiation of Fetal and Adult Human Hemoglobin: Its Medicolegal Importance, Especially in Connection with Alkali Test for Carbon Monoxide of Blood, Arch. Path. 35:776, 1943.

Lecks, H., and I. J. Wolman, Fetal Hemoglobin in the Human: A Review, Am. J. M. Sc. 219:684, 1950.

Nomenclature for the Varieties of Human Hemoglobin: Report of a Committee of the Hematology Study Section of the Division of Research Grants of the National Institutes of Health, Blood 8:386, 1953.

Schulman, I., and C. H. Smith, Fetal and Adult Hemoglobins in Hemolytic Disease of the Newborn, A.M.A. Am. J. Dis. Child. 87:167, 1954.

Singer, K., A. I. Chernoff, and L. Singer, Studies on Abnormal Hemoglobins. I. Their Demonstration in Sickle Cell Anemia and Other Hematologic Disorders by Means of Alkali Denaturation. II. Their Identification by Means of the Method of Fractional Denaturation, Blood 6:413, 1951.

White, J. C., and G. H. Beaven, A Review of the Varieties of Human Haemoglobin in Health and Disease, J. Clin. Path. 7:175, 1954.

CONGENITAL METHEMOGLOBINEMIA

Breakey, V. K., Q. H. Gibson, and D. C. Harrison, Familial Idiopathic Methaemoglobinaemia, Lancet 1:935, 1951.

Eder, H. A., C. Finch, and R. W. McKee, Congenital Methemoglobinemia: A Clinical and Biochemical Study of a Case, J. Clin. Invest. 28:265, 1949.

Gasul, M., E. H. Fell, R. Casas, and R. Pereiras, Congenital Methemoglobinemia Simulating Tricuspid Atresia, J.A.M.A. 149:258, 1952.

Gibson, Q. H., The Reduction of Methaemoglobin in Red Blood Cells and Studies on the Cause of Idiopathic Methaemoglobinaemia, Biochem. J. 42:13, 1948.

Kravitz, H., L. D. Elegant, E. Kaiser, and B. M. Kagan, Methemoglobin Values in Premature and Mature Infants and Children, A.M.A. J. Dis. Child. 91:1, 1956.

Waisman, H. A., J. A. Bain, J. B. Richmond, and F. A. Munsey, Laboratory and Clinical Studies in Congenital Methemoglobinemia, Pediatrics 10:293, 1952.

ACQUIRED METHEMOGLOBINEMIA

Brieger, H., and J. E. Mazur, A Note on Poisoning Due to Ingestion of Wax Crayons, J. Pediat. 33:742, 1948.

Chen, K. K., and *C. L. Rose,* Nitrate and Thiosulfate Therapy in Cyanide Poisoning, *J.A.M.A.* **149:**113, 1952.

Cornblath, M., and *A. F. Hartmann,* Methemoglobinemia in Young Infants, *J. Pediat.* **33:**421, 1948.

Etteldorf, J. N., Methylene Blue in the Treatment of Methemoglobinemia in Premature Infants Caused by Marking Ink, *J. Pediat.* **38:**24, 1951.

Ewing, M. C., and *R. M. Mayon-White,* Cyanosis in Infancy from Nitrates in Drinking-water, *Lancet* **1:**931, 1951.

Howarth, B. E., Epidemic of Aniline Methaemoglobinaemia in Newborn Babies, *Lancet* **1:**934, 1951.

Jones, J. A., and *H. Brieger,* Poisoning Due to Ingestion of Wax Crayons, *J. Pediat.* **30:**422, 1947.

Kagan, B. M., B. Mirman, J. Calvin, and *E. Lundeen,* Cyanosis in Premature Infants Due to Aniline Dye Intoxication, *J. Pediat.* **34:**574, 1949.

MacDonald, W. B., Methaemoglobinaemia Resulting from Poisoning in Children, *M. J. Australia* **1:**145, 1951.

Marcus, H., and *J. R. Joffe,* Nitrate Methemoglobinemia, *New England J. Med.* **240:**599, 1949.

Maxcy, K. F., Relation of Nitrate Nitrogen Concentration in Well Water to the Occurrence of Methemoglobinemia in Infants, *U.S. Armed Forces M. J.* **1:**1007, 1950.

McLetchie, N. G. B., and *H. E. Robertson,* Nitrate Poisoning from Well-water, *Canad. M. A. J.* **60:**230, 1949.

Rieders, F., and *H. Brieger,* Mechanism of Poisoning from Wax Crayons, *J.A.M.A.* **151:**1490, 1953.

Robertson, H. E., and *W. A. Riddell,* Cyanosis of Infants Produced by High Nitrate Concentration in Rural Waters of Saskatchewan, *Canad. J. Pub. Health* **40:**72, 1949.

Stening, S. E. L., Methaemoglobinaemia Due to Aniline, *M. J. Australia,* **1:**578, 1951.

Wallace, W. M., Methemoglobinemia in Infant as Result of Administration of Bismuth Sulfate, *J.A.M.A.* **133:**1280, 1947.

SULFHEMOGLOBIN

Fichter, E. G., Sulfhemoglobinemia, *A.M.A. Am. J. Dis. Child.* **88:**749, 1954.

Finch, C. A., Methemoglobinemia and Sulfhemoglobinemia, *New England J. Med.* **239:**470, 1948.

Reynolds, T. B., and *A. G. Ware,* Sulfhemoglobinemia Following Habitual Use of Acetanilid, *J.A.M.A.* **149:**1538, 1952.

PAPER ELECTROPHORESIS OF HEMOGLOBINS

Larson, D. L., and *H. M. Ranney,* Filter Paper Electrophoresis of Human Hemoglobin, *J. Clin. Invest.* **32:**1070, 1953.

Motulsky, A. G., M. H. Paul, and *E. Durrum,* Paper Electrophoresis of Abnormal Hemoglobins and Its Clinical Applications. A Simple Semiquantitative Method for the Study of the Hereditary Hemoglobinopathies, *Blood* **9:**807, 1954.

Smith, E. W., and *C. L. Conley,* Filter Paper Electrophoresis of Human Hemoglobins with Special Reference to the Incidence and Clinical Significance of Hemoglobin C, *Bull. Johns Hopkins Hosp.* **93:**94, 1953.

Zuelzer, W. W., J. V. Neel, and *A. R. Robinson,* Abnormal Hemoglobins, chap. 5 in L. M. Tocantins (ed.), "Progress in Hematology," vol. 1, Grune & Stratton, Inc., New York, 1956.

CHAPTER 10

Erythrocyte Sedimentation Rate

The speed of erythrocyte sedimentation becomes increased in the presence of more than minimal tissue destruction or exudative reactions anywhere in the body. Absorbed products from the site of injury alter the plasma in some way not well understood, so that when the subject's blood is mixed with an anticoagulant and permitted to stand in a vertical column the red cells exhibit an unusual tendency to form large aggregates of the character of rouleaux. The larger the aggregates, the faster the sedimentation rate. The top of the sedimenting column is usually clear and horizontal, but fuzzy and indistinct when the reticulocyte content is high.

UNDERLYING MECHANISMS

The exact nature of the changes in the plasma which bring about this tendency to increased rouleaux formation are as yet not clear. The theoretical explanations have been variously couched in terms of stickiness, surface tension, electric charge, plasma viscosity, and hydration reactions. An elevation in the serum content of fibrinogen or globulin will increase the sedimentation rate. At body temperature ($37°C$) the rate is higher than at room temperatures. Slight fluctuations in room temperature exert little influence. Excessive cold has a retarding action. The oxygen–carbon dioxide relationships have little influence. An excess of bile salts may cause acceleration.

When readings are taken at intervals of every few minutes the rate of sedimentation exhibits an S-shaped curve, no matter what technique is employed. This S shape is a reflection of three phases which take place successively:

1. The phase of agglomeration or rouleaux formation, during which the rate of fall accelerates as the aggregates grow larger. This phase usually takes 10 to 15 minutes and gives the first bend of the curve. It may not be demonstrable if considerable time elapses between the collection of the blood and the setting up of the test.

2. The phase of constant rate of fall, responsible for the linear part of the curve. The aggregates have attained their maximum size and density and settle

119

at a regular rate. As they move downward the supporting plasma is displaced upward, giving rise to retarding currents.

3. The phase of packing, the decelerating bend in the curve, portrays the piling up of the aggregates at the bottom of the tube.

Tall columns sediment more rapidly than short ones. Tubes with diameters between 1.5 and 10 mm (Cutler, Wintrobe, Westergren) give about the same rates of fall, provided the columns are of the same height to begin with. Diameters less than 1.5 mm occasionally inhibit and occasionally promote the rate of settling.

Sources of error must be avoided if comparable results are to be secured on repeated testing. The anticoagulant should be added as soon as possible after securing the blood. The test is best performed within 1 hour after collection of the sample. The column should be kept exactly vertical, for an inclination of as little as 5 degrees will set up accelerating currents at the dependent side of the tube. Care should be taken not to wet the glass above the top of the blood column, or else large aggregates may form in the wet film above the blood column. There are no significant differences in the sedimentation rate between arterial and venous blood specimens drawn at the same time.

CRITIQUE OF METHODS

The procedures used for determining the sedimentation rate, though differing in significant details from each other, all portray rouleaux formation. There is no unanimity as to which procedure does this the most effectively. The method employed should always be stated when results are given. Despite many attempts it has not been feasible to find a simple formula for comparing the results obtained by one method with those obtained by another.

The "inclined tube" test is performed in a tube held at a 45-degree angle. This accelerates the settling of the red cells. The reading is taken at the end of 15 minutes instead of at 1 hour, thereby conserving time. A pertinent set of "normal" values is of course needed.

Most of the more widely used procedures (Cutler, Wintrobe, Westergren) express their results in terms of the number of millimeters in which the top of the red cell column fails in a specified unit of time, usually 60 minutes. The Rourke-Ernstene and the modified Cutler methods report the maximum rate of fall per unit of time. The Linzenmeier method measures the number of minutes required for the top of the column to fall a distance of 18 mm.

Several "micro" methods have been proposed for use with infants and young children whose blood vessels do not lend themselves to ready venipuncture. These utilize blood obtained by skin puncture and drawn into narrow capillary tubes in the presence of an anticoagulant. Because of surface tension and related phenomena the rates of fall are different than with the "macro" tubes, so that separate ranges for normal have to be established for each type of procedure. The influence of contaminating tissue fluid is an unmeasurable factor. Most workers do not like these so-called micromethods because occasional clotting and technical and other difficulties may give ambiguous or misleading readings.

In their study of methodology, Hollinger and Robinson found that repeated 1-hour readings on blood from the same individuals may vary by as much as ±5 mm with the Wintrobe method; ±7 mm with the Landau-Adams microtechnique; and ±4 mm with the Westergren technique. The accuracy of a single report must therefore be considered with respect to this rather wide zone of technical variation.

There is difficulty in defining the "normal" to serve as the standard of comparison. It is a zone rather than a range of distribution.

Within the so-called normal zone, children who appear to be in excellent health and free of disease show wide differences in readings among themselves. The upper limits of readings tend to be somewhat higher than those for adults, regardless of the method used. There are no significant sex differences prior to puberty. The best index of "normality" for any convalescent child whose accelerated sedimentation rate is subsiding gradually is to assume that the level for health of this particular child is that within the normal zone beyond which no further recession occurs. Many normal adolescents, especially girls, exhibit an increased rate during the years of the growth spurt.

Diseases unaccompanied by much absorption of products of tissue breakdown seem not to alter the sedimentation rate. Examples are appendicitis, early acute or chronic; chronic tonsillitis, laryngitis, or sinusitis; abscessed teeth; colitis; allergic reactions; malnutrition; nonnecrotic benign tumors; psychiatric disturbances; most skin diseases; uncomplicated pertussis; inactive heart disease.

Generally speaking, for children the upper limit of normal with the Westergren method is approximately 15 or even 20 mm in 1 hour; with the Wintrobe method 10 mm; with the Cutler method 15 mm. With the Rourke-Ernstene the maximal rate of fall is 0.5 mm per minute; with the Cutler modification, 1 mm in 5 minutes.

SIGNIFICANCE OF INCREASED SEDIMENTATION

An increased sedimentation rate may be viewed as an indicator of some internal disorder associated with tissue injury, or of some severe inflammation, or of some toxemic disturbance of general nature. It is not diagnostic of any specific disease. Pregnancy induces an acceleration after the third month. Normochromic normocytic anemia of itself may result in an apparent minor increase.

Development of an increased rate in the presence of an acute infection, whether local or generalized, seems to depend upon the intensity and duration of the accompanying inflammation. Generally speaking, catarrhal reactions usually result in no increase, whereas tissue necrosis or suppuration of appreciable degree will elicit a rise. Such inflammation occurs in pneumonia, septicemia, osteomyelitis, pericarditis, peritonitis, pleurisy, mastoiditis, diphtheria, etc. Detectable changes however, do not occur even in severe acute infections unless these last more than a few days. Hence the determination of sedimentation rate is of little value in the early study of acute illnesses, but can be of value in supporting the diagnosis of complications.

Rises which attend a brief generalized infection often persist for several weeks afterward, even when complications have not occurred. Hence an accelerated rate may reflect some recent illness; it does not necessarily connote a disorder actually active at the time of the test. An increase in rate during an infection which usually does not evoke an increase should make one suspicious of some other concurrent disorder. A rapid rate may be encountered also in the presence of malignant tumors, leukemia, active nephritis, hyperthyroidism, severe acute hepatitis, inflammatory forms of arthritis, acute poisonings, and miscellaneous other systemic diseases.

In uncomplicated poliomyelitis and other viral infections of the nervous system, the sedimentation rate is often elevated at the beginning of the disease, but the test is of no value in differentiating between poliomyelitis and other infections of the nervous system which may simulate it. No correlation could be established by Hartman and Weinstein between the elevation of the sedimentation rate and the clinical type of poliomyelitis, the severity of the attack, or the degree of reaction in the cerebrospinal fluid.

In asthmatic children the rate tends to rise when the disturbance is precipitated by an infection, but to remain unaltered when the asthma is noninfectious (allergic) in origin (Livingston).

Chorea in the presence of active rheumatic fever is usually accompanied by an elevated rate, whereas when there are no signs of rheumatic activity the rate is usually normal.

The rate ordinarily rises during such subacute and chronic infections as rheumatic fever, atypical pneumonia, active tuberculosis, malaria, histoplasmosis, coccidioidomycosis, and untreated congenital syphilis. The degree of abnormality may vary from patient to patient, but in any one case the trend of change on serial repetitions will mirror the advance or subsidence of the disease process. In primary atypical pneumonia the rate tends to return to normal some days slower than the clearing of the roentgen shadows. In the recovery stages of acute nephritis the rate subsides more or less parallel with the disappearance of the erythrocytes from the urinary sediment.

In rheumatic myocarditis with circulatory insufficiency the rate often subsides paradoxically to normal levels while the patient is in congestive heart failure, to become rapid again when the circulatory congestion is relieved. Lack of appreciation of this phenomenon may lead one to adjudge a rheumatic patient as improving when in reality his status is becoming worse.

In childhood tuberculosis the sedimentation rate typically attains its maximum increases between the second and sixth week after the recognized onset of the disease and returns to normal between the third and fifth months as the patient improves. The rate rises and returns to normal a little earlier than the changes in level of serum gamma globulin. In cases which end fatally or develop miliary or meningeal tuberculosis, the rate tends to rise further as the disease progresses. An occasional child, however, may maintain a rapid sedimentation long after subsidence of all other signs of clinical activity.

With all these illnesses one must be certain when evaluating the reading that the patient does not have and has not had any acute coincidental infection within the preceding 2 or 3 weeks. One must also bear in mind that healthy children between 9 and 15 years of age, and notably girls, will often exhibit an increased rate. With convalescent children in this age period the rate may remain elevated long after all other evidence of disease has gone.

Many practitioners use the sedimentation test as a screening device for advance information concerning patients. Blood specimens are collected and run through this test in the anterooms to the doctor's office. Any child with a rapid sedimentation test for no immediately obvious cause is checked carefully for deep-seated lesions. As a rule, however, thorough studies of such children usually fail to uncover any pathologic disturbance which is not already apparent from other examinations.

Conversely, normal rates are occasionally encountered in the presence of diseases which customarily give abnormal readings. In this circumstance a suggested explanation is that absorption of toxic products is not occurring.

CORRECTIONS FOR ANEMIA

Sedimentation proceeds somewhat faster when the proportion of red cells to plasma has been reduced artificially after a blood sample has been collected. This has led to the widespread adoption of *correction factors for anemia,* on the thesis that anemia may at times cause an otherwise normal red cell population to sediment sufficiently rapidly to suggest the presence of some active disease.

In the author's opinion, the introduction of such a correction factor is an arbitrary manipulation which is as likely to distort as to rectify a reading. It does not take into account the abnormalities of shape, size, and hemoglobin content of the erythrocytes which exist in many forms of childhood anemia. It ignores also the alterations in plasma proteins and other plasma components which may attend the anemia and which perhaps may act to enhance the suspension stability.

Good examples of the difficulties which may ensue when "corrections" are introduced are iron deficiency anemia and the hereditary dystrophies of the red cells. Readings on such patients with red cell counts as low as 2 million or less usually show normal or even slow rates of sedimentation unless a serious infection is superimposed. Adding a correction factor results in figures which if valid would indicate an ascension of the red cells out of the plasma.

"Corrections" are employed most often with patients suffering from chronic disorders such as rheumatic fever, nephritis, or active tuberculosis, which typically induce both an increased sedimentation rate and an anemia. In such disorders the anemia is usually of normochromic normocytic character, more nearly resembling the artificial situations from which the correction factors were derived. Since both the anemia and the influences responsible for faster sedimentation are more or less proportional to the activity of the disease process, the physician who utilizes serial sedimentation rates for following the clinical progress of his patients will receive the necessary information without "correcting" the results.

RELATION TO SLUDGED BLOOD

Increased sedimentation, an in vitro reaction, has been found to be closely though not invariably correlated with the intravascular agglomeration of the circulating blood known as *sludging*. The common denominator in both of these phenomena appears to be clumping of the red cells. Sludging has been shown by Knisely to be one of the major factors in the shock syndrome which follows severe trauma and thermal burns, and in many thromboembolic disturbances. The process has two steps: (1) formation of small masses of agglutinated blood cells—the so-called "basic masses" of a sludge—which do not break up as they pass through the progressively narrowing arterioles and the cylindrical capillaries, and (2) agglutination of these basic masses into larger cohering aggregates which dissociate as they pass through arterioles and capillaries and reunite in the widening venules to form new aggregates. The size, internal rigidity, and external stickiness of these masses are related to the damage to tissues taking place in the body when sludging occurs.

Direct observation of clumping in the capillaries of the human conjunctiva has been described. The degree seemed proportional to the rapidity of the sedimentation rate, as a rule. Whether these apparent agglutinations represent true sludging of red cells or are clumps of white cells or platelets, or combinations of these, is still unsettled.

SLIDE TESTS

There are two other approaches to the estimation of the sedimentation rate when only a drop or two of blood is available, in addition to the so-called "micro" methods. One is to place as large a drop as possible from the finger tip or venipuncture needle on a clean glass slide and permit the drop to dry slowly. If the sedimentation rate is much increased, the dried deposit of blood will have a coarsely grained appearance due to aggregates which form during the drying. The other approach is to examine the red cells in thin smears of the peripheral blood stained with Wright's or similar stain. If the red cells have a strong propensity to rouleaux formation, this will be apparent in the smears. Mild rouleaux formation is often seen in blood from children whose sedimentation rate seems to be unaltered.

These slide methods are qualitative rather than quantitative and have fair reliability. Cold autoagglutinins operative at room temperature cause similar clumping and have to be thought of.

BIBLIOGRAPHY

SEDIMENTATION RATE

Bayrd, E. D., The Clinical Significance of Increased Rouleau Formation in Smears of the Peripheral Blood, *Am. J. Clin. Path.* 21:777, 1951.

Eastham, R. S., The Erythrocyte Sedimentation Rate and the Plasma Viscosity, *J. Clin. Path.* 7:164, 1954.

Ham, T. H., and *F. C. Curtis,* Sedimentation Rate of Erythrocytes, *Medicine* 17:447, 1938.

Harris, T. N., Erythrocyte Sedimentation Rate in Rheumatic Fever, *Am. J. M. Sc.* 210:173, 1945.

Hartman, R. L., and *L. Weinstein,* Erythrocyte Sedimentation Rate Determinations in Poliomyelitis and Other Infections of Central Nervous System and Meninges, *J. Pediat.* 33:462, 1948.

Hollinger, N. F., and *S. J. Robinson,* A Study of the Erythrocyte Sedimentation Rate for Well Children, *J. Pediat.* 42:304, 1953.

Knisely, M. H., An Annotated Bibliography on Sludged Blood, *Postgrad. Med.* 10:15, 1951.

————, *E. H. Bloch, T. S. Eliot,* and *L. Warner,* Sludged Blood, *Science* 106:431, 1947.

Landau, A., Microsedimentation (Linzenmeier-Raunert Method), *Am. J. Dis. Child.* 45:691, 1933.

Levy-Solal, E., J. Badin, and *K. Djazmati,* Un nouveau mode d'étude clinique du sang du cordon: la mesure del la vitesse de sédimentation en tube incliné, *Gynéc. et obst.* 49:329, 1950.

Livingston, S., Sedimentation Rate in Asthma in Children, *Bull. Johns Hopkins Hosp.* 82:385, 1948.

Perry, C. B., The Sedimentation Rate in Rheumatic Carditis, *Arch. Dis. Childhood* 9:285, 1934.

Rogatz, J. L., A Simple Micrometric Apparatus for Determining the Sedimentation Rate of the Erythrocytes, *J. Lab. & Clin. Med.* 28:1842, 1943.

Smith, C. H., A Method for Determining the Sedimentation Rate and Red Cell

Volume in Infants and Children with the Use of Capillary Blood, *Am. J. M. Sc.* **192**:73, 1936.

————, Sedimentation Rate in Nutritional Anemia of Infants and Children, *Am. J. Dis. Child.* **56**:510, 1938.

Trought, H., Micro-method for Estimation of Sedimentation Rate of Red Cells, *Arch. Dis. Childhood* **17**:136, 1942.

Wolman, I. J., Office Use of the Sedimentation Test, *Clin. Medicine* **52**:41, 1945.

CHAPTER 11

Blood Group Systems

RED CELL AGGLUTINOGENS

The red cell agglutinogens of importance in blood grouping are genetically determined independent mucoprotein complexes situated on the surface of the cells. There is one major system (ABO), numerous minor systems of lesser clinical importance, and a few weak "private" systems occurring within single families. "Naturally occurring" antibodies in significant potency against any of these antigens are ordinarily absent, except in the case of the ABO system.

The ABO System

The distribution of the antigens of this major blood group system within the white population of the United States is approximately as follows:

O	45 per cent	B	10 per cent
A	41 per cent	AB	4 per cent

About 85 per cent of persons with A, B, or O antigen in their red cells are referred to as *secretors* because the same substances appear in the saliva, urine, tears, gastrointestinal juices, and other body fluids. Both secretors and nonsecretors possess the respective blood group factors in all body cells in lipid-soluble form. Only when these mucoid substances are also water-soluble do they occur in the body fluids and secretions. The characteristic is transmitted genetically as a simple mendelian dominant, independently of the inheritance of the other factors which determine blood groups and types.

AGGLUTINOGEN A. This is a spectrum of subgroup factors of which the principal ones are A_1 and A_2. Other more weakly reacting forms such as A_3 and perhaps A_4 have also been described. A_1 as an antigen reacts much more strongly with most anti-A sera than does A_2, and A_3 is the weakest of all. When these occur together, as is usual, A_1 is dominant to A_2, and A_2 is dominant to A_3, so that the individual is constitutionally considered as belonging to A_1 or A_2. In newborn infants the differentiation between A_1 and A_2 cannot be made readily. Approximately one-fifth of all A individuals are in subgroup A_2.

Serum for specific A_1 testing is prepared by taking group B serum containing both anti-A_1 and anti-A_2 agglutinins and absorbing away the anti-A_2 component by adding known A_2 cells. After centrifuging the serum contains only anti-A_1 antibodies and is referred to as *absorbed anti-A* or *absorbed-B* serum.

Such A or AB subgrouping is not necessary in blood grouping for routine transfusions. It is useful, however, in medicolegal situations or when an irregular or unexplained agglutinin is encountered during cross matching. Erythroblastosis fetalis due to subgroup A incompatibility between mother and fetus is possible theoretically but occurs rarely if ever.

AGGLUTINOGEN B. The B agglutinogen appears to be a single substance, no subtypes having been discovered. It may occur in combination with either A_1 or A_2, giving rise to the specific subgroups A_1B and A_2B.

AGGLUTINOGEN O. The O substance was defined originally as a purely negative characteristic of the red cells. It is recognized now that distinct O antigens may occur, bearing a mendelian recessive relation to A_1, A_2, and B when studied with currently available serums.

There appear to be two varieties of anti-O antibodies. One variety occurs spontaneously in the serum of cattle, rabbits, rats, eels, and guinea pigs, and in goats immunized with *Shigella dysenteriae*. These anti-O agglutinins tend to react with A_2 cells almost as strongly as with O cells, but weakly and inconstantly with A_1 cells. The other variety of anti-O antibodies, known as *anti-H*, is similar serologically, but appears to unite with a ubiquitous heterophile H substance distributed widely through human and animal tissues and perhaps related to the Forssman heterophile antigen.

INHERITANCE OF ABO. It has been established by studies of family groups with specific sera of types anti-A, anti-A_1, and anti-B that the antigens A_1, A_2, B, and O are transmitted genetically. Each A_1, A_2, and B phenotype may represent any of several constitutional genotypes as follows:

Phenotype		Genotypes
A	A_1	A_1A_1, A_1A_2, A_1O
	A_2	A_2A_2, A_2O
B		BB, BO
AB	A_1B	A_1B
	A_2B	A_2B
O		OO

Until a satisfactory laboratory method can be developed for recognizing the presence or absence of the O factor in any given A or B individual, the only practical method to determine whether he is homozygous or heterozygous must be by a blood grouping survey of his parents and siblings. An individual's ABO grouping is determined by the reactions of his red cells to potent anti-A and anti-B testing serums:

Red cells agglutinated by		
Anti-A	*Anti-B*	*ABO group*
—	—	O
+	—	A
—	+	B
+	+	AB

Minor Blood Group Systems

RH·HR SYSTEM. Clinically the most important of the minor systems, this is discussed at length in Chap. 13.

MN·S SYSTEM. The M and N antigens are allelic, giving rise to MM, MN, and NN types of individuals. Variants M_2 or N_2 in place of M or N have been recognized. Potent anti-M and anti-N serums can be prepared from the serum of rabbits selectively immunized with human red cells. A few human cases of acquired anti-M antibodies have been reported, but these almost never lead to transfusion reactions or erythroblastosis fetalis. N is so much weaker as an antigen that no clinical difficulties ascribable to it are known to have occurred.

Linked closely with the MN system are the two subdividing factors S and s. About 55 per cent of the white population is S-positive, and 90 per cent s-positive. The result is an intricate system of genetic combinations even more complex than the Rh·Hr system. The most frequent hereditary combinations appear to be MM·S, MN·S, MsMs, MsNs, NN·S, and NsNs. Anti-S antibodies, acquired following antigenic stimulation from transfused blood or fetal red cells, have seemed responsible for a few instances of erythroblastosis fetalis.

DUFFY SYSTEM. This is of more importance in transfusion reactions than in erythroblastosis fetalis. The two antigens thus far found are known as Fy^a and Fy^b. Approximately 65 per cent of the British population has been found to be Fy^a-positive, and 35 per cent Fy^b-positive.

KELL SYSTEM. The Kell (K) and k (Cellano) antigens give rise to three combinations which occur in the white population with the following frequencies: kk, 88 per cent; Kk and KK, 12 per cent. The anti-K antibody may be associated with erythroblastosis fetalis or transfusion reactions.

KIDD SYSTEM. This contains two antigens termed Jk^a and Jk^b. About 75 per cent of the white population is Jk^a-positive, and 25 per cent is Jk^b-positive.

LEWIS (LE) SYSTEM. The existence of at least two distinct members of this group, namely, Le^a and Le^b, has been established by the discovery of the corresponding antiserums. The phenotypes and their approximate prevalence in the population are: Le $(a^+ b^-)$, 22 per cent; Le $(a^- b^+)$, 70 per cent; Le $(a^- b^-)$, 8 per cent.

LUTHERAN (LU) SYSTEM. This system, clinically unimportant, comprises the two genes Lu^a and Lu^b. Less than 10 per cent of the population appears to be Lu^a-positive.

P SYSTEM. Approximately 80 per cent of individuals are P-positive, and 20 per cent are P-negative. This antigen is of almost no clinical importance.

PRIVATE SYSTEMS. A number of weak grouping antigens have been described whose presence (or absence) has been responsible for red cell sensitivity phenomena in single families. Because of their rarity they have been termed blood factors. Among those which have been reported to date are the *Levay, Gr., Jobbins, Miltenberger, Jay, Cavaliere,* and *Berrens*. To test for the corresponding antibody it is often necessary to employ red cells from the donor if the immunizing mechanism was transfusional, or from the father or erythroblastotic infant if the immunizing mechanism was gestational.

Medical Importance of the Blood Groups

The principal applications of knowledge concerning the respective blood groups are (1) blood transfusions and transfusion reactions, (2) fetal sensitization leading to erythroblastosis fetalis, (3) genetic investigations, including problems of disputed parentage and similar medicolegal situations, (4) study of population groups in relation to ethnic and anthropologic classifications, (5) determination of red cell survival times in the study of patients with hemolytic anemias. The blood group characteristics have the great utility of being universally distributed, unaffected by environmental influences, and easy to recognize and chart. In the study of phenomena exhibited by twins, for example, it is possible to establish monozygosity or dizygosity by grouping studies of the respective pairs. Blood grouping may some day be as valuable as fingerprinting in the identification of individuals; over 300,000 combinations can already be constructed from the known red cell antigens.

STUDY OF PATERNITY. The courts of most states will accept as evidence the results of blood grouping tests in legal disputes dealing with the question of paternity. The utilization of these tests is based on the accepted principle that in the offspring the blood group characteristics are determined unalterably by the corresponding characteristics of both parents. The ABO, MN, and Rh·Hr determinations are the ones which are currently utilized in the study of paternity. A child cannot possess any of the agglutinogens of any of these series unless the corresponding characteristic is present in the blood of at least one parent. A group O parent cannot have an AB child or a homozygous M parent a homozygous N child. Since a man who is not the father may chance to possess the same blood characteristics as the man who is the true father, the results of blood grouping tests can serve solely to exclude paternity; they cannot establish it.

The tests are carried out with red cells which are first washed with isotonic sodium chloride solution and then prepared in 2 per cent suspensions. The suspensions are tested in duplicate with specific antiserums for the A, A_1, B, M, N, D, C, E, c, and perhaps e factors. Each test is checked with known control cells. In addition, the serum of each individual is tested against known red cells of types O, A, A_2, and B. Extreme care is taken to avoid errors in labeling. Some workers identify each adult by fingerprints, and newborn infants by footprints.

Because of the importance and implications of the findings, blood grouping studies with medicolegal implications should be undertaken only by qualified experts who are in charge of adequate specialized laboratories. Every step in every test must be carried out with meticulous care, and often in duplicate. Potent reliable serums must be available for detecting weakly reacting antigens, including the variant forms of the Rh factors and the N variant known as N_2. The latter, found only in association with M, gives rise to the type MN_2; if this weakly reacting antigen is missed, the blood may be classified erroneously as group M. An understanding of genetics as well as experience with immunohematology is obviously essential.

SPECIFIC ANTI–RED CELL ANTIBODIES

These seem to fall into different classes. One class, such as the familiar anti-A and anti-B hemagglutinins, is *saline-active*. Another related class —the *albumin-active* agglutinins—causes no visible changes in saline solutions but agglutinates incompatible red cells suspended in human or bovine albumin. They are of smaller molecular size, are transmissible across the placenta, and play the major role in the production of erythroblastosis fetalis.

Blocking antibodies, a less well defined group, are so named because they coat the red cells and thereby block the activity of the saline-active agglutinins. Still another poorly defined class of weak antibodies, the *cryptagglutinoids,* do not cause agglutination in either saline or albumin solutions and do not elicit the blocking phenomenon; the Coombs antiglobulin procedure is needed for their demonstration.

"Naturally Occurring" Anti–Red Cell Antibodies

The specific hemagglutinin anti-A or b is found regularly in individuals of blood groups B and O. Anti-B or a is found in individuals of groups A and O. Neither occurs in blood group AB. These so-called naturally occurring antibodies are of great clinical importance in that they can give rise to severe and even fatal transfusion reactions when mismatched blood is given. They seem to be able at times to induce a hemolytic disorder in newborn infants born of heterospecific pregnancies (p. 167).

The ABO antibodies will agglutinate red cells suspended in saline into masses which resist shaking and further diluting. Most older children and adults give anti-A and anti-B titer readings between 1:16 and 1:32 at room temperatures, though values as high as 1:1,024 are not uncommon. Some A_1 and A_1B individuals contain a hemagglutinin in their serum against both A_2 and O.

Although the A and B antigens develop in the red cells of the fetus as early as the third gestational month, the reversely corresponding hemagglutinins anti-A and anti-B are detectable in only about 60 per cent of normal infants at birth. They occur only when the mother possesses these antibodies, and they are not antagonistic to the blood group of the fetus. The saline-active antibodies tend to be present in weaker concentrations than the albumin-active ones. Titers rarely exceed 1:128 and are ordinarily considerably lower than the maternal levels of the same antibodies. This neonatal activity usually fades away at a few weeks of age, indicating a maternal origin. Similar neonatal hemolysins are found much less frequently. Hemagglutinins actively produced by the infant himself begin to appear in the middle of the first year, rise gradually to a maximum in the second decade, and diminish slowly through adult life. Those against A are usually in higher titer than those against B.

In about 30 per cent of individuals the anti-A or anti-B hemagglutinins are accompanied by anti-A or anti-B hemolysins, in lower titer. These require the presence of complement for their demonstration. Serums prepared for blood grouping purposes have their contained complement inactivated by warming, in order to prevent any hemolysin activity from confusing the readings.

The serum concentrations of anti-A and anti-B hemagglutinins and hemolysins may be enhanced by the antigenic excitation induced by mismatched transfusions or injection of purified A and B substances. Children injected intramuscularly with incompatible red cells after 2 to 10 days may exhibit fever, malaise, leukocytosis, and painful swelling of the injection site as well as a more permanent rise in these antibodies.

Naturally occurring hemagglutinins against the minor blood group antigens are rare. When present their activity tends to be manifest at refrigerator temperature and low or absent at 37°C.

Acquired ("Immune") Antibodies

These differ from the natural occurring antibodies in that one or more exposures to type-incompatible red cells in the form of successive transfusions or pregnancies are required for their production. They are more active at 37°C than at lower temperatures. If of weak titer they usually cannot be demonstrated without the aid of the Coombs antiglobulin technique. As the stimulatory excitants continue, however, their potency may increase to an extent sufficient to give rise to erythroblastosis fetalis or clinically evident transfusion reactions.

The possibility always exists that a fetus that inherits an antigenic minor blood group factor from the father may be affected by erythroblastosis fetalis if the mother has already become sensitized to that factor. It is essential, therefore, *never* to use the husband as a blood donor for any woman still in the child-bearing age, in order to safeguard her from such sensitization. Absence of ABO and Rh·Hr incompatibility between husband and wife is no protection against the danger of sensitization by a member of some other blood group system.

When hemolytic phenomena are found in a newborn infant, and maternal sensitization to any of the usually responsible red cell antigens cannot be demonstrated by screening tests, the maternal serum should be tested carefully for specific hemagglutinins against the red cells of both husband and infant.

BLOOD GROUPING

The first essential in the proper conduct of a blood transfusion is to ascertain the exact ABO and Rh grouping of the recipient, and then cross-match with blood from donors of the same group. Save with group O blood as discussed below, the inadvertent administration of blood of a different ABO group may have the most tragic consequences. The first transfusions of Rh-incompatible donor blood of the same ABO grouping can be given with immediate safety, but serial repetitions will result not infrequently in the recipient becoming sensitized to one of the Rh·Hr antigens.

Blood for grouping and cross matching may be taken by a skin prick if all tests are to be done in the next few hours. Collection of undiluted specimens by venipuncture and refrigerator storage are essential if the specimens are to be held for a longer period, since the risk of bacterial contamination is minimal by this method and any organisms which are introduced do not proliferate rapidly inside of blood clots. Clotted, oxalated, citrated, or heparinized blood may be used as the source of the red cells.

In the blood grouping procedure the anti-A and anti-B hemagglutinins of potent serums unite with the corresponding antigens of the red cells almost immediately, but the clumping may take a little time. When employing the slide test, therefore, it is important to agitate the serum-cell mixture continuously for 10 to 15 minutes to ensure full contact of the antibody-coated cells with each other. With the tube test, the centrifuging for 1 minute at 500 to 1,000 rpm adequately achieves the same end. If a centrifuge is not available, the tubes may stand for 1 hour at room temperature.

For ABO identification of red cells it is important to use standardized anti-A and anti-B grouping serums of high potency. The slide test gives best results with a thick suspension of red cells and a reading taken at 3 minutes. The tube test is carried out according to the standard technique, using a freshly prepared 2 per cent saline red cell suspension. When there is any question about the readings, or if confirmation is desired, one can look for the serum isohemagglutinins which correspond reversely with the red cell antigens.

For Rh grouping the slide test is satisfactory in emergencies and in statistical surveys of populations, provided the testing serums have a high content of albumin-active antibodies. The tube test has a lesser margin of error and is preferred when time and facilities allow.

Red cells of donors in subgroup D^u sometimes fail to react with anti-D serum and appear erroneously to be D-negative (p. 156). Repeated giving of such blood to D-negative recipients may evoke antibodies against anti-D. Anti-D^u testing serum is scarce. To forestall such inadvertent sensitization, apparent D-negative donors may be typed with serums containing anti-C and anti-E, since the most common genetic patterns which contain D^u are CD^u and CD^uE. Another approach is to apply the Coombs technique to the donor red cells after they have been exposed to a strong anti-D serum (see below).

CROSS MATCHING

Proper cross matching rules out the possibility of the presence of intra-group natural or acquired antibodies in either donor or recipient which might cause transfusion reactions. It is also an indispensable check on the accuracy of the preliminary blood grouping. The absence of agglutination or hemolysis in both "major" and "minor" serum-cell mixtures indicates compatibility.

Both the slide and the test tube procedures are satisfactory for cross matching, though the latter is preferred when a centrifuge is available. When the slide technique is used, the test with the mixtures of donor's serum should be done in duplicate on two slides, one being warmed over a light source. Anti-A and anti-B isohemagglutinins are more active at room temperature; Rh-antibodies are more active at 45 to 50°C. Possible confusion from cold isohemagglutinins and other autoagglutinins is eliminated by warming. If clumping is seen within 3 minutes, 1 or 2 drops of normal saline solution is added to rule out pseudoagglutination due to rouleaux formation.

The test tube cross match is done with 2 per cent suspensions of donor and recipient red cells in normal saline, mixed with the opposite serums. The mixtures are centrifuged slowly for 10 minutes, and the tubes then gently agitated to observe for clumping. If the reading is questionable a drop of the cell suspension is placed on a slide and inspected with a microscope. Cross-matching preparations must always be inspected for agglutination at exactly the recommended time, before any hemolysin has opportunity to act.

Though often the only techniques employed, neither the slide nor the saline cross-matching procedures can be relied upon to always detect weak hemagglutinins and related antibodies against the minor blood group antigens other than those of the Rh·Hr system. The addition of a small amount of 20 to 30 per cent bovine albumin to the serum–red cell test tube mixtures before centrifuging will aid in the detection of antibodies in low titer.

Even more sensitive cross matching can be achieved by applying the indirect Coombs technique. A suspension of donor red cells is mixed with recipient serum; the reverse is also done. The mixtures are incubated at 37°C for 1 hour, then centrifuged slowly. If macroscopically recognized clumping has not occurred as a sign of incompatibility, the red cells are washed three times with sterile normal saline, and then resuspended as 2 per cent suspensions. A few drops of Coombs antiglobulin serum are then added to each. After 15 minutes the mixtures are centrifuged slowly, and then agitated gently while being examined for signs of clumping. Prior trypsinization of the red cells facilitates the demonstration of weak antibodies against some of the red cell antigens, and hampers the demonstration of others.

When cross matching appears to demonstrate incompatibility between the serum of the potential recipient and red cell samples from numerous donors who are apparently compatible with respect to ABO and Rh·Hr, the blood grouping procedures should be repeated to check on the accuracy of the original identification. Cold autoagglutination, pseudoagglutination, and false agglutination due to contamination of the specimens by unclean glassware or bacteria must also be considered. Cold isohemagglutinins acting at room temperature can be bypassed by carrying out all stages of the tests at 37 to 42°C.

Pseudoagglutination due to rouleaux formation gives difficulty in techniques which utilize serum-cell mixtures on slides. Rouleaux are almost never a problem when the tests are done with saline suspensions of red cells in test tubes, though they may appear in patients with severe liver disease or other profound illnesses or who are in a state of partial shock consequent to prolonged hemorrhage. Microscopy in this circumstance shows the donor red cells piled in twisted columns rather than clumped in shapeless aggregates. If this phenomenon is the sole cause of the apparent incompatibility, the donor blood can be given with safety.

SPECIAL IMMUNOHEMATOLOGIC SITUATIONS

ABO Problems

Demonstrable incompatibility on the major side of a cross matching, indicating the presence of antibodies in the recipient's serum against the red cells of the prospective donor, will lead to a serious hemolytic reaction if this blood is given. Donor blood with incompatibility on the minor side only may be given with immediate safety in an emergency, provided its content of serum antibodies against recipient red cells is of low titer. This is the situation which obtains when group O blood is transfused into a recipient of any other ABO group or when A or B blood is given to an AB recipient (see comment on p. 144).

Cells of group A_2 may react like those of group O during cross matching if they happen to be of low agglutinability or if the anti-A hemagglutinins in the serum of the other individual happen to be of weak potency. The mistaking of group A_2 blood for universal group O donor blood and administering it to a recipient of group B or group O can result in severe posttransfusion hemolysis, since many such recipients possess natural anti-A_2 agglutinins. Similar dangers attend the giving of O blood to the rare recipient of subgroup A_1B who has agglutinin anti-A_2, because the latter reacts with cells of group O even more readily than with cells of A_2.

Newborn Infants

The absent or feeble titer of most hemagglutinins in early infancy and the low antigenicity of the agglutinogens at this early age make blood grouping and cross matching more difficult than in adults. An infant's serum during cross matching will often fail to agglutinate erythrocytes from a prospective donor belonging to some other group. Erythrocytes from a group A_2 infant are readily mistaken for those of group O, and A_2B erythrocytes for those of group B, unless the testing serums are of high potency. Once such a transfusion has been given, the presence of red cells from the donor will confuse further the identification of the blood group of the infant.

Because of the poor hemagglutinin production by newborn infants, one or two transfusions of blood of an incompatible group may not result in any clinically recognizable hemolytic reactions. Eventual sensitization may be anticipated, however, with further transfusions from donors of the same incompatible type leading to serious complications. Despite this risk, in an obstetric emergency the blood of either parent may be transfused immediately into a newborn infant with safety when no other donors are available, with the exception of using maternal blood when the infant has erythroblastosis fetalis.

Minor Blood Group Systems

A hemolytic transfusion reaction in a recipient of the same ABO and Rh·Hr type as the donor may be due to previous sensitization by one or more of the minor blood group factors, the most frequent being those of the MN·S, Duffy, Kell, and Kidd systems (p. 129). This phenomenon is becoming more important with the growing use of frequent regular transfusions to sustain adequate hemoglobin levels in children with chronic blood disorders (p. 142). Patients with acquired hemolytic anemia, lupus erythematosus, lymphoma, Wilm's tumor, and related allergic and malignant diseases seem especially susceptible to sensitization by the minor blood group antigens. Cross matchings for all such patients should always be done with the indirect Coombs procedure after preliminary screening with the saline techniques. There is a growing trend for all cross matchings to be done with this precaution, regardless of whether the recipient has ever received a prior transfusion.

Since atypical autoantibodies may appear suddenly in any child who is seriously ill or receiving potent medications, all cross matchings for such a recipient should be done with a sample of his blood collected within 24 hours of the contemplated transfusion. If the latter is postponed, the cross matching should be repeated. This precaution is less necessary with a well child being prepared for an elective operation.

BIBLIOGRAPHY

THE ABO SYSTEM

Axtrup, S., Iso-immunization in the A B O System and Morbus Haemolyticus Neonatorum, *Acta paediat.* 38:45, 1949.

Chown, B., and *M. Lewis,* A-B-O and Rh Blood Antigens of Fetuses of about Forty-five and Fifty-five Days, *Canad. M. A. J.* 58:504, 1948.

Davidsohn, I., A Method for Recognition of Blood Subgroups A₁ and A₂ as a Means of Avoiding Transfusion Reactions, *J.A.M.A.* 112:713, 1939.

Diamond, L. K., and *F. H. Allen, Jr.,* Rh and Other Blood Groups, *New England J. Med.* 241:867, 907, 1949.

Hervey, G. W., L. K. Diamond, and *V. Watson,* Geographic Blood Group Variability in the United States, *J.A.M.A.* 145:80, 1951.

Jakobowicz, R., and *L. M. Bryce,* Some Observations on Anti-O Agglutinins, *M. J. Australia* 2:373, 1949.

Sickles, G. R., and *P. P. Murdick,* Isoagglutinin Response to Injections of Specific Substances A and B Derived from Animal Sources and from Meconium, *Am. J. Clin. Path.* 23:322, 1953.

Young, L. E., Studies of the Subgroups of Blood Groups A and AB. I. The Active and Passive Acquisition of Alpha (α₁) Agglutinins by A₂ Patients as a Result of Blood Transfusion, *J. Immunol.* 51:101, 1945.

——— and *E. Witebsky,* Studies of the Subgroups of Blood Groups A and AB. II. The Agglutinogen A₃: Its Detection with Potent B Serum and an Investigation of Its Inheritance, *J. Immunol.* 51:111, 1945.

Zuelzer, W. W., and *E. Kaplan,* ABO Heterospecific Pregnancy and Hemolytic Disease: A Study of Normal and Pathologic Variants. II. Patterns of A and B Isoantibodies in the Cord Blood of Normal Infants, *A.M.A. Am. J. Dis. Child.* 88:179, 1954.

THE MINOR BLOOD GROUP SYSTEMS

Brendemoen, O. J., Further Studies of Agglutination and Inhibition in the Leᵃ-Leᵇ System, *J. Lab. & Clin. Med.* 36:335, 1950.

Davidsohn, I., K. Stern, R. Strauser, and *W. Spurrier,* Be, A New "Private" Blood Factor, *Blood* 8:747, 1953.

de Vries, S. I., and *H. S. Smitskamp,* Haemolytic Transfusion Reaction Due to an Anti-Lewis Agglutinin, *Brit. M. J.* 1:280, 1951.

Gilbey, B. E., A New Blood Antigen, "Jobbins," *Nature* 160:362, 1947.

Graydon, J. J., A Rare Isohaemagglutinogen, *M. J. Australia* 2:9, 1946.

Grubb, R., and *W. T. J. Morgan,* The "Lewis" Blood Group Characters of Erythrocytes and Body-fluids, *Brit. J. Exper. Path.* **30:**198, 1949.

Levine, P., A Brief Review of the Newer Blood Factors, *Tr. New York Acad. Sci.* ser. II, **13:**205, 1951.

————, *M. Backer, M. Wigod,* and *R. Ponder,* A New Human Hereditary Blood Property (Cellano) Present in 99.8% of All Bloods, *Science* **109:**464, 1949.

————, *A. H. Stock, A. B. Kuhmichel,* and *N. Bronikovsky,* A New Human Blood Factor of Rare Incidence in the General Population, *Proc. Soc. Exper. Biol. & Med.* **77:**402, 1951.

Miller, E. B., H. D. Tannor, and *C. F. Hsu,* The P. Factor and Its Variants in Caucasians, Negroes and Chinese, *J. Lab. & Clin. Med.* **36:**230, 1950.

Race, R. R., and *R. Sanger,* "Blood Groups in Man," 2d ed., Charles C Thomas, Springfield, Ill., 1954.

Rosenfield, R. E., P. Vogel, N. Gibbel, G. Ohno, and *G. Haber,* Anti-JK^a: Three New Examples of the Isoantibody, *Am. J. Clin. Path.* **23:**1222, 1953.

Sanger, R., and *R. R. Race,* The MNSs Blood Group System, *Am. J. Human Genet.* **3:**332, 1951.

Wiener, A. S., Heredity of the M-N-S Blood Types: Statistical Considerations, *Am. J. Human Genet.* **4:**37, 1952.

Zoutendiyk, A., and *P. Levine,* A Second Example of the Rare Serum Anti-jay, *Am. J. Clin. Path.* **22:**630, 1952.

GROUPING AND CROSS MATCHING

Dausset, J., The Agglutination Mechanism of Trypsin Modified Red Cells, *Blood* **7:**816, 1952.

Grove-Rasmussen, M., N. Driesler, R. S. Shaw, and *E. Casna,* D^u Bloods in Routine Rh-Typing and Cross-Matching Procedures, *Am. J. Clin. Path.* **26:**736, 1956.

Hunter, B., Jr., and *J. B. Ross,* Newer Methods of Detection of Incompatibilities in Blood Transfusion, *Am. J. Clin. Path.* **23:**27, 1953.

Jakobowicz, R., and *L. M. Bryce,* Iso-agglutinins in Cord Blood, *M. J. Australia* **1:**669, 1948.

Jones, B. B., Isohemolysins in Human Blood, with Especial Reference to the Blood of the New-born, *Am. J. Dis. Child.* **22:**598, 1921.

Landsteiner, K., "The Specificity of Serological Reactions," Harvard University Press, Cambridge, Mass., 1946.

MacCready, R. A., and *M. C. Manin,* A Typing Study of One Hundred Fifty Thousand Bloods, *J. Lab. & Clin. Med.* **37:**634, 1951.

Rosenthal, M. C., W. Dameshek, and *R. Burkhardt,* Trypsin-modified Erythrocytes: Their Use as Test Cells in Acquired Hemolytic Anemia, *Am. J. Clin. Path.* **21:**635, 1951.

Smith, C. H., Iso-agglutinins in the Newborn, *Am. J. Dis. Child.* **36:**54, 1928.

Unger, L. J., Blood Grouping Tests for Exclusion of Paternity, *J.A.M.A.* **152:**1006, 1953.

Vogel, P., Current Problems in Blood Transfusion, *Bull. New York Acad. Med.* **30:**657, 1954.

Witebsky, E., N. C. Klendshoj, and *C. McNeil,* Potent Typing Sera Produced by Treatment of Donors with Isolated Blood Group Specific Substances, *Proc. Soc. Exper. Biol. & Med.* **55:**167, 1944.

CHAPTER 12

Transfusions

Every indirect transfusion should be started by an experienced physician, except perhaps in situations where a nurse working under medical supervision has been specially trained for the procedure. Until the transfusion is completely over the recipient should be under constant observation for the first sign of a reaction or other potentially serious accidents. The slower any transfusion is given the better is it tolerated.

The amount of blood to be given a child in any one transfusion depends upon weight, state of circulation, and need. The maximums which may be given with safety (in the absence of frank bleeding when more may be required) are as follows: (1) for infants in good physical condition, up to 20 ml per kg body weight, (2) for ill infants in poor physical condition, up to 10 ml per kg body weight, (3) for older children weighing over 15 kg and in good physical condition, up to 15 ml per kg, (4) for older children in poor physical condition, up to 10 ml per kg. These maximal amounts refer to the total volumes of whole blood in the acid-citrate-dextrose (ACD) solution currently popular, in which 4 parts of whole blood from the donor are mixed with 1 part of the anticoagulant solution.

When seriously ill patients are in need of considerable quantities of blood, it is best to give several small transfusions on successive days. Every precaution must always be taken against hematologic incompatibilities, clerical errors, bacterial contamination, and manipulations which may injure or lyse the red cells while in the transfusion equipment.

WHOLE-BLOOD TRANSFUSIONS

The usual transfusion container prepared according to NIH specifications and containing whole blood collected from a normal adult consists of 480 ml of blood mixed with 120 ml of a citrated (ACD) anticoagulant solution. When transfusing this mixture, 100 ml is equivalent to 80 ml of whole blood. The usual blood donation taken from a normal adult can be assumed for calculation purpose to contain approximately 15 gm of hemoglobin per 100 ml or 5 million red cells per cu ml before citration.

139

One hundred milliliters of such citrated blood will therefore furnish about 12 gm of hemoglobin.

There is ordinarily not enough surplus citrate in blood or plasma rendered noncoagulable by ACD solution to give rise to clinically significant derangements attributable to the citrate. However, when large amounts of such citrated blood are infused in a short space of time, as occurs in exchange transfusion and during thoracic surgery, a transitory hypocalcemia may be induced. This may give rise to muscle tremors and prolonged Q-T interval, depression of the T waves, and related electrocardiographic changes. Injections of a solution of a calcium salt will alleviate the complication. In infants receiving exchange transfusion, experience has shown that 1 or 2 ml of 10 per cent calcium gluconate solution should be given after each 100 ml of citrated donor blood. When too much calcium is given, the heart rate may slow and the blood pressure fall. If a patient has been receiving digitalis, calcium may potentiate the action of the digitalis. Hypocalcemia due to citrate does not occur with ordinary transfusions given at a slow rate, because the citrate iron is rapidly catabolized and removed by the liver.

Whole blood is the most appropriate therapy (1) for replacement of blood loss after sudden massive hemorrhage, (2) for support during surgical operations attended by bleeding, (3) for maintenance of effective blood volume in dehydration or vascular collapse when shock is present or impending, (4) for the therapy of anemia associated with severe malnutrition, and (5) for other special conditions such as exsanguination procedures in erythroblastosis fetalis. Once a reduced blood volume has been restored, red cell concentrates may be given subsequently if indicated to correct a still low hemoglobin level and red cell count.

Blood which has been stored in the cold for 1 or 2 weeks is about as effective as freshly collected blood when the purpose is to replace the amount lost by bleeding, to restore or support blood volume in dehydrative and shocklike states, or to correct anemia in acute infections. However, for anemias which are chronic and of hypoplastic origin so that the patient requires repeated supportive transfusions, the fewer the days that have passed since collection of the donor blood, the longer will be its survival in the recipient.

Chelating agents such as calcium disodium ethylenediaminetetraacetic acid (CaEDTA) are used at times as the anticoagulant in place of citrate or oxalate. The survival of red cells in storage with such preparations is about the same as with citrate, though platelets may remain intact longer. With multiple transfusions, the risk of hypocalcemia is greater since the chelating agents circulate for some time before being excreted by the kidneys, whereas citrate is metabolized rapidly.

Fresh whole blood or plasma is preferable for therapy of most hemorrhagic disturbances. The coagulation factors are the significant moiety here. The diverse specific coagulating factors in the blood diminish at variable rates after blood or plasma are placed in storage at 4°C. An appreciable portion of the antihemophilic thromboplastinogen will disappear in the first 24 hours. Platelets, though sturdy, adhere to rubber tubing and glass surfaces, so that more than half of those originally present are no longer functional after the first day, and by 3 to 5 days all that remain have undergone spontaneous lysis. Ac-globulin deteriorates more slowly, being at about 75 per cent concentration at 1 week and 50 per cent at 2 weeks. Loss of prothrombin is negligible even after 3 weeks. Fibrinogen persists indefinitely.

The administration of freshly collected blood, preferably if handled in plastic or siliconized equipment, may alleviate a hemorrhagic tendency due to platelet inadequacy for a day or more, except with the idiopathic form of thrombocytopenic purpura in which transfused platelets seem to survive but a few hours.

As a rule, banked blood may be taken from the refrigerator and infused directly into a patient, provided it is run in slowly. Preliminary warming is necessary only when the recipient is in shock or incipent shock, such as a dehydrated or erythroblastotic infant, or when the recipient's serum contains cold isohemagglutinins or the atypical antibodies of acquired hemolytic anemia in high titer. The container of donor's blood may be given a preliminary warming by letting it stand at room temperature for several hours or by placing it in a basin of water whose temperature, *when tested by a thermometer,* is not more than 37°C.

CONCENTRATED RED CELL SUSPENSIONS

When one transfuses with the thoroughly sedimented or centrifuged portion of blood in the transfusion bottle, one gives approximately double the concentration of red cells and hemoglobin of the original whole blood. Such suspensions flow into the veins more slowly than whole blood itself. They should be given within 6 hours of preparation.

Red cell suspensions are preferable to whole blood when there is need to raise the blood hemoglobin content in the presence of a total blood volume which is already normal or near normal. Among such circumstances are (1) anemic states in which the patient is in no immediate distress, such as iron-deficiency anemia, Mediterranean anemia, aplastic anemia, leukemia; (2) anemia in conditions where an increase in blood volume is contraindicated, such as cardiac disease, hypertension, nephritis; (3) severe acute hypohemoglobinemic situations in which it is important to rapidly increase the oxygen-carrying capacity of the blood, such as methemoglobinemia, carbon monoxide poisoning, erythroblastosis fetalis after the first day; and (4) preparation for surgery of anemic patients whose blood volume is normal. Fewer transfusions need be given, and the risk of overload reactions is minimized. Another advantage in the use of sedimented red cell suspensions is that reactions due to allergens or other toxic factors residing in the plasma are greatly reduced.

The plasma of whole blood preserved with citrate solution accumulates excess potassium during storage, derived by diffusion out of the red cells. Even though neither the citrate nor the extra potassium in such whole blood is sufficient to induce toxic changes in a recipient's metabolism, except perhaps when hypocalcemia or hyperpotassemia is already present, the metabolic burdens on the recipient are lessened by administering a concentrate.

The content of sodium chloride in a red cell suspension is only 4 gm per liter, compared with 9 gm per liter in plasma or nonsedimented whole blood preserved with the usual acid-citrate dextrose solution. This lower content is of importance with patients having cardiac or related ailments for which the intake of sodium chloride is being restricted. If such a recipient is in circulatory failure, keeping him upright in a chair while giving the transfusion slowly will reduce the strain on the circulation and minimize the possibility of edema.

Red cell suspensions may have to be administered at regular intervals of 3 weeks or more to patients whose bone marrow does not produce enough red cells to permit ambulatory activity or perhaps even to sustain life itself. The patients in our transfusion clinic include instances of Mediterranean anemia, leukemia, congenital aregenerative anemia, and hypoplastic anemia due to chronic nephritis. About a dozen of these have received over 50 transfusions to date, and several others have had over 300. The children report for transfusions approximately every 3 to 6 weeks and receive concentrated red cell suspensions. Reactions are kept to a minimum by permitting the transfusion to flow in very slowly, over a few hours' period. It has been observed that when the donor blood has been stored more than 2 or 3 days its survival in the recipient seems to be reduced significantly, so that the next transfusion becomes necessary after a shorter interval of time.

Calculation of Transfusion Requirement in Anemia

This can be computed simply:

Example: It is desired to raise the hemoglobin level from 5 to 11 gm per 100 ml by transfusion, in a child weighing 25 lb, with nutritional anemia.

Calculations

a. 25 lb = 11.4 kg body weight.

b. Blood volume = approximately 7.5 per cent of body weight.

$$0.075 \times 11.4 = 0.855 \text{ kg of blood}$$

The specific gravity of blood in severe anemia can be estimated as 1.040 (normal: 1.045).

$$\frac{0.855}{1.040} = 0.822 \text{ liter} = 822 \text{ ml}$$

c. There is now 5 gm of Hb per 100 ml of blood.

$$5 \times 8.22 = 41.1 \text{ gm Hb present in body}$$

d. Desired level of Hb: 11 gm per 100 ml of blood.

$$11 \times 8.22 = 90.4 \text{ gm}$$
$$90.4 - 41.1 = 49.3 \text{ gm of Hb needed}$$

e. Whole blood from adult donors may be assumed to contain 15 gm of Hb per 100 ml before dilution with anticoagulant fluid. The usual proportion in donor bottles is 80 per cent blood and 20 per cent anticoagulant solution.

$$0.80 \times 15 \text{ gm} = 12 \text{ gm Hb per 100 ml}$$

$$\frac{49.3 \text{ gm}}{12 \text{ gm per 100 ml}} = 411 \text{ ml whole blood needed from donor bottle}$$

f. 20 ml of transfused blood per kilogram body weight is the accepted maximum compatible with safety. The body weight is 11.4 kg.

$$20 \times 11.4 = 228 \text{ ml maximum for one transfusion}$$

One would therefore give two transfusions of whole blood, of approximately 205 ml each.

g. Sedimented red cell preparations are usually a little less than twice as rich in hemoglobin as is whole citrated blood. Hence a single transfusion of 210 to 225 ml of such a preparation will be adequate.

By actual checks on infants and children we have been able to verify the validity of this form of computation. The correction factor for specific gravity is a refinement which may be omitted in practice without significant distortion of the results.

After a whole-blood transfusion the full expected increase in hemoglobin concentration may not be immediately demonstrable. The plasma proteins contained in whole blood tend to raise the blood volume transitorily, and readjustment to the pretransfusion volume may not take place for 12 to 24 hours. Fluctuations in blood volume of spontaneous character or due to illness or bleeding may also influence the adjustment process. Concentrated red cell suspensions, on the other hand, contain so little plasma that within an hour the physiologic readjustment of blood volume is accomplished.

PLASMA TRANSFUSIONS

Intravenous plasma may be administered (1) as an emergency substitute for whole blood in shock following hemorrhages, burns, crushing wounds, and related disturbances in which plasma is lost into the tissues with resulting hemoconcentration, (2) to repair the hypoproteinemia which follows an insufficient intake or excessive urinary loss of protein, (3) in prophylaxis or treatment of circulatory failure resulting from a diminution in blood volume, (4) as an adjunct in the correction of the dehydration and intoxication which attend severe diarrhea, diabetic acidosis, and related prostrating illnesses (p. 623).

Plasma when taken from a single donor should be demonstrated by cross matching to be compatible with the red cells of the recipient with respect to the ABO blood group system. For example, a patient of group A may receive plasma from a donor of group A or AB with safety whereas a donor of group B or O may have naturally occurring anti-A antibodies which may give rise to hemolytic phenomena in the recipient. When units of plasma from several donors of different groups are mixed together, however, dilution and some cross neutralization of the antibodies results. Such pools of plasma are administered to recipients of any blood group without preliminary cross matching. Hemolytic reactions need not be feared, so long as exceptionally large amounts are avoided.

The value of plasma as a carrier of protective immune substances for therapy of any of the bacterial diseases is negligible. Antibiotics or sulfonamides when specifically applicable are immeasurably more effective.

Infusions of plasma are only of minor benefit for protein feeding. One hundred milliliters of donor blood in anticoagulant solution contains only about 3 gm of protein per 100 ml; the concentration is doubled in separated plasma. For an infant whose 24-hour protein requirement will approximate 30 gm normally, 500 ml of intravenous plasma or 1,000 ml of preserved whole blood is needed for a day's supply. The parenteral feeding of 600 ml of a 5 per cent amino acid solution will provide the equivalent of 30 gm of protein much more economically and without danger of enlarging the blood volume.

USE OF GROUP O Rh-NEGATIVE BLOOD IN EMERGENCIES

In many hospitals group O Rh-negative whole blood (*universal donor blood*) is kept available for any patient who may develop a need for a transfusion while the blood bank is closed. Where this is the practice it is important for the bank to determine the anti-A and anti-B agglutinin titers of all O bloods which may be intended for this purpose. Excluded are those with anti-A or anti-B saline isoagglutinin titers of 1:200 or more, or the 25 per cent with the highest anti-A and anti-B titers. Any which contain anti-A or anti-B hemolysins should be given only to recipients of compatible type. The absence of antibodies to the Rh·Hr antigens donor plasma should be demonstrated by specific testing.

Some blood banks routinely add a mixture of soluble A and B substances, purified from animal sources, to group O bloods intended for recipients of other blood groups. These substances have their greatest utility with O donor bloods of high anti-A or anti-B saline titers; they do not seem necessary when these isohemagglutinins are low. A theoretical objection to their use is the fear of sensitizing the recipient when multiple transfusions containing an excess of these substances have to be given. Another is that rare donors possess high titers of albumin-active antibodies against A or B, which are not neutralized by the addition of group-specific substances.

As a rule, transfusing with universal donor blood without prior grouping or cross matching is unattended with immediate difficulties. Many blood bank directors, however, look with disfavor upon this practice. Blood from donors who have had previous transfusions or who possess atypical antibodies can give rise to hemolytic reactions. The possibility exists of sensitizing an Rh-positive recipient to the c(hr′) antigen when Rh-negative blood, which always contains this antigen, is given. This consideration, even though remote, makes it preferable that Rh-positive children, and especially females, be always transfused with Rh-positive rather than Rh-negative blood except in grave emergencies.

A minority of recipients who belong to blood group AB already have naturally occurring anti-O antibodies, and these may increase under the stimulation of transfused O cells. Preliminary testing of all recipients for saline anti-O hemagglutinins, though usually omitted, is an important safeguard, but even with this a few instances have been reported in which difficulties resulted because the recipient had albumin-active anti-O hemagglutinins in his serum without any of the saline-active class.

Group O donor red cells when followed by the Ashby technique in an A, B, or AB recipient will usually exhibit the same survival time as do cells of the recipient's own blood group. Careful studies have shown, however, that the proportion of recipient cells often diminishes slightly in the first 24 hours after such a transfusion, suggesting destruction of some of these cells by the transfused anti-A or anti-B antibodies. Occasionally one finds also a mild posttransfusion hyperbilirubinemia or an elevated fecal urobilinogen.

After large transfusions of universal donor blood the patient's blood stream contains a mixture of red cells of two blood groups and may also carry some isohemagglutinins transferred from the donor. Endeavors to perform cross-matching tests then become subject to confusing complications. Hence, even if a satisfactory cross matching can be done, such a patient who needs further transfusions should continue to receive O blood until at least 2 weeks have passed.

Because of all the above considerations, a transfusion from a donor of the same ABO and Rh·Hr blood group is always to be preferred. The transfusion needs of hospital patients and the availability of blood-bank service should be so regulated that the giving of group O Rh-negative blood is limited solely to those true emergencies where need for whole blood is immediate and completely unforeseeable. Perhaps the only exceptions to this rule in the pediatric field lie in the management of newborn infants with erythroblastosis fetalis, and of older children with hemolytic anemia due to circulating autoantibodies, in whom blood grouping and cross-matching procedures cannot be performed with reliability.

TRANSMISSION OF DISEASE BY TRANSFUSION

While isolated instances have been reported of other infections such as measles, typhus, and brucellosis transmitted by transfusions, the major diseases which may be spread by the transfer of blood are serum hepatitis, syphilis, and malaria. An obvious preliminary in collecting blood is to exclude would-be donors who have had hepatitis or malaria at any time in their lives or untreated syphilis within the preceding 2 years. Unreliability of histories and unrecognized subclinical illnesses ending in a carrier state keep such a survey of donors from being more than a desirable precaution.

The chance of transmission of hepatitis from a single donor to a single recipient is comparatively insignificant provided that the donor has never had known hepatitis. A possible risk does exist, however. Attacks of acute hepatitis inferentially spread by transfusion are not unprecedented in hospital practice.

The use of plasma from large pools to support the circulation in conditions associated with shock has in the past been associated with a high risk of serum hepatitis (5 to 22 per cent in numerous reported series). Such pooled plasma was preserved by lyophilizing, freezing, or storage in the liquid state under refrigeration. Recent reports (Allen, Murray) have indicated that storage of such plasma at room temperature for 6 months reduces to less than 1 per cent the risk of transmitting serum hepatitis.

The likelihood of introducing a complicating disease due to a viral or bacterial contaminant in plasma is also reduced, though not wholly eliminated, by preliminary ultraviolet irradiation after the plasma has been separated. Since one infected donor can contaminate all fractions of a plasma pool regardless of size, it is preferable that such pools be prepared from small groups of donors, no more than about six.

The risk of syphilis can be practically eliminated by (1) performing pretransfusion serologic tests for syphilis and discarding all positive reactors (such seropositive blood can be safely used for production of plasma), or (2) storing the blood at 4°C for at least 4 days, which is adequate for killing off any contained spirochetes. A spirocheticidal drug such as penicillin should be added in dilute concentration when fresh blood from a seropositive or doubtful donor must be transfused in an emergency.

We have seen a number of cases of malaria transmitted to children by fresh transfusions. The donor in each instance was a parent or relative whose symptoms had been quiescent for so many years that the actual occurrence of the disease had been forgotten at the time the pretransfusion inquiry was made. Such latent malaria is almost always caused by tertian forms of the parasite and can be eradicated quickly in the recipient by modern therapy. Malarial parasites when present in blood collected from a donor may remain viable for several days during storage at refrigerator temperature.

TRANSFUSION REACTIONS

These may be classified as hemolytic, plasmogenic, allergic, pyrogenic, embolic, or "speed." After every reaction the effort to track down the cause should be made. The bottle of blood or plasma along with the tubing and needle should be kept sterile and without further handling be referred back to the blood bank for study of the contents serologically and bacteriologically. A review should also be made of the entire performance of the transfusion, in order to uncover possible deviations from the usual routine. One may find that the container of blood after leaving the blood bank had been subjected to changes in temperature conditions, which can injure stored red cells. It may have been overwarmed by being placed in a basin of hot water, or alternately warmed and chilled by being taken out of and replaced in the refrigerator several times before use. The refrigerator used for temporarily storing the blood after its removal from the blood bank may be functioning poorly. Large amounts of 5 or 10 per cent warm glucose, or water of condensation, may have been permitted to mix with donor blood in the apparatus prior to the transfusion. An aspirating needle may have been introduced into the original container previously, with resulting bacterial contamination of the contents.

It is a wise precaution to note the temperature, pulse rate, and blood pressure of every child before a transfusion, immediately afterward, and again an hour later. When feasible one may also collect a urine specimen just before the transfusion; if reactionlike symptoms develop, a second specimen may then be compared with it for color, protein, free hemoglobin, hemoglobin-containing casts, and hematin crystals.

Hemolytic Reactions

The blood bank should always preserve the residues of cells and serum used in grouping and cross matching for at least 1 week after the transfusion is given. This permits a later check on accuracy should the need arise. The bottle which contained the donor blood should be returned to the blood bank after use.

Any headache, chilly feeling, nausea, vomiting, abdominal or back pain, fever, or other untoward complaints are danger signals, and the transfusion should be stopped at once.

Following a transfusion, the finding of a low blood pressure, the physical appearance of shock, and the passage of red or brown hemoglobin-containing urine are indicative of a severe hemolytic reaction. All such patients must be kept under close observation, with body temperature, blood pressure, and pulse rate recorded at frequent intervals. Salicylates may be given if the temperature rises more than 2°F above the pretransfusion reading. Chills may be treated with blankets and the application of heat externally. It is most important to administer large amounts of fluid by mouth or intravenously as soon as a hemolytic reaction is suspected. Infusion of compatible plasma is advisable if shock develops. Later, if oliguria or anuria ensue from renal tubular damage, the problem becomes fundamentally one of adjustment of parenteral salts and fluids in order to keep the patient alive until kidney function returns (p. 426). Jaundice if it occurs is proportional to the amount of blood destroyed, but is of less concern prognostically than the severity and duration of the renal suppression.

Whenever a transfusion reaction is suspected, a specimen of blood should be withdrawn from the recipient as soon as possible, using a clean dry syringe and removing the tourniquet before the blood is withdrawn. Some of this is placed in a tube containing an anticoagulant, and the remainder in a clean dry tube and permitted to clot. A urine specimen should be obtained immediately, and further specimens at frequent intervals.

To track down the cause of a hemolytic reaction, one should first recheck the ABO and Rh·Hr groupings and the cross matching itself, using the few drops left in the donor bottle and pre- and posttransfusion specimens taken from the recipient. These cross matchings should be done in an albumin-containing medium and also with the indirect globulin (Coombs) test. If all results are negative but a hemolytic reaction is still suspected, the plasma or serum of both donor and recipient should be tested for cold isohemagglutinins and for atypical or weakly acting antibodies, after enzyme treatment of the cells (p. 96).

The blood in the donor bottle should be centrifuged to see whether it has become partially hemolyzed because of mishandling. It should also be cultured aerobically and anaerobically. The serum from the posttransfusion specimen of blood is separated by centrifugation and examined for free hemoglobin or an increase in bilirubin. Visual comparison is usually adequate, though chemical analysis may have to be performed in doubtful situations. Nonclotted posttransfusion blood of the patient is inspected grossly and microscopically for the possible occurrence of red cell clumping indicative of intravascular agglutination. A rise in serum bilirubin level in several tests some hours apart confirms the interpretation. Another corroboration is to find hemoglobin, red cells, or red cell casts in the first specimen of urine passed after the reaction. The peripheral blood smear displays spherocytosis and leukocytosis, followed by reticulocytosis. The spherocytes are sometimes recognizable for many days after the other hemolytic symptoms are gone. Should all these procedures prove negative, a hemolytic reaction can be excluded.

The hemolytic character of a mild reaction can be confirmed by measuring the titer of the recipient's serum against the donor's red cells and other A and B red cells posttransfusionally and a week later. Should a pronounced rise occur, an unusual incompatibility may be presumed.

Mild reactions frequently attend the regular giving of transfusions for the maintenance of adequate hemoglobin levels in children with Mediterranean anemia, aplastic anemia, leukemia, and other chronic blood disorders. Exceptionally, these reactions tend to become progressively more severe. Some are due to presumed incompatibilities referable to the minor blood group antigens, known or unknown. Others may be a response to some substance in the donor plasma—the plasmogenic transfusion reactions discussed below. Identification of the causative factor is beyond the scope of most clinical laboratories. By meticulous cross matching based on the application of a modified Coombs technique, it is feasible to eliminate those donors whose minor red cell antigens are incompatible with weak antibodies already present in the recipient (p. 135).

Plasmogenic Reactions

Plasma transfusion reactions are believed to be caused by a heat-labile component of the plasma. Red cell suspensions containing little plasma can usually be transfused with impunity into such susceptible patients, but washing the red cells with normal saline solution may be needed before attacks can be prevented.

Mild plasmogenic reactions consist of a chilly feeling or headache, with a slight drop in body temperature and blood pressure. More severe reactions consist of a shaking chill, often with abdominal pain, nausea, vomiting, headache, or even diarrhea. These reactions may occur unpredictably in patients with febrile illnesses or hematologic and other disorders. A similar set of symptoms occurs with anaphylactic and peptone shock, intravenous administration of foreign proteins such as tuberculin and typhoid bacilli, too rapid intravenous injection of iron compounds, and during the hemolytic paroxysms of cold hemoglobinuria, favism, and blackwater fever.

Pyrogenic Reactions

Fever, pallor, anorexia, shivering, or diarrhea may result from contamination of the blood or transfusion equipment by bacteria themselves or products of their growth. Such reactions typically begin during or within 2 hours after the transfusion and last from 30 minutes to 8 hours. Mild reactions consist merely of a slight increase in body temperature of short duration; more severe ones may be accompanied by a chill. To detect these reactions, especially in young children and infants who may make no complaint, it is advisable to take a body temperature reading every half hour for the first few hours and every hour thereafter for 8 hours.

Scrupulous attention must always be directed toward prevention of contamination of the anticoagulant fluid before the collection of blood, or of the blood in the container during its later withdrawals. Skin bacteria which are accidentally introduced into blood for transfusion are ordinarily unable to proliferate to any extent because of the low temperatures of storage and the bactericidal properties of blood itself. Many of the contaminating bacteria which give rise to severe or even fatal pyrogenic reactions are nonpathogenic strains of micrococci, Pseudomonas, Gram-negative bacilli, spore formers, or diphtheroids which are able to survive or even proliferate at refrigerator temperatures. Some of these grow poorly if at all at the standard 37°C obtaining in most hospital incubators. Setting the thermostat at between 25 and 30°C makes it feasible to demonstrate practically all blood contaminants.

When investigating the possibility of bacteria in a container of blood one should also examine stained smears of centrifuged portions for bacterial bodies. Live organisms may no longer grow out in culture, but their dead forms and the products of their growth may still produce severe reactions when injected intravenously.

Massive bacterial contamination of blood produces a characteristic shocklike syndrome. Chill, fever, vomiting, diarrhea, and peripheral vascular collapse commence suddenly. The outcome may be quickly fatal. In most reported instances the contaminating organism has been a strain of coliform bacilli, derived apparently from unsterile glassware.

Not every febrile reaction can be ascribed to pyrogens. Occasional patients who receive sustaining transfusions at periodic intervals regularly experience posttransfusion fever with or without chills. Most of these reactions are presumably plasmogenic in origin. Nevertheless, when episodes of fever follow more than 1 or 2 per cent of all transfusions given in an institution, it is advisable to carry out a thorough investigation of all practices related to the preparing of anticoagulant solutions and cleansing and sterilizing of the glassware, tubing, and needles. A frequent source of difficulty is improper processing or storage of the distilled water used for rinsing the apparatus and preparing the solutions.

Allergic Reactions

These usually take the form of urticarial lesions, which may begin to appear soon after the transfusion is started. Treatment is with epinephrine or antihistamine drugs. The transfusion need not be discontinued, but the child should be kept under the closest observation for the development of further symptoms. If angioneurotic edema, asthma, or edema of the larynx appear, the transfusion should be stopped immediately and medications given; these latter complications are rare. Such recipients nearly always prove to be individuals known to have allergic hypersensitivities.

When the recipient is known to be allergic or has had allergic transfusion reactions previously, an antihistamine drug in standard dosage may be given by mouth 1 hour before the transfusion and repeated when the transfusion is started. These substances are sometimes added directly to the bottle of donor blood immediately before transfusion, but this is in conflict with the sound doctrine that the addition of any medication to blood is undesirable.

Allergic reactions are responses to some allergen in the blood of the donor. This is the main reason why the donor should be in a fasting state when bled.

When the donor himself is highly allergic, his blood or plasma may transfer his sensitivities passively. The recipient will then experience an allergic response any time during the course of the next few weeks when exposed to an allergen that the donor is sensitive to. It is best, therefore, to avoid using any individual afflicted with major allergies as a donor.

Embolic Reactions

Difficulties from clots of blood entering the recipient's circulation from a faulty donor bottle will be almost nonexistent if a fine filter is placed in the infusion system and a narrow needle used in the vein. Any clot which passes these safeguards is too small to cause tissue damage.

Fatalities from air embolism are undoubtedly more frequent than medical literature would indicate, since most instances are never reported. Air may enter the recipient's circulation (1) through an incised exposed vein when a "cut-down" approach is used unless ligatures are properly applied and the distal segment of vein fully tied off; (2) through a leaky connection near the hub of the needle in the vein if the patient has a negative venous pressure; (3) through air bubbles caught in the tubing and elsewhere before the transfusion is begun or as one bottle of blood is replaced by another; (4) through leaks in the drip chamber if the clip controlling the rate of flow is placed by mistake above this chamber instead of below where it belongs; (5) if the filter is covered with clots, so that a reserve of blood appears to remain in the bottle even though air is being drawn into the tubing beneath it; or (6) if air has to be forced under positive pressure into the donor bottle in order to drive the blood into the veins, as is sometimes necessary in shock states. If this last is done a continuous close watch must be kept to ensure that the transfusion is discontinued before all the blood has been forced from the infusion tubing.

Speed Reactions

A safe infusion rate for blood should not exceed 2 ml per minute for young infants, up to 10 ml per minute for adolescents. With severe shock it may be administered more rapidly.

In the presence of chronic severe anemia, pulmonary edema, or a strained or diseased myocardium the rate should be much slower. Otherwise serious or even fatal symptoms from collapse, acute circulatory failure, or disturbed cardiac function may result. The ability of the cardiovascular system to withstand the added amount of blood being given may be evaluated by examining the heart and lung bases at frequent intervals, or even taking serial venous pressure measurements. Another precaution consists of keeping the child in a sitting position throughout the transfusion. If circulatory failure is already present it may be advisable to first withdraw from the patient's vein a volume of his own blood equal to that about to be given; in this circumstance the transfusion had best consist of sedimented red cells.

COAGULATION DEFECTS FOLLOWING LARGE TRANSFUSIONS

After receiving large amounts of stored blood as replacement during prolonged major surgery, or of plasma as therapy for a bleeding ulcerated lesion, some patients may exhibit a tendency to bleed for the first 2 days after the transfusions. The multiple mechanisms which underly this phenomenon are still not fully understood. One influence is the loss of the patient's own coagulating elements during the bleeding period, another is the diluting effect of the transfused fluid, and a third is the transitory depression of the platelet level. There is also a rise in the antithrombin content of blood after 2 weeks of storage, though this is of minimal importance.

These changes, ordinarily not significant, may give rise to bleeding phenomena if the patient already has a pretransfusion thrombocytopenia or a low plasma content of accelerator factors. The plasma accelerator factors often diminish significantly 24 to 36 hours postoperatively, so that a transfusion of stored blood low in these factors may cause difficulty at this time.

BIBLIOGRAPHY

TRANSFUSIONS

Alton, O. M., and *W. R. Platt*, An Evaluation of the Use of Group-specific Substances in Group O Blood Transfusions, *Am. J. Clin. Path.* 19:536, 1949.

De Gowen, E. L., R. C. Hardin, and *J. B. Alsever,* "Blood Transfusion," W. B. Saunders Company, Philadelphia, 1949.

Donohue, D. M., B. W. Gabrio, and *C. A. Finch,* Preservation and Transfusion of Blood, *J.A.M.A.* 161:784, 1956.

Gabrio, B. W., C. A. Finch, and *F. M. Huennekens,* Erythrocyte Preservation: A Topic in Molecular Biochemistry, *Blood* 11:103, 1956.

Keynes, G., "Blood Transfusion," J. Wright, Bristol (England), 1949.

Mollison, P. L., "Blood Transfusion in Clinical Medicine," Basil Blackwell & Mott, Ltd., Oxford (England), 1951.

Sloviter, H. A., Preservation of Whole Blood and Red Cells, *Am. J. M. Sc.* 225:197, 1953.

Smith, D. W., and *J. Elliott,* Red Blood Cell Suspension Transfusions, *J.A.M.A.* 147:737, 1951.

Smith, R. M., Blood Replacement in Thoracic Surgery for Children, *J.A.M.A.* 161:1124, 1956.

Soutter, L., F. H. Allen, Jr., and *C. P. Emerson, Jr.,* Blood Grouping, Blood Banking and Blood Transfusion, *New England J. Med.* 245:367, 410, 456, 1951.

Strumia, M. M., and *J. J. McGraw, Jr.,* "Blood and Plasma Transfusions," F. A. Davis Company, Philadelphia, 1949.

Weiner, A. S., D. N. W. Grant, L. J. Unger, and *W. G. Workman,* Medicolegal Aspects of Blood Transfusion, *J.A.M.A.* 151:1435, 1953.

TRANSFUSION REACTIONS

Allen, J. G., D. M. Enerson, E. S. G. Barron, and *C. Sykes,* Pooled Plasma with Little or No Risk of Homologous Serum Jaundice, *J.A.M.A.* 154:103, 1954.

Brande, A. I., J. P. Sanford, J. E. Bartlett, and *O. T. Mallery, Jr.,* Effects and Clinical Significance of Bacterial Contaminants in Transfused Blood, *J. Lab. & Clin. Med.* 39:902, 1952.

Bunker, J. P., J. B. Stetson, R. C. Coe, H. C. Grillo, and *A. J. Murphy,* Citric Acid Intoxication, *J.A.M.A.* 157:1361, 1955.

Chown, B., Never Transfuse a Woman with Her Husband's Blood, *Canad. M. A. J.* 61:419, 1949.

Crosby, W. H., and *M. Stefanini,* Pathogenesis of the Plasma Transfusion Reaction with Especial Reference to the Blood Coagulation System, *J. Lab. & Clin. Med.* 40:374, 1952.

—— and *J. N. Howard,* The Hematologic Response to Wounding and to Resuscitation Accomplished by Large Transfusions of Stored Blood: A Study of Battle Casualties in Korea, *Blood* 9:439, 1954.

Davidsohn, I., and *K. Stern:* Diagnosis of Hemolytic Transfusion Reactions, *Am. J. Clin. Path.* 25:381, 1955.

Davison, W. C., Viral Hepatitis and Its Risk from Blood and Plasma Transfusions, *J. Pediat.* 46:717, 1955.

Ervin, D. M., R. M. Christian, and *L. E. Young,* Dangerous Universal Donors, Further

Observations on In Vivo and In Vitro Behavior of Isoantibodies of Immune Type Present in Group O Blood, *Blood* 5:553, 1950.

Hill, L. F., and *Associates,* Transfusion Reaction, Dangerous Universal Donor, *J. Pediat.* 38:518, 1951.

Hutcheson, J. B., J. M. Haber, and *A. Kellner,* A Hazard of Repeated Blood Transfusions: Hemolytic Reaction Due to Antibodies to the Duffy (Fy^a) Factor, *J.A.M.A.* 149:274, 1952.

Keitel, H. G., and *J. Wich,* Hemolysis in Infants Following Administration of Pooled Plasma, *A.M.A. Am. J. Dis. Child.* 87:537, 1954.

Klendshoj, N. C., and *E. Witebsky,* Reactions to Single and Multiple Transfusions, Comparison between Homologous and Conditioned O Blood Transfusions, *Blood* 5:123, 1950.

Krevans, J. R., and *D. P. Jackson,* Hemorrhagic Disorder Following Massive Whole Blood Transfusions, *J.A.M.A.* 159:171, 1955.

Mollison, P. L., Blood Transfusion in Clinical Medicine, chap. 2 in "Blood Volume," Basil Blackwell & Mott, Ltd., Oxford (England), 1951.

Murray, R., J. W. Oliphant, J. T. Tripp, B. Hampil, F. Ratner, W. C. L. Diefenbach, and *H. Geller,* Effect of Ultraviolet Radiation on the Infectivity of Icterogenic Plasma, *J.A.M.A.* 157:8, 1955.

Pittman, M., A Study of Bacteria Implicated in Transfusion Reactions and of Bacteria Isolated from Blood Products, *J. Lab. & Clin. Med.* 42:273, 1953.

Rapoport, M., and *J. Stokes, Jr.,* Reaction Following the Intramuscular Injection of Whole Blood, *Am. J. Dis. Child.* 53:471, 1937.

CHAPTER 13

Rh·Hr and Erythroblastosis Fetalis

THE Rh·Hr BLOOD GROUP SYSTEM

Most of the clinical problems with respect to the Rh·Hr blood group system can be traced to the interactions between the Rh and Hr antigens which are inherited and the specific antibodies produced by sensitization which are transmitted from the mother in erythroblastosis fetalis or which develop postnatally in transfusion reactions. The full exposition is intricate and involved, but the major phenomena which are operative in the great majority of the cases can be stated somewhat simply.

One source of difficulty is the existence of two sets of terminologies, reflecting in part the controversy between the supporters of Wiener's theory of multiple alleles at a single gene locus, and of Fisher's theory that the pertinent chromosomes each carry three related allelomorphic sets of genes.

The many Rh·Hr combinations are built up from three "major" or Rh genes (C, D, and E) and three "minor" or Hr genes (c, d, and e). These occur in multitudinous combinations. The following designations are used for referring to the individual antigens or factors:

Fisher terminology	Wiener terminology
C	rh'
D	Rh_0
E	rh''
c	hr'
d	hr^0
e	hr''

D (Rh_0) is the most highly antigenic and is responsible for most of the transfusion and erythroblastotic disturbances resulting from Rh·Hr incompatibility. The occurrence of any of the antigens in tissues other than mature and immature erythrocytes has not been established.

Gene Interrelations

The Wiener theory postulates that the individual Rh and Hr genes are situated in allelic arrangement on a pair of chromosomes, often in

155

specific groupings such as the combination Rh_0 rh' (Rh_1) and the combination Rh_0 rh'' (Rh_2). These are inheritable double units which almost never divide into their component parts. "Triple-action" units such as Rh_0rh'rh'' (Rh_2) have also been postulated.

The alternative Fisher or CDE theory of inheritance portrays the Rh·Hr factors as triads of closely linked genes stretched along a pair of chromosomes—for example, CDE/cde. Capital letters are used to portray the Rh genes and small letters the reciprocally related Hr genes. Each chromosome can carry either the C or c gene, D or d gene, and E or e gene. The members of each pair—C and c, D and d, and E and e—are genetic allelomorphs. An individual who possesses a gene is said to be *positive* for that gene; if it is absent, he is *negative*. The term *Rh-positive*, as commonly used, refers to the presence of an Rh gene, usually D or Rh_0. *Rh-negative* is applied to persons who are cde/cde.

Several allelomorphic forms replacing D and C and E have been demonstrated. These can be represented by substituting D^u for D; C^w, C^u, or C^x for C; E^u for E. Another Rh antigen termed f appears to belong to a fourth set of allelomorphic genes; as an antigen this is very weak.

Of the allelomorphs, D^u is of the most practical importance. Not all anti-D testing serums possess anti-D^u activity, and hence many individuals who are D^uD^u or D^ud have been considered as being D-negative. Red cells from such individuals, when given in transfusion to D-negative recipients, may stimulate the formation of anti-D antibodies.

Racial Distribution

The clinically important D (Rh_0) factor occurs in nearly 85 per cent of the white population, in about 90 per cent of American Negroes, and in 98 to 100 per cent of ethnically unmixed American Indians, Mexican Indians, Filipinos, Chinese, Japanese, Eskimos, Fijians, and Siamese. D^u appears to be more frequent in Negroes than in whites.

In England, according to Mollison, Mourant, and Race (1948), the comparative frequencies of the chromosomal pairs (genotypes) are as shown in Table 13-1. It is now believed, from tests with more recently obtained anti-D^u serum, that some of the individuals previously typed as d are in reality D^u.

Inheritance

Every heritable character in the body has a two-gene origin, one from each parent. When both of a pair of genes are identical the inheritance pattern for the character is "pure" or homozygous. When the genes are dissimilar the character is "hybrid" or heterozygous. None of the Rh·Hr genes appear in a child unless possessed by one or both parents.

One method of determining whether a given individual is homozygous or heterozygous with respect to any of the Rh·Hr genes is to make a blood group survey of all close blood relatives. For example, with a D-negative (dd) mother and a homozygous D-positive (DD) father, every child will inherit one D and one d gene and be heterozygous D-positive (Dd). With a D-negative mother (dd) and a heterozygous D-positive father(Dd), half the children should be heterozygous D-positive (Dd) and half D-negative (dd). The exact fifty-fifty ratio in the latter situation is encountered only with statistically large numbers of offspring. In small families the ratio is often different, reflecting the action of chance. When

Table 13-1. The Comparative Frequency of Rh Chromosomal Genotypes among Residents of England

Genetic and antigenic constitution	Short symbol	Percentage frequency
CDe/cde	R₁r	31.68
CDe/CDe	R₁R₁	16.61
cde/cde	rr	15.10
CDe/cDE	R₁R₂	11.50
cDE/cde	R₂r	10.97
CDe/cDe	R₁R₀	2.09
cDe/cde	R₀r	2.00
cDE/cDE	R₂R₂	1.99
CDe/CʷDe	R₁R₁ʷ	1.05
CʷDe/cde	R₁ʷr	1.00
Total of all other combinations		6.01
		100.00

SOURCE: Adapted from Mollison, Mourant, and Race, The Rh Blood Groups and Their Clinical Effects, *Med. Res. Council (London) Mem.* 27, 1952.

both the father and the mother are D-negative, all their children must be D-negative. Finding a D-positive child when both parents seem D-negative indicates either an error in the tests or an extrafamilial paternity.

Immunoserologic studies of the individual are another means of determining homozygosity or heterozygosity. If an individual's red cells contain an antigen, they will be agglutinated by the corresponding antiserum. For example, if the red cells are agglutinated by anti-C but not by anti-c, the c factor must be absent; if by anti-c serum only, the C factor must be absent. Agglutination by both anti-C and anti-c serums is an indication of heterozygosity.

Rh·Hr TYPING

Fresh venous blood should be collected sterilely without anticoagulant and stored as whole clotted blood in a refrigerator until tested. Hemolysis from air bubbles, wet syringes, skin disinfectants, and other causes must be avoided at all costs.

Typing methods in current use fall into several categories: (1) slide agglutination, (2) saline test tube incubation, (3) albumin test tube incubation, and (4) capillary tube agglutination. Instructions for performance usually accompany the serums purchased for that purpose. Many laboratories test with two separate methods in order to check on accuracy.

All methods of Rh·Hr typing are delicate and difficult. For dependable results they must be performed with high-quality serums by technicians experienced in the procedure. A tendency of the erythrocytes to form rouleaux may simulate Rh agglutination. Blood which has clotted imperfectly may also exhibit small clumps. Cold agglutinins usually do not produce error, since the standard procedures are carried out at 37°C.

Detailed examination for antibodies is difficult also and calls for special techniques (p. 131). With problem cases the blood specimens should be submitted to a reference laboratory which specializes in Rh testing. Such laboratories possess skilled personnel and scarce test reagents not available generally.

Because many typing serums in the past have been weak and unsatisfactory by modern standards, and because even the best techniques sometimes go astray, it is advisable to redetermine the Rh status of all patients and donors whenever another transfusion is being projected or a woman returns for prenatal care in another pregnancy.

The red cells of an infant ill with erythroblastosis fetalis will sometimes be so saturated with maternal antibody as no longer to react with specific typing serum. Washing or trypsinizing the red cells will usually assist in revealing the true Rh status.

SENSITIZATION INDUCED BY TRANSFUSIONS

One or two transfusions of Rh-positive blood given to an Rh-negative recipient serve mainly to sensitize the recipient. The erythrocytes need not be given intravenously to produce sensitization; an intramuscular injection, even of as little as a few milliliters, can serve as a potent immunizer. After sensitization has been induced, the reactions which attend each successive mismatched transfusion grow progressively more severe and may ultimately prove fatal. D is the strongest of the antigens in this regard. No D-negative subject, male or female, should be given D-positive blood even though at the time only a single transfusion is contemplated. Other transfusions may be needed later in life.

All the other weaker antigens have at times been found to be capable of inducing sensitization. It is most important, therefore, that all blood typing prior to cross matching be done with a full battery of Rh·Hr serums. It is dangerous to employ simply a pure anti-D serum as a short cut to determining whether either a recipient or prospective donor is Rh-positive or Rh-negative. Ignoring the tests for Cc and Ee factors may result in sensitization of a wholly Rh-negative (cde/cde) recipient by

C- or E-positive blood or of a C- or E-positive recipient with c-positive or e-positive blood. Anti-e and particularly anti-d testing serums are scarce.

Husband's blood, even when strictly ABO- and Rh·Hr-compatible, should *never* be transfused into his wife except in direst emergency or unless she has had no children and can no longer bear them. The husband's erythrocytes may possess some minor blood group antigen which is lacking in his wife. Transfusion may result in sensitization, which in turn may lead to erythroblastosis in later pregnancies if the fetuses inherit the paternal antigen. Reversely, if she has already had pregnancies, one of the infants possessing the father's antigen may have transplacentally immunized the mother, so that a later transfusion of husband's blood may eventuate in a serious or even fatal hemolytic reaction.

D-SENSITIZATION AND PREGNANCY

About 1 of every 10 white pregnancies taken at random will result in a D-positive infant being born to a D-negative mother. In the first pregnancy none of these infants will have erythroblastosis fetalis unless the mother had been already sensitized to D by a previous mismatched transfusion. After one or more such pregnancies, however, antibodies which can tranverse the placenta and injure D-positive fetal red cells may begin to be produced by the mother. The probability of the first D-positive pregnancy sensitizing a mother sufficiently for her to deliver an erythroblastotic infant in the second pregnancy is only about 2 per cent —that is only 1 in 50. Third and later pregnancies result in erythroblastosis in 25 to 30 per cent of families in which the father is homozygously D-positive. With a heterozygous father the number of pregnancies before erythroblastosis appears will be greater. The first infant born with the disease is usually less seriously affected than those born subsequently, but there are many exceptions to this rule. In some families the severity of the symptoms is much greater than in others. There is no proof that disorders which arise in the first few months of pregnancy, such as abortions or congenital anomalies, have their origin in Rh incompatibility.

D-negative women need not fear having another child just because their husbands are D-positive, unless a previous erythroblastotic pregnancy or the detection of an anti-D antibody titer indicates otherwise. Two major variables seem to determine whether sensitization will occur: the extent of entry of fetal red cells into the mother and the capacity of the mother to produce antibodies. Contemporary attempts to forestall erythroblastosis in D-negative pregnant women are directed against these possibilities, but thus far none have led to conclusive results. Abelson's data indicate that about 1 of every 17 Rh-negative women become Rh-sensitized during pregnancy.

Within the Rh·Hr blood group system the anti-D antibodies, with or without associated anti-C or anti-E antibodies, appear to be responsible for nearly all instances of erythroblastosis fetalis. Anti-c antibodies are the next most common cause of difficulty. Exceptional instances may be encountered of erythroblastosis due to incompatibility related to Kell, Kidd, Duffy, or other weakly antigenic factors.

Serologic studies for possible sensitization to one of these other antigens should be begun immediately whenever an infant with erythroblastosis fetalis is born to a D-positive mother or whenever both mother and infant appear to be D-negative. Sensitization of the mother usually proves to be through a prior blood transfusion. The illness in the infant resembles that of erythroblastosis fetalis due to D sensitization and is treated similarly.

ERYTHROBLASTOSIS-PRODUCING Rh·Hr ANTIBODIES

Anti-Rh and anti-Hr serums contain diverse specific antibodies, not necessarily in equal titer. The component principles, which still need more elucidation, seem to be separable into several main classes: (1) saline-active antibodies which can clump erythrocytes in saline suspensions, (2) albumin-active antibodies which clump erythrocytes only when suspended in a viscous medium such as human serum or bovine albumin; and (3) cryptagglutinoids which can be demonstrated only by the indirect Coombs test (see below). The saline-active antibodies are sometimes termed *complete* or *bivalent* or *conglutinins;* the albumin-active antibodies, *incomplete* or *univalent* or *glutinins.* Those which induce agglutination only with the Coombs test are also termed incomplete. Saline agglutinins ordinarily remain in the circulation but a few months, whereas albumin agglutinins may persist for many years. All antibody titrations are subject to considerable error unless scrupulously done, with adequate controls at each stage of the process.

Related Immunohematologic Phenomena

The so-called "blocking phenomenon" is caused by absorption of albumin-active antibodies on the red cells. Their presence inhibits the reactivity of the cells on later exposure to potent agglutinating serums.

Anti-D antibodies, often in combination with anti-C or anti-E, are responsible for most of the cases of erythoblastosis fetalis. Occasional instances of an identical illness prove referable to c or to the Kell, Kidd, or other minor blood group antigen.

Conglutination refers to the tendency of packed sensitized red cells to clump spontaneously when suspended in normal adult serum or a 20 to 30 per cent solution of bovine or human albumin. *Autoconglutination* describes this phenomenon when elicitable with the infant's own cells and serum. The tests are usually made on a slide by mixing a drop of infant's cells from a clot with an equal-sized drop of serum or albumin solution. Rouleaux formation should be ruled out by microscopic examination. *Autoagglutination* is a related phenomenon in which a small drop of cells added to a relatively large drop of saline results in clumping.

Coombs Antiglobulin Tests

In 1945 Coombs, Mourant, and Race reported that serum from rabbits immunized with human globulin would agglutinate human erythrocytes coated with Rh antibodies. This is the direct Coombs test, in which erythrocytes which carry absorbed antibody become agglutinated when mixed with such immune antiglobulin rabbit serum. The strength of the reaction is recorded as strong, moderate, or weak, depending upon the size and tenacity of the clumps.

The direct reaction is positive nearly always in erythroblastosis fetalis due to Rh incompatibility. This is both the most sensitive and the most reliable of the serologic methods for detecting Rh sensitization. The reaction is occasionally weakly positive in cases of ABO incompatibility between mother and child.

In the indirect Coombs test a serum suspected of containing an anti-Rh antibody is incubated with corresponding Rh-positive erythrocytes of a compatible ABO group. The red cells, after being washed with normal saline solution, are tested with antiglobulin rabbit serum as in the direct test. If the patient's serum contains anti-Rh antibodies, the erythrocytes absorb the antibody and are then agglutinated by the rabbit serum. This method is highly sensitive and detects antibodies in minimal concentrations. It can be made quantitative by progressive dilution of the serum with saline solution, and even more sensitive by prior exposure of the red cells to trypsin.

Relation of Maternal Rh Antibodies to Erythroblastosis Fetalis

Migration of the anti–blood group antibodies across the placenta results in erythroblastosis fetalis if the infant's red cells can react with these antibodies. The wide clinical differences in the resulting erythroblastotic process may be ascribed to several determinants: (1) the potency and character of the antibodies of the mother; (2) the extent to which these antibodies make their way across the villous barrier into the infant; and (3) the constitutional susceptibility of the erythrocytes of the fetus and the responsivity of his organ systems. Saline-active agglutinins do not pass the placental barrier as readily as the other varieties of antibodies.

Serums from sensitized mothers and transfusion recipients show great diversity in the titers of the various anti–red cell antibodies which have developed. Many of these serums are multispecific and will react with more than one of the Rh factors. The most frequent is mixed anti-C and anti-D, produced by cde/cde individuals who have been immunized by C and D. Mixed anti-D and anti-E is not uncommon, produced also by cde/cde individuals.

Application of Serologic Findings to Pregnancy

Knowledge concerning Rh sensitization has progressed to the stage where the birth of an erythroblastotic infant due to Rh incompatibility can almost always be predicted prior to delivery. It is most important to have this information in advance, since the prognosis for the affected baby is much better when treatment is begun within the first few hours after birth.

The first precaution is to determine the Rh status of every pregnant woman who reports for prenatal care. Should she be D-positive there is almost no likelihood of erythroblastosis due to Rh incompatibility developing in the fetus. Should she be D-negative, however, the Rh status of the husband must next be ascertained. If he too prove D-negative, the prospect for an erythroblastotic infant is also minimal. It is best to make these tests with anti-DC serum.

Every pregnant woman who has had a transfusion in the past should be tested for the possible presence of the various kinds of anti–red cell antibodies, employing a panel, when feasible, of red cells representing the major and minor blood types.

If the husband of a D-negative unsensitized pregnant woman is D-positive, the maternal serum should be tested for anti-D antibodies in the fourth, seventh, and ninth months, inasmuch as these antibodies may not appear until late in pregnancy. The tests should be made immediately with every D-negative mother who reports to a maternity hospital in labor and whose serum has not been tested in the preceding 5 weeks. When this cannot be done, the infant should have blood tests and be watched especially carefully during the first few days for early signs of erythroblastosis.

A rise in maternal antibody titer during pregnancy usually means progressive sensitization of the mother by a D-positive fetus and probable damage to the fetus. Erythroblastosis may develop, however, in the absence of a rise in titer.

It is unwise to make an absolute antepartum prognosis with respect to the fetus from the status of the maternal antibodies. Rh antibodies found in the maternal serum may antedate the present pregnancy. The fetus now in gestation in a D-negative woman may also be D-negative and not susceptible to the action of these antibodies. A slight rise in titer during pregnancy may be nonspecific or anamnestic in nature and may take place even with a D-negative fetus.

Rh·Hr ERYTHROBLASTOSIS FETALIS

Statistical evaluations have made it clear that most infants with Rh·Hr erythroblastosis have poorer survival rates when delivered 1 to 2 months prematurely by induced labor or elective cesarean section. It is deemed best, therefore, to permit pregnancy to continue until about the due date. An exception is made when there are reasons to expect the infant to be affected severely. During the delivery itself the maternal analgesia and anesthesia should be so regulated as to avoid even minimal anoxia or central nervous depression in the infant. Should signs of fetal distress become apparent, a cesarean section is usually advisable.

Preparations for the care of the infant should always be made ahead of time whenever maternal serologic studies give warning of probable erythroblastosis. Personnel and equipment should be ready at the time of delivery—for resuscitation, for immediate study of the baby for signs of hemodestruction, and for exchange transfusion if necessary. Unless the physician looking after the mother is well skilled in newborn care including the performance of exchange transfusion he would be wise to transfer to a pediatrician, in advance, the responsibility for management of the infant. Once an erythroblastotic infant has been delivered alive (only a minority are stillborn), the advances in therapy have reduced greatly the risk of neonatal death or permanent nervous system injury.

A tubeful of cord blood may be collected from every newborn infant in whom erythroblastosis is a possibility, including those whose prenatal care had failed to include maternal Rh studies. An unusually small clot and an unusually icteric tint in the overlying serum will be apparent if anemia and hemolysis are pronounced.

Specific treatment of erythroblastosis fetalis consists fundamentally of exchange transfusion. Other constitutional measures include oxygen, stimulants, external warmth, vitamin K, antibiotics, and similar measures.

Clinical Manifestations

Fetal hydrops is the most severe form. Such babies are usually premature and stillborn and may be born macerated; if alive when delivered they rarely survive more than a few hours. The amniotic fluid is likely to be bile-stained and excessive in amount and the placenta relatively large and heavy.

The majority of affected infants are not recognizably jaundiced at birth but become so within the first hours thereafter. This briefness of the time interval is a most important differentiating feature, since physiologic jaundice of the newborn and other causes of neonatal jaundice rarely become evident before the second day. Every infant who becomes icteric in the first 24 hours should have careful blood studies for erythroblastosis fetalis and the ABO hemolytic syndrome. Anemia in mild degree is usually demonstrable and rapidly progressive. The spleen almost always becomes palpable and the liver grows large. Bile appears in excess in the urine. After a few days the stools may become very pale or pigment-free. Hemorrhages may appear in the skin, gastrointestinal discharges, and terminally in the lungs. The jaundice may be prominent and the anemia less striking, or vice versa.

Erythroblastosis fetalis may be complicated by irritation or destruction in the central nervous system (kernicterus). Affected infants may have opisthotonus, unusual drowsiness, excessive restlessness, or crying. If death occurs, autopsy shows focal yellow staining in the nuclear masses of brain and spinal cord and in the gray matter of the cortex. Survivors are usually but not necessarily left with cerebral damage in the form of idiocy, spasticity, incoordination, or similar nervous disorders. High serum bilirubin levels seem a most significant predisposing influence (p. 165). Nuclear jaundice in early infancy may develop occasionally in other illnesses unrelated to blood group incompatibility.

Laboratory Features

Laboratory testing is of much greater assistance than clinical observation for the early diagnosis of erythroblastosis fetalis. Immediately after birth, every potentially erythroblastotic infant should receive a thorough physical examination for splenomegaly and other signs and have a blood specimen collected for determinations of Coombs responses, serum bilirubin, red cell and hemoglobin levels, and Rh typing. Venous blood is better than cord blood for these purposes, inasmuch as the latter may be contaminated by Wharton's jelly or amniotic contents. If clear signs of erythroblastosis are not apparent in the initial examinations, the studies should be repeated every few hours during the first day and at least once daily over the next few days to detect a more slowly developing process.

RH TYPING. If such an infant appears D-positive at birth, it is likely that erythroblastosis is present. However, many affected D-positive infants appear to be D-negative on initial typing because of heavy coating of the red cells with antibodies. One must remember also that erythroblastosis may be caused by blood factors outside of the Rh system.

Following an exchange transfusion or multiple simple transfusions with D-negative blood, a D-positive infant's red cells may appear D-negative for a month or more. Hyman and Sturgeon found the maximal return of D-positive reactivity was attained in the third or fourth month.

ANTIBODIES IN THE INFANT. The usual newborn D-positive infant with erythroblastosis fetalis exhibits circulating antibodies derived from the mother. The closer the infant titer approaches that of the mother, the more severe is the disease likely to be. Albumin-active agglutinins are usually, though not always, present in moderate to severe cases, and their titer is ordinarily not high. Saline agglutinins are almost never found except when the disturbance is extremely severe. Interestingly, in D-negative infants born to sensitized D-negative mothers the passively transferred maternal antibodies circulate but produce no ill effects.

The most dependable test for anti-D antibodies in the blood of the newborn is the direct Coombs test applied to the infant's washed red cells. This procedure should always be utilized, with the readings made macroscopically. A weak reading is as significant as a strong one. The finding of a positive Coombs test in association with the presence of anti-D antibodies in the maternal circulation is presumptive evidence of erythroblastosis fetalis, even when all other findings in the infant are negative. Ideally, the physician who is interested in the management of erythroblastosis fetalis and the giving of exchange transfusions should be able to carry out the Coombs test himself, since decisions frequently have to be made at night and at other times when trained technicians are not available.

The presence of *blocking* antibodies which coat the surfaces of the erythrocytes and may inhibit their agglutination will often result in clumping together (conglutination) of sensitized erythrocytes when these are suspended in vitro in an albumin preparation or the patient's own serum.

The D-positive red cells in erythroblastosis fetalis treated by simple transfusion may continue to give a positive Coombs direct test for at least 10 days after birth, and sometimes for as long as 60 days. Persistence of this reaction is not correlated with the development of late anemia. Within a few days after exchange transfusion with D-negative blood, in contrast, the test usually becomes negative.

SERUM BILIRUBIN LEVELS. The pathologically increased rate of red cell destruction in erythroblastosis fetalis is portrayed in the tendency for the serum content of bilirubin and related pigments to be enhanced at the time of delivery and to mount rapidly during the first day. These increases are in the total bilirubin; 1-minute readings are almost never elevated. In 34 infants with erythroblastosis fetalis, Hsia and associates found in cord blood a range of 2.1 to 10.3 mg per 100 ml for total serum bilirubin, with a mean of 5.1 mg. In 99 control full-term infants the cord blood content ranged from 0.2 to 5.9 mg with a mean of 1.9 mg, and in 9 premature infants was questionably less (p. 485).

With erythroblastosis fetalis the serum bilirubin typically rises with unusual rapidity and may attain levels higher than 50 mg per 100 ml within the first 24 hours when exchange transfusion is not done. The serum content of other hemoglobin pigments is elevated concomitantly. Normal full-term infants, in contrast, usually reach a peak of not more than 7 or 8 mg by the second day, and normal premature infants a peak of no more than 12 to 15 mg by about the third or fourth day.

Elevations and alterations in the serum levels of the related circulating heme pigments, derived from hemoglobin destruction, portray accurately the clinical severity of the erythroblastosis (Boggs and Abelson).

A close correlation between the development of kernicterus and the height of the bilirubin level in the first day or two has been shown by many authors. For example, Hsia and associates noted that kernicterus was not seen in infants whose initial levels before exchange transfusion were between 0 and 5 mg per 100 ml. The disturbance developed in 18 per cent with levels between 16 and 30 mg and in 50 per cent with levels above 30 mg.

Accordingly, every effort should be made to keep the serum bilirubin level below 20 mg, when necessary by repeating the exchange transfusion one or more times. In fact, current opinion is that one should not wait until the serum bilirubin level approaches this level. Any newborn infant who has a history of maternal Rh·Hr sensitization and who exhibits a positive Coombs test and abnormal serum bilirubin level at birth is best treated by an exchange transfusion within the next few hours. This precautionary management is especially necessary when anemia is also present early, or when delivery has been premature, or when a previous affected sibling has had kernicterus.

ERYTHROCYTE AND HEMOGLOBIN LEVELS. In about half the cases the blood at birth shows hemoglobin and erythrocyte levels in the low normal range. In the remainder these levels are subnormal, the reductions being related to the severity of the hemodestructive process. Severely affected hydropic infants may have hemoglobin levels as low as 4 or 5 gm per 100 ml and erythrocyte counts of 1 million per cu mm. Their serum proteins are extremely low also.

In the usual affected infant the hemoglobin and erythrocyte levels begin to decline within the first few hours. A drop of 3 to 6 gm in hemoglobin level and of 2 to 3 million in erythrocyte count during the first day is not unusual. When the hemoglobin is being measured by the Sahli or related methods, icterus of the serum may add to the pigment intensity and give a misleading high reading for hemoglobin. Mild cases when left untransfused subside more gradually; the hemoglobin may not reach a low point of, say, between 7 or 8 gm until 1 month of age. The hemoglobin and erythrocytes may drop suddenly in the second or third week after having been relatively stable for some days preceding.

ERYTHROCYTE MORPHOLOGY. Normoblasts and even the more primitive megaloblasts may be found in the peripheral blood at birth. Their number, stage of maturity, and persistence depend upon the severity of the illness and the degree of coexistent prematurity.

Nucleated erythrocytes are indistinguishable from nucleated leukocytes when doing the leukocyte count; hence a correction factor must be introduced. In the normal newborn infant the nucleated erythrocytes in the circulation rarely number more than 1 per 20 leukocytes or exceed 300 per cu mm in absolute count. In prematurity the ratio of nucleated erythrocytes to leukocytes may rise to 1:10, and the absolute count to 1,000 per cu mm. In the milder cases of erythroblastosis fetalis the nucleated erythrocytes in the circulation will often remain within normal limits. Severely affected infants may have as many as 5 or 10 nucleated erythrocytes for every leukocyte, a 5:1 or 10:1 ratio.

Correlation studies with postmortem material support the belief that the nucleated red cells in the circulation have their origin in foci of extramedullary hemopoiesis and that their disappearance coincides with the subsidence of these foci. The nucleated red cells in the bone marrow may be in normal or increased amounts.

The reticulocytes tend to be elevated and may amount to as many as 40 per cent of all the circulating red cells. Their numbers decline gradually during the first week, whether transfusions are given or not. Marked differences are seen from patient to patient with respect to the degree of anemia, the proportion of nucleated erythrocytes, and the severity of the reticulocytosis.

Another characteristic of the erythrocytes is marked variation in size. Cell diameters may range from 4 to 11 μ or more. The smaller cells often seem pale at the centers, whereas many of the largest tend to be hyperchromic and somewhat basophilic. The latter forms are the reticulocytes, which by special stains can be shown to be unusually abundant. Even in mild cases the polychromasia and unequal size distribution can be prominent. The irregularities in cell size and shape subside gradually and are no longer recognizable beyond 2 to 3 weeks of age, even when stubborn anemia persists.

ERYTHROPHAGOCYTOSIS. Phagocytosis of erythrocytes by circulating neutrophils or monocytes, usually minimal, can be demonstrated in nearly every erythroblastotic infant if exhaustive studies are made of the stained slides. The examiner should first scan the stained smear of the peripheral blood with the low-power objective, and then scrutinize all large cells with irregular outlines and suspicious contours of ingested erythrocytes with the oil-immersion lens. The phenomenon is more prominent with anti-A or anti-B than with anti-Rh or other sensitization.

OTHER LABORATORY CHANGES. In all but minimally affected cases a moderate leukocytosis is found. The platelet count is occasionally reduced. The bone marrow typically shows excessive erythropoietic hyperplasia. The bleeding and clotting times may be prolonged, in part because of reduction in blood prothrombin. The urobilinogen content of the urine may or may not be elevated; bile pigment is regularly present when the serum bilirubin is elevated.

The liver tests—serum cholesterol, alkaline phosphatase, cephalinflocculation, and galactose tolerance—usually give readings in erythroblastosis fetalis which are similar to those exhibited by normal newborns. The cholesterol ester level is sometimes very low during the height of the illness. The serum gamma globulin level, as measured by zinc sulfate turbidity, is often subnormal.

HEMOLYTIC DISEASE OF THE NEWBORN ASSOCIATED WITH MOTHER-CHILD ABO INCOMPATIBILITY

The term *heterospecific pregnancy* has been applied to those pregnancy situations in which the fetal red cells possess an A or B agglutinogen not present in the mother's red cells. These relations exist in the American population in approximately one out of every five pregnancies. As an example: when a woman is in blood group O, she will regularly have in her circulation both anti-A and anti-B antibodies (p. 131).

Diagnosis

Serologic studies have demonstrated that in most heterospecific pregnancies the titers of maternal anti-A and anti-B antibodies do not increase during gestation or after delivery. In a minority of such mothers Zuelzer and Kaplan noted a rise in titer of the antibodies antagonistic to the fetal blood group antigen with infants who were secretors belonging to subgroup A_1. These same authors found that anti-A and anti-B antibodies normally pass the placenta and are demonstrable in the infant's blood stream after birth, except when the infant possesses an A or B factor and the mother does not. This suggests that the A and B factors in the tissues of the fetus normally will neutralize any antagonistic maternal antibody which reaches them.

Occasionally, however, newborn infants will exhibit a hemolytic disturbance which inferentially seems attributable to placentally transmitted anti-A or anti-B antibodies. These disturbances occur most frequently in infants of blood group A and may be due in part to the greater prevalence of this group within the general population. As a rule the mother belongs to blood group O. It is possible theoretically for the disease to occur when a group A mother has a B or AB child or when a B mother has an A or AB child, though such instances appear to be rare. Severe disturbances ascribable to such heterospecific pregnancies are unusual, but no one knows how prevalent are the milder or subclinical instances of ABO fetal sensitization which escape detection. Many instances have been known to occur in first-born children.

Jaundice beginning in the first day of life is the most prominent symptom. Anemia is often absent, or when present tends to be mild. The red cell count often falls steadily over the ensuing few weeks, and this may lead to the need for a supportive transfusion. Hepatomegaly is minimal, and splenomegaly unusual. Kernicterus is an uncommon sequel, even in untreated cases. The disease is much less severe than erythroblastosis resulting from Rh incompatibility. Fetal hydrops is almost unknown.

Laboratory studies of the infant's peripheral smear typically reveals an easily recognized spherocytosis, a reticulocytosis up to 30 per cent, and occasional nucleated red cells. The osmotic and mechanical fragility of the red cells is increased. All such infants who develop pronounced jaundice beginning on the first day of life should be followed with repeated determinations of the total serum bilirubin. The level is usually above 5 mg per 100 ml. It is recommended that exchange transfusion be performed when the level seems to be rising near 20 mg per 100 ml, on the thesis that higher levels are conducive to brain injury and kernicterus. Group O blood (perhaps with added A or B substance) is given, provided it has a low titer or is low in anti-A or anti-B antibodies.

Symptoms ordinarily do not increase in severity with succeeding pregnancies when more than one infant is affected, unlike what occurs in erythroblastosis fetalis caused by D sensitization. Heterospecific pregnancy appears to be the most common cause of pronounced neonatal jaundice in the absence of complications—the so-called "icterus neonatorum praecox."

At present there is no single test which will establish the existence of neonatal icterus or anemia caused by ABO incompatibility. ABO differences between mother and child must be demonstrated, of course. As mentioned, the mother is typically in group O and the infant in A or B. More than half the mothers have anti-A or anti-B isohemagglutinins in the blood in a titer of 1:1,024 or higher. These differ from the normally occurring antibodies in being of higher titer at incubator than at refrigerator temperature (naturally occurring anti-A and anti-B hemagglutinins tend to show the reverse). The titer of hemagglutinins in colloid mediums may be higher than in saline. These agglutinins persist after heating or addition of Witebsky's A or B substances. Blocking antibodies may also appear. Maternal hemolysins (*isolysins*) and other complement-fixing antibodies may develop against the A or B cell group of the infant. However, none of these phenomena are sufficiently distinctive to permit of antenatal prediction of hemolytic symptoms in the infant.

With most techniques the titer of maternal isohemagglutinins is normally in the range of 1:16 to 1:256, with no relation to whether the mother is a primipara or multipara. The presence of a rise or a higher level in tests conducted during the postpartum period is not proof of an etiologic relationship to jaundice in the infant, since most women with heterospecific pregnancies exhibit rises in their anti-A or anti-B hemagglutinin titers in the few weeks after pregnancy. These rises may be from 4- to 64-fold and are thought to be more frequent with infants who are secretors. Levels of 1:12,000 or even higher by the third week of the puerperium have been reached in the absence of any recognizable effect upon the child.

The best serologic evidence for an anti-A or anti-B origin of the disturbance is the finding in the circulation of antibodies, presumably derived from the mother, which are incompatible with the infant's own ABO blood group. Typically these are in low titer and are demonstrable as saline agglutinins or by means of the indirect Coombs test using adult A or B cells. The direct Coombs test usually gives no or a questionably positive response, suggesting that the cells are only weakly coated if at all.

EXCHANGE TRANSFUSIONS

The most important measure in the treatment of Rh·Hr erythroblastosis fetalis, when the condition is recognized early, is to replace the infant's own circulating blood with that from an adult donor. The rationale is to take from the baby's circulation the maternal antibodies, the antibody-injured erythrocytes which will soon be destroyed, and especially the excess of bilirubin and toxic derivatives of hemoglobin derived from erythrocyte breakdown. For best results the exchange transfusion should be started within the first few hours after birth, and a total volume up to 500 ml of blood interchanged.

Because recognition of blood groups is difficult in the first few days of life, fresh O Rh-negative blood is advisable. Preliminary cross matching is not necessary if the donor blood can be fully established as Rh-negative by typing with anti-C, anti-D, and anti-E serum. Otherwise, donor's group O red cells may be cross-matched by the indirect Coombs technique (p. 161) with the mother's serum. The latter contains much more anti-Rh antibody then the infant's serum and has the further advantage of being available before the birth of the baby. Transfused Rh-negative red cells are much less likely to break down in the infant's circulation when Rh antibodies are present than are Rh-positive red cells.

Hypocalcemia with tetany may develop during exchange transfusions, in part as the result of the large amounts of sodium citrate or oxalate present in the donor blood. Hence calcium salts are generally given during the procedure.

To avoid the possibility of inducing hyperpotassemia, the donor blood should be no more than 5 days old. The concentration of potassium in the plasma of a stored bottle containing anticoagulant may increase from 5 up to 8 mEq per liter after 4 days and up to 12 to 20 mEq per liter after 9 to 21 days. After an exchange transfusion with old stored blood having a high potassium content, the plasma potassium level of the infant, normal at the beginning of the procedure, may be elevated to 8 mEq or more. Fresh blood has the additional advantage of surviving longer in the recipient's circulation.

The exchange transfusion may have to be repeated daily or oftener if the indications for possible injury to the central nervous system continue. Indications for repeating are (1) appearance or recurrence of signs of nervous system irritation; (2) recurrence of a rise in serum bilirubin level which promises to approach 20 mg per 100 ml, or a rise of related heme pigments; or (3) other signs of persistent hemolysis after the first exchange.

The only situation in which exchange transfusion may be omitted in early-recognized cases of Rh·Hr erythroblastosis fetalis is when a healthy-appearing full-term infant maintains, for the first 2 days, a normal hemoglobin value (above 15 gm per 100 ml) and unelevated serum bilirubin levels (less than 2.5 mg per 100 ml at birth, 6 mg at 24 hours, and 7.5 mg at 48 hours).

Exceptionally the mother of an erythroblastotic infant proves to be Rh-positive. The most frequent immunologic background is a homozygous CDE or CDe mother sensitized to c. Donor blood lacking in c is best for the exchange transfusion. If one has already been given with O Rh-negative blood, a second should be given as soon as a suitable donor can be found and cross-matched, using the mother's serum and the Coombs procedure (Boggs).

With hemolytic phenomena due to ABO incompatibility, exchange transfusions are not deemed necessary except when the serum bilirubin level approaches 20 mg per 100 ml within the first 5 days. Matched O blood of a compatible Rh type should be given.

SIMPLE TRANSFUSIONS

An exchange transfusion is of less benefit when the existence of erythroblastosis is not recognized until after the third day of life or when the symptoms after the first day are still mild and the serum pigments not appreciably elevated. A good rule is to transfuse whenever the hemoglobin level falls to 8 gm per 100 ml or the red cell count to 2.5 million. Whole blood is probably superior to red cell concentrates at this early age because of the contained normal plasma. One may administer 10 ml per kg body weight for severely ill infants, or as much as 20 ml per kg for milder cases with anemia as the prominent symptom. Sedimented or even saline-washed red cell suspensions may be given if whole-blood transfusions are followed by reactions.

The bone marrow of most infants after recovery from the acute symptoms of the first week passes through a period of erythropoietic aregeneration lasting 1 to 2 months or occasionally longer. Further transfusions become advisable if the infant becomes listless and anorexic, contracts an intercurrent infection, or develops a hemoglobin level below 7 gm per 100 ml or an erythrocyte count below 2.5 million. A mild peripheral reticulocytosis usually begins after the fourth week and reaches a peak in the second month, heralding return of bone marrow activity.

TRANSITORILY PROLONGED JAUNDICE

In about 2 per cent of infants with erythroblastosis fetalis the jaundice becomes obstructive in character. It may continue for 3 to 8 weeks and occasionally for as long as a half year. This complication is sometimes called the "inspissated bile syndrome," though parenchymal cell injury is a more likely cause. An early sign is a high in excess of 1.5 mg per 100 ml at birth or a rise in the 1-minute serum bilirubin level which becomes evident by the third or fourth day. The ratio of the 1-minute to the total serum bilirubin reading typically becomes more than 33 per cent. The stools remain steadily or intermittently bile-free for several weeks or months, and bile persists in the urine. The serum alkaline phosphatase may rise to 10 to 25 Bodansky units (normal 5 to 12 units). The results of the cephalin flocculation tests are as a rule negative. The results of the thymol turbidity test become positive in about 20 per cent of the cases. Recovery is spontaneous and complete, and the prognosis good.

ANEMIA

An infrequent sequel of erythroblastosis is a state of anemia which may last for several weeks up to 4 or 5 months before subsiding spontaneously. The onset may be insidious, with no recognizable signs of illness in the first days after delivery. Bone marrow studies show a transient erythrocytic hypoplasia of the bone marrow. Supportive transfusions may be needed. Because of the possibility of this complication the hemoglobin level should be determined once or twice weekly for several months in all Rh-positive infants with a history of maternal Rh sensitization, even when the infant was not detectably ill during the first few days.

BIBLIOGRAPHY

Rh AND Hr BLOOD TYPES

Boyd, W. C., Present Status of Rh Blood Types and Nomenclature, Am. J. Phys. Anthropol. 7:519, 1949.

DeNatale, A., A. Cahan, J. A. Jack, R. R. Race, and R. Sanger, V, a "New" Rh Antigen, Common in Negroes, Rare in White People, J.A.M.A. 159:247, 1955.

Diamond, L. K., and F. H. Allen, Jr., Rh and Other Blood Groups, New England J. Med. 241:867, 907, 1949.

Jones, A. R., L. K. Diamond, and F. H. Allen, Jr., A Decade of Progress in the Rh Blood-group System, New England J. Med. 250:283, 324, 1954.

Malone, R. H., and I. Dunsford, The Rhesus Antibody Anti-E in Pregnancy and Blood Transfusion. I. The Frequency of Occurrence of Pure Anti-E: Report of Twelve Cases, Blood 6:1135, 1951.

Marsters, R. W., The Occurrence of Erythroblastosis Fetalis in American Negroes, J. Lab. & Clin. Med. 35:544, 1950.

Mollison, P. L., A. E. Mourant, and R. R. Race, The Rh Blood Groups and Their Clinical Effects, Med. Res. Council (London) Mem. 19, 1948.

———, ———, and ———, The Rh Blood Groups and Their Clinical Effects, Med. Res. Council (London) Mem. 27, 1952.

Potter, E. L., "Rh: Its Relation to Congenital Hemolytic Disease and to Intragroup Transfusion Reactions," Year Book Publishers, Inc., Chicago, 1947.

Race, R. R., A. E. Mourant, S. D. Lawler, and R. Sanger, The Rh Chromosome Frequencies in England, Blood 3:689, 1948.

────── and R. Sanger, "Blood Groups in Man," 2d ed., Charles C Thomas, Springfield, Ill., 1954.

Rosenfield, R. E., P. Vogel, B. Miller, and G. Haber, Weakly Reacting Rh Positive (Dᵘ) Bloods, Blood 6:23, 1951.

SEROLOGY OF ERYTHROBLASTOSIS FETALIS

Chown, B., M. Lewis, and A. Bryce, On the Detection, Differentiation and Titration of Anti-Rh Antibodies, Canad. M. A. J. 59:379, 1948.

Coombs, R. R. A., A. E. Mourant, and R. R. Race, A New Test for the Detection of Weak and "Incomplete" Rh Agglutinins, Brit. J. Exper. Path. 26:255, 1945.

Davidsohn, I., and K. Stern, Interpretation of Rh Antibodies, Am. J. Clin. Path. 18:690, 1948.

Diamond, L. K., The Production and Proper Use of Rh Typing Reagents, Am. J. Pub. Health, 38:645, 1948.

Grundorfer, J., Latent Hemolytic Disease of the Newborn Infant: The Variable Quantitative Relationship between the Amount of Maternal Rh Antibodies and the Extent of Damage to the Rh-positive Infant, J. Pediat. 40:172, 1952.

──────, Hemolytic Disease of the Newborn Infant Caused by Maternal Sensitization to the Blood Factor HR′ (C): Report of Two Cases with Special Reference to the Etiologic Significance of Multiple Blood Transfusions in Rh Positive Women Prior to Gestation, Blood 7:609, 1953.

Hartmann, O., and O. J. Brandemonen, Incidence of Rh Antibody Formation in First Pregnancies: Outcome of Pregnancies in 23 Cases Not Previously Sensitized to Rh Antigens, Acta paediat. 42:20, 1953.

Jakobowicz, R., V. I. Krieger, and R. T. Simmons, The Value of the Coombs Test in Detection of Iso-sensitization of the Newborn, M. J. Australia 2:143, 1948.

Kelsall, G. A., and G. H. Vos, The Antibody Titre in Maternal and Infants Serum as an Indication for Treatment in Haemolytic Disease of the Newborn, M. J. Australia 39:349, 1952.

Krieger, V. I., and E. J. Williams, Experimental and Statistical Studies on Rh Antibodies, J. Lab. & Clin. Med. 46:199, 1955.

Rosenthal, R. E., P. Vogel, and N. Rosenthal, The Antiglobulin Test: Technic and Practical Applications, Am. J. Clin. Path. 21:301, 1951.

Wheeler, W. E., A. L. Luhby, and M. L Scholl, The Action of Enzymes in Hemagglutinating Systems. II. Agglutinating Properties of Trypsin-modified Red Cells with Anti-Rh Sera, J. Immunol. 65:39, 1950.

SERUM BILIRUBIN AND KERNICTERUS

Boggs, T. R., Jr., and N. M. Abelson, Plasma Pigments in Erythroblastosis Fetalis. II. The Level of Heme Pigment: An Early Guide to Management of Erythroblastosis Fetalis, Pediatrics 17:461, 1956.

Erythroblastosis Fetalis, Report of the Seventh M & R Pediatric Research Conference, M & R Laboratories, Columbus 16, Ohio, 1954.

Hsia, D. Y., F. H. Allen, Jr., L. K. Diamond, and S. S. Gellis, Serum Bilirubin Levels in the Newborn Infant, J. Pediat. 42:277, 1953.

──────, ──────, S S. Gellis, and L. K. Diamond, Erythroblastosis Fetalis. VIII. Studies of Serum Bilirubin in Relation to Kernicterus, New England J. Med. 247:668, 1952.

Mollison, P. L., and M. Cutbush, A Method of Measuring the Severity of a Series of Cases of Hemolytic Disease of the Newborn, Blood 6:777, 1951.

Vogel, F. S., Studies on the Pathogenesis of Kernicterus with Special Reference to the Nature of Kernicteric Pigment and Its Deposition under Natural and Experimental Conditions, J. Exper. Med. 98:509, 1953.

Waters, W. J., D. A. Richert, and *H. H. Rawson,* Bilirubin Encephalopathy, *Pediatrics* 13:319, 1954.

NEONATAL DISTURBANCES ASSOCIATED WITH ABO INCOMPATIBILITY

Crawford, H., M. Cutbush, and *P. L. Mollison,* Hemolytic Disease of the Newborn Due to Anti-A, *Blood* 8:620, 1953.

Dunn, H. G., Hemolytic Disease of the Newborn Due to ABO Incompatibility, *A.M.A. Am. J. Dis. Child.* 85:655, 1953.

Halbrecht, I., Icterus Precox: Further Studies on Its Frequency, Etiology, Prognosis and Blood Chemistry of Cord Blood, *J. Pediat.* 39:185, 1951.

Hsia, D. Y., and *S. Gellis,* Studies on Erythroblastosis Due to ABO Incompatibility, *Pediatrics* 13:503, 1954.

Robinson, G. C., R. M. Phillips, and *M. Prystowsky,* Spherocytosis and Increased Fragility Occurring in Erythroblastosis Fetalis Associated with ABO Incompatibility, *Pediatrics* 7:164, 1951.

Rosenfield, R. E., A-B Hemolytic Disease of the Newborn: Analysis of 1480 Cord Blood Specimens, with Special Reference to the Direct Antiglobulin Test and to the Group O Mother, *Blood* 10:17, 1955.

Shumway, C. N., G. Miller, and *L. E. Young,* Hemolytic Disease of the Newborn Due to Anti-A and Anti-B, *Pediatrics* 15:54, 1955.

Van Loghem, J. J., Jr., M. van der Hart, and *A. M. H. Paulussen,* Quelques considérations sur la pathogénie de la maladie hemolytique du nouveau-né, en particulier sur le mecanisme sérologique d'iso-immunization par les antigènes A et B, *Rev. hémat.* 5:371, 1950.

von Grumbach, A., and *C. Gasser,* ABO Inkompatibilitäten und Morbus Haemolyticus Neonatorum, *Helvet. paediat. acta* 3:447, 1948.

Zuelzer, W., and *E. Kaplan,* ABO Heterospecific Pregnancy and Hemolytic Disease. IV. A Study of Normal and Pathologic Variants, *A.M.A. Am. J. Dis. Child.* 88:158, 179, 307, 319, 1954.

ERYTHROBLASTOSIS FETALIS CAUSED BY OTHER BLOOD GROUPS

Davidsohn, I., K. Stern, E. R. Strauser, and *W. Spurrier,* BE, A New "Private" Blood Factor, *Blood* 8:747, 1953.

Diamond, L. K., F. H. Allen, and *W. O. Thomas, Jr.,* Erythroblastosis Fetalis: Treatment with Exchange Transfusion, *New England J. Med.* 244:39, 1951.

Levine, P., L. R. Ferraro, and *E. Koch,* Hemolytic Disease of the Newborn Due to Anti-S: A Case Report with a Review of 12 Anti-S Sera Cited in the Literature, *Blood* 7:1030, 1952.

Mollison, P. L., "Blood Transfusion in Clinical Medicine," pp. 150–179, Basil Blackwell & Mott, Ltd., Oxford (England), 1951.

MANAGEMENT OF ERYTHROBLASTOSIS FETALIS

Abelson, N. M., Erythroblastosis Fetalis, *M. Clin. North America* 37:609, 1953.

————, Erythroblastosis Fetalis, *Postgrad. Med.* 18:319, 1955.

Allen, F. H., Jr. (ed.), Erythroblastosis Fetalis: Report of the Seventh M. & R. Pediatric Research Conference, M & R Laboratories, Columbus 16, Ohio, 1954.

———— and *L. K. Diamond,* Prevention of Kernicterus; Management of Erythroblastosis Fetalis According to Current Knowledge, *J.A.M.A.* 155:1209, 1954.

Boggs, T. R., Jr., Exchange Transfusion as a Therapeutic Measure with Special Reference to Its Use in Erythroblastosis Fetalis, in "Progress in Hematology," vol. I, chap. 3, Grune & Stratton, Inc., New York, 1956.

Bolande, R. P., H. S. Traisman, and *H. F. Philipsborn, Jr.,* Electrolyte Considerations in Exchange Transfusions for Erythroblastosis Fetalis, *J. Pediat.* 49:401, 1956.

Davies, B. S., J. Gerrard, and *J. A. H. Waterhouse,* The Pattern of Hemolytic Disease of the Newborn, *Arch. Dis. Childhood* **28**:466, 1953.

Hyman, C. B., and *P. Sturgeon,* Observations on the Convalescent Phase of Erythroblastosis Fetalis, *Pediatrics* **16**:15, 1955.

Marsters, R. W., The Occurrence of Erythroblastosis in American Negroes, *J. Lab. & Clin. Med.* **35**:544, 1950.

Mollison, P. L., and *M. Cutbush,* Haemolytic Disease of the Newborn: Criteria of Severity, *Brit. M. J.* **1**:123, 1949.

—— and *M. Cutbush,* A Method of Measuring the Severity of a Series of Cases of Hemolytic Disease of the Newborn, *Blood* **6**:777, 1951.

—— and *W. Walker,* Controlled Trials of the Treatment of Hemolytic Disease of the Newborn, *Lancet* **1**:429, 1952.

Pickles, M. M., "Haemolytic Disease of the Newborn," Charles C Thomas, Springfield, Ill., 1949.

Sturgeon, P., Immunohematologic Observations on Erythroblastotic Infants. I. Diagnosis and Prognosis, *Pediatrics* **3**:318, 1949.

CHAPTER 14

Leukocytes

The leukocytes not only use the blood stream as a means of transportation, but perform a multitude of enzymatic and other functions within its current. Unfortunately the studies of their metabolism are not yet far enough along to make it possible to correlate morphologic appearances with physiologic activities. Lymphocytes found in the blood are produced chiefly, if not entirely, by the lymph nodes and other lymphatic tissues; they may be one source of antibodies. Neutrophils and other granulocytes are produced by the bone marrow; in infections and other conditions attended with necrosis of tissue one of their activities is to ingest and destroy bacterial and other foreign particles. Monocytes seem to come from the reticuloendothelial system, although their precise origins are in doubt.

The life span of the leukocytes is a matter of days. The prevailing view is that in the normal human these cells require 3 to 15 days to reach maturity in the bone marrow or lymph nodes, and then survive from a few hours to a few days after release into the circulation.

Motility, chemotaxis, phagocytosis, enzyme liberation, and antibody production are all expressions of leukocyte functioning. Diverse staining methods are being developed which can identify and localize the contained proteins, lipids, carbohydrates, inorganic substances, enzyme systems, and related substances. In unstained living cells the cytoplasmic formations which stain as granules appear as fluid droplets and may be derivatives of mitochondria. With Sudan black B the granules of granulocytes and monocytes stand out prominently, whereas those of the lymphocytes do not take the stain. Nuclear material reacts with the stains for desoxyribonucleic acids and with those for acid and alkaline phosphatase.

The lungs sequester great numbers of leukocytes. The spleen likewise has a reservoir function and is probably one graveyard for effete cells. The prompt leukocytosis and thrombocytosis which follow intravenous epinephrine were viewed in the past as manifestations of splenic contraction, but sudden emptying of the lung may participate in the phenomenon.

176

TOTAL AND DIFFERENTIAL LEUKOCYTE COUNTS

These counts are requested clinically (1) to assist in making the specific diagnosis when an illness which may induce leukocyte changes is suspected; (2) to screen every new patient, even when apparently well, to make sure he is free from some unsuspected disease involving the leukocytes such as infectious mononucleosis, leukemia, or toxic agranulocytosis from drugs; (3) as indexes to evaluate and follow the severity of any infection or other disease a patient may have.

Fluctuations in the total number of leukocytes per unit volume of blood are due to alterations in any or several major cell systems. For example, bacterial infections of more than minimal severity often begin with a neutrophilia with increase in immature forms, along with a lymphocytopenia and eosinopenia. Then, when recovery begins, these changes subside and a mild absolute monocytosis and eosinophilia may supervene.

The leukocyte and the differential counts are subject to broad variation as a consequence of four independent influences: (1) normal physiologic fluctuations in the circulating white cell population, (2) possible imperfections in the apparatus used or the technique of performance, (3) the statistical or chance error inherent in the procedures, and (4) individual deviations in the leukocytic responses to disease processes. Any suspected quantitative change in the white cells of the peripheral blood must always be interpreted with these variables in mind. Every variety of leukocyte in the circulating blood (with the possible exception of basophils) may be found also in inflammatory exudates.

The leukocyte count in the absence of a coincident differential count is useful only for detecting conditions which may lead to unusually high or unusually low total numbers. By itself it will fail to detect any disturbance which alters the morphology of the leukocytes or their differential distribution without distorting the total count beyond normal variation. More often than not, in leukemia and infectious mononucleosis the total count falls within normal limits.

Each cell strain tends to maintain its own basal zone in conditions of health and to swing up or down independently of the others in abnormal states. A moderate increase in one variety such as the neutrophil in infections or the lymphocyte in pertussis may pass unnoticed if other varieties of leukocytes chance to be low when the total is counted.

With children receiving potentially toxic drugs which may depress the granulocytes, such as sulfonamides in rheumatic fever prophylaxis or tridione for epilepsy, simple scanning of a stained blood film will give an experienced worker the necessary information with respect to possible toxic depression of the neutrophils. If the granulocytes do not seem diminished in relation to the red cells, it may be concluded that their production is not being interfered with.

Technical Variability

The same technical factors which lead to statistical variations in the red cell count are operative with leukocyte counting. The standard error of the usual total leukocyte count as made by approved methods is about 10 per cent. This means that 95 per cent of counts of mean value of 10,000 per cu mm lie within the range of 8,000 to 12,000. The normal physiologic fluctuations are so great that minor technical errors in leukocyte counting, unlike those in erythrocyte counting, are of comparatively little practical significance.

Physiologic Variability

It is highly misleading to present the expected normal leukocyte counts for children in terms of single figures. In every healthy child, and especially during the neonatal and infancy periods, the quantitative status of each leukocyte strain fluctuates erratically from hour to hour, day to day, and week to week. These fluctuations have no consistent rhythms and are not related to hour of the day, physical activity, meals, or other routine happenings. Sudden changes in total numbers may be brought about by redistribution of cells between the peripheral capillaries and the main blood vessels, or between the vascular spaces themselves and the production reservoirs of bone marrow and lymphatic system. During infancy the lymphocytes fluctuate the most widely, and the granulocytes thereafter. The extent and limits of these variations differ in different children. Hence deviations in total and differential counts must be of considerable magnitude before they can be interpreted as significantly abnormal. The average must not be viewed as being the ideal or the normal.

These generalizations are exemplified in Washburn's account of 908 serial leukocyte counts made with 20 healthy infants 2 to 26 weeks of age. The lowest total leukocyte count in the group was 5,700 per cu mm; the highest, 24,150; the average 12,196. If the top and bottom 10 percentiles are omitted in order to exclude abnormal stimuli or responses, the remaining 80 per cent of the counts spread from 8,000 to 16,500. Osgood, Baker, and associates described a range of 4,000 to 13,000 in total counts in children 8 to 14 years of age, with a mean of 8,370. Benjamin and Ward from similar experiences proposed a normal range of 7,000 to 13,000 total leukocytes for children 1 to 6 years of age; 5,000 to 12,000 for those 6 to 10 years; and 5,000 to 11,000 for those 10 to 12 years.

There seem to be no significant differences related to sex or population group in infancy and childhood. The means show only minor trends of change after 3 years of age (Table 14-1).

NEWBORN PERIOD. At the moment of birth the total count averages about 18,000 per cu mm, with a high content of neutrophils. This rises to about 20,000 or 22,000 in the first few hours and remains at this level until the

Table 14-1. Approximate Normal Values for Leukocyte Counts
in Childhood: Absolute Values

(*Number of cells per cubic millimeter*)

Age	Total leukocytes		Total neutrophils		Lymphocytes		Monocytes		Eosinophils		Blasts and unclassifiable cells		Basophils	
	Range	Av.	Range	Av.	Range	Av.	Range	Av.	Range	Av.	Range	Av.	Range	Av.
1 day	7,000–35,000	18,000	2,500–27,000	11,000	1,500–10,000	5,400	200–2,500	850	100–1,000	400	0–1,000	300	0–300	50
2 days	8,000–40,000	22,000	3,000–32,000	14,000	1,500–12,000	6,400	200–2,500	850	100–1,000	400	0–800	300	0–300	50
7–14 days	4,000–20,000	10,000	1,000–10,000	3,000	1,200–13,000	5,500	200–2,500	850	100–800	300	0–800	200	0–300	50
2 weeks–6 months	5,500–20,000	12,500	1,000–8,000	3,700	1,500–13,000	7,500	200–2,500	800	100–700	300	0–600	100	0–300	50
6 months–1 year	6,000–16,000	11,000	1,500–7,000	3,800	3,000–10,000	5,900	400–2,000	750	100–700	300	0–600	100	0–250	50
1–2 years	6,000–15,000	10,300	1,500–7,000	4,000	3,000–8,000	5,000	400–2,000	700	100–600	300	0–600	100	0–200	50
2–3 years	5,500–14,000	9,500	1,500–7,000	4,100	2,500–7,000	4,200	400–2,000	600	100–600	250	0–600	100	0–200	50
4–6 years	5,000–13,000	9,000	1,500–7,500	4,300	1,500–7,000	4,000	300–1,800	350	100–600	250	0–600	100	0–200	50
7–12 years	4,000–13,000	8,500	1,500–8,000	4,300	1,000–6,500	3,300	300–1,500	500	100–600	250	0–600	100	0–200	50
Adults (after Wintrobe)	5,000–10,000	7,000	3,200–6,200	4,300	1,500–3,000	2,000	300–500	400	100–300	200	0–600	100	15–50	25

second day. In 73 counts of 6 healthy infants studied by Washburn during the first 10 days of life the minimum was 6,400 per cu mm; the maximum 34,450; the average 15,208. The excess neutrophils are gone by the end of the first week.

THE DIFFERENTIAL COUNT

Procedure

Most routine laboratories prepare their blood films for differential counting on glass slides rather than on cover slips. For satisfactory counting the drop of blood should have spread over the greater part of the slide and be thin enough for the leukocytes to be flattened rather than rounded. Neutrophils and other large cells tend to be more abundant at the edges and tail of the film, whereas lymphocytes are more numerous in the central areas. To correct for this irregular distribution the technician should zigzag across the slide. Should preliminary inspection show an uneven spread with many of the leukocytes clumped or broken, or poorly stained so that the leukocytes are over- or undercolored, the report of percentages will not be accurate.

It is most important to scan all edges of the film. Large and unusual cells tend to be accumulated along the edges, and their presence or comparative numbers may be overlooked if merely 100 or 200 leukocytes are hastily counted. Needless to say, the oil-immersions lens and a high-power ocular are essential for conscientious scrutiny of individual cells.

Because the slide method leads to unequal dispersion of leukocytes, the more difficult cover-glass method is preferred by many experts. With this procedure the blood spreads by capillary action between the two thin cover glasses and the leukocytes are dispersed by chance distribution.

Random Variation

It has been shown statistically that when 100 cells are counted differentially on a blood film in which the white cells are distributed homogeneously (which is not always true), the statistical error is inversely proportional to the number of cells counted. Enumerating four times as many cells doubles the precision. The maximal chance error of three standard deviations is ±15 per cent when 100 cells are counted, ±11 per cent with 200 cells, and ±7.5 per cent with 400 cells. Nevertheless, in considering these limits of accuracy one must remember that approximately two-thirds of a series of counts on the same specimen will fall within ±5 per cent of the mean result and 95 per cent within ±10 per cent.

At least several hundred leukocytes must be identified before much reliance can be placed on minor deviations in the differential percentages of cell varieties which are ordinarily present in small numbers, such as monocytes, eosinophils, basophils, myelocytes, blast cells, and plasma cells. When only 100 leukocytes are studied a chance grouping of these cells may convey the misleading impression of an inordinately high proportion, or their absence may be misconstrued as a quantitative depression. The reported differences in percentages of neutrophil cells observed in vitally stained preparations as compared with films fixed with Wright's stain appear to be the result of random distribution. The dried films may contain more injured and smudged cells, but there is a question whether adult lymphocytes or adult granulocytes are more prone to rupture. Immature, injured, and abnormal cells are more fragile than mature and normal cells.

Normal Percentage Distributions

When the total of circulating leukocytes is *neither elevated nor depressed* beyond the normally wide range, the *usual* values for the different cell series are as summarized below:

NEUTROPHILS

First few days:	50–85 per cent
1 week–1 year:	30–50 per cent
1–6 years:	35–55 per cent
7–12 years:	40–60 per cent
Adolescence:	45–65 per cent

LYMPHOCYTES

First few days:	15–45 per cent
1 week–1 year:	45–65 per cent
1–6 years:	40–60 per cent
7–12 years:	35–55 per cent
Adolescence:	30–50 per cent

MONOCYTES

First few days:	1–5 per cent
1 week–6 years:	2–7 per cent
Over 6 years:	1–6 per cent

EOSINOPHILS (all ages): 1–5 per cent

BASOPHILS (all ages): Rarely exceed 1 per cent

BLAST FORMS (all ages): Rarely exceed 1 per cent

UNIDENTIFIED CELLS (all ages): Rarely exceed 1 per cent

Absolute vs. Relative Counts

The newer trend is to present the distribution of leukocytes in a blood sample in terms of absolute counts (Table 14-1). These values are derived by multiplying the percentages from the differential distribution into the total leukocyte count. A total count of 10,000 per cu mm with 60 per cent neutrophils and 40 per cent lymphocytes becomes 6,000 neutrophils and 4,000 lymphocytes. Time-consuming computations can be avoided by referral to tables calculated in advance, as in the handy brochure compiled by Waugh. The extra calculations and the chore of learning what is essentially a new vocabulary are compensated for by the much more precise information obtained.

Percentages always have to be considered in relation to the total number of leukocytes. A 20 per cent content of lymphocytes when the total count is 20,000 is numerically the same as an 80 per cent content when the total is 5,000. An eosinophil count as high as 12 per cent is well within the normal zone when the total leukocyte count is only 5,000, whereas 4 per cent represents a clearly abnormal increase when the total is 20,000 or higher. Comparisons between serial differential counts must always take into account any associated variations in the total counts.

EVALUATION OF THE BLOOD LEUKOCYTES

Neutrophils (Neutrophilic Granulocytes, Polymorphonuclear Neutrophils)

Neutrophils are subclassified according to apparent degree of maturity. Mature neutrophils measure 9 to 12 μ in diameter, usually have four nuclear segments connected by thin filaments of chromatin, and their cytoplasm contains fine refractile lipid granules which stain palely with a neutral dye. Immature neutrophils are slightly larger, with unsegmented nuclei and poorly defined granules. There is doubt whether Schilling's distinction between the so-called "degenerative" irregularly stained stab nucleus and the "regenerative" plumper and straighter nucleus with more homogeneous nucleoplasm has any validity in the pediatric period. Metamyelocytes and myelocytes are larger, have kidney-shaped or rounded nuclei, and exhibit greater basophilia of the faintly granular cytoplasm; the gradations between these two growth stages are so continuous that they are usually tabulated together as myelocytes.

Neutrophils exposed to anticoagulants such as sodium citrate or mixed oxalates very quickly undergo vacuolization, distortion of the nuclei, and other evidences of injury. For this reason films for microscopy should be prepared directly from freely bleeding skin punctures. There are no consistent differences in the total and differential counts between venous and capillary blood.

NORMAL RANGES (Table 14–1). In six healthy newborn infants Washburn found the neutrophils to vary during the first 10 days from 2,740 to 27,328 per cu mm in absolute count, or from 36.5 to 86.5 per cent of all the leukocytes, with up to one-fourth being immature cells and myelocytes. The latter forms decline rapidly during the first week. Throughout childhood the immature cells constitute less than 10 per cent and usually less than 5 per cent of all the neutrophils in the absence of stimulating disorders. Myelocytes are seen in normal blood films only sporadically.

The average absolute count of neutrophils rises slowly from about 3,700 in early infancy to about 4,300 in older childhood and adolescence. The approximate limits of normal variation for the absolute count throughout postneonatal infancy and childhood are 1,000 to 8,000 per cu mm.

NEUTROPHILIA. The absolute count of the neutrophils is high physiologically in the first 2 days of life or after protracted exercise at any age. It customarily rises in immediate response to necrosis of tissue, as in burns, abscesses, infarctions, or necrobiosis of poorly vascularized tumors. It usually mounts also in acute bacterial infections, acidosis, poisonings, dehydrative states, uremia, intestinal obstructions, and granulocytic (myelocytic) leukemia; after operations or hemorrhages or convulsive seizures; as an accompaniment to hyperactive hemopoiesis in the hereditary anemias and the more acute hemolytic disturbances; in the course of paroxysmal tachycardia; and as a complication of emotional reactions associated with pain, fear, and related stimuli.

In hospital practice the most frequent cause of neutrophilic leukocytosis is an infection with the so-called pyogenic bacteria, whether such organisms are free in the circulation or localized in an inflamed area. Staphylococci, streptococci, pneumococci, meningococci, influenza, colon and Proteus bacilli, and other less common pathogens are familiar causative agents. The stimulus appears to be a cellular product such as *leukotaxine*, and the purpose is phagocytosis of the bacteria. The leukocytosis usually begins within a few hours after the onset of the infection and continues for its duration. A steadily rising or persistent neutrophilia usually means localization and good resistance. A marked decline after an initial rise denotes either the beginning of recovery, a poor bone marrow response, or excessive demand of the inflamed tissue for more cells.

Whenever a leukocytosis is severe or prolonged the percentage of immature neutrophils increases—the so-called "shift to the left"—and toxic granules or vacuoles may appear within the cells. In general, the intensity of these changes reflects the severity of the infection. An extreme degree of neutrophilic leukocytosis is often termed a "leukemoid reaction"; the bone marrow in this circumstance typically displays a pronounced granulocytic hyperplasia. In the leukocytosis associated with hemorrhage or increased blood destruction immature forms are abundant but toxic granulations and vacuoles are lacking.

In adult patients, a neutrophilic increase is believed to confirm the diagnosis of acute appendicitis whenever the history and physical findings are suggestive. Not much reliance can be placed on this test during childhood. The dehydration and acidosis which accompany many nonappendiceal gastroenteritides also call forth a neutrophilia; conversely, inflammation in the appendix often fails to evoke this response.

Neutrophilia is seen in less than half the children with typhoid fever. Most viral diseases do not cause neutrophilia unless bacteria become secondary invaders. Chronic low-grade bacterial inflammation of the skin, tonsils, nasal sinuses, or kidneys and infections with brucella, tuberculosis, syphilis, malaria, and most other parasitic diseases usually are not accompanied by neutrophilia.

Granulocytic leukemia in childhood is characterized as much by qualitative abnormalities in cellular appearance and infiltrations of organs as by any striking increase in total granulocyte count (p. 212). One is as likely to encounter a depression as an elevation of the total neutrophil count.

NEUTROPENIA (NEUTROPHILOPENIA). With hypoplastic or infiltrative states of the bone marrow, depression of the peripheral neutrophil count may be a manifestation either of imperfect or inadequate granulocyte formation or of failure of the release mechanisms in the bone marrow. With overwhelming infection, anaphylactic shock, and splenic hyperactivity this may be ascribable, at least in part, to the accelerated removal of these cells in peripheral structures. The pathogenesis of the chronic neutrophilopenia sometimes seen in thyrotoxicosis, brucellosis, typhoid fever, and disseminated lupus erythematosus is as yet not well understood. A low neutrophil count rarely will accompany severe malnutrition.

Severe depression of granulocyte formation or release (*agranulocytosis*) may be seen in or in association with lymphocytic leukemia; treatment with nitrogen mustards, radioactive phosphorus, or irradiation; severe bacterial infections; or exposure to compounds of gold, arsenic, or bismuth or to radium or other radioactive substances. It has been observed also as a sign of sensitization to drugs of organic nature such as sedatives, salicylates, amidopyrine, sulfonamides, diuretics, thiouracil, nitrogen mustard, antiepileptic drugs, and chloramphenicol. Some instances cannot be attributed to any drug or toxin.

In agranulocytosis the pattern of bone marrow response is not constant. Most often one finds hypercellularity of the granulocyte precursors with arrest of cell development at the myelocyte level—the so-called "maturation arrest." When the marrow has an aplastic appearance the outcome is likely to be fatal. The dissimilarities in the reported marrow patterns of drug-sensitivity states are due both to individual variations in the severity of the disease and to differences in the times at which specimens have been examined in relation to the course of the disease.

Symptoms which should lead the clinician to suspect the development of sensitization in a patient receiving medications or exposed to potential poisons are fatigue, malaise, fever, or acute sore throat. The symptoms develop later than the reduction of the neutrophils and are frequently irreversible; hence the importance of doing frequent blood counts in all such patients. There is usually little or no anemia, and the platelets are normal at first.

Frequent examinations of the neutrophil status are advisable while potentially hemotoxic drugs are being administered, in order to guard against the complication of agranulocytosis or aplastic anemia. Such supervision is obligatory when the history states that the drug had been given previously and had had to be discontinued because of a probable sensitivity reaction. Agranulocytosis is usually the first overt sign of a beginning generalized bone marrow depression.

The author has set up the following principles for his own guidance: (1) Almost never are a child's granulocytes sensitive congenitally to a potentially injurious drug. Hence any such drug, if never before received, may be taken for a short span of 3 to 7 days without immediate anxiety or need for special blood counts. (2) If such a drug has to be given continuously for a protracted period, or intermittently on repeated occasions, it is advisable to survey peripheral blood smears for granulocytes at intervals of once or twice a week for the first few weeks. Should no granulocyte depression appear during this period the counts may then be done every 2 to 4 weeks. The patient and his parents should be informed that if a sore throat, fever, or hemorrhagic rash develops, the drug should be stopped and the physician notified at once. (3) It has been argued that agranulocytosis-producing drugs injure the bone marrow before the peripheral blood undergoes detectable changes and that serial leukocyte counts not only fail to prevent the development of the condition but induce a false sense of security. In answer to this objection, which is essentially sound, one replies that late is better than never and that the outlook for the patient is better if the agranulocytosis or bone marrow aplasia is detected in its earliest phase. The outlook for recovery from agranulocytosis is better than from complete bone marrow aplasia, provided the offending agent can be identified and removed. (4) During the height of a period of neutropenia there is unusual susceptibility to bacterial infections. The child should be shielded as much as possible and given some antibiotic prophylactically to which he is not sensitive.

MORPHOLOGIC CHANGES. Qualitative peculiarities in the circulating granulocytes often appear in fluid imbalances and related conditions. The changes which are important features of granulocytic leukemia and are seen at times in some anemias are discussed under those headings. In dehydration and acidosis the nuclei may become compact and irregularly deeply staining. The so-called "vacuoles" are small unstainable rounded aggregations of lipid or mucoprotein which may appear in either the nucleus or cytoplasm of almost any variety of leukocyte during disease states. In lupus erythematosus the granulocytes and sometimes the monocytes can be shown to be able to engulf and destroy leukocytes in vitro (p. 225). Some nuclear changes relate to sex (p. 753).

Toxic granulations are deeply staining basophilic granules of varying size which may appear in the cytoplasm of the neutrophils, and sometimes of monocytes also, in infective, toxemic, and neoplastic states. They are intermingled with the normal granules. When very abundant the cell may simulate a basophil. Such affected neutrophils may exhibit also some pyknotic changes in the nucleus, vacuoles in nucleus or cytoplasm, or irregular blue-staining cytoplasmic areas known as Dohle bodies. Toxic granulations do not react with the peroxidase stain.

Granulocytes with nuclei hypersegmented into 6 to 12 lobes—so-called polycytes—may be seen during recovery from infections and in macrocytic or chronic anemias. Such cells may be extremely large, unusually small, or irregular in shape.

The Pelger-Huët anomaly of the neutrophils is characterized by permanently defective or absent lobulation of the nuclei in individuals otherwise asymptomatic. It is transmitted genetically as a simple mendelian dominant, not sex-linked.

In lipochondrodystrophy (gargoylism), the neutrophils and even a few of the lymphocytes sometimes contain coarse azurophilic granules. These are not present in all cases, but when seen are distinctive of this disease.

Lymphocytes

Lymphocytes are produced within the innumerable foci of lymphoid tissue in all regions of the body. They reach the blood stream directly from these sites or indirectly by way of the thoracic ducts. Once in the circulation they survive for a few days.

Enormous numbers of lymphocytes are distributed through the bone marrow spaces in childhood (10 to 40 per cent of all nucleated cells), where the absence of mitotic figures and the scanty cytoplasm suggest that these are senile forms of hematogenous origin rather than proliferating locally. The relationships between the lymphocytes of the connective tissue and those of the blood stream are obscure. Lymphocytes occur in abundance in the mucosa and submucous tissues of the stomach and intestines and are excreted therefrom into the intestinal lumen, but total surgical excision of the stomach and intestines in animals is not followed by a rise in the content of these cells in the blood.

One major function of the lymphocytes in the body economy seems to be the formation and later release of beta and gamma globulins related to immune and hypersensitivity reactions. A peripheral lymphocytopenia and shrinkage of the lymphatic structures including the thymus gland may follow acute stimulation of the adrenal cortex either pharmacologically or by some infections. Diminution in production of the adrenocortical hormones may be followed by hyperplasia and increase in weight of the lymphoid structures.

NOMENCLATURE. The small or so-called "adult" lymphocyte measures only 7 to 10 μ in stained films and is only slightly larger than a red cell. Its round nucleus has deeply staining chromatin of variable pattern, and its scanty cytoplasm may stain either light or dark blue with Wright's stain. A few azurophilic or deep-blue lipid granules may be seen in the cytoplasm.

The large lymphocyte varies in size from 10 to 18 μ. The nucleus is rounded, and its chromatin less deeply stained. In older children and adult subjects some authors differentiate "large" from "young" lymphocytes. Large forms are said to have a nucleus slightly bigger than that of the small lymphocytes; their cytoplasm is more abundant, stains a clear light blue, and also may contain azurophilic granules. Young forms are said to be those having a larger nucleus which fills most of the cell and scanty cytoplasm which stains deep blue and is free of granules. So many gradations and intermediate forms are to be found in the blood stream of infants and small children that this morphologic distinction seems impractical in pediatrics. The frequent occurrence of "atypical" large forms in the childhood years confuses the differentiation further. Because it has not been established that greater size or proportion of cytoplasm always means an earlier stage of maturity or a different origin or function, we prefer to subclassify the normal lymphocytes simply as "large" and "small."

Lymphoblasts are not seen in the circulation except in lymphocytic leukemia or in leukemoid reactions involving this cell series. The lymphoblast is of inconstant size and has a red-purple-staining nucleus with fine chromatin and one or several nucleoli. The cytoplasm may be abundant or scanty, stains dark blue, and may have a clear perinuclear zone. Granules are not present.

NORMAL RANGES. (Table 14–1). Lymphocytes are at their maximum during the first half year of life and recede gradually as the child grows. The normal range is extremely wide in early infancy, extending from about 1,200 up to 13,000 per cu mm. At 1 to 2 years the usual range is 2,000 to 8,000; at 7 to 12 years, 1,000 to 6,500. The proportion of large to small lymphocytes is also greatest in early infancy, where the larger forms may comprise up to 50 per cent or more of the total. Beyond infancy these larger forms become less numerous and above 6 years constitute a negligible percentage.

LYMPHOCYTOSIS. The usual childhood conditions which evoke a lymphocytosis are pertussis, infectious mononucleosis, acute infectious lymphocytosis, hyperthyroidism, lymphocytic leukemia, and leukosarcoma. The lymphocytosis which is described as accompanying typhoid fever, brucellosis, tuberculosis, rickets, and malnutritional states usually proves to be relative—a comparative neutrophilopenia makes the lymphocyte percentage seem high in the differential count, yet on calculation the absolute lymphocyte count falls within normal limits.

In many viral diseases the lymphocytes fall during the initial febrile period, and then rise sharply above normal during the first week of convalescence. During and immediately after the illness many of these cells may have an "atypical" appearance (see p. 188).

In pertussis the lymphocytes usually amount to 7,000 to 20,000 per cu mm in absolute numbers, though readings as high as 120,000 are not rare. The cells are of the small or "mature" type, with scanty cytoplasm and deeply staining nuclei. Discussed elsewhere are the lymphocytosis of infectious mononucleosis (p. 203), acute infectious lymphocytosis (p. 223), and lymphocytic leukemia (p. 213).

LYMPHOCYTOPENIA. The administration of cortisone, or of corticotropin in the presence of functioning adrenals, is usually followed by a diminution in lymphocyte count, though the lymphocytopenia will not be as marked as the eosinophilopenia produced simultaneously. Generally speaking, the lymphocyte count reaches approximately half its former level in an hour or two after an injection of such hormone and returns gradually to normal over 6 to 8 hours. Lymphocytes within the lymph nodes may be similarly affected.

Many stimuli of nonspecific character have been shown experimentally to stimulate the adrenal cortex. The liberated secretions then serve to decrease the number of blood lymphocytes and induce involution of the lymphoid organs. This is what appears to take place at times in diverse constitutional disturbances associated with shock or stress states, such as acute appendicitis, acute cholecystitis, acute pancreatitis, and intestinal obstruction. Lymphocytopenia may also be induced by excessive irradiation, nitrogen mustard administration, Hodgkin's disease, circulatory failure, overwhelming toxic states, and terminal nephritis or tuberculosis.

ATYPICAL LYMPHOCYTES (TOXIC OR IMMATURE LYMPHOCYTES, "STRESS" LYMPHOCYTES, "TÜRK" CELLS, "VIROCYTES"). Variations in size and appearance of some of the large lymphocytes often become apparent during or immediately after some viral diseases. The nuclear contours tend to become irregular, and the chromatin may have an evenly granular distribution. The cytoplasm may be deeply basophilic and coarsely granular or clear and pale-staining; vacuolations or fenestrations or fine red-staining granules may be present. The margins may be irregular, as if the cell substance were unusually flexible. Similar cells are often found in the peripheral sinuses of biopsied lymph nodes, suggesting the site of origin. A blood film which contains these cells in large numbers may be suggestive of infectious mononucleosis or even leukemia. The differentiation may have to be established by heterophil antibody response or bone marrow examination. The so-called "irritation forms of Türk" resemble plasma cells or large lymphocytes in having homogeneous basophilic cytoplasm and a round nucleus with fine chromatin. It has been suggested by Frank and Dougherty that this type of large lymphocyte appears in the circulation as a response to stress.

Atypical lymphocytes are not restricted to the virus diseases. Serum sickness, miliary tuberculosis, and assorted other illnesses will sometimes evoke them in appreciable numbers. Occasional ones are seen at times in the blood of apparently well children; inquiry will often elicit a history of a respiratory tract infection a week or so previously. Some authors deem that such patients are having unsuspected attacks of infectious mononucleosis even when the heterophil antibody responses are negative. It is our opinion that the diagnosis of infectious mononucleosis should be restricted to patients having characteristic symptoms including lymph node enlargement and at least 1,000 atypical lymphocytes in the absolute count. With these criteria a positive heterophil reaction is nearly always found. We have several times seen children who during a respiratory tract infection had small numbers of atypical lymphocytes in the blood and who a year or two later experienced an unequivocal attack of infectious mononucleosis. Their heterophil antibody reactions were negative during the first illness, but positive during the second.

Monocytes

MORPHOLOGY. Monocytes measure 12 to 20 μ in a blood smear. The nucleus tends to be round, oval, branched or kidney-shaped, with lacy, lightly staining chromatin. The cytoplasm is gray or gray-blue with Wright's stain and may contain fine pink or purple granules in groups. Most of these granules will not take the peroxidase stain. During infancy many of the monocytes have coarse azurophilic cytoplasmic granules and deeply staining nuclei of inconstant shape and may resemble the myelocyte or immature neutrophil. Another variant less frequently seen is an agranular monocyte with round, kidney-shaped, or bilobed nucleus. This may be mistaken for a large or atypical lymphocyte, but its nucleus is paler-staining and the cytoplasm less blue and homogeneous.

NORMAL RANGES (Table 14-1). The absolute count ranges from 1,500 to 2,000 per cu mm during infancy and childhood. The mean subsides slowly from about 850 in the early years to 500 at the beginning of adolescence.

MONOCYTOSIS. An increase above normal range sometimes takes place in tuberculosis, brucellosis, subacute bacterial endocarditis, staphylococcal sepsis, typhoid fever, poisonings, chronic malaria and other protozoan diseases, Vincent's stomatitis, Gaucher's disease, monocytic leukemia, agranulocytosis, and the monocytoid variant of lymphocytic leukemia. During the acute stage of many viral and bacterial infections, the total number of monocytes is usually moderately depressed and young and binucleated or dividing monocytes may appear in the peripheral blood. Immediately after, during recovery, a mild increase above normal may occur. In tuberculosis the monocytosis may amount to as much as 1,000 to 3,000 absolute count, with or without an accompanying neutrophilic leukocytosis. The monocytes in this disease may be irregular and epithelioid in appearance.

A monocytosis is generally regarded as an unfavorable prognostic sign in tuberculosis, whereas a lymphocytosis is believed to indicate that the lesions are healing. The monocyte-lymphocyte relation has thus been employed to follow the progress of tuberculosis patients. The average M:L ratio or "index" is approximately 2.9; an increase above 3.2 is regarded as "favorable," whereas a decline to below 2.6 is regarded as "unfavorable."

Basophils

These are 10 to 12 μ in size and have lobulated nuclei similar to those of the neutrophils. Their cytoplasm is filled with large rounded granules of unequal size which stain purple or blue-black and may overlap the nucleus in the stained film. They vary from 0 to 300 per cu mm in absolute count, though usually about 50. Their function is not known but may have something to do with the formation of heparin-like substances. Basophilia is seen occasionally in smallpox, chickenpox, Hodgkin's disease, leukemoid responses, and chronic granulocytic leukemia.

Blast Cells

These appear in the blood films as immature leukocytes too undifferentiated to be subclassifiable as lymphoblasts, myeloblasts, or monoblasts. From 12 to 30 μ in diameter, they have large round or oval deeply staining nuclei with one to four nucleoli and deep-blue-staining blurred cytoplasm which is often scanty in amount. They are seen most often in infancy and may be evoked by all disturbances which induce highly abnormal leukocytic pictures. Normally they constitute less than 1 per cent of all circulating leukocytes.

Endothelial Cells and Histiocytes

These large irregular or elongated cells of the reticuloendothelial system are often classified as and grouped with monocytes. Their nuclei, occasionally eccentric, are round or oval and may contain one or more nucleoli. Their cytoplasm with Wright's stain is pale blue and finely granular. They appear not uncommonly in the blood stream during subacute bacterial endocarditis and other chronic infections. In hemolytic disorders an occasional cell may contain phagocytosed red cells or hemosiderin pigment.

When found in normal blood, they may be derived from the endothelial lining of blood vessels, torn away by the puncturing needle. Hence it is advisable to wipe away and discard the first drop of blood oozing from a skin puncture or always to use a sharp needle when smears are being made from venous blood.

Megakaryocytes

Rarely one will find in the blood film an overlarge leukocyte with pale-staining gray-blue cytoplasm which may be studded with tiny clumps of azurophilic granules. The nucleus is vesicular and irregular and stains purple or lavender with Wright's stain. Such cells presumably are megakaryocytes escaped from the marrow. They are not uncommon in the blood of infants in the first month or two of life.

Plasma Cells

Plasma cells are small and oval; they have eccentric round nuclei with coarse chromatin clumping and gray-blue-staining cytoplasm which may contain acidophil mucoproteinous inclusions known as Russell bodies. Almost never present in the peripheral blood during health, they appear occasionally in German measles, scarlet fever, chickenpox, multiple myeloma, and leukemoid or aplastic states of the bone marrow. Plasma cell leukemia is almost unheard of before adult life.

Rieder Cells

These are large monocyte-like cells, 14 to 20 μ across, which appear in the blood in small numbers in chronic infections. The nuclei are lobulated or convoluted with fine pale-staining chromatin. The cytoplasm is homogeneous and moderately basophilic and may contain fine azurophilic granules.

BIBLIOGRAPHY

LEUKOCYTE COUNTING AND NORMAL VARIATION

Barnett, C. W., The Unavoidable Error in the Differential Count of the Leukocytes of the Blood, *J. Clin. Invest.* **12**:77, 1933.

Berkson, J., T. B. Magath, and *M. Hurn,* The Error of Estimate of the Blood Cell Count as Made with the Hemocytometer, *Am. J. Physiol.* **128**:309, 1940.

Finch, S. C., J. E. Ross, and *F. G. Ebaugh,* Immunologic Mechanisms of Leukocyte Abnormalities, *J. Lab. & Clin. Med.* **42**:555, 1953.

First Report of the Committee for Clarification of the Nomenclature of Cells and Diseases of the Blood and Blood-forming Organs Sponsored by the American Society of Clinical Pathologists and the American Medical Association, *Am. J. Clin. Path.* **18**:443, 1948.

Gordon, A. S. (ed.), Leukocytic Functions, *Ann. New York Acad. Sci.,* vol. 59, art. 5, 665–1070, 1955.

Kato, K., Leukocytes in Infancy and Childhood: A Statistical Analysis of 1,081 Total and Differential Counts from Birth to Fifteen Years, *J. Pediat.* **7**:7, 1935.

Kowalski, H. J., W. E. Reynolds, and *D. D. Rutstein,* Changes in White Blood Cell Counts after Administration of Cortisone Acetate to Healthy Ambulatory Individuals, *J. Lab. & Clin. Med.* **40**:841, 1952.

Lippman, H. S., A Morphologic and Quantitative Study of the Blood Corpuscles in the New-born Period, *Am. J. Dis. Child.* **27**:473, 1924.

Lucey, H. C., Fortuitous Factors Affecting the Leucocyte Count in Blood from the Ear, *J. Clin. Path.* 3:146, 1950.

MacGregor, R. G. S., W. Richards, and *G. L. Loh,* The Differential Leukocyte Count, *J. Path. & Bact.* 51:337, 1940.

Menkin, V., and *M. A. Kadish,* Studies on Physiological Effects of Leukotaxine, *Am. J. Physiol.* 124:524, 1938.

Osgood, E. E., R. L. Baker, I. E. Brownlee, M. W. Osgood, D. M. Ellis, and *W. Cohen,* Total, Differential and Absolute Leukocyte Counts and Sedimentation Rates for Healthy Children, *Am. J. Dis. Child.* 58:282, 1939.

Rebuck, J. W., The Functions of the White Blood Cells, *Am. J. Clin. Path.* 17:614, 1947.

Schilling, V., "The Blood Picture and Its Clinical Significance," 7th and 8th eds., The C. V. Mosby Company, St. Louis, 1929.

Small, C. S., and *G. G. Hadley,* Leukocytes in "Virus X" Infection, *California Med.* 70:205, 1949.

Squier, T. L., Variations in Circulating White Blood Cells after Specific and Nonspecific Stimuli, *J. Allergy* 22:82, 1951.

Valentine, W. N., Quantitative Biochemical Studies on Leukocytes in Man: A Review, *Blood* 6:845, 1951.

Washburn, A. H., Blood Cells in Healthy Young Infants. I. The Leukocyte Picture during the First Three Months with Special Reference to Hourly and Daily Variations, *Am. J. Dis. Child.* 47:993, 1934.

——, Blood Cells in Healthy Young Infants. III. A Study of 608 Differential Leukocyte Counts, with a Final Report on 908 Total Leukocyte Counts, *Am. J. Dis. Child.* 50:413, 1935.

Waugh, T. R., "White Blood Cell Differential Tables," Appleton-Century-Crofts, Inc., New York, 1943.

Wegelius, R., On the Changes in the Peripheral Blood Picture of the Newborn Infant Immediately after Birth, *Acta paediat.,* vol. 35, suppl. 4, 1948.

GRANULOCYTES

Allen, J. G., P. V. Moulder, and *D. M. Enerson,* Pathogenesis and Treatment of the Postirradiation Syndrome, *J.A.M.A.* 145:704, 1951.

Bierman, H. R., R. L. Byron, Jr., and *K. H. Kelly,* The Role of the Spleen in the Leukocytosis Following the Intra-arterial Administration of Epinephrine, *Blood* 8:153, 1953.

——, *K. H. Kelly, F. L. Cordes, R. L. Byron, J. A. Polhemus,* and *S. Rappoport,* The Release of Leukocytes and Platelets from the Pulmonary Circulation by Epinephrine, *Blood* 7:683, 1952.

——, ——, ——, *N. L. Petrakis, H. Kass,* and *E. L. Shpil,* The Influence of Respiratory Movements upon Circulating Leukocytes, *Blood* 7:533, 1952.

Bruck, E., Agranulocytosis in Childhood: Report of a Case with Serial Bone Marrow Studies, *Am. J. Dis. Child.* 73:186, 1947.

Doan, C. A., The White Blood Cells in Health and Disease, *Bull. New York Acad. Med.* 30:415, 1954.

Haunz, E. A., J. D. Cardy, and *C. M. Graham,* Agranulocytosis Due to Gantrisin: Report of a Case with Recovery, *J.A.M.A.* 144:1179, 1950.

Hilts, S. V., and *C. C. Shaw,* Leukemoid Blood Reactions, *New England J. Med.* 249:434, 1953.

Jonsson, E., L. Boström, and *B. Bringel,* Pelger-Huët's Anomaly of the Nuclei of the Leucocytes, *Acta med. scandinav.* 131:380, 1948.

Kostmann, R., Infantile Genetic Agranulocytosis: A New Recessive Lethal Disease in Man, *Acta paediat.* suppl. 105, 1956.

Lawrence, J. S., W. S. Adams, and *W. N. Valentine,* White Blood Cell Changes in Clinical Disorders, *J.A.M.A.* 150:454, 1952.

Meranze, D. R., T. H. Mendell, and *T. Meranze,* Cytoplasmic Changes in the Peripheral Neutrophil as an Aid in Diagnosis and Prognosis, *Am. J. M. Sc.* 189:639, 1935.

Ponder, E., The Polycyte, *J. Lab. & Clin. Med.* 27:866, 1942.

────── and *R. Ponder,* The Cytology of the Polymorphonuclear Leukocyte in Toxic Conditions, *J. Lab. & Clin. Med.* 28:316, 1942.

Price, W. C., and *M. E. Frank,* Accidental Acute Dilantin Poisoning: Report of a Case with Complete Recovery in a Nonepileptic Child, *J. Pediat.* 36:652, 1950.

Reilly, W. A., The Granules in the Leukocytes in Gargoylism, *Am. J. Dis. Child.* 62:489, 1941.

Sanford, H. N., The Polymorphonuclear Count in the Newborn. I. Preliminary Report, *Am. J. Dis. Child.* 38:271, 1929.

──────, *D. F. Eubank,* and *F. Stenn,* Chronic Panniculitis with Leucopenia (Weber-Christian Syndrome), *A.M.A. Am. J. Dis. Child.* 83:156, 1952.

Slobody, L. B., H. Abramson, and *L. S. Loizeaux, Jr.,* Agranulocytosis of the Newborn Infant, *J.A.M.A.* 142:25, 1950.

Sutro, C. J., Cytoplasmic Changes in Circulating Leukocytes in Infection, *Arch. Int. Med.* 51:747, 1933.

Yamasowa, Y., T. Fujii, and *K. Tsuchitori,* The Pelger-Huët Familial Anomaly of Leukocytes, *Blood* 8:370, 1953.

Young, C. J., Leucocyte Counts in the Prevention of Drug Agranulocytosis, *Brit. M. J.* 2:261, 1949.

LYMPHOCYTES

Benjamin, B., and *S. M. Ward,* Leukocytic Response to Measles, *Am. J. Dis. Child.* 44:921, 1932.

Frank, J. A., and *T. F. Dougherty,* The Assessment of Stress in Human Subjects by Means of Quantitative and Qualitative Changes of Blood Lymphocytes, *J. Lab. & Clin. Med.* 42:538, 1953.

Hirst, A. E., Jr., and *V. J. Johns,* Lymphopenia in Diagnosis of the Acute Abdomen, *Am. J. M. Sc.* 223:548, 1952.

Keuning, F. J., The Role of Immature Plasma Cells, Lymphoblasts and Lymphocytes in the Formation of Antibodies, as Established in Tissue Culture Experiments, *J. Lab. & Clin. Med.* 36:167, 1950.

Litwins, J., and *S. Leibowitz,* Abnormal Lymphocytes ("Virocytes") in Virus Diseases Other Than Infectious Mononucleosis, *Acta haemat.* 5:223, 1951.

Shillitoe, A. J., The Common Causes of Lymphopenia, *J. Clin. Path.* 3:321, 1950.

Valentine, W. N., C. G. Craddock, and *J. S. Lawrence,* Relation of Adrenal Cortical Hormone to Lymphoid Tissue and Lymphocytes, *Blood* 3:729, 1948.

Williamson, R., The Production of Cytoplasmic Bodies by Lymphocytes, *J. Path. & Bact.* 62:47, 1950.

Wiseman, B. K., Lymphopoiesis, Lymphatic Hyperplasia and Lymphemia: Fundamental Observations Concerning the Pathologic Physiology and Interrelationships of Lymphatic Leukemia, Leukosarcoma and Lymphosarcoma, *Ann. Int. Med.* 9:1303, 1936.

Yoffey, J. M., The Mammalian Lymphocyte, *Biol. Rev.* 25:314, 1950.

MONOCYTES AND HISTIOCYTES

Falkenberg, T., Macrophages in the Peripheral Blood in Staphylococcic Sepsis, *Acta path. et microbiol. scandinav.* 24:1, 1947.

Orchard, N. P., Letterer-Siwe's Syndrome: Report of a Case with Unusual Peripheral Blood Changes, *Arch. Dis. Childhood* 25:151, 1950.

Shanberge, J. N., Accidental Occurrence of Endothelial Cells in Peripheral Blood Smears, *Am. J. Clin. Path.* 25:460, 1955.

Tompkins, E. H., The Response of Monocytes to Adrenal Cortical Extract, *J. Lab. & Clin. Med.* 39:365, 1952.

CHAPTER 15

Eosinophils and Eosinophilia

PHYSIOLOGY

The eosinophils of the peripheral blood are normally derived from the eosinophilic myelocytes of the bone marrow, though it has been suggested that an increased peripheral count in some disturbances may be caused in part by an overflow from local proliferation in the tissue spaces.

The principal physiologic functions of eosinophils seem to be in connection with removal, detoxication, or protection against certain poorly defined classes of foreign substances. The pituitary-adrenal mechanisms play a role in regulating their level in the circulation. They possess the power of phagocytosis and are more sluggish in movement than neutrophils. Iron oxides, peroxidase, and histamine have been described in their substance. Charcot-Leyden crystals appear to be crystalline proteins derived from the nuclei.

Eosinophils in the blood can be enumerated either (1) by indirect calculation from the differential count and the total leukocyte count, or (2) by direct counting with a hemocytometer, using special diluting and staining fluids. The hemocytometric method is more rapid and by far the more accurate in experienced hands. The absolute level of eosinophils is unrelated to the total leukocyte count.

Experiments by Essellier and associates indicate that the total life span of the normal eosinophil from formation in the bone marrow to disappearance from the circulation is about 6 days, and the life expectancy once they have passed into the tissues 1 to 2 days.

With peripheral eosinophilia of any duration the marrow usually shows an increased content of eosinophilic myelocytes, but the correlation between the intensity of eosinophilia in blood and bone marrow is not always close. When a shocklike stimulus or a specific tissue injury causes the circulating eosinophils to fall, the bone marrow responds by an enhanced rate of production about 12 hours later. After the stimulus or tissue need has subsided the blood level tends to remain unusually elevated for a week.

NORMAL VALUES

There is marked daily fluctuation in the absolute eosinophil level. In the mean curves from a large series of adult studies, Rud found a mid-morning drop of about 20 per cent from the 8 A.M. level. This was followed by a return to that level at noon and a steady rise thereafter to approximately 30 per cent higher after midnight. The rise then gradually disappeared. With single individuals, however, the variations in the eosinophil levels usually show no consistent diurnal trend. Occasional normal subjects will spontaneously exhibit an increase or diminution of more than 50 per cent within a 4-hour period for no apparent reason. Meals and physical activity seem to have no relation to these fluctuations.

Most healthy infants and children in random tests show absolute counts between 80 and 500 per cu mm. About 600 or 700 per cu mm may be taken as the approximate top normal. This is 6 or 7 per cent of the differential when the total leukocyte count is 10,000. It is apparent that the diagnosis of eosinophilia in childhood is made more often than actually warranted.

When the eosinophil count is in the normal range the forms in the circulation are typically mature and multilobulated, with only 1 or 2 per cent being immature or stab forms. When eosinophilia exists, however, the number of immature forms is proportional to the increase in the absolute count. When the eosinophils number over 10,000, as many as 20 per cent may be immature.

During the neonatal period the counts of these cells are possibly a little higher than later in childhood. The values for newborn infants in the first 24 hours of life in published series have spread from 200 to 600 per cu mm, with extreme single readings from 20 to 1,150.

Minor traumatic experiences such as lumbar punctures and intramuscular and intravenous injections are followed by mild transitory drops in the eosinophil count, according to the studies of Naiden and Ross. These eosinophil falls last an hour or two and range in magnitude from 10 to 100 cells per cu mm.

EOSINOPHILIA

This may develop now and then in almost every morbid condition, but in only a few classes of disturbances does it occur with fairly consistent regularity. The basic stimuli are not fully understood.

Allergy and Atopy

Most true hypersensitive disturbances appear to be associated with local or systemic eosinophilia or both. Abnormal or split foreign proteins seem the responsible incitants. Eosinophilia can be demonstrated intermittently, if not consistently, during asthma, hay fever, atopic eczema, and related manifestations of true hereditary atopy while there is contact with irritating antigens. The absolute count as a rule is between 400 and 4,000 eosinophils per cu mm. In such patients nonspecific stimuli tend to evoke a higher eosinophil rise than in normal persons.

Elevated eosinophil counts are also seen in a large percentage of the cases of serum sickness, angioneurotic edema, drug reactions, urticaria, allergic skin rashes, polyarteritis nodosa, anaphylactoid purpura, and related disorders whose pathogenesis is associated with acquired hypersensitivity.

Infestations with metazoan parasites almost always induce an eosinophilia except when the parasites do not penetrate the body tissues. This is well shown in hookworm, roundworm, and trichinal parasitism. Enterobiasis usually fails to induce an eosinophilia. Protozoan diseases such as malaria and amebiasis, and also scabies and other forms of dermatitis caused by insects, will often evoke a local or circulatory eosinophilia.

Eosinophils are usually numerous in affected tissues in those disorders which are associated with eosinophilia. They occur in abundance in the nasal discharge of allergic sinusitis, the sputum of bronchial asthma, the intramuscular lesions of trichinosis, and the focal cellular reactions of polyarteritis nodosa. During quiescent periods the eosinophilia usually subsides, both at local sites and in the peripheral blood.

Visceral Larva Migrans

Prolonged eosinophilic leukocytosis with or without constitutional symptoms with transitory pulmonary infiltrations can attend invasion of the lungs by the larvae of roundworms, hookworms, or trichinae. Paroxysms of coughing may lead to expectoration of sputum rich in eosinophils.

Larvae of nematodes which ordinarily are parasitic only for lower animals may sometimes invade human beings. Liver infiltrations and peripheral eosinophilia are prominent symptoms. The parasites thus far identified in reported cases have been the dog and cat ascarids of the genus Toxocara. The larvae cannot complete their life cycle within the human, but may survive in the viscera for many months. Before these causative agents were recognized the symptom-complex was referred to as Loeffler's syndrome, tropical eosinophilia, or chronic eosinophilia with visceral manifestations.

Children acquire Toxocara while ingesting dirt which has been contaminated with feces from infected pets. The ova, after being swallowed, hatch in the gastrointestinal tract and penetrate the portal blood and lymphatic vessels. Thence they migrate widely through the body, entering abdominal organs, muscles, and even the central nervous system. Symptoms of fever and eosinophilia of obscure nature may be produced. The small focal granulomas which form at the sites of tissue lodgement are made up of larvae encapsulated by fibroblasts, epithelioid cells, and masses of phagocytes containing many eosinophils. Ova do not appear in the feces of the human host. The only known approach to establishing the diagnosis in a suspected case is by liver biopsy.

Infectious Diseases

Circulating eosinophils are diminished in the early stages of most severe acute infections. Their numbers return as the patient improves, often before the total leukocyte count subsides, and for a time may reach hypernormal levels. It has been said that this pattern of response is a valuable prognostic sign: persistence of eosinophils in the peripheral blood heralds a mild illness at the beginning of an infection but is of grave import once the patient has become severely ill. The return of eosinophils usually precedes the clinical improvement by one or more days.

Eosinophilia is a regular occurrence in scarlet fever, with or without an initial drop. It reaches a maximum, usually between 7 and 10 per cent of the total leukocyte count, at about the sixth day, several days after the outbreak of the rash. Toward the end of convalescence it may temporarily return.

Miscellaneous

Bites of the black widow spider frequently evoke a peripheral eosinophilia. This rise is of diagnostic importance, inasmuch as the remainder of the clinical picture usually simulates an acute abdominal inflammation.

The rare sarcoma-like disease known as Kaposi's hemangiosarcoma is usually attended by eosinophilia.

An indefinite syndrome of familial eosinophilia has been described in which affected members habitually and persistently exhibit these cells. Before making this diagnosis care must always be taken to rule out hereditary allergy and a familial epidemic of parasitism.

In granulocytic leukemia the eosinophils sometimes are increased. Rarely they have outnumbered the neutrophils in the peripheral blood, bone marrow, and infiltrated organs. A satisfactory remission has been reported in such a case following administration of adrenocorticotropic hormone (ACTH).

Eosinophilia occurs with fair consistency during infectious mononucleosis, Hodgkin's disease, penicillin reactions, intensive gold treatment of rheumatoid arthritis, chronic lead poisoning, protracted drug therapy, and assorted chronic skin disorders. It is a frequent concomitant of adrenocortical insufficiency, whether in the chronic form of dyscorticism or the acute Waterhouse-Friderichsen syndrome.

After severe body burns the eosinophil count falls to low or zero value within a few hours; this is often accompanied by a lymphocytopenia and a neutrophil leukocytosis of degree proportional to the severity of the burn. The eosinopenia lasts from 1 to 7 days, as a rule, after which normal values return.

Tropical eosinophilia, as the name implies, is an acute or chronic febrile disease with splenomegaly and pronounced eosinophilia seen in the tropics. The cause is unknown. A similar syndrome is sometimes seen in residents of temperate climates.

Not infrequently an apparently well child is encountered in whom a differential count reveals the existence of an unusually high percentage of eosinophils without obvious cause. The first step when faced with such an occurrence is to calculate the absolute count of eosinophils from the differential percentage and the total leukocyte count. Often, as already mentioned, the absolute value will prove to be within normal limits. Should the count be well above 700, however, the next step is to search for common stimulatory disturbances, which in temperate climates are atopic and hypersensitivity states, intestinal parasitism, and convalescence from acute infections. After these have been excluded the rarer causes may be looked for. As a rule no pathogenetic mechanism can be elicited. Over the past 10 years the author has seen several dozen apparently healthy children, from the neighborhood of Philadelphia, whose eosinophilia has remained unexplained despite very thorough clinical and laboratory investigations. Under observation this eosinophilia usually disappeared after several weeks or months, but in a few instances it has persisted for over a year without emergence of any attendant disorders which might have been considered the incitant.

RESPONSE OF EOSINOPHILS TO STRESS

Acute stress or an injection of corticotropin or cortisone may be followed by a fall in both circulating eosinophils and lymphocytes, that of the eosinophils being more prominent (p. 745). The exact doses of the hormones are not significant. The higher the initial count, the longer the time interval required for absolute eosinopenia to develop. A similar response but of lesser intensity is often induced by epinephrine, ephedrine, or insulin. The eosinopenia in these situations is believed by Essellier and associates to be the result of an enhanced destruction of the eosinophils by the reticuloendothelial system, combined with an inhibition of release of eosinophils from the bone marrow.

The eosinophil level usually subsides during sustained therapy of nearly all disorders with corticotropin or cortisone and remains low until the therapy is discontinued. This obtains with allergic as well as nonallergic children.

BIBLIOGRAPHY

EOSINOPHILS

Ayres, W. W., and N. M. Starkey, Studies on Charcot-Leyden Crystals, Blood 5:254, 1950.

Beaver, P. C., C. H. Snyder, G. M. Carrera, J. H. Dent, and J. W. Lafferty, Chronic Eosinophilia Due to Visceral Larva Migrans: Report of Three Cases, Pediatrics 9:7, 1952.

Best, W. R., R. M. Kark, R. C. Muehrcke, and M. Samter, Clinical Value of Eosinophil Counts and Eosinophil Response Tests, J.A.M.A. 151:702, 1953.

———— and M. Samter, Variation and Error in Eosinophil Counts of Blood and Bone Marrow, Blood 6:61, 1951.

Bonner, C. D., Eosinophil Levels as an Index of Adrenal Responsiveness, J.A.M.A. 148:634, 1952.

Brill, R., J. Churg, and P. C. Beaver, Allergic Granulomatosis Associated with Visceral Larva Migrans, Am. J. Clin. Path. 23:1208, 1953.

Burrell, J. M., A Comparative Study of the Circulating Eosinophil Level in Babies, Arch. Dis. Childhood 27:337, 1952.

Essellier, A. F., R. L. Jeanneret, and L. Morandi, The Mechanism of Glucocorticoid Eosinopenia: Contribution to the Physiology of Eosinophile Granulocytes, Blood 9:531, 1954.

Friedman, M., I. J. Wolman, and H. H. Tyner, Eosinophil Leukemia, with Report of a Case, Am. J. M. Sc. 208:333, 1944.

Hain, K., Circulating Eosinophils in Children in Health and Disease, Pediatrics 7:408, 1951.

Hodes, H. L., R. E. Moloshok, and M. Markowitz, Fulminating Meningococcemia Treated with Cortisone: Use of Blood Eosinophil Count as a Guide to Prognosis and Treatment, Pediatrics 10:138, 1952.

Jailer, J. W., A. S. H. Wong, and E. T. Engle, Pituitary-Adrenal Relationship in Fullterm and in Premature Infants as Evidenced by Eosinophil Response, J. Clin. Endocrinol. 11:186, 1951.

Mercer, R. D., H. Z. Lund, R. A. Bloomfield, and F. E. Caldwell, Larval Ascariasis as a Cause of Chronic Eosinophilia with Visceral Manifestations, Am. J. Dis. Child. 80:46, 1950.

Milburn, C. L., Jr., and K. F. Ernst, Eosinophilia-Hepatomegaly Syndrome of Infants and Young Children: Report of a Case Due to Invasion of Liver by Nematode Larvae, Pediatrics 11:358, 1953.

Morf, H., Das "Eosinophile Leukämoid," Helvet. paediat. acta 5:505, 1950.

Muehrcke, R. C., E. L. Eckert, and R. M. Kark, A Statistical Study of Absolute Eosinophil Cell Counts in Healthy Young Adults Using Logarithmic Analysis, J. Lab. & Clin. Med. 40:161, 1952.

Naiden, E., and S. Ross, The Total Circulating Eosinophil Count under Environmental and Stress Stimuli, J. Pediat. 44:145, 1954.

Nemir, R. L., A. Heyman, J. D. Gorvoy, and E. N. Ervin, Pulmonary Infiltration and Blood Eosinophilia in Children (Loeffler's Syndrome), J. Pediat. 37:819, 1950.

Rud, F., The Eosinophil Count in Health and in Mental Disease, Acta psychiat. et neurol., suppl. 40, 1947.

Silver, H. K., P. Henderson, and A. Contopoulos, Extreme Eosinophilia, Increased Blood Heterophile Agglutination Titer, and Hyperglobulinemia, A.M.A. Am. J. Dis. Child. 83:649, 1952.

Squier, T. L., Variations in Circulating White Blood Cells after Specific and Nonspecific Stimuli, *J. Allergy* 22:82, 1951.

Stickney, J. M., and *F. J. Heck,* Clinical Occurrence of Eosinophilia, *M. Clin. North America* 28:915, 1944.

Van Meirhaeghe, A., Eosinophilia and Scarlatina, *Acta paediat. belg.* 1:70, 1946–47.

Visscher, M. B., and *F. Halberg,* Daily Rhythms in Numbers of Circulating Eosinophils and Related Phenomena, *Ann. New York Acad. Sc.* 59:834, 1955.

Weiner, H. A., and *D. Morkovin,* Circulating Blood Eosinophils in Acute Infectious Disease and the Eosinopenic Response, *Am. J. Med.* 13:58, 1952.

Wolman, I. J., The Eosinophil Count in Pediatrics, *Quart. Rev. Pediat.* 6:287, 1951.

Zuelzer, W. W., and *L. Apt,* Disseminated Visceral Lesions Associated with Extreme Eosinophilia: Pathologic and Clinical Observations on a Syndrome of Young Children, *Am. J. Dis. Child.* 78:153, 1949.

CHAPTER 16

Infectious Mononucleosis

Typical cases of infectious mononucleosis give little difficulty in diagnosis, but the high prevalence of atypical and mild cases makes it one of the most protean and imitative of all the infectious diseases. Most patients have, if only briefly, some malaise, fever, headache, enlarged superficial lymph nodes, pharyngitis, and characteristic blood changes. Less commonly there may be pneumonitis, anemia, electrocardiographic abnormalities, skin rashes, gastrointestinal disturbances, liver involvement, splenomegaly, or even encephalitis-like symptoms. Overlapping of the diverse manifestations makes it impractical to subgroup the cases according to symptom complexes.

Pathologically the lymph nodes and spleen exhibit reticuloendothelial proliferation, hyperplasia of the follicles, and accumulation of abnormal leukocytes within the sinuses and throughout the pulp. Other organs such as the lungs, liver, kidneys, or brain may contain perivascular aggregates of normal and abnormal lymphocytes. Histologic sections of bone marrow, liver, lung, myocardium, and other tissues often reveal foci of "granulomatous" proliferation of mononuclear cells. The bone marrow shows no other significant changes; this is an important point in the differential diagnosis of infectious mononucleosis from leukemia.

The occurrence of the disease in epidemics, coupled with failure of all efforts to isolate a causative microorganism and the absence of benefit from chemotherapy, support the suspicion that an as yet undiscovered virus-like agent is responsible. Some of the manifestations suggest that hypersensitivity to abnormal substances may be one component in pathogenesis.

Recovery is usually complete within a few weeks or months after the onset of an attack, but the weakness and distinctive leukocytes in the blood may last several months, subsiding gradually. Relapses or recurrences are unusual. A few deaths with generalized infiltrations have been reported. When the liver is affected the illness may be mistaken at first for acute hepatitis, since the latter may also evoke abnormal lymphocytes; the subsequent course will make the distinction clear.

202

Monocytosis, lymphocytosis, and an outpouring of abnormal cells develop during the illness. The monocytosis subsides first, leaving most convalescents with a relative lymphocytosis. The high count of normal monocytes in the early phases exceeds the limits seen in almost every other variety of monocytosis.

TOTAL LEUKOCYTE COUNT

The total count tends to remain below 15,000 per cu mm throughout the illness, though an occasional patient may show a rise to 20,000 or higher. Increases are due chiefly to neutrophils or abnormal lymphocytes or both. The leukocytosis recedes as the fever and constitutional symptoms subside. About 2 per cent of cases have a leukocytopenia of less than 5,000 in the early phases, which later may be succeeded by a lymphocytic leukocytosis. The characteristic atypical cells begin to make their appearance within the first few days, but may not be recognizable in definitive numbers until the second week, or rarely as late as the third week from the onset of symptoms.

DIFFERENTIAL COUNT

This is far from constant. All the cell systems may seem disturbed. The patterns may fluctuate widely as the illness runs its course. A relative eosinophilia of 6 to 12 per cent develops in about 10 per cent of patients during convalescence.

The neutrophils may rise during the first few days if secondary bacterial complications are developing or the attack is severe. Should they become extremely depressed, as occurs rarely, an erroneous preliminary diagnosis of typhoid fever may be made if the patient displays fever, splenomegaly, extreme malaise, and a fine rash. The neutrophils exhibit no alterations other than "toxic" granules occasionally.

ABNORMAL MONONUCLEAR CELLS (ATYPICAL LYMPHOCYTES)

The origin of the abnormal large-nucleated cells in this disease is still unsettled. They appear to originate from metaplastic proliferation of primitive reticuloendothelial or lymphocyte progenitors and are generally interpreted as atypical lymphocytes.

These cells are often referred to by the Downey classification of types I, II, and III. In all three types the cells are at least 10 to 15 μ in diameter, of the size of an immature lymphocyte or small monocyte. The blood films of most patients show cells of all three types, usually totaling more than half of all the mononuclear cells present. Type I cells predominate in about half the cases, and type II cells nearly as often, whereas type III cells are only occasionally numerous. There are no highly significant correlations between the character of the predominating cells and the severity or duration or other clinical manifestations of the disease.

The type I atypical lymphocyte has an eccentric nucleus which is oval or indented or even lobulated. The chromatin is coarse and not sharply differentiated from the parachromatin. The cytoplasm is foamy or mottled and may stain deeply or be faintly basophilic. There is often a clearer area next to the indentation of the nucleus. Azurophilic granules may or may not be present.

The type II atypical lymphocyte has an eccentric or central nucleus which is often irregular in shape but less than that of type I. The chromatin is very coarse and in clear contrast with the parachromatin, giving rise to what is known as a "basket-weave" appearance. The cytoplasm is less mottled and flaky.

The type III atypical lymphocyte is the largest and most primitive in appearance and may be confused with a leukemic cell. Its nucleus tends to be extremely large, with nucleoplasm arranged in a fine network. Nucleoli are common. The cytoplasm tends to be deeply basophilic.

Intermediate cell forms may be numerous. There may be small mature lymphocyte-like cells with clear nuclear areas which give the nucleus a fenestrated appearance. Vacuoles are not uncommon in nucleus or cytoplasm. The cell outlines may spread out irregularly. The cytoplasm is usually free of granules and may stain with a gray tint.

Abnormal lymphocytes resembling those of infectious mononucleosis make their appearance in small numbers in the peripheral blood during various other diseases (p. 188).

HETEROPHIL ANTIBODY TESTS

Hemagglutinins ("heterophil antibodies") against sheep and beef erythrocytes usually develop in appreciable concentration whenever the attack is of more than minimal severity. Similar but serologically differentiable antibodies may appear in serum sickness, infectious hepatitis, vaccinia, Hodgkin's disease, leukemia, and lymphosarcoma. The original impression was that the antigen in sheep or beef erythrocytes which reacts with patient's serum is the Forssman heterophil antigen, common to the tissues of such diverse species as guinea pigs, horses, mice, and chickens. It has been shown, however, that the serum antibodies which arise in infectious mononucleosis, though absorbable with either sheep or beef erythrocytes, are absorbable only partially or negligibly by guinea pig kidney. Reversely, the somewhat similar antibodies which appear in the serum from patients with serum sickness and leukemia-like diseases, or in low titer in normal individuals, can be absorbed almost entirely by guinea pig kidney.

The heterophil antibody test as customarily performed consists of two parts, the "presumptive" test and the "differential" test. The presumptive, or screening, test is performed with sheep erythrocytes alone. The differential test includes an additional agglutination with a suspension of guinea pig kidney and sometimes also with beef red cells. In most laboratories the differential test is not made unless a prior presumptive reading has been 1:56 or higher.

The presumptive test consists of setting up uniform suspensions of sheep erythrocytes in a row of 10 test tubes and then adding graded dilutions of serum. The results are reported according to the highest dilution in which agglutination occurred, after all diluents and reagents have been added. In the Davidsohn procedure the readings are expressed in multiples of 1:14. With the Davidsohn method, in our laboratory, titers up to 1:28 or 1:56 with sheep cells are often given by normal children, and trace reactions up to 1:112 are not uncommon among those hospitalized for other illnesses. These antibodies in normal serum are nearly always absorbed partially or completely by sheep or beef cells, and usually completely by guinea pig kidney. Rarely, however, a normal subject may be encountered who exhibits the serologic pattern characteristic of infectious mononucleosis—complete absorption with sheep or beef cells and incomplete with guinea pig kidney.

In infectious mononucleosis in the early active stages, most of the readings fall between 1:112 and 1:1,792 but may be higher. After absorption with guinea pig kidney the titer typically falls only two or three dilutions, for example, from 1:896 to 1:112. A titer of 1:28 or more after absorption by guinea pig kidney is generally interpreted as diagnostic for infectious mononucleosis provided all other findings are compatible, and a titer of 1:14 may be suspicious. When beef red cells are used for the preliminary absorption in infectious mononucleosis, the titer with sheep red cells will be reduced to a negligible level, for the reason that beef and sheep red cells react with the same antibody.

In serum sickness from horse serum, and in a minority of cases of viral hepatitis and lymphocytic leukemia or lymphosarcoma with prominent swelling of the lymph nodes, the titer before preliminary absorption with guinea pig kidney antigen may be 1:224 or more, but after absorption the titer falls markedly, for example, from 1:448 down to 1:28.

With the Paul-Bunnell test procedure, which employs different concentrations of reagents and ignores some of the added saline in its computation of dilutions, normal serums may agglutinate sheep erythrocytes in final dilutions up to 1:8. After horse serum injections or in leukemia the titer may increase to 1:32 or even higher. Readings of 1:16 or 1:32 are deemed suggestive of infectious mononucleosis, and higher ones are taken as diagnostic.

The heterophil reaction typically becomes positive in the first or second weeks of illness, but occasionally not until later. When a negative reaction is secured in a suspected case it is advisable to repeat the determination in a week or so. Should there be no rise from the preceding reading, other diagnostic possibilities should be explored. Rises in titer, once begun, continue to a maximum and then subside. Most children maintain positive levels for 1 to 3 months or a little longer. Sometimes the elevations in titer are so transitory as to escape detection unless frequent tests are made.

The frequency with which positive heterophil reactions are encountered in infectious mononucleosis depends in large measure upon the rigidity of the other criteria used in identifying the disease. If one is unwilling to make the diagnosis except when clear-cut signs and symptoms are present and the absolute count of abnormal leukocytes numbers at least 1,000 per cu mm, then positive heterophil tests are encountered in nearly all cases, especially if the test is repeated when early reports are negative. In other words, the serologic tests tend to give positive results when the clinical features and blood smears are highly characteristic, but tend to give negative or borderline results when the diagnosis is otherwise in doubt.

LIVER INVOLVEMENT

Liver biopsies of patients with infectious mononucleosis have shown infiltrations of normal and atypical lymphocytes in the periportal areas. Jaundice is recognizable in only 1 or 2 per cent of cases, however, and usually lasts but a week or two. The total and 1-minute-reacting serum bilirubin levels may be elevated. The liver function tests frequently give abnormal findings, which may be due to alterations in serum proteins from sources other than the liver. The flocculation reactions may remain abnormal for many months after the results of the other tests have returned to normal and clinical recovery appears complete.

In addition to the clinical differences, the proportion of abnormal lymphocytes and the severity of the cellular changes are much higher in infectious mononucleosis than in primary liver disease. Furthermore, in the latter a positive heterophil response is uncommon; when present, it is of low titer and is removed by the guinea pig antigen.

MISCELLANEOUS LABORATORY FINDINGS

A moderate normochromic anemia may appear, from which recovery is often slow even when iron and vitamins are administered liberally. The red cell sedimentation rate may be elevated. The urine at the height of the illness occasionally contains protein, bile, glucose, casts, or red cells. The serum proteins, and especially the globulin fractions, often deviate from the normal. In patients exhibiting neck stiffness the cerebrospinal fluid may show a moderately elevated protein content or even a mononuclear pleocytosis and may give a positive heterophil reaction when the serum level rises. Beta-hemolytic streptococci are frequently found in throat cultures early in the illness.

Some patients have temporary signs of splenic hyperactivity in the form of hemolytic anemia or leukocytopenia or thrombocytopenia, with or without hemorrhages. Acute swelling of the spleen may lead to sudden rupture and abdominal hemorrhage.

Peculiar serologic responses may take place transitorily during infectious mononucleosis. Positive reactions may be observed in the serologic tests for syphilis, the flocculation tests for liver disturbances, the

Weil-Felix agglutination with *Proteus vulgaris* antigen, the titers of anti-streptolysin and staphylococcic antitoxin, and agglutination reactions with *Listeria monocytogenes*. Human group O erythrocytes modified by exposure to the virus of Newcastle disease virus are agglutinated by the serum of approximately half of the cases of infectious mononucleosis. Cold hemagglutinins for sheep erythrocytes often develop also.

These serologic abnormalities appear to be the products of the reticuloendothelial hyperplasia, which is one of the major reactions to the disease. The hyperplasia of this tissue system in general runs parallel to the quantitative titer of the heterophil agglutinins in the serum.

BIBLIOGRAPHY

INFECTIOUS MONONUCLEOSIS

Bender, C. E., Diagnosis of Infectious Mononucleosis, *J.A.M.A.* **149**:7, 1952.
Custer, R. P., and *E. B. Smith,* The Pathology of Infectious Mononucleosis, *Blood* **3**:830, 1948.
Davidsohn, I., Infectious Mononucleosis, *J.A.M.A.* **143**:1360, 1950.
Downey, H., and *C. A. McKinlay,* Acute Lymphadenosis Compared with Acute Lymphatic Leukemia, *Arch. Int. Med.* **32**:82, 1923.
Evans, A. S., Liver Involvement in Infectious Mononucleosis, *J. Clin. Invest.* **27**:106, 1948.
Evans, F. A., and *T. P. Sprunt,* Mononuclear Leukocytosis in Relation to Acute Infections, *Bull. Johns Hopkins Hosp.* **31**:410, 1920.
Hunt, J. S., The Pathogenesis of Infectious Mononucleosis, *Am. J. M. Sc.* **228**:83, 1954.
Isaacs, R., Chronic Infectious Mononucleosis, *Blood* **3**:858, 1948.
Limarzi, L. R., J. T. Paul, and *H. G. Poncher,* Blood and Bone Marrow in Infectious Mononucleosis, *J. Lab. & Clin. Med.* **31**:1079, 1946.
Paul, J. R., and *W. W. Bunnell,* The Presence of Heterophile Antibodies in Infectious Mononucleosis, *Am. J. M. Sc.* **183**:90, 1932.
Schultz, L. E., Heterophile Antibody Titer in Diseases Other Than Infectious Mononucleosis, *Arch. Int. Med.* **81**:328, 1948.
Simmonds, W. L., and *A. Markowitz,* Heterophile Antibodies of Infectious Mononucleosis, *Am. J. Clin. Path.* **22**:730, 1952.
Small, C. S., and *G. G. Hadley,* Acute Hemolytic Anemia Complicating Infectious Mononucleosis, *Am. J. Clin. Path.* **20**:1056, 1951.
Stevens, J. E., E. D. Bayrd, and *F. J. Heck,* Infectious Mononucleosis: A Study of 210 Sporadic Cases, *Am. J. Med.* **11**:202, 1951.
———, ———, and ———, Infectious Mononucleosis: The Prognostic Significance of Various Changes of the Blood Leukocytes, *Blood* **7**:31, 1952.
Watson, J., P. Johnson, J. Kahn, and *F. M. Stone,* Subclinical Infectious Mono-

nucleosis with Hepatitis, Epidemic in a Class of One Hundred Two Medical Students: A Two-year Study, *A.M.A. Arch. Int. Med.* 88:618, 1951.

Walker, S. H., The Failure of Antibiotic Therapy in Infectious Mononucleosis, *Am. J. M. Sc.* 226:65, 1953.

Zarafonetis, C. J. D., H. L. Oster, and *V. F. Colville,* Cold Agglutination of Sheep Erythrocytes as a Factor in False-Positive Heterophile Agglutination Tests, *J. Lab. & Clin. Med.* 41:906, 1953.

CHAPTER 17

Childhood Leukemia

Leukemia may be defined as a disease in which one class of circulating leukocytes becomes anarchistic and proliferates irreversibly until the death of the patient. The cause is not known. Mortality statistics record about 1,200 childhood cases a year in the United States. Genetic factors probably exert some influence, as illustrated by the rarity of the disease in the colored race. Closely similar diseases in mice and chickens can be transferred experimentally by virologic techniques, but the human disease has never been indisputably transmitted to other humans or to animals.

NATURAL HISTORY

Pallor, fever, weakness, enlargement of lymph nodes, splenomegaly, hemorrhages, skeletal changes, and unusual susceptibility to the common infections are the most familiar clinical features. Swelling of a joint may simulate rheumatic fever. The sequence of development varies markedly from patient to patient. In untreated children the expectation of life is 1 to 8 months from onset of symptoms, with less than half surviving over 4 months, though exceptional cases have survived as long as a year or more with transfusions and simple supportive measures. The development and utilization of the folic acid antagonists, mercaptopurine, steroid hormones, and related chemotherapeutic agents in the past decade have extended the life expectancy to at least a year in half the cases; a considerable minority survive for 2 years or more.

Septicemia, exhaustion states, infiltrations of important organs, acute hemorrhages, or cardiac failure are the common terminal events. Spontaneous remissions are infrequent; these may be induced by a superimposed acute infection.

Since most parents today know the hopeless outcome of leukemia, it is wise to keep them in ignorance of this possibility until the existence of the disease has been clearly established. The diagnosis should never be made with finality until either a bone marrow aspiration or an adequate period of observation has corroborated the impression given by the clinical findings and the peripheral blood studies. Once the diagnosis has been established indisputably, emotional support of the parents becomes most important.

The blood changes in leukemia must be differentiated from other disturbances which give rise to superficially similar reactions of the circulating white cells. Lymphocytosis may be evoked by pertussis, infectious lymphocytosis, some viral diseases, and infectious mononucleosis. Neutrophilic granulocytosis occurs in infectious diseases, infarctions, traumatic injuries, polyarteritis nodosa, etc. Granulocytopenia may be confused with aplastic anemia. The appearance of many immature cells in the peripheral blood, sometimes with a few granulocytoblasts, may be seen at times in so-called leukemoid reactions following splenectomy and in disturbances of the bone marrow with or without extramedullary hemopoiesis.

TERMINOLOGY

Leukemic changes are typically limited to one leukocytic strain. In many childhood cases, when first seen, the abnormal cells may be so aberrant or so immature that they simulate blast or stem cells and the exact identification must await later developments. In our own series of several hundred cases, approximately 80 per cent at first have appeared to be lymphocytic ("lymphogenous"), 13 per cent have been neutrophil granulocytic ("myelogenous, myelocytic"), 5 per cent have been stem cell blast (or "undifferentiated"), and 2 per cent have been monocytic. About 60 per cent of the cases of each type occur in boys. The most frequent age is 2 to 4 years. The majority of instances of blast cell leukemia have ultimately proved to be of lymphocytic character. Plasma cell, eosinophilic, and basophilic leukemia are rare before adult life.

By the time that symptoms appear the abnormal leukocytes in the circulation seem to be derived principally from the bone marrow, though there may be infiltrative foci in the spleen, lymph nodes, and other organs. In very early lymphocytic leukemia, however, the abnormal proliferation may seem to be centered in the lymph nodes or spleen and later spread diffusely into the bone marrow.

LEUKOCYTE COUNTS

Peripheral leukocyte counts may range from a low of 100 per cu mm to a high of 500,000 or higher. In 20 per cent of childhood patients when first seen the total leukocyte count is below 5,000 per cu mm; in 40 per cent between 5,000 and 20,000; and in 20 per cent over 100,000. There are no highly significant correlations between morphologic abnormalities in the cells, total leukocyte count, or intensity of marrow infiltration, as related to prognosis, clinical course, or response to any of the therapeutic agents. Hence there is no great pertinence in describing those cases with low counts as "aleukemic" as if this were a special subvariety. The qualifying phrases "with leukopenia" or "with leukocytosis" may be used if one desires to direct attention to the level of the count.

The peripheral cellular responses in children with leukemia differ so widely from case to case that it is difficult to outline a typical blood reaction in categoric terms. Immature and abnormal cell forms become more numerous as the disease progresses, both in the marrow and the peripheral blood. If morphologically the leukemic cells in the peripheral blood closely simulate the normal, their presence may escape detection for a time unless the absolute numbers are increased. The clinical course tends to be more fulminating when the percentage of primitive-appearing cells is high. The content of leukocytes per unit of circulating blood represents the balance between liberation and destruction. If the cells are entering the blood from their sites of origin more rapidly than they are being destroyed, the result will be a high peripheral count, and vice versa. With lymphocytic leukemia the response to chemotherapy cannot be prognosticated from the cytology or peripheral count; with granulocytic leukemia the response is usually less satisfactory when the cells appear primitive and the count is high.

MORPHOLOGY OF LEUKEMIC LEUKOCYTES

Leukemic leukocytes almost always show aberrations, though only a few may be recognized and escape detection unless especially looked for. These aberrations can be deviations and inequalities in cell size or contours; unequal maturity of nucleus and cytoplasm; nuclear coarseness or irregularity; presence of one or several nucleoli; abnormalities in size, number, or distribution of cytoplasmic granules; abnormal staining quality in the background substance; presence of abnormal vacuoles in nucleus or cytoplasm.

Immature cells, often somewhat abnormal, usually but not invariably appear in the blood stream. In granulocytic leukemia these will be chiefly promyelocytes and myelocytes; in lymphocytic leukemia, large "prolymphocytes." Nucleated blast forms in inconstant numbers are not uncommon. These abnormal immature cells are sometimes termed micromyelocytes or microlymphocytes. Should it be desirable to make a careful study of abnormal cells when their number in the direct blood smear is very low, one may prepare a film from the buffy coat of a centrifuged sample.

Diagnostic aspiration or biopsy of the bone marrow from any site customarily reveals overcrowding from excessive proliferation of leukocytes (Chap. 27). These either are obviously related to one of the major cell series or are so immature or atypical as to be unclassifiable. In general, leukemic cells in bone marrow aspirates show more abnormalities than do those in the circulation.

"ACUTE" VS. "CHRONIC"

In adults with leukemia the dividing line between acute and chronic as applied to the disease is based chiefly on life expectation in the absence of treatment. The minimum has been set somewhat arbitrarily for chronic leukemia at 12 months, though such patients may survive for many years. Another distinguishing feature is the tendency for the numerically predominant cell, whether of the lymphocyte, granulocyte, or some other cell series, to appear nearly identical with the specific mature cell found in the peripheral blood and bone marrow and to circulate in large numbers. Spontaneous partial remissions are frequent also. In acute leukemia, in contrast, the survival time is short, the predominant cells are undifferentiated or only partly differentiated, and spontaneous remissions are uncommon. In both varieties the extent and character of the infiltrations in bone marrow and other organs are independent of the cell type.

When these criteria are applied to the untreated disease as it occurs in infancy and childhood, nearly all lymphocytic and monocytic cases and the great majority of granulocytic cases fit into the "acute" category. Most childhood cases have a high percentage of immature cells in the circulation and the bone marrow, regardless of whether the total leukocyte count is high or low. Few affected children will survive more than 6 months with supportive transfusions in the absence of chemotherapy.

GRANULOCYTIC (MYELOCYTIC) LEUKEMIA

In the so-called acute forms of this disease the immature and abnormal neutrophilic granulocytes are unusually abundant in both bone marrow and peripheral blood. Many of the leukemic cells in the bone marrow may exhibit nuclei at the metamyelocyte stage but with retarded cytoplasmic maturation as shown by poorly developed or even absent specific granules. Eosinophilic cytoplasmic rods simulating tubercle bacilli—the so-called Auer bodies—are often found in the myeloblasts. These rods are also seen in the monoblasts of acute monoblastic leukemia, but are rare in the lymphoblasts of acute lymphocytic leukemia. Mitotic figures are more frequent in granulocytic leukemia than in lymphocytic leukemia. Granulocytic myeloblasts may have three or four nucleoli, whereas lymphoblasts tend to have only one or two. Circulating eosinophils or basophils, often atypical, may be coincidentally prominent. A few unquestionable instances of true eosinophilic leukemia in childhood have been reported. Thrombocytosis may occur in the early stages.

As already mentioned, the diagnosis of "chronic" granulocytic ("chronic" myelogenous) leukemia sometimes is applied when there is a high peripheral count of granulocytes with the majority being mature cells, a relatively long duration of the disease, absence of peripheral glandular enlargement, and early toxic symptoms. In this disturbance there is often pronounced infiltration of the spleen and other organs. Hemorrhagic manifestations associated with thrombocytopenia are especially common in the infancy years and in the terminal stages. Such patients can sometimes be supported by transfusions and simple supportive measures until the hemorrhagic tendency abates, despite failure of the thrombocytopenia to disappear wholly and provided an intercurrent infection does not supervene.

Attempts to depress the hyperplastic granulocytic cells by toxic agents such as arsenic, urethane, benzol, radioactive phosphorus, or irradiation by x-ray have at times been of temporary benefit. Radiotherapy is probably the best of these latter measures since the dosage can be readily controlled. For the most prolonged results the therapy should be given intermittently and only to eradicate pain or other disabling symptoms.

So-called "panmyelosis," characterized by pleomorphic proliferations, is an unusual variant of chronic granulocytic leukemia. A congeries of granulocytes, megakaryocytes, erythrocytes, reticulum cells, and connective tissue cells in apparently random combination proliferates in the bone marrow, spleen, and lymph nodes. The peripheral blood shows normal and abnormal granulocytes, often with many nucleated red cells.

LYMPHOCYTIC (LYMPHATIC) LEUKEMIA

In lymphocytic leukemia the cytologic abnormalities are variability in size or shape of the entire cell or of the nucleus only; uneven staining of the nuclear chromatin; notched or irregular nuclear margins; scanty or unusually abundant cytoplasm which stains unevenly and may be rich in vacuoles or azurophil granules. Changes are detected more readily when lymphocytosis raises the suspicion of leukemia. In most childhood cases of lymphocytic leukemia the proportion of primitive-appearing cells is appreciable.

The bone marrow typically is infiltrated with abnormal lymphocytes including some lymphoblasts. Exceptionally the marrow aspirate may be markedly hypocellular and simulate aplastic anemia. In one recently studied case, four marrow aspirations from different vertebrae exhibited this phenomenon; the fifth from an iliac crest revealed aggregates of lymphocytic leukemic cells. Early in the disease the lymphocytic infiltration of the marrow may not seem prominent even when the peripheral blood shows numbers of these cells; in this circumstance the leukemic cells in the circulation are believed to enter from the lymph follicle system.

STEM CELL LEUKEMIA

Many cases of childhood leukemia are not identifiable morphologically in the early stages because the immature or bizarre appearance of the abnormal cells reminds one only of blast cell forms. After remissions induced by chemotherapy, however, the cell type almost always proves to be lymphocytic.

RED CELLS

Nearly all children with leukemia are anemic when first seen, though this is not invariable. The anemia is typically of the normochromic normocytic type with approximately parallel diminution in hemoglobin and erythrocytes. It seems to result from massive displacement or toxic depression of the erythropoietic marrow elements by leukemic cells and their metabolic products, along with an enhanced rate of hemodestruction. During vigorous therapy with folic acid antagonists, and in some prolonged cases without such treatment, the red cells may take on a macrocytic change. The reticulocyte count tends to be normal or below normal as the disease advances, but may be elevated slightly. A rise in reticulocytes is an early sign of a favorable therapeutic effect from chemotherapy; this reticulocytosis may transiently amount to as much as 30 per cent. When red cells are being destroyed rapidly, the serum bilirubin may be slightly elevated and urobilinogenuria will appear.

PLATELETS

The platelet count may be normal or low in the early stages; as the disease advances it is almost invariably low. Interestingly, the threshold for bleeding is often less than the 60,000 level noted in most other forms of thrombocytopenia; the count may be 10,000 or 20,000 without petechiae or ready bruising becoming evident.

The influence which depresses the circulating platelets and marrow megakaryocytes is chiefly depression of the marrow megakaryocytes by leukemic encroachment. A resurgence of platelets in the peripheral blood is an early and reliable sign of benefit from chemotherapy.

BLOOD COAGULATION

In advanced cases the blood coagulation mechanisms are often defective, as evidenced by spontaneous ecchymoses and other hemorrhagic phenomena. The finger tip bleeding time becomes prolonged, and sometimes the venous coagulation time as well. Clot retraction is often imperfect. This bleeding tendency seems due in part to the diminution in circulating platelets and in part to an increased permeability of the smaller vessels. In some children a heparin-like substance may appear in the blood stream during exacerbations of the disease. Transfusions with fresh blood, corticotropin intramuscularly or by slow intravenous infusion, or platelet concentrates given intravenously are the best measures for immediate control of a hemorrhagic episode.

THERAPY

Folic acid antagonists, mercaptopurine and related substances, and corticotropin, cortisone, and related adrenal cortical hormones are more effective in childhood than in adult leukemia. At least one of these agents will induce at least one remission in most affected children. A remission, whether partial or complete, is never permanent. The duration of these remissions varies from 1 to 2 months with the hormones up to many months with the other agents. It is feasible at times to induce a repetition of a remission by a later course of therapy with the same agent, and particularly with a hormone, but each remission will be shorter than its predecessor.

Folic Acid Antagonists (Antifolic Substances, Antifolates)

The folic acid antagonists (Aminopterin, A-methoperin, Amino-an-fol, and related substances) all act by interfering with folic acid metabolism. Strains of leukemic cells which need folic acid as an essential metabolite will fail to proliferate if the responsive intracellular mechanisms become blocked at a dosage level which does not produce serious deficiency symptoms in the tissues of the patient. When one folic acid antagonist no longer produces improvement it is futile to change to another. The dosages have to be adjusted continually to fit the responses of the patient. If too little is given, the desired therapeutic benefit will not be had; if too much, toxic symptoms may develop. The margin between therapeutic effectiveness and toxicity is narrow.

Aminopterin is usually administered in single oral doses of 0.5 to 1 mg daily, after an initial dosage of 2 mg for a few days. A-methopterin (Methotrexate) is given similarly in doses of 2.5 to 10 mg daily.

The early manifestations of toxicity from the folic acid antagonists are hemorrhagic atrophy along the mucocutaneous borders of the lips, erosions of the oral mucosa, and gastrointestinal hemorrhages. Later developments may be bone marrow depression, affecting primarily the white cell series and megakaryocytes. Bleeding, when it occurs as a sign of overdosage, has been ascribed to local atrophy of the mucous membranes, blood vessel wall damage, further depression of platelets, or other unknown mechanisms. Gastrointestinal hemorrhages do not develop, as a rule, when a dosage schedule is maintained which keeps the stomatitis at the level of dry lips or one or more small sores in the mouth. Severe toxic changes may be counteracted more rapidly by giving corticotropin preferably, or the citrovorum factor. If an overdosage of Aminopterin is inadvertently given, an injection of 3 to 6 mg of this latter substance should be administered within 4 hours.

Mercaptopurine (6-Mercaptopurine, Purinethol)

This purine derivative, which acts as a purine antimetabolite with certain forms of bacteria, has been found able to produce clinical and hematologic remissions in children with acute leukemia. Its mode of action in this disease is not known. The dosage is 2.5 mg per kg body weight daily.

The most serious toxic effect is bone marrow depression. Oral lesions are unusual, but nausea, vomiting, and anorexia may appear as secondary effects.

When the bone marrow is depressed one may encounter leukocytopenia, thrombocytopenia, anemia, and bleeding. With patients receiving this drug leukocyte studies should accordingly be made at least once weekly and the administration discontinued if the neutrophils become significantly reduced. Treatment may be resumed after the count has ceased falling or begins to rise. Remissions are usually short-lived when the drug is withdrawn. When the inevitable exacerbation begins, the dosages may be doubled or even trebled in the hope of prolonging its effect, but the child's leukocyte count must then be kept under closer supervision.

Hormones

The hormones which are of most established benefit in childhood leukemia are corticotropin and cortisone. Cortisone can be given orally and produces fewer side effects and is therefore preferable to corticotropin as a general rule. The susceptibility of the disease is about the same with either substance. When one is no longer effective, the other will sometimes still be able to induce a short further remission.

A patient who has become refractory to hormone therapy may still exhibit a remission to a folic acid antagonist or mercaptopurine if these had not been given previously, and vice versa. Because of the higher cost of the hormones, the briefer duration of the improvement, the enhanced susceptibility to infections while receiving steroid hormones, and the likelihood of endocrinal side effects, these other substances are preferably administered first, except when the patient is severely ill when first seen. It is advisable to supplement hormone therapy with an antibiotic for prophylaxis against infections.

The daily dosage of cortisone, divided into two to four portions, varies from 50 to 200 mg depending upon the age of the child and the severity of symptoms. The dosage of corticotropin is usually 40 to 80 mg per day, given intramuscularly. The amounts should be kept to the minimum compatible with satisfactory remission. Acute episodes of thrombocytopenic bleeding can often be arrested temporarily by slow daily intravenous infusions of 20 mg of corticotropin. Some children have been maintained in relative good health for a prolonged period by combined therapy with cortisone, a chemotherapeutic agent, supportive transfusions, and a prophylactic antibiotic.

Undesirable effects of corticotropin therapy may be a Cushing-like syndrome, abdominal distention, glycosuria, hypertension, acne, mental aberrations, cerebral edema, peripheral edema, and adrenal cortical involution. An Addison-like syndrome may appear on withdrawal of corticotropin. With cortisone these disturbances are less frequent and less marked.

Transfusions

Frequent transfusions may be advisable when the leukemic process is active in the marrow or when excessive hemodestruction is occurring. The interval between needed transfusions is highly variable and may be anywhere from a few days to many months. The principal indication for transfusion is anemia. Transfusions associated with liberal use of antibiotics can be of great value in significantly prolonging life, even in the absence of drug or hormone therapy. Posttransfusion hemolytic reactions are seen much less frequently than before testing for Rh compatibility was introduced. Atypical agglutinins or hemolysins which give rise to intragroup incompatibility difficulties are found more frequently than in normal children.

Splenectomy

This operation is of no value in the management of most children with leukemia. The main problems for which splenectomy may be considered are (1) marked pancytopenia or thrombocytopenia far out of proportion to the infiltration of the marrow spaces by leukemic cells, or (2) extremely rapid red cell destruction regardless of whether circulating anti–red cell antibodies are present. These situations are more likely to be seen in granulocytic leukemia and in older children. Cortisone or corticotropin should be tried first, with splenectomy kept in reserve. In rare individuals the existence of leukemia may not be recognized until after a splenectomy has been done for relief of hypersplenic anemia or pancytopenia.

Miscellaneous

Roentgen irradiation, urethane, splenectomy, Myleran, nitrogen mustard, and other procedures are effective in rare and special situations; when used indiscriminately they are more likely to aggravate the symptoms. Remissions have been induced by radioactive phosphorus. Mild roentgen irradiation of infiltrated bones may alleviate pain when present in these structures. Thymectomy has proved of no value. Essential elements of therapy in every case are continous medical supervision, transfusions for anemia, and sympathetic understanding and support of the problems borne by the family.

REMISSIONS

The onset of a remission following initiation of therapy is heralded by increased strength, subsidence of overt signs and symptoms, diminution in the total quantity and relative proportion of circulating abnormal leukocytes, shrinkage of enlarged organs, fading away of abnormal infiltrations in the bone marrow and their replacement by regenerating normal cells, greater resistance to infections, and rises in the red cell and platelet counts. A transitory reticulocytosis is an encouraging sign. Improvements may be noted in the blood picture as soon as a few days following the onset of the therapy. An early sign is an increase in number of shattered cells in the blood smear, coincident with a decline in the count of abnormal circulating leukocytes. Along with the abnormal cells, the morphologically normal segmented neutrophils sometimes become diminished for a few days. It is difficult, at times, to distinguish between the leukopenia induced by a chemotherapeutic agent as the leukemic cells disappear from the bone marrow and the leukopenia which is a manifestation of the acute leukemia itself.

A remission may be termed *complete* when all clinical disturbances subside, the peripheral blood picture returns to normal, and the marrow aspirates show less than 10 per cent primitive or abnormal cells. In a *partial* remission the symptoms and signs regress but reversion of the leukocytic and bone marrow changes is incomplete. In a "minimal" remission the symptoms improve slightly for a brief period but the bone marrow pattern remains unchanged. Partial return of the marrow to normal activity can maintain the red cell and hemoglobin levels. When leukemic cells continue to crowd the marrow spaces, monthly or semimonthly blood transfusions may be needed.

The first evidences of relapse after a remission are an increasing percentage of abnormal cells in the differential count and in the marrow, a beginning fall in the red cell and platelet levels, and often a leukemic leukocytosis. These hematologic exacerbations typically precede by some days or weeks the return of clinical manifestations such as fever and enlargement of organs.

Spontaneous remissions occur in less that 5 per cent of untreated childhood cases, usually as a sequel to an acute infection or several blood transfusions. Antifolic therapy or mercaptopurine will each induce a remission in about 50 per cent of children, and the hormones in about 90 per cent.

With chemotherapeutically induced remissions there may occur for some days a preliminary period of anemia, leukocytopenia, neutrophilopenia, and hypocellularity of the bone marrow. This may be accompanied by an exacerbation of hemorrhages and other symptoms and may even prove fatal. Hormone therapy should therefore be given coincidentally with the folic acid antagonists and mercaptopurine when a patient is already seriously ill when treatment is initiated.

Sometimes in untreated leukemia or in the terminal stages, a clinical and hematologic picture may be presented which simulates acute idiopathic aplastic anemia.

Complete blood counts, including platelet counts, should be taken every 2 or 3 days during the first few weeks of any form of therapy, until the proper maintenance dosage has been established. These will provide information as to the results of therapy. Rises in hemoglobin, red cells, reticulocytes, and platelets are signs of reversal of the infiltrated bone marrow toward normal. Downward trends, on the other hand, especially when accompanied by fading away of all granulocytes both normal and abnormal, are indications of overdosage and call for temporary discontinuance of the drug.

Once a good remission has been established, laboratory observations are not needed more often than every week or two. Hemoglobin and platelet levels which persist in the normal range are adequate indications that normal bone marrow function is not significantly depressed. The leukocyte and differential counts give information as to the proliferation activity of the leukemic process. Often, in skilled hands, simply a hemoglobin determination and a blood smear examination are adequate to convey the information that the disease is quiescent.

ERYTHROLEUKEMIA (DI GUGLIELMO'S DISEASE)

This is in essence a malignant progressively advancing blood cell dyscrasia which is characterized by a persistent severe normochromic anemia; presence in the blood stream of an abundance of nucleated red cells which frequently are basophilic, multinucleated, or otherwise atypical; extreme proliferation of the erythropoietic tissue in the marrow, and often also in extramedullary sites, with numerous bizarre or blast-like cell forms; enlargement of the spleen; and a propensity for the development of leukemia-like changes in the granulocytes of the bone marrow, peripheral blood, spleen, and elsewhere. The leukocytic abnormalities may not become apparent at the same time as those of the red cells.

This disorder is believed to be a variant form of granulocytic leukemia, with the primitive or blast cell strain evolving in the direction of the erythrocyte more than the leukocyte. Only a few childhood cases have been reported, under such names as "immature cell erythremia," "erythremic myelosis," and "erythroblastic leukemia." It is probable, however, that careful scrutiny of the smears of peripheral blood and of marrow aspirates, whenever a child has an otherwise unexplained refractory anemia with splenomegaly and red cell marrow hypercellularity, would show that the disorder is more common than believed.

BIBLIOGRAPHY

DIAGNOSIS AND NATURAL HISTORY

Anderson, R. C., Familial Leukemia: A Report of Leukemia in Five Siblings with a Brief Review of the Genetic Aspects of this Disease, *A.M.A. Am. J. Dis. Child.* 81:313, 1951.

Bassen, F. A., and *J. L. Kohn,* Multiple Spontaneous Remissions in a Child with Acute Leukemia, *Blood* 7:37, 1952.

Bernhard, W. G., I. Gore, and *R. A. Kilby,* Congenital Leukemia, *Blood* 6:990, 1951.

Best, W. R., L. R. Limarzi, and *H. G. Poncher,* White Blood Cell Counts in the Leucemias, *J. Lab. & Clin. Med.* 38:789, 1951.

Bierman, H. R., P. Cohen, J. N. McClelland, and *M. B. Shimkin,* The Effect of Transfusions and Antibiotics upon the Duration of Life in Children with Lymphogenous Leucemia, *J. Pediat.* 37:455, 1950.

Block, M., L. O. Jacobson, and *W. F. Bethard,* Preleukemic Acute Human Leukemia, *J.A.M.A.* 152:1018, 1953.

Cooke, J. V., The Occurrence of Leukemia, Blood 9:340, 1954.

Falkenstein, D., and W. M. Fowler, Acute Lymphatic Leukemia in Childhood, Am. J. Dis. Child. 65:455, 1943.

Furth, J., Analytical Review: Recent Studies of the Etiology and Nature of Leukemia, Blood 6:964, 1951.

Gessler, C. J., Monocytic Leukemia, Blood 3:960, 1948.

Gilliam, A. G., Age, Sex and Race Selection at Death from Leukemia and the Lymphomas, Blood 8:693, 1953.

Gross, L., Is Leukemia Caused by a Transmissible Virus? A Working Hypothesis, Blood 9:557, 1954.

Heen, R. C., Congenital Lymphatic Leukemia, Am. J. Dis. Child. 80:800, 1950.

Karpinski, F. E., Jr., The Skeletal Lesions of Leucemic Children Treated with Aminopterin, J. Pediat. 37:208, 1950.

Kelsey, W. M., Jr., and D. H. Anderson, Congenital Leukemia, Am. J. Dis. Child. 58:1268, 1939.

Lanman, J. T., H. R. Bierman, and R. L. Byron, Transfusion of Leukemic Leukocytes in Man: Hematologic and Physiologic Changes, Blood 5:1099, 1950.

Maloney, W. C., and R. D. Lange, Leukemia in Atomic Bomb Survivors. II. Observations on Early Phases of Leukemia, Blood 9:663, 1954.

Moody, E. A., and R. W. Davis, Duration of Acute Leukemia in Children: Review of Literature and Report of a Case of Unusually Long Survival, Am. J. Dis. Child. 80:955, 1950.

Rosenthal, N., The Lymphomas and Leukemias, Bull. New York Acad. Med. 30:583, 1954.

Southam, C. M., L. F. Craver, H. W. Dargeon, and J. H. Burchenal, A Study of the Natural History of Acute Leukemia with Special Reference to the Duration of the Disease and the Occurrence of Remissions, Cancer 4:39, 1951.

Tivey, H., Prognosis for Survival in the Leukemias of Childhood, Pediatrics 10:48, 1952.

GRANULOCYTIC LEUKEMIA

Aballi, A. A., J. M. Labourdette, and L. Barreras, Dos Casos de Leucemia Mieloide Cronica en Niñes, Rev. cubana pediat. 18:630, 1946.

Black-Schaffer, B., and L. D. Stoddard, Panmyelosis and Chronic Granulocytic Leukemia, Am. J. Path. 29:413, 1953.

Cooke, J. V., Chronic Myelogenous Leukemia in Children, J. Pediat. 42:537, 1953.

Eisenberg, A. A., and H. Wallerstein, Chronic Myelosis in Children with Report of a Case, J. Lab. & Clin. Med. 19:713, 1934.

Friedman, M., I. J. Wolman, and H. H. Tyner, Eosinophil Leukemia with Report of a Case, Am. J. M. Sc. 208:333, 1944.

Keith, H. M., Chronic Myelogenous Leukemia in Infancy, Am. J. Dis. Child. 69:366, 1945.

Laha, P. N., Chronic Myeloid Leukemia in a Girl Aged Eight Years, Antiseptic 43:56, 1946.

Ruiz, E. P., Reporte de un caso de leucemia mieloide cronica en un lactante tratado con uretano, Rev. cubana pediat. 12:751, 1950.

Scarizza, P. M., Un caso di leucemia mieloide cronica in un bambino trattato con uretano, Minerva pediat. 2:278, 1950.

THERAPY OF LEUKEMIA

Adams, W. S., W. N. Valentine, S. H. Bassett, and J. S. Lawrence, The Effect of Cortisone and ACTH in Leukemia, J. Lab. & Clin. Med. 39:570, 1952.

Burchenal, J. H., The Clinical Management of Leukemias, Cancer Res. 14:615, 1954.

Burchenal, J. H., The Treatment of Leukemia, *Bull. New York Acad. Med.* 30:429, 1954.

———, *M. L. Murphy,* and *C. T. C. Tan,* Treatment of Acute Leukemia, *Pediatrics,* 18:643, 1956.

Creskoff, A. J., T. Fitz-Hugh, Jr., and *J. W. Frost,* Urethane Therapy in Leukemia, *Blood* 3:986, 1948.

Earle, A. M., Thymectomy and ACTH in Lymphatic Leucemia, *J. Pediat.* 38:63, 1950.

———, *W. A. Reilly,* and *W. G. Lawson,* Citrovorum Factor in Leucemia: Two Cases with Autopsy Findings, *J. Pediat.* 39:560, 1951.

Farber, S., Some Observations on the Effect of Folic Acid Antagonists on Acute Leukemia and Other Forms of Incurable Cancer, *Blood* 4:160, 1949.

Leikin, S., The Treatment of Acute Leukemia in Children, *J. Pediat.* 41:40, 1952.

Poncher, H. G., H. A. Waisman, J. B. Richmond, O. A. Horak, and *L. R. Limarzi,* Treatment of Acute Leukemia in Children with and without Folic Acid Antagonists, *J. Pediat.* 41:377, 1952.

Proc. Conf. on 6-Mercaptopurine, *Ann. New York Acad. Sc.* 60:183, 1954.

Schulman, I., J. T. Lanman, O. E. Laxdal, and *L. E. Holt, Jr.,* Effects of ACTH and Cortisone on Leukemia in Childhood, *Pediatrics* 8:34, 1951.

Snelling, C. E., et al., Pituitary Adrenocorticotropic Hormone (ACTH) and 11-Dehydro-17-Hydroxy Corticosterone (Cortisone) Therapy in the Leukemias and Lymphonas of Children, *Pediatrics* 8:22, 1951.

Wolman, I. J., Current Therapy of Childhood Leukemia, *Quart. Rev. Pediat.* 10:203, 1955.

———, *J. H. Githens, Jr., B. Dickstein, P. G. Eglick, B. C. Slaughter, H. E. Butson,* and *A. N. Evans,* The Folic Acid Antagonists in Acute Leukemia of Childhood, *Quart. Rev. Pediat.* 7:121, 1952.

ERYTHROLEUKEMIA

Martin, W. J., and *E. D. Bayrd,* Erythroleukemia, with Special Emphasis on the Acute or Incomplete Variety: Report of Five Cases, *Blood* 9:321, 1954.

Menten, M. L., and *P. C. Gaffney,* Immature Cell Erythremia, *Am. J. Dis. Child.* 80:982, 1950.

Oropeza, P., M. Layrisse, and *J. Barnola,* Mielosis Eritremica, *Arch. venez. de puericult. y pediat.* 16:177, 1953.

Wegelius, R., and *T. Peltonen,* Erythraemic Myelosis (di Guglielmo) in an Infant, *Acta paediat.* 43:280, 1954.

CHAPTER 18

Miscellaneous Disorders of the Leukocytes

LEUKEMOID REACTIONS

An extreme degree of neutrophilic leukocytosis with a total count of 50,000 to 150,000 or higher occasionally develops during the course of severe infections or intoxications or systemic diseases. This reaction is perhaps more common during infancy but may be seen at any age. Band forms, metamyelocytes, myelocytes, and even more primitive cell forms are often numerous, and "blast" cells and atypical cells may appear. Bone marrow aspiration typically shows great numbers and proliferative activity of the granulocyte precursors. The blood and marrow findings may simulate acute granulocytic leukemia. If the causative disease is one that has an associated anemia, splenomegaly, and fever, differentiation from leukemia may be impossible at the time, and later developments must be awaited. A leukemoid reaction typically subsides quickly (provided the patient recovers), whereas true leukemia does not.

Leukemoid reactions have been observed in a wide diversity of diseases, including septicemia, pneumonia, congenital syphilis, diphtheria, malaria, osteomyelitis, diabetic coma, acute poisonings, and after sudden hemorrhages. Large numbers of immature and distorted cells may enter the circulation terminally in patients dying of any cause.

Nucleated erythrocytes and increased number of platelets usually accompany the great outpouring of granulocytes and may serve to confuse the recognition of the disturbance. If the nucleated red cells are in considerable numbers, a proper correction in the observed leukocyte count should be made in order to obtain the true figure.

To be considered as having leukemoid reactions are those occasional children whose total leukocytes are not disturbed significantly but whose differential studies of blood and bone marrow temporarily show an unusual number of blast cells and dystrophic cells of either the lymphocytic or granulocytic series. When this condition is suspected it is best to withhold the diagnosis of leukemia and manage the patient solely with frequent blood counts and physical examinations. The passage of time will answer the question whether these cellular changes are benign or malignant.

222

CYCLIC NEUTROPENIA (PERIODIC SYNDROME)

This is a peculiar disorder of unknown cause, in which 5- to 10-day periods of infections, fever, and neutrophilopenia recur at approximately 3-week intervals over many years. The infective phenomena, highly variable, may consist of pharyngitis, tonsillitis, otitis media, furunculosis, gastroenteritis, oral ulcers, arthralgia, abdominal pain, bronchopneumonia, or related manifestations.

Most of the recorded cases have had their onset in infancy or childhood. Careful examination has demonstrated that the first sign of a recurrent episode is a virtual disappearance of maturing granulocytes from the bone marrow. One or two days later the peripheral neutrophils fall to less than 1,000 and often to practically zero. In another day or two the fever and signs of infection develop. During the height of the agranulocytosis the lymphocytes and monocytes may show a slight absolute increase. After the attack it takes 1 to 2 weeks for the neutrophils to rise slowly to normal or subnormal levels in both blood and bone marrow.

Closely related, if not of identical origin, is the syndrome of recurrent abdominal pain and fever without overt infection. Between episodes the patients appear in good health. The leukocyte count may not change. Antiepileptic drugs and other forms of therapy are of no benefit.

Apart from the frequent granulocytopenia and an elevated red cell sedimentation rate, there are no other characteristic laboratory abnormalities.

ACUTE INFECTIOUS LYMPHOCYTOSIS

This is a benign infectious disease of unknown origin which typically produces no symptoms. Attacks seem to occur more often in infants and children than in adults and are characterized by a marked leukocytosis due to a marked increase in lymphocytes. Many epidemics are on record. The incubation period is tentatively thought to be 12 to 21 days. An occasional patient at the onset of an attack may have for a day or two some abdominal discomfort, diarrhea, vomiting, neck rigidity, nasal discharge, or low fever. When siblings or institutional contacts of a case are surveyed, other asymptomatic individuals with similar blood changes are often discovered.

The total leukocyte count may range from 15,000 to as much as 150,000 per cu mm but usually falls between 20,000 and 50,000. The responsible lymphocytes are identical morphologically with normal small lymphocytes. The hemoglobin levels, blood sedimentation rates, and heterophil antibody responses are undisturbed. There are no other known laboratory abnormalities. The bone marrow shows no significant increase in these cells, and the superficial lymph nodes over the body are not swollen. The lymphocytosis lasts from 2 to 8 weeks, as a rule, and then subsides gradually. This peculiar illness may be highly prevalent within a child-hood population but will go unrecognized unless screening blood studies are made. The writer suggests this diagnosis whenever lymphocytosis with morphologically unaltered cells is discovered in a child who has no indications of any other disease which is known to evoke such a cellular reaction. The physical examination and blood counts should always be repeated 2 to 4 weeks later to rule out leukemia and infectious mononucleosis.

PRIMARY SPLENIC GRANULOCYTOPENIA

This is a disturbance in which the peripheral absolute count of neutro-phils becomes depressed in consequence of splenic humoral activity or so-called hypersplenism (p. 295). The erythrocytes or platelets are some-times also moderately depressed. The bone marrow displays hypercellu-larity of the myelocytes and granulocytes, often with an unusual propor-tion of highly immature cells. The disturbance, if it continues and is refractory to cortisone or corticotropin or other hemopoietic stimulants, will nearly always be relieved by splenectomy.

CHRONIC HYPOPLASTIC GRANULOCYTOPENIA

This is a rare syndrome of unknown cause which is characterized pri-marily by a prolonged and severe depression of the neutrophils. Patients have an unusual propensity to infections which may occur in any part of the body, but the skin and oral cavity are involved most frequently. Between infections there are no symptoms. The spleen is often moderately enlarged. The absolute count of granulocytes usually remains below 1,000 per cu mm and rarely exceeds 2,000 even transiently. Some patients have an absolute lymphocytosis or monocytosis or a slight anemia or thrombo-cytopenia. In the bone marrow there is a paucity of cells in the granulo-cytic series, with a relatively undisturbed appearance and cellularity of the rubricytes and megakaryocytes. Splenectomy does not affect the dis-ease. Antibiotic and supportive measures are needed for infections when present. The major hematologic differentiation is from granulocytopenia caused by splenic hyperactivity.

In what appears to be a less advanced variety of this syndrome the marrow may show an abundance of myelocytes and other immature granulocytes, rather than a diminution in numbers. These patients often have no splenomegaly and no unusual susceptibility to infection. The condition may be chronic and persistent or recede spontaneously after several months or years.

INFANTILE GENETIC AGRANULOCYTOSIS

Kostmann has described a hereditary disorder in which marrow maturation of granulocytes appears to be blocked, resulting in a peripheral agranulocytosis or granulocytopenia. Affected newborn infants have a pronounced susceptibility in infections, especially those caused by staphylococci.

TRANSITORY GRANULOCYTOPENIA OF THE NEWBORN

A transitory granulocytopenia lasting a few weeks has been observed during the neonatal period in successive sibling infants, along with a marrow pattern of maturation arrest at the premyelocyte stage.

ALYMPHOCYTOSIS

This is an unusual and fatal disease, seen most often in infancy or early childhood, and characterized by fever, hepatomegaly, splenomegaly, and lymphocytopenia. Postmortem examination reveals widespread atrophy and necrosis of the lymphoid tissue. Lymphocytes disappear almost entirely from the circulating blood and bone marrow during life, but the granulocytes, erythrocytes, and other cell forms are not much diminished, if at all.

FAMILIAL HEMOPHAGOCYTIC RETICULOSIS

This is a rare familial disorder in which a tremendous proliferation and overgrowth of reticuloendothelial cells take place in the lymph nodes, spleen, liver, bone marrow, and kidneys. The patients exhibit a progressive reduction in all the cellular elements of the blood other than the lymphocytes, despite a marked compensatory hyperplasia of the uninvaded areas of the bone marrow. Fever, jaundice, purpura, and signs of systemic intoxication appear, and death usually follows the onset of symptoms by a few months. The proliferating reticuloendothelial cells have a diffuse rather than granulomatous distribution and ingest and destroy red cells, leukocytes, and platelets.

LUPUS ERYTHEMATOSUS

In this poorly understood form of what is believed to be a hypersensitivity reaction, the neutrophils and sometimes other cell strains demonstrate the property of being able to phagocytize other leukocytes on in vitro incubation. The characteristic LE (lupus erythematosus) cell is a neutrophil from the peripheral blood or bone marrow which contains a basophilic inclusion body in the cytoplasm, or a group of neutrophils encircling and engulfing similar amorphous masses. These inclusion bodies and extracellular material give a positive reaction with Feulgen's stain and appear to be depolymerized desoxyribose nucleic acid derived from the nuclei of other cells. With Wright's stain their color varies from deep reddish purple to light bluish purple.

Often accompanying LE cells are so-called "tart" cells, which are monocytes or reticuloendothelial cells with a nucleus-like body in the curve of the main nucleus.

LE cells are usually not apparent in smears made immediately from aspirated material. To bring out the phenomenon a time lag of 15 minutes to 2 hours is required between securing of the blood or marrow sample and its fixation upon the glass slide. The property of inducing this cellular change resides in the serum, as shown by the observation that serum from lupus erythematosus patients will induce this change in the leukocytes from fresh heparinized bone marrow or peripheral blood of normal individuals or even of experimental animals. The converse does not obtain. Splenectomy does not alter the reactivity of the serum. The plasma factor has been shown by electrophoresis to be part of the gamma globulin complex.

Test Procedure. Numerous relatively simple methods for demonstrating the lupus erythematosus phenomenon have been described. Mathis's instructions follow, in modified form:

1. Collect 5 ml of blood from a vein or the bone marrow and transfer to a sterile centrifuge tube containing an anticoagulant. Mix by gentle shaking.

2. Stand the tube upright at room temperature for 30 minutes, until the blood cells have settled to the bottom.

3. With a sterile long-stemmed narrow pipet, transfer the supernatant plasma and uppermost level of the underlying cells to a sterile centrifuge tube or Wintrobe sedimentation tube. This is kept at 37°C for 45 minutes in an incubator or water bath, or for 2 hours at room temperature.

4. After this incubation, centrifuge the specimen for a few minutes at 1,500 to 2,000 rpm.

5. Remove the supernatant plasma with a narrow pipet and discard all but approximately 0.5 ml. Retain the latter for subsequent use as a diluent.

6. Remove the sediment with the pipet, and prepare smears on glass slides in the usual way. The slides should be kept in 95 per cent alcohol and wiped dry just before using. Search the interior of the centrifuge tube for small cartilage-like masses, composed mainly of collections of packed platelets. These should be picked up with a small wire loop, placed on a slide, emulsified with a drop of the plasma diluent, and smears should be made.

7. Stain with any of the Romanowsky stains such as Wright's stain. Mathis recommends tetrachrome (MacNeal) stain.

8. Examine the films microscopically with "high-dry" and oil-immersion objectives. LE and tart cells will be most abundant at the edges of the smears and in the platelet masses.

PELGER-HUËT ANOMALY

This is a hereditary disturbance of the segmentation of the granulocytes. Most of these cells are monolobed or bilobed. There is a high percentage of band cells and even more immature cells in the circulation.

The marrow may show an unusual abundance of myelocytes and meta-myelocytes. The granulocyte nuclei at all stages of maturation have an unusually coarse chromatin structure. The disorder may be mistaken for low-grade chronic granulocytic leukemia.

GARGOYLISM (DYSOSTOSIS MULTIPLEX)

In this generalized constitutional disturbance, the granulocytes or other circulating leukocytes may contain dark-staining granules or be otherwise distorted.

BIBLIOGRAPHY

CYCLIC NEUTROPENIA

Borne, S., Cyclic Neutropenia in an Infant, *Pediatrics* 4:70, 1949.
Coventry, W. D., Cyclic Neutropenia: Report of a Case Treated By Splenectomy, *J.A.M.A.* 153:28, 1953.
Moncrieff, A., Recurrent Neutropenia, *Arch. Dis. Childhood* 26:438, 1951.
Owren, P. A., Cyclic Agranulocytosis, *Acta med. scandinav.* 134:87, 1949.
Periodic Syndrome. *Case Reports of The Children's Memorial Hospital, Chicago, Ill.* 14:3932, 1956.
Reimann, H. A., and *C. T. DeBerardinis,* Periodic (Cyclic) Neutropenia, an Entity: A Collection of 16 Cases, *Blood* 4:1109, 1949.

ACUTE INFECTIOUS LYMPHOCYTOSIS

Barnes, G. R., Jr., A Clinical Study of an Institutional Outbreak of Acute Infectious Lymphocytosis, *Am. J. M. Sc.* 218:646, 1949.
Lemon, B. K., and *D. H. Kaump,* Infectious Lymphocytosis: A Report of an Epidemic in Children, *J. Pediat.* 36:61, 1950.
Moyer, J. B., and *G. S. Fisher,* Acute Infectious Lymphocytosis, *Blood* 5:677, 1950.
Smith, C. H., Acute Infectious Lymphocytosis, *Advances Pediat.* 2:64, 1947.
Waldman, S., and *A. M. Frumin,* Infectious Lymphocytosis: A Report of Two Cases Noted Following Trauma, *J. Pediat.* 39:455, 1951.

LUPUS ERYTHEMATOSUS

Beerman, H., The L. E. Cell and Phenomenon in Lupus Erythematosus, *Am. J. M. Sc.* 222:473, 1951.
Cornelia, M., Demonstrating L. E. (Lupus Erythematosus) Cells in Blood, *Canad. J. Med. Technol.* 16:60, 1954.
Hargraves, M. M., Systemic Lupus Erythematosus and L.E. Cell Phenomenon, *Postgrad. Med.* 16:164, 1954.
Holman, S., The Lupus Erythematosus Cell Inclusion Phenomenon, *J. Clin. Path.* 4:290, 1951.
Mathis, H. B., A Simple Office Procedure for Demonstrating Lupus Erythematosus Cells in Peripheral Blood, *Blood* 6:470, 1951.

MISCELLANEOUS

Begemann, N. H., and *A. V. L. Campagne,* Homozygous Form of Pelger-Huët's Nuclear Anomaly in Man, *Acta haemat.* 7:295, 1952.

Donohue, W. L., Alymphocytosis, *Pediatrics* 11:129, 1953.

Farquhar, J. W., and *A. E. Claireaux,* Familial Haemophagocytic Reticulosis, *Arch. Dis. Childhood* 27:519, 1952.

Kostmann, R., Infantile Genetic Agranulocytosis (Agranulocytosis infantilis hereditaria): A New Recessive Lethal Disease in Man, *Acta paediat.* Suppl. 105, 1956.

Reilly, W. A., The Granulocytes in the Leukocytes in Gargoylism. *Am. J. Dis. Child.* 62:489, 1941.

Spaet, T. H., and *W. Dameshek,* Chronic Hypoplastic Neutropenia, *Am. J. Med.* 13:35, 1952.

Stahlie, T. D., Chronic Benign Neutropenia in Infancy and Early Childhood, *J. Pediat.* 48:710, 1956.

Young, C. J., Leucocyte Counts in Prevention of Drug Agranulocytosis, *Brit. M. J.* 2:261, 1949.

CHAPTER 19

Physiology of Coagulation of the Blood

Children with an unusual tendency to hemorrhage present intriguing laboratory problems. Almost no single test is pathognomonic for any one disorder, with the possible exception of absent fibrinogen in congenital afibrinogenemia. Elucidation of the disturbance calls for a careful history and physical examination and critical testing of the many physiologic mechanisms which protect normal individuals from abnormal bleeding.

From the standpoint of classification, the hemorrhagic disorders can be subdivided somewhat empirically on the basis of being attributable primarily to (1) abnormalities in the thrombocytes or platelets, (2) disturbances in the chemoserologic systems related to blood clotting, or (3) defects in vascular integrity.

The integration and overlapping of the various hemostatic mechanisms and their surplus or reserve capacities make it possible for a defect to exist in a single mechanism without any resulting bleeding, provided all other mechanisms are normal. Symptoms which go back to early infancy are more characteristic of congenital and hereditary disturbances, whereas a comparatively late onset is more typical of a nonhereditary disease. Spontaneous hemorrhages in the absence of recognizable trauma are usual in platelet and vascular deficiencies, whereas bleeding related to injury is more typical of a blood clotting disturbance such as hemophilia. The spleen may be enlarged in thrombocytopenic purpura and leukemia, but not in uncomplicated hemophilia, vascular defects, and prothrombin deficiencies.

COAGULATION OF THE BLOOD

This extremely complex phenomenon results from the interaction of many chemical and enzymatic influences. Most of these represent equilibria between dynamically balanced components rather than single substances.

Coagulation is best presented as a sequence of three interdependent steps or phases (Table 19-1). Inherent in each successive step is one or several chain reactions, in which intermediate substances as soon as produced serve as accelerators of their own further production.

229

PHYSIOLOGIC FACTORS WHICH FAVOR COAGULATION

Platelets (Thrombocytes)

These are the trigger stimuli for the formation of thrombi within blood vessels and the gel-like coagulation of blood at sites of tissue injury. Were it not for their natural tendency to be attracted to rough spots and to disintegrate promptly thereafter with the liberation of clotting enzymes, the innumerable small tears of blood vessels constantly produced by body activities could not be sealed off immediately. Petechiae, ecchymoses, and related manifestations of imperfect hemostasis would then be of everyday occurrence, as takes place in active thrombocytopenic states (Chap. 23).

Table 19-1. Stages in the Coagulation of Blood (Simplified Outline) *

Stage I

THROMBOPLASTINOGEN (AHF)—————————————→THROMBOPLASTIN
　　　　　　　　　　　　　　　　Platelet factor,
　　　　　　　　　　　　　　　　PTC, PTA, others

Stage II

　　　　　　　　　　THROMBOPLASTIN
PROTHROMBIN—————————————→THROMBIN
　　　　　　　　　Calcium
　　　　　　　　　Labile factor (V)
　　　　　　　　　Stable factor (VII)

Stage III

　　　　　　　　　THROMBIN
FIBRINOGEN—————————→FIBRIN
　　　　　　　Platelet factor

* See text for explanation.

Platelets lyse spontaneously whenever blood comes in contact with a rough or foreign surface, whether in traumatized blood vessels or on glass surfaces. Disintegrating platelets liberate substances which attract other platelets and hasten their dissolution in turn. One substance is the factor which activates thromboplastinogen, the plasma precursor of thromboplastin. Some authors hold that the platelets release thromboplastin itself. Platelets also give rise to at least two other platelet accelerator factors which enter into later phases of the coagulating reaction. One of these facilitates the conversion of prothrombin to thrombin, and the other enhances the reaction between thrombin and fibrinogen to form fibrin. It is probable also that platelets are responsible for a vasoconstrictor agent, termed serotonin, which aids in the hemostatic sealing off of traumatized blood vessels.

Platelets normally survive in the circulation for 5 or 6 days. New ones are being liberated constantly in great numbers from the marrow megakaryocytes.

In hemophilia the platelets and platelet enzymes are normal, as shown by unimpaired coagulation of normal deplateletized plasma when washed hemophilic platelets are added to it. The clotting time of recalcified hemophilic plasma is longer when the plasma has been prepared by rapid centrifugation to remove the platelets. Some cases of hemophilia-like disease are believed due, at least in part, to a circulating anticoagulant which seems to oppose this platelet enzyme.

Enumeration of Platelets

Platelets are highly fragile. They attach themselves with great speed to the surfaces of glass or debris in laboratory equipment and disintegrate rapidly during handling. They are usually counted by means of the so-called direct approach of Rees and Ecker. Finger tip blood is mixed with a solution containing sodium citrate, formaldehyde, and brilliant cresyl blue dye and the platelets enumerated in a counting chamber.

Reported ranges for normal individuals vary considerably. The accuracy of the procedure depends greatly upon the skill of the technician. Furthermore, physiologic variability appears to be somewhat more pronounced in children than in adults. The values for healthy children counted by the Rees and Ecker method in our laboratory spread from 200,000 to 300,000 per cu mm. The average is approximately 250,000. Deviations in serial readings are not deemed of much significance unless greater than 10 per cent of each other.

Many normal infants exhibit counts as low as 100,000 at birth; as a rule these rise to the level for older children within 3 months. Otherwise there are no pronounced trends of change with respect to age or sex during childhood. In adolescent girls the count may decrease by as much as 50,000 during the first few days of menstruation.

Thromboplastin (Thrombokinase, Cytozyme, Thromboplastic Protein, Thrombokinin)

This term is applied collectively to a group of phospholipid protein compounds which occur in tissue juice and organ extracts and are liberated by traumatized or altered vascular endothelium. Preparations for use in laboratory testing can be extracted from rabbit brain, human brain, rabbit lung, beef lung, and other tissues. Standardized preparations are available from commercial sources.

A precursor form, thromboplastinogen or antihemophilic factor (AHF), exists in the plasma perhaps in combination with an inhibitor. Thromboplastinogen is converted into plasma thromboplastin by the enzyme liberated from disintegrating platelets, provided the plasma thromboplastin component (PTC; "Christmas factor") and related substances such as plasma thromboplastin antecedent (PTA) are present in adequate amounts (Chap. 21). Some workers suggest that all these combine to form an intermediate product which in turn unites with factors V and VII (see below) to produce thromboplastin.

Prothrombin Complex

Prothrombin, a globulin contained normally in plasma, becomes converted to thrombin by thromboplastin when calcium ions and other activators are present. Prothrombin is continually being synthesized by the liver, with vitamin K as an essential ingredient. When the liver is damaged seriously or the intake or absorption of vitamin K suddenly curtailed, the blood prothrombin level will fall within a day or two. There is evidence that prothrombin occurs in the plasma partly as a free form and partly as a precursor which has to be activated.

Several components of the plasma, in addition to the platelet accelerator and calcium, promote the conversion of prothrombin to thrombin. One of these is serum Ac-globulin (serum accelerator factor, labile factor, accelerin, thrombinogenase, or factor VI). Another is its inactive precursor, plasma Ac-globulin (plasma accelerator factor, unconverted labile factor, proaccelerin, prothrombinogenase, or factor V). Together these are known as accelerator factor or labile factor. Still another component is factor VII (convertin, prothrombin conversion factor, or stable factor). The precise character of these and their interrelations among each other and to prothrombin is still far from agreed upon, and the distinctions between them may be somewhat artificial. They appear to be consumed during the formation of thrombin. Normal subjects seem to possess ample reserves of all these factors.

Blood coagulation appears to be initiated by the liberation of platelet components. Some of the intermediate products which first form have an autocatalytic action. For example, it has been postulated that when prothrombin reacts with thromboplastin (in the presence of calcium ions), thrombin develops very slowly at the beginning. The first thrombin to form converts the hitherto inactive plasma Ac-globulin into the active serum Ac-globulin. The serum Ac-globulin then speeds up the interaction of prothrombin and thromboplastin, so that thrombin is yielded with accelerating speed. The latter in turn may facilitate the disintegration of platelets still intact, thereby releasing more thromboplastinogenase and accelerating the entire reaction chain.

Calcium

This occurs in plasma in such abundance that relevant coagulation defects and difficulties do not ensue even in the most extreme of clinical hypocalcemic states. The calcium must be in a diffusible ionized form, perhaps in combination with an organic cofactor, for coagulation to take place.

Soluble citrates or oxalates, when added to blood, inhibit clotting by combining with the calcium or suppressing its ionization. This phenomenon is utilized in the collection of blood for indirect transfusions and in the preparation of plasma for laboratory procedures.

Fibrinogen

An unstable soluble protein of high molecular weight, this occurs in plasma in a concentration of 0.2 to 0.4 gm per 100 ml. In the blood it is continually being destroyed and renewed, with a complete turnover every few days. A threshold concentration of at least 0.06 gm per 100 ml is believed necessary for clotting to be detectable.

Fibrinogen is converted to solid fibrin by the action of thrombin. A solid clot becomes detectable when somewhat less than half the fibrinogen has been converted to fibrin.

In vitro, as more and more fibrin is produced the clot becomes firmer and soon begins to contract. The measurable thrombin and prothrombin activity diminish rapidly, either from neutralization or more probably by absorption onto the surface of the fibrin. By virtue of being able to absorb unused thrombin and prothrombin from the circulating blood, fibrin itself is somewhat of a clotting antagonist.

Disorders characterized by inadequate fibrin formation are congenital afibrinogenemia (p. 275), congenital or acquired hypofibrinogenemia (p. 275), and purpura fibrinolytica (p. 288).

PHYSIOLOGIC FACTORS WHICH COUNTERACT COAGULATION

Nearly every coagulating influence seems to be matched by a corresponding inhibiting mechanism. Were this not so, any small clot commencing anywhere in an injured terminal vessel would spread and involve ultimately the entire vascular system. The more important of these counteracting mechanisms are as follows:

The Blood Current

This is a most important safeguard against intravascular clotting. The incessant wearing out of platelets, prothrombin, and fibrinogen within the blood stream would shift the fluid equilibria in the direction of coagulation if the flowing stream did not dilute and inactivate these coagulant products before they might accumulate.

Intact Vascular Endothelium

The smooth lining of the blood vessels protects against local adhesion of platelets whose ensuing disintegration would otherwise spark the process of coagulation into activity. Intravascular clotting does not occur except after local injury or extreme stagnation of the stream.

Antithromboplastin

Substances antagonistic to plasma thromboplastic activity are extractable from blood, plasma, brain tissue, and lung. Hemophilic blood is stated by Tocantins to contain more antithromboplastin than does normal blood. Abnormal antithromboplastins may develop in lupus erythematosus, pemphigus, and in hemophilia after multiple transfusions.

Antithrombin

Substances exhibiting activity antagonistic to the formation of both prothrombin and thrombin have been uncovered in the albumin fraction of normal plasma by special methods. Poorly understood, these agents are believed to occur in concentrations just adequate to neutralize the beginning phases of intravascular clot formation. Pharmaceutic agents of varying potency which may act as coagulation inhibitors are heparin, hirudin, Dicumarol, Tromexan, penicillin, and salicylates in high dosages.

Fibrinolysin

Clotted blood or plasma from a normal individual will ordinarily remain intact for days or weeks if kept sterile. In some disturbances, however, the clot may liquefy spontaneously and dissolve within a few hours. This has been observed to occur in blood specimens collected during or soon after exposure of the subject to a variety of stimuli—violent physical activity, states of fear, anxiety, or other violent emotions, hemorrhage, shock, trauma, anesthesia, surgical operations, injections of epinephrine, hemolytic transfusion reactions, severe parenchymal liver disease, and extensive pulmonary surgery.

Such lysis of fibrin clots is effected by the enzyme fibrinolysin (plasmin) which is capable of attacking not only fibrin but also fibrinogen and the members of the prothrombin complex. Fibrinolysin is ordinarily present in the circulating blood as an inert proenzyme (profibrinolysin, plasminogen). Activation of the conversion of profibrinolysin into fibrinolysin requires stimulation by a specific enzyme provisionally termed fibrinokinase (fibrinolysokinase), which normally is present in both tissues and plasma. In ordinary circumstances this enzyme appears to be depressed or neutralized by inhibitors in the plasma. The biochemical circumstances which stimulate it into activity are not yet understood. Also contained in the blood are powerful antifibrinolysins (antiplasmin) capable of destroying fibrinolysin and thereby protecting fibrinogen, fibrin, and prothrombin.

OTHER FACTORS INFLUENCING COAGULATION

Agreement is fairly universal as to the actuality of the components of the coagulation reaction thus far mentioned. The platelets, in addition to initiating or influencing the action of thromboplastin, seem to potentiate the reaction between fibrogen and thrombin. There may be a thrombocytolysin factor in plasma to shatter the platelets. Heparin itself or heparin-like substances known as antithrombins may not function normally as physiologic anticoagulants, but appreciable quantities are sometimes demonstrable in the serum after prolonged irradiation or exposure to nitrogen mustards.

When fibrin is deposited in the presence of an abundance of platelets its strands are long and thin, whereas if platelets are scanty the strands are thick and shorter.

CLOT RETRACTION

Changes continue in clotted blood in vitro after solidification first becomes evident. Intact platelets, activated by thrombin, combine with or pull upon the precipitated fibrin strands and cause them to twist and shrink. In normal blood this process of retraction begins soon after the clot is fully solidified and is completed by 1 or 2 hours thereafter. Clot retraction is incomplete in platelet disorders such as purpura hemorrhagica; it is inadequate also when fibrin formation is defective. There is a question whether clot retraction occurs within the body. The phenomenon is nevertheless very helpful in the laboratory study of hemorrhagic disturbances (p. 249).

CONTRACTION AND OCCLUSION OF SMALL BLOOD VESSELS

Injured small blood vessels participate in hemostasis by almost immediate vasoconstriction at sites of trauma. The vascular lumens then become occluded by plugs of platelets, followed soon by precipitation of supporting threads of fibrin.

Initial contraction of blood vessels is mediated in part through the sympathetic nervous system. One stimulus for this response may be a vasoconstricting agent released by the first platelets to adhere to the traumatized edges of the vessels. This cohesive aggregation of platelets at a site of injury is encouraged by tissue thromboplastin seeping in from the contiguous tissue spaces. Fibrin is deposited later, in response to the thrombin produced within the platelet clot after the platelets have disintegrated and their thromboplastinogen has been released. It has been suggested that plugging of injured small vessels by tenacious plugs fails to occur in thrombocytopenic states, hyperheparinemia, and Dicumarol-produced hypoprothrombinemia.

Bleeding disturbances attributable to dysfunctioning or fragile blood vessels include such conditions as hereditary hemorrhagic telangiectasia, scurvy, congenital capillary weakness, and some forms of pseudohemophilia.

BIBLIOGRAPHY

HEMOSTASIS AND COAGULATION

Allen, G. W., and *A. M. Attyah*, A Rational Approach to the Problems of the Coagulation Time, *J. Lab. & Clin. Med.* 41:767, 1953.

Biggs, R., and *R. G. Macfarlane*, "Human Blood Coagulation and Its Disorders," Charles C Thomas, Springfield, Ill., 1953.

Budtz-Olsen, O. E., "Clot Retraction," Charles C Thomas, Springfield, Ill., 1951.

DeRobertis, E., P. Paseyro, and *M. Reissig*, Electron Microscopic Studies of the Action of Thrombin on Blood Platelets, *Blood* 7:587, 1953.

Donovan, T. J., and *B. Zimmermann*, The Effect of Artificial Surfaces on Blood Coagulability, with Special Reference to Polyethylene, *Blood* 4:1310, 1949.

Laurell, C.-B., Synonyms for Components Influencing Blood Coagulation, *Blood* 7:555, 1952.

Lewis, M. L., and *A. G. Ware*, The Mechanism of Action of Human Accelerator Globulin and Its Relation to Other Clotting Factors, *Blood* 9:520, 1954.

Quick, A. J., Clot Retraction: Its Physiological and Clinical Significance, *Am. J. M. Sc.* 220:538, 1950.

———, "The Physiology and Pathology of Hemostasis," Lea & Febiger, Philadelphia, 1951.

Stefanini, M., Basic Mechanisms of Hemostasis, *Bull. New York Acad. Med.* 30:239, 1954.

——— and *W. Dameshek*, "The Hemorrhagic Disorders: A Clinical and Therapeutic Approach," Grune & Stratton, Inc., New York, 1955.

CHAPTER 20

Hemorrhagic Disorders: Laboratory Approaches

A goodly array of tests have been standardized to study the integrity of the mechanisms of hemostasis in patients with a tendency to hemorrhage. Because of the complexity of the interrelationships, however, practically all these tests assay not one but several of these mechanisms simultaneously. A normal result with any one test means that all the several pertinent factors are in good functional condition. An aberrant result, though indicating that something is wrong, requires further studies to elucidate the nature of the disturbance. Interpretation may be difficult because of (1) great physiologic reserves, so that minor quantitative deficiencies are not easily apparent, and (2) absence of "pure" preparations of most of the constituents of blood clotting, making it difficult or impossible to set up accurate laboratory systems to control the comparisons or titrations.

In the childhood years, thromboses and lesser manifestations of hypercoagulability are exceptional. Clinical disturbances related to hemostasis and blood clotting nearly always are in the direction of hemorrhagic phenomena.

The succeeding pages discuss the laboratory features of the various hemorrhagic disorders in approximately the same order as they relate to the major steps in the coagulation of the blood. Should all tests give normal results one must conclude that (1) the hemostatic dysfunction is inactive at the time of the test; (2) it is of minor severity and needs to be investigated by more sensitive and delicate tests if available; or (3) no true hemorrhagic dyscrasia exists in the patient, and the bleeding phenomena result from anatomic, traumatic, or other local factors.

CLOT-FORMING CAPACITY OF WHOLE BLOOD

Peripheral Clotting Time (Capillary Tube Technique)

A warmed finger tip is first cleansed with alcohol or similar sterilizing fluid and permitted to dry. The ear lobe may be used, but gives less reliable results in childhood. The site should not be rubbed vigorously during the preliminary cleansing, else vascular damage may release some thromboplastin. The lateral side of the finger tip (or ear lobe) is pricked with a sharp needle and the time noted. The blood should flow rapidly and spontaneously. Squeezing or other manipulations negate the value of the test. The first drops of blood to appear are drawn by capillary action into an open glass tube 1.5 to 2 mm in diameter and about 5 cm in length. Small segments of the tube are then broken off at half-minute intervals until coagulation is detected. The period from the appearance of blood on the skin until a thread of clot forms is taken as the clotting time. Though the test is commonly done at room temperature, it is better to keep the tubes warm by holding in the hand until coagulation has occurred.

In the Dale and Laidlaw modification, segments of capillary tubing 1.5 to 2 mm in diameter and 15 mm in length and containing a small movable lead shot are filled with blood, placed in a glass beaker containing water at 37°C, and gently tilted until the shot fails to move.

Blood specimens collected peripherally coagulate more rapidly than do venous specimens in test tubes because surface contact between blood and glass is much more extensive and glass is a coagulation accelerator.

The normal limits for peripheral clotting are somewhat variable, being influenced by the bore and cleanliness of the tube, the finger temperature, and the rate of flow of the blood. In our own laboratory, using finger tip blood and empty new capillary tubes which are hand-warmed, most normal infants and children give readings between 3 and 5 minutes. The Dale and Laidlaw clotting times tend to fall between 1½ and 3 minutes.

It has been suggested that clotting times of unusual shortness are indicative of increased coagulability and a prethrombotic state and that operative patients in whom thrombosis is suspected should be observed with serial repetitions of this test. When hypercoagulability is feared, however, it is best sought for by methods which explore the resistance to added heparin.

Prolonged peripheral clotting times have the same clinical implications as those obtained with venous blood. Mild degrees of hemophilia or neonatal hypoprothrombinemia with only partial depletion of thromboplastin or prothrombin often show normal results with the peripheral clotting test, whereas with more severe deficiencies the readings are prolonged.

The peripheral clotting time is most useful as a means of following the progress of a patient with a chronic coagulation defect, once the diagnosis has been established by more precise procedures and treatment is under way. As a screening test for major coagulation difficulties it is helpful, but it fails to detect most lesser abnormalities.

Venous Clotting Time

Investigation of the clotting time of venous blood is much more amenable to standardization than the capillary tube approach. The longer interval required for the blood to clot in the broader tube enables one to detect the precise moment of mass coagulation more precisely and thereby uncover minor prolongations. Furthermore, blood collected by venipuncture is much less likely to be contaminated by tissue juices containing thromboplastin. All steps should be carried out with a minimum of trauma, utilizing scrupulously clean glassware and needles and following a standard procedure such as that outlined below.

VENOUS CLOTTING TIME (LEE-WHITE TEST). The skin over the antecubital or some other superficial vein is sterilized and permitted to dry. (Because of the possibility of serious or even fatal hemorrhage in derangements of hemostasis, deep jugular or deep femoral or longitudinal sinus punctures should never be made to secure a blood sample for this test, except by the very expert.) A tourniquet is applied just prior to venipuncture. At least 2 ml of blood is withdrawn with a sharp broad needle into a dry clean syringe. If blood is not obtained immediately and without manipulation, a new puncture should be made of another vein with a second needle and syringe. One milliliter of blood is transferred into each of two scrupulously cleaned serologic test tubes (Pyrex 100 × 13 mm). The tubes are kept warm at 37°C by being held in the hand or placed in a water bath. A vacuum bottle containing water at 37°C, fitted with a hole in which the test tube can be inserted, may also be used. The first tube is tilted gently every 30 seconds until the blood no longer moves on tilting. The second tube is then similarly tilted and watched. The clotting time is recorded as the interval between the moment when blood first enters the syringe and the longer of the intervals required for the blood in the tubes (usually the second tube) to become solidified.

With this procedure the normal range for children in our laboratory is 6 to 12 minutes, with the majority of specimens clotting between 7 and 11 minutes. Firming of the clots requires only a few more minutes with normal blood, but may take 2 or more hours in abnormal conditions.

When borderline or subclinical disturbances are suspected, the "three-tube test" may be performed. After a neat venipuncture, three syringes in succession are used to withdraw three separate specimens of blood, leaving the needle in place within the vein while the changes are made. Should thromboplastin from skin or subcuteaneous tissue have contaminated the needle point during its introduction, the blood in the third and usually in the second tube will have longer clotting times than that in the first tube.

Venous clotting times are much longer when these tests are performed in plastic, paraffined, or silicone-coated test tubes. In these circumstances, readings of 25 to 40 minutes are ordinarily obtained with normal subjects. Blood from individuals with clotting defects requires disproportionately longer periods. Blood from patients with minor coagulation defects which give normal or nearly normal clotting reading in glass tubes may require several hours to clot. Should minute amounts of tissue thromboplastin come in contact with hemophilic blood during its collection into such special tubes, however, the readings may be the same as those of normal blood. Clean glass tubes of fixed size are preferred for routine testing because of economy, greater ease of handling, and shorter time required for the readings.

Prolonged clotting times of whole blood tend to be encountered in hemophilia and hemophilia-like diseases, fibrinogen deficiencies, extreme prothrombin deficiencies, severly toxic diphtheria, in the presence of circulating anticoagulant antibodies, after large doses of therapeutic anticoagulants or of poisons such as snake venom, and sometimes in newborn infants with florid erythroblastosis fetalis. Normal readings are met with in thrombocytopenic disturbances, capillary defects, fibrinogenopenia, scurvy, and anaphylactoid purpura. In any prothrombin deficiency, regardless of cause, the prothrombin activity must be reduced to near 20 per cent of normal before the clotting readings become appreciably prolonged. In hemophilia, as already discussed, any carelessness in venipuncture which permits admixture of tissue thromboplastin may obscure the thromboplastinogen defect of the circulating blood. Furthermore, in mild forms of this disease the clotting time may be prolonged only slightly if at all when the blood is faultlessly withdrawn, even while frank hemophilic bleeding is taking place.

BLEEDING TIME

This simple procedure tests the responsivity of the combined hemostatic mechanisms when the skin tissue is injured by an incision. With children, a small cut approximately 2 mm long and 2 mm deep is customarily made in the finger tip or ear with a sharp lancet. With adults the volar surface of the forearm is often chosen. The rate of flow of blood from the incised skin, at first brisk, gradually ceases. Since clot formation may distort the result, the ooze from the cut is blotted away lightly with clean filter paper at 15-second or half-minute intervals. The interval between the moment the cut is made and the moment when bleeding stops represents the reading. The paper with its series of blood spots can be saved as a record of the time taken, shown by the number of blots, and of the rate of diminution of blood flow, shown by their progressively smaller size; it furnishes also a rough record of the quantity of blood lost. In the Macfarlane modification of the bleeding-time test the tip of the incised finger or ear is immersed in a glass cylinder containing normal saline solution at 37°C. The drops of blood descend through the saline, and the termination of bleeding can be precisely noted. The normal bleeding time with either method is 1½ to 4 minutes.

Results from normal and abnormal subjects exhibit wide variability, even in the same subject on the same day in the same finger or ear. Some workers make two to five cuts simultaneously and consider the mean of the time intervals as a more definitive reading. Skin thickness, skin and environmental temperatures, vascular contractility, depth and smoothness of the incision, number of open vessels cut, extent of tissue tearing, and platelets and other anticoagulant factors in the tissue juices or flowing blood—all affect the time required for the incised small vessels finally to cease bleeding.

An incision which penetrates only slightly into the subcutaneous tissue will throw the responsibility for repair largely upon the contractility of the capillary bed. A deeper cut, on the other hand, calls heavily upon the clotting principles of the blood as well as the reactivity of the local tissue and is much more likely to evoke a prolonged bleeding time in a patient with some abnormality in the coagulation factors.

Inconstant depth of the cuts and differences in skin thickness account for the variations in bleeding times reported for hemophilic patients. The bleeding time is usually normal with a superficial incision but may be prolonged with a deeper one.

The bleeding time is prolonged most typically in the various forms of thrombocytopenic purpura and severe hypoprothrombinemia, less regularly in conditions associated with widespread capillary disturbances, and occasionally in severe rheumatic fever, scarlet fever, and chronic nephritis. Prolonged bleeding time and even hemorrhages due to diminished prothrombin activity may be demonstrable when the clotting time is still within normal limits. In the afibrinogenemias the bleeding time may be normal or prolonged.

THROMBIN FORMATION FROM PROTHROMBIN (PLASMA PROTHROMBIN ACTIVITY)

The prothrombin time is prolonged when there are deficiencies, singly or in combination, of prothrombin itself, of the prothrombin activators or accelerators, or of fibrinogen. In addition, conversion of prothrombin to thrombin may be counteracted by heparin or circulating heparin-like anticoagulants, by Dicumarol and related drugs, and by antibody-like and other antithrombic substances. A variety of forms have been recognized in children, including (1) "physiologic" hypoprothrombinemia of the newborn, (2) hepatic hypoprothrombinemia, (3) enteral hypoprothrombinemia, (4) hypoprothrombinemia induced by drugs, (5) congenital hypoprothrombinemia, and (6) as a complication of major operations. In the nephrotic syndrome the plasma prothrombin activity may be augmented or diminished. Study of the prothrombin-thrombin phase of coagulation is therefore of assistance in the differential diagnosis of hemorrhagic disorders, in the detection of certain prehemorrhagic conditions, and as a guide for the administration of Dicumarol and other therapeutic anticoagulants which act by depressing the prothrombin level. The tests are much more sensitive than the bleeding and clotting times, and any abnormalities are pathogenetically more sharply defined.

Whole-blood Prothrombin Time

BEDSIDE TEST. A simple screening test for determining whether the plasma prothrombin activity is normal or prolonged is that of Smith, Ziffren, Owen, and Hoffman. In a small glass tube a measured amount of freshly drawn venous blood (usually 1 ml) is thoroughly mixed with a standard amount of thromboplastin. The elapsed number of seconds between the moment of mixing and the moment of clotting is compared with the mean interval for normal blood as previously determined. The percentage content of prothrombin in the blood is then approximated from the formula:

$$\frac{\text{Standard prothrombin time} \times 100}{\text{prothrombin time of patient's blood}} = \% \text{ prothrombin in patient's blood}$$

Though less precise than the one-stage test, the bedside test will detect any deficiency of prothrombin severe enough to be responsible for overt bleeding.

Plasma Prothrombin Time

ONE-STAGE TEST. This procedure expresses prothrombin activity in terms of the time needed for coagulation to occur after an excess of thromboplastin and an optimal amount of calcium have been added under standardized conditions to a unit volume of citrated or oxalated plasma. With the widely used method of Quick, which employs acetone-extracted rabbit brain as the source of thromboplastin, plasma from normal venous blood will form a coagulum in almost precisely 12 seconds. With other sources of thromboplastin such as animal lung, Russell viper venom, or human brain, somewhat different time readings may be obtained.

Minor variations in the routine of the procedure can affect the result. It is essential that every step in the procedure, even to the emptying of the pipets, be always carried out in precisely the same manner. With every new batch of reagents a series of determinations on normal subjects should be carried out in order to establish the mean normal value and its range of deviation. Blood specimens are best taken at the same time each day, because the diurnal variation in the readings from normal subjects can be as great as 2 seconds. Since formation of serum enhances prothrombin action, care should be taken to avoid partial coagulation during collection of the blood specimens to be tested.

Mention may be made of numerous micro modifications of the prothrombin determinations, such as those of Kato or of Hoffman and Custer. These employ drops of whole capillary blood obtained by punctures of the heel, toe, ear lobe, or finger and have been designed particularly for infants and small children. They employ essentially the same reagents as the macro procedures but are somewhat more involved in performance. The procedure must be standardized and the normal range determined at each laboratory.

When the coagulation time with the one-stage prothrombin test proves to be longer than in normal controls, the reading is compared with normal by reference to a "standardized" dilution curve and expressed as "per cent of normal activity." This practice may be criticized on the grounds that the dilution curves of normal and abnormal or of childhood and adult plasma do not always have the same slope or contour. This may explain why many apparently healthy children appear to have somewhat less than "100 per cent concentration" of plasma prothrombin when tested.

Numerous modifications of the one-stage prothrombin activity test have been developed for special purposes. Diluting the plasma sample to 12.5 per cent with added saline or processed serum is useful in the control of anticoagulant therapy.

The content of the individual accessory factors may be determined by proper adjustment of all variables. For example, fresh normal serum is a rich source of accelerator substances, yet will contain but little prothrombin if left in contact with the clot for several hours before separation. If the difficulty in a patient with persistent hypoprothrombinemia is a deficiency of an accelerator factor, the addition of fresh normal serum to the patient's fresh plasma before performing the one-stage test will reduce the prothrombin time of the mixture almost to normal. Adjusting the proportions of added serum to the patient's plasma brings about corresponding alterations in the readings.

The one-stage test is best viewed as what it is: a test procedure in which an excess of the thromboplastin factor is added to plasma or whole blood in order to initiate and accelerate the precipitation of fibrin. A prolonged one-stage reading indicates either primary lack in the activity of prothrombin itself or the plasma prothrombin accelerators, some difficulty in the formation of thrombin from prothrombin, or an unusually low plasma content of fibrinogen. Since the latter are rare, the chief usefulness of the one-stage test is as an index for the detection and study of clinical disturbances related to prothrombin deficiency. In both hemophilia and thrombocytopenic purpura the readings are normal, since the plasma in these diseases has an adequate content of prothrombin.

TWO-STAGE TESTS. These procedures, which dissociate the coagulation reaction in vitro into separate steps, are believed to give more precise information regarding the prothrombin concentration in the blood than does the one-stage test. The first step aims to quantitate the conversion of prothrombin to thrombin. Prothrombin-containing plasma is incubated under standardized conditions with a mixture composed of thromboplastin in excess and calcium and known accessory factors in the proper concentrations. After measured time intervals the content of converted thrombin which has formed is determined by adding a standardized fibrinogen solution and noting the exact interval required for clotting. Comparison of the clotting time with the reading from a parallel experiment using standardized thrombin of known activity indicates the original prothrombin concentration. One prothrombin unit in these methods is the amount which yields one unit of thrombin. This latter, in turn, is the minimal amount which coagulates 1 ml of a standardized fibrinogen solution. The usual prothrombin level in healthy adults is 300 to 360 units per ml, which is taken as 100 per cent.

Prothrombin Consumption Test (Serum Prothrombin Time)

The free prothrombin initially present in normal blood tends to be converted or "consumed" during and for some time after visible clotting has taken place. Conversion of prothrombin is defective in the hemophilic and thrombocytic groups of disorders.

Methods for performance of this test vary in details. As a rule, 2 ml of the patient's blood is collected without tissue juice contamination in a dry syringe and transferred to a clean test tube. This is placed in a water bath or incubator at 37°C and the clotting time noted. After 1 hour the serum is separated and residual prothrombin activity assayed with the Quick one-stage method by the addition of thromboplastin and other pertinent substances. Readings are recorded in seconds, which may be converted if desired into prothrombin concentration.

With normal serum the prothrombin time as assayed by the above procedure usually falls between 35 and 60 seconds or longer. Typical readings in diseases in which determination of the rate of prothrombin consumption is clinically useful are listed below:

	Seconds		Seconds
Normal	35–60	Deficiency in prothrombin complex	15–35
Hemophilia, severe	12–20	Thrombocytopenic states and thrombasthenia	12–40
Hemophilia, mild	15–50	Circulating anticoagulant	12–40

In hemophilia the prothrombin consumption rate is roughly but not consistently proportional to the clinical severity of the disorder. In thrombocytopenic states, whether idiopathic or secondary, the rate of prothrombin consumption is usually not as much retarded as in severe hemophilia and, as a rule, is inversely proportional to the platelet count when less than 70,000 cu mm. With counts above this threshold level the prothrombin consumption is as a rule normal.

Thrombin Generation Test

When blood is collected cleanly and transferred to a glass vessel, the contact with the glass initiates the chain of clotting reactions, with production of thrombin as an intermediate phase. The rate of production or "generation" of thrombin can be utilized for the recognition of hemophilic coagulation disturbances.

Two milliliters of freshly collected venous blood is mixed with 0.2 ml of saline in a glass centrifuge tube and placed in a water bath at 37°C. At 1-minute intervals, 0.1-ml portions are transferred to a series of tubes containing 0.4 ml of a previously prepared fibrinogen solution. After the blood in the original tube has clotted, further 0.1 portions of serum are procured by pushing aside the clot. The coagulation times of the mixtures are compared with a standardized curve and used as indexes of thrombin liberation. By a simple modification the process can be studied in recalcified citrated plasma.

Normally, the concentration of free thrombin rises to attain a peak in about 6 minutes, and then subsides gradually to disappear in 9 to 15 minutes. In hemophilia of all varieties, except when of minimal degree, the rate of thrombin generation is much retarded.

Thromboplastin Generation Test

This measures the efficiency of the individual factors which enter into the conversion of thromboplastinogen to thromboplastin, by performing a clotting test in which all the factors have been standardized except the one to be tested. The procedure is more sensitive and accurate than the prothrombin consumption test for detecting disturbances in the formation of thromboplastin but is still too involved for routine use in the average clinical laboratory. It is helpful in detecting and differentiating minimal and even subclinical states of hemophilia. Poor thromboplastin generation is found also with platelet deficiencies, thromboplastin inhibitors, and inadequacies of the prothrombin accessory factors.

Clotting Time of Recalcified Oxalated Plasma

This modification of the coagulation-time determination is designed to study the clotting phenomenon under controlled conditions. Venous blood is collected with a siliconized needle and syringe, then oxalated and chilled. The tubes are centrifuged for 5 minutes at 750 rpm (revolutions per minute) to spin down the red cells and leukocytes, or at 3,000 rpm to eliminate the platelets also. The supernatant is removed, placed in a water bath at 37°C, a measured amount of calcium chloride solution added, and the time required for clotting noted. Normal plasma subjected to rapid centrifugation and therefore comparatively free of platelets will have a clotting time not more than 15 seconds longer than when subjected to slow centrifugation. The usual range for normal subjects is 75 to 125 seconds. In hemophilia the clotting time after recalcification may not only require many minutes, but a platelet-poor specimen may take even longer.

In thrombocytopenic states the clotting time tends to be moderately prolonged when the platelet count is 40,000 to 60,000 per cu mm, and more so when the count is below 10,000. After the first few months of illness there may be a nearly normal clotting time despite a low platelet count.

FIBRIN FORMATION

Plasma Fibrinogen

The concentration of fibrinogen in blood is much the same at birth as in infancy and childhood and ranges from 250 to 400 mg per 100 ml. The concentration can be measured by coagulating the fibrinogen and measuring the nitrogen content of the coagulum, by ascertaining the difference in protein content of plasma before and of serum after coagulation, or by other equally good methods.

In acute and chronic nephritis the blood fibrinogen level may be somewhat elevated, and individual readings greater than 1 gm of fibrinogen per 100 ml of blood have been noted in the nephrotic syndrome.

In congenital afibrinogenemia the blood does not clot, even after the addition of thromboplastin or thrombin (p. 275). In hypofibrinogenemia the clotting time of whole blood appears to be normal unless the depletion is profound. Quantitative defects in fibrinogen are best looked for by chemical analysis for this protein.

A defective reactivity of fibrinogen has been described. This rare qualitative disturbance can be demonstrated by adding highly concentrated thrombin to oxalated plasma and noting the delayed clotting.

UNUSUAL ANTICOAGULANT ACTIVITY

Increase in Heparin-like Substances

Heparin and heparin-like substances are highly potent anticoagulants extractable from lungs, liver, and mast cells. There is considerable question whether these are of physiologic importance in the blood of normal subjects. Minor changes in the direction of an increase have been described in acute leukemia, idiopathic thrombocytopenic purpura, aplastic anemia, during nitrogen mustard therapy, in anaphylactic shock, and after total body irradiation. To uncover a presumed increase a variety of procedures has been proposed.

The heparin retardation test is performed by adding increasing quantities of a dilute heparin solution containing a uniform amount of calcium to oxalated plasma and timing the clotting of the mixture, just as is done in the venous clotting time test. The protamine titration consists of ascertaining how many milligrams of protamine are needed to counteract the coagulation-prolonging effect of heparinized plasma. The normal range is 0.10 to 0.14 mg. The toluidine titration tests measure the effect of toluidine blue on the clotting time of recalcified oxalated plasma.

Elevated readings are not uncommon with these tests in many blood disturbances. The extreme variability in the values, the lack of parallelism of the abnormalities in the different approaches, and the fact that many patients exhibit readings within normal limits have made these procedures useful only rarely in arriving at clinical diagnoses in the hemorrhagic diseases.

The hemorrhages which follow massive irradiation are of complex origin. Increase in heparin-like substances is erratic, yet may be sufficient to inhibit coagulation of a mixture of patient's and normal blood. Platelets fall during the first week after exposure, generally to below 50,000 per cu mm, which is the threshold for bleeding. Prothrombin activity is not altered significantly, so that administration of vitamin K cannot be expected to be of great value. Capillaries seem unusually permeable. Leukocytes, erythrocytes, and concentrations of antibodies in the circulation become much diminished.

ANTITHROMBIN EXCESS

Many adults with acute pancreatitis, obstructive jaundice, and thrombotic lesions have been found to have elevated plasma antithrombin levels. One method of performing the test is to incubate defibrinated plasma from the patient with a known quantity of weak thrombin in solution and then add fibrin in the form of normal plasma. The rate of inhibition of clotting by the defibrinated plasma is taken as the measure of antithrombin activity. The plasma antithrombin level is undisturbed in nearly all childhood disturbances, including chronic diarrhea, celiac disease, and marasmus. Plasma antithrombin rises may take place in cystic fibrosis of the pancreas.

BLOOD MIXTURE TESTS

There is a simple office procedure for studying the coagulation defect in a patient whose whole-blood hemorrhagic tendency is sufficiently altered to give rise to prolongation of the venous clotting time. Two operators withdraw simultaneously, from both the patient and a normal control, 1 or 2 ml of blood by clean venipuncture. The precise times of the first appearance of blood in the syringes is noted. In a small test tube, 0.5 ml of the patient's blood and 0.5 ml of the normal blood are mixed by a single inversion of the tube. The remaining contents of the syringes are placed separately in other tubes. All clotting times are determined at 37°C. Since clumping or lysis of red cells occurs occasionally when patient and subject are of different ABO blood groups, it is preferable (though not essential) that both be of the same blood group.

For more accurate results, a titration procedure may be employed. Venous blood is collected simultaneously from the patient and a healthy control subject, employing two syringes and placing the contents separately in glass tubes. Serial dilution mixtures are then prepared as indicated below and kept at 37°C. Listed also are representative observations in two types of disturbances:

	PATIENT'S BLOOD/CONTROL BLOOD (ML)					
	1/0	0.8/0.2	0.6/0.4	0.4/0.6	0.2/0.8	0/1
Hemophilia, clotting time (minutes)						
Uncomplicated	90	40	12	11	11	10
Complicated by presence of a circulating anticoagulant	90	85	60	30	14	10

When a circulating anticoagulant is responsible for the patient's coagulation difficulty, the clotting times of the mixtures fall between the readings for the individual specimens. When the defect is of hemophilic character, the clotting time of the mixtures become approximately the same as that of the healthy control, since normal blood contains enough excess thromboplastinogen to replace the deficiency in that from the patient.

A mixture of blood from two hemophilic patients, each having prolonged coagulation, will show a normal clotting time when the defects are different, but no rectification when the defects are the same (Chap. 21).

The above phenomena can be reproduced with specimens of recalcified plasma (p. 245).

INCREASED FIBRINOLYSIN ACTIVITY

Procedure. Blood obtained by venipuncture is diluted 1:10 with added sterile 3.8 per cent sodium citrate solution under aseptic conditions, and the plasma separated by centrifuging for a few minutes. Of this diluted fibrinogen-containing plasma 0.2, 0.1, and 0.05 ml are introduced into duplicate sets of three tubes and sufficient normal saline solution added to make a total volume of 2.9 ml in each tube. One set is clotted by addition of 0.1 ml of 0.35 per cent $CaCl_2$ solution, and the other by 1.0 ml of 1:250 solution of topical thrombin. Both sets of tubes are incubated at 37°C and observed for a 24-hour period. Fibrinolysis is said to be brisk when all clots lyse spontaneously within an hour or two, and absent if there is no fibrinolysis in any tube. Longer incubation is needed to demonstrate minimal fibrinolytic activity. The thrombin-clotted dilutions of plasma lyse faster than the recalcified.

STUDY OF PLATELET ADEQUACY

The functional capacity of the platelets (thrombocytes) can be sought in several ways. The count or number per unit volume of blood is the most direct approach. The cytologic appearances can be scrutinized in a stained film of peripheral blood. Their capacity to disintegrate in freshly clotted blood becomes reflected in the prothrombin consumption rate. Their activity with respect to fibrin is portrayed in the rate of retraction of the clot. Their "adhesiveness" can be estimated by exposing heparinized fresh blood collected in siliconized glassware to glass wool or other glass surfaces and noting what proportion becomes attached to and retained by the glass.

The bleeding time test, tourniquet test, and negative pressure test become abnormal in the presence of pronounced platelet inadequacy, except perhaps when the inadequacy is chronic. These tests can be used to evaluate the functional efficiency of platelets, provided vascular integrity and the other coagulation variables which participate in the phenomenon being observed are otherwise intact.

Thrombocytosis

Platelets may become transitorily abundant in leukemoid reactions, in early rheumatic fever, immediately after violent exercise or hemorrhage, and for several weeks after severe trauma or surgical operations. Protracted thrombocytosis may also be encountered in early granulocytic leukemia, Hodgkin's disease, and polycythemia vera. Splenectomy for whatever cause is nearly always followed by a thrombocytosis which may last for months or years. A few cases of idiopathic thrombocytosis have been described, with platelet counts above 1 million and splenomegaly, thromboses, and a tendency to bleed.

Thrombocytopenia

Diminution of circulating platelets is a distinguishing feature of the various thrombocytopenic states (Chap. 23). The correlation is not close between low platelet counts and the thresholds for bleeding, but the count must be below about 60,000 per cu mm before hemorrhagic symptoms appear. A form of functional "thrombasthenia" has been described in which the platelets are normal in number but seem qualitatively incompetent (p. 287).

CLOT RETRACTION

The clot formed from normal blood in a test tube will begin to contract within 1 or 2 hours, expressing serum in the process. Retraction is usually maximal by 12 hours, though the clot may grow smaller after that time as a consequence of fibrinolysis.

When the fibrinogen and red cell content of the blood are normal, the extent of clot retraction is related directly to the number and adhesiveness of the intact platelets present. In the absence of platelets no retraction occurs, even when platelet suspensions of extracts have been added. After first serving as foci for the cohesive precipitation of fibrin, the thrombocytes later shrink by agglutination and shortening of pseudopodia, thereby drawing the fibrin web into a more compact mass. In disturbances in which the proportion of adhesive thrombocytes is reduced, a higher total platelet count is needed to promote adequate clot retraction. When the thrombocyte count is below about 80,000 per cu mm, with thrombocytes qualitatively normal, retraction begins to be inadequate, as is readily obvious on simple inspection of the clot after 12 hours standing. With counts below 20,000 the clot may not retract at all.

Clot retraction is characteristically incomplete or defective in thrombocytopenic states. The clot which forms in this group of diseases differs from the normal in being weak and friable, with many uncaught red cells. The clotting time of the blood is nevertheless normal, for the reason that even a few thrombocytes can liberate enough enzyme to initiate the coagulation chain reactions and cause the blood to solidify within the usual period of time. Full precipitation of the fibrin may be much delayed. Retraction may be defective also in hypofibrinogenemia, severe hypoprothrombinemic states, and functional thrombasthenia. Retraction is hindered passively in erythrocytosis and hyperfibrinogemia (as in kidney or liver disease).

Clot retraction is difficult to estimate quantitatively, with no agreement as to the best method. Direct inspection of the extent of retraction after a test tube containing blood has been left to stand for several hours at 37°C is a reliable though rough approach when the blood is otherwise normal. With the usual clinical problems there is little need for quantitative estimations. The latter is helpful only when there is an excess or a diminution of the red cells or of the fibrinogen.

STUDY OF VASCULAR ADEQUACY

The capacity of the minute skin vessels to withstand abnormal strain and prevent leakage of blood through their walls can be tested by several different approaches. There is the positive pressure test, the suction or negative pressure test, the bleeding tests, the study of blood vitamin C, skin tests which employ snake venom or histamine, and direct microscopic observation of the vessels of the nail beds after minor injury.

Arterioles and venules as well as capillaries contract after injury. It is somewhat of a misnomer to refer to such as tests for "capillary" fragility.

Vascular inadequacy may be uncovered with fair consistency in thrombocytopenic states. It is a regular feature of scurvy, hereditary hemorrhagic telangiectasia, and the poorly defined condition known as diffuse capillary permeability of unknown etiology. It may become manifest transitorily during many of the acute infectious diseases of childhood, chronic nephritis, and leukemia. The principal infections in which the vascular endothelium may show toxic weakening include scarlet fever, typhoid fever, rickettsial diseases, diphtheria, rheumatic fever, pneumonia, subacute bacterial endocarditis, meningococcemia, and other septicemias of diverse origins. "Infectious purpura" or "purpura fulminans" are the names frequently applied to the bleeding in these disorders. The Waterhouse-Friderichsen syndrome is the result of bilateral necrosis or hemorrhage into the adrenal glands during the course of meningococcemia or other severe septicemias. With practically all of these conditions corticotropin or cortisone can cause transitory strengthening of the vascular walls by direct local action. Rutin, hesperidin, and related bioflavonoids may exert a similar effect in some instances but are much less potent and their results unpredictable. They are of no benefit when the results of vascular tests are normal.

Kerpel-Fronius and associates followed 233 healthy infants over a year with vascular fragility tests. A marked seasonal variation was noted with heightened fragility most common during the winter and spring with the peak in March. This incidence curve exactly paralleled the curves for the incidence of cephalhematoma, cerebral hemorrhage, and conjunctival bleeding. They found no similar seasonal variation of permeability in patients with other diseases.

Even normal blood vessels may rupture under sudden or extraordinary strain. So-called "mechanical purpura" may be induced in an extremity by local trauma, in the conjunctivae or nose or eyelids by the increased venous pressure of whooping cough, in the face and neck by convulsions or violent screaming, and so on. The epistaxes in rheumatic fever, the retinal and other hemorrhages in uremia, and the purpuric lesions in frostbite are produced by vascular injury related to the underlying disease.

Of the various methods to be described, the tourniquet test is the simplest to perform and gives consistently reliable results. The negative-pressure test is useful when it is desired to explore the vascular fragility in various parts of the body. It is helpful also when tests are to be repeated on the same patient in therapeutic experiments, since petechiae at any one site may take several days to fade away.

In hemorrhagic disturbances the resistance tends to run parallel to exhibition of overt symptoms. Unusual vascular fragility may not be demonstrable in thrombocytopenic states when the bleeding tendency is inactive. After splenectomy for idiopathic thrombocytopenic purpura the vascular resistance returns to normal immediately following the operation, several days before a rise in platelet count can be detected.

Postive-pressure Methods

TOURNIQUET (RUMPEL-LEEDE) TEST. A circular area 2.5 cm in diameter (the size of a quarter of a dollar) is marked in one antecubital space a few centimeters below the antecubital fold. A blood-pressure cuff is placed on the arm and a pressure of 80 mm Hg or midway between systolic and diastolic is maintained for 3 minutes. The cuff is then removed, and all the petechiae which appear within the circular area are counted. Normally 1 or 2 small petechiae may appear; a borderline (probably increased) reading is 3 to 5 petechiae; an increased reading is 6 or more petechiae.

GÖTHLIN INDEX. Blood-pressure cuffs are placed on the arms and the pressure maintained at 35 mm Hg for 15 minutes. The resulting petechiae in a 6-cm circle in the antecubital fossae are counted with a magnifying lens. The determinations are repeated in an hour at 50 mm pressure. The Göthlin index is then computed by adding twice the number of petechiae at 35 mm to the number produced after 50 mm inflation. Eight or less is given by normal subjects, whereas thirteen or more is taken as a sign of abnormal capillary fragility.

Suction (Negative-pressure) Test

Suction is applied to the interior of a small cup placed on the skin, and increasing negative pressures applied for successive one-minute periods. The pressure which first evokes two petechiae is taken as the capillary resistance. The site for performing the test which gives the most uniform results is the surface of the forearm about 2 cm below the antecubital fossa.

Normal capillary resistance for infants under 2 years of age is −20 to −25 cm Hg or higher; for older children, −15 to −20 cm. If hemorrhages can be produced by pressures weaker than −20 cm, the capillary fragility is said to be increased.

Moccasin Venom Test

Fragile capillaries are believed to be highly sensitive to toxins such as snake venom. An injection is given of 0.1 ml of 1:3,000 standardized moccasin venom into one forearm intradermally and of normal saline into the other as a control. The response is positive when a hemorrhage 1 cm or greater in diameter appears at the site of the venom injection and not at the control.

Pinching Test

Pinching of the skin in the infraclavicular region with the examiner's thumb and forefinger will usually give rise to local ecchymoses when capillary resistance is seriously impaired.

CONCLUDING REMARKS

Infants and children being studied for a bleeding tendency for the first time may be subjected first to the following battery of screening tests: (1) blood-clotting time (venous clotting preferred), (2) clot retraction, (3) bleeding time, (4) capillary fragility, (5) platelet count, (6) prothrombin activity (bedside or one-stage test), (7) determination of the red cell and leukocyte counts and hemoglobin level, and (8) microscopy of the stained blood film. The results of these, when coupled with the past and family histories and the physical and other findings, nearly always will provide a working diagnosis. On this basis one can start immediate therapy or carry out further studies along the paths indicated. The latter line of attack includes more complete blood cell studies (if abnormalities in the red cells or leukocytes are found); x-rays of the bones and a therapeutic trial with vitamin C (if scurvy seems probable); determination of fibrinogen level or fibrinolysin (if the blood clot seems defective); blood mixture tests (if the disease is hemophilia-like); estimation of prothrombin consumption and related phenomena (if hemophilia or thrombasthenia is suspected); tests for circulating anticoagulants (if the disturbance resembles hemophilia); bone marrow aspiration and examinations of the platelet mechanisms if the platelets seem diminished or imperfect); liver function tests or estimation of accelerator factors (if the prothrombin activity is diminished); direct microscopy of the capillaries (if these appear to be at fault); and so on. Most of these approaches fall within the capacity of a good clinical laboratory.

Interpretation of abnormal findings in single tests is made difficult by the tendency for disturbances primary to one component to involve other phases of coagulation. This overlapping occurs more often than one would expect from the recognized coagulation schemas.

BIBLIOGRAPHY

SEROLOGIC FACTORS IN BLOOD COAGULATION

Alexander, B., Coagulation, Hemorrhage and Thrombosis, *New England J. Med.* 252:432, 1955.

Biggs, R., and *A. S. Douglas,* The Thromboplastin Generation Test, *J. Clin. Path.* 6:23, 1953.

———— and *R. G. Macfarlane,* "Human Blood Coagulation and Its Disorders," Charles C Thomas, Springfield, Ill., 1953.

Brinkhous, K. M., R. D. Langdell, G. D. Penick, J. B. Graham, and *R. H. Wagner,* Newer Approaches to the Study of Hemophilia and Hemophiloid States, *J.A.M.A.* 154:481, 1954.

DeNicola, P., Factor VII (SPCA): Its Physiopathologic Significance, *Blood* 8:947, 1953.

Hoffman, O. D., and *R. P. Custer,* A Micro Method for Determining Prothrombin Time on Fresh Capillary Blood Using Standard Physical Conditions, *Am. J. M. Sc.* 204:420, 1942.

Kato, K., Micro-prothrombin Test with Capillary Whole Blood, *Am. J. Clin. Path.* 10:147, 1940.

Laki, K., The Clotting of Fibrinogen, *Blood* 8:845, 1953.

Macfarlane, R. G., and *R. Biggs,* Fibrinolysis: Its Mechanisms and Significance, *Blood* 3:1167, 1948.

———— and ————, A Thrombin Generation Test: The Application in Haemophilia and Thrombocytopenia, *J. Clin. Path.* 6:3, 1953.

Mann, F. D., Clinical Assay of Blood Coagulation Factors, *Am. J. Clin. Path.* **23**:623, 1953.

Quick, A. J., The Coagulation Mechanism with Specific Reference to the Interpretation of Prothrombin Time and a Consideration of the Prothrombin Consumption Time, *Am. J. Clin. Path.* **19**:1016, 1949.

———, "Hemorrhagic Diseases," Lea & Febiger, Philadelphia, 1957.

Rapoport, S., New Formula for Dilution Curve of Plasma Prothrombin: Normal Standards and Changes in Pathologic Conditions, *Proc. Soc. Exper. Biol. & Med.* **64**:478, 1947.

Smith, H. P., S. E. Ziffren, C. A. Owen, and *G. R. Hoffman,* Clinical and Experimental Studies on Vitamin K, *J.A.M.A.* **113**:380, 1939.

Stefanini, M., Fibrinolysis and "Fibrinolytic Purpura," *Blood* **7**:1044, 1952.

——— and *W. H. Crosby,* Serum Prothrombin Time, A Composite Effect: An Analysis of the Factors Involved, *Am. J. Clin. Path.* **20**:1026, 1950.

——— and *W. Dameshek,* "The Hemorrhagic Disorders: A Clinical and Therapeutic Approach," Grune & Stratton, Inc., New York, 1955.

Sussman, L. N., and *I. B. Cohen,* The Serum Prothrombin Consumption Test in Infancy and Childhood, *Pediatrics* **17**:652, 1956.

———, ———, and *R. Gittler,* Clinical Application of Simplified Serum Prothrombin Consumption Test, *J.A.M.A.* **156**:702, 1954.

Tocantins, L. M. (ed.), "The Coagulation of Blood: Methods of Study," Grune & Stratton, Inc., New York, 1955.

Unger, P. N., M. Weiner, and *S. Shapiro,* The Vitamin K Tolerance Test, *Am. J. Clin. Path.* **18**:835, 1948.

Ware, A. G., and *W. H. Seegers,* Plasma Accelerator Globulin: Partial Purification, Quantitative Determination, and Properties, *J. Biol. Chem.* **172**:699, 1948.

——— and ———, Serum Ac-Globulin: Formation from Plasma Ac-Globulin; Role in Blood Coagulation; Partial Purification; Properties; and Quantitative Determination, *Am. J. Physiol.* **152**:567, 1948.

Warren, R., and *J. S. Belko,* Deficiency of Plasma Prothrombin Conversion Accelerators in the Postoperative State with a Description of a Simple Method of Assay, *Blood* **6**:544, 1951.

Waugh, T. R., and *D. W. Ruddick,* A Test for Increased Coagulability of the Blood, *Canad. M. A. J.* **50**:547, 1944.

Wiener, M. J., and *S. Shapiro,* Fibrin Appearance Time: A Rotating Tube Method for Estimating the Clotting Time of the Blood, *J. Lab. & Clin. Med.* **32**:1037, 1947.

PLATELETS

Adams, E., Observations on the Influence of the Hypophysis and the Adrenal Cortex on Blood Platelet Levels, *Blood* **4**:936, 1949.

Carr, T. L., and *W. M. Fowler,* Observations on the Coagulation Defect in Thrombocytopenic Purpura, *J. Lab. & Clin. Med.* **34**:1227, 1949.

Moolten, S. E., and *L. Vroman,* The Adhesiveness of Blood Platelets in Thromboembolism and Hemorrhagic Disorders, *Am. J. Clin. Path.* **19**:701, 1949.

Sloan, A. W., The Normal Platelet Count in Man, *J. Clin. Path.* **4**:37, 1951.

Stefanini, M., and *W. Dameshek,* Collection, Preservation and Transfusion of Platelets, with Special Reference to the Factors Affecting the "Survival Rate" and the Clinical Effectiveness of Transfused Platelets, *New England J. Med.* **248**:797, 1953.

Tocantins, L. M., Counting Platelets in the Blood, chaps. 1–5, in "The Coagulation of Blood: Methods of Study," Grune & Stratton, Inc., New York, 1955.

VASCULAR ADEQUACY

Glass, W. H., Rutin Therapy in Diffuse Capillary Bleeding: Ineffectiveness When Fragility Tests Are Normal, *Am. J. M. Sc.* **220**:409, 1950.

Hare, F. W., Jr., and *A. J. Miller,* Capillary Resistance Tests, *A.M.A. Arch. Dermat. & Syph.* **64**:449, 1951.

Martin, G. J., and *A. Szent-Gyorgyi* (eds.), Bioflavonoids and the Capillary, *Ann. New York Acad. Sc.* **61**:3, 637–736, 1955.

O'Brien, J. R., The Bleeding Time in Normal and Abnormal Subjects, *J. Clin. Path.* **4**:272, 1951.

Zweifach, B. W., R. Chambers, R. E. Lee, and *C. Hyman,* Reactions of Peripheral Blood Vessels in Experimental Hemorrhage, *Ann. New York Acad. Sc.* **4**:553, 1948–1949.

CHAPTER 21

Hemophilia and Related Disturbances

As outlined in Table 19-1 (p. 230), the defect in hemophilia lies in stage 1 of blood coagulation (formation of thromboplastin); the components of stage 2 (prothrombin complex) and stage 3 (fibrinogen) remain unaltered.

Thromboplastin activity requires a plasma precursor beta$_2$ globulin known as thromboplastinogen, or antihemophilic factor (AHF), or antihemophilic globulin (AHG). Elaboration of thromboplastin from thromboplastinogen is initiated by a platelet enzyme, and requires the participation of other normal plasma constituents of which the chief known ones are PTC, PTA, and PTF-D (see below). Any of these may be defective in a patient with hemophilia. The comparative incidence of these various disorders in several hospital clinics is shown in Table 21-1.

Since the majority of children with a congenital coagulation defect suffer from AHF deficiency, emphasis in the ensuing discussion is centered on this disease. The differences between hemophilia and related disorders and the prominent features of the latter will be commented upon separately.

AHF DEFICIENCY (HEMOPHILIA A, AHG DEFICIENCY)

Genetic Aspects

This defect is transmitted genetically as a sex-linked mendelian dominant. Asymptomatic female carriers married to normal males transmit the gene to 50 per cent of sons (who exhibit clinical symptoms) and to 50 per cent of daughters (who remain well but pass the gene to 50 per cent of their offspring). A hemophilic male married to a healthy female has normal sons and carrier daughters. A hemophilic male married to a carrier female has an equal likelihood of having a normal son, a hemophilic son, a carrier daughter, and a hemophilic daughter. (The last-named is rare in humans, perhaps because this gene combination may be lethal.)

With only 70 per cent of affected males, however, can a positive family history be elicited. With the remainder the disease either has been

256

transmitted only through the females for some generations or has arisen from mutant genes. It is most prevalent in whites, but does occur in the Negro and Oriental population groups. In severity, symptoms tend to be much the same in members of an affected family.

Clinical Aspects

The disturbance usually becomes evident in infancy or early childhood and almost always before puberty. The first signs are contusions and hematomas after minor blows or bumps, or persistent oozing following lacerations or minor operations. At any age a patient may experience a hemarthrosis, muscle or tissue hematoma, hematuria, buccal or gastrointestinal bleeding, subdural or subarachnoid hemorrhage, or oozing into a body cavity or elsewhere. Surgical operations and dental extractions

Table 21-1. Comparative Incidence of Forms of Hemophilia

	Frick	*Rosenthal*	*Spaet*	*Wolman*
AHF deficiency	45	36	44	45
PTC deficiency	6	7	8	6
PTA deficiency	4	4	0	1
PTF-D deficiency	0	0	1	0
Circulating anticoagulant	0	1	1	1
Unclassified	0	0	2	1
Total abnormal	55	48	56	54
(Total males)	(54)	(47)	(not stated)	(52)

are attended by excessive blood loss unless precautionary measures are used. Periods of comparative good health may alternate with intervals in which hemorrhages are common. The highest incidence of hospitalization is between 1 and 10 years of age, being related to the lively agility and immature judgment of growing boys.

Hemophilia is sometimes classified according to intensity as severe, moderate, mild, or minimal. These grades are not clearly delimited and shade into each other. Clinical manifestations and coagulation abnormalities are usually but not necessarily parallel in intensity. With cases exhibiting only minor symptoms, when the existence of a hemophilic coagulation defect cannot be clearly established at one laboratory examination, studies should be repeated when symptoms are more prominent.

The procedures used in the study of a patient with a hemorrhagic disorder are described in Chap. 20. Only the pertinent findings in hemophilia are discussed here.

Venous Clotting Time

Approximately three-fourths of all hemophiliacs have venous clotting times which are prolonged above the normal limit of 12 minutes with the standard Lee-White venous clotting test done in glass tubes. Readings tend to remain at about the same level with individual cases—they may fall between 1 and 2 hours in one patient over months and years, for example, and between 12 and 20 minutes in another.

Peripheral Clotting Time

This is a less sensitive test for diagnostic studies than the venous clotting time. A prolonged reading in a child suspected of having a coagulation difficulty has considerable reliability, whereas a reading within the normal range does *not* exclude this possibility.

Blood Mixture Tests

When 1 ml of fresh blood or recalcified plasma from a patient with uncomplicated hemophilia is added to a similar fresh specimen from a normal subject or from a patient with some other coagulation defect, the clotting time of the mixture will be approximately the same as that of a normal subject. The corrective effect becomes evident when as little as 10 per cent of normal blood is added, though 20 to 50 per cent may be needed to obliterate the defect completely. On the other hand, with two hemophiliacs having the same disturbance, the clotting time of the mixture will fall between their individual clotting times, even when the clotting time of one patient is normal or nearly normal. Silicone-lined glassware may be needed for this demonstration.

Bleeding Time

Bleeding from shallow superficial cuts seems controllable by platelet thrombi and small vessel contractility, which are not altered in hemophilia. When the test is performed properly the bleeding time rarely exceeds a few minutes. With deep jabs these hemostatic mechanisms may be overtaxed, and oozing continue for many minutes.

Prothrombin Tests

In hemophilia the plasma prothrombin activity is normal. This is a most significant differentiating feature between the hemophilic and hypoprothrombinemic groups of disorders (Table 21-2). The prothrombin consumption rate (serum prothrombin time), which is a measure of the disappearance of serum prothrombin after a clot has formed, is exceptionally slow except in the mildest cases. After 24 hours as much as 90 per cent of the original serum prothrombin activity may still remain. The more protracted the venous clotting time the greater tends to be the retention of prothrombin activity by the serum on standing, but this parallelism is far from close. The prothrombin consumption test is more sensitive than the venous clotting time, and the new thromboplastin generation test even more so.

Table 21-2. Differentiation of Coagulation Defects Due to Plasma Abnormalities

| | THROMBOPLASTIN COMPLEX | | | PROTHROMBIN COMPLEX | | | FIBRINOGEN | |
| | HEMOPHILIA | | | | | | | |
	AHF deficiency	PTC deficiency	PTA deficiency	Hypoprothrombinemia	Ac-globulin (factor V) deficiency	Factor VII deficiency	Afibrinogenemia	Circulating anticoagulant
Character of missing substance	Labile	Stable	Stable	Labile	Labile	Stable	Stable	Stable
Sex	M	M	M-F	M-F	M-F	M-F	M-F	M-F
Venous coagulation time *	Prolonged	Prolonged	Prolonged	Prolonged	Prolonged	Prolonged	Prolonged	Prolonged
Bleeding time	Normal	Normal	Normal	Variable	Variable	Variable	Variable	Variable
Prothrombin time	Normal	Normal	Normal	Prolonged	Prolonged	Normal	Prolonged	Variable
Prothrombin consumption	Slow	Slow	Slow	Variable	Variable	Variable	Variable	Variable
Defect corrected in vitro by:								
Fresh normal oxalated plasma †	Yes	Yes	Yes	Yes	Yes	Yes	Partial	Partial
Old normal plasma or serum	No	Yes	Yes	Yes	No	Yes	Partial	Partial
BaSO$_4$-treated fresh plasma	Yes	No	Yes	No	Yes	No	Partial	Partial
Duration of benefit from transfused fresh plasma	6–48 hours	1–3 weeks	1 week	Indefinite	1–3 days	1–3 weeks	Indefinite	Indefinite

* When deficiencies are partial, coagulation time may be normal and other abnormalities may not appear.
† Each defect will be corrected by fresh plasma (less than 24 hours old) from a patient with any other defect, but not by fresh plasma from a patient with the same defect.

Other Laboratory Findings

The platelets in hemophilia are quantitatively normal, as are fibrinogen, serum calcium, and all other components of the coagulation complex. The capillary fragility is almost always unaltered. Clot retraction, once the blood has coagulated, is normal. Circulating anticoagulant activity is not demonstrable by the usual tests, save in the rare child who develops such antibodies as a sequel to prolonged therapy with blood or blood concentrates. Normochromic anemia follows pronounced hemorrhages. The bone marrow shows no changes except for unusual proliferation of the rubricytes after a bleeding episode. The megakaryocytes are morphologically normal and may even seem increased in number.

If the plasma prothrombin level appears diminished, vitamin K may be prescribed in high dosage for several weeks. The determination should then be repeated to see whether the hypoprothrombinemia remains, since, as mentioned, in true hemophilia there is no abnormality in the prothrombin complex.

PTC DEFICIENCY (PLASMA THROMBOPLASTIN COMPONENT DEFICIENCY); HEMOPHILIA B; "CHRISTMAS DISEASE"; SCHULMAN-SMITH SYNDROME

Distinguishable from AHF deficiency by coagulation studies is a clinically identical hemorrhagic dyscrasia due to diminution in the specific PTC factor. As in AHF deficiency, the more severely affected patients exhibit bruising on trauma, normal platelets, normal bleeding time, normal plasma prothrombin, and retardation of prothrombin consumption and thromboplastinogen generation. The whole-blood clotting time and plasma recalcification time are prolonged except in the mildest cases. The other coagulation factors are not reduced. Blood from these patients, just as from normal subjects, will correct the delayed coagulation time and other defects of AHF deficiency, and vice versa. Patient's blood mixed with specimens from other patients with PTC deficiency will have no mutually corrective action. The disorder is hereditary, limited to males, and transmitted as a sex-linked trait. The missing coagulation factor is stable and will remain active in serum stored for some days in a refrigerator.

The PTC factor is absorbed by barium sulfate or calcium phosphate gel added to fresh oxalated plasma, whereas the AHF factor is not. In PTC deficiency the poor prothrombin consumption of the plasma will not be corrected by the addition of fresh oxalated plasma which has been treated with the above substances, unlike what occurs in AHF deficiency. The poor prothrombin consumption of PTC deficient plasma will be corrected by normal or AHF deficient serum which is several days old or by the eluate from barium sulfate or calcium phosphate gel added to fresh or old plasma (Table 21-2).

PTA DEFICIENCY (PLASMA THROMBOPLASTIN ANTECEDENT DEFICIENCY; HEMOPHILIA C)

In this hemophilia-like familial disease, first described by Rosenthal, Dreskin, and Rosenthal, the missing substance is as stable as the PTC factor, but unlike it is not absorbed by calcium $BaSO_4$ or $Ca_3 (PO_4)_2$ gel (Table 21-2). Blood from such patients will correct the coagulation defect of blood deficient in AHF or PTC, and vice versa. The disease appears in both sexes, is hereditarily transmitted, and is clinically not severe.

IDENTIFICATION OF THE DEFECT

Understanding of the physiology of blood coagulation, techniques for recognizing and separating defects by laboratory means, and improvements in hemotherapy have advanced in recent years to a point where it has become essential that the nature of the defect be identified in every patient. Accordingly, arrangements should be made at a patient's very first visit to perform the battery of hematologic tests which characterize the defect. Knowledge of the "coagulogram" aids in determining the therapeutic course to be followed when a serious hemorrhage occurs, and also in prognosticating the outcome. As will be brought out, patients with AHF deficiency need a much more aggressive program of therapy than those with the PTC or PTA defects. When PTA is lacking, all other members of the family of both sexes should be surveyed by coagulograms to determine which are affected similarly, since this disturbance may remain subclinical and unsuspected for years until a tissue-lacerating procedure such as tonsillectomy or dental extraction is done.

If a previously unstudied patient appears for medical attention with a severe bleeding lesion which requires immediate management, he should be presumed to have AHF deficiency, the most troublesome variety, and treated accordingly. Later, after the acute situation has been treated, a period of 3 to 6 weeks should be allowed to pass in order for all passively transfused coagulation factors to be eliminated, and a coagulogram then done.

PRACTICAL MANAGEMENT OF AHF DEFICIENCY

Hemotherapy

With oxalate as the anticoagulant, the antihemophilic (AHF) activity of fresh blood collected from a normal donor will deteriorate to subtherapeutic levels within 24 hours even during storage at 4°C. With citrate as the anticoagulant, in contrast, some AHF activity may persist for days or weeks. Citrate of course is the effective anticoagulant in the ACD (acid-citrate-dextrose) solution used for blood preservation by most blood banks. When the usual AHF-deficient patient is transfused with blood or plasma that is only a few hours old, the venous coagulation time will be brought down partially or fully to normal for 6 to 24 hours, and then will become prolonged again.

Antihemophilic activity can be preserved indefinitely by separating the plasma from fresh blood by centrifugation, and freezing and storing it at a low temperature. Normal plasma lyophilized within a few hours after collection will also retain its potency. Many hospitals keep a supply of such preserved plasma on hand, ready for emergencies in hemophilic patients. It is important to administer plasma of an ABO and Rh blood group compatible with the recipient's red cells. Rh-negative recipients may become sensitized to an Rh antigen when plasma from an Rh-positive donor contains residual red cells.

With a child 2 to 5 years of age the coagulation defect in AHF deficiency usually can be corrected temporarily with 200 to 250 ml of fresh whole blood, or half that volume of properly preserved plasma. With infants the dosage is proportionately less and with older children proportionately more. The amounts needed are dependent upon body weight and severity of the disorder. With pronounced bleeding problems it is often advisable to give double this amount in the first few hours. A transfusion of blood or plasma every 6 to 12 hours thereafter is ordinarily adequate. It is often wise to give plasma, perhaps in lesser amounts, for 1 or 2 days after the bleeding has ceased. Clotting studies are advisable every few hours to regulate the amounts administered when the lesion is internal; when the bleeding is superficial, as from a cut or dental socket, visual observation of the oozing is a helpful adjunct.

Fresh whole blood is advisable as therapy when the red cell count and blood volume have fallen because of marked bleeding. Fresh plasma is preferred when there is no anemia. In an emergency, citrated blood which has been stored for a week or more may still have an appreciable AHF content and can be given with benefit.

All transfusions and concentrates must be administered intravenously or intramedullarly. Intramuscular injections produce negligible improvement.

Also effective but not recommended for therapy is an "antihemophilic globulin" concentrate. When prepared from fresh human plasma this is rich in thromboplastinogen. Unfortunately this seems to facilitate the development of a "refractory state" in some patients (see below).

Infection and tissue necrosis at an involved area may counteract hemostatic therapy; hence antibiotics should be given locally or systemically when infection is suspected. Salicylates do not aggravate the bleeding tendency.

Surgery

Should a surgical operation be necessary, fresh blood or plasma are first given in large amounts until the coagulation reactions have become fully normal. The patient is then operated on like any other patient. Transfusions should be administered during the procedure and continued for a number of days thereafter, the schedule being regulated by the extent of the surgery, the severity of the hemophilia, and other individual circumstances. Adjuvant hemostatic agents such as alum, fibrin foam, or commercial thrombin are applied locally as required.

Local Treatment

When bleeding occurs at a site near the body surface, cold applications combined with local pressure are often successful in contracting the traumatized blood vessels and stopping the hemorrhage. An elastic bandage may be applied if feasible. These measures must not be pushed to such an extent that tissue necrosis results. The affected area should be immobilized. Complete rest on the part of the patient is of value in reducing the systemic blood pressure. Fibrin foam or packs saturated with epinephrine or thrombin can be useful if the bleeding site is approachable. Hot applications are contraindicated, since they cause vasodilatation and promote bleeding.

Hemarthroses

Extravasations of blood into joint cavities occur frequently, especially after 2 years of age. The areas most often affected are the knees, ankles, hips, shoulders, and elbows. Distinctive symptoms usually seen with a beginning hemarthrosis are (1) distention of the joint capsule and (2) pain on weight-bearing or movement. Extraarticular hematomas permit minor movements and weight-bearing. One should give plasma, aspirate the joint, inject hyaluronidase, and immobilize for a few days.

Dental Complications

Hemophilic children seem more prone to develop dental caries and dental root abscesses than other children. If an extraction is necessary the child is hospitalized a day earlier, and enough fresh plasma is transfused in advance to correct the coagulation defect. After the extraction the cavity is plugged with gelfoam which contains topical thrombin, and overlying pressure applied if feasible. Hemotherapy is continued several times daily for some days. Tooth sockets often bleed intermittently for 4 to 10 days postoperatively even when this is done.

Patients with PTC or PTA deficiency are as likely to have postoperative bleeding as those with the AHF defect. (This similarity among the three defects does not hold for surgery with well-sutured incisions; major operations may be done without postoperative bleeding complications on PTC and PTA patients if the hemotherapy is well regulated.)

MANAGEMENT OF PTC AND PTA DEFICIENCIES

Since these factors are more stable, the coagulation status of such patients are typically restored to normal for longer periods of time by one or two transfusions. Stored blood or plasma which is 1 or more days old will correct the defect almost as well as very fresh material. Good correction ordinarily lasts for 3 to 10 days. It is feasible also to alleviate the propensity of these patients to hemorrhage by giving prophylactic transfusions of fairly fresh plasma every 7 to 14 days.

REFRACTORY STATE

Rarely, hemophiliacs become refractory to hemotherapy. This refractory state is due apparently to the development of anticoagulant antibodies against the antihemophilic substance present in the plasma. It appears to be more likely to follow the giving of plasma fractions than of fresh blood or plasma. Patients with mild or moderate forms of the disease are less prone to experience this immunologic difficulty, presumably because they already possess trace amounts of the deficient plasma coagulation factor and are therefore unlikely to develop antibodies against a substance naturally present in their own blood. Existence of an anticoagulant can be made evident by the blood mixture test; blood from the hemophiliac prolongs the coagulation time of the normal. Precipitins to plasma protein derivatives possessing antihemophilic activity have been described.

A refractory state, once developed, sometimes can be overcome temporarily by very large transfusions of fresh whole blood or plasma; 500 ml of fresh plasma may be required to achieve what 50 ml was able to accomplish earlier. The large volumes neutralize the anticoagulant principles first and then furnish enough supplementary thromboplastinogen to effect the desired response. In extreme instances an exsanguination transfusion may be necessary.

Once an anticoagulant has developed, the original disturbance may no longer be identifiable by standard laboratory tests. It is advisable that every hemophilic child who has received transfusions be tested by the blood mixture procedure about once a year, in order that management can be modified if an anticoagulant has developed.

The anticoagulant itself and the refractory state often subside spontaneously if blood and plasma therapy can be withheld for a year or two. Conversely, repeated hemotherapy seems to aggravate this undesirable complication. Corticotropin and the cortisone-like hormones do not usually depress these anticoagulants, but may be tried therapeutically.

OTHER HEMOPHILIA-LIKE DISORDERS

Plasma Thromboplastic Factor D (PTF-D) Deficiency

A fourth substance which participates in plasma thromboplastin formation has been described by Spaet, Aggeler, and Kinsell; their patient
with this deficiency exhibited typical symptoms of hemophilia.

Hageman Factor (HF) Deficiency

In this rare deficiency disturbance the venous coagulation time is prolonged and the prothrombin consumption is deficient despite a full complement of all the previously described antihemophilic factors involved
in the generation of thromboplastin. It is named after the first individual
in whom the deficiency was discovered. Affected persons have no symptoms. They do not bleed excessively during or after trauma or surgical
operations. Preoperative transfusions are not needed. A transfusion of as
little as 50 ml of 3-week-old blood will correct the abnormal clotting
tests for about 2 days.

Vascular Hemophilia (Pseudohemophilia B)

Another newly recognized hereditary hemorrhagic dyscrasia is that
in which there is a plasma deficiency of AHF along with a morphologic
abnormality of the capillaries. The pattern of inheritance is different
from classical AHF-deficiency hemophilia in that both males and females
may be affected. Reports have been published recently by Singer and
Ramot (1 case), Schulman, Smith, Erlandson, Fort, and Lee (7 cases),
and other workers.

This disturbance simulates hemophilia. Symptoms may begin in infancy. Nosebleeds, skin ecchymoses, and bleeding after trauma or dental
extractions are frequent. Peripheral bleeding time is nearly always in excess of the top normal of 6 or 7 minutes. Venous coagulation time is
usually normal but may be minimally prolonged. Prothrombin consumption is moderately retarded.

Schulman, Smith, and associates studied the capillaries of the finger-
nail beds and bulbar conjunctivae of 5 of their children with the 100X
magnification of the standard binocular microscope. The capillaries,
instead of appearing as normal smooth parallel loops, were coiled, tortuous, and irregular; many were dilated.

This disease is now classified as one subvariety of the syndrome first
described by von Willebrand in 1926, and bearing his name. The other
subvariety is that in which the vascular defect is not associated with any
demonstrable anomaly of coagulation. Therapeutic management is the
same as for hemophilia. Transfusion of fresh plasma or blood transitorily
corrects the bleeding time and coagulation defect.

BIBLIOGRAPHY

HEMOPHILIA

Biggs, R., and *R. G. Macfarlane,* "Human Blood Coagulation and Its Disorders," Charles C Thomas, Publisher, Springfield, Ill., 1953.

Brennan, M. J., R. W. Monto, and *H. C. Shafer,* Hemorrhagic Diathesis Due to Ac-Globulin Deficiency, *Am. J. Clin. Path.* 22:150, 1952.

Brinkhous, K. M., Hemophilia, *Bull. New York Acad. Med.* 30:325, 1954.

Dameshek, W., and others, Symposium: What is Hemophilia? *Blood* 9:244, 1954.

De Palma, A. F., Guiding Principles in the Surgery of Hemophilic Patients, chap. 9 in "Progress in Hematology," L. M. Tocantins (ed.), vol. 1, Grune & Stratton, Inc., New York, 1956.

Frick, P. G., The Relative Incidence of Anti-Hemophilic Globulin (AHG), Plasma Thromboplastic Component (PTC), and Plasma Thromboplastin Antecedent (PTA) Deficiency: A Study of Fifty-Five Cases, *J. Lab. & Clin. Med.* 43:860, 1954.

Graham, J. B., Biochemical Genetics of Blood Coagulation, *Am. J. Human Genet.* 8:63, 1956.

————, *W. W. McLendon,* and *K. M. Brinkhous,* Mild Hemophilia: An Allelic Form of the Disease, *Am. J. M. Sc.* 225:46, 1953.

Lewis, J. H., J. H. Ferguson, and *T. Arends,* Hemorrhagic Disease with Circulating Inhibitors of Blood Clotting: Anti-AHF and Anti-PTC in Eight Cases, *Blood* 11:846, 1956.

MacMillan, R. L., C. Ezrin, and *A. Butler,* Prothrombin Consumption in Haemophiliac Kindred, *J. Clin. Path.* 4:460, 1951.

Merskey, C., The Occurrence of Haemophilia in the Human Female, *Quart. J. Med.* 20:299, 1951.

National Hemophilia Foundation, "Proceedings of International Hemophilia Symposium, New York City, Aug. 24, 25, 1956." The University of North Carolina Press, Chapel Hill, N.C. (in press).

Ramot, B., B. Angelopoulos, and *K. Singer;* Variable Manifestations of Plasma Thromboplastin Component Deficiency, *J. Lab. & Clin. Med.* 46:80, 1955.

————, *K. Singer, P. Heller,* and *H. J. Zimmerman,* Hageman Factor (HF) Deficiency, *Blood* 11:745, 1956.

Rosenthal, M. C., Deficiency in Plasma Thromboplastin Component. II. Its Incidence in a Hemophilic Population: Critique of Methods for Identification, *Am. J. Clin. Path.* 24:910, 1954.

Rosenthal, R. L., O. H. Dreskin, and *N. Rosenthal,* New Hemophilia-like Disease Caused by Deficiency of a Third Plasma Thromboplastin Factor, *Proc. Soc. Exper. Biol. & Med.* 82:171, 1953.

Schulman, I., and *C. H. Smith,* Hemorrhagic Disease in an Infant Due to Deficiency of a Previously Undescribed Clotting Factor, *Blood* 7:794, 1952.

————, ————, *M. Erlandson, E. Fort,* and *R. E. Lee,* Vascular Hemophilia: A Familial Hemorrhagic Disease in Males and Females Characterized by Combined Antihemophilic Globulin Deficiency and Vascular Abnormality, *Pediatrics* 18:347, 1956.

Singer, K., and *B. Ramot,* Pseudohemophilia Type B: Hereditary Hemorrhagic Diathesis Characterized by Prolonged Bleeding Time and Decrease in Antihemophilic Factor, *A.M.A. Arch. Int. Med.* 97:715, 1956.

Spaet, T. H., Recent Progress in the Study of Hemophilia, *Stanford Med. Bull.* 13:24, 1955.

——, Studies on the Storage Lability of Human Antihemophilic Factor, *J. Lab. & Clin. Med.* 46:111, 1955.

Stefanini, M., and *W. Dameshek,* "The Hemorrhagic Disorders: A Clinical and Therapeutic Approach," Grune & Stratton, Inc., New York, 1955.

Tocantins, L. M., R. T. Carroll, and *R. H. Holburn,* The Clot Accelerating Effect of Dilution on Blood and Plasma. Relation to the Mechanism of Coagulation of Normal and Hemophilic Blood, *Blood* 6:720, 1951.

Van Creveld, S., P. G. Hoorweg, and *M. M. P. Paulssen,* Researches on a Circulating Anticoagulant in a Hemophiliac. II. Effect of Administration of ACTH and Cortisone, *Blood* 8:125, 1953.

Wolman, I. J., Management of Hemophilia, *Quart. Rev. Pediat.* 11:183, 1956.

CHAPTER 22

Hypoprothrombinemias
and Related Diseases

NEONATAL HYPOPROTHROMBINEMIA

Coagulation Factors in the Newborn Infant

Even when vitamin K is administered to the mother just before birth, or to the infant just afterward, the prothrombin activity in the blood of the infant at birth and during the first week is much below the adult level. This is demonstrable with both the one-stage and two-stage methods of measurement. The bleeding time is usually 4 or 5 minutes and may be much more protracted. The clotting time in both capillary and glass test tubes is slightly prolonged, the usual reading in the latter being 10 to 15 minutes. The protamine and toluidine blue titrations occasionally indicate an excess of heparinlike substances. The platelets as a rule are qualitatively normal and in the same quantitative range as those of older children and adults, but a minority of newborns have unusually low counts (p. 283). The plasma fibrinogen level may be slightly lower than later, but not sufficiently to affect coagulation. Unusual susceptibility of the fine vascular network to trauma is another contributing factor, especially in infants prematurely born. With all the blood coagulation factors the variability is greater than in later infancy and seems independent of birth weight.

These changes remain prominent for about a week, and then begin to subside. Diminished prothrombin activity is the most prominent, especially when vitamin K has been withheld, but the hypocoagulability of newborn infants cannot be adequately explained as a deficiency of prothrombin alone. There is considerable evidence that the plasma of the newborn is deficient also in Ac-globulin and perhaps other factors which accelerate the conversion of prothrombin to thrombin.

Plasma Prothrombin Activity

With normal newborn infants not treated with vitamin K, the plasma prothrombin activity exhibits wide variability. At the moment of birth the usual prothrombin level is 20 to 50 per cent of normal adult values, regardless of whether the mother was given vitamin K shortly before birth. By the second day most infants show a beginning fall, which typically reaches a low point on the third to fifth day and then rises again. In many of these the prothrombin activity is well below the level for hemorrhage of approximately 20 per cent of adult values. Infants with severe intrauterine asphyxia as the result of difficult labor seem more likely to develop low prothrombin values unless vitamin K is given.

The prothrombin activity recovers steadily until it attains a level of approximately 50 per cent of that of the child on the seventh or eighth day.

When vitamin K is given parenterally or orally to a normal pregnant woman 12 to 24 hours prior to delivery, or to her infant immediately afterward, the prothrombin level of the infant may still undergo a significant drop during the first few neonatal days.

Relation to Vitamin K

Vitamin K is a generic term applied to all naphthoquinone derivatives whose entry into the body is essential for prothrombin synthesis and blood coagulation. The two naturally occurring substances are vitamin K_1, present in the chloroplasts of green leaves, and vitamin K_2, produced by bacterial action or the putrefaction of protein. Both forms are soluble in fats but insoluble in water and require the presence of bile salts for absorption from the intestine. Numerous pharmaceutic compounds with vitamin K activity, not found in nature, have been synthesized. Their parent substance is 2-methyl-1, 4-naphthoquinone, also known as vitamin K_4. Most of these are sufficiently soluble in water to permit of safe parenteral injection or of absorption from the intestine despite absence of bile salts.

During intrauterine life the prothrombin activity of the fetus seems to be of maternal origin, transmitted by diffusion across the placenta. The prompt fall after delivery is ascribed to the absence of a reserve supply. The infant liver is capable of converting vitamin K to prothrombin, as evidenced by its prompt activity once this vitamin reaches it from gastrointestinal absorption or parenteral injection, but this function is not assumed until after separation from the mother.

The rise after the first few days is due to synthesis of vitamin K by the intestinal bacteria as they act upon ingested milk. The vitamin is absorbed almost instantly. It is carried to the liver, converted into prothrombin, and discharged into the circulation. The earlier the milk feedings are begun, the quicker the rise begins.

As noted earlier, the lower prothrombin activity during infancy appears to be due to a partial lack of some conversion or other coagulation factor. Addition of small amounts of adult serum or plasma to an infant's plasma in vitro boosts the prothrombin activity toward the adult level, whereas the feeding or injection of vitamin K will not force it above that of other normal infants. The presence of jaundice does not affect the prothrombin activity.

Newborn infants with intestinal abnormalities who are not treated with vitamin K are unusually prone to develop a low prothrombin level, and this may be maintained for a longer period than in comparable infants without such abnormalities. This deficiency results from either defective intestinal synthesis or poor absorption of the vitamin. Sound management calls for the liberal administration of vitamin K parenterally both before and after surgery.

Prematurity

The prothrombin activity in premature infants when vitamin K is withheld from them or from their mothers during labor behaves much like that of full-term infants, except that the neonatal decrease tends to reach a low point 1 or 2 days earlier and to terminate more rapidly. Neither age of gestation nor weight at birth seems to influence the initial prothrombin levels or the rate of change in the first few days.

Administration of vitamin K to infant or mother may retard the neonatal fall.

For some as yet unexplained reason, in about 5 per cent of premature infants the blood at birth does not clot or give any prothrombin reactions. After the first day, however, the coagulation reactions become the same as those of other premature infants. No unusual propensity to hemorrhagic manifestations seems to be associated with this phenomenon.

Older Infants

Plum studied with a one-stage method a group of 256 infants and children aged 1 week to 14 years. During the third and fourth weeks the prothrombin activity was still consistently reduced lower than that of adults. The prothrombin activity level of normal adults was attained by 50 per cent of the infants between the second and twelfth months. After the first year nearly all were at the adult level. Brinkhous, Smith, and Warner similarly found a blood prothrombin activity below 50 per cent of the adult during the newborn period, 60 per cent at 2 months, and a gradual rise to 100 per cent by the first birthday.

Hemorrhagic Disease of the Newborn Infant

This general diagnosis is applied to newborn infants who exhibit hemorrhagic oozing in the absence of gross anatomic injuries. Hematemesis, melena, umbilical hemorrhage, or persistent bleeding from a skin cut or finger prick are the usual symptoms. The common practice of administering vitamin K to mothers during labor or to the infants immediately after birth appears to have reduced the frequency of the milder and more slowly developing forms of this symptom complex. Acute cerebral hemorrhages and other gross bleeding disturbances which have their origin in obstetric lacerations of large vessels remain unreduced by this prophylaxis. With hypoprothrombinemic infants whose mothers did not receive vitamin K during delivery, a parenteral injection of this substance usually puts an end to such bleeding within an hour or two.

Other factors which may contribute to hemorrhages in occasional newborns are trauma, sepsis, prematurity, afibrinogenemia, thrombocytopenic purpura, undue capillary fragility, and related disturbances of hemostasis.

Erythroblastosis Fetalis

In newborn infants with active erythroblastosis fetalis the clotting time of venous blood may range from 7 minutes to an hour, or even fail to show any coagulation at all. In 10 such infants reported by Heyn and associates the prothrombin activity in the first hours of life ranged from 56 to 100 per cent of normal, essentially in the normal range. Of 8 who were treated with exchange transfusion, 6 had a higher prothrombin concentration after the procedure. On the third day of life the average prothrombin concentration in those 8 was 77 per cent of normal, higher than the 65 per cent observed in a series of normal control infants. By the fifth day all infants had 100 per cent levels.

Therapy

The best immediate therapy for a newborn infant with hemorrhagic symptoms is transfusion supplemented with vitamin K. The transfusion should consist either of fresh whole blood or of fresh or freshly frozen serum or plasma, since the coagulation-promoting activity deteriorates on storage. Liberal amounts are advisable, up to the physiologic capacity of the infant. Correction of any prothrombin defect will be achieved immediately and will persist long enough for vitamin K to take effect. Intramuscular or intraperitoneal injections of plasma or serum will not raise the plasma prothrombin.

The plasma prothrombin activity will rise to safe levels within 1 to 2 hours if vitamin K therapy is given intravenously or intramuscularly. Oral therapy will take only an hour or two longer, provided there is no biliary tract block and intestinal absorption is normal. One- or two-milligram doses are adequate. In the presence of hemorrhagic symptoms associated with hypoprothrombinemia, vitamin K should be continued until the bleeding ceases, provided other possible causative mechanisms for the disturbance have been ruled out.

HYPOPROTHROMBINEMIA OF LIVER DISEASE

The liver must receive a continuous supply of vitamin K for the maintenance of a normal plasma prothrombin level. The plasma level begins to fall within a day or two after failure of prothrombin production. In diseases of the liver or bile ducts, whether acute or chronic, not enough bile may be eliminated to permit adequate absorption of vitamin K from the intestine, or the prothrombin-forming capacity of the liver itself may be damaged, or both. Among the liver diseases which can produce hypoprothrombinemia are erythroblastosis fetalis, obstructive jaundice, Laennec's cirrhosis, viral hepatitis, congenital obstruction of the bile ducts, postanesthetic liver damage, chloroform, bismuth and related poisonings, and syphilis of the liver.

The response of plasma prothrombin activity to vitamin K given parenterally can be used diagnostically to test for liver disease. A large dose of water-soluble vitamin K is given intravenously for 4 consecutive days. The prothrombin concentration is estimated daily during this period and for several days thereafter. An initially prolonged reading which reverts to normal following the vitamin K administration denotes absorptive deficiency rather than liver damage. Negligible or transitory rises are positive signs of poor liver function.

Bleeding and coagulation defects in liver disease occasionally persist after the hypoprothrombinemia has been eliminated, presumably as the result of other defects in the hemostatic equilibrium. In obstructive jaundice there is believed to occur some increased antithrombin activity. In hepatocellular jaundice, Ac-globulin production may be impaired and fibrinolysis seems unusually active. A prolonged bleeding time is often encountered, suggesting that the integrity of the vascular walls is impaired.

ENTERAL HYPOPROTHROMBINEMIA

Hypoprothrombinemia of intestinal origin can result from impaired formation of vitamin K by the intestinal microorganisms, hypermotility of the intestine, or altered absorptive capacity of the mucosa. Among the causative disturbances may be mentioned intestinal obstruction; cystic fibrosis of the pancreas and related disorders of the celiac syndrome; depression of intestinal tract bacteria by chemotherapy; ulcerative colitis; intestinal and biliary fistulas; persistent diarrhea; and any other disorder accompanied by prolonged hyperperistalsis or mucosal injury. When the depression of blood prothrombin is marked, hemorrhagic manifestations may become evident as nosebleeds, skin petechiae, blood in the stools, prolonged bleeding from needle punctures or other incisions, etc.

With infants having marked diarrhea lasting more than a few days the plasma prothrombin activity almost invariably becomes low. The extent of the depression tends to parallel the severity of the diarrhea. Readings between 5 and 40 per cent of normal are the rule. There may be a rise with clinical improvement, and a progressive fall in fatal cases. Overt bleeding, however, is the exception rather than the rule. Of interest is Matoth's observation that in such infants the oral administration of streptomycin or unabsorbable sulfonamides does not depress the prothrombin level further. These drugs sometimes seem to raise the prothrombin level a little, probably by helping to restore a more normal bowel flora. This is opposite to what happens in preoperative patients thus treated.

Therapeutic doses of vitamin K in enteral hypoprothrombinemia are followed by cessation of bleeding phenomena if present and a prompt return of the prothrombin readings to normal or near normal. For this reason it is advisable to include vitamin K in the therapeutic program of all severe intestinal diseases and to give it preferably by the parenteral route.

HYPOPROTHROMBINEMIA INDUCED BY DRUGS

Salicylates administered orally for therapeutic purposes will depress prothrombin activity in most individuals after 2 to 5 days, but not to any great extent. There is no correlation between the reduction in prothrombin activity and the serum levels of salicylate. If the salicylate therapy is continued in children, the prothrombin levels return to normal pretreatment levels by about the ninth day. Hemorrhagic symptoms rarely appear, though some otolaryngologists believe that children given aspirin after tonsillectomy are more prone to postoperative bleeding complications. Large doses of salicylates enhance the activity of Dicumarol and its derivatives.

The sulfonamides and common antibiotics, in dosage levels adequate to maintain therapeutic blood concentrations, do not alter the coagulating mechanisms to any significant clinical degree.

The dicoumarin drugs depress prothrombin or its activators in the recipient's blood. These are used widely in adult medicine to forestall intravascular thrombosis and other thromboembolic complications, but have almost no applicability to pediatrics. Administration is usually regulated by the prothrombin test.

DEFECTS IN THE PROTHROMBIN COMPLEX

These are comparatively rare disturbances in which coagulation is imperfect as a consequence of a persistent deficiency of either prothrombin itself or a prothrombin accelerator. Early in life, or later, the tendency to easy bruising and bleeding after minor trauma becomes apparent, though hemarthroses are uncommon. Either sex may be affected. Significant findings in the initial screening tests are prolongation of venous clotting and a low plasma "prothrombin time" (Table 21-1). The clot may or may not retract well. Results of the tourniquet test, platelet count, fibrinogen concentration, and antithrombin titer are usually normal. The bleeding time may be normal or prolonged. A circulating anticoagulant and spontaneous fibrinolysis are not demonstrable. Liver disease is not present. Addition of fresh normal or hemophilic plasma in vitro to the plasma of an individual with this defect will correct the coagulation disturbance.

Some of these cases—the so-called "parahemophilia" group—may be shown to have a specific deficiency of the labile accessory factor V (p. 232). As with hemophilia, this deficiency is relieved promptly by administration of fresh normal blood or fresh citrated plasma which has been preserved by freezing or is less than a few days old. Fresh blood or plasma when administered intravenously restores the labile factor activity for only 1 or 2 days, so that repeated daily transfusions are advisable for control of hemorrhagic symptoms.

Other cases—"hypoconvertinemia," "stable factor deficiency"—have been traced to a congenital deficiency of factor VII (p. 232). The patient's coagulation status can be temporarily restored to normal by transfusions of fresh or stored normal blood, plasma, or serum, inasmuch as the defective factors are comparatively stable and do not disappear during coagulation.

Sometimes the hemorrhagic symptoms date back to birth and are clearly of congenital nature. Other asymptomatic family members may be found who have had a bleeding tendency or who exhibit laboratory evidences of subclinical deficiency of the same factor.

When the disturbance does not become evident until later in life the origin is then more ambiguous and familial prevalence may not be found. The "acquired" cases are usually ill with some systemic disturbance such as chronic leukemia or severe liver disease and have hypoprothrombinemia as a secondary manifestation.

HEMOPHILIA-LIKE DISEASES (HEMOPHILIOID DISEASE)

This term is applied to a miscellaneous group of patients with spontaneous hemorrhagic manifestations somewhat similar to hemophilia whose blood, when mixed with normal blood or recalcified citrated plasma, will lengthen the clotting time of the normal. This is evidence of the presence of a circulating anticoagulant. There is usually a prolonged venous coagulation time, normal bleeding time, normal platelets, normal fibrinogen, and diminished capillary strength. The disturbance occurs in both sexes.

The anticoagulants discoverable in these patients are not all identical. There may be neutralization or destruction of thromboplastinogen, with retardation in the formation or utilization of thromboplastin. Sometimes the transformation of prothrombin to thrombin has seemed inhibited. An excess of circulating heparin-like substances may be found. There may be a systemic disease such as amyloidosis, multiple myeloma or other "dysproteinemia" in which an excess of normal or abnormal proteins seem to bind the calcium, prothrombin, or other factors and inhibit their participation in the coagulation reaction. The anticoagulants are generally stable, resistant to storage, and not inactivated by refrigeration or by warming to 60°C.

Differentiation must be made from hemophilia in which a patient, after receiving repeated transfusions of blood or blood derivatives, develops antibodies against the clotting component missing from his own circulation (p. 264). It may not be possible in a male subject with apparent hemophilia to be certain of the exact nature of the disorder if the family history is negative for the disease and if no tests had been done earlier in childhood to demonstrate that a circulating anticoagulant was not then present.

FIBRINOGEN DEFICIENCIES

Congenital Afibrinogenemia

Complete absence of fibrinogen from the blood plasma is rare. Several dozen childhood cases have been recorded, nearly always of congenital origin. The defect occurs in both males and females and appears to be recessive. Hemorrhages typically become apparent early in life, often from the umbilical stump. The severity of the disturbance is not as severe as in hemophilia, despite complete incoagulability of the blood. Bleeding does not occur spontaneously, but only after direct trauma or with ulceration of the gastrointestinal tract. Hemarthroses do not develop in congenital afibrinogenemia.

The usual laboratory findings are complete incoagulability of the blood as a consequence of complete absence of fibrinogen; occasional undue capillary fragility; slow blood sedimentation rate; intermittent thrombocytopenia. No clotting occurs in the one-stage prothrombin test. The fibrinogen peak is absent in the electrophoretic recordings of the plasma.

The absence of fibrinogen from the blood can be confirmed by several simple tests. Incubation of the patient's fresh whole blood at 37°C for 3 days results in no clot formation. Heating of the plasma to 60°C or one-fourth saturation of the plasma with ammonium sulfate fails to bring down a precipitate of fibrin.

Bleeding from shallow finger tip punctures will usually stop in 2 to 3 minutes, whereas deeper punctures or incisions may ooze for several days. The bleeding may stop and then recur, presumably as the small vessels contract and relax.

Congenital Fibrinogenopenia

Closely related to the above disturbance is congenital fibrinogenopenia which may represent the heterozygous condition. Some of the cases have been found in families in which an infant has been born with afibrinogenemia. Affected individuals show a tendency to easy bleeding and bruising, after trauma, but their bleeding and clotting times, capillary resistance, sedimentation rates, and platelet counts are normal or nearly normal. Blood-clotting studies may or may not show an imperfection. The plasma fibrinogen level fluctuates typically between 50 and 250 mg per 100 ml, as compared with the normal range of variation of 250 to 400 mg per 100 ml.

Acquired Fibrinogenopenia

The fibrinogen level of the blood may become chronically reduced in severe liver disease and starvation states. An acutely developing hypo- or afibrinogenemia of obscure pathogenesis is an infrequent but serious hemorrhagic complication of transfusion reactions and of severe crushing injuries and burns.

Therapy

All varieties of fibrinogen deficiency can be corrected temporarily by large transfusions of blood or plasma or concentrates of human fibrinogen. Normal coagulation can be restored by raising the plasma fibrinogen above a critical level of approximately 80 mg per 100 ml. Transfusions may have to be repeated at approximately daily intervals to maintain this level in congenital afibrinogenemia.

A study was conducted by Frick and McQuarrie on the rate of disappearance of injected fibrinogen in a 7-year-old boy with this disease. After approximately 4 gm of human fibrinogen was infused rapidly, a plasma concentration of 161 mg per 100 ml was noted ½ hour afterward. The plasma level fell gradually, and after 12 days no fibrinogen could be detected.

DIFFUSE SMALL-VESSEL FRAGILITY

Structural weakness of the vascular walls which permits them to break and ooze blood under strain which normal vessels can withstand is a rare cause of hemorrhagic disturbances in childhood. In the few children we have recognized with this disturbance the diagnosis has been based on (1) superficial ecchymoses or deeper skin hematomas occuring singly or in crops, with or without hemorrhages in other regions of the body, (2) increased fragility of the small vessels as shown by the pressure procedures, regularly or intermittently present, and (3) normal findings in all tests for impairment of the clotting and platelet mechanisms. The disorder may be familial. Rutin or hesperidin (bioflavonoids) are sometimes helpful in therapy.

BLEEDING IN CONGENITAL HEART DISEASE

Patients with cyanotic congenital heart disease, through mechanisms which are not clear, often have platelet counts below 200,000 per cu mm (p. 105). Prothrombin consumption tests show that in this respect platelet function is normal. The plasma fibrinogen concentration may be somewhat reduced also. Clot retraction is frequently defective. The prothrombin time may be prolonged slightly to moderately, from a reduction in prothrombin itself rather than a deficiency of any accessory plasma component. This hypoprothrombinemia does not improve after the intravenous administration of large amounts of potent vitamin K preparations.

Transfusing of large quantities of blood in the course of a prolonged cardiovascular operation tends to depress the platelet count further and also reduces the plasma Ac-globulin level. Postoperative hemorrhage sometimes follows. When this complication develops, the pouring of more blood into the circulation aggravates the defect. It is important during such operations to keep the infused blood to the minimum compatible with maintaining blood pressure and other physiologic equilibria.

BIBLIOGRAPHY

HYPOPROTHROMBINEMIA IN THE NEWBORN INFANT

Brinkhous, K. M., H. P. Smith, and *E. D. Warner,* Plasma Prothrombin Level in Normal Infancy and in Hemorrhagic Disease of the Newborn, *Am. J. M. Sc.* 193:475, 1937.

Dam, H., H. Dyggve, H. Larsen, and *P. Plum,* The Relation of Vitamin K Deficiency to Hemorrhagic Disease of the Newborn, *Advances Pediat.* 5:129, 1952.

De Sousa, C. A., A propos de la tendance hemorragique du nouveau-né, *Arch. franç. pediat.* 9:482, 1952.

Fanconi, G., "Die Störungen der Blutgerinnung beim Kinde mit besonderer Berucksichtigung des K-Vitamins und der Neugeborenenpathologie," Georg Thieme Verlag, Leipzig, 1941.

Garces, S. H., Contribucion al estudio de la coagulacion sanguinea en el recien nacido, *Rev. chilena de pediat.* 21:191, 1950.

Grossman, B. J., R. M. Heyn, and *I. H. Rozenfeld,* Coagulation Studies in Newborn Infant. I. Normal Infants, *Pediatrics* 9:182, 1952.

Heyn, R. M., I. H. Rozenfeld, B. J. Grossman, and *J. D. Stuart,* Coagulation Studies in the Newborn Infant. II. Erythroblastosis Fetalis, *Pediatrics* 9:327, 1952.

Israels, L. G., A. Zipursky, and *C. Sinclair,* Factor V Levels in the Neonatal Period, *Pediatrics* 15:180, 1955.

Kato, K., and *H. G. Poncher,* Prothrombin in the Blood of Newborn, Mature and Immature Infants as Determined by a Micro Prothrombin Test, *J.A.M.A.* **114:**749, 1940.

Kerpel-Fronius, E., F. Varga, and *E. K. Pál,* Cause and Significance of Seasonal Variation in the Haemorrhagic Tendency in the Newborn, *Arch. Dis. Childhood* **23:**87, 1948.

Kove, S., and *C. Benton,* Prothrombin in the Newborn Infant, *J. Pediat.* **37:**78, 1950.

Plum, P., The Prothrombin Content of the Blood during the First Years of Life, *Acta paediat.* **38:**526, 1949.

Randall, A., IV, and *J. P. Randall,* Prothrombin Deficiency of the Newborn, *Proc. Soc. Exper. Biol. & Med.* **70:**215, 1949.

Reich, C., R. L. McCready, and *H. Chaplin,* Parenteral Vitamin K Therapy during the Antepartum Period and Its Effects on the Infants' Prothrombin Levels, *Am. J. Obst. & Gynec.* **53:**300, 1947.

Sanford, H. N., M. Kostalik, and *B. Blackmore,* Prothrombin Studies on the Blood of the Premature Infant and the Value of Vitamin K Therapy, *Am. J. Dis. Child.* **78:**686, 1949.

Waddell, W. W., Jr., and *G. M. Lawson,* Hemorrhagic Diathesis in the Newborn: Further Observations Concerning Prevention and Treatment, *J.A.M.A.* **115:**1416, 1940.

DEFICIENCY OF PROTHROMBIN ACCELERATOR FACTORS

Brennan, M. J., R. W. Monto, and *H. C. Shafer,* Hemorrhagic Diathesis Due to Ac-Globulin Deficiency, *Am. J. Clin. Path.* **22:**150, 1952.

Brink, A. J., and *C. S. Kingsley,* A Familial Disorder of Blood Coagulation Due to Deficiency of the Labile Factor, *Quart. J. Med.* **21:**19, 1952; *ibid.* **23:**323, 1954.

Goldstein, A. R., G. Landwehr, and *C. D. Cook,* Congenital SPCA Deficiency: A Hitherto Unrecognized Coagulation Defect with Hemorrhage Rectified by Serum and Serum Fractions, *J. Clin. Invest.* **30:**596, 1951.

Halliwell, H. L., and *L. Brigham,* Pseudohemophilia, *Ann. Int. Med.* **29:**803, 1948.

Owren, P. A., Parahemophilia: Hemorrhagic Diathesis Due to Absence of a Previously Unknown Clotting Factor, *Lancet* **1:**446, 1947.

Redner, B., H. Scalettar, and *M. Weiner,* Parahemophilia (Owren's Disease), *Pediatrics* **12:**5, 1953.

Sacks, M. S., and *G. Raccuglia,* Hereditary Deficiency of Proaccelerin (Parahemophilia): A Family Study, *J. Lab. & Clin. Med.* **46:**98, 1955.

Wurzel, H. A., K. Roth, and *S. Zubrow,* Mild Familial Hypoproconvertinemia, *J. Lab. & Clin. Med.* **44:**403, 1954.

MISCELLANEOUS FORMS OF HYPOPROTHROMBINEMIA

Biggs, R., and *A. S. Douglas,* The Measurement of Prothrombin in Plasma; A Case of Prothrombin Deficiency, *J. Clin. Path.* **6:**15, 1953.

Freeman, G., and *J. S. Hyde,* Roles of Prothrombin Activity, Heparin-Protamine Titer and Platelet Concentration in Bleeding of Leukemia, *Blood* **7:**311, 1952.

Harrington, W. J., R. H. Manheimer, J. F. Desforges, H. P. Minkel, C. B. Crow, and *F. Stohlman,* The Bleeding Tendency in Hepatocellular and Obstructive Jaundice, *Bull. New England M. Center* **12:**121, 1950.

Hartmann, R. C., A Hemorrhagic Disorder Occurring in Patients with Cyanotic Congenital Heart Disease, *Bull. Johns Hopkins Hosp.* **91:**49, 1952.

Heindl, I. S., B. G. Anderson, and *R. D. Friedlander,* Acute Idiopathic Hypoprothrombinemia: Response to Massive Doses of Vitamin K, *Ann. Int. Med.* **29:**347, 1948.

Ley, A. B., G. G. Reader, C. W. Sorenson, and *R. S. Overman,* Idiopathic Hypoprothrombinemia Associated with Hemorrhagic Diathesis, and the Effect of Vitamin K, *Blood* 6:740, 1951.

Matoth, Y., Plasma Prothrombin in Infantile Diarrhea, *A.M.A. Am. J. Dis. Child.* 80:944, 1950.

Rapoport, S., and *K. Dodd,* Hypoprothrombinemia in Infants with Diarrhea, *Am. J. Dis. Child.* 71:611, 1946.

———, *M. Wing,* and *G. M. Guest,* Hypoprothrombinemia after Salicylate Administration in Man and Rabbits, *Proc. Soc. Exper. Biol. & Med.* 53:40, 1943.

Schlesinger, B., W. W. Payne, and *E. D. Burnard,* Liver Damage in Gastroenteritis, *Arch. Dis. Childhood* 24:15, 1949.

CIRCULATING ANTICOAGULANTS

Allen, J. G., P. V. Moulder, R. M. Elghammer, B. J. Grossman, C. L. McKeen, M. Sanderson, W. Egner, and *J. M. Crosbie,* A Protamine Titration as an Indication of a Clotting Defect in Certain Hemorrhagic States, *J. Lab. & Clin. Med.* 34:473, 1949.

Bell, W. N., A Coagulation Defect Due to an Anticoagulant Possessing Antithromboplastic and Antithrombic Properties, Probably Heparin, *Blood* 6:1199, 1951.

Griffith, W. H., Plasma Antithrombin in Thrombosis, Hemorrhage and Liver Disease, *J. Lab. & Clin. Med.* 40:367, 1952.

Klein, P. D., and *W. H. Seegers,* The Nature of Plasma Antithrombin Activity, *Blood* 5:742, 1950.

Nilsson, I. M., and *A. Wenckert,* Hyperglobulinemia as the Cause of Hemophilia-like Disease, *Blood* 8:1067, 1953.

Pons, E. R., Jr., and *M. V. de Torregrosa,* Hemorrhagic Diathesis Due to a Circulating Anticoagulant: Report of Case with Laboratory Observations, *Blood* 7:20, 1952.

Speer, R. J., J. M. Hill, M. Maloney, and *A. Roberts,* Hemorrhagic Diathesis Associated with Hyperheparinemia, *J. Lab. & Clin. Med.* 45:730, 1955.

FIBRINOGEN DEFICIENCY

Alexander, B., R. Goldstein, L. Rich, A. G. Le Bollo'h, L. K. Diamond, and *W. Borges,* Congenital Afibrinogenemia: A Study of Some Basic Aspects of Coagulation, *Blood* 9:843, 1954.

Allibone, E. C., and *H. S. Baar,* Fibrinogen Deficiency as a Factor in Haemorrhagic Disease, *Arch. Dis. Childhood* 18:146, 1943.

Frick, P. G., and *I. McQuarrie,* Congenital Afibrinogenemia, *Pediatrics* 13:44, 1954.

Gitlin, D., and *W. H. Borges,* Studies on the Metabolism of Fibrinogen in Two Patients with Congenital Afibrinogenemia, *Blood* 8:679, 1953.

Henderson, J. L., G. M. M. Donaldson, and *H. Scarborough,* Congenital Afibrinogenemia: Report of a Case with a Review of the Literature, *Quart. J. Med.* 14:101, 1945.

Lewis, J. H., and *J. H. Ferguson,* Afibrinogenemia, *A.M.A. Am. J. Dis. Child.* 88:711, 1954.

Prichard, R. W., and *R. L. Vann,* Congenital Afibrinogenemia, *A.M.A. Am. J. Dis. Child.* 88:703, 1954.

CHAPTER 23

Thrombocytopenic States

The thrombocytopenic states may be divided into several varieties on the basis essentially of pathogenesis and relation to other diseases. All have in common the clinical evidences of (1) an abnormal tendency to bleed into the skin, mucous membranes, gastrointestinal tract, and internal organs, and (2) a diminished thrombocyte count and associated hematologic changes. These changes, as discussed in detail under idiopathic purpura, hold for the other varieties except as specifically noted.

IDIOPATHIC THROMBOCYTOPENIC PURPURA

This variety of the disorder appears to arise spontaneously and suddenly and in children is often of comparatively short duration. Unlike what happens in adults, the disorder is not much more common in females than in males. One can often elicit a history of a recent infection, therapy with an antimicrobial or other drug, or probable exposure to a toxic agent such as an insecticide or organic solvent.

Fragmentary evidence is at hand which indicates that different physiologic mechanisms, individually or in diverse combinations, may lead to thrombocytopenic purpura. Sometimes the production of platelets in the bone marrow seems to be arrested, possibly as the result of some splenic hormone which arrests the maturation of megakaryoblasts and promegakaryocytes. In other cases the elaboration of platelets by the marrow megakaryocytes appears to be normal or accelerated, but they seem to be sequestered or removed at an unduly rapid rate in the lungs, spleen, or other parts of the reticuloendothelial system. Antiplatelet substances are sometimes demonstrable in the circulation. An attendant unusual propensity for capillary oozing is demonstrable in most cases. The parents of every affected child should be queried with respect to the possibility of contact with any potential incitant, and further exposure to this substance discontinued at once.

In typical cases, transfused foreign platelets are destroyed within a few hours. This is in contrast with the thrombocytopenia of bone marrow aplasia or infiltration, in which transfused platelets tend to persist for the normal 5 days or a little longer.

Clinical Aspects

Almost invariably the prominent symptoms are easy bruising and the spontaneous occurrence of petechiae and ecchymoses into the skin, mouth, or conjunctivae. Melena, hematuria, menorrhagia, or bleeding into the central nervous system and other organs are uncommon. The patient is usually not aware of any local trauma as a precipitating cause. Excessive bleeding may follow operative procedures such as tonsillectomy or tooth extractions. Vaginal bleeding may be prominent in girls during the menarche. Hemarthroses are most uncommon. Most of the affected children are between 3 and 7 years of age. More than one case in the same family is most unusual. The disturbance is sometimes seen in children with large hemangiomas in chronic form.

Physical examination usually reveals no positive findings other than hemorrhages. The spleen is as a rule not palpable, or only barely so. If it is unduly large some other cause of the splenomegaly must be looked for and will usually be found. Generalized lymphadenopathy and liver enlargement are most exceptional. Gastrointestinal bleeding is not accompanied by abdominal pain, as in anaphylactoid purpura. Central nervous system hemorrhages are the most dreaded complications.

Laboratory Features

The most characteristic finding is a diminution in the circulating platelets. The count is practically always less than the lower limit of normal—i.e., below 150,000 per cu mm. Peripheral hemorrhages do not occur in early cases except when the count is lower than about 60,000; when it rises above this level the bleeding ceases. After some weeks the count may fall to lower levels without any exhibition of bleeding.

The venous clotting time is not increased, but the clotting time of recalcified oxalated plasma tends to be prolonged. The prothrombin time is unimpaired. The prothrombin consumption rate may be diminished, more or less proportionately to the reduction in platelet count. When the platelet count is below about 60,000, the peripheral bleeding time is typically prolonged and the capillary permeability as determined with the tourniquet test is increased. There are no anemia or red cell changes except what can be attributed to blood loss. A moderate eosinophilia or lymphocytosis is not infrequent. A transitory granulocytic leukocytosis may follow an internal hemorrhage. Clot formation and retraction are almost invariably impaired during active phases. The blood fibrinogen level is undisturbed. Atypical lymphocytes and even lymphoblasts sometimes become prominent in the peripheral blood and in the tissues.

In bone marrow aspirates the megakaryocytes may occur in normal numbers and usually seem more numerous (p. 324). A significant eosino-philia (more than 5 per cent of all granulocytes) is seen in about half the marrow specimens (p. 318).

Prognosis

The usual episode of purpura hemorrhagica is mild or moderate, lasting only one or several months and then subsiding spontaneously. In approximately 15 per cent of childhood attacks, however, the clinical course is more serious or the thrombocytopenia may continue for months or even several years. When this occurs the disturbance is sometimes called chronic idiopathic purpura hemorrhagica; such cases are far less frequent than among adults. Bruising and bleeding usually (but not invariably) become less prominent and the tourniquet test may give negative results.

Sometimes a relapse occurs after the purpura has subsided and the platelets have risen to normal or nearly normal levels. This quiescent interval may last a few months to 10 or 20 years. Hence the wisdom of routine checkups of the blood status at regular intervals of all apparently fully recovered cases. Recurrences often seem related to an acute infection.

Less than 1 per cent of affected children exhibit protracted severe bleeding, often with complete absence of megakaryocytes from the marrow. These have a poor prognosis and usually receive no benefit from splenectomy.

Therapy

Transfusions may be given for anemia. When feasible it is best to give fresh blood which has had a minimum of handling. It is of little help to use siliconized or plastic equipment or to give direct transfusions, since transfused platelets are destroyed by the recipient within a few hours.

Splenectomy is necessary only exceptionally. Most childhood cases recover spontaneously or with hormone therapy. The surgery is both costly and not entirely without risk. Not all patients are improved, or the improvement may be only transitory. When the purpura is chronic or recurrent or the bleeding uncontrollable, however, splenectomy is usually followed by a prompt increase in platelets and a disappearance of symptoms. The platelet count may rise well above normal limits during the first week and may remain between 400,000 and 1 million for several months postoperatively.

Splenectomy usually improves capillary fragility whether the thrombocyte count rises or not. It is suspected that the early phases of improvement are related to the nonspecific stimulation of operative interference.

Adrenal cortical steroids or corticotropin will frequently relieve bleeding symptoms. The immediate action is through improving vascular integrity. In those patients in whom continuous benefit is to be obtained from these hormones, the platelets will commence to rise sharply in the first week, as a rule. Corticotropin in large doses may be more effective than the other hormones, but the ease of administration of the latter is much greater. Improvement may not be complete or lasting, but these hormones can support a patient through the early period when the possibility of a fulminating hemorrhage is greatest.

THROMBOCYTIC PURPURA CAUSED BY DRUGS OR TOXINS

Depressed thrombocyte counts and hemorrhagic symptoms in the absence of generalized bone marrow depression may be provoked in sensitized individuals by a wide diversity of drugs—Sedormid, gold salts, DDT, benzol, Tridione, quinidine, amidopyrine, chloramphenicol, sulfathiazole, etc. In view of the widespread use of many of these agents, this toxic reaction in the exceptional case must be viewed as due to individual idiosyncrasy. The clinical and laboratory findings are much the same as in the idiopathic variety. Acute thrombocytopenia with superimposed hemorrhages may develop within a few hours after a severe generalized burn or as a complication of severe sunstroke.

When drug sensitivity is at fault the removal of the offending substance when feasible will often, but unfortunately not always, result in prompt recovery. Severe or stubborn cases may be treated with transfusions, corticotropin, or adrenal cortical steroids. Hemopoietic stimulants and the antihistamines may be of benefit. Administration of BAL may facilitate recovery when gold or arsenic compounds are responsible.

Should the marrow injury continue, agranulocytosis or hypoproduction of the red cells or both may soon be superimposed. The therapeutic problem then becomes that of the management of aplastic anemia (p. 79). Sometimes the hemorrhages, leukocytopenia, and thrombocytopenia are the first overt signs of toxic marrow suppression, while the disturbances secondary to absent red cell regeneration do not become manifest until later.

THROMBOCYTOPENIC PURPURA OF THE NEWBORN

Infants with this disorder exhibit purpuric hemorrhages into the skin, mucous membranes, gastrointestinal tract, and other organs. Symptoms usually begin on the first day, with 50 per cent of the cases showing evidences of purpura at the moment of birth. In routine laboratory studies these infants have the same changes as do older children with thrombocytopenic purpura—diminished platelet count, increased bleeding time, unusual capillary fragility, normal coagulation time, poor clot retraction, and so forth. The bone marrow may show normal or increased megakaryocytes, often atypical or immature in appearance. Sometimes the bone marrow has been hypoplastic or even aplastic. The spleen is ordinarily not palpable. The symptoms tend to subside spontaneously before the end of the first month of life as a rule, and the infant remains well thereafter. Transfusions are usually adequate as therapy. In a few infants with severe generalized hemorrhages and prominent marrow megakaryocytosis, improvement has followed splenectomy. Corticotropin or cortisone should be given a trial before this operation is considered seriously.

Of extreme interest in unraveling the pathogenesis of thrombocytopenic purpura in the newborn is the finding that many of the mothers have or have had the disease, either in the idiopathic form or secondary to sensitization to some known drug or toxin. It has been suggested that platelets may contain antigens of differing types, in a manner analogous to that of the ABO and Rh types of the red cells, and that the purpura in some of these infants results from transplacental transfer of incompatible maternal antibodies. This hypothesis receives substantiation from the fact that successive newborn infants may be affected. The majority of mothers with the disease give birth to unaffected infants.

In a minority of infantile cases the purpura persists indefinitely instead of regressing spontaneously. Some congenital anomaly in the platelet-forming mechanisms must then be hypothesized. With most of these the megakaryocytes have been absent or permanently reduced. A few families have been reported in which all or nearly all the offspring have had this form of the disturbance.

Affected infants may be misdiagnosed as having hypoprothrombinemia of the newborn unless thorough blood studies are done. The differential diagnosis must also exclude other hemorrhagic diseases such as those caused by drug sensitivity, severe infection, or inclusion body disease.

THROMBOCYTOPENIC PURPURA SECONDARY TO SPLENOMEGALY

Almost any condition which leads to splenomegaly can induce thrombocytopenic purpura through the route of hypersplenism (p. 295). The bone marrow in these cases tends to be hypercellular with respect to the megakaryocytes, with a preponderance of immature forms. It has been surmised that a majority of childhood cases of idiopathic thrombocytopenic purpura are caused primarily by splenic dysfunction, as evidenced by the prompt recovery which usually follows removal of this organ. Since some apparently identical cases are not much relieved by the operation, or only transitorily, the relation between the spleen and the "idiopathic" disease remains far from clear. In line with the principle that the spleen may depress the liberation or longevity of granulocytes or red cells simultaneously with or independently of that of the platelets, in thrombocytopenic purpura one sometimes finds a concomitant peripheral granulocytopenia or anemia or even pancytopenia.

THROMBOCYTOPENIC PURPURA DURING INFECTIONS AND OTHER SYSTEMIC DISEASES

Almost any viral or bacterial infection in a child may lead to the extraordinary complication of thrombocytopenia with purpura. This is perhaps more likely to occur after upper respiratory tract infections, measles, mumps, chicken pox, German measles, scarlet fever, septicemia, typhoid fever, influenza, typhus, miliary tuberculosis, and infectious mononucleosis. Thrombocytopenic purpura may develop also during the course of nephritis, lupus erythematosus, and sundry other noninfectious systemic diseases of the internal organs. When the patient is an infant the prognosis is especially grave.

Purpuric symptoms beginning during the height of an acute infection tend to subside as the latter improves. The thrombocytopenia pursues a similar course. Should the hemorrhages continue, the presumption is strong that the infection was but the trigger mechanism for an "idiopathic" disturbance which had been smoldering previously at a subclinical level. With purpura and thrombocytopenia which develop 1 or 2 weeks after an infection, the duration and other characteristics are indistinguishable from the idiopathic variety.

It is possible that the association of thrombocytopenic purpura with infectious disease is an extreme expression of a marrow depression which takes place much more often to a lesser and clinically unrecognizable extent (p. 56). During many infectious illnesses the platelet count tends to fall moderately (say from 250,000 to 150,000 per cu mm). This is sometimes followed by a transitory rise above the normal.

PURPURA HEMORRHAGICA SECONDARY TO BONE MARROW INVOLVEMENT

Mechanical displacement or local dysnutrition of the megakaryocyte series within the bone marrow itself can hamper formation of platelets along with the other types of cells and give rise to the thrombocytopenic syndrome. This takes place chiefly in leukemia, aplastic anemia, myelofibrosis, and metastatic sarcoma, but may evolve also in other blood dyscrasias or other hypoplastic states of the marrow. Heavy exposure to x-ray or other radiations can be responsible.

When the marrow is suddenly and acutely damaged the purpura may precede recognizable anemia by an appreciable interval. Failure of production of platelets, whose average duration in the circulation is only 5 days, will result in pertinent symptoms long before the absence of new red cells of 110 days average survival becomes apparent. Conversely, when the marrow lesion develops slowly the anemia may be noted first or be more prominent. In this circumstance the gradual subsidence of the platelet level may be compensated for by corrective influences. Granulocytes exist in the circulation for only a few days, but their acute disappearance will not be followed by any overt symptoms unless infection supervenes.

Transfusion in thrombocytopenic purpura of aplastic origin replaces the red cells but does not correct the deficiencies in leukocytes and thrombocytes except when the blood passes almost immediately from donor to recipient through siliconized or plastic apparatus. Splenectomy is of no value whenever the marrow megakaryocytes are crowded out. Corticotropin or adrenal hormones or other nonspecific bone marrow stimulants will sometimes promote the partial return of megakaryocytes and thrombocytes and suppress the purpura, at least for a time. Chemotherapy of an underlying malignancy may also arrest the process.

In the blood of children with leukemia one may find some subsidence in prothrombin activity, an increase in heparin-like substances, or rarely a diminished fibrin content. The prothrombin deficiency can be ascribed to the anoxia or infiltrations of the liver and the malnutrition and partial vitamin deficiencies which attend the advanced stages of the disease. The major factors in the bleeding of childhood leukemia appear to be the integrity of the capillary network and the content of circulating platelets. Generalized hemorrhages are almost never seen in these patients until the platelet level is much below the apparently critical level of 50,000 to 60,000 per cu mm of the capillary blood (p. 214).

THROMBOCYTOPENIA FOLLOWING MASSIVE TRANSFUSIONS OF WHOLE BLOOD

Mention has been made in Chap. 12 that abnormal hemorrhage may follow transfusions of exceptionally large amounts of compatible blood. This is due in part to depression of the peripheral platelet count which is a regular occurrence in this circumstance and lasts for several days. The same phenomenon has been observed occasionally in newborn infants with erythroblastosis fetalis after an exchange transfusion. The extent of the depression is roughly proportional to the comparative quantities of blood transfused and the rate in hours over which these are given.

THROMBOTIC THROMBOCYTOPENIC PURPURA (DIFFUSE DISSEMINATED PLATELET THROMBOSIS)

This disease, most common among young adult females, has been observed in both sexes at all ages. Onset is usually abrupt with malaise, weakness, fever, nausea, diarrhea, and joint and other pains. A purpuric rash appears, most prominent on the legs and abdomen. Hematemesis or melena are common, and bleeding may occur at any part of the body. Microscopic hematuria is constant; this is believed to be a manifestation of acute glomerulitis. Transient focal neurologic disturbances (facial weakness, aphasia, headache, disturbed reflexes, apraxia, etc.) are brought about by lesions in the cerebral vessels, and progress to stupor and death.

The thrombocyte count declines rapidly and may become virtually absent in the advanced stages. There is also a rapidly developing hemolytic anemia, with reticulocytosis, bilirubinemia, undue osmotic fragility, and rapid destruction of transfused blood. Spherocytosis has been noted in a few patients. Normoblasts may appear in the circulation. The granulocytes may show transient leukemoid reactions. Endothelial proliferation and vascular thrombi should be looked for in bone marrow, skin sections or muscle biopsy when the diagnosis is suspected. Marrow megakaryocytes are adequate in numbers and regular in appearance.

The course is rapid and fatal, rarely lasting more than 2 months. Necropsy reveals hyaline thrombi widespread through terminal arterioles, capillaries, and venules. The primary injury seems to begin in the vascular endothelium, often in conjunction with necroses of the vessel walls.

THROMBASTHENIC NONTHROMBOCYTOPENIC PURPURA (GLANZMANN'S THROMBASTHENIC PURPURA)

This is a variant type of purpura hemorrhagica, not sex-linked, in which the thrombocytes are not so much reduced in number as impaired in functioning capacity. Affected children exhibit easy bruising, spontaneous hemorrhages, a prolonged bleeding time, a normal clotting time, a positive tourniquet test, usually impaired clot retraction, and a diminished prothrombin consumption rate. The platelets are reduced only slightly if at all, so that bleeding symptoms can be prominent even when the count is between 100,000 and 300,000 per cu mm. The platelets themselves when examined in a stained smear often stain weakly and may be smooth-bordered, abnormally large, and devoid of granules. Megakaryocytes are found in the marrow in normal numbers but with agranular poorly staining cytoplasm suggestive of an intrinsic defect.

VON WILLEBRAND'S DISEASE (PSEUDOHEMOPHILIA A)

This hereditary disease affecting both sexes is characterized by a propensity to bleed, prolonged bleeding time, normal blood coagulation, efficient clot retraction, and no demonstrable reduction in count, morphology, or physiology of the platelets. The condition, once thought to be a platelet disturbance, is now viewed as an inherited defect of the capillaries of the skin and mucous membranes.

ANAPHYLACTOID PURPURA

This is a syndrome in which nontraumatic hemorrhages with or without urticarial edema occur in the skin, subcutaneous tissue, joints, or gastrointestinal tract, while the blood platelets remain normally abundant and no coagulation defect can be demonstrated. A macular exanthem, antecedent streptococcic pharyngitis, abdominal colic, and generalized listlessness are common symptoms. The passage of a bloody stool soon after the onset of abdominal symptoms is a valuable diagnostic sign. Attacks may be single or recurrent. Each episode usually lasts for a few weeks. Proteinuria lasting some months or years may be the sole sequel. Chronic nephritis sometimes follows.

NONTHROMBOCYTOPENIC PURPURA
ASSOCIATED WITH RENAL DYSFUNCTION

A group of children were described by Clement and Diamond who had a nonthrombocytopenic bleeding state in association with pallor, hematuria, marked proteinuria, and nitrogen retention. One had hypertension. The illnesses lasted 2 to 6 months and then faded away. Skin biopsy of one child showed an acute perivascular inflammation.

FIBRINOLYTIC PURPURA

This is an unusual condition in which bleeding symptoms develop as a manifestation of undue liberation of the enzyme (fibrinolysokinase, fibrinokinase) from damaged tissues. This stimulates the fibrinolysin, normally in the circulating blood as an inert proenzyme, into activity. Excessive fibrinolysis should always be suspected in a patient with a sudden and otherwise unexplainable bleeding disorder, especially when many coagulation elements appear to be simultaneously disturbed. Expected benefits from transfusion may not occur if the fibrinolysin attacks the proteinous coagulant factors in the administered blood.

BIBLIOGRAPHY

IDIOPATHIC THROMBOCYTOPENIC PURPURA

Clement, D. H., and L. K. Diamond, Purpura in Infants and Children: Its Natural History, A.M.A. Am. J. Dis. Child. 85:259, 1953.

Faloon, W. W., R. W. Greene, and E. L. Lozner, The Hemostatic Defect in Thrombocytopenia as Studied by the Use of ACTH and Cortisone, Am. J. Med. 13:12, 1952.

Greene, R. W., W. W. Faloon, and E. L. Lozner, The Use of ACTH in Preparing Patients with Idiopathic Thrombocytopenic Purpura for Splenectomy, Am. J. M. Sc. 226:203, 1953.

Heinild, S., and L. Lindgren, Thrombopenia in Childhood, Acta pediat. suppl. 77:149, 1949.

Hirsch, E. O., and *W. Dameshek,* "Idiopathic" Thrombocytopenia, *A.M.A. Arch. Int. Med.* 88:701, 1951.

────── and *F. H. Gardner,* The Transfusion of Human Blood Platelets with a Note on Transfusion Granulocytes, *J. Lab. & Clin. Med.* 39:556, 1952.

Newton, W. A., and *W. W. Zuelzer,* Idiopathic Thrombopenic Purpura in Childhood, *New England J. Med.* 245:879, 1951.

Pisciotta, A., V. Stefanini, and *W. Dameshek,* Studies on Platelets. X. Morphologic Characteristics of Megakaryocytes by Phase Contrast Microscopy in Normals and in Patients with Idiopathic Thrombocytopenic Purpura, *Blood* 8:703, 1953.

Presley, S. J., W. R. Best, and *L. R. Limarzi,* Bone Marrow in Idiopathic Thrombocytopenic Purpura: Analysis of 100 Cases with Reference to the Prognostic Significance of Eosinophils and Megakaryocytes, *J. Lab. & Clin. Med.* 40:503, 1952.

Schwartz, S. O., and *S. R. Kaplan,* Thrombocytopenic Purpura: The Prognostic and Therapeutic Value of the Eosinophil Index: An Analysis of 100 Cases, *Am. J. M. Sc.* 219:528, 1950

Sprague, C., W. J. Harrington, R. D. Lange, and *J. B. Shapleigh,* Platelet Transfusions and the Pathogenesis of Idiopathic Thrombocytopenic Purpura, *J.A.M.A.* 150:1193, 1952.

Stefanini, M., J. B. Chatterjea, W. Dameshek, L. Zannos, and *E. P. Santiago,* Studies on Platelets. II. The Effect of Transfusion of Platelet-rich Polycythemic Blood on the Platelets and Hemostatic Function in "Idiopathic" and "Secondary" Thrombocytopenic Purpura, *Blood* 7:53, 1952.

────── , *G. I. Plitman, W. Dameshek, J. B. Chatterjea,* and *I. B. Mednicoff,* Studies on Platelets. XI. Antigenicity of Platelets and Evidence of Platelet Groups and Types in Man, *J. Lab. & Clin. Med.* 42:723, 1953.

Tullis, J. L., Identification and Significance of Platelet Antibodies, *New England J. Med.* 255:541, 1956.

Wilson, S. J., G. Eisemann, and *J. H. Chance,* The Effect of the "Thrombocytopenic Factor" of Idiopathic Thrombocytopenic Purpura on Platelet Levels as Measured by Direct and Indirect Methods, *J. Lab. & Clin. Med.* 40:498, 1952.

Zarafonetis, C. J. D., W. A. Steiger, and *S. K. Cary,* Compounds E and F, and ACTH in the Management of Idiopathic Thrombocytopenic Purpura, *Am. J. M. Sc.* 228:1, 1954.

THROMBOCYTOPENIC PURPURA IN THE NEWBORN

Barclay, P. E., Congenital Thrombocytopenic Purpura, *Arch. Dis. Childhood* 20:94, 1945.

Bluestone, S. S., and *H. L. Maslow,* Essential Thrombocytopenic purpura, *Pediatrics* 4:620, 1949.

Gruber, S., B. Redner, and *B. Kogut,* Congenital Idiopathic Thrombopenic Purpura in a Premature Infant with Splenectomy, *New York J. Med.* 51:649, 1951.

Landolt, R. F., Congenital (Neonatal) Thrombocytopenia (Kongenitale [Neonatale] Thrombopenien), *Helvet. paediat. acta* 3:3, 1948.

Litchfield, H. R., S. D. Sternberg, and *B. M. Zweifler,* Congenital Thrombocytopenic Purpura of the Newborn Infant, *J. Pediat.* 37:94, 1950.

Roberts, M. H., and *M. H. Smith,* Thrombopenic Purpura: Report of Four Cases in One Family, *Am. J. Dis. Child.* 79:820, 1950.

Robson, H. N., and *C. H. M. Walker,* Congenital and Neonatal Thrombocytopenic Purpura, *Arch. Dis. Childhood* 26:175, 1951.

Talmadge, J., and *B. Berman,* Congenital Thrombocytopenic Purpura, *J. Pediat.* 30:691, 1947.

THROMBOTIC THROMBOCYTOPENIC PURPURA

Blackman, N. S., B. M. Cohen, and *J. Watson,* Thrombotic Thrombopenic Purpura, *J.A.M.A.* 148:546, 1952.

Meacham, G. C., J. L. Orbison, R. W. Heinle, H. J. Steele, and *J. A. Schaefer,* Thrombotic Thrombocytopenic Purpura: A Disseminated Disease of Arterioles, *Blood* 6:706, 1951.

Wedgwood, R. J. P., and *M. H. Klaus,* Anaphylactoid Purpura (Schönlein-Henoch Syndrome). A Long-term Follow-up Study with Special Reference to Renal Involvement, *Pediatrics* 16:196, 1955.

Wile, S. A., and *P. Sturgeon,* Thrombotic Thrombocytopenic Purpura: Review of the Subject with a Report of Three Cases in Children, *Pediatrics* 17:882, 1956.

ANAPHYLACTOID PURPURA

Derham, R. J., and *M. M. Rogerson,* The Schönlein-Henoch Syndrome and Collagen Disease, *Arch. Dis. Childhood* 27:139, 1952.

Gairdner, D., The Schönlein-Henoch Syndrome (Anaphylactoid Purpura), *Quart. J. Med.* 17:95, 1948.

Philpott, M. G., and *J. N. Briggs,* Treatment of the Schoenlein-Henoch Syndrome with Adrenocorticotrophic Hormone (A.C.T.H.) and Cortisone, *Arch. Dis. Childhood* 28:57, 1953.

Stefanini, M., C. A. Roy, L. Zannos, and *W. Dameshek,* Therapeutic Effect of Pituitary Adrenocorticotrophic Hormone (ACTH) in a Case of Henoch-Schönlein Vascular (Anaphylactoid) Purpura, *J.A.M.A.* 144:1372, 1950.

THROMBOCYTOPENIC STATES

Angle, R. M., and *H. L. Alt,* Thrombocytopenic Purpura Complicating Infectious Mononucleosis, *Blood* 5:449, 1950.

Bogin, M., and *J. Thurmond,* Hemangioma with Purpura, Thrombocytopenia and Erythrocytopenia, *A.M.A. Am. J. Dis. Child.* 81:675, 1951.

Bolton, F. G., and *R. V. Young,* Observations on Cases of Thrombocytopenic Purpura Due to Quinine, Sulphamezathine and Quinidine, *J. Clin. Path.* 6:320, 1954.

Fisher, O. D., and *T. M. Kraszewski,* Thrombocytopenic Purpura Following Measles, *Arch. Dis. Childhood* 27:144, 1952.

Franklin, A. W., and *D. A. J. Williamson,* Haemangio-Endothelioma with Haemorrhage and Thrombocytopenia, *Arch. Dis. Childhood* 28:490, 1953.

Holoubek, J. E., J. V. Hendrick, and *W. J. Hollis,* Toluidine Blue in Bleeding Associated with Thrombopenia, *J.A.M.A.* 139:214, 1949.

Kelin, E., S. Farber, I. Djerassi, R. Toch, G. Freeman, and *P. Arnold,* The Preparation and Clinical Administration of Lyophilized Platelet Material to Children with Acute Leukemia and Aplastic Anemia, *J. Pediat.* 49:517, 1956.

Krevans, J. R., and *D. P. Jackson,* Hemorrhagic Disorder Following Massive Whole Blood Transfusions, *J.A.M.A.* 159:171, 1955.

Lozner, E. L., Differential Diagnosis, Pathogenesis and Treatment of the Thrombocytopenic Purpuras, *Am. J. Med.* 14:459, 1953.

———, The Thrombocytopenic Purpuras, *Bull. New York Acad. Med.* 30:184, 1954.

Madison, F. W., The Role of Allergy in the Pathogenesis of Purpura and Thrombocytopenia, *Blood* 3:1083, 1948.

Mills, S. D., Purpuric Manifestations Occurring in Measles in Childhood, *J. Pediat.* 36:35, 1950.

———, Purpura in Childhood: Observations in 187 Cases, *J. Pediat.* 49:306, 1956.

Reichelderfer, T. E., P. H. Pearson, and *S. Livingston,* Thrombocytopenic Purpura

Occurring in Association with Paradione (Paramethadione) and Dilantin Sodium (Phenytoin Sodium) Therapy, *J. Pediat.* **43**:43, 1953.

Savitsky, J. P., A Plasma Factor for Platelet Adhesiveness and Clot Retraction Acceleration, *Blood* **12**:1091, 1953.

Southard, S. C., A. G. DeSanctis, and *R. J. Waldron,* Hemangioma Associated with Thrombocytopenic Purpura, *J. Pediat.* **38**:732, 1951.

Whitesell, F. B., Jr., and *A. M. Snell,* Thrombopenia and Increased Capillary Fragility in Hepatic Disease, *J.A.M.A.* **140**:1071, 1941.

CHAPTER 24

Disturbances of the Spleen

SPLENOMEGALY

When trying to elucidate the cause of an obscure enlargement of the spleen, a logical approach is to determine first whether this reflects (1) some systemic disease in which the tissues of the spleen are responding to stimuli originating elsewhere in the body, or (2) some local disease of the organ or its nutrient blood vessels. The disturbances produced can be *mechanical,* with postural difficulties resulting from size and weight; *hematologic* ("hypersplenic") affecting blood cell destruction and production; *shocklike,* should the organ rupture spontaneously; or *gastrointestinal hemorrhages* if there is hypertension in a distended collateral venous circulation.

Splenic enlargement and palpability are not necessarily synonymous. An enlarged organ weighing 100 to 300 gm or higher (normal, 20 to 80 gm, depending on age) may escape detection on abdominal examination if it is bound to the diaphragm by adhesions or displaced backward and upward behind a distended stomach or a prominent left hepatic lobe. Abdominal roentgenography sometimes helps to discover large but clinically undetectable spleens, but a negative finding does not rule out enlargement.

Splenomegaly Secondary to Systemic Diseases

Diseases originating elsewhere which can evoke splenomegaly fall into a number of major etiologic classes:

1. ACUTE INFECTIONS. Subacute bacterial endocarditis, meningococcemia, salmonellosis, and other forms of septicemia associated with circulating microorganisms are well-known causes of splenomegaly. The swelling may be due to proliferation of the reticuloendothelial or lymphocytic elements or both, to stasis and destruction of injured red cells, or to focal metastatic abscesses. Some viral and rickettsial infections and infectious mononucleosis may also produce enlargement of the organ.

2. CHRONIC INFECTIONS. Among these may be listed malaria, miliary tuberculosis, brucellosis, histoplasmosis, echinococcus disease, leishmaniasis, schistosomiasis, moniliasis, and congenital syphilis. In most of

292

these the enlargement is produced by inflammatory responses to the specific organisms within the cells or tissue spaces of the organ. The presence of these organisms can often be demonstrated, if necessary, by splenic puncture and microscopic study or bacteriologic culture of the aspirate. Rarely in a chronic infection the splenic enlargement may be due wholly or in part to interstitial deposit of amyloid.

3. MALIGNANT DISEASES AND GENERALIZED DISEASES OF THE RETICU-LOENDOTHELIAL SYSTEM. A prominent feature of the reticuloendothelioses —Gaucher's disease, Niemann-Pick disease, Letterer-Siwe disease, and, less regularly, the Hand-Schüller-Christian syndrome—is splenomegaly. Likewise in Hodgkin's disease, leukosarcoma, giant follicular lymphoblastoma, and related disorders of the lymph node system, the organ may become infiltrated and swollen. If the spleen is involved in the systemic pseudomalignant disease known as Kaposi's hemangiosarcoma, its size can be reduced by roentgen irradiation of the organ.

4. HYPERTENSION OF THE PORTAL CIRCULATION. Chronic cardiac failure, whether of rheumatic, congenital, or other origin or due to chronic constrictive pericarditis, usually leads to congestive splenomegaly; and the enlargement subsides as the visceral congestion is relieved by digitalis and other supportive therapy. Since both the portal and peripheral venous systems are affected by increased venous pressures, a prominent collateral circulation does not develop in these cases. The rare postnatal persistence of the umbilical vein associated with hypoplasia of the liver, a very large spleen, and portal hypertension is sometimes called the Cruveilhier-Baumgarten syndrome.

5. BLOOD DYSCRASIAS. Of the chronic genetically transmitted anemias, active Mediterranean anemia tends to give rise to the largest spleen, which is firm and fibrous. Hereditary spherocytosis (congenital hemolytic anemia) as a rule also produces enlargement, the consequence of accelerated lysis of red cells, though in asymptomatic or minimally affected cases the organ may not be palpable. In active sickle cell anemia and the related disorders caused by hemoglobin or stroma anomalies the spleen is usually not swollen except when hypersplenic red cell destruction is going on. In erythroblastosis fetalis, the acquired hemolytic anemias, the hemoglobinurias, and all nonhereditary anemias associated with accelerated red cell destruction, enlargement of variable degree is often apparent. In the carrier states of Mediterranean anemia and sicklemia the organ is minimally enlarged if at all. In iron-deficiency anemia, megaloblastic anemia, aplastic anemia, and pure red cell anemia, splenomegaly is exceptional.

With thrombocytopenic purpura the spleen is palpable in about one-third of the cases. In childhood leukemia the spleen tends to grow in size as other organs are infiltrated and the differential count has a high percentage of abnormal cells, and to shrink away during remissions. Ex-

tramedullary hemopoiesis secondary to bone marrow hypoplasia, myelofibrosis, or infiltration may also cause splenic swelling; a leukemia-like
variant of this disorder is the poorly understood entity of agnogenic
myeloid metaplasia of the spleen. True polycythemia vera is not seen in
the pediatric age period. Splenic neutropenia and splenic pancytopenia
may have an associated enlargement of the organ.

6. MISCELLANEOUS SYSTEMIC CONDITIONS. The explanations for the
splenic enlargement in such diverse and unrelated disturbances as advanced rickets, hyperthyroidism, Felty's syndrome, rheumatoid arthritis,
Stevens-Johnson disease, disseminated lupus erythematosus, and Boeck's
sarcoid are as yet not well understood.

Splenomegaly Due to Local Diseases

TUMORS, CYSTS, AND MALFORMATIONS. All of these are rare. Fibromas,
myomas, and angiomas are typical forms of benign spontaneously
arising splenic tumors. Hamartoma (splenadenoma, splenoma, lymphoma
of the spleen) is a benign tumorous congenital anomaly composed of
abnormal mixtures of normal splenic elements. Dermoid cysts, primary
and metastatic sarcomas, and posthemorrhagic, postinfarction, and post-
inflammatory cysts of various kinds may also occur.

LOCALIZED CONGESTIVE SPLENOMEGALY (BANTI'S SYNDROME). In addition
to liver disease and cardiovascular failure, obstruction of venous outflow
with resulting local hypertension can be caused by thrombosis of the
splenic or portal veins, anomalous venous valves, external compression of
the vein by nodes, tumors, or adhesions, and other more obscure
mechanisms. Careful inquiry when splenomegaly of obscure origin is
present will frequently elicit a history of severe trauma to the abdomen
or neonatal venous omphalitis several years prior to the onset of splenomegaly and related disturbances. These can initiate splenic or portal
vein thrombosis and the subsequent evolution of secondary symptoms.
Thrombotic processes originating anywhere in the portal system tend
to spread slowly and ultimately occlude all the major branches. There
is sound pathologic evidence for viewing *cavernous transformation of the
splenic veins* as the terminal stage of thrombus organization and recanal-
ization.

IDIOPATHIC (NONSPECIFIC) SPLENOMEGALY. Enlargement for no evident
reason and with no detectable secondary disturbance is seen at times in
children. This category has been invented as a cover for ignorance. The
diagnosis is always provisional.

BANTI'S SYNDROME

When portal hypertension accompanies splenomegaly the clinical picture is sometimes referred to as Banti's syndrome. Splenic infarcts or
overlying peritonitis may stir up abdominal pain. Anemia, leukocyto-

penia, and thrombocytopenia of hypersplenic origin are not uncommon (see next section). Hemorrhagic symptoms—epistaxis, hematemesis, melena, purpura—can be traced to hypertension in the portal system, overloaded gastric or esophageal varices, peripheral thrombocytopenia, hypoprothrombinemia from impaired liver anabolism of vitamin K. The spleen may shrink down and cease to be palpable for a few days after a bleeding episode, and then enlarge again.

Florid liver cirrhosis with or without ascites is a not infrequent termination. Sometimes a liver disease seems to be the initiating disturbance, but more often the chronic splenic enlargement at times seems to stir up liver derangements.

A recent diagnostic suggestion is to inject some radiopaque water-soluble substance directly into the spleen through a needle while the sedated or anesthetized patient lies on the x-ray table. A roentgenogram taken a few seconds later will make visible the venous drainage of the spleen and reveal any obstructions, varicosities, or development of collateral circulation. This procedure is not without danger in the pediatric age group because of respiratory and other movements.

The disease tends to run a chronic course. There is no good conservative treatment. Whenever the return of portal blood to the liver is obstructed the resulting portal hypertension favors the development of splenomegaly and later of esophageal and gastric varices. Irreversible situations of this type may be treated by surgical excision of the spleen followed by anastomosis of the portal vein to the inferior vena cava (portocaval shunt) or of the splenic to the left renal vein. A successful operation of this type will reduce the size of the collateral circulation and the probability of ascites or gastrointestinal tract hemorrhages. The hypersplenic phenomena which may or may not be coincidentally present will also be relieved. Life expectancy in cases operated on is much better when the splenic vein alone is involved than when the portal vein is thrombosed or narrowed beyond the reach of the surgeon. The pathologic findings in the spleen are those of a congestion with secondary fibrotic changes in the more advanced cases. It usually is not feasible to differentiate clinically between splenic vein and portal vein lesions.

HYPERSPLENISM

Pathogenesis

One normal task of the spleen is to participate in the destruction and elimination of effete or injured red cells, granulocytes, and platelets. When these and related functions become overactive, numerous secondary and compensatory mechanisms are set in motion. Anemia, granulocytopenia, or thrombocytopenia or any combination of these may be produced. Several processes may go on separately or concurrently: (1) excessive destruction within the parenchyma of one or more of the blood cell series, (2) splenic elaboration of a humoral substance that arrests blood cell formation within the marrow or blocks the release of formed cells, and (3) undue stimulation by the spleen of other pathways of blood cell destruction. The bone marrow nearly always shows proliferative changes with respect to the affected cell systems. With terminal liver failure it may become hypocellular.

The disturbances which result are grouped together under the category of primary hypersplenism when limited to the spleen and the blood cells, with no cause evident. Secondary hypersplenism refers to cytopenic syndromes as a result of splenic hyperactivity, but with a prior splenomegaly from some other known disease. In this category may be placed essentially every one of the disorders which can cause splenomegaly. The mediating stimuli which excite this form of splenic overactivity are not known. Physical weakness and susceptibility to infections are customary manifestations and tend to be restored to normal after splenectomy. Some affected children have had associated anomalies of bodily structure. The administration of cortisone or corticotropin, or of antibacterial therapy of specific infections when present, will often cause symptoms to recede.

The entity of hypersplenism is difficult to delimit. The spleen itself is not necessarily enlarged, or even though enlarged may not be palpable. Many times the hematologic disturbances associated with splenic hyperactivity have arisen in the absence of enlargement of the organ as verified at the operating table. It has been aptly said that the ultimate criterion for the diagnosis is to demonstrate that an existing cytopenia is affected favorably by the removal of the spleen. Tiny accessory spleens may induce a recurrence after removal of the spleen itself.

Manifestations

Hereditary spherocytosis is a classical example of splenic hyperactivity limited to the red cell series. Removal of the spleen puts an end to the excessive red cell destruction, even though the defect in the cells remains unaltered. Splenic hyperactivity with respect to the red cell series may also become evident in some cases of active sickle cell anemia, acquired hemolytic anemia, congenital porphyria, and rare instances of Mediterranean anemia and other more unusual forms of hereditary anemia. In some patients with acquired hemolytic anemia the circulating autoantibodies or other pathogenetic mechanisms seem attributable to disturbed splenic function, at least in part (p. 94).

Idiopathic thrombocytopenic purpura is a hypersplenic disorder in which the spleen retains and destroys platelets directly (splenic cytolysis) or suppresses their formation or maturation through hormonal control of the bone marrow.

Splenic neutropenia is a persistent condition in which the circulating neutrophils are diminished in number due to sequestration and phagocytosis of granulocytes to an abnormal degree by the spleen. The bone marrow shows hypercellularity of the granulocytic series, and immature band forms are released into the circulation at an excessive rate. A humoral substance which can lyse normal white cells in vitro in the presence of complement—a so-called "leukocidin"—has been found in the circulation in some of these patients. Fever, pain in the splenic area, and palpable splenomegaly are common findings in the early stages. An injection of epinephrine may result in a transitory rise in circulating granulocytes, though these cells may come from the pulmonary or peripheral capillaries rather than the spleen.

SPLENECTOMY

Operative removal always comes into consideration in the management of any patient with progressive splenomegaly, hypersplenism, or Banti's syndrome. For rupture of the organ, regardless of cause, removal becomes an urgent and lifesaving measure. The operation, *if indicated,* will usually be followed by cessation of symptoms in hereditary spherocytosis (p. 57), idiopathic thrombocytopenic purpura (p. 282), acquired hemolytic anemia (p. 97), Mediterranean anemia (p. 60), Gaucher's disease (p. 335), and local cysts and tumors. The hyperhemolysis which develops infrequently in active sickle cell anemia is usually relieved by the operation (p. 66).

When there is thrombosis of the splenic vein or other local causes of Banti's syndrome, removal of the spleen relieves only those disturbances due to splenic overfunction. Splenectomy combined with a successful anastomosis of the portal, splenic, or mesenteric vein to the systemic circulation may relieve the portal hypertension as well and can be of much greater benefit to the patient (p. 295).

The operation is of little benefit in subacute bacterial endocarditis, most forms of leukemia, and other disturbances in which the enlargement is only part of a generalized process.

A few cases of congenital pure red cell anemia which have had associated depression of granulocytes seem to have been helped by surgery (p. 91). In the rare disorders in which the spleen is a source of blood formation and the bone marrow is hypocellular and hypoplastic, the operation is strongly contraindicated (p. 311). In chronic malaria, hypersplenism if present may be cured by splenectomy, but the infection itself often relapses soon afterward. A prominent change in the peripheral blood which follows splenectomy for any cause, even in cases without a hereditary anemia, is the occurrence of target cells and irregular crenated fragments derived from fission of larger cells (schizocytes). Other red cells may assume a "pincered" structure, as if part of their substance had been contracted and pulled outward by a pair of pincers. Pappenheimer bodies, which are deep-staining granular formations detected by the Leishman stain, sometimes appear in abundance.

Splenic puncture is done with much more confidence in foreign clinics than in this country. Fear of inducing hemorrhage from the needle-puncture wound is the major deterrent. The fact that chronic latent malaria is uncommon in this country eliminates one of the major diseases which can be recognized by this approach.

SPLENIC ASPIRATION

The purpose of this maneuver is to obtain additional information for establishing the nature of the splenomegaly or related constitutional disturbance in difficult cases. The spleen must be large and the child old enough to cooperate by remaining motionless and momentarily holding his breath. Any constitutional bleeding tendency is a strong contraindication.

The operator stands at the left side of the patient and with one hand grasps the spleen firmly through the abdominal wall. While the patient holds his breath a 20-gauge needle attached to a dry syringe is introduced through the abdominal wall, close to the costal margin at the midclavicular line. The aspiration is done swiftly followed by immediate removal of the needle. The total procedure should take about 10 seconds. The aspirate (usually a tiny drop) is then spread on a glass slide and stained.

With a normal spleen the aspirated leukocytes consist almost entirely of small lymphocytes (85 per cent) and large lymphocytes (15 per cent). A few reticulum cells arranged singly or in syncytial masses may be seen, along with some sporadic neutrophils, eosinophils, and monocytes. In suppurative lesions, whether caused by pyogenic organisms or tubercle bacilli, aspirated fluid will be rich in fibrin and debris, with numerous neutrophils and other phagocytic cells. Special stains for bacteria may succeed in visualizing the causative organism. Bacterial identification may also be performed by rinsing the needle and syringe with liquid culture medium which is then incubated. In malaria the pattern is that of reticuloendothelial proliferation, with some neutrophils and intra- and extracellular parasites in all stages of development. In Hodgkin's disease many monocytoid and other variations of Reed-Steinberg cells appear, together with eosinophils, neutrophils, and a higher percentage of large lymphocytes. In lymphosarcoma involving the spleen one finds large lymphocyte-like malignant cells with scant cytoplasm and no nucleoli. In acute lymphocytic leukemia there are nucleolated lymphoblasts, occasionally in mitosis. In chronic lymphocytic leukemia the Grumelée cells appear—small lymphocytes whose nuclear chromatin stains with a "checkerboard" or mosaic appearance. In granulocytic leukemia the predominant cells are atypical variants of the granulocytic series.

In giant follicular lymphoblastosis, rare in the childhood years, there are lymphosarcoma-like cells, monocytoid cells, and small lymphocytes. In the reticuloendothelioses (Gaucher's, Niemann-Pick, Letterer-Siwe, etc.) the characteristic cells are seen in the aspirate, sometimes when the bone marrow examination has been negative. In acquired hemolytic anemia the splenic reticuloendothelial cells may show erythrophagocytosis. In splenic neutropenia or pancytopenia the reticuloendothelial cells are sometimes increased in numbers and may exhibit phagocytosis of red cells or leukocytes. In all the chronic anemias with unusual blood destruction, hemosiderin granules are prominent.

With extramedullary hemopoiesis the aspirate contains immature rubricytes, granulocytes, and megakaryocytes. This process occurs at times when the marrow is osteosclerotic or aplastic and is not uncommon in congestive splenomegaly of whatever cause, with or without alterations in the bone marrow. It does not occur in the dystrophic anemias such as sickle cell anemia and Mediterranean anemia.

CONGENITAL ABSENCE OF THE SPLEEN

This anomaly, when uncomplicated, is usually not productive of symptoms in the childhood years. In later life there has seemed to be an unusual susceptibility to diseases involving the lymphatic system, such as tuberculosis, typhoid fever, malaria, and lymphosarcoma. An appreciable number of infants have been reported in whom absence of this organ was associated with other congenital defects in a syndrome comprising a persistent atrioventricular septal defect, accessory lobes of the lung, partial situs inversus of the abdominal viscera, and anomalies of major blood vessels.

The peripheral blood often exhibits abnormalities of the erythrocytes in the form of basophilic inclusions, target cells, Howell-Jolly bodies, and related changes.

BIBLIOGRAPHY

SPLEEN

Blakemore, A. H., Portocaval Shunt for Portal Hypertension, *J.A.M.A.* 145:1335, 1951.

Cole, W. H., J. D. Majarakis, and *L. R. Limarzi,* Surgical Aspects of Splenic Disease, *A.M.A. Arch. Surg.* 71:33, 1955.

Coller, F. A., A. Blain, III, and *G. Andrews,* "Indications for and Results of Splenectomy," American Lecture Series 86, Charles C Thomas, Springfield, Ill., 1950.

Dameshek, W., and *S. Estren,* "The Spleen and Hypersplenism," Grune & Stratton, Inc., New York, 1947.

Doan, C. A., Hypersplenism, *Bull. New York Acad. Med.* 25:625, 1949.

―――― and *C. Wright,* Primary Congenital and Secondary Acquired Splenic Pan-hematopenia, *Blood* 1:10, 1946.

Farber, S., The Spleen and Reticulo-endothelial System, in C. G. Grulee and R. C. Eley (eds.), "The Child in Health and Disease," 2d ed., The Williams & Wilkins Company, Baltimore, 1952.

Greene, R., W. W. Faloon, and *E. L. Lozner,* The Use of ACTH in Preparing Patients with Idiopathic Thrombocytopenic Purpura for Splenectomy, *Am. J. M. Sc.* 226:203, 1953.

Hsia, D. Y.-Y., and *S. S. Gellis,* Portal Hypertension in Infants and Children, *A.M.A. Am. J. Dis. Child.* 90:290, 1955.

Limarzi, L. R., L. H. Sloan, C. B. Puestow, and *W. H. Cole,* Indications for Splenec-tomy, *Am. Pract.* 4:25, 1949.

Linton, R. R., and *D. S. Ellis,* Emergency and Definitive Treatment of Bleeding Esophageal Varices, *J.A.M.A.* 160:1017, 1956.

Mahoney, E. B., and *L. Hogg, Jr.,* Congenital Stricture of the Portal Vein, *Arch. Surg.* 61:713, 1950.

Moeschlin, S., "Spleen Puncture," Grune & Stratton, Inc., New York, 1952.

Morrison, M., A. A. Samwick, J. Rubinstein, H. Morrison, and *L. Loewe,* Splenic Aspiration, *J.A.M.A.* 146:1575, 1951.

Moschcowitz, E., The Pathogenesis of Splenomegaly in Hypertension of the Portal Circulation: "Congestive Splenomegaly," *Medicine* 27:187, 1948.

Polhemus, D. W., and *W. B. Schafer,* Congenital Absence of the Spleen, *Pediatrics* 16:495, 1955.

Tocantins, L. M., The Hemorrhagic Tendency in Congestive Splenomegaly (Banti's Syndrome), *J.A.M.A.* 136:616, 1948.

Von Haam, E., and *A. J. Awny,* The Pathology of Hypersplenism, *Am. J. Clin. Path.* 18:313, 1948.

Williams, N. L., and *W. M. Kelsey,* Splenic Panhematopenia in Children, *Am. J. Dis. Child.* 79:862, 1950.

Wolman, I. J., Disturbances of the Spleen, *Quart. Rev. Pediat.* 7:179, 1952.

Wright, C., C. A. Doan, B. A. Bouroncle, and *R. M. Zollinger,* Direct Splenic Arterial and Venous Blood Studies in the Hypersplenic Syndromes before and after Epinephrine, *Blood* 6:195, 1951.

Wyss, R., The Clinical Picture of Stenosis of the Splenic and Portal Veins in Child-hood (Das Klinische Bild der Milzvenen und Pfortaderstenose im Kindesalter), *Helvet. paediat. acta* 7:452, 1952.

Young, L. E., R. F. Platzer, M. Ervin, and *M. J. Izzo,* Hereditary Spherocytosis. II. Observations on the Role of the Spleen, *Blood* 6:1099, 1951.

CHAPTER 25

General Features of Bone Marrow Examination

Cytologic study of the bone marrow has become a well-recognized procedure in the study of suspected blood dyscrasias or possible neoplastic or infiltrative diseases. Indeed, no examination of a child with an obscure anemia or bleeding tendency or bizarre leukocytic picture, an enlarged liver or spleen or lymph nodes, or a palpable visceral tumor can be deemed complete until after the marrow has been examined. Aspiration of a specimen and preparation of a smear are not difficult once the techniques have been mastered and can be carried out in the office or dispensary. When the physician himself is unfamiliar with marrow cytology the smears are then forwarded to someone more skilled.

A bone marrow specimen cannot as a rule be evaluated competently in the absence of accompanying information. The examiner should be informed of the age and clinical findings; the disease suspected; the peripheral blood picture; the bone from which the marrow specimen comes; the manner in which the specimen was collected and prepared; the probable degree of dilution of the marrow sample with blood. He must also be familiar with the morphology of blood and marrow cells and the standard criteria for their identification and be on the alert for uneven distribution and other possible sources of error which attend the study of stained preparations.

The line between normal and questionably abnormal cellular distribution is far from sharp. Many variables, physiologic and technical, are responsible for the wide divergences among the sets of so-called normal standards proposed by different authorities. Despite these limitations, however, the bone marrow examination can be of great usefulness when attention is paid not so much to precise numerical percentages as to any qualitative changes which may be present. Results are most consistent when all phases of the examination are carefully carried out by the same workers, observing recognized precautions in a uniform routine way.

301

SITES FOR PROCURING MARROW SPECIMENS

In the older child, active hemopoiesis is restricted largely to the so-called short bones—vertebrae, ribs, sternum, skull, innominate bones, and proximal epiphyses of the femur and humerus. In long bones such as the tibia or femur, after age 18 months to 2 years, the bulk of the aspirated specimen consists of scattered lymphocytes, segmented neutrophils and fat cells, with nucleated red cells usually less than 1 per cent. On histologic study of particles obtained by aspiration of the tibia, Sturgeon found hemopoietic areas occupying about 50 per cent of the marrow area in the second year and less than 20 per cent in the sixth year, in contrast to 100 per cent at birth.

All the actively hemopoietic areas in the skeleton are similar cytologically. Hence specimens procured from any cellular area may be deemed representative, except when from (1) fatty areas in the long bones of older children, (2) focal infiltrations in metastatic malignancy, or (3) patches of unusual change in some cases of aplastic anemia or myelofibrosis.

With adult subjects the sternum is a favorite site for aspiration, since it lies immediately under the skin and has a comparatively thin cortex. With younger children and infants, however, sternal punctures are less satisfactory than other routes. The bone is thin, so that there is risk of forcing the needle point into the epicardial mediastinum if the child should make a sudden forward movement during the procedure. Apprehension invariably attends the watching of perforative manipulations over the cardiac area. In early infancy the paired pattern of the sternal ossification centers may create difficulty because of their irregular growth and variable location.

Since only the manubrium is already fused at the time of birth, sternal puncture when called for with infants is best made opposite the first interspace. The most satisfactory site for sternal puncture with older children is between the second and third ribs, with the needle inserted slightly to one side of the mid-line.

The vertebral column is suitable at all ages. The spinous and lateral processes are easy of access and out of the patient's range of visibility. The needle may be introduced at any level, though the lumbar vertebrae are largest and perhaps most accessible. This approach is particularly useful when serial aspirations are needed; the needle can be inserted sequentially at various levels.

The crest of the ilium is also satisfactory at all ages. The bone is entered approximately 3 to 5 cm posterior to the anterior superior iliac crest and about 2.5 cm below the superior margin, depending on age. The needle is forced through the cortex in a direction perpendicular to the bone surface. When the overlying tissue is abundant the plane of the bone can be ascertained by probing with the needles used for preliminary periosteal anesthetization or for the aspiration itself.

The tibia and femur are satisfactory until about 1½ years of age (p. 302). In fact, these sites are preferable during the first months of life. The needle may be inserted into the mid-portion of the femur from the lateral aspect of the thigh or into the anterior tibial surface, slightly below the tubercle, without risk of accidentally traumatizing a major blood vessel.

Whenever a disease process is suspected which may have a patchy distribution, samples of marrow from several places may furnish more information than single specimens. We have had several experiences where examination at one site yielded nearly normal marrow, whereas another examination elsewhere, made almost simultaneously, revealed obvious metastatic sarcoma or focal inflammatory reactions.

BIOPSY

Needle trephine or biopsy consists of the surgical removal of a segment of bony cortex and attached marrow. General anesthesia may be advisable. The skin is not incised. A large compound needle of the Turkel type is used. The outer guiding needle is driven to the surface of the bone. The inner trephine needle with a hollow bore then drills through the cortex and excises a cylindrical cone. A marrow aspirating needle is next introduced through the aperture in the cortex and some of the marrow withdrawn, followed if feasible by insertion of a curet and scooping out of fragments of marrow. The aspirate is spread on glass slides, and the bone segment and marrow fragments are sectioned histologically.

Biopsy specimens have some advantages over those obtained by aspiration. The sections reveal all the contained cells, in true proportions to each other. Reticulum cells and their derivatives, such as the giant fat-containing cells of the xanthomatoses, tend to be bound to the reticulum fibers of the marrow and may fail to come away in any abundance when marrow is aspirated. The same sometimes seems true of megakaryocytes; hence with cases of thrombocytopenic purpura in which aspirates show few or no such cells, their paucity should be verified by examination of sections. Granulomas and aggregates of abnormal cells tend to be broken or distorted by smearing, thereby masking valuable information concerning the architectural arrangements including whether any lesions are situated within the tissue interstices or the lumens of the blood vessels. Sections are also more dependable indicators of the cellularity of the marrow. A liberal admixture of peripheral blood in an aspirate can give an apparently hypocellular picture when the original marrow is rich in cells.

Unfortunately, trephine biopsy has certain disadvantages. The procedure is more troublesome, often requires a general anesthetic, and may be attended by bleeding if the patient has a hemorrhagic tendency. Preparation of histologic sections entails some delay. Recognition of individual cell types is often difficult, especially when abnormal cells are present. Biopsy, therefore, is best reserved for those situations where aspiratory specimens have been unsatisfactory or where one wishes to examine an undisturbed representation of the marrow architecture. It is of particular assistance in the study of suspected hypoplastic states, tumor metastases, reticuloendothelioses, and lipid storage diseases.

The biopsy approach can be utilized for study of abnormal bone lesions. Roentgenologic control may be needed to make certain that the needle tip lies in the involved area. The needle may withdraw a plug of tissue, purulent exudate, gelatinous material, blood, or other fluid. If the aspirate is extruded into a glass jar containing sterile normal saline solution, fragments of tissue if present will sink to the bottom and be readily identified. Should only blood clots or shreds of fat appear, another specimen may be taken. By this approach one can secure sufficient tissue to identify not only leukemia and metastatic sarcoma, but giant cell tumors, pyogenic granulations, tuberculous tissue, histoplasmosis, etc.

NEEDLE ASPIRATION

Needle aspiration of bone marrow is easier to perform than biopsy and can be repeated as frequently as desired. Preparations can be stained and studied immediately, giving cellular appearances which are clear and distinct. For most problems involving the bone marrow an aspirated sample furnishes all the information desired.

Needle aspiration has certain technical disadvantages. All cells may not be equivalently aspirated. There may be failure to remove all primitive cells, organized formations such as tubercles and tumor nodules, or even large megakaryocytes. The anatomic positions of the various cells in relation to each other are not preserved or reconstructable. Most importantly, an undetermined amount of peripheral blood is withdrawn from the vascular sinusoids along with the marrow cells; when dilution is considerable the specimen is unsatisfactory.

At times, some small articles of solid marrow come away during aspiration. Study of such particles in conjunction with the smeared aspirate is most satisfactory.

Procedure. Any special marrow aspirating needle may be used, so long as it is fitted with an easily removable stylet and possesses a collar which will cling tightly to the syringe. Shortened lumbar puncture needles have proved satisfactory for the procedure. The bore should be of sufficient breadth to permit passage of bits of tissue. Number 20 gauge is ordinarily adequate with children. The bevel should be sharp but short, to avoid piercing and injuring the underlying structures.

Preliminary sedation is helpful. Asepsis is essential. Sterilized gloves should be worn. The skin is first cleansed and sterilized. Through a small syringe with a fine needle, 1 or 2 ml of a local anesthetic solution is injected successively into the skin, the subcutaneous tissues, and the overlying periosteum. After a few minutes the needle with stylet in place is forced vertically forward through the overlying structures and bone cortex with a slow twisting motion. When aspirating the sternum the needle may be directed obliquely with the plane of the bevel parallel to the outer surface of the bone. A sudden "give" will be detectable on passage through the cortex. The stylet is not removed until the medullary cavity has been entered; otherwise a bit of cortical bone or cartilage may plug the needle and block the flow of marrow fluid. After the stylet is withdrawn a large dry syringe with tightly fitting plunger is applied for gentle suction. If no fluid comes away the syringe is removed, the stylet restored, and the needle advanced or moved back slightly for another try.

Aspirates which consist of only a few drops of marrow regularly prove the most satisfactory for direct microscopic examination. The attempt to withdraw 0.5 to 1.5 ml of marrow contents, as sometimes recommended, favors dilution of the sample with sinusoidal blood (it has been shown that when 0.1-ml portions of medullary contents are aspirated in series, each successive portion will have a lower nucleated cell count than its predecessor). A smear of peripheral blood from the finger tip may be taken at the time of the aspiration, for study purposes. A nucleated cell count of the aspirate may be made when dilution with peripheral blood is in question (p. 309), or bacteriologic specimens may be prepared if desired.

Direct Smears of Aspirate

This method of study, which is also the simplest, nearly always provides the information necessary for diagnosis. Single droplets of marrow are deposited at one end of each of six to eight alcohol-washed scrupulously clean dry slides, and the droplets smeared into a thin film with the end of another slide. Or one may place the droplets between cover slips and then pull the cover slips apart. These must be made immediately, before the marrow fluid has time to clot. The best preparations are secured when the syringe and needle are passed to a skilled assistant while the operator is still dressing the puncture wound.

Particle Smears

With older children, some workers make an attempt to procure small particles of solid marrow. Approximately 0.5 ml of bloody marrow fluid is aspirated and distributed in large drops on separate slides. The blood itself is immediately sucked off with a fine pipet applied to the edges of the drops. Films are quickly spread from any tiny marrow fragments which are left behind. The marrow fragments when dragged by the spreader leave trails of cells behind them. The differential counts are made on these trails, commencing at the marrow fragments and moving toward the head of the film.

The undisturbed marrow architecture may be studied by histologic sectioning of these fragments. A few drops of the aspirate are used for direct smears, and the remaining fluid deposited on a piece of unglazed blotting paper. The serum is absorbed by the paper, and a clot of concentrated marrow tissue remains. The paper with the adherent clot is immersed in Zenker's fixative, allowed to remain for ½ to 1 hour, and washed with running tap water for 1 hour. It is then placed in formalin solution for sectioning.

Volumetric Approach

To obtain blood for volumetric studies a snug aspirating syringe of 20- to 30-ml capacity is used. When the needle is in place the plunger is pulled out vigorously to the graduated end. Two to five milliliters of marrow fluid will flow into the syringe, except with newborn infants from whom only about 1 ml may be obtained. The aspirated fluid is mixed immediately with powdered heparin in a test tube lined with paraffin or silicone. Then 1.0 ml of the fluid is transferred to a narrow graduated hematocrit tube such as that of Wintrobe and sedimented by centrifuging at 2,000 to 3,000 rpm for 5 minutes. Fat forms the uppermost layer; next is plasma; then comes a gray-red buffy layer of nucleated cells; and finally, a column of packed red cells. The comparative volumes of the respective layers are measured and expressed in percentages. The buffy layer with some of the overlying plasma is removed and mixed on a paraffin-covered watch glass, then smeared and stained in the usual manner.

With aspirates from short bones such as vertebrae, iliac crest, or sternum, the fat layer normally constitutes less than 2.5 per cent of the total volume in the first decade but measures 6 or 8 per cent above 10 years of age. Percentages above 3 to 5 per cent in children indicate usually a comparatively fatty or hypocellular condition. Such higher values, however, are customary with marrow specimens from the long bones after 2 years of age. With infants during the first few months of life and in hypercellular situations the fatty layer is usually too thin to be measured.

The plasma and the erythrocyte layers each constitute 20 to 50 per cent of the total volume in normal circumstances, though the variability is great. The nucleated cell layer normally varies from 0.5 to 5 per cent, with most readings between 0.5 and 3 per cent. The thickness of this layer conveys essentially the same information as would a count of total nucleated cells. When no cellular layer is seen, sufficient fluid to prepare 1 or 2 slides is aspirated from the zone of transition between plasma and red cells.

Microscopic Examination

A direct smear if well prepared will show numerous marrow cells within each oil-immersion field. A scanty content of mature erythrocytes will indicate a negligible admixture of leukocytes from peripheral blood. Preparations which seem very dilute, except from a patient with aplastic anemia, may lead to an erroneous diagnosis and should not receive much consideration.

Staining for routine surveys is best done with the Wright, Wright-Giemsa, Jenner-Giemsa, or May-Grünwald-Giemsa stain. As a rule, with any batch of stain, films of bone marrow require about twice as long a period for staining as do those of peripheral blood. Other stains are employed for specialized purposes: Sudan IV for lipids, Prussian blue for iron-containing hemosiderin, pyronin-methyl green for nucleoli and cytoplasmic basophilia, or Fuelgen's staining process for chromatin and chromosomes.

In our laboratory the usual marrow aspirate is spread over 5 to 10 slides. Of these, 2 are stained at first; if these prove under- or overcolored, another pair is stained with the time schedules adjusted to correct the faults in the first set. The aspirate should dry for at least a half hour before being stained; otherwise tiny bubblelike artefacts may appear in the erythrocytes and other cells.

The differential count is best done with the oil-immersion objective. Before commencing, however, one should first scan the stained slide with the low power of the microscope in order to discover groups of tumor or other cells or lipid- or pigment-filled macrophages. If scattered in small numbers these may be missed in an examination limited to random oil-immersion fields alone. Such a survey will also convey information with respect to the structure and comparative number of megakaryocytes, which normally are not numerous. When malaria, histoplasmosis, or leishmaniasis is suspected but no organism is seen in thin smears of marrow, a careful low- or high-power survey of thick preparations for the parasites is advisable.

The drop originally placed on the slide should be small enough so that the smear made from it does not extend to the ends or edges of the slide. Since larger cells and cell masses tend to be more numerous at the margins, the preliminary scanning and the later detailed counting should include representative areas from both edges as well as scattered central portions of the smear. It is preferable to include several slides in the examination.

Counting

When making the count, the cells should be tabulated according to the recognized cell series—granulocytes, rubricytes (nucleated erythrocytes), lymphocytes, megakaryocytes, reticulum cells, and primitive or stem cells—and subgrouped in accordance with stages of development. Search should also be made for abnormal findings such as parasites or crystals and for the abnormal cell forms of leukemia, sarcoma, xanthoma, and other diseases. All disintegrated ("smudge," "basket") cells must be included and recorded as such in the differential count.

When changes are not extreme the percentage distribution should be determined by a differential count of at least 300 cells. The mental discipline demanded by identification of every cell encountered aids in the recognition of aberrant changes. Simple inspection of a slide may overlook minor but significant deviations in cell content and lead to an erroneous diagnosis.

There is a timesaving method of determining the percentage of cells which may be present in small numbers, such as megakaryocytes, plasma cells, xanthoma cells, and the like. The relative percentages of the common cellular types are noted by differential counting of several hundred cells. The proportion of the unusual cell type is then calculated by noting the total number of these per 5,000 nucleated marrow cells, examining areas from all regions of the smear.

CELLULARITY

The bone marrow as an organ stays constantly in what may be termed a state of dynamic equilibrium. Its activity is determined largely by the shifting demands constantly being made upon it. Its histologic architecture may be conceived of as a vascular mosaic containing rubricytes, granulocytes, lymphocytes, megakaryocytes, monocytes, reticuloendothelial cells, primitive or stem cells, and supportive adipose and other connective tissue elements.

In biopsy sections the marrow of normal fetuses and stillborns seems to be more cellular than in later infancy, and in younger children more than in older children or adults. Crowding with cells is also prominent in some diseases; for example, in the congenital hemolytic anemias, in cyanotic heart disease, and in leukemia. In aspirated smears the unmeasurable degree of dilution with peripheral blood makes recognition of hyper- or hypocellularity less reliable, but an experienced hematologist can often gain a fairly accurate impression from the degree of ease with which the aspiration was performed and the abundance or sparsity of marrow cells seen in the smears.

The bone marrow is highly labile and can respond to stimuli by active proliferative changes in as brief a period as a few hours. Thus, the myelogram of extreme "megaloblastic" crowding due to vitamin deficiency can be restored practically to normal within 48 hours by restoration of the missing nutrients.

With the exception of the supportive elements, each class of cells responds to outside stimuli with a fair degree of autonomy. Any class can separately exhibit hyperplasia or hypoplasia, though irritation of one frequently overflows to the others. Hemorrhages, for example, will often stimulate proliferation in the platelet- and granulocyte-forming elements as well as accelerating the production of erythrocytes. Drug reactions and toxins may depress several or all cell groups.

The adipose tissue of the bone marrow is related more or less reciprocally to the hemopoietic components. Its function seems to be chiefly space-occupying—it increases when the cellular elements become less active and diminishes when cellular hyperplasia begins again. Adipose tissue is well preserved in histologic sections. Intact marrow fat cells are usually not seen in smears of aspirates; when present they are large, with small eccentric reticular nuclei and delicate poorly staining cytoplasm.

Considerable variability may be found in the cellular distribution patterns of marrow specimens procured from different sites of the same patient on the same day, or even in successive slides from the same sample of aspirate. Some of these differences reflect fluctuations in response to stimulation, but technical factors are more important. The cells do not always come away in exactly the same proportions, nor do they distribute themselves uniformly and homogeneously when smeared on a glass slide. Furthermore, unless at least several thousand cells from all parts of a slide have been counted, the cytologic distribution is represented only approximately in the differential count. Hence too great importance cannot be placed on minor deviations from the so-called "normal" figures. In fact, the percentages expressing cell-type distribution are best viewed as semiquantitative approximations rather than as precise measurements.

Total Cell Counts

One would often like to know the functional status of the marrow as a whole—whether the medullary spaces are heavily, normally, or only sparsely filled with reactive cells. The answer is immediately evident in biopsy specimens.

One method of obtaining this information from aspirates is to employ the volumetric approach described on page 306. Another technique is that of total cell counts. The nucleated cells in a drop of *aspirate which must be comparatively undiluted* are counted in a hemocytometer chamber in the same manner as leukocytes are counted. The normal range is usually between 150,000 and 400,000 cells per cu mm though it may be as low as 40,000 or as high as 1 million. The normal variation is so extreme as to detract from the value of this measurement. Megakaryocytes or foam cells when present are readily recognized in this procedure and may be counted separately.

A hypercellular reaction that can be recognized in the direct smear is of more hematologic significance than is the appearance of hypocellularity. The latter may result from dilution with peripheral blood.

Myeloid-Erythroid Ratio

Some workers express the apparent comparative activity of the granulocyte and erythrocyte series as the so-called M/E (myeloid-erythroid) ratio. Lymphocytes are not included in this computation. With normal children the M/E ratio displays considerable variability. With newborn infants it rises from about 2 in the first day of life to about 10 or 12 at the second week, reflecting the increase in granulocyte production and the decline in erythrocyte production which occurs in this period. During the latter half of the first month the ratio subsides to between 4 and 3 and remains there for the rest of the first year. Beyond infancy it usually falls between 2.5 and 3.5.

The chief diffiulty in the clinical application of this ratio is that a shift in values does not convey any information as to whether one type of cell has become unusually abundant or another type unusually sparse. The ratio is nevertheless helpful in portraying the changes which occur in successive studies of a patient with a blood disturbance.

PROLIFERATION AND MATURATION

Multiplication of the marrow cells takes place largely, if not entirely, through mitotic division. Mitotic figures are not infrequent in marrow specimens, being perhaps a little more common in cells of the granulocytic than of the erythrocytic series. As a rule the daughter cells appear to be in the same stage of physical development as the mother cells.

As a rule, also, the structural changes in maturation of nuclear and cytoplasmic components advance at approximately the same rate. Under conditions of injury or unusual demand, however, the nucleus or cytoplasm may attain full development or retain primitive characteristics somewhat independently of each other. In severe iron-deficiency anemia, for example, the nuclei of the erythrocytes may be overmature and pyknotically ready for extrusion, while the hemoglobin is still scanty or underdeveloped and markedly basophilic. The converse seems to occur in the megaloblastic forms of anemia.

CELLULAR ACTIVITY IN THE BONE MARROW AS REFLECTED IN PERIPHERAL COUNTS

Marrow hyperplasia in any cell system is often but not necessarily accompanied by a corresponding increase in the absolute count of the more mature cells of this system in the peripheral blood. One such exception occurs in so-called "aleukemic" leukemia, in which, despite a crowded marrow, the peripheral leukocyte count can be very low. In some of these cases the abnormal cells seem to be extremely short-lived peripherally.

Erythrocytes enter the circulation at a retarded rate in many forms of anemia. The marrow spaces may be filled with unmatured erythrocytes awaiting the needed stimulation for full ripening and release.

Not all hyperplastic reactions in the peripheral blood are due to bone marrow hyperactivity. The outpouring of lymphocytes in whooping cough, or of peculiar cells in infectious mononucleosis, are usually not associated with significant alterations in marrow appearance.

RELATION BETWEEN BONE MARROW AND SPLEEN

Certain hematologic disturbances such as the excessive erythrocyte destruction in hereditary spherocytosis and acquired hemolytic anemia and the bleeding tendency in idiopathic thrombocytopenic purpura may be relieved by splenectomy, at least for a time, but the mechanisms remain to be elucidated. There is considerable evidence that the spleen produces hormones which regulate the formation and emission of cells by the bone marrow. In such hypersplenic conditions the marrow is usually overactive with respect to one, several, or all cell series. Splenectomy is contraindicated in suspected hypersplenism if the marrow proves to be hypoplastic (p. 295).

EXTRAMEDULLARY HEMOPOIESIS

During the latter months of pregnancy the fetal liver and spleen possess blood-forming islets in large numbers, with less abundant aggregations in the adrenals, pancreas, thymus, kidneys, lymph nodes, intestinal wall, and other organs. Within the first day or two after birth this extramedullary blood formation ceases abruptly. The marrow then remains the sole organ of blood formation, save that the lymph nodes, spleen, thymus, and related structures continue to discharge lymphocytes and perhaps monocytes into the circulation throughout the whole life span.

In newborn infants the postnatal disappearance of these extramedullary blood-forming islands can be delayed by an exceptionally great demand for new blood cells as occurs with severe infections, erythroblastosis fetalis, severe congenital syphilis, pronounced prematurity, and cyanotic malformations of the heart or great vessels.

In later life these foci can become reactivated under the stimulation of leukemoid reactions, congenital or acquired hemolytic anemia, and severe Mediterranean anemia. Extramedullary "myelophthisic" proliferation may occur also when fibrotic changes or massive infiltrations occupy the normal marrow spaces, as in leukemia, metastatic sarcoma, Gaucher's or Niemann-Pick disease, osteosclerotic bone disorders, poisonings, or the obscure disturbance known as generalized myelofibrosis. This response may occur even when the bone marrow itself seems normally hyperplastic, or is perhaps invaded in comparatively small foci only. Extramedullary hemopoiesis in response to stress is seen more often in infancy than in older children, and during both age periods more often than in adult life.

Extramedullary hemopoiesis is attended typically by an altered cellular pattern in the peripheral blood—the so-called leukoerythroblastotic reaction. This consists of chronic progressive anemia, a leukocyte count which may be low or excessively high, and circulating immature granulocytes and erythrocytes in inconstant numbers. Myelocytes and progranulocytes may number 20 per cent of all the white cells, and reticulocytes and more primitive rubricytes make their appearance in showers. The platelet count tends to be low despite prominence of megakaryocytes in the marrow and extramedullary foci. Giant-sized platelets and fragments of megakaryocytes may be seen in the blood smear (*megakaryocytic reaction*). Severe peripheral blood changes of this character may be mistaken for granulocytic leukemia, hemolytic anemia, leukemoid reaction, or thrombocytopenic purpura. Such a peripheral blood picture, when associated with two or more unsuccessful or "dry" marrow punctures, should rouse a diagnostic suspicion of marrow infiltration, osteopetrosis, or connective tissue replacement. Confirmation should be sought by roentgenography or biopsy.

The lymph nodes over the body, and usually the spleen or liver, become noticeably enlarged when this disturbance continues for more than a few weeks.

In the rare and fatal disorder known as agnogenic myeloid metaplasia of the spleen the marrow spaces become filled chiefly with fibroblasts while centers of extramedullary hemopoiesis make their appearance in the enlarging spleen, liver, and lymph nodes. The peripheral blood shows leukocytosis and thrombocytosis with immature granulocytes and rubricytes in large numbers. Small doses of x-ray over the spleen may alleviate local pain if present, but splenectomy or heavy irradiation of the spleen are contraindicated. This condition, rare in childhood, usually proves to be a variant form of granulocytic leukemia.

BIBLIOGRAPHY

PROCEDURES AND GENERAL FEATURES

Dacie, J. V., and *J. C. White,* Erythropoiesis with Particular Reference to Its Study by Biopsy of Human Bone Marrow: A Review, *J. Clin. Path.* 2:1, 1949.

Diwany, M., Sternal Marrow Puncture in Children, *Arch. Dis. Childhood* 15:159, 1940.

Downey, H., The Megaloblast-Normoblast Problem: A Cytologic Study, *J. Lab & Clin. Med.* 39:837, 1952.

Downing, V., Bone Marrow Examination in Children, *Pediat. Clin. North America* 2:243, 1955.

Fadem, R. S., and *R. Yalow,* Uniformity of Cell Counts in Smears of Bone Marrow Particles, *Am. J. Clin. Path.* 21:541, 1951.

Gairdner, D., Blood Formation in Infancy. I. The Normal Bone Marrow, *Arch. Dis. Childhood* 27:128, 1952.

Glaser, K., L. R. Limarzi, and *H. G. Poncher,* Cellular Composition of the Bone Marrow in Normal Infants and Children, *Pediatrics* 6:789, 1950.

Kato, K., Sternal Marrow Punctures in Infants and in Children, *Am. J. Dis. Child.* 54:209, 1937.

Leitner, S. J., C. J. C. Britton, and *E. Neumark,* "Bone Marrow Biopsy: Hematology in the Light of Sternal Puncture," Grune & Stratton, Inc., New York, 1949.

Limarzi, L. R., Evaluation of Bone Marrow Concentration Techniques: Modified Method for Simultaneous Preparation and Staining of Blood and Bone Marrow Films, *J. Lab. & Clin. Med.* 32:732, 1947.

Osgood, E. E., and *A. J. Seaman,* Cellular Composition of Normal Bone Marrow as Obtained by Sternal Puncture, *Physiol. Rev.* 24:46, 1944.

Pease, G. L., Bone Marrow Findings in Disorders of the Hemopoietic System: A Review, *Am. J. Clin. Path.* 25:654, 1955.

Poncher, H. G., Diagnostic Application of Study of Bone Marrow in Infants and in Children, *Am. J. Dis. Child.* 76:227, 1948.

Rohr, K., "Das menschliche Knochenmark," George Thieme Verlag, Leipzig, 1940.

Smith, C. H., Bone Marrow Examination in Blood Disorders of Infants and Children, *M. Clin. North America* 31:525, 1947.

Sturgeon, P., Volumetric and Microscopic Pattern of Bone Marrow in Normal Infants and Children. I. Volumetric Pattern, *Pediatrics* 7:577, 1951. II. Cytologic Pattern, *ibid.* 7:642, 1951. III. Histologic Pattern, *ibid.* 7:774, 1951.

Turkel, H., and *F. H. Bethell*, Biopsy of Bone Marrow Performed by a New and Simple Instrument, *J. Lab. & Clin. Med.* 28:1246, 1943.

Wolman, I. J., and *B. Dickstein*, Clinical Applications of Bone Marrow Examination in Childhood, *Am. J. M. Sc.* 214:677, 1947.

Zuelzer, W. W., Normal and Pathologic Physiology of the Bone Marrow, *Am. J. Dis. Child.* 77:482, 1949.

CHAPTER 26

Marrow Cell Systems and Their Responses

Within each cell series the process of maturation seems to proceed continuously from less differentiated to more differentiated stages. The categories utilized for classification are based on size, staining characteristics, and nuclear and cytoplasmic appearances. When a cell seems to be transitional between two categories it is customarily classified as the more differentiated form. When the nucleus and cytoplasm exhibit unlike degrees of maturation the status of the nucleus should be utilized for the identification.

The very primitive or "blast" cells morphologically are very similar in all cell series. They are usually 8 to 15 μ across, exhibit a fine nuclear chromatin structure, usually contain one or more nucleoli, and have basophilic cytoplasm often with azurophil granules. Series identification may have to be made from the associated cells which are more mature and readily recognized.

Azurophil granules are small dark-staining formations which occur in the cytoplasm of mature lymphocytes and monocytes and the promyelocyte and myelocyte stages of the granulocytes.

THE MYELOGRAM IN HEALTHY CHILDREN

The proportions of the various cell types in normal children of the same ages may exhibit wide fluctuations, even in the same child at different periods of the day. These variations, along with differences in techniques and lack of a standardized nomenclature, explain why published averages for normal children submitted by different investigators often show wide divergences.

In any one laboratory the hematologists should agree on a uniform system of criteria for cell identification. Reliance can be placed on trends displayed by individual patients on successive examinations only when a constant nomenclature is adhered to strictly.

On differential counting of aspirated marrow the various series of cells from normal children will group themselves in approximately the proportions shown in Table 26-1. These figures represent the expected

314

ranges for healthy normal children of all ages, from after the neonatal period up through puberty. The extremes of normal variation are occasionally even broader.

Infants and children differ from adults in having more erythrocytic cells and lymphocytes, proportionately speaking. There is also a trend for greater immaturity in the respective cell series. Early stages of red cells, myelocytes, and megakaryocytes are more abundant in the first year of life, and mature forms correspondingly fewer. These differences are most prominent in the first month of life, and especially so in premature infants.

Table 26-1. Approximate Percentage Distribution of Cell Types in Active Bone Marrow Values for Normal Infants and Children above 2 Months of Age *

	Range, %	Average, %
ERYTHROCYTES		
Rubriblasts	0–1	0.5
Megaloblasts	1–3	2
Normoblasts	10–35	20
Total		22
GRANULOCYTES		
Myeloblasts	0–4	1
Promyelocytes	0–8	3
Myelocytes, neutrophilic	10–40	20
Metamyelocytes, neutrophilic	8–25	13
Band and lobulated neutrophils	3–30	15
Eosinophils, all stages	1–10	3
Total		55
LYMPHOCYTES (almost entirely small forms) †	5–40	20
MISCELLANEOUS (megakaryocytes, plasma cells, monocytes, basophils, reticulum cells, primitive cells, etc.)	0–5	3

* Under 2 months the cellular distribution is more highly variable.

† During infancy the lymphocytes are more abundant than at later ages, and larger forms more numerous. During the first 2 years the lymphocytes usually average about 25 per cent, whereas above 6 years they are closer to 15 per cent.

Neonatal Period

On the day of birth the nucleated red cells are relatively numerous: 30 to 65 per cent, with an average of about 35 per cent. They become much reduced during the first 2 weeks; by the fourteenth day they are only 8 to 30 per cent, with an average of about 10 per cent. They then increase gradually and attain the usual childhood level of around 20 per cent at 3 to 4 weeks of age. The granulocytes rise to about 70 per cent in the first week, and then fall again. The lymphocytes, which number about 10 per cent at birth, rise slowly to 40 per cent at 3 weeks and subside to about 30 per cent at 1 month.

All the cell systems in premature and newborn full-term infants have as efficient a capacity to react to injurious processes by accelerated hemopoiesis as do older infants and children.

GRANULOCYTE CELLS

Granulocyte is an inclusive term applied to the neutrophils, eosinophils, basophils, and their precursors.

The most primitive granulocyte, the myeloblast, ranges from 12 to 20 μ in width. It has a large round or oval nucleus with fine reddish-staining chromatin containing one or more pale-staining nucleoli. The scanty nongranular cytoplasm is faintly basophilic, stains more lightly near the nucleus, and may contain a few azurophilic granules. The progranulocyte (promyelocyte) has coarser chromatin and perhaps one or more nucleoli. The cytoplasm is more abundant and moderately basophilic or even polychromatophilic. It typically contains azurophilic granules and sometimes a few early specific granules.

The myelocyte is distinguished from the progranulocyte by having no nucleoli and faintly basophilic or acidophilic cytoplasm which contains neutrophilic, eosinophilic, or basophilic granules and few or no azurophilic granules. Eosinophilic or basophilic granules when present are larger than in the corresponding adult form. Occasional myelocytes may exhibit all three types of specific granules mingled together. Eosinophilic and basophilic myelocytes are more numerous in normal marrow than are the corresponding mature forms in the peripheral blood. The majority of new granulocytes are produced by swelling, mitosis, and division at the myelocyte and promyelocyte levels. In the so-called "early" myelocyte the cytoplasm is still basophilic, the azurophilic granules numerous, and specific granules are beginning to appear in the inner curve of the nucleus where the cytoplasm is clearer. The latter is sometimes referred to as the "sunburst effect."

In the metamyelocyte the nucleus is deeper-staining, elongated, and kidney-shaped. There are many specific granules—neutrophilic, eosinophilic, or basophilic—lying in faintly eosinophilic cytoplasm.

The band cell (staff or juvenile cell) has a nucleus that appears as a curved or coiled band with parallel sides. The granules are small, numerous, and stain with shades of faint pink or blue. The segmented granulocyte (neutrophil, eosinophil, basophil) has the lobes of the nucleus connected by a threadlike filament. The number of lobes is believed to reflect the age of the cell.

Hyperplasia and Alterations in Appearance

Hyperplasia of maturing neutrophilic or eosinophilic granulocytes may occur in a variety of diseases and disturbances. Hyperplasia of the basophilic granulocytes (mast cells) is practically never seen except in the very rare basophilic leukemia. The totals for marrow eosinophils or basophils at all stages have such low normal limits that it is very difficult to recognize hypoplastic states should they occur.

Toxic granules are abnormal azurophilic or pyknotic deposits which occur in the cytoplasm of mature granulocytes in severe toxemic illnesses. *Toxic vacuoles* are lipid-like nonstaining droplets which appear in the nucleus or cytoplasm of any variety of leukocyte during leukemia, infectious mononucleosis, and diverse other disease states.

The term *toxic neutrophils*, followed by a 1-plus to 4-plus sign, has been recommended for the grading of toxic granules and vacuoles and condensation of nuclear chromatin. The grading depends more on the degree of change than on the percentage of cells involved. Toxic changes should be noted in the report whenever the change exceeds 2 plus in degree.

PYOGENIC INFECTIONS. In most acute bacterial infections of any severity the peripheral leukocytosis is accompanied by proliferation of the neutrophilic elements in the bone marrow. The younger cell forms tend to be disproportionately increased, in numbers which parallel the severity of the infection and the increase of immature cells in the circulation ("shift to the left"). These changes are more easily evoked in the newborn period and young infant than later in childhood. Vacuoles and toxic granulations are evident in the marrow metamyelocytes when present in the circulating neutrophils. In severe chronic infections the same neutrophilic proliferation may obtain, along with a plasma cell increase. In typhoid fever and other Salmonella infections the granulocytes in the marrow are increased even when the peripheral leukocyte count is low.

LEUKEMOID REACTIONS. An extreme degree of peripheral granulocytosis represents an exceptional response to pyogenic stimulation and may not be immediately differentiable from granulocytic leukemia of the chronic variety (p. 212). The most significant difference in the bone marrow is that in leukemoid reactions the displacement by atypical or blast cells, as in leukemia, does not occur. The immature granulocytes of the marrow, though increased in number, are normal in appearance, apart from the presence of toxic granules and related changes to suggest the influence of an infection.

HYPERSPLENISM. In occasional instances of chronic splenomegaly (p. 297), a granulocytic hyperplasia may be seen in the early stages when the peripheral blood exhibits a moderate anemia and leukopenia. Later, when the peripheral blood changes become more marked, the accumulations of myelocytes and promyelocytes in the marrow may suggest a maturation arrest of the neutrophil precursors. Megakaryocytes become more numerous as the circulating platelets diminish. Erythrocytic hyperplasia may also develop.

LEUKEMIA. In acute granulocytic leukemia the majority of the cells may clearly belong to the granulocytic series, but often with appearances which are immature or bizarre (p. 212). In chronic granulocytic leukemia the proportions of immature eosinophil or basophil granulocytes in the marrow may increase even when most of the cells in the blood seem of the neutrophil series. In the rare eosinophil leukemia the marrow displays marked infiltration or proliferation of atypical eosinophilic myelocytes.

EOSINOPHILIA. Marrow eosinophilia can develop within the space of but a few days and disappear just as rapidly. At times the granules may stain immaturely gray-blue or be multicolored when the nuclei are already banded or segmented, indicating a more rapid rate of nuclear than of cytoplasmic maturation.

Eosinophilia in the marrow does not necessarily coincide or run parallel to eosinophilia in the blood: the blood eosinophils may be elevated and the marrow eosinophils low, or vice versa. In idiopathic thrombocytopenic purpura hemorrhagica more than half the children have an increase in marrow eosinophils. Marrow eosinophilia may be seen in measles, scarlet fever, and other infections, at times when these cells are numerous in the peripheral blood.

In allergic and parasitic diseases and in many other diseases associated with peripheral eosinophilia one may find marrow hyperplasia of the eosinophilic myelocytes and possibly other granulocytes, though the rises are usually less striking than in comparable diseases which evoke neutrophilic stimulation. Eosinophils sometimes rise to as high as 35 per cent of all the marrow leukocytes, occasionally for no obvious cause.

MALNUTRITIONAL STATES. In the majority of cases of mild malnutrition the granulocytes of the bone marrow appear normal or nearly so, even when there is an accompanying iron deficiency which disturbs the red cell series. In the macrocytic or "megaloblastic" anemias, however, and in pernicious anemia, changes in the granulocytes of the nature of disturbed maturation are often seen. Retarded mitoses, giant metamyelocytes, binucleated myelocytes, and 5- or 6-lobed neutrophils may make their appearance.

Agranulocytosis

Mild degrees of granulocyte depression are known as neutropenia or granulocytopenia, more severe forms as agranulocytosis. The marrow pattern is found inconstant and variable even when the peripheral granulocytes seem entirely absent. The appearance may suggest interference with or arrest of maturation, in that there may be an abundance of granulocytes either in normal distribution or with a shift to excess promyelocytes. When the injury seems more advanced, practically all the granulocytes may be progranulocytes or younger forms, or even these may disappear, leaving lymphocytes and plasma cells as almost the sole leukocytes in the marrow. When the erythrocytes and thrombocytes are coincidentally depressed, the cellular pattern corresponds to that of aplastic anemia.

As remission begins the marrow spaces fill up with regenerating granulocytes in all stages of development. Promyelocytes appear first, to be followed soon by more mature forms. The marrow may pass through a phase of becoming crowded with maturing granulocytes while the peripheral leukocyte count is still in a comparative agranulocytosis.

Granulocytic hypoplasia may appear without apparent cause (idiopathic) or be secondary to a drug, to irradiation, or to some focal or general infection (p. 184). The marrow seems to be the primary site of injury. When granulocyte production ceases, granulocytes already developing may continue to progress to maturity and sustain the peripheral blood count for a few days. Serial leukocyte counts during the administration of drugs which tend to suppress granulocytes are therefore not absolute safeguards against agranulocytosis, because the information given may come too late. The granulocytopenia may continue to progress to agranulocytosis whether the sensitizing drug is stopped or not. When drug therapy is being given as treatment for an infection the depressant effect of the infection itself upon the granulocyte count may not be immediately differentiable from a possible sensitization reaction to the drug.

The prognosis is better when there is maturation arrest than when the process has gone on to almost complete aplasia. Treatment consists of discontinuance of all suspected toxic agents, a vigorous attack an any underlying infection or other possible cause, and administration of all hematopoietic stimulants. Serial bone marrow examinations are of great assistance in evaluating the effects of the therapy given.

Cases of idiopathic agranulocytosis have been recorded in which no drugs appear to have been taken and no obvious cause could be found. Some such cases ultimately prove to have acute leukemia. Others may be resistant to all forms of stimulant therapy and succumb to a progressive and complete aplasia involving the red cells as well as the megakaryocytes.

Infiltration of the marrow spaces by leukemic or other foreign cells can depress granulocytopoiesis and give rise to low marrow and peripheral neutrophil counts. If chemotherapy succeeds in destroying or depressing these abnormal elements, the normal cell series usually regenerate in appreciable numbers within a week or less. There may, however, be an interval phase during which an aplastic marrow pattern will be found.

LYMPHOCYTIC CELLS

The lymphoblast has a fine chromatin structure in a large nucleus, one or more nucleoli, and basophilic scanty cytoplasm; it ranges in width from 10 to 20 μ. Cells of blast morphology occurring with an abundance of lymphocytes are classified by association as lymphoblasts.

The "large" lymphocyte is typically 10 to 18 μ in width. It has coarser nuclear chromatin and no nucleoli. Some authors separate the large lymphocytes into two types. One type has a smaller nucleus with coarse deep-staining chromatin and a comparatively large amount of clear light-blue cytoplasm which may contain a few haphazardly distributed azurophilic granules. The other, sometimes called "young lymphocyte," differs in having a comparatively larger nucleus with less clumping of the chromatin and deep-blue cytoplasm without granules.

The "small" lymphocyte usually measures 8 to 10 μ and rarely exceeds 12 μ. Its nucleus is small, round, central, and deeply staining. The cytoplasm is scanty, stains light or dark blue with Wright's stain, and may contain azurophilic granules.

The great majority of the lymphocytes occurring in the marrow are of the small variety, except in the first few months of life. When a high percentage of young or large lymphocytes is found in the aspirate from a child or older infant one should be suspicious of some blood dyscrasia.

During the first 2 months of life the lymphocytes often outnumber the granulocyte elements in the bone marrow as well as in the peripheral blood.

Hyperplasia

The lymphocytes range from 10 to 40 per cent or occasionally higher in normal marrow. Since lymph follicles do occur in the bone marrow, though rare, one should not be sure of the existence of a marrow lymphocytic hyperplasia unless goodly numbers are encountered on repeated aspirations and preferably from different sites.

In acute infectious lymphocytosis the normal lymphocytes may seem a little increased. Myeloid elements and nucleated red cells are normal in quantity. In other infections which may induce lymphocytosis in the blood, such as measles, chickenpox, and especially whooping cough, the marrow shows no excessive lymphocytosis. Lymphocytic leukemia is the most striking disturbance in which a marrow lymphocytosis occurs (p. 213).

Hypoplasia

Because of normal variation, the diagnosis of lymphocytopenia cannot be made from bone marrow aspiration except when there is complete alymphocytosis (p. 225).

MONOCYTIC CELLS

The monoblast is a large blast cell. Its nucleus may be uneven, with fine chromatin and several nucleoli. The cytoplasm stains uniformly deep blue or gray-blue with Wright's stain and may contain red-purple granules or rod-shaped Auer bodies. The promonocyte ("young monocyte") has an irregular or folded-appearing nucleus with coarse chromatin structure and perhaps one or more nucleoli. Its cytoplasm resembles that of the mature cell. The monocyte measures 12 to 20 μ. Its nucleus is large and round or indented, with fine reticulated chromatin but no nucleoli. The cytoplasm stains an uneven gray-blue; it may contain an inconstant number of azurophilic granules and sometimes a few vacuoles. Deviations from this typical appearance are not uncommon, especially in the first few months of life.

Monocytes are infrequent in normal marrow. One or two per cent is the usual count, but occasionally as many as 5 per cent may be found without apparent cause.

Hyperplasia

In monocytic leukemia, which is rare in childhood, marked infiltration with monocytoid cells may occur. In granulomatous infections and in refractory cases of aplastic anemia, primary or secondary, the monocyte content of the marrow may seem proportionately increased.

In infectious mononucleosis the marrow smear may contain small numbers of abnormal cells similar to those in the blood stream. Otherwise the lymphocytes and monocytes are not increased and all appearances are normal. The source of the abnormal cells is presumably the lymph tissue. The absence of cellular infiltrations in infectious mononucleosis is in striking contrast to the replacement with abnormal cells which takes place in leukemia.

RETICULOENDOTHELIAL CELLS

The reticuloendothelial cell (histiocyte, endothelial leukocyte, mesenchymal cell, macrophage, clasmatocyte) is variable in size and appearance, not always distinguishable from an adult monocyte. Its nucleus is large, eccentric, and pale-staining, with thin strands of chromatin and usually some nucleoli. The cytoplasm is abundant and palely basophilic, and the cell boundaries irregular or indistinct. Vacuoles or phagocytosed granules may lie within the cell. The maturation pattern is not clearly established. Daland and Ham have subclassified these cells into several types: (1) ameboid form, (2) phagocytic form, (3) basophilic or "blast" form, (4) lymphocytic form, (5) lipid-storage forms, (6) "hemohistioblasts of Ferrata." When encountered in the peripheral blood they may be derived from the spleen, lymph nodes, or vascular endothelium rather than from the bone marrow.

These cells are recovered from healthy marrow in small numbers only and rarely exceed 3 per cent of the aspirate.

Hyperplasia

Reticuloendothelial cells are found in increased numbers in the marrow in aplasia or hypoplasia of the marrow due to any cause. They may be unusually abundant in subacute bacterial endocarditis and other protracted chronic infections, reticulum cell sarcoma, Letterer-Siwe disease, Hodgkin's disease, the rare histiocytic leukemia, and after heavy exposure to irradiation. The large cells seen in Gaucher's disease and Niemann-Pick disease are lipid-containing reticuloendothelial cells.

Reticuloendothelial cells are phagocytes. They are likely to exhibit hemosiderin deposits in hematologic disorders attended by undue destruction of red cells, or when the iron stores of the body as a whole are in great excess of normal.

OSTEOBLASTS

These are seen exceptionally in aspirates. They are large (20 to 30 μ) elongated oval cells with basophilic mottled cytoplasm and rounded nuclei. Ordinarily single, they may occur in groups and be mistaken for tumor cells.

PLASMOCYTIC CELLS

The plasmoblast, 25 to 40 μ in width, has a large irregular nucleus and a thin rim of cytoplasm. The nuclear chromatin is fine and reticular and contains one to three nucleoli. The cytoplasm stains more opaquely than that of other blast cells. The proplasmocyte, a little smaller, has a central or eccentrically placed nucleus with coarse irregularly clumped chromatin and usually no nucleoli. Its cytoplasm is more abundant, unevenly basophilic, and frequently vacuolated. The adult plasma cell or plasmocyte is 8 to 25 μ in diameter. It has an eccentric nucleus with deeply staining coarse clumps of chromatin, a heavy nuclear membrane, and no nucleoli. Multinucleated forms are not uncommon. The cytoplasm stains diffusely blue-gray or purple-gray, often with a pale perinuclear zone. There are no granules but occasional nonstaining vacuoles of inconstant size. In the so-called "senile" plasma cell, the nucleus is pyknotic or fragmented; the cytoplasm stains unevenly and lightly and may contain violet-red–staining intracytoplasmic inclusions—so-called Russell bodies.

The plasma cell content of normal marrow is less than 1 per cent, usually in the neighborhood of 0.5 per cent. They are diminished in numbers or absent in agammaglobulinemia. The primitive plasmoblasts become numerous in plasmocytic leukemia and multiple myeloma.

Plasma cells are believed to originate from the reticulum cells of the marrow and of the lymphoid tissue. Hence it is possible to have a peripheral plasmocytosis of lymph follicle origin without proliferation in the marrow.

Hyperplasia

The more mature forms of marrow plasma cells may become more numerous in such apparently unrelated diseases as measles, rubella, mumps, chickenpox, aplastic and other anemias, rheumatoid arthritis, roseola infantum, infectious mononucleosis, polyarteritis nodosa, hepatic cirrhosis, Hodgkin's disease, lupus erythematosus, and miscellaneous other acute and chronic diseases. Levels above 1 per cent may be considered a significant elevation. The reticulum cells of the marrow are usually increased coincidentally. The plasma globulin level is usually elevated when marrow plasmocytosis is prominent, suggesting that the hyperglobulinemia is a product of these cells. In sections of biopsied marrow the plasma cells lie characteristically in the walls of the arterial capillaries but may be found in clumps or spread diffusely.

Multiple myeloma is the classic situation in which the marrow becomes heavily infiltrated with plasma cells. During the early stages the infiltration may be spotty, giving inconstant counts in repeated punctures. Myelomatous plasma cells are abnormal in appearance, with double nuclei, multiple nucleoli, uneven staining, and vacuolization of the cytoplasm. Multiple myeloma is almost unknown in the early years, though it has been observed in older children near or at puberty.

THROMBOCYTIC CELLS

Four stages have been identified in the maturation of the platelets or thrombocytes. The megakaryoblast is larger than the other blast cells but resembles them otherwise. The promegakaryocyte, the next stage, has a nucleoli-containing irregular nucleus with a coarse chromatin structure and fine azurophilic granules scattered through the cytoplasm.

The megakaryocyte is ordinarily gigantic, up to 60 μ in width. It has a dense homogeneous deeply staining nucleus, usually lobulated, without nucleoli. The cytoplasm displays masses of azurophilic platelet-like formations. The cell borders are often jagged and indefinite. Platelets are nonnucleated fragments of megakaryocytic cytoplasm containing azurophilic granules of variable size.

Counting of Megakaryocytes

The megakaryocyte content of marrow is extremely difficult to ascertain with any accuracy. Coincident examinations of stained smears of aspirate, of suspensions of marrow in a hemocytometer, and of sections of marrow tissue prepared histologically ordinarily give different results. Study of bone marrow sections obtained by biopsy seems to be the most dependable approach to determining the content of megakaryocytes in questionable cases. Since in stained aspirates these cells tend to accumulate at the sides and far edges of the smears, one should survey the entire slide under low-power magnification, and when checking on the content of megakaryocytes, report them as "absent," "decreased," "normal," or "increased."

Thrombocytopenic States

In "idiopathic" thrombocytopenic purpura hemorrhagica (Chap. 23), the marrow megakaryocytes are typically in abundance. Many are young and immature, with or without a corresponding diminution of the well-developed platelet-producing forms. The number or cytologic maturity of these cells does not seem to have much direct correlation with either the ultimate prognosis or the severity of the bleeding manifestations. When much blood has been lost by hemorrhage, the erythrocytic and granulocytic elements of the marrow may also be hyperplastic. A marrow eosinophilia, usually not mirrored in the peripheral blood, is often present also.

Megakaryocytes are few or even undemonstrable in many diseases which interfere with platelet formation. Among these are aplastic anemia, myelofibrosis, osteopetrosis, and leukemic, sarcomatous, or reticuloendothelial infiltrations. Drug-induced or hypersplenic thrombocytopenia may be attended either by normal or reduced numbers of megakaryocytes. Because of the possibility of some infiltrative or hypoplastic change in the bone marrow, it is imperative to make a careful marrow study of every thrombocytopenic patient with purpura hemorrhagica before considering a possible splenectomy. The operation can be expected to have a much more favorable influence when the number of megakaryocytes is adequate or high.

If the first aspirated marrow specimen suggests impaired megakaryocytogenesis and one wishes to corroborate this impression, a second aspiration should be done from another site. In doubtful cases a biopsy with study of a marrow section may be necessary to establish the quantitative status of the megakaryocytes. On the other hand, a liberal sprinkling of these cells in smear or counting chamber can only mean a megakaryocyte-rich marrow.

ERYTHROCYTIC CELLS

The rubriblast (proerythroblast, erythrogone) is 12 to 15 μ or more in width. It is not seen in any quantity except in severe forms of anemia and may then have irregularities in nucleus or cytoplasm. The nuclear chromatin is finely granular or stippled and perhaps a little different from the lacy pattern of other blast cells. Several nucleoli are usually present. The cytoplasm is variable in amount and strongly basophilic, without granules.

The megaloblast (prorubricyte, early erythroblast), also a large cell, represents the next stage in maturation. Its nucleus is comparatively large, with a coarse clumped chromatin structure and an occasion ill-defined nucleolus. The cytoplasm is deeply basophilic.

The normoblast (rubricyte, late erythroblast) is smaller, 8 to 12 μ in width. Its nucleus is comparatively small with the chromatin in coarse clumps, sometimes like the spokes of a wheel; nucleoli are not present. Well-formed double nuclei are occasionally seen in swollen megaloblasts and normoblasts as a preliminary to cell division. Very mature normoblasts show a tiny pyknotic or fragmented nuclear mass which may be autolyzed or partially extruded. As hemoglobin develops within the normoblast its cytoplasm matures from weakly basophilic through muddy gray to the orthochromic orange-pink of the fully hemoglobinized cell. Hence these cells may be subclassified as basophilic, polychromatic, and orthochromic (normochromic).

The reticulocyte is a little larger than the mature erythrocyte. It has lost its nucleus but is still faintly basophilic because of the persistence of traces of the primordial cytoplasm. Supravital staining—usually with brilliant cresyl blue—brings out these remnants as fine granules or a diffuse network of fibrils. Mitoses may be seen at the megaloblast and early normoblast level of maturation, with the greatest number normally in the normoblasts.

The usual pattern of red cell formation, seen in normal states and the minor forms of most anemias, is *normoblastic*. The maturing cells past the rubriblast stage tend to be small. As they divide and hemoglobinize the chromatin becomes aggregated early into dense clumps and the nucleoli disappear.

The *megaloblastic* pattern of red cell growth, interpreted as pathologic, appears when folic acid, vitamin B_{12}, or related essential nutrients other than iron are deficient. Large megaloblasts accumulate in the marrow as a manifestation of abnormal formation or maturation arrest. The myelocytes and metamyelocytes become unusually large, with bandlike or multipronged nuclei and poorly granulated abundant cytoplasm.

The large *pernicious anemia* type of nucleated erythrocytes measure 15 to 25 μ in diameter. The nuclei have a relative increase in the pale-staining portions of the nuclear chromatin, and nucleoli which vary in size and number. The cytoplasm is usually basophilic but may show partial hemoglobinization while the nuclei remain highly immature. Intermediate cells of this type are indicative of a minor deficiency of these hemopoietic factors.

In advanced deficiencies, as in the megaloblastic anemia of infancy (p. 47), one may find atypical mitoses, displaced chromosomes, fragmented nuclei, and cytoplasmic vacuoles. The more severe the nutritional disturbance, the greater these distortions. Unstained granules may seem to be imbedded in the dark-staining chromatin of the nuclei. A significant characteristic is the retention of nucleoli for much longer than in normoblastic maturation. When corrective dietary therapy is begun these cells mature and transform themselves either into normoblasts or macrocytes.

Macronormoblasts are unusually large prorubricytes and rubricytes which otherwise resemble their normal counterparts. They appear in the marrow when erythropoiesis is accelerated and a reticulocytosis and macrocytosis exist in the peripheral blood and are presumably the precursors of the macrocytes. Macronormoblasts are seen in active hereditary spherocytosis and other chronic hemolytic anemias, during recovery from hemorrhage, and in patients with iron deficiency receiving restorative iron therapy.

Hyperplasia

Proliferation of the marrow erythrocytic elements is characteristic whenever there is recurrent loss or excessive destruction of blood. As many as 60 to 90 per cent of the nucleated marrow cells may be in the erythrocyte series, in place of the more customary 8 to 40 per cent. Along with the increase in numbers the proportion of megaloblasts and other immature cells goes up also, and mitoses at these more primitive levels become more abundant. Generally speaking, the greater the need for more red cells, the more prominent the erythropoiesis and the number of younger and dividing forms. The other constituents of the marrow often share in the hyperplasia to some extent, so that there may be an accompanying peripheral granulocytosis or thrombocytosis.

Chronic heart failure, congenital cardiac anomalies of the cyanotic group, and other disorders which cause anoxemia, such as emphysema and chronic methemoglobinemia, may evoke moderate erythrocytic hyperplasia. This response is different from what occurs in the polycythemia vera of adult life, in which hyperplasia of the granulocyte and thrombocyte elements occurs as well.

The broadening and demineralization of the skeletal bones or thickening of the roof of the skull, typical of the florid case of Mediterranean anemia, may be seen also in severe sickle cell anemia and congenital pure red cell anemia.

In hereditary spherocytosis the erythrocyte hyperplasia is predominantly at the normoblast level, though more immature forms are increased also. There is no close correlation between the cytologic changes in the marrow, the degree of peripheral reticulocytosis, and the severity of the anemia. Some orthochromic normoblasts may display the abnormal spherocytic shape of the mature erythrocytes. Following splenectomy the marrow hyperplasia becomes less intense and the immature cells less numerous.

In the active sickle cell anemias the marrow similarly shows exaggerated activity, with a shift to immaturity. The aspirate consists largely of normoblasts and megaloblasts, usually with a moderate increase in myelocytes. Eosinophils and megakaryocytes also may be more numerous. The reticuloendothelial cells may contain ingested red corpuscles and nuclear fragments. Pigment granules may be scattered about.

In florid Mediterranean anemia the bone marrow is extraordinarily hyperplastic, whether the spleen has been removed or not. There seem to be innumerable rubriblasts, megaloblasts, and normoblasts. Some of these may have stippled or vacuolated cytoplasm. Myelocytes and megakaryocytes are increased as well. Reticuloendothelial cells are numerous and rich in hemosiderin. Small islands of foam cells may give an appearance suggestive of Gaucher's cells.

In erythroblastosis fetalis due to Rh incompatibility the bone marrow is usually hyperplastic at birth, though when the disturbance is mild the appearance may be indistinguishable from that of an unaffected newborn. Irregular areas may be found in which blood-forming cells are completely absent and the spaces between the trabeculae filled with mucoid connective tissue. Extramedullary foci of hemopoiesis may be responsible for the many immature cells found in the blood at the time of birth. The low erythrocyte and hemoglobin levels sometimes seen after the first few weeks in convalescent infants are usually associated with transitory hypocellularity of the red cell elements.

In anemia due to iron deficiency the bone marrow typically exhibits an accumulation of normoblasts with a minor increase in megaloblasts. Most of the normoblasts seem small, with a decrease in the quantity of cytoplasm. Iron deficiency may be inferred when these cell forms are abundant. After treatment is begun, mitosis and more immature forms increase rapidly to reach a peak synchronous with the maximal reticulocytosis in the peripheral blood. In protracted anemia associated with iron deficiency the erythrocytic elements are occasionally diminished in number.

Hypoplasia

In congenital hypoplastic or "pure red cell" anemia, with symptoms dating back to birth (p. 90), the primitive red cell forms frequently number only about 1 per cent or less of all the nucleated cells in the aspirate. Some of these are small primordial cells, known as hematogones, which are smaller than but resemble lymphocytes; they have dense homogeneous nuclear chromatin and a narrow rim of nongranular cytoplasm. More mature rubricytes tend to be scanty or absent and may have but little cytoplasm which stains deeply basophilic.

At times the erythropoietic cells in the marrow may seem within normal numerical limits. Rubriblasts and megaloblasts are more abundant than the more mature cell forms. The latter may show finely granular nuclear chromatin and irregular amounts of fragile cytoplasm. More advanced normoblasts tend to be scanty and may have scanty deeply basophilic cytoplasm. In culture studies of marrow from these patients, Cathie observed that maturation of the hemoglobinizing normoblasts seems to be arrested at that stage, instead of continuing through to the reticulocyte and the adult erythrocyte.

Production of the other cell constituents of the marrow—platelets, granulocytes, and other leukocytes—appears normal. Plasma cells may seem unusually abundant.

In the constitutional diseases which lead to the normochromic normocytic form of anemia (Chap. 5), as for example in chronic infections or hypothyroidism, erythropoiesis in the bone marrow may appear approximately normal or a little depressed. No distinctive qualitative changes in cell appearance or maturation pattern can be identified.

In chronic renal diseases the pattern of erythropoiesis ordinarily appears unimpaired, unless the nonprotein nitrogen level of the blood is above approximately 150 mg per 100 ml. Hypocellularity of the erythrocytic elements may then ensue and be proportional roughly to the degree of nitrogen retention. The cells of the granulocytic and thrombocytic series may be either hyperplastic or hypoplastic. We have twice seen children with the presenting complaint of hypoplastic anemia who were found on exploratory study to have unsuspected chronic renal disease as the cause of the anemia. A cellular bone marrow in chronic nephritis is not in itself evidence of hemopoietic activity and does not carry prognostic significance. The bleeding of terminal uremia is apparently not due to injury of marrow megakaryocytes, for the platelets in the blood are adequate. It seems to be caused by a combination of toxic capillary injury and prothrombin deficiency, both induced by toxic retention products.

Acute Erythroblastopenia (Aplastic Crisis)

Erythrocyte production may slow down for a week or more during or after an infectious or allergic disease process. With hematologically normal individuals whose red cell survival time is approximately 120 days, the temporary suppression of red cell production results in a slight fall in peripheral red cell and hemoglobin levels which is within the limits of error of the counting procedures. With patients having hemolytic disorders, however, in whom the red cell survival time may be only 15 to 30 days, an acute cessation of red cell production for only a few days can cause already depressed red cells and hemoglobin to fall to symptomatic levels.

Examination of aspirated bone marrow during a period of erythroblastopenia shows a marked reduction in most of the red cell precursors. A few large megaloblast-like cells up to 60 μ in diameter may be observed. Rubriblasts are not increased. Eosinophils may be prominent in patients with allergic backgrounds, or the plasma cells increased in chronic infections or some virus infections. Atypical lymphocytes may be found in infectious mononucleosis. The other marrow constituents usually appear unaltered, even though there may be peripheral thrombocytopenia or leukocytopenia. As recovery begins, the red cell forms in the bone marrow become abundant again and a reticulocytosis and polychromatophilic and other immature erythrocytes become evident in the circulation within a few days.

Since the period of red cell hypoproduction is usually brief, no specific treatment is needed for the patient without underlying hematologic disturbances. With a complicating hemolytic process, however, transfusions are advisable as soon as the condition is recognized.

HYPOPLASIA OR APLASIA OF THE ENTIRE BONE MARROW (PANMYELOPHTHISIS)

Acute toxic injury can inhibit all the hemopoietic elements of the bone marrow, either transiently or permanently. This is reflected in the peripheral blood as anemia, granulocytopenia, and thrombocytopenia. The precipitating cause may be an overwhelming infection, a chemical agent such as benzol or organic arsenical or gold compounds, or exposure to roentgen rays or radioactive substances. Similar marrow hypoplasia has been observed in cirrhosis of the liver. Idiosyncratic sensitivity must be hypothesized to explain this lesion on the rare occasions when it follows exposure to Tridione, chloramphenicol, insecticides, and similar substances which are not toxic to most individuals. Acute leukemia and other blood disturbances must be ruled out by marrow examination and continued observation of the patient.

"Idiopathic" refractory aplastic anemia is a progressive disease of unknown cause characterized by profound anemia, thrombocytopenia, leukopenia, multiple hemorrhages, and a marrow which is hypoplastic or sclerotic (p. 79).

Starvation or severe chronic malnutrition may be attended by diminished activity and reduction in cellular content of the marrow. When the von Jaksch syndrome associated with malnutrition and rickets is treated by a good diet high in vitamins, the hepatosplenomegaly, anemia, and peripheral signs of extramedullary hemopoiesis fade away gradually as the marrow reverts to normal cellularity.

Familial chronic pancytopenic anemia has been reported. In this the marrow has shown an orderly but quantitatively diminished formation of all families of cells.

Bone marrow aspirates in clear-cut cases of bone marrow aplasia, regardless of cause, have a scanty content of marrow cells and tend to resemble smears of peripheral blood. When this finding is encountered it is important to repeat the examination, utilizing another site, since islets of functioning tissue may be scattered through aplastic areas. Care should be taken that the aspirations are made from short bones such as the vertebra or ileum in which hemopoiesis is normally active, rather than one of the long bones which are ordinarily fatty and poor in cells beyond infancy.

Should a generalized hyperplasia of the bone marrow be found in the presence of a peripheral pancytopenia, the probability of a hypersplenic disturbance should be considered (p. 295).

Erythropoiesis may be inhibited mechanically when infiltrations from leukemia or metastatic sarcoma, or osteosclerotic alterations, become widespread and displace the usual hemopoietic elements.

BIBLIOGRAPHY

RESPONSES OF THE BONE MARROW CELL SYSTEMS

Abt, A. F., Aplastic Anemias in Childhood: Report of a Primary Idiopathic Refractory Type, with Splenectomy, in an Eleven Year Old Girl, *Am. J. Dis. Child.* 78:516, 1949.

Axelrod, A. R., and *L. Berman,* The Bone Marrow in Hyperthyroidism and Hypothyroidism, *Blood* 6:436, 1951.

Braun, K., The Bone Marrow in Secondary Polycythemia Associated with Cor Pulmonale, *Clin. Path.* 21:149, 1951.

Buetler, E., W. Drennan, and *M. Block,* The Bone Marrow and Liver in Iron-deficiency Anemia, *J. Lab. & Clin. Med.* 43:427, 1954.

Callen, I. R., and *L. R. Limarzi,* Blood and Bone Marrow Studies in Renal Diseases, *Am. J. Clin. Path.* 20:3, 1950.

Castle, W. B., Erythropoiesis: Normal and Abnormal, *Bull. New York Acad. Med.* 30:827, 1954.

Cathie, I. A. B., Erythrogenesis Imperfecta, *Arch. Dis. Childhood* 25:313, 1950.

Cook, J. E., J. W. Franklin, H. E. Hamilton, and *W. M. Fowler,* Syndrome of Myelofibrosis: Report of Eight Cases, *A.M.A. Arch. Int. Med.* 91:704, 1953.

Custer, R. P., "An Atlas of the Blood and Bone Marrow," W. B. Saunders Co., Philadelphia, 1949.

Daland, G. A., and *T. H. Ham,* "A Color Atlas of Morphologic Hematology with a Guide to Clinical Interpretation," Harvard University Press, Cambridge, Mass., 1951.

Dameshek, W., and *E. B. Miller,* The Megakaryocytes in Idiopathic Thrombocytopenic Purpura: A Form of Hypersplenism, *Blood* 1:27, 1946.

Diggs, L. W., D. Sturm, and *A. Bell,* "The Morphology of Human Blood Cells," W. B. Saunders Company, Philadelphia, 1956.

Doan, C. A., and *C. S. Wright,* Primary Congenital and Secondary Acquired Splenic Panhematopenia, *Blood* 1:10, 1946.

Good, R. A., and *B. Campbell,* Relationship of Bone Marrow Plasmacytosis to the Changes in Serum Gamma Globulin in Rheumatic Fever, *Am. J. Med.* 9:330, 1950.

Goulding, A. J., M. J. Rowen, and *L. M. Meyer,* Transient Hyperglobulinemia and Plasmacytosis of Bone Marrow during an Acute Infection, *Am. J. Clin. Path.* 20:779, 1950.

Klein, H., and *M. Block,* Bone Marrow Plasmocytosis, *Blood* 8:1034, 1953.

Louis, J., M. H. Lepper, and *L. R. Limarzi,* Bone Marrow Studies in Infectious Disease, *J. Lab. & Clin. Med.* 40:920, 1952.

Presley, S. J., W. R. Best, and *L. R. Limarzi,* Bone Marrow in Idiopathic Thrombocytopenic Purpura: Analysis of 100 Cases with Reference to the Prognostic Significance of Eosinophils and Megakaryocytes, *J. Lab. & Clin. Med.* 40:503, 1952.

Rhoads, C. P., and *D. K. Miller,* Histology of the Bone Marrow in Aplastic Anemia, *Arch. Path.* 26:648, 1938.

Schwartz, S. O., and *S. R. Kaplan,* Thrombocytopenic Purpura, the Prognostic and Therapeutic Value of the Eosinophil Index: An Analysis of 100 Cases, *Am. J. M. Sc.* 219:528, 1950.

Zuelzer, W. W., and *F. N. Ogden,* Megaloblastic Anemia in Infancy: A Common Syndrome Responding Specifically to Folic Acid Therapy, *Am. J. Dis. Child.* 71:211, 1946.

—— and *J. Rutzky,* Megaloblastic Anemia of Infancy, *Advances Pediat.* vol. 6, 1953.

CHAPTER 27

Infiltrations and Miscellaneous Disorders
of the Bone Marrow

LEUKEMIA

Abnormal cells are regularly demonstrable in the bone marrow in leukemia. In the advanced stages, all marrow areas including the fatty tissue become diffusely replaced by leukemic cells and the erythrocytic, megakaryocytic, and other cell series are associatedly depressed. Prolonged intramedullary proliferation may distort the trabeculae and cortex, leading to roentgenologically detectable changes. Terminally, in rare instances, the marrow may become hypoplastic or aplastic in appearance.

There is no consistent relation between the peripheral count of abnormal leukocytes and the marrow cellularity. The medullary interstices may be crowded with cells whether the peripheral blood film has an abundance of leukemic cells or contains so few as to be missed on superficial examination.

Leukemic cells in the bone marrow resemble those in the circulation (p. 211), though in the bone marrow the proportion of primitive forms is higher. It is usually no easier to make a hematologic identification of the responsible cell series from marrow aspirates than from peripheral blood smears, except when the peripheral leukocyte count is extremely depressed or the percentage of abnormal cells extremely low. It is ordinarily not easy to distinguish between lymphoblasts, myeloblasts, and monoblasts, and the problem becomes more difficult when the primitive leukemic cells show morphologic abnormalities. Accompanying cells of intermediate maturity assist in the identification.

Confusion may arise also when questionably leukemic cells are few in number or simulate normal cells. Careful study of both marrow and peripheral smears is then necessary, in order to search for more atypical and blast cell forms than would be expected in other leukocytic disorders.

332

In untreated lymphocytic leukemia the majority of infiltrating cells may so deviate from the customary appearance of the lymphocyte as to simulate blast cells or be unidentifiable. Nearly always the children with unidentifiable or "stem cell" leukemia on further study prove to have lymphocytic leukemia.

In rapidly advancing granulocytic leukemia the myeloblasts tend to be adundant in the prolifierations, with a relative paucity of more differentiated granulocyte forms. In the more chronic granulocytic leukemia the dense and homogeneous prolifierations contain an abundance of myelocytes, metamyelocytes, and apparently mature neutrophils which show few morphologic abnormalities. Eosinophils in various stages of development may be numerous. Erythropoiesis and platelet production vary from case to case.

A variant of chronic granulocytic leukemia called panmyelosis exhibits a pleomorphic proliferation of granulocytes, erythrocytes, megakaryocytes, reticulum cells, fibroblasts, and osteoblasts in various combinations. This pleomorphism may be found in proliferations within the liver and spleen as well as the bone marrow. The spleen is typically very large. Osteosclerosis sometimes appears. Nucleated red cells may appear in the circulation, presumably from extramedullary foci. Death is commonly produced by inanition and cachexia, as contrasted with the more usual hemorrhage or infection in chronic granulocytic leukemia.

Responses to Chemotherapy

When the leukemic process begins to be suppressed by any drug (p. 214), the bone marrow may exhibit changes as early as 3 days or as late as 3 weeks. The first response ranges from a reduction in numbers to an apparently complete dissolution of the leukemic infiltration. A minimal diminution will often take place even in the absence of any recognizable clinical or peripheral hematologic improvement. There may be an interval of a few days in which the marrow appears aplastic, followed by regeneration and proliferation of the normal cell elements. With the folic acid antagonists the marrow megaloblasts occasionally become moderately increased in numbers and the circulating neutrophils may exhibit excessive lobulation. An overdosage of mercaptopurine during a remission results in a temporary depression of all the normal cells.

In therapeutically induced remissions the extent of disappearance of leukemic cells and regeneration of normal cells varies from patient to patient. Even when the return toward normal is impressive in all other respects, a few leukemic cells can always be found in the marrow. The persisting cells may so closely resemble the few primitive or blast cells found in every normal marrow specimen that the existence of a leukemic state may be no longer recognizable. After an indefinite time, however, the leukemic infiltrations begin to reappear despite the continuance of therapy and precede the recurrence of peripheral blood changes and leukemic symptoms by one or more weeks.

NEOPLASMS

Almost any variety of visceral sarcoma with a tendency to dissemination may metastasize to the bone marrow. The most common invaders are neuroblastoma and lymphosarcoma.

These cells often have the size and general appearance of lymphocytes and individually may be mistaken for normal or leukemic lymphocytes. Sometimes they exhibit large acidophilic nuclei with irregular chromatin and nucleoli. Their cytoplasm is variable and usually scanty. Vacuoles filled with translucent material may be present in nucleus or cytoplasm. Sarcoma cells are often fragile and may become "smudged" and unrecognizable during the preparation of a smear.

When differentiating between sarcoma and leukemia in bone marrow aspirates it is helpful to find small particles of undistorted marrow. Metastatic tumor cells tend to be aggregated into clusters, which in neuroblastoma are sometimes circular and rosettelike. In biopsy specimens they lie inside or outside the blood vessel spaces. When aspirates are smeared on glass sides these groupings are usually demolished, causing the tumor cells to become mixed with the other cellular constituents of the marrow. In smear preparations the entire slide should be scanned with the low-power objective, and especially the smear margins, in the search for persistent clusters. In doubtful cases a biopsy may be taken of a segment of bone cortex, supplemented by direct curettage of the medullary contents.

RETICULOENDOTHELIAL PROLIFERATIONS

The lipid storage disturbances and the reticuloendothelioses usually show themselves in the bone marrow when involvement is widespread. However, the spleen may be enlarged as a manifestation of one of these disorders but the bone marrow aspirate seem negative for abnormal cells. A trephine biopsy should be done in such circumstances before ruling out the diagnosis.

When searching marrow spreads for lipid-filled cells (see below) one should first scan the entire slide with the low power objective. The characteristic cells stand out clearly at this low magnification, even when few and widely scattered, whereas they may be missed if oil immersion study of restricted fields is begun immediately. The cells often seem unduly fragile, and may appear as large "smudged" forms of ambiguous nature. In suspected cases, when only such forms are seen, a second marrow aspiration may be performed with more gentleness in manipulation of the aspirate. Marrow altered by other severe diseases such as leukemia may occasionally contain scattered large vacuolated cells simulating those of the xanthomatoses.

Niemann-Pick Disease

In this disorder the marrow may contain hypertrophied prominent reticuloendothelial cells 20 to 60 microns in width. These are round, oval, or polyhedral, have 1 or 2 small nuclei, and occur singly or in small groups. Their cytoplasm is filled with masses of fine droplets supported by web-like pale-staining cytoplasm, and assumes a pale blue-black color when stained for myelin by the Smith-Dietrich method.

Gaucher's Disease

Altered large reticuloendothelial cells are often but not always found in the bone marrow aspirate. These measure 20 to 80 microns in width, are rounded or polyhedral in contour, and may contain several nuclei eccentrically placed. Their cytoplasm, which appears finely wrinkled, stains faintly or not at all with fat stains; chemical study shows the cells to be rich in the cerebroside known as kerasin.

Patients with florid Gaucher's disease have widespread involvement of organs with these abnormal cells. Survey of the parents and siblings by bone marrow studies sometimes reveals that several other members of the family, though superficially well, are carrying these Gaucher cells in their marrow in small numbers.

A few scattered Gaucher cells usually induce no other changes in the bone marrow, whereas a heavy proliferation may crowd the normal maturing cells. Very often the hypertrophied spleen induces a generalized bone marrow hyperplasia by a hypersplenism mechanism, with coincidental depression of the cellular elements of the peripheral blood.

Reticuloendothelial Granulomas

The best opinion at this time prefers to interpret what were once deemed three separate diseases as progressively severe grades of the same fundamental but obscure process. Eosinophilic granuloma, occurring most often in bone, is deemed the most benign form; Hand-Schüller-Christian disease as somewhat more advanced; and Letterer-Siwe disease as the most severe and malignantly progressive. There is considerable overlapping in the histologic features displayed by these three conditions. Some patients may show lesions characteristic of two or even of all three in different portions of the body or at different times.

EOSINOPHILIC GRANULOMA OF BONE. The skeletal lesions, which may be single or multiple, are characterized histologically by granulomatous accumulations made up of reticuloendothelial cells, multinuclear giant cells, fibroblasts, and eosinophils. The reticuloendothelial cells infrequently contain small lipid deposits. The eosinophils are numerous at the beginning, but disappear as the lesions become older. The diagnosis is best made by surgical biopsy of an affected area of bone as found on roentgen study.

HAND-SCHÜLLER-CHRISTIAN DISEASE. In this disorder, slowly progressive destructive lesions may develop in almost any bone of the skeleton. The typical lesion is a granuloma made up of large reticuloendothelial cells, eosinophils, foreign body giant cells, and scar tissue. The reticuloendothelial cells become distended with cholesterol and other lipids, which gives them a foamy appearance; mitoses may be numerous. As the lesions age they become necrotic and hemorrhagic, and lipid may lie free in the tissues surrounded by monocytes with lipid-filled cytoplasm. Aspirated marrow from other parts of the skeleton in this disease and in eosinophilic granuloma usually shows no reticuloendothelial hyperplasia or xanthoma-like cells. Sometimes the process is extremely widespread, resembling Letterer-Siwe disease.

LETTERER-SIWE DISEASE. In this disorder the reticuloendothelial cells throughout the body, including the bone marrow, grow large and proliferate. These cells are round, oval, irregular, or polyhedral, with single small nuclei which are eccentric and vesicular. They typically are 10 to 30 μ in length. Their cytoplasm is pale-staining and faintly acidophilic and usually with no granules or lipid droplets. In the focal lesions of the bones and other structures they may be very numerous and accompanied by eosinophils or multinucleated giant cells suggestive of Hodgkin's disease.

Other Granulomatous Formations

Small organized granulomatous formations are found not infrequently in bone marrow particles in many disturbances, especially infectious mononucleosis, lupus erythematosus, syphilis, erythema nodosum, acute and chronic infectious diseases, and the various blood dyscrasias. They are especially prevalent in patients with lymphocytic disorders of the malignant lymphoma class. There is a background of proliferating reticulum cells and fibroblasts, with infiltration by variable numbers of lymphocytes, eosinophils, plasma cells, and other wandering cells. In tuberculosis and histoplasmosis the cellular arrangements may be sufficiently characteristic to permit a morphologic diagnosis. In Hodgkin's disease some of the larger cells may have the appearance of Reed-Sternberg cells.

UNORGANIZED DEPOSITS

Cystine Disease

The finding of cystine crytals in aspirated marrow is of great diagnostic value in suspected cases and probably the most rapid method of recognition of this disease. Crystals should be looked for in unstained marrow films, since otherwise many will dissolve and disappear in the process of staining. They are characteristically flat and hexagonal, but may be rectangular or irregular. They may occur as pillar formations like a pile of coins, either free in the tissues or imbedded in reticulum cells. Doubly refractile, they can be identified as cystine by testing for sulfur with an alkaline lead acetate solution (Sullivan's test). After alcohol extraction, they can be made to change from hexagonal shape into long needles grouped in bundles by addition of strong hydrochloric acid.

Hemosiderin

Hemosiderin is one of the two forms in which the iron reserves of the body are kept, the other being ferritin which is a soluble iron-protein complex not morphologically identifiable. In older children the amount of hemosiderin deposited in the marrow reticuloendothelium and other connective tissue elements is a rough indicator of the status of the iron reserves.

Fragments of marrow are secured by means of a broad puncture needle. About 4 ml of mixed marrow and blood is drawn into a 20-ml syringe containing 6 ml of 4 per cent sodium citrate. The mixture is ejected onto a large watch glass, from which marrow fragments are picked with a capillary pipet for microscope examination. On unstained slides under reduced illumination the hemosiderin stands out as discrete golden-yellow granules. On slides stained with potassium ferrocyanide and hydrochloric acid (Prussian blue reaction) the granules assume a blue color. The amount of iron is assessed as none, slight, moderate, heavy, and very heavy. Familiarity with the normal is essential. Anemic patients shown to have adequate or increased marrow hemosiderin by this method are less likely to be helped by iron therapy.

Amyloid

In amyloidosis the bone marrow aspirate may display rounded fragments of pink eosinophilic amorphous material, situated intra- or extracellularly.

BACTERIOLOGIC EXAMINATIONS

Marrow puncture can be utilized to search for organisms in obscure bacterial infections in which blood cultures have been negative. Success has been reported in the demonstration of the specific bacterium in typhoid fever, brucellosis, streptococcic septicemia, histoplasmosis, subacute bacterial endocarditis, lobar pneumonia, tuberculosis, and other infections. The superiority of this approach is attributable to the probability that in some if not all of these infections, organisms are viable despite being held within the reticuloendothelial cells and commence to multiply after these cells have lysed within the culture bottles.

PROTOZOAN DISEASES

Protozoan parasites are sometimes demonstrable in aspirated marrow when the peripheral blood seems free of their presence. This approach has been successful with kala-azar, malaria, trypanosomiasis, and toxoplasmosis. The parasites are largely contained in the reticuloendothelial cells. A concomitant proliferation of eosinophils is usually observed. When searching for protozoa a marrow puncture will give a higher percentage of positive results than splenic or hepatic puncture.

In chronic malaria the marrow shows many more sexual forms of the parasites than does the blood. In subtertian malaria the gametocytes may be numerous in the marrow though absent from the blood. Active mitosis may be observed as well. A granulocytic and an erythrocytic increase have also been described—the latter change in response to the anemia. Proliferation of rubricytes and prorubricytes may be suggestive of the findings in pernicious anemia. Gigantic band forms or hypersegmented leukocytes may appear.

MYCOTIC DISEASES

In generalized histoplasmosis the fungus parasites may be seen inside granulocytes, megakaryocytes, or enlarged reticuloendothelial cells and lying free in the tissue fluid as well. Focal bone lesions in actinomycosis, blastomycosis, and coccidioidomycosis will show the presence of the invading parasite, both intra- and extracellularly and singly or in small colonies.

Cultures of the bone marrow on special media for fungi and other mycotic organisms are often successful. Bone marrow is aspirated in the usual way from any of the bones and may be heparinized or citrated to prevent clotting. About 0.1 ml of the liquid material is permitted to flow over a Sabouraud slant or blood agar, and the preparation is incubated at room temperature. The organism usually grows out in 7 to 10 days and can be identified by its gross and microscopic appearances. At times, the colonies do not become evident until 3 or 4 weeks have passed.

INTRAMEDULLARY THERAPY

In situations where it is not feasible to use the intravenous route, therapeutic fluids or blood can be supplied by intramedullary administration. The sternum is a convenient site in patients older than 4 years of age. With infants and younger children the tibia or femur are the sites of choice, though the humerus or pelvic bones may be used. The same needles are utilized as for marrow aspiration.

Sequellae after intramedullary therapy may occur despite careful technique and surgical asepsis. Osteomyelitis, subcutaneous abscesses, arterial thrombosis, and mediastinitis (following intrasternal injections) have been described. The bone marrow approach is therefore not recommended for administration of parenteral fluids except in special difficulties such as circulatory collapse, unusable veins, unskilled personnel, or emergencies outside of hospitals where parenteral fluids are urgently needed.

MARROW TRANSPLANTS

Attempts have been made to transfer healthy bone marrow from normal donors into the medullary cavity of patients with blood dyscrasias. This has been done on an experimental basis with agranulocytosis and aplastic anemia, with equivocal results thus far. The same precautions as to sterility, blood group compatibility, and absence of infection in the donor are employed as when giving blood transfusions. The donor and recipient are placed on parallel tables near each other. Aspirating needles are introduced into the respective bony sites of both subjects. Five to ten milliliters of marrow are then withdrawn from the donor, sometimes from multiple sites, and injected immediately but slowly into the recipient. We have treated a child with congenital hypoplastic anemia by this method, with no benefit.

BONE MARROW EMBOLISM

Fragments of bone marrow as well as fat may be found in the branches of the pulmonary artery at postmortem examination following fracture or crushing injuries of the skeletal system.

BIBLIOGRAPHY

BONE MARROW INFILTRATIVE REACTIONS

Abt, A. F., and E. J. Denenholz, Letterer-Siwe's Disease: Splenohepatomegaly Associated with Widespread Hyperplasia of Nonlipoid-storing Macrophages: Discussion of So-called Reticulo-endothelioses, Am. J. Dis. Child. 51:499, 1936.

Blanchard, A. J., and F. H. Boone, Reticuloendothelial Granulomatosis: Report of Two Cases of Hand-Schüller-Christian Disease, Am. J. Dis. Child. 76:1, 1948.

Canmann, M. F., Niemann-Pick's Disease, J. Pediat. 24:335, 1944.

Havard, E., L. J. Rather, and H. K. Faber, Nonlipoid Reticuloendotheliosis (Letterer-Siwe's Disease), Pediatrics 5:474, 1950.

Jaffe, H. L., and L. Lichtenstein, Eosinophilic Granuloma of Bone, Arch. Path. 37:99, 1944.

Klingberg, W. G., Generalized Histoplasmosis in Infants and Children, J. Pediat. 36:728, 1950.

Pease, G. L., The Significance of Granulomatous Lesions in Bone Marrow Aspirations, Am. J. Clin. Path. 22:107, 1952.

Rath, C. E., and C. A. Finch, Sternal Marrow Hemosiderin: A Method for the Determination of Available Iron Stores in Man, J. Lab. & Clin. Med. 39:946, 1951.

Reed, J., and M. C. Sosman, Gaucher's Disease, Radiology 38:579, 1942.

Schafer, E. L., Non-lipid Reticulo-endotheliosis—Letterer-Siwe's Disease: Report of Three Cases, *Am. J. Path.* 25:49, 1949.

Schmid, R., and *C. J. Watson,* A Study of the Prophyrins of Bone Marrow and Liver in the Various Forms of Porphyria, *J. Lab. & Clin. Med.* 38:946, 1951.

Smith, C. H., and *W. R. Bell,* Aminopterin in Treatment of Leukemia in Children: Serial Aspirations of Bone Marrow as a Guide to Management and Appraisal of Treatment, *Am. J. Dis. Child.* 79:1031, 1950.

CHAPTER 28

Urine: Physical Characteristics

Unsuspected irregularities are uncovered by urine analysis often enough to warrant carrying out this procedure at least once a year with every child. Abnormalities point the way for further investigations, but normal findings are equally significant for ruling out possible disorders. With presumably well children the so-called "routine urine analysis" should include tests for (1) color, (2) specific gravity, (3) pH, (4) protein, (5) sugar, (6) acetone, and (7) microscopic sediment. With ill or hospitalized children, additional tests can be made for the distinctive substances which may be excreted in the disease or diseases whose presence is being looked for (Table 28-1).

Urine should be tested as soon as possible after voiding. The lapse of a few hours can be sufficient for partial or complete lysis of casts and of erythrocytes or other cells which may be present, for bacterial decomposition of some of the urea to ammonia, and for conversion of urobilinogen to urobilin. If delay is unavoidable the urine should be collected in a sterile container and stored in a refrigerator.

SECURING URINE SPECIMENS FROM INFANTS AND CHILDREN

There are a score of devices and schemes for the collection of urine specimens from children too young to void voluntarily into a specimen bottle. An older infant can be left on a toilet or high chair with a hollow seat and a wide pan placed underneath to catch the urine as it comes. With younger infants a test tube or bottle can be slipped over the penis, or a wide-mouthed bottle or a feeding receptacle of the type used in bird cages placed over the vulva, and bound in place by adhesive tape until a sample is collected. It is most important beforehand to clean all smegma and debris from under the foreskin and around the labia. Infants can often be made to void by placing them supine on a cold surface such as an examining table.

Continuous urine collections from infants, as in metabolism studies, are done more easily with males. The infant is restrained in a sitting or supine position, with one end of a flexible tube strapped on the penis by adhesive or held in place by a belt around the abdomen. The other end of the tube leads to a bottle hung below the level of the mattress.

Table 28-1. Abnormal Urinary Substances in Specific Disturbances

Prominent symptom or suspected disease	Substances which may be found in the urine
Abnormal color	Assorted metabolic pigments
Anemia	Urobilinogen
Calculus in genitourinary tract	Crystals, stone fragments, red cells
Coma	Glucose, acetone bodies, barbiturates, findings of nephritis
Cystinosis	Protein, glucose, excess amino acids
Cystinuria	Cystine crystals
Cytomegalic inclusion disease	Epithelial cells containing inclusion bodies
Diabetes mellitus	Glucose, acetone, diacetic acid
Genitourinary tract infection	Leukocytes, red cells, protein, bacteria, occasional casts
Hemosiderosis of kidney	Cells containing hemosiderin granules
Hyperparathyroidism	Calcium-containing casts
Intravascular hemolysis	Free hemoglobin, hemoglobin casts
Jaundice, liver disease	Bilirubin, urobilinogen, bile salts
Lead poisoning	Coproporphyrin, protein, casts, glucose, excess amino acids
Mental deficiency (one variety)	Phenylpyruvic acid
Nephritis (various forms)	Red cells, leukocytes, casts, protein, bacteria
Nondiabetic mellituria	Pentose, fructose, galactose, higher sugars
Oxalosis	Calcium oxalate crystals
Photosensitive skin rash	Porphyrins, porphyrinogens
Renal tubular dysfunction	Abnormal amino acids, glucose or other sugars

Catheterization should be avoided when securing specimens for routine urine studies because of the danger of starting an infection if some urinary tract anomaly is present. Should catheterization be necessary, it must always be done with strict aseptic precautions. The major indications are (1) to procure an uncontaminated sample of female urine for bacteriologic study, (2) to rule out vaginitis in girls whose voided urine contains pus cells, (3) to measure residual urine volume when this is urologically indicated, and (4) to secure accurately timed and measured specimens during renal function tests.

THE URINARY SOLIDS

The urine is 90 to 98 per cent water. With seven of Macy's children, 8 to 12 years of age, the mean ratio between water and total urinary solids was approximately 19:1 (882.46 gm). The mean energy value per day was 92 calories; of this, 51 calories, or 55 per cent, was in the urea.

Of the dissolved solids roughly three-fourths are products of protein metabolism—urea, ammonia, uric acid, creatine, creatinine, and other nitrogen- or sulfur-containing compounds. The mean daily excretions per day for a large group of children were as follows (Macy):

	mg			mg	
Ammonia	290 ±	90	Creatinine	221 ±	64
			Undetermined nitrog-		
Urea	8,074 ±	1,597	enous products	461 ±	382
Uric Acid	132 ±	22	Inorganic sulfate	643 ±	36
Creatine	133 ±	74	Ethereal sulfate	48 ±	12

The remaining urinary solids, apart from trace amounts of pigment and miscellaneous other substances, are mineral salts, largely ionized.

The higher the rate of urine flow, the lower the concentration of solids. Hot weather reduces the volume and raises the concentration, whereas diuretic substances and emotional states have the opposite effect.

NORMAL DAILY VOLUME

In infancy, 150 to 500 ml per 24 hours is the usual spread of the total 24-hour urinary volume, though it may be as little as 20 ml per day in normal newborn infants before oral fluids are given. In a series of children aged 3 to 15 years on unrestricted diets studied by Macy, the total daily output ranged from 150 to 2,100 ml with a mean of 948 ml.

The amount of the individual voidings is highly variable, of course, with age being a major factor. Young infants may excrete as little as 5 or 10 ml at a time. Above 4 years of age the usual child will accumulate 300 to 500 ml of urine before insisting on voiding, with girls being able to retain much more than boys. In children with nocturnal enuresis, however, the habitual capacity is often much less than 300 ml.

The total daily excretion can become almost nil in dehydrative states or mount to many liters in diabetes insipidus. In acute nephritis the secretion of urine may become scanty or even cease altogether for a few days at the peak of symptoms; then, coincident with recovery, the urine flow for a time may be exceptionally abundant. In nephrosis the flow is usually scanty save for occasional bouts of diuresis. In chronic glomerulonephritis the daily output lies at or above that for normal children.

SPECIFIC GRAVITY

This is the most practical approach to determining the concentration of solids in urine. In healthy infants the specific gravity ordinarily varies from 1.001 to 1.026. In healthy children above 1 or 2 years of age the ceiling rises to approximately 1.032, and occasionally to 1.035. Higher concentrations may be attained in early infancy when normal kidneys are placed under severe strain (Pratt, Bienvenu, and Whyte).

Noting the maximum that specific gravity can attain when water intake is restricted while the usual urinary solute load is being delivered to it is one of the simplest and best means of estimating renal function.

Solutes cannot be concentrated efficiently when renal function is inadequate. One of the best tests for renal function is to withhold fluids for 12 or more hours and observe how concentrated the urine will become. A reading in the range from 1.026 and 1.032 in a urine specimen free from abnormalities is an almost unfailing sign that renal function is good. Minor degrees of parenchymal damage, or constitutional disturbances such as fever or dehydration, will result in inability to concentrate urine over 1.024 in young children, as a rule. With untreated diabetes insipidus, of pituitary or renal origin (p. 423), the specific gravity of the urine is ordinarily between 1.001 and 1.004 and almost never above 1.006.

Small infants when ill do not concentrate solutes to any great extent. With diarrhea or vomiting or diminished fluid intake, or when they are given large amounts of salt solution parenterally, the urinary specific gravity tends to remain low even though the output be scanty.

In active sickle cell anemia, because of a defect of unknown nature, the kidneys are unable to excrete as concentrated or as dilute a urine as the normal. Random urine specimens from such children generally fall between 1.006 and 1.016.

Abnormal urinary constituents if in any abundance may raise the specific gravity. Each 1 per cent of protein in urine increases the specific gravity reading by approximately 0.003. Each 1 per cent of glucose increases the reading by approximately 0.004, explaining why values up to 1.050 may be encountered in poorly treated diabetes mellitus.

In the early stages of acute nephritis the urine, though of scanty volume, may have a high specific gravity as the result of a high content of nitrogenous components, including protein. In chronic nephritis the combination of a low daily output and a low specific gravity indicates very severe kidney damage.

Determination of Specific Gravity of Small Amounts of Urine

Diminutive urinometers and similar devices are available for measurement of specific gravity when only a few milliliters can be procured.

After the other tests are done (with proper reagents it is not difficult to carry out a complete urine analysis using one or two drops for each constituent test), the amount left over may be measured and placed in the smallest available urinometer cylinder. A measured amount of distilled water is added, enough to float the spindle and permit a reading to be taken. Multiplying the last two figures of the reading by the ratio of the total volume after addition of water to the initial volume before dilution gives an approximation of the original specific gravity.

Another maneuver, more efficient for a busy laboratory, is to prepare an appropriate set of mixtures of organic solvents which are immiscible with water (Table 28-2). A single drop of urine is added to these mixtures, individually placed in clear glass bottles. The one in which the drop neither floats nor sinks indicates the specific gravity. Interpolation is sometimes necessary.

Table 28-2. Composition of Mixtures of Organic Solvents Used for Determining Specific Gravity of Urine

Specific gravity	Xylene, ml	Brombenzine, ml
1.005	75	22.5
1.010	75	23.5
1.015	75	24.5
1.020	75	25
1.025	75	27
1.030	75	28
1.035	75	29
1.040	75	30
1.050	75	32
1.060	75	35

These mixtures are prepared freshly every day or two and placed in clean glass jars or tubes. They are kept tightly corked between tests.

OSMOTIC PRESSURE

The osmotic pressure exerted by the urine reflects its content of ionized and non-ionized solutes, chiefly electrolytes and urea. Electrometric and other devices are available for measuring this characteristic, based on the principle of freezing-point depression. Determining the urine osmotic pressure after some hours of water deprivation is actually a physiologically sounder approach to the investigation of renal concentrating power than is the specific-gravity reading, but technical reasons have kept the osmotic pressure from being widely used.

The unit of osmotic pressure exerted in water by one mole of non-ionized solute is known as an osmol (Osm). A milliosmol (mOsm) is one one-thousandth of an osmol. Electrolytes which split into two ions exert an osmotic pressure equivalent to twice the molar value.

The upper limit of solute concentration by the healthy child is 1,200 to 1,400 mOsm per liter, corresponding roughly to a specific gravity of 1.032 to 1.034. This is nearly fourfold that of the osmotic pressure of the plasma. In kidney diseases, and in circulatory and other generalized disturbances in which renal function is reduced, the solute concentration may fall to the neighborhood of 400 mOsm per liter, corresponding roughly to a specific gravity of 1.010.

HYDROGEN-ION CONCENTRATION

The ionic balance among the mineral and organic metabolites cast off by the kidney determines the pH of the urine. The physiologic limits for urinary pH are about 4.5 on the acid side and 8.4 on the alkaline side. It is not possible to force the pH beyond these limits by giving large amounts of acid- or alkali-forming substances.

The average American diet is nearly neutral in ionic content, but the body metabolism tends to result in an excess of anions. Because of this, and because more cations than anions are excreted into the feces, the urine in infancy and childhood is ordinarily acid in character.

In the 112 normal boys and girls 3 to 15 years of age followed hourly for 24 hours by Kenyon, Wilson, and Macy, the urinary pH fluctuated between 4.8 and 8.4 and averaged 6.0 for the entire series of specimens. The urine of infants fed breast milk exclusively is about pH 7.0, whereas the urine of infants fed cow's milk is more acid.

Change to alkaline urine takes place (1) with foods rich in alkaline ash, such as oranges, (2) after vomiting of hydrochloric acid–containing gastric juice, as in pyloric stenosis, (3) in response to hyperventilation, or (4) after ingestion of salts of strong bases and weak acids, such as the citrate, bicarbonate, or lactate salts of potassium or sodium. Conversely, salts of strong acids and weak bases such as the chloride or sulfate of ammonium, calcium, or magnesium have a urine-acidifying effect. These salts can give rise to systemic acidosis when given in larger amounts than the kidneys can handle.

In upsets of acid-base equilibrium within the body the urinary pH reflects the attempt by the kidney to correct the disturbance. In alkalosis the urine is generally alkaline, while in acidosis it is on the acid side. This rule has so many exceptions, however, that it is not safe to regulate the acid-base content of intravenous fluids by following the pH of the urine.

NEWBORN URINE

Thomson's studies of normal newborns, fluid intake unspecified, showed the following average characteristics:

	1	2	3	4	5	6	7	8	9
					Age in days				
Volume (ml)	19.5	20.6	36.	64.8	103.3	124.5	146.6	151.	175.4
Specific gravity	1.012	1.015	1.013	1.010	1.009	1.009	1.009	1.008	1.008
pH	5.7	5.8	6.1	6.2	6.4	6.4	6.5	6.5	6.5
Urea (mg per 100 ml)	670	956	690	497	324	286	272	282	250

BIBLIOGRAPHY

PHYSICAL CHARACTERISTICS

Corcoran, A. C., Electrometric Urinometry: A Note on Comparative Determinations of Urinary Osmolarity and Specific Gravity, J. Lab. & Clin. Med. 46:141, 1955.

Darrow, D. C., R. E. Cooke, and W. E. Segar, Water and Electrolyte Metabolism in Infants Fed Cow's Milk Mixtures during Heat Stress, Pediatrics 14:602, 1954.

Dean, R. F. A., and *R. A. McCance,* Renal Responses of Infants and Adults to the Administration of Hypertonic Solutions of Sodium Chloride and Urea, *J. Physiol.* **109**:81, 1949.

Dogramaci, I., Measuring the Specific Gravity of Small Amounts of Urine, *J. Pediat.* **30**:672, 1947.

Eggleton, M. G., Some Factors Affecting Acidity of Urine in Man, *J. Physiol.* **106**:456, 1947.

Hawks, J. E., M. M. Bray, and *M. Dye,* Effects of Diet on Constancy of Urinary Nitrogen Constituents Excreted Daily by Pre-school Children, *J. Nutrition* **13**:179, 1937.

Kenyon, F., C. A. Wilson, and *I. G. Macy,* Daily Fluctuations in Urinary pH, *Arch. Pediat.* **51**:490, 1934.

Kunz, H. W., E. L. Pratt, G. W. Mellin, and *M. W. Cheung,* Impairment of Urinary Concentration in Sickle Cell Anemia, *Pediatrics* **13**:352, 1954.

Macy, I. G., "Nutrition and Chemical Growth in Childhood," vol. I, Charles C Thomas, Springfield, Ill., 1942.

McCance, R. A., and *M. A. von Finck,* The Titratable Acidity pH, Ammonia and Phosphates in the Urines of Very Young Infants, *Arch. Dis. Childhood* **22**:200, 1947.

Newberry, N., and *J. J. Van Wyk,* A Technique for Quantitative Urine Collection in the Metabolic Study of Infants and Young Children, *Pediatrics* **16**:667, 1955.

Poncher, H. G., and *J. C. Ricewasser,* Quantitative Collection of Urine from Infants and Young Children, *J. Pediat.* **20**:759, 1942.

Pratt, E. L., B. Bienvenu, and *M. M. Whyte,* Concentration of Urine Solutes by Young Infants, *Pediatrics* **1**:181, 1948.

Shohl, A. T., "Mineral Metabolism," Reinhold Publishing Corporation, New York, 1939.

Smith, H. W., "The Kidney: Structure and Function in Health and Disease," Oxford University Press, New York, 1951.

Thomson, J., (a) Observations on the Urine of the New-born Infant, *Arch. Dis. Childhood* **19**:169, 1944. (b) Urinalysis in Dehydration Fever, *Arch. Dis. Childhood* **22**:226, 1947.

Wolman, I. J., Urine Analysis in Pediatrics: Ten Years' Progress, *Am. J. M. Sc.* **208**:767, 1944.

Yun-Chen, M. K., and *M. M. Steiner,* Diabetes Insipidus in Infancy Resistant to Pitressin, *Pediatrics* **12**:400, 1953.

CHAPTER 29

Urinary Pigments

UROCHROME

The color of normal urine, ranging from straw to yellow-brown, reflects its content of the obscure pigment urochrome which is always being excreted. Every urine specimen with a color different from that of urochrome should be subjected to special tests for identification of the pigment.

The 24-hour output of urochrome by a healthy individual is approximately the same from day to day, indicating its derivation from endogenous metabolism rather than from food or other sources. The rate of excretion goes up in fever, hyperthyroidism, starvation states, and other conditions which elevate metabolism or accelerate tissue breakdown. Administration of acids may enhance the excretion temporarily, whereas alkalis cause it to diminish. The comparative constancy of excretion per unit of time explains why dilute urine produced during diuresis is pale in color and why concentrated specimens of high specific gravity are much darker. Measurements of urochrome output show such good correlation with other estimations of basal metabolism that the rate of excretion has been proposed as a measure of basal metabolism.

ANTHOCYANIN

The redness of urine which occasionally follows the feeding of red beets is due to anthocyanin, the principal substance of the beet. This pigment can be quickly differentiated from hemoglobin by adding potassium or sodium hydroxide to the urine. The color becomes deep yellow when alkalinized and reverts to the original red when reacidified.

Anthocyanuria is almost never seen beyond babyhood. It appears most often in infants of a few months of age after their first few feedings of puréed beets.

UROBILINOGEN AND UROBILIN

Urobilin represents a mixture of bilirubin derivatives which give fluorescence in solutions of alcoholic zinc acetate (Schlesinger's test).

348

Some of these derivatives are voided as urobilinogen, but become converted within a few hours to urobilin on exposure to light and air.

Urobilinogen and its derivatives originate from the bilirubin of the bile which is excreted into the intestinal tract and there acted upon by the colon bacteria. In healthy subjects whose liver is functioning properly, the intestinal urobilinogen is picked up by the mucosa, carried to the liver by the portal circulation, and reexcreted into the bile. Only when urobilinogen is being brought to the liver in extraordinary amounts, or when this organ has been injured or is otherwise functioning poorly, will enough excess escape in the general circulation to be excreted by the kidney. The rate of production increases when hemoglobin catabolism and bilirubin excretion are increased. Urobilinogenuria can thus be a manifestation of liver cell insufficiency, excessive hemolysis, or both. Indeed, in most hemolytic disorders the hypoxia caused by the anemia itself induces imperfect liver function. In liver or bile duct disturbances which hamper the flow of bile into the intestine, and in the anemias accompanied by a slowed rate of blood destruction, the intestinal production of urobilinogen is diminished.

The scanty amount of urobilinogen which may be found in normal urine produces no color recognized with the unaided eye. When in excess it may impart a pink tint to the urine.

The test for urobilinogen is easier to perform than the test for urobilin and leads to more consistent results in quantitative studies. This reagent contains 2 gm per 100 ml of para-dimethylaminobenzaldehyde (Ehrlich's reagent) in 20 per cent hydrochloric acid. With the Wallace and Diamond modification, progressive dilutions of urine and water are prepared in a row of test tubes, each tube containing 5 ml. The test solution is then added in 0.5-ml amounts, and the tubes inspected after 5 minutes. The color reaction is pink when weakly positive, red when strongly positive. A pink tint in dilutions of 1:10 to 1:20 of concentrated urine is interpreted as still within normal limits. Positive reactions may be given also by indole, skatole, and the porphobilinogen which is characteristic of acute porphyria. The urine should be tested while fresh and preferably while still warm.

Most of the urobilinogen produced in the intestine is excreted into the stools. The urinary output normally constitutes only about 5 per cent of all that is formed. During infancy and early childhood this is usually less than 2 mg daily; in later years and puberty, less than 6 mg. These comparatively negligible amounts escape detection in the usual urine tests.

With anemias of hemolytic origin the total production of urobilinogen increases strikingly and is often twenty to thirty times the normal. The ratio between stool and urine urobilin remains about the same as in normals. Random specimens of urine give a positive reaction except when highly dilute.

In the presence of severe liver damage, the proportion of urinary to fecal urobilin may rise to 10 to 20 per cent or higher. Should blood destruction and liver function be only mildly altered, as occurs often in bacterial infections, an increased stool content of urobilinogen may be the sole indicator of excessive hemodestruction, with the urinary output remaining within normal limits.

The output of urine urobilinogen even when increased is erratic and irregular from hour to hour and day to day, in response presumably to fluctuations in the activity of the liver.

It is wise, when searching for urobilinogenuria in a patient suspected of having undue hemolysis, to repeat the test daily for several days and preferably with 24-hour specimens. Each day's urine should be collected in a brown bottle containing 5 gm of sodium carbonate to keep it alkaline and 40 ml of petroleum ether to protect from oxidation. Bilirubin if concomitantly present can be removed by mixing a portion of the urine with an equal volume of 10 per cent barium chloride solution. The precipitated barium is filtered off, and the test performed on the filtrate.

In the early stages of viral hepatitis the urobilinogen output is increased, reflecting initial involvement of the parenchyma. If the disease progresses so that bile is no longer excreted into the stools, the urine urobilinogen will disappear completely. Later, during recovery, it may or may not return in excess.

The excretion of urobilinogen in the stool and urine after transfusion with stored blood is directly proportional to the length of blood storage and becomes prominent with blood more than a week old.

The urinary urobilinogen test may be of assistance when tracking down the cause of jaundice in the first few months of life. Infants with complete congenital block of the biliary channels excrete urine free from urobilinogen, whereas infants with hemolytic disorders or partially damaged liver cells usually have an augmented excretion. Unfortunately for this argument, infants with excessive hemodestruction or with hepatitis may pass through a phase of full hepatocellular obstruction during which urobilinogen formation and excretion also fall temporarily to zero (inspissated bile syndrome).

BILIRUBIN

Bilirubin appears in the urine in detectable concentrations whenever the serum bilirubin becomes sufficiently elevated. With an elevated 1-minute serum level (p. 477) the threshold for renal passage seems to be at or above 1.6 mg bilirubin per 100 ml. When only the 30-minute reading is elevated the threshold is variably higher. Coincident retention of bile salts seems to facilitate diffusibility.

Para-aminosalicylic acid (PAS) gives a strong color reaction with

Ehrlich's aldehyde reagent. Urine from children with tuberculosis who are receiving aminosalicylic acid may accordingly appear to contain urobilinogen.

Tests for Bilirubin

The familiar nitric acid and iodine ring tests often react with other substances unrelated to bilirubin. They are useful in routine urine analysis as screening tests, but positive reactions should be confirmed with a diazo spot test (see below).

The quantitative methylene blue test for bile pigment in urine is performed by first diluting 5 ml of urine (preferably prebreakfast) with 20 ml of tap water, and then adding 0.2 per cent of fresh methylene blue chloride solution, drop by drop. The first drop or two change the urine color to green, and subsequent drops bring out a blue color. Normal urine will attain blue color after 2 to 3 drops. When 5 drops or more is needed the reaction is interpreted as positive. Stokes, Gambill, and Osterberg found this methylene blue test to become positive at a minimal concentration of 2.0 mg bilirubin per 100 ml of urine. Gmelin's nitric acid test was slightly more sensitive, with a threshold level of 1.7 mg per 100 ml.

The methylene blue test is usually strongly positive in the preicteric stage of infectious hepatitis, while the serum bilirubin is still in the normal zone, and remains positive throughout the acute phase of the disease. The degree of positivity of the test in jaundiced patients runs parallel to the clinical disturbance, so that the test can be of value in following the progress of recognized cases. It often becomes negative during the convalescent period while the serum bilirubin is still elevated. Misleadingly positive results may be given by concentrated oliguric specimens, ammoniacal urine, and the excretory end products of penicillin, riboflavin, Atabrine (quinacrine), or vitamin B complex.

The diazo spot tests are the most specific and sensitive, particularly when carried out in conjunction with concentration measures such as selective adsorption by barium chloride, calcium chloride, or talc. With concentration methods positive tests may be obtained with urines containing as little as 0.025 mg bilirubin per 100 ml. At very low concentrations the test becomes difficult to read.

Procedure for Harrison diazo spot test for bilirubin.

1. To 10 ml of acid urine add 5 ml 10 per cent barium chloride solution. If urine is alkaline, acidify with a few drops of weak glacial acetic acid. Strain through filter paper.

2. Wash precipitate with 10 ml of 0.2 per cent barium chloride solution.

3. Unfold filter paper; spread on paper towel.

4. Add one or two drops of Fouchet's reagent. Bile pigment is present if precipitate turns blue, blue-green, or green.

5. Readings vary from 1 plus to 4 plus, depending upon the intensity of the color and the rapidity of its appearance.

BILE ACIDS AND SALTS

Cholic and tauric acids also appear in the urine in obstructive jaundice and in the more severe cases of infectious hepatitis. During recovery from hepatitis the bilirubin often disappears from the urine while the bile salt excretion and the clinical icterus are still persisting. Bile acids are not easy to test for, but their presence may be inferred when excess foam follows shaking of the specimen.

Hay's test is widely used for this purpose: Sprinkle a pinch of finely powdered sulfur (flowers of sulfur) on the surface of cold urine in a bottle or test tube. Immediate sinking of the sulfur suggests a concentration of bile acids of 0.01 per cent or more; sinking after mild shaking, between 0.0025 and 0.01 per cent. Bile salts are absent if the sulfur floats.

ALKAPTON BODIES

Alkaptonuria is a rare asymptomatic anomaly of tyrosine and phenylalanine metabolism in which some homogentisic acid is excreted in the urine. This substance, colorless itself, oxidizes on standing to become brown and then black. In enuretics the wet bed linen turns dark after some hours have passed. Should pigmentation of the sclera and ears develop, with or without arthritis, the condition is known as ochronosis.

Homogentisic acid reacts with hydroquinone. When a drop of urine which has been made alkaline is placed on sensitized photographic paper the paper promptly becomes black. This does not happen with normal urine. Homogentisic acid reacts with Fehling's and Benedict's solutions, but not with alkaline bismuth reagents, and is not fermented by yeast.

When the urine is clear, the adding of 10 per cent sodium hydroxide solution brings out a brownish-black ring at the surface which gradually penetrates downward. Ferric chloride solution evokes a transitory blue color with each drop, and silver lactate or ammoniacal silver nitrate turns rapidly black. Specific methods are available for quantitative estimation.

HEMOGLOBIN

Free hemoglobin will appear in the urine to give it a red or dark-brown color in renal infarction or whenever red cells are being broken down within the circulation rapidly enough to raise the plasma content above the approximately 100-mg level which is the renal threshold for hemoglobin. With rapid hemodestruction an immediate sequel may be anuria with symptoms of anemia and shock. The anuria is now believed to be due to necrosis of portions of the renal tubular epithelium. Hemoglobin-containing casts are excreted during recovery.

The urine will be dark red, purple, brown, or brownish black, depending on the proportions of oxyhemoglobin (red), bilirubin (yellow), methemoglobin (chocolate brown), and reduced hemoglobin (black) which are present. The hand spectroscope will reveal the characteristic absorption spectra when the quantity is sufficient to give a decided color to the urine. Or the photoelectric colorimetric method of Evelyn and Mallory may be utilized. To exclude red cell hemolysis outside of the body, the urine specimen should be examined soon after being passed and have a specific gravity above 1.007. The benzidine and orthotolidine tests will detect free hemoglobin if over 150 mg per 100 ml and will not react with bilirubin or urobilinogen (p. 706).

MELANIN

Malignant melanomas are extremely rare before puberty. When they occur they may be associated with the urinary excretion of dark brown or brownish-black melanin. If the pigment is in the colorless precursor state known as melanogen, the urine will turn dark when exposed to light for some days or when ferric chloride solution is added. The giving of thiouracil to melanuric patients may stop for a time the excretion of pigment, presumably by inhibiting melanin formation within the tumor itself.

PORPHYRINS

The porphyrins are a family of stable metal-binding pigments derived from porphin, which is a heterocyclic compound composed of four pyrrole rings united by methene bridges. Hemoglobin, myoglobin, cytochrome, catalase, and peroxidase are built up of combinations of protoporphyrin III with iron and other substances.

The porphyrin pigments are reddish brown in alkaline solution, purple or reddish violet when dissolved in mineral acids, and dull red in organic acid solutions. They give a reddish fluorescence in ultraviolet light.

Coproporphyrins and uroporphyrins in microgram quantities can be detected by highly sensitive methods in the urine of all normal subjects. The coproporphyrin in normal urine is excreted largely as a colorless precursor or chromogen, which Schwartz, Ziene, and Watson have found to be fully convertible to the pigmented fluorescent form by an iodine solution if the urine as soon as passed is made alkaline by added sodium carbonate.

The term *porphyrinuria* is applied to those situations in which a coproporphyrin with perhaps a little uroporphyrin is excreted in excess of normal. Porphyrinuria of mild degree often develops in hemorrhagic states, sickle cell anemia, hereditary spherocytosis, pellagra, severe infections, liver diseases, lead poisoning, poliomyelitis, acute rheumatic fever, disseminated lupus erythematosus, rheumatoid arthritis, and after diverse drugs and anesthetics.

Porphyria is a rare constitutional error of porphyrin metabolism in which abnormal uroporphyrin is formed and excreted.

Of the various classifications of porphyria the simplest is that which lists two types: (1) the congenital or erythropoietic form, (2) the acquired or hepatic form. The first is seen most commonly in childhood and may subside during adolescence (p. 92). The other does not ordinarily begin until the adult age period; while perhaps also of congenital origin it is only occasionally associated with sensitivity to light.

Children with congenital porphyria will early in life exhibit photosensitivity of the skin with blistering, necrosis and scarring, gastrointestinal pain, hirsutism, and familial occurrence. Exacerbations may be precipitated by exposure to a toxic factor, such as lead, barbital, Trional, sulfonal, acetanilid, nitrobenzol, sulfonamides, or other drugs. The urine tends to be pink, wine red, or dark brown; if colorless when passed it darkens on standing. The blood serum, teeth, and urine may exhibit red or reddish-orange fluorescence in ultraviolet light. Along with the porphyrins the urine may contain melanin, urofuscin, and other colored substances. Siblings, parents, and other members of the family should be investigated also as possible asymptomatic cases of the disorder. Several instances have been recorded of an entirely symptomless idiopathic coproporphyrinuria (isomer III).

Several infants have been reported, born to mothers with clinical porphyria, who had "passive porphyrinuria." The porphyrinuria was asymptomatic, lasted only a few days, and was believed to be due to placental transmission of porphyrins and their precursors.

Tests for Porphyrins

At times the porphyrins are excreted in a precursor or porphobilinogen state and may not be evident at first. In such cases the color is brought out by permitting the urine to stand in the light or by adding an oxidizing agent. Watson and Schwartz's test for porphobilinogen is indicated here:

Equal parts of urine and modified Ehrlich's reagent are mixed in a test tube. An equal volume of saturated solution of zinc acetate is added. A few milliliters of chloroform is added and thoroughly mixed. The aldehyde compound of urobilinogen is removed by the chloroform, while that of porphobilinogen, insoluble in chloroform, remains in the supernatant and colors it red.

The presence of porphyrins in urine can be demonstrated with the aid of a simple spectroscope. Direct examination of a suitably deep layer of urine may show a two-banded absorption spectrum similar to that of oxyhemoglobin but due to a porphyrin-metal complex. Moreover, when a few drops of concentrated hydrochloric acid are added to the urine, this compound and free neutral porphyrin are converted into the acid porphyrin, which shows a band of medium width in the green dilute and another narrower and less intense band in the yellow when stronger. If a portion of the urine is acidified with acetic acid and shaken with ether, the coproporphyrin present will pass into the ether, which then exhibits a complex five-banded spectrum with one band in the red. Uroporphyrin will not dissolve in ether. Identification of the individual porphyrins is a complex technical procedure.

A simpler approach to diagnosis is direct inspection of fresh urine in ultraviolet light. A dermatologist's Wood's lamp such as is used for examination of the scalp for tinea capitis is satisfactory for this purpose. Normal urine in ultraviolet light has a greenish-blue or greenish-yellow fluorescence, possibly with a faint pinkish tint if highly concentrated or if containing trace amounts of coproporphyrin. When uroporphyrin is present the fluorescence will be pink red or red.

A fluorescence test for porphyrins should always be done when a patient has dermatologic, hematologic, or gastrointestinal symptoms suggestive of porphyria, or the urine is pink, red, or brown or assumes such a color on standing.

Lead Poisoning

The urinary content of coproporphyrin type III is often many times greater in lead poisoning than in normals. Coproporphyrin is searched for by extracting the urine with ether and examining it under ultraviolet light for fluorescence. One starts with either a 24-hour collection or, less preferably, a concentrated random specimen of urine. Unless the urine can be examined within a few hours after passage, a few drops of thymol should be added and the specimen stored in a cool dark place.

Five milliliters of urine is placed in a large test tube, and about 5 drops of chemically pure glacial acetic acid is run in, sufficient to make the specimen strongly acid. Five milliliters of ether is next added, and the mixture shaken vigorously. The ether layer is then scrutinized for reddish fluorescence under ultraviolet light in a dark room. The ultraviolet radiation must contain rays of wave length of 3,660 angstrom units else the coproporphyrin may not fluoresce.

The fluorescence varies in intensity from faint or doubtful pink to a very deep red, in proportion to the coproporphyrin and lead present. Johnson and Whitman found the fluorescent color to have semiquantitative significance, as follows:

	Coproporphyrin per liter (mg, approximately)	Mean values for lead (mg per liter)
Faint or doubtful pink	0.50	0.060
Pink	0.75	0.074
Strong pink to definite red	1.00	0.087
Red	1.25	0.100
Deep red	1.50	0.115
Very deep red	1.75	0.132

The data of Bradley and associates indicate that one-third of children with blood lead levels of 0.05 mg per 100 ml or higher (p. 975) may not exhibit coproporphyrins in single urine samples. Chisolm and Harrison have found that the urinary coproporphyrin output of children with symptoms of lead poisoning seems to be related to the concentration of lead in the soft body tissues.

HEMOSIDERIN

This iron-containing pigment may be found in the urine in small amounts in Mediterranean anemia, active sickle cell anemia, erythroblastosis fetalis, and other forms of chronic hemolytic anemia or hemochromatosis. It is apparently more prominent in paroxysmal nocturnal hemoglobinuria, a condition which may first become evident during adolescence (p. 101).

Urine may be tested for hemosiderin by the Prussian blue reaction. Fifteen milliliters of urine is centrifuged, and the sediment stirred up in 1 ml of the supernatant. To this is added 1 ml of 5 per cent hydrochloric acid and 0.5 ml of a 10 per cent aqueous solution of potassium ferrocyanide. Blue-stained hemosiderin granules may be found in casts, renal epithelial cells, or the amorphous sediment.

MYOGLOBIN

This is a red proteinous pigment which occurs in abundance in skeletal and cardiac muscle. A limited number of otherwise well individuals have been described who exhibited one or more paroxysmal crises of myoglobinuria, usually after extreme physical activity.

The typical paroxysm begins abruptly with weakness and pain in some muscles, malaise, fever, and the passage of dark-red or mahogany-brown urine. Renal damage may ensue, presumably from injury to the tubules. The myoglobin in the urine gives a positive reaction with the reagents for hemoglobin, but can be differentiated by spectroscopic analysis.

BIBLIOGRAPHY

UROCHROME

Drabkin, D., Normal Pigment of Urine: Relationship of Basal Metabolism to Output of Normal Urinary Pigment, J. Biol. Chem. 75:443, 481, 1927.

Fennel, E. A., Urinary BMR Determination, Proc. Staff Meet. The Clinic, Honolulu 17:51, 1951.

Ostow, M., and S. Philo, Chief Urinary Pigment: Relationship between Rate of Excretion of Yellow Urinary Pigment and Metabolic Rate, Am. J. M. Sc. 207:507, 1944.

Vorzimer, J., I. B. Cohen, and J. Joskow, The Use of Urinary Pigment Execretion for the Measurement of Basal Metabolic Rate, J. Lab. & Clin. Med. 34:482, 1949.

ANTHOCYANIN

Matheson, A., Anthocyaninuria, *Am. J. Dis. Child.* 51:226, 1936.
Poole, M. W., Anthocyaninuria: Report of a Case, *Am. J. Dis. Child.* 33:784, 1927.

UROBILINOGEN AND UROBILIN

Wasserman, L. R., M. Volterra, and *N. Rosenthal,* Quantitative Urobilinogen Execretion Following Transfusions of Stored and Fresh Blood, *Am. J. M. Sc.* 204:356, 1942.
Wilson, T. M., and *L. S. P. Davidson,* Ehrlich's Aldehyde Test for Urobilinogen, *Brit. M. J.* 1:884, 1949.

BILIRUBIN

Abbasy, A. S. A., Efficiency of Loeffler's Methylene Blue Test as a Liver Function Test, *Arch. Pediat.* 64:235, 1947.
Bryant, D., and *F. V. Flynn,* An Assessment of New Tests for Detecting Bilirubin in Urine, *J. Clin. Path.* 8:163, 1955.
Foord, A. G., and *C. F. Baisinger,* Comparison of Tests for Bilirubin in Urine, *Am. J. Clin. Path.* 10:238, 1940.
Franklin, M., New Tablet for Urinary Bilirubin, *J. Lab. & Clin. Med.* 34:1145, 1949.
Gellis, S. S., and *J. Stokes, Jr.,* The Methylene Blue Test in Infectious (Epidemic) Hepatitis, *J.A.M.A.* 128:782, 1945.
Klatskin, G., Some Observations on Liver Function Tests, *Yale J. Biol. & Med.* 21:127, 1946.
Stokes, G. D., E. E. Gambill, and *A. E. Osterberg,* Methylene Blue Test for Bilirubinuria: Clinical and Spectrophotometric Observations, *J. Lab. & Clin. Med.* 37:924, 1946.
Watson, C. J., The Bile Pigments, *New England J. Med.* 227:665, 705, 1942.
―――, Some Newer Concepts of the Natural Derivatives of Hemoglobin; General Considerations; Serum Bilirubin and Bilirubinuria; Erythrocyte Protoporphyrin, *Blood* 1:99, 1946.

ALKAPTON BODIES

Baldwin, E., "Dynamic Aspects of Biochemistry," Macmillan & Co., Ltd., London, 1947.
Haldane, J. B. F., "New Paths in Genetics," George Allen & Unwin, Ltd., London, 1942.
Mauser, C. L., Alkaptonuria, *J.A.M.A.* 146:815, 1951.
Medes, G., New Error of Tyrosine Metabolism; Tyrosinosis; the Intermediary Metabolism of Tyrosine and Phenylalanine, *Biochem. J.* 26:917, 1932.
Neuberger, A., C. Rimington, and *J. M. G. Wilson,* Studies on Alcaptonuria: Investigations on Case of Human Alcaptonuria, *Biochem. J.* 41:438, 1947.

HEMOGLOBIN

Crosby, H. W., and *W. Dameshek,* The Significance of Hemoglobinemia and Associated Hemosiderinuria, with Particular Reference to Various Types of Hemolytic Anemia, *J. Lab. & Clin. Med.* 38:829, 1951.
Ham, T. H., Hemoglobinuria, *Am. J. Med.* 18:990, 1955.
Melohn, M. J., et al., A Consideration of Some Factors in Urine Which Cause the Precipitation of Hemoglobin in Vitro, *J. Lab. & Clin. Med.* 34:936, 1949.
Rous, P., Urinary Siderosis, *J. Exper. Med.* 28:645, 1918.

Schaar, F. E., Paroxysmal Myoglobinuria: Description of a Case and a Review of the Literature, *A.M.A. Am. J. Dis. Child.* 89:23, 1955.

Stats, D., L. R. Wasserman, and *N. Rosenthal,* Hemolytic Anemia with Hemoglobinuria, *Am. J. Clin. Path.* 18:757, 1948.

White, A. G., Effect of Tyrosine, Tryptophane and Thiouracil on Melanuria, *J. Lab. & Clin. Med.* 32:1254, 1947.

PORPHYRINS

Aldrich, R. A., R. A. Labbe, and *E. L. Talman,* A Review of Porphyrin Metabolism with Special Reference to Childhood, *Am. J. Med. Sc.* 230:675, 1955.

Bradley, J. E., A. E. Powell, W. Niermann, K. R. McGrady, and *E. Kaplan,* The Incidence of Abnormal Blood Levels of Lead in a Metropolitan Pediatric Clinic, with Observation on the Value of Coproporphyrinuria as a Screening Test, *J. Pediat.* 49:1, 1956.

Chisolm, J. J., Jr., and *H. E. Harrison,* Quantitative Urinary Coproporphyrin Excretion and Its Relation to Edathamil Calcium Disodium Administration in Children with Acute Lead Intoxication, *J. Clin. Invest.* 35:1131, 1956.

Gibson, Q. H., and *D. C. Harrison,* A Note on the Urinary Uroporphyrin in Acute Porphyria, *Biochem. J.* 46:154, 1950.

Hsia, D. Y., and *M. Page,* Coproporphyrin Studies in Children. I. Urinary Coproporphyrin Excretion in Normal Children, *Proc. Exper. Biol. & Med.* 85:86, 1954.

Johnson, W. S., and *N. E. Whitman,* Coproporphyrinuria as an Index of Lead Absorption, *Arch. Indus. Hyg.* 2:170, 1950.

Lysaught, J. N., and *J. M. McCleery,* Acute Intermittent Porphyria: Report of a Case in an Infant Aged Eight Months, with Discussion of Porphyrin Metabolism, *J. Pediat.* 46:552, 1955.

Rosenthal, I. M., E. L. Lipton, and *G. Asrow,* Effect of Splenectomy on Porphyria Erythropoietica, *Pediatrics* 15:663, 1955.

Schwartz, S., L. Zieve, and *C. J. Watson,* An Improved Method for the Determination of Urinary Coproporphyrin and an Evaluation of Factors Influencing the Analysis, *J. Lab. & Clin. Med.* 37:843, 1951.

Sunderman, F. W., Jr., and *F. W. Sunderman,* Practical Considerations of Porphyrin Metabolism: Porphyria and Porphyrinuria, *Am. J. Clin. Path.* 25:1231, 1955.

Watson, C. J., and *E. A. Larson,* Urinary Coproporphyrins in Health and Disease, *Physiol. Rev.* 27:478, 1947.

Woody, N. C., Porphyrinuria: Report of an Unusual Case, *Pediatrics* 4:47, 1947.

Zeligman, I., Red Fluorescence of Urine in Wood's Light as Aid in Office Diagnosis of Porphyria, *Arch. Dermat. & Syph.* 61:853, 1950.

CHAPTER 30

Normal Soluble Constituents

CALCIUM

Only a small proportion of the calcium in the food appears in the urine. With the 29 normal children studied by Macy, an average of 10 per cent of ingested calcium was excreted in the urine and 70 per cent in the feces; the remainder was retained.

Calcium is ordinarily not excreted in liberal amounts except after ingestion of milk, cheese, or acidifying agents. However, even when the dietary intake is low, excretion is increased in metabolic disorders associated with a high blood calcium level. An increase may also be seen in the Fanconi syndrome and in chronic base-losing nephritis with renal acidosis resulting from a decreased ability of the kidneys to make ammonia. Some adults who have come to clinical attention with the complaint of stones in the urinary tract have been found to be excreting excessive calcium without obvious cause.

The extent of urinary calcium excretion can be assayed roughly with the Sulkowitch reagent, which is a buffered oxalate solution of the following composition (Albright and Reifenstein):

Oxalic acid	2.5 gm	Glacial acetic acid	5.0 ml
Ammonium oxalate	2.5 gm	Distilled water to make	150 ml

When shaken with urine the reagent precipitates the calcium as a cloud of calcium oxalate, provided the calcium is in more than minimal concentration. The test is carried out by mixing 5 ml of urine with 2 ml of reagent in a test tube. The density of the precipitate and the speed of its appearance (3 to 30 seconds) determine the reading, which is expressed as negative or 1 plus or 2 plus, 3 plus, or 4 plus.

The Sulkowitch reagent will often react with the calcium excreted by normal children if the urine is of high specific gravity. After several cupfuls of water are taken by children whose urine gives a strong reaction, the next specimen may be found negative. Conversely, the drinking of a large amount of milk may elicit a 3 plus or 4 plus reaction. Because of such normal fluctuations the Sulkowitch test is not very reliable as a screening test for abnormal calcium metabolism in childhood.

359

Albright has recommended the Sulkowitch test for regulation of medication in patients receiving treatment for hypoparathyroidism (p. 576). The intake of calcium and medication should be so adjusted that the urine consistently displays a light cloud of precipitate. This will keep the serum calcium at a safe slightly subnormal level and will guard the patient against both under- and overtreatment.

Calcium may not appear in the urine when the blood calcium level is near or below the renal threshold of 7.5 to 9 meters per 100 ml of serum. Hence, the Sulkowitch test has been suggested as a bedside aid in the differential diagnosis of tetany. In alkalotic tetany the urine with a normal serum calcium level should contain calcium, whereas in hypocalcemic tetany none should be demonstrable. Occasional individuals, however, will excrete calcium even when their blood level is subnormal, and vice versa.

With patients having kidney stones and rarefaction of bones in whom the serum calcium and phosphorus levels are equivocally abnormal, a persistently strong Sulkowitch reaction will be in favor of hyperparathyroidism, whereas a negative or weakly positive reaction will point in the other direction.

CHLORIDES

The daily output of urine chlorides in the healthy child is proportional to the amount ingested. Expressed as sodium chloride, this is usually 2 to 6 gm, being roughly proportional to age.

The urinary chlorides usually drop in the presence of diarrhea, vomiting, excessive perspiration, edema, drainage from a surgical wound, or when the salt intake is cut down by illness or for other reasons. When the plasma chloride level falls to 95 per cent of normal the excretion of chloride into the urine practically comes to a stop. In nephritis there may be either retention or undue excretion ("salt-losing nephritis"). In untreated bacterial pneumonia the excretion falls to unusually low levels just prior to the crisis, reaches its lowest level during the crisis, rises abruptly to supernormal levels for 1 to 2 days, and then promptly returns to normal. Early chemotherapy cuts this cycle short.

Observing the urinary chloride excretion is a crude means of detecting salt depletion in postoperative dehydrative states in older children. The test of Fantus is said to be accurate to within 0.5 gm NaCl per liter of urine. The necessary apparatus and solutions are a test tube, a medicine dropper, 20 per cent potassium chromate, 2.9 per cent silver nitrate, and distilled water. Ten drops of urine is placed in a test tube and one drop of potassium chromate solution mixed in. The silver nitrate solution is then added drop by drop, with shaking, until the solution changes suddenly from yellow to brick red. The same dropper is used throughout and rinsed with distilled water between solutions. The number of drops of silver nitrate needed to bring out the red color change approximates the urinary sodium chloride concentration in grams per liter.

CREATINE

Creatine is physiologically present in childhood urine until about puberty; above that age period it is not seen in men, though small amounts are eliminated periodically by women. In normal children the rate of creatine excretion fluctuates widely from day to day and seems to be comparatively greater in younger than in older children. The output per kilogram of body weight per day falls gradually from about 10 to 12 mg at 2 years to about 2 mg at 14 or 15 years.

Unusually high creatine excretion is seen following exercise and in myasthenia gravis and pseudohypertrophic muscular dystrophy and also when endogenous protein catabolism goes up, as in fever, malnutrition, and hyperthyroidism. In contrast, the excretion falls or ceases altogether in cretinism and hypothyroidism, but can be restored by therapy with thyroid substance. It becomes diminished or absent in prematurity and in myotonia congenita. The giving of glycine to patients with progressive muscular dystrophy may result in marked augmentation of the excretion. In all these circumstances the child's urine has to contain either extremely large or nearly infinitesimal amounts of creatine before it can be evaluated as "abnormal."

CREATININE

Creatinine (creatine anhydride) is formed almost exclusively during muscle catabolism. The rate of excretion is a direct reflection of the total weight of the muscle tissue and remains remarkably constant from hour to hour and day to day, unaffected by activity. Reynolds and Clark found the mean 24-hour excretion in 100 children to increase from 0.36 gm at 5 years of age to 1.58 gm at 17 years. Boys began to excrete significantly higher amounts than girls after the age of 11 years. The creatinine–body weight ratio (milligrams per 24 hours per kilogram) remained at about 21± for girls but rose to 25±1 for boys. Talbot has calculated that 1 gm of urinary creatinine per day corresponds to a muscle mass of 17.8 kg for the infant and 17.9 kg for the adult man.

The creatinine coefficient (milligrams of urinary creatinine per 24 hours divided by the body weight in kilograms) is higher when the muscles are well developed and the fat scanty, and lower with obesity or poorly developed musculature. The coefficient for the average child ranges from 3 to 12 at birth; from 14 to 30 in infancy; and 18 to 35 at older ages. It rises most rapidly when muscle growth is at a peak. Talbot, Worcester, and Stewart have worked out a set of creatinine standards for basal metabolism when body build is abnormal.

GLYCOCYAMINE

Glycocyamine (guanidoacetic acid) is an intermediary product in the synthesis of creatinine. The rate of urinary output of glycocyamine in 17 normal children ranging in age from prematurity to 13 years was found by Flood and Pinelli to range from 0.68 to 1.70 mg per kg per 24 hours at all ages. Nephrotic children had a striking increase in output, with a range from 3.5 to 3.7 mg per kg per 24 hours.

ENZYMES

The content of amylase (diastase) in urine and blood becomes unusually high during mumps. An increase may be detectable as early as the second day of the glandular swelling and continues for 5 to 7 days or sometimes longer. The source of the excess is presumably the affected glands—submaxillaries, parotids, and sublinguals—rather than the pancreas. Determination of amylase in blood or urine can be helpful in distinguishing between mumps and other localized enlargements of the neck such as bacterial infection of lymph nodes. Elevated values occur also in obstructive pancreatic diseases such as acute pancreatitis and blocking of the common duct by stone, but such disorders are rare in the childhood age period.

A number of other related principles make their appearance in the urine, but their appearance and degree of activity have been too erratic and irregular to be of much service in pediatrics. There is a protein-digesting principle related to gastric pepsin and presumably derived from it, known as uropepsin. There is a thromboplastin which will clot hematuric extravasations of blood, even in hemophilics.

Carbonic anhydrase is not contained in normal urine, but appears during acute hemolytic illnesses associated with intravascular hemolysis. Urinary lysozyme, a bacteriolytic agent which causes lysis of the bacterium *Micrococcus lysodeikticus*, was found by Wilson in 26 per cent of 595 healthy children and infants, in small amounts.

INDICAN

Indican has its origin in tryptophane, which when it reaches the colon is broken down by bacterial action into indole. Indole is absorbed locally, oxidized by the liver, and conjugated with sulfuric acid to form potassium indoxyl sulfate, which is indican. Detectable amounts of indican can be found in the urine of most infants, especially those fed cow's milk mixtures.

The appearance of large amounts of indican in the urine is accepted as meaning inordinate bacterial destruction of protein within the large intestine. It can be tested for with Obermayer's hydrochloric acid–ferric chloride reagent which gives rise to an indigo-blue or sometimes an indigo-red color. The extent of excretion of indican has not been shown to be of significance in disease of infants and children.

NEUTRAL 17-KETOSTEROIDS

These urinary steroids with an oxygen atom at the 17-position of the nucleus are derived in the male from both adrenal and testicular androgens, but in the female from the adrenal androgens almost entirely. The quantitative measurement of the excretion of these substances is utilized as a rough index of the amounts of androgens being elaborated in the body. Measurement is done on a 24-hour pooled specimen of urine.

Attempts at separation of the individual components, except in research laboratories, are restricted currently to differentiation between the so-called alpha and beta components. The output of the beta fraction, normally about one-tenth of the total, becomes increased markedly in the presence of androgen-producing adrenal tumors.

Normal Values

These may be summarized as follows:

Age	Range	Average
Up to 1 year	0.1–1.2	0.8
4–7 years	0.8–2.6	1.3
7–12 years	1.8–5.0	4.0
12–15 years	5.0–12.0	8.2
Females over 15 years	5.0–17.0	10.0
Males over 15 years	8.0–20.0	15.0

Disease States

The excretion of neutral 17-ketosteroids may fall to minimal amounts in debilitating illnesses, starvation, pituitary failure, and advanced adrenocortical insufficiency.

The output may go up whenever there is excess secretion of androgens or related substances by either adrenal cortex or testicles. Testicular hypersecretion is seen in precocious puberty and some tumors of the testis. Adrenal cortical hypersecretion is seen in Cushing's syndrome, some tumors of the adrenal, the adrenogenital syndrome, and congenital adrenal hyperplasia. Increased amounts appear for a few days after acute trauma such as fractures and surgical operations and after exposure to cold. In a child with pseudohermaphroditism or virilism, a high neutral 17-ketosteroid excretion suggests that the adrenal is at fault; if the beta fraction is high the lesion is probably tumor rather than hyperplasia.

CORTICOSTEROIDS (CORTICOIDS)

Numerous corticosteroid metabolites (corticoids) can be demonstrated within the urine after suitable hydrolysis by chemical assay methods.

These substances are not included in the results when the neutral 17-ketosteroids of the urine are determined. When referred to total body surface the total daily output of urinary 11-17-oxycorticosteroids tends to be approximately the same regardless of age, whereas that of 17-ketosteroids when judged by the same standard goes up rapidly with increasing years. Corticosteroid output goes down or disappears in Addison's disease; rises usually in hyperadrenocorticism and in disturbances which throw a strain on the body such as infections, operations, fever, heart failure, and burns.

Bongiovanni and Eisenmenger encountered elevated values for urinary corticosteroids in chronic hepatic disease (Laennec cirrhosis) with ascites. This may represent an overflow of steroids not normally disposed of by the liver, rather than actual adrenal cortical hyperactivity.

BIBLIOGRAPHY

CALCIUM

Albright, F., and *E. C. Reifenstein, Jr.,* "The Parathyroid Glands and Metabolic Bone Disease: Selected Studies," The Williams & Wilkins Company, Baltimore, 1948.

Linder, G. C., and *J. M. Latsky,* Urinary Calcium in Nutrition Surveys: Sulkowitch Test, *Lancet* 1:105, 1942.

Macy, I. G., "Nutrition and Chemical Growth in Childhood," vol. I, "Evaluation," Charles C Thomas, Springfield, Ill., 1942.

Shohl, A. T., "Mineral Metabolism," Reinhold Publishing Corporation, New York, 1939.

Yoshina, T., The Sulkowitch Test in Diagnosis and Management of Hypocalcemic Tetany of Newborns and Infants, *Hawaii Med. J.* 5:327, 1946.

CHLORIDES

Fantus, B., Fluid Postoperatively: a Statistical Study, *J.A.M.A.* 107:14, 1936.

Macy, I. G., "Nutrition and Chemical Growth in Childhood," vol. I, "Evaluation," Charles C Thomas, Springfield, Ill., 1942.

Sherman, H. W., and *N. Corbin,* Significance of Urinary Chlorides in Pneumonia and Other Conditions, *Arch. Pediat.* 59:223, 1942.

Shohl, A. T., "Mineral Metabolism," Reinhold Publishing Corporation, New York, 1939.

Van Slyke, K. K., and *E. I. Evans,* Significance of Urine Chloride Determination in Detection and Treatment of Dehydration with Salt Depletion, *Ann. Surg.* 128:391, 1948.

Wilder, T. S., and *T. G. H. Drake,* Metabolism of Chloride and Total Fixed Base in Pneumonia and Relation to Salt and Water Retention, *J. Clin. Invest.* 7:353, 1929.

CREATINE, CREATININE, AND GLYCOCYAMINE

Flood, R. G., and *R. W. Pinelli,* Urinary Glycocyamine, Creatine and Creatinine: Their Excretion by Normal Infants and Children, *Am. J. Dis Child.* 77:740, 1949.

—— and ———, Urinary Glycocyamine, Creatine and Creatinine: Their Excretion in Children with the Nephrotic Syndrome, *Am. J. Dis. Child.* 78:67, 1949.

Magee, M. C., Excretion of Creatine and Creatinine: Hourly Excretion in Normal Children and in Children with Progressive Muscular Dystrophy, *Am. J. Dis. Child.* 43:322, 1932.

Marples, E., and *S. Z. Levine,* Creatinuria of Infancy and Childhood; Normal Variations; Creatine Tolerance Tests and Effect of Amino-Acetic Acid in Normal Infants, *Am. J. Dis. Child.* 51:30, 1936.

Poncher, H. G., I. P. Bronstein, H. W. Wade, and *J. C. Ricewater,* Creatine Metabolism in Hypothyroid Infants and Children: Further Observations, *Am. J. Dis. Child.* 63:270, 1942.

Reynolds, E. L., and *L. C. Clark,* Creatinine Excretion, Growth Progress and Body Structure in Normal Children, *Child Develop.* 18:155, 1947.

Roche, M., J. D. Benedict, T. F. Yu, E. Bien, and *D. W. Stettin,* Origin of Urinary Creatine in Progressive Muscular Dystrophy, *Metabolism,* 1:13, 1952.

Talbot, N. B., Measurement of Obesity by the Creatinine Coefficient, *Am. J. Dis. Child.* 55:42, 1938.

———, *J. Worcester,* and *A. Stewart,* New Creatinine Standards for Basal Metabolism and Its Clinical Application, *Am. J. Dis. Child.* 58:506, 1939.

ENZYMES

Dillard, G. H., The Trypsin Inhibitor of the Urine in Health and Disease, *J. Lab. & Clin. Med.* 36:266, 1950.

Duffin, J. D., and *K. Kowalewski,* An Improved Technique for Uropepsin Assay, *J. Lab. & Clin. Med.* 43:165, 1954.

Janowitz, H. D., M. H. Levy, and *F. Hollander,* The Diagnostic Significance of Urinary Pepsinogen Excretion in Diseases of the Upper Gastrointestinal Tract, *Am. J. M. Sc.* 220:679, 1950.

Nothman, Martin M., Urinary Diastase in Mumps, *New England J. Med.* 244:13, 1951.

Olmstead, E. G., and *J. S. Hirschboeck,* Significance of Urorennin Excretion in Pernicious Anemia, *Am. J. M. Sc.* 226:84, 1953.

Peak, W. P., E. Viergiver, E. J. Van Loon, and *G. G. Duncan,* The Determination and Clinical Value of Uropepsinogen, *J.A.M.A.* 162:1441, 1956.

Robinson, J. R., Urinary Excretion of Carbonic Anhydrase: A Simple Test for the Detection of Intravascular Haemolysis, *J. Clin. Path.* 3:142, 1950.

Wilson, A. T., Urinary Lysozyme. I. Identification and Measurement, *J. Pediat.* 36:39, 1950. II. Lysozymuria in Healthy Children and in Children with Miscellaneous Diseases (a Sex Difference), *ibid.* 36:45, 1950. III. Lysozymuria in Children with the Nephrotic Syndrome, *ibid.* 36:199, 1950.

URINARY 17-KETOSTEROIDS AND CORTICOSTEROIDS

Bongiovanni, A. M., Evaluation of Adrenal Cortical Function in Pediatrics: Methods, *Am. J. Med. Sc.* 220:697, 1950.

———, A Method Adapted for the Determination of Urinary 17-Ketosteroids in Children, *J. Pediat.* 39:606–610, November, 1951.

Hamburger, C., Normal Urinary Excretion of Neutral 17-ketosteroids with Special Reference to Age and Sex Variations, *Acta endocrinol.* 1:19, 1948.

Jailer, J. W., Virilism, *Bull. New York Acad. Med.* **29:**377, 1953.

Landau, R. L., Diagnostic Significance and Laboratory Methods in Determination of the 17-Ketosteroids, *Am. J. Clin. Path.* **19:**424, 1949.

Read, C. H., E. H. Venning, and *M. P. Ripstein,* Adrenal Cortical Function in Newlyborn Infants, *J. Clin. Endocrinol.* **10:**845, 1950.

Sandberg, A. A., D. H. Nelson, E. M. Glenn, F. H. Tyler, and *L. T. Samuels,* 17-Hydroxycorticosteroids and 17-Ketosteroids in Urine of Human Subjects: Clinical Application of a Method Employing β-Glucuronidase Hydrolysis, *J. Clin. Endocrinol.* **13:**1445, 1953.

Ulstrom, R. A., and *D. Doeden,* Chromatographic Studies of Urinary Steroids in Term and Premature Infants, chap. 3 in L. I. Gardner (ed.), "Adrenal Function in Infants and Children: A Symposium," Grune & Stratton, New York, 1956.

Wood, M. E., and *E. H. Gray,* The Urinary Excretion of Neutral 17-Ketosteroids in Childhood, *J. Endocrinol.* **6:**111, 1949.

CHAPTER 31

Glycosuria

Minute amounts of reducing substances can be detected in every urine specimen by employing highly sensitive tests. Dextrose is the most common, but traces of other substances may be found also. Among these latter are ascorbic acid, pentoses, numerous glucuronic acids, uric acid, creatinine, di- and polysaccharides derived from dextrinous foods, and derivatives of salicylates, cinchophen, or para-aminobenzoic acid when these are being taken. The nonsugar reducing substances almost never show themselves when Benedict's test is performed accurately. Benedict's qualitative reagent, when used in the recommended proportions and boiled over a flame *for no more than 2 minutes,* or heated *for only 3 minutes in a water bath,* has a threshold sensitivity of about 0.05 gm of sugar per 100 ml of urine (0.05 per cent).

Indicator-type paper strips are now available for urine testing which are impregnated with an enzyme specifically active against glucose. In use, the end of the strip is dipped into the urine and then allowed to dry in the air for 1 minute. A color change denotes the presence of glucose, and the intensity of the change hints at the concentration per 100 ml.

Clinical interest in urinary reducing substances becomes aroused when these are excreted in sufficient amounts to be demonstrable by the standard tests. As a rule the reacting substance proves to be dextrose. Lactose, pentoses, galactose, fructose, sucrose, or more complex polysaccharides are infrequent.

The term melituria designates the appearance of any sugar in the urine in amount sufficient to be detectable by the usual tests. *Pseudomelituria* designates the presence of a reducing substance other than a sugar. The best way to avoid pseudomelituric readings is to apply the test procedures correctly.

IDENTIFICATION OF URINE SUGARS

Most of the reducing substances encountered in urine can be identified by routine laboratory procedures. The primary differentiation is by fermentation with baker's yeast at a temperature of 37°C for 2 to 8 hours.

Yeast destroys dextrose and fructose, but does not attack the pentoses, lactose, or galactose (the latter perhaps a little). Levulosuria (fructosuria) is so rare that any yeast-fermentable reducing substance found in urine may be regarded as being dextrose without further study, except when the attendant circumstances are peculiar. Penicillin or streptomycin given intravenously in high dosage may be excreted in the urine and react with Benedict's reagent.

The simpler chemical tests for differentiating lactose, galactose, and the pentoses and for confirming the presence of dextrose or fructose are outlined in Table 31-1. Descriptions of these and other more involved procedures for identifying the urinary sugars—paper chromatography, polariscopy, phenylhydrazine osazones, and fermentation with specific bacteria or fungi—will be found in texts on clinical pathology. Paper chromatography is now the method of choice.

Yeast fermentation should be applied to at least one urine specimen from any patient with a reducing substance in the urine. This precaution is especially important when the active principle of the testing reagent is bismuth, as in the commercial powders which take on a black color. The testing reagents which employ copper, such as Benedict's or Fehling's solutions, give many fewer nonglucose positive reactions.

Table 31-1. Useful Tests for Differentiating Urinary Sugars

	Benedict's test		Room temp. (3 hr.)	Yeast fermentation	Glucose-specific indicator paper	Bial test	Seliwanoff test
	Boiling temp. (3 min.)	55°C (10 min.)					
Glucose	+	0 *	0 *	+	+	0	0
Pentose (except ribose)	+	+	+	0	0	+	0
Galactose	+	0	0	Trace or negative	0	0	0
Fructose	+	±	+	+	0	0	+
Sucrose	Trace or negative	0	0	+	0	0	0
Ribose	Trace or negative	0	0	0	0	0	0

* May be positive if over 4 per cent concentration.

GLYCOSURIA (DEXTROSURIA)

This may be due to diabetes mellitus, to low renal threshold for glucose, or to a transient excretion of glucose. Whenever more than a trace of glucose is found in the urine, unless some other cause is immediately obvious, a careful history, urine studies for ketose bodies, and determinations of blood sugar status are called for.

The concomitant presence of acetone with or without diacetic acid in a specimen of urine does not always signify the existence of diabetes mellitus. A child with a low renal threshold or other form of glycosuria may have a ketosis superimposed from an acute infection or other causes.

DIABETES MELLITUS

The glycosuria of diabetes is due to overflow from the high blood glucose. In the first weeks after onset of this disease the blood level may remain abnormally high for 3 or more hours after each meal, yet drop to the normal range during the night fasting period. Hence when searching for diabetes it is best to examine a urine specimen passed some hours after a meal, rather than immediately on arising. In unregulated patients the amount of glucose in the urine typically exceeds 2 gm per 100 ml, whereas in most nondiabetic glycosuric conditions the concentrations are lower.

The management of diabetic children with diet and insulin aims for the middle ground between hyperglycemia with poor nutrition, on the one hand, and hypoglycemia accompanied by collapse attacks, on the other. It is universally agreed that hypoglycemic attacks are bad for the patient, but opinion is far from unanimous with respect to the need for keeping the blood sugar low enough to prevent glycosuria. Many men with wide experience have taken the stand that a therapeutic regimen which permits occasional glycosuria will guard against hypoglycemic reactions, should the food intake become temporarily less than usual or unusual physical activity be indulged in. Most patients so treated seem to do well as judged by immediate health and well-being. But some long-range follow-up studies, such as those of Jackson and associates, are indicating that laxness in metabolic control and duration of the disease are the two known variables in diabetic patients most associated with ultimate development of retinopathy, calcification of the arteries, hypertension, proteinuria, and related degenerative phenomena. High values for serum cholesterol and total lipids are more common in patients with a free diet regimen.

The onset of diabetes is ordinarily much more precipitous in children than in adults. The existence of unsuspected diabetes in a child is rarely recognized by routine screening of the urine. Weakness, loss of weight, excessive thirst and urinations, and perhaps stupor or coma are usually well established by the time a physician is called.

Before treatment is started, or if it is omitted, the diabetic child excretes impressive amounts of glucose—up to 5 or 10 gm per 100 ml of urine. The urine will also contain acetone and diacetic acid; the blood glucose level will be between 120 and 600 mg per 100 ml, or perhaps higher; and the cerebrospinal fluid if withdrawn for study because of central nervous system depression may have a glucose content well over 100 mg per 100 ml.

The content of glucose in the urine, once treatment has been begun, can be quite informative for evaluating the efficiency of treatment and the cooperation of the patient. A scheme for rating the control of the disease if under strict regulation has been suggested by Jackson:

Good control	Freedom from glycosuria except for occasional slight traces; approximately normal blood sugar levels; no ketonuria
Fair control	Less than half the urine specimens are free from sugar; only small amounts of sugar and no ketonuria in the rest; slightly elevated blood sugar levels
Poor control	Continuous but varying amounts of sugar in the urine; intermittent ketonuria; elevated blood sugar levels
Very poor control	Continuous prominent glycosuria, usually witn ketonuria; elevated blood sugar levels

When a child is first home after the initial hospitalization for diabetes his urine may have to be tested for glucose three times daily by the parents or by the child himself if old enough. Later, as the carbohydrate metabolism becomes better regulated, this may be reduced to once a day. A written record should be kept, to be brought to the physician at each regular visit. The finding of acetone signifies that the insulin dosage is too low, with risk of more serious derangement. A positive reaction for diacetic acid is a sign of impending ketosis, and the physician should be notified at once.

RENAL GLYCOSURIA AND LOW RENAL THRESHOLD

These conditions may be defined as the harmless chronic nondiabetic excretion of glucose. Hyperglycemia does not occur during fasting or after a meal; in fact, the tolerance test often yields an unusually low curve. Injections of insulin may transiently inhibit the glycosuria by reducing the blood sugar level. The metabolic utilization of carbohydrate and fat are normal. Symptoms are nonexistent, and treatment is not needed. Many subjects have been followed for as long as two decades without ever demonstrating any signs of diabetes or other disease attributable to the glycosuria. Nevertheless every newly discovered case should be followed medically for some years, inasmuch as beginning diabetes mellitus rarely can simulate benign glycosuria.

In *renal glycosuria* the excretion of dextrose proceeds continuously through day and night. In *low renal threshold*, which is a lesser degree of the same process, the subjects have sugar-free urine when fasting but excrete sugar following a meal containing carbohydrate. The blood sugar threshold for glucose excretion may range from 50 to 160 mg per 100 ml, the latter figure being the commonly accepted lower limit of normal.

The quantity of dextrose excreted may fluctuate with the diet but in the more pronounced cases is largely independent of diet. Random urine specimens only exceptionally contain more than 2 gm of glucose per 100 ml.

Renal glycosuria in childhood is nearly always of hereditary origin. The youngest reported case has been a 1-month-old infant. There is some sex linkage; males seem to be affected more frequently than females. Once established the sugar excretion can be expected to persist. Many of the childhood cases have been detected in family surveys made after another member has been found with the complaint.

Tests of renal function in these subjects give normal results, the only demonstrable defect being a selective impairment of glucose reabsorption. Specific loading tests may or may not demonstrate defects in the maximum reabsorptive capacity for glucose during periods of hyperglycemia.

TRANSITORY GLYCOSURIA

In hospital laboratories the glucose found in the majority of urine specimens proves to be derived from recently given intravenous infusions.

In private practice with well children a good proportion of positive specimens seem to be related in some way to fright or excitement attending the visit to the physician. Studies for diabetes and low renal threshold are negative, and the glycosuria is not seen again. The term "emotional glycosuria" is sometimes given to these cases, on the theory that excessive secretion of some endocrine hormone in response to the stress of the emotion has inhibited temporarily the reabsorption of glucose within the renal tubules. The few studies that have been done on such individuals have uncovered normal blood sugar levels.

When a child who seems otherwise in excellent health produces a sugar-containing urine specimen in the physician's office and the yeast fermentation test points to glucose (or fructose) as the excreted sugar, there may be some question as to whether to go ahead with blood chemistry investigations. Under such circumstances the next step should be to collect and test successive urine specimens passed in midday, about 2 hours after carbohydrate-rich meals. If two or three such specimens contain no sugar, the child may be instructed to return in 2 months for another medical examination and urine test, or earlier if unusual symptoms develop. Or else the blood sugar level may be determined about 2 hours after a heavy meal, in search of the elevation characteristic of diabetes mellitus (p. 510).

Intermittent glycosuria may be encountered in children with lead poisoning, hyperthyroidism, glycogen storage disease, chronic nephritis, subarachnoid hemorrhage, encephalitis, meningitis, brain tumor, or during the therapeutic administration of corticotropin (ACTH) or cortisone. Hyperglycemia may also be present, but more often the blood sugar level is not elevated. A beginning meningitis may be mistaken at first for diabetic acidosis because of the combination of sudden coma, glycosuria, and ketosis.

The concentration of sugar in the urine in most individuals with transitory glycosuria is usually below 1 gm per 100 ml, but occasionally may be 2 gm per 100 ml or higher.

The Fanconi Syndrome

Glycosuria is an essential component of the Fanconi syndrome, which includes also hypophosphatemic rickets, polyuria, and acidosis with extreme reduction of the serum bicarbonate (p. 424). The concentration of reducing substances in the urine may vary from trace amounts up to 4 to 5 per cent. The reducing substance is usually dextrose, though fructose, glycuronic acid, and other sugars may be excreted along with the dextrose. The glucosuria may be intermittent and disappear for considerable periods of time, but in the more severe cases is likely to be continuous.

FRUCTOSURIA

This may be congenital or symptomatic. The congenital or "essential" excretion of fructose (levulose) is a rare error of metabolism, often familial. Affected subjects cannot catabolize fructose normally, whether it be ingested as the simple sugar or incorporated in a more complex carbohydrate such as sucrose. The excretion continues whenever fructose or one of its precursors is being taken; it ceases temporarily on withdrawal of these substances from the diet. The disturbance is benign and continues throughout life without complications. The concentration of fructose in the urine is typically of the magnitude of 1 to 3 gm per 100 ml.

Symptomatic or "acquired" fructosuria may be seen in cirrhotic liver disturbances or in conjunction with glycosuria in severe protracted diabetes mellitus. In these circumstances the fructosuria may persist even when fructose has been entirely eliminated from the diet—a differentiating point from the essential form.

A feeding test can be utilized for confirming congenital fructosuria. On the evening before the test the supper should consist of foods free of fructose, excluding fruits, vegetables, salads, sugar, cakes, and other sweets. Meat, fish, cheese, bread, and milk products may be taken. Breakfast next morning should consist only of milk or coffee or tea without sugar. The patient empties his bladder, takes 50 gm of glucose in water, and voids again 90 minutes later. Portions of both urine specimens, in 100-ml amounts, are saved. Twenty-four hours later the same procedure is repeated except that 50 gm of sucrose is taken instead of the glucose. Fasting urine and a 90-minute voiding are again taken. All urine specimens are collected in sterilized containers, stored in a refrigerator, and analyzed for sugar on the second day of the test.

In congenital fructosuria the first three specimens will be free of reducing substances, whereas the last will contain 2 to 3 gm of fructose. With small children smaller doses of the sugars may be given.

Special treatment is not required for essential fructosuria, except that it may be wise to keep the intake of sucrose, fruits, and honey to a minimum. The therapy of symptomatic fructosuria is directed toward the underlying disturbance.

GALACTOSURIA

Galactose in the urine is usually a manifestation of a profound constitutional error of metabolism, known as galactosemia, in which the body is lacking in some enzyme or enzymes necessary for the metabolism of galactose. The disease begins to show itself in early infancy and gives rise to retarded growth, hepatomegaly, galactosuria, and cataracts in about half of the cases. The urine contains also an excess of amino acids. While the infant receives a milk-containing diet the fasting blood sugar level will appear elevated (100 to 250 mg per 100 ml) by standard testing methods. Fermentative and other identification studies, however, will reveal that a significant fraction of the total blood sugar is galactose and that the glucose fraction is normal or even depressed. Removal of lactose from the diet (a milk-free diet) is followed by disappearance of the galactose from the urine within 1 or 2 days.

LACTOSURIA

Lactose may appear in the urine of women who are pregnant or actively lactating. Lactosuria is not a problem in the pediatric age period.

SUCROSURIA

Very few instances of idiopathic sucrosuria (saccharosuria) have been reported. In such individuals the sucrosuria occurs either when saccharose itself is given in excess or when fed in lesser amounts along with other sugars. Transitory sucrosuria of alimentary origin may also be seen. Perhaps one reason for its apparent rarity lies in the fact that sucrose (and maltose) will not react with Benedict's solution unless the urine is first acidified and boiled to hydrolyze the sugar into its constituent hexoses.

Whenever sucrosuria is encountered, deception and malingering should always be ruled out by collecting a urine specimen under direct supervision and testing it personally.

PENTOSURIA

Pentosuria may be divided into two types, alimentary and essential. It is important to make the distinction.

Alimentary pentosuria refers to the transient or occasional excretion of pentoses following the ingestion of foods rich in pentoses or their polymers the pentosans. Fruits are chiefly responsible, such as cherries, apples, grapes, plums, berries, and prunes and derivatives such as cider and wines. The condition may be seen in children of any age. Dunsky and Lawrence described an unusual Negro boy with a low renal threshold for both glucose and pentoses. He excreted pentoses in considerable amounts whenever given fruits in ordinary servings.

Essential pentosuria is a hereditary metabolic anomaly characterized by continuous excretion of small amounts of pentose in the urine. The condition has an estimated incidence of approximately 1:50,000 in the general population. There is a strong familial tendency. The pentose most often excreted seems to be levorotatory xylulose, known also as L-xyloketose. The output is not influenced by changes in the carbohydrate or protein content of the diet, by exercise or bed rest, or by the eating of fruit, but can be increased by ingestion of its metabolic precursor, D-glucuronic acid. The concentration in a random urine specimen is ordinarily from 0.5 to 1 gm per 100 ml, which corresponds to a weakly positive reaction.

Essential pentosuria can persist unchanged throughout life. It is more common in males and in individuals of Jewish extraction. It does not predispose to diabetes mellitus or other metabolic disorders. No essential differences have been found in the absorption or excretion of pentoses between normal controls and pentosuric children. A family survey should always be made whenever a case is encountered. The defect seems to lie in the renal mechanisms, since the nonfermentable reducing substances of the blood are not increased. The blood dextrose and pentose tolerance curves following ingestion of test amounts of these sugars are normal.

Essential pentosuria may be confused with renal glycosuria or even diabetes mellitus. It should be thought of whenever a child exhibits persistent melituria of mild degree, uninfluenced by diet or starvation. The possibility of pentosuria is the principal reason for performing at least one identification of urinary sugar with every child who exhibits persistent melituria.

The simplest test for differentiating between glucose and pentose (L-xyloketose) is to let a mixture of 1 ml of urine and 5 ml of qualitative Benedict's solution stand at room temperature for about 3 hours or in a water bath at 55°C for 10 minutes. L-xyloketose being an active ketose sugar will reduce Benedict's solution under these circumstances, whereas glucose will not (Table 31-1).

The only other urinary sugar which would give a positive test in similar concentrations is levulose, but this is found in the urine only rarely. Levulose is fermented by yeast, whereas the pentoses are not. Bial's orcinol-HCl reagent gives a green color with pentoses. Another identifying characteristic is that urine containing L-xyloketose keeps its reducing power almost indefinitely, whereas a glucose-containing urine (unless strongly acid) tends spontaneously to lose much or all of its reducing power when the specimen stands for 12 to 24 hours at 37°C or for a longer period at room temperature. Paper chromatography for identification should be applied whenever feasible (Fales).

RIBOSURIA

Ribose (a pentose) may appear in the urine of patients with progressive muscular dystrophy, dystrophia myotonica, myotonia congenita, or amyotonia congenita. When ribosuria is suspected, the patient should be given a diet free of fruit and fruit juices for 24 hours before a urine specimen is collected. Add 8 drops to 5 ml of Benedict's solution in a test tube and place in a boiling water bath for 45 minutes. A positive reaction is presumptive of ribose provided a muscular dystrophy is present, though with a specimen of high specific gravity a positive reaction may be given also by nonsugar reducing substances as discussed in the first paragraph of this chapter.

BIBLIOGRAPHY

GLYCOSURIA

Bayer, L. M., and *J. H. Davis,* Nondiabetic Glycosuria in Children: Report of 9 Cases, Am. J. Dis. Child. 60:580, 1940.

Bland, J. H., Renal Glycosuria: A Review of the Literature and Report of Four Cases, Ann. Int. Med. 29:461, 1948.

Bock, J. C., Benign Meliturias, Physiol. Rev. 24:169, 1944.

Fales, F. W., Identification of Urinary Sugar, Am. J. Clin. Path. 25:336, 1955.

Ferguson, F. C., and *D. P. Barr,* Glycosuria in Meningitis, Ann. Int. Med. 21:173, 1944.

Fischer, A. E., Intermittent and Continuous Renal Glycosuria: Report of 3 Cases, Am. J. Dis. Child. 50:166, 1935.

Goettsch, E., and *H. H. Mason,* Glycosuria in Lead Poisoning: Report of Case and Study of Pathogenesis, Am. J. Dis. Child. 59:119, 1940.

Horowitz, L., and *S. Schwarzer,* Renal Glycosuria: Occurrence in Two Siblings and a Review of the Literature, J. Pediat. 47:634, 1955.

Jackson, R. L., R. C. Hardin, G. L. Walker, A. B. Hendricks, and *H. G. Kelly,* Degenerative Changes in Young Diabetic Patients in Relationship to Level of Control, Pediatrics 5:959, 1950.

Lichtenstein, A., The Treatment of Diabetes in Childhood, Arch. Dis. Childhood 24:237, 1949.

Neuberg, H. W., Streptomycin as a Cause of False-Positive Benedict Reaction for Glycosuria, Am. J. Clin. Path. 24:245, 1954.

Watson, B. A., The Clinical Significance of Glycosuria in the College Age Group, Bull. Am. Stud. Health A. 22:31, 1938.

Whipple, R., and *W. Bloom,* The Occurrence of False Positive Tests for Albumin and Glucose in the Urine and during the Course of Massive Penicillin Therapy, J. Lab. Clin. Med. 36:635, 1950.

Wolman, I. J., Urine Analysis in Pediatrics: Ten Years' Progress, Am. J. Med. Sc. 208:767, 1944.

Wolman, I. J., Melituria in Healthy American Men with Special Reference to Transitory Glycosuria, *Am. J. Med. Sc.* 212:159, 1946.

Zarafonetis, C. J. D., and *J. P. Chandler,* Reducing Substance in Urine of Patients Treated with Para-aminobenzoic Acid, *J. Lab. & Clin. Med.* 37:425, 1951.

FRUCTOSURIA

Broman, B., Essential Fructosuria: Report of a Case, *Acta paediat.* suppl. 75, 1949.

Cohen, A. S., and *N. Kantor,* A Simplified Paper Chromatographic Method for Separation of Glucose and Fructose in Urine, *Am. J. Clin. Path.* 25:1328, 1955.

Sachs, B., L. Sternfield, and *G. Kraus,* Essential Fructosuria: Its Pathophysiology, *Am. J. Dis. Child.* 63:252, 1942.

Trivette, D., and *K. Anderson,* Essential Fructosuria in 2 Siblings, *Am. J. Dis. Child.* 75:88, 1948.

GALACTOSURIA

Bell, L. S., W. C. Blair, S. Lindsay, and *S. J. Watson,* Galactose Diabetes (Galactosemia), *J. Pediat.* 36:427, 1950.

Goldstein, E. O., and *J. M. Ennis,* Galactosemia, *J. Pediat.* 33:147, 1948.

Greenman, L., and *J. C. Rathbun,* Galactose Studies in an Infant with Idiopathic Galactose Intolerance, *Pediatrics* 2:666, 1948.

Hsia, D. Y., H. Hsia, S. Green, M. Kay, and *S. S. Gellis,* Amino-aciduria in Galactosemia, *A.M.A. Am. J. Dis. Child.* 88:458, 1954.

SUCROSURIA

Elmer, A. W., M. Krasowska, and *L. Ptaszek,* Sucrosuria: Rare Metabolic Error, *Acta med. scandinav.* 101:596, 1939.

Masserman, J. H., Effects of Intravenous Administration of Hypertonic Solutions of Sucrose, with Special Reference to Cerebrospinal Fluid Pressure, *Bull. Johns Hopkins Hosp.* 57:12, 1935.

Reiner, M., and *S. B. Weiner,* Saccharosuria in Infant, *Am. J. Dis. Child.* 57:590, 1939.

PENTOSURIA

Dunsky, I., and *G. Lawrence,* Renal Glycosuria Associated with Pentosuria, *J. Pediat.* 30:416, 1947.

Fischer, A. E., and *M. Reiner,* Pentosuria in Children, *Am. J. Dis. Child.* 40:1193, 1930.

Lasker, M., The Question of Arabinosuria, with a Scheme for Identifying Reducing Substances in Urine, *Am. J. Clin. Path.* 20:485, 1950.

Peterman, M. G., Pentosuria with Diabetic Symptoms, *J. Pediat.* 26:296, 1945.

Sunderman, F. W., B. E. Copeland, R. P. MacFate, V. E. Martens, H. N. Naumann, and *G. F. Stevenson,* Manual of American Society of Clinical Pathologists Workshop on Glucose, *Am. J. Clin. Path.* 26:1355, 1956.

CHAPTER 32

Proteinuria

The proteins which appear in the urine are conventionally known as "albumin," though actually they are a mixture of serum albumin with the various serum globulins. Serum albumin usually accounts for from 50 to 95 per cent of the total urinary protein, and ω_1 globulin for the most of the remainder. The fractional distribution is never identical from specimen to specimen, no matter how severe any renal damage may be. Experimental evidence indicates that some serum protein normally leaks constantly through the glomerular tufts, in concentrations up to 25 mg per 100 ml of glomerular filtrate, and that this is reabsorbed within the tubules.

Minute traces of protein can be found in every urine if looked for by refined techniques. Such content rarely exceeds 5 mg per 100 ml and is usually less than 2 mg per 100 ml. Since the thresholds of sensitivity for the tests which employ heat or strong acids lies at or above 10 or 15 mg per 100 ml, these lesser quantities ordinarily escape detection. More pronounced proteinuria in the absence of disease is not uncommon in childhood and adolescence. The prostate and seminal vesicles are not sources of urinary protein in boys before puberty, as at times in adult males. Penicillin in the urine may react with the chemical reagents for protein when above 8,000 units per ml—a concentration ordinarily not seen except after intravenous infusions of large doses.

It is ordinarily not very helpful to express the quantity of urinary protein as 1 plus, 2 plus, 3 plus, or 4 plus. These subjective terms are used differently by different workers. More importantly, the content of protein per unit volume of urine is integrally related to the state of dilution or concentration of the urine as reflected in specific gravity.

The scale of comparative values as popularly understood is about as follows:

Negative	No perceptible cloudiness
Trace	Less than 20 mg per 100 ml
+	20 to 50 mg per 100 ml
++	Approximately 100 mg per 100 ml
+++	Approximately 300 mg per 100 ml
++++	500 mg per 100 ml and higher

Urine containing 3,000 mg (3 gm) per 100 ml will show a solid precipitate when boiled.

When the initial qualitative test is positive for protein, many laboratories make an additional quantitative measurement by photoelectric turbidity or by comparison with opalescent standards such as those of Kingsbury and Clark.

In addition to the circumstances discussed in this and the two following chapters, proteinuria is frequent in such constitutional disorders as dehydration, febrile illnesses, burns, intoxications, and congestive heart failure. As a rule its severity and duration reflect the intensity of the systemic responses. The specific Bence-Jones urinary protein, evoked by multiple myeloma, is rare in childhood. Somewhat similar proteins, which precipitate between 50 and 56°C, redissolve on boiling and reappear on partial cooling, and appear occasionally during osteomalacia, leukemia, metastatic bone lesions, and in young persons with hypertension.

INTERMITTENT PROTEINURIA

This variety of proteinuria is often referred to also as functional, lordotic, benign, postural, adolescent, physiologic, or orthostatic. The most characteristic feature is lack of constancy, which is why the term *intermittent* seems preferable. Disease of the kidney should not be diagnosed unless other signs of renal damage are demonstrable.

Intermittent proteinuria is exceptional under 6 years of age. It begins to become frequent thereafter, reaching a peak at 14 or 15 years and then declining; it is rarely seen above age 20. It usually escapes detection in examinations of single casual specimens of urine. Successive tests on the same subjects make the chances of finding it much higher. Of a series of 110 active young adult males tested by the author eight times within a 5-day period, 62 (56 per cent) exhibited at least one protein-containing specimen of urine and 14 (13 per cent) had protein in more than half of the specimens collected.

In intermittent proteinuria the protein content of the urine may vary from 10 mg up to 3 gm per 100 ml or higher. The excretion is accelerated by an erect body posture or vigorous physical activity and subsides or ceases altogether when the patient is seated or stretched out; hence *orthostatic* or *postural.* Occasional individuals may exhibit the reverse situation: the urine is protein-free when upright but protein-containing when lying down.

The frequency with which intermittent proteinuria is uncovered in groups of children and adolescents will depend upon their ages, recent physical activity, season of the year, delicacy of the test approach, number of tests done, specific gravity of the urine, and other indeterminate factors. It can be aggravated by emotional or vasomotor disturbances and by prolonged immobilization in erect or lordotic positions. It has been found as a persistent residual defect after an attack of acute glomerulonephritis.

That intermittent proteinuria is harmless and benign is based on sound evidence. The highest incidence is at puberty, despite the comparative rarity of kidney diseases at this period. There is also the universal propensity to spontaneous disappearance, attested to by a number of long-range follow-up studies. Nearly always the clinical story, urine analysis, and physical examinations are otherwise negative, both at the time the proteinuria is found and when later studies are made. With every case, nevertheless, it is important to carry out a thorough physical examination and several careful microscopic studies of the urine.

To establish the diagnosis the posture test is essential. When the results are equivocal, the test should be repeated.

Posture Test

In the evening, 1 hour after the child has been put to bed, he is roused to void at the bedside and the specimen is discarded. This gets rid of the urine which had been secreted in the period before bedtime, when he was about and active. The child is kept lying in bed all night and given water or food if requested. The next morning, immediately on awakening, he voids again. The specimen is saved for analysis for protein and sediment. A glass of water is now taken. He then leans backward over the side of the bed, keeping his feet on the floor and his buttocks on the edge of the mattress, while back, head, and shoulders rest upon the bed itself. This lordotic position is maintained for at least 30 minutes and as long thereafter until a second specimen of urine can be furnished. This is also saved. If the first or overnight specimen proves to be protein-free while the second or lordotic specimen contains a demonstrable cloud of protein and both are free from abnormal sediment, intermittent proteinuria can be said to be present.

A few nonbenign conditions may give rise to a positive posture test. These are subclinical chronic glomerulonephritis and the recovery phase of acute nephritis. With such patients, however, red cells or casts are customary in the urinary sediment and a history of nephritis is elicitable.

The large life-insurance companies have learned from experience that young healthy individuals with intermittent proteinuria possess as good an expectation of life as do those who have no proteinuria. With children and young adults these companies ordinarily attach no significance to protein in amounts less than 50 or 75 mg per 100 ml, though sometimes they request studies to exclude urologic disease. Intermittent proteinuria is not a valid reason for excluding an adolescent boy from athletic endeavors or a military academy.

TRANSITORY PROTEINURIA

Protein may appear temporarily in the urine of any individual during intense physical activity, acute infections, emotional strain, exposure to

cold, or head injuries (including encephalography). Thus of 37 boys
7 to 13 years of age tested by Nackagawa and Kowamo, 35 showed
proteinuria following a long race (1,200 meters). The concentration of
protein which appears during physical activity may be as high as 6 gm
per 100 ml.

CONTINUOUS PROTEINURIA

Occasionally an individual is seen who continually excretes protein in
all urine specimens but seems otherwise free of kidney or urologic disease. Lying down or physical inactivity may reduce the intensity of the
proteinuria but does not stop it. During World War II, the author encountered seven such individuals among 22,000 otherwise healthy young
male recruits, nearly all 16 and 17 years of age. Regular follow-up examinations for signs of more serious renal disturbances seem indicated as
long as the disturbance persists. Intravenous urography and repeated
Addis counts will not infrequently uncover an anatomic renal defect or a
mild latent chronic glomerulonephritis.

UROLOGIC PROTEINURIA

Protein found in the urine does not necessarily come from the kidney.
Proteinuria of extrarenal origin may be derived from an inflamed bladder,
ureter, renal pelvis, prostate, or urethra. One usually finds accompanying
microscopic evidences of inflammation, with leukocytes outnumbering the
erythrocytes. Casts are ordinarily not seen in the absence of pyelonephritis.

The proteinuria is usually irregular and not heavy unless an abundance
of pus is also present; the content is usually in the neighborhood of 100
mg per 100 ml. Simple bleeding from the urinary mucous membranes
can give a positive protein test, but coincident erythrocytes or hemoglobin point to the origin of the protein.

NEPHRITIC PROTEINURIA

Acute nephritis leads to inconstant excretion of protein into all urine
specimens, regardless of posture, with quick inexplicable changes seem-
ingly unrelated to diet or activity or the amounts of accompanying water.
In general, the concentrations are higher than with the other forms of
proteinuria, apart from nephrosis, and may be as much as 6 or 7 gm per
100 ml in severe acute nephritis.

During chronic nephritis or the recovery phase of acute nephritis, in
contrast, the rates of excretion tend to remain more or less the same
from hour to hour, with transient rises during active exercise or after a
meal rich in protein. Hence, depending upon whether there is diuresis
or a scanty concentrated urine, the amount of protein per 100 ml of
urine will exhibit marked fluctuations through the day. If the period
between voidings is known and the bladder completely emptied each

time, the total protein excretion for 24 hours can be approximated from the quantitative study of a single specimen.

Quantitative studies of the 24-hour excretion of protein, erythrocytes, and casts in nephritis have shown that in general the amounts excreted per unit of time reflect the severity of the disease. The rate of protein excretion may therefore be taken as a guide to clinical progress. It must be remembered, however, that patients with marked edema, hypertension, and hematuria are occasionally seen in whom proteinuria may be mild or even cease for a time.

It is possible to make an otherwise constant nephritic proteinuria of mild degree disappear temporarily by forcing fluids to dilute the urine, while at the same time giving alkali by mouth in large doses to render the urine alkaline and its protein more soluble.

A sudden increase in the rate of excretion of protein by a patient who seems to be recovering from an active episode of acute nephritis is suggestive evidence that a turn for the worse is at hand. Such patients should be watched carefully, both clinically and by frequent urine tests, for early signs of further kidney damage. An exacerbation of proteinuria may herald the beginning of a nephrotic phase.

During recovery from acute nephritis the proteinuria gradually becomes milder and may take on a postural character. The proteinuria may last from a few weeks to many months after all clinical symptoms have gone. As the kidneys heal the various evidences of injury disappear independently of each other. The excretion of erythrocytes, casts, and epithelial cells as seen microscopically and measured quantitatively by the Addis method should all be back to normal before recovery can be adjudged as complete.

NEPHROTIC PROTEINURIA

The most prominent manifestations of the nephrotic syndrome in childhood are peripheral edema, low serum protein, lipemia, copious proteinuria, and minimal or absent hematuria. The total of protein lost in the urine may amount to as much as 10 to 20 gm per day, though it is usually between 0.5 and 5 gm daily. In terms of concentration this represents a spread from 0.3 to about 2 gm of protein per 100 ml of urine, though it may be as high as 6 gm per 100 ml. Fractional studies indicate that the urinary protein in the nephrotic syndrome is 80 or 90 per cent albumin. In more severe cases the globulin may become more abundant.

The excretion of protein in nephrosis fluctuates markedly from day to day. It mounts during relapses and diminishes during remissions. Balance studies on nephrotic patients receiving plasma protein concentrates intravenously have shown that all or nearly all such injected protein is lost in the urine within a matter of hours afterward. A sudden drop in the degree of proteinuria is one of the first signs of improvement and usually precedes diuresis by several days.

At the onset of an attack of kidney disease, when it is not clear whether a child is developing "pure" nephrosis or nephritis with a nephrotic component, the relation between the proteinuria and the excretion of casts and erythrocytes can be of aid in making the differentiation. In early nephritis, blood cells and casts tend to be as prominent as the proteinuria, whereas in beginning nephrosis these formed elements may be so few as to be missed in hasty examinations. However, the urine may be scanty and of high specific gravity in the early stages of either condition.

Electrophoretic data on urinary proteins in the various kidney diseases have shown the predominant component to be plasma albumin, though excretion of plasma globulin is increased also. However, in all forms of kidney diseases the fractional components vary so widely that it not feasible to associate any characteristic electrophoretic pattern with any single disease entity.

BIBLIOGRAPHY

PROTEINURIA

Addis, T., "Glomerular Nephritis: Diagnosis and Treatment," The Macmillan Company, New York, 1948.

Ek, J., Is Urinary Protein Excreted by the Renal Tubular Epithelium? *Scandinav. J. Clin. & Lab. Invest.* 2:72, 1950.

Greiner, Capt. T., and *J. P. Henry*, Mechanism of Postural Proteinuria, *J.A.M.A.* 157:1373, 1955.

King, S. E., Proteinuria Variations in the Differentiation of Renal Disorders, *J.A.M.A.* 155:1023, 1954.

Lippman, R. W., Effect of Antibiotic Agents on the Tests for Protein and Reducing Sugar in Urine, *Am. J. Clin. Path.* 22:1186, 1952.

Nakagawa, I., and *K. Kawamo*, Metabolism in Children during Muscular Work: Effect of Racing on Urinary Constituents in Boys, *Am. J. Dis. Child.* 49:594, 1935.

Nowak, H., Uber die Ursache und die Häufigkeit der Eiweissausscheidung im Harne Jugendlicher, *Monatsschr. Kinderh.* 59:341, 1933–1934.

Preston, L. S., Report of Intensive Laboratory Studies of High-school Athletes, *New York J. Med.* 40:1599, 1940.

Prince, C. L., Orthostatic Albuminuria, *J. Urol.* 50:608, 1943.

Rigas, Demetrios A., and *Carl G. Heller*, The Amount and Nature of Urinary Proteins in Normal Human Subjects, *J. Clin. Invest.* 30:853, August, 1951.

Routh, J. I., E. L. Knapp, and *C. K. Kobayashi*, Electrophoretic Studies of Plasma and Urinary Proteins in Children with Lipoid Nephrosis, *J. Pediat.* 33:688, 1948.

Wang, C. F., and *H. Wu*, Method for Determination of Protein in Normal Urine with Some Observations, *Chinese J. Physiol.* 12:371, 1937.

Wolman, I. J., Incidence, Causes and Intermittency of Proteinuria in Young Men, *Am. J. M. Sc.* 210:86, 1945.

CHAPTER 33

Microscopic Examination

Among the structures recognizable by urine microscopy are red cells, leukocytes, epithelial cells, casts, crystals, mucus shreds, talc or starch granules from dusting powders, oil globules from catheter lubricants, pinworm or other ova washed down from the vulvar area, and formed and amorphous crystals of various sorts. The number of such structures in a microscopic field depends upon the quantities originally present, their capacity to resist disintegration within the bladder before voiding or in the collection receptacle after voiding, the degree of concentration of the urine, and the technical handling of the specimen.

For most satisfactory results the microscopic examination should be made as soon as possible after voiding. Cellular elements and casts disintegrate rapidly and may disappear within a few hours, especially when the urine is alkaline or of low specific gravity. All specimens should be kept in a refrigerator until tested. When delay is unavoidable the formed structures can be preserved by adding 1 drop of formalin solution for each 30 ml of urine.

Erythrocytes, epithelial cells, leukocytes, and even casts are found occasionally in the urine of healthy individuals, particularly when it is of high specific gravity (i.e., concentrated) and examined soon after being passed. Should these occur with any frequency in uncentrifuged specimens, irritation or inflammation in the kidneys or urologic tract must be suspected. Strenuous exercise will often evoke a transitory appearance of red cells and assorted casts in the urine.

The most satisfactory specimen for the study of suspected nephritis is one passed after an interval of fluid deprivation, such as the first voiding of the morning. Such urine is richest in cells and casts. The specific gravity reading taken concurrently is another valuable indicator of renal status, since concentrating ability is one of the first functions to be lost in early parenchymal disease and one of the last to return during convalescence. Failure to find formed elements does not exclude renal disease except when the urine specimen is fresh, concentrated, and acid.

The usual method for determining whether the formed elements are increased is by noting the count of cells per high power field. This approach is far from accurate, since the number of cells is contingent upon many variables, including the cleanliness in collection. It is best to first scrutinize a shaken preparation and to centrifuge only when the urine appears cell-free by this approach. We have found it a good working rule, in the absence of clinical indications to the contrary, to view one or two nonepithelial leukocytes or erythrocytes in uncentrifuged urine from males or catheterized girls, or slightly more in younger uncatheterized girls, as the usual upper limits of normal. Counting the number of red or white cells in a known volume of uncentrifuged urine with a hemocytometer has been recommended; it is unusual to find more than 10 cells per cu mm in specimens from males or catheterized young girls (p. 393). Significant pyuria or hematuria is not excluded with fewer cells when the urine is excessively dilute as indicated by a low specific gravity. A catheterized specimen should be procured when there is doubt about the significance of leukocytes in voided urine from a girl.

In urologic disorders there are often periods in which the urine is rich in both erythrocytes and leukocytes and other periods in which it appears normal and cell-free. For this reason, when symptoms are suggestive of renal disease but corroboration is not found in the urine, several examinations should be made. Sometimes x-ray studies or cystoscopy reveal the presence of lesions despite negative urinary findings.

ERYTHROCYTES

Erythrocytes may enter the urine anywhere from the glomeruli to the urethral meatus. Their origin is frequently suggested by the attendant findings. For example, accompanying casts are a feature of nephritis; sulfonamide crystals suggest renal irritation; colicky lower abdominal cramps suggest a calculus; leukocytes or stainable microorganisms in a freshly voided specimen are evidences of renal or infrarenal inflammation. Absence of accompanying red cell casts suggests that the source of bleeding is below the kidney. The urethral orifice should always be examined, particularly in boy babies, since the site of the bleeding may be a marginal ulcer secondary to diaper or enuretic irritation.

Gross hematuria can be produced by nephritis, urologic lesions, stones, blood dyscrasias, medicaments, tumors, trauma, or local infection. Sometimes the cause is not apparent. Red cells in small numbers may be seen in any illness characterized by fever or toxemia.

Oil droplets or yeast cells may be mistaken for erythrocytes. A drop of glacial acetic acid added to the microscopy preparation will lyse red cells, but not yeast cells or oil.

Confirmatory checks for the occurrence of hematuria are the various chemical tests for hemoglobin. The orthotolidine test for blood in urine seems to be more sensitive than the others. To the centrifuged sediment of 15 ml of urine resuspended in 1 ml of urine is added 2 drops of 1 per cent orthotolidine (not orthotol*u*idine) solution in pure methyl alcohol and 2 drops of a mixture of glacial acetic acid 1 part and commercial hydrogen peroxide 2 parts. A transient blue color represents a positive result, the intensity of the color paralleling roughly the number of red cells present.

This test cannot be used with specimens preserved with formalin as in the Addis sediment-count technique. Formalin, iodides, and bromides will react with the reagent. If the color produced is due to blood, it will decrease or disappear after the urine is boiled for 1 minute, whereas if due to a halide it is unaffected by boiling.

The chemical tests respond to either red cells or free hemoglobin. Urine containing 2,000 red cells per ml will give a slight positive reaction with orthotolidine; 5,000 red cells per ml will give a comparatively strong reaction. With benzidine and phenolphthalin, a faintly positive reading is given by approximately 3,000 red cells per ml; at least 10,000 cells are needed for a strong reaction. Guaiac gives a faint positive reading with 5,000 cells and a strong reaction with 50,000 cells. The other components of urine seem to inhibit these test substances, rendering them much less sensitive than when used for stool studies.

Erythrocytes are ordinarily detectable with the high power of the microscope when their number exceeds 5,000 per ml of uncentrifuged urine. The microscopic search for red cells in fresh urine after centrifugation is therefore much more sensitive than chemical tests for detecting minimal numbers. The chemical tests are nevertheless useful when no microscope is at hand and moderate to severe hematuria is suspected. They are valuable in establishing the identity of hemoglobin in an old urine specimen whose red cells have become lysed.

EPITHELIAL CELLS AND LEUKOCYTES

Large flat cells of the squamous variety come from surface linings of the urethra, bladder, ureters, and renal pelves and calcyes. The deeper layers of the mucous membrane yield cells which are more rounded; these are not always distinguishable from tubular epithelial cells, wandering phagocytes from the blood stream, and cells from some extraurinary locus such as the vagina. All cells tend to change in appearance and size after being shed, because in osmotic pressure and pH the urine is usually quite different from blood and tissue fluid. Adding a drop of 1 per cent methylene blue solution to the microscopic preparation will assist in outlining the character of the nucleus.

The only cells which can be confidently ascribed to the kidney itself are the rounded or oval epithelial cells with prominent nuclei. When loaded with fat globules these are characteristic of renal disease or systemic disease involving the kidney. Those with only a few fat droplets may be seen also in febrile and other constitutional disturbances. Tumor cells may be excreted in small numbers in neoplasms originating within the kidney, but escape recognition in routine examinations.

Pus cells with polymorphic nuclei are called out whenever there is inflammation or other irritation in either the urogenital tract or the kidneys. When in small numbers they are typically discrete and separate, whereas when in abundance some may adhere in clumps. In girls they may be of vulvar rather than of urologic origin.

CASTS

Casts can develop in the tubules and in the collecting ducts. They are seen most often in nephritis in its various forms, but may appear also in congenital renal polycystic disease, anaphylactoid purpura, mercury poisoning, chronic pyelonephritis, hypercalcemia, polyarteritis nodosa, and obstructive uropathy. The long cylindrical casts come from the distal segments of damaged tubules, whereas those that are broader and perhaps shorter are derived from the collecting duct system. Casts may be conveniently grouped into several classes—hyaline, cellular or epithelial, blood-containing, cylindroids, and calcium-containing.

Hyaline Casts

These are pale and homogeneous and have sharp straight contours. They are believed to be formed by leakage and precipitation of proteinous material into the lumens of tubules containing weakly acid urine rich in dissolved salts. The more slender forms are believed to come from tubules with swollen epithelium.

Hyaline casts and their derivatives dissolve spontaneously in water and in acid urine and may be digested by the proteolytic enzymes normally present in urine. They are best sought for in freshly passed specimens.

Hyaline casts appear in a wide variety of conditions and may be found in otherwise normal individuals. They often form during periods of dehydration or inhibition of urine formation, as in fever and after exercise. Their presence does not necessarily signify the existence of acute nephritis, but only that the local environment in the distal tubules with respect to pH, dialyzable solutes, and stasis is favorable for protein precipitation. They have been observed in chronic congestion of the kidneys associated with circulatory failure, in diabetes which is not well regulated, in dehydration, in marasmus, and in jaundice even when proteinuria is not present. They are a regular feature of nephritis and may persist long after the proteinuria has disappeared.

Hyaline casts may contain red cells, epithelial cells, fat droplets, or cell debris. During nephritis, as Addis points out, the variants in hyaline cast structure depend upon the differences in tubular fluid content at the time the casts are forming. Trapped erythrocytes indicate glomerular damage, whereas epithelial cells and cell derivatives denote tubule cell degeneration or death.

Epithelial Casts

Casts of this variety may contain clearly recognizable segments of tubules, though more often they seem made up of packed agglomerations of separately desquamated cells. When the cells have disintegrated so that only debris and granules lie packed together, the appearance is that of the so-called granular cast. On further degeneration and autolysis, according to Addis, the granular casts become waxy. Waxy casts usually predominate in the first specimens obtainable from patients with tubule degeneration after a period of anuria.

Generally speaking, granular casts or their derivatives testify that tubular injury and desquamation are taking place. They occur abundantly in all forms of nephritis in which the tubules are affected. In the acute phases of glomerulonephritis they may be less numerous than later on. In febrile illnesses and circulatory congestion of the kidney they may be passed in small numbers. Epithelial casts and their granular and waxy derivatives do not dissolve in water, as will pure hyaline casts.

Renal Failure Casts

In terminal nephritis or uremia of any variety the so-called renal failure casts make their appearance. These may be epithelial, granular, or waxy; their significant characteristic lies in being two to six times broader than ordinary casts.

Blood-containing Casts

Made up largely of fibrin which has seeped through the glomerular walls and become precipitated within the tubules are casts which contain trapped erythrocytes or hemoglobin or partially broken down blood pigment. They are not water-soluble. Their presence is a sign of glomerular bleeding.

Cylindroids

Cylindroids are transparent formations of precipitated matter which resemble hyaline casts somewhat but differ in being longer and less clearly delimited. They are slender and may be branched or tapering. They are usually seen in acute nephritis during the recovery stage and in the same conditions which give rise to hyaline casts. They may be sufficiently plentiful to form a tangled mass at the bottom of the centrifuge tube.

Calcium-containing Casts

Casts containing calcium appear in the urine in hyperparathyroidism, vitamin D overdosage, and related disturbances which give rise to hyperphosphaturia and hypercalcinuria. They are granular in appearance, with a hyaline matrix containing precipitated calcium salts. They appear when the urine is close to neutrality or on the alkaline side. When urine containing these casts is acidified, they dissolve; the granules disappear first and the hyalin matrix soon afterward. Their continuing excretion is a sign of progressive kidney damage.

CRYSTALS

Crystals are frequently found in urine, especially when the specimen has been permitted to stand for some hours at low temperatures before examination. Triple phosphates, calcium phosphate, calcium carbonate, and ammonium urate crystallize out in alkaline urines. Calcium oxalate, sodium, calcium, magnesium, and potassium urates and uric acid crystals appear in acid urines. Sulfonamides may settle out when these are being taken. Cholesterol may be found in the nephrotic syndrome. Textbooks of clinical pathology carry illustrations and descriptions of these various crystals. Those which form in alkaline urine will generally redissolve when a little acid is added. Uric acid crystals are soluble in sodium hydroxide solution. The other urates can be made to disappear by simple heating of the specimen. The octahedral and dumbbell-shaped crystals of calcium oxalate are insoluble in acetic acid and in sodium hydroxide but will dissolve in strong hydrochloric acid.

These generalizations are helpful to remember when trying to examine centrifuged sediment which is rich in crystals. A drop of sodium hydroxide solution or of hydrochloric or acetic acid, depending on the urine pH, will usually clear away the interfering crystals.

The ready precipitation of urate crystals in the urine of newborn infants, and in the collecting ducts of the kidney as *uric acid infarcts,* results from physicochemical conditions rather than a higher concentration of urinary urates.

PARASITES

Trichomonas vaginalis is recognizable occasionally in fresh urine from adolescent girls who happen to have trichomoniasis. In very fresh and warm specimens these protozoa may still be motile. Under high-power magnification they appear as round or oval structures superficially resembling leukocytes and may be mistaken for such. Ova of the pinworm (*Oxyuris vermicularis*) may enter from vulvar contamination of the voided specimens in female children of all ages. The blood fluke (*Schistosoma hematobium*) deposits ova in the urine accompanied by blood and leukocytes; this infestation is endemic in some parts of Africa.

CYTOMEGALIC INCLUSION DISEASE

This is a poorly understood syndrome in which affected newborn infants exhibit jaundice, purpura, hepatomegaly, anemia, and splenomegaly. The urine is usually normal, but sometimes may contain epithelial cells, derived presumably from exfoliated renal tubular epithelium, which have large intracytoplasmic or intranuclear inclusionlike bodies. One method for their demonstration is to fix the smears of urine sediment in a mixture of equal parts of ether and 95 per cent ethyl alcohol for 20 minutes and then stain with hematoxylin and eosin.

BIBLIOGRAPHY

MICROSCOPIC EXAMINATION

Addis, T., "Glomerular Nephritis, Diagnosis and Treatment," The Macmillan Company, New York, 1948.

Albright, F., and *E. Bloomberg,* Hyperparathyroidism and Renal Disease with a Note as to the Formation of Calcium Casts in this Disease, *Trans. Am. A. Genito-Urin. Surgeons* **27**:195, 1934.

Boyle, H. H., C. A. Aldrich, A. Frank, and *S. Borowsky,* Addis Count in Children Following Clinical Recovery from Post Infectious Nephritis, *J.A.M.A.* **108**:1496, 1937.

Brewer, D. B., A Simple Technique for the Demonstration of Urinary Casts, *J. Clin. Path.* **6**:251, August, 1953.

Friedman, I. S., S. Zuckerman, and *T. D. Cohn,* The Production of Urinary Casts during the Use of Cation Exchange Resins, *Am. J. M. Sc.* **221**:672, 1951.

Gardner, K. D., Jr., "Athletic Pseudonephritis"—Alteration of Urine Sediment by Athletic Competition, *J.A.M.A.* **161**:1613, 1956.

Giles, M. G., Addis Count in Prognosis of Acute Nephritis in Childhood, *Arch. Dis. Childhood* **22**:232, 1947.

Larcom, R. C., Jr., and *G. H. Carter,* Erythrocytes in Urinary Sediment: Identification and Normal Limits, *J. Lab. & Clin. Med.* **33**:875, 1948.

Lippman, Richard W., "Urine and the Urinary Sediment: A Practical Manual and Atlas," Charles C Thomas, Springfield, Ill., 1951.

Lyttle, J. D., Addis Sediment Count in Normal Children, *J. Clin. Invest.* **12**:87, 95, 1933.

Margileth, A. M., The Diagnosis and Treatment of Generalized Cytomegalic Inclusion Disease of the Newborn, *Pediatrics* **15**:270, 1955.

Rofe, P., The Cells of Normal Human Urine, *J. Clin. Path.* **8**:25, 1955.

Rubin, M. I., M. Rapoport, and *A. D. Waltz,* Comparison of Routine Urinalysis, Addis Count and Blood Sedimentation Rate as Criteria of Activity in Acute Glomerulonephritis, *J. Pediat.* **20**:32, 1942.

Snoke, A. W., Normal Addis Sediment Count in Children, *J. Pediat.* **12**:473, 1938.

Sternheimer, R., and *B. Malbin,* Clinical Recognition of Pyelonephritis, with a New Stain for Urinary Sediments, *Am. J. Med.* **11**:312, September, 1951.

Wedgwood, R. J. P., and *H. K. Marshall,* Anaphylactoid Purpura (Schonlein-Henoch Syndrome). A Longterm Follow-up Study with Special Reference to Renal Involvement, *Pediatrics* **16**:196, 1955.

CHAPTER 34

Other Abnormal Constituents

EXCESS AMINO ACIDS

Arginine, cystine, glycine, histidine, leucine, methionine, phenylalanine, serine, threonine, tryptophane, tyrosine, valine, proline, lysine, and iso-leucine—each in small amount—may occur in normal human urine. The total 24-hour output of amino acids by the average healthy child ranges from 100 to 400 mg, calculated as amino nitrogen.

Excessive or abnormal excretions of amino acids have been described in phenylpyruvic idiocy, cystine storage disease, cystinuria, acute necrosis of the liver, severe chronic liver disease, galactosemia, hepatolenticular degeneration (Wilson's disease), after intravenous infusion of amino acids, in premature infants not receiving ascorbic acid, and in various renal disorders. The aminoaciduria which accompanies severe diseases of the liver (usually with extensive cellular destruction) is associated with an increased content of amino acids in the blood. In cystinuria and most of the other disturbances, on the other hand, the excretion seems to be a renal phenomenon since the blood level of these substances is not elevated.

Microbiologic Assay

The amino acids in urine or other body fluids can be identified and even quantitatively estimated by microbiologic techniques or by paper partition chromatography. The microbiologic method employs selected bacterial strains which require certain of the amino acids for growth. *Streptococcus faecalis* is used for leucine, isoleucine, valine, methionine, tryptophane, threonine, lysine, arginine, and histidine. *Lactobacillus delbrueckii* is utilized for phenylalanine, serine and tyrosine, *L. arabinosus* for glutamic acid, and *Leuconostoc mesenteroides* for cystine, aspartic acid, proline, and glycine. For each determination the urine or other unknown fluid and the test bacterium are added to a synthetic medium which is complete with respect to every essential nutrient except the respective amino acid to be assayed. The extent of growth of the organism is a measure of the quantity of specific amino acid present.

Paper Partition Chromatography

This approach is based upon the differential solubility of the respective amino acids in solvents of different properties. In practical operation, a few droplets of very dilute urine are placed at one end of a strip of moisture-saturated filter paper or at the center of a paper disk. A solvent, preferably not water-miscible, is then allowed to creep slowly along the paper. The individual amino acids, having distinctive solubilities for the water held in the cellulose fibers of the paper and for the moving solvent, are drawn along at definite speeds and arrange themselves characteristically at various spots along the way. The paper is then sprayed with a reagent such as 0.1 per cent Ninhydrin in butyl alcohol. Drying causes the amino acids to show themselves as purple spots. The location of each is then denoted by the so-called Rf value, which is the ratio of the distance of a spot from the starting point to the total distance traveled by moving solvent. Interpretations may be confirmed and unknown spots identified by parallel tests with synthetic mixtures of known chemicals, by addition of known amino acids as "markers" to the specimen, or by removal of a spot through destruction with specific enzymes. The precise concentrations are indicated roughly by comparison of the size and intensity of developed color spots with those from known amounts of pure amino acids applied at the same time.

In unhydrolyzed urine, fewer free amino acids are found with paper partition chromatography than with microbiologic assay. After hydrolysis, however, results with the two methods are essentially identical.

CYSTINOSIS (CYSTINE STORAGE DISEASE WITH AMINOACIDURIA, LIGNAC-FANCONI DISEASE)

This is a congenital disorder of amino acid metabolism in which cystine crystals are widely distributed through the reticuloendothelial system. During life the crystals may be demonstrated in bone marrow and lymph node aspirates and in the cornea and conjunctiva of the eyes.

The disease may be transmitted hereditarily as a mendelian recessive or dominant and shows itself soon after birth. There may be stunting of growth, refractory rickets, polyuria, polydipsia, aminoacidemia, acidosis, hypopotassemia, hypophosphatemia, dehydration, hypocalcemia, or allied metabolic imbalances. Involvement of the kidneys aggravates the condition; lactose, glucose, or other sugars may be excreted intermittently. Uremia is a common cause of death.

Paper partition chromatography of the urine is a ready way of establishing the diagnosis. The urine typically contains 10 to 20 normal and abnormal amino acids in excess, including some cystine. Cystine crystals, however, are rarely demonstrable in microscopic study of the urinary sediment, and cystine calculi do not become deposited in the urologic tract.

CYSTINURIA

Many otherwise normal-appearing individuals continuously excrete unusual amounts of cystine in the urine. This defect appears to be different from the more severe cystinosis with associated growth defects described above. The fault seems to lie in the internal metabolism of cysteine, homocysteine, or methionine. Lewis found 4 instances among

11,000 healthy college students. Nearly always the condition is benign and not suspected.

Normal urine always contains small amounts of cystine, 0.01 to 0.8 gm per 24 hours. Patients with cystinuria may excrete as much as 0.5 or even 1.0 gm per 24 hours. Paper chromatography has revealed that lysine and usually arginine may also be excreted in excess, despite normal plasma levels of these and the other common amino acids. The urinary loss of these substances seems due to a specific impairment of renal tubular reabsorption. The condition is hereditary, being a mendelian recessive, and is present at birth. When one member of a family is affected, several others can usually be found with the disturbance. The subjects are clinically normal, though a small percentage ultimately develops urinary stones. The urine is supersaturated with respect to cystine when excreted, so that the characteristic crystals tend to separate out after voiding, especially when the reaction is acid. These crystals are flat, colorless, and hexagonal. If the reaction is alkaline, addition of acid will often induce further crystal formation after several hours. Most effected individuals go through life unaware of their metabolic anomaly unless cystine stones develop in the kidney or bladder (p. 402), perhaps with a hydronephrosis or urinary tract infection.

FREE AMMONIA

The most common rash in the diaper region during the infancy years, and with enuresis of older ages, is an irritative dermatitis caused by free ammonia. The ammonia forms in the diaper or other garments *after* they have become wet, as the result of decomposition of the urinary urea by the bacteria on the perineal skin. *Alkaligenes faecalis, Al. ammonia-genes, Proteus vulgaris,* diphtheroids, and micrococci are the chief offenders. Urine is a good culture medium for organisms, and the body warmth favors their growth. The wet diapers must remain in contact with the skin for at least a half hour and usually much longer before enough ammonia can form to be irritating.

The reason that ammoniacal diaper rash is not seen in the newborn period or the first few months of life is probably related to the absence of these organisms in the feces at this age period. Once they become established in the colon they appear to persist throughout life.

Ammoniacal diaper dermatitis is best treated by prevention. Commonly employed measures include (1) boiling of the diapers between usings in order to sterilize them, (2) application of salves to the affected areas to promote healing and prevent further exposure to the irritant should ammonia continue to form, (3) sprinkling or impregnation of the diapers with some antiseptic or boric acid. Boric acid both inhibits the growth of the urea-splitting bacteria and neutralizingly combines with any ammonia which is produced.

When an obstructed urinary tract is infected internally with any of the urea-splitting organisms, as in pyuria or pyelonephritis, local liberation of ammonia may cause an irritative cystitis or serve as the basis for the formation of calculi.

BACTERIA AND URINARY TRACT INFECTIONS

Urinary tract infections in children are caused by organisms which enter from the bowel, skin, or circulation. These infections may be transitory, persistent, or recurrent. Recent studies indicate that pyelonephritis is more common than previously thought and that most instances of acute and chronic urinary tract infection in childhood originate in or are associated with a pyogenic focus within the kidney parenchyma itself. The pyelonephritis may be secondary to some urinary tract malformation, especially in boys, or it may develop in the absence of any demonstrable obstructive lesion.

Chills, fever, lumbar pain, dysuria, pyuria, proteinuria, and bacilluria are the usual manifestations in the early stages. Uremia and anemia may be late complications. Symptoms are often intermittent. Repeated urine analyses and cultures may be necessary to establish the diagnosis, since single urine specimens may be cell-free, protein-free, and bacteriologically sterile.

The leukocytes are usually more increased than the erythrocytes. Excessive protoplasmic motion within the leukocytes in freshly passed urine has been said to be a sign of active bacterial infection. The few casts which may be seen tend to be granular. The protein output is often less than 100 mg per 100 ml of urine.

Differentiation of pyelonephritis from glomerulonephritis and the other nephropathies rests upon the history of recurrent urinary tract infections, the roentgen demonstration of distortion in the urologic tract, and the recovery of pus cells and bacteria from the urine itself. Treatment must consist both of correction of all discoverable anatomic irregularities and of a chemotherapeutic attack on the offending bacteria.

The possibility of urinary tract infection must always be entertained whenever a child, and especially a girl, exhibits fever for which no cause is apparent on careful physical examination. That pyuria may be absent must be kept in mind since even when heavy with organisms the urine at times may appear crystal-clear. After a course of treatment the urine should be demonstrated to be free of bacteria by culture rather than simply by microscopic study for leukocytes. One is more likely to recover organisms if diuresis exists at the time the culture is made.

Aseptic Collection of Urine Specimens

No antibacterial medication should be given for 3 days prior to taking the culture. Urine cultures from boys are usually satisfactory if the prepuce is retracted, the urethral meatus cleansed with soapy water or a mild antiseptic, and the first portion of the voiding discarded before a sample is caught in a sterile test tube.

Cultures from girls must always be obtained by catheterization. Metal catheters are preferable to those of flexible rubber or plastic, though either type may be used. Glass catheters may break and should not be used. Catheters about 10 cm long with about 4 cm of rubber tubing attached at the far end can be sterilized within the test tubes which will be later used to hold the urine and carried in the physician's bag for emergency use. After every catheterization, and particularly when a urinary tract anomaly with stasis is suspected, it is advisable to give an antibiotic or sulfonamide for at least 3 days in order to guard against implantation of contaminating infection by the procedure itself.

Identification of Organisms

The urine when collected should be cultured first and then spun in a centrifuge to procure sediment for microscopic examination. The sediment may be fixed on a slide with heat and stained. Gram stain is preferable to methylene blue because the differentiation between Gram-positive and Gram-negative bacteria is an essential first step in the identification. Microorganisms if present in large numbers will be readily detectable, and their appearances and staining responses will give preliminary information as to identity.

In our experience, the stained smears of centrifuged fresh sediment will reveal recognizable organisms in about half of all urine specimens which later yield positive cultures. The occurrence of leukocytes in the sediment has borne no direct correlation with the presence or absence of demonstrable bacteria or later cultural results. Bacteriologic cultures are necessary even when the smears show organisms, in order to identify the species and determine its antibiotic sensitivities.

Bacteria multiply rapidly in nonsterile specimens, especially if not refrigerated. Discovery of bacteria in urinary sediment is of no significance unless the examination is made within a few minutes after voiding.

Urinary tract infections may be caused by a diversity of organisms. The most frequent invaders are *Escherichia coli, Proteus ammoniae* or *vulgaris, Streptococcus faecalis, Aerobacter aerogenes,* or *Pseudomonas aeruginosa.* Less frequently found are *Alcaligenes faecalis, Escherischia intermedium* or paracolon (the "coliform" bacilli), *Staphylococcus areus, Streptococcus haemolyticus, Mycobacterium tuberculosis,* nonhemolytic streptococci, diplococci, *Klebsiella pneumoniae* or pneumococci. Co-agulase-negative staphylocci are occasionally recovered; these are usually interpreted as contaminants. Multiple species may be found in 10 to 20 per cent of cultures. Pseudomonas, Proteus, colon bacilli, and other Gram-negative bacilli are, at the time of writing, among the most refractory to therapy of all the organisms mentioned.

The choice of culture media depends upon the organism whose presence is suspected. The Gram-negative bacilli, and particularly *Esch. coli, A. aerogenes, Pr. vulgaris,* and *Ps. aeruginosa,* grow well on eosin–methylene blue agar. *Str. faecalis* is the only Gram-positive streptococcus that will grow on this medium, so that, according to Helmholz, any Gram-positive coccus growing on an eosin–methylene blue agar plate becomes thereby identifiable. Blood agar plates or tubes are the best to bring out the other Gram-positive organisms. *M. tuberculosis* requires its own special media or guinea pig inoculation.

Coliform organisms when present tend to overgrow staphylococci and streptococci on culture plates, so that the coincident presence of the latter may be overlooked at first. If therapy suppresses the coliform strains, the remaining bacteria in the mixture become revealed when resistant.

Pleuropneumonia-like organisms have at times been isolated from inflamed genitourinary tracts by special selective media. These organisms appear to be components of the normal flora of females, so that more critical information must be accumulated before their pathogenicity can be accepted.

A simple office procedure for urine culture has been described by Helmholz. Sterile agar in a culture tube is melted over a flame or in boiling water. This is permitted to cool sufficiently so that the tube can be held comfortably against the cheek. Three drops of urine is then introduced, under strict precautions. The tube is kept warm in an incubator or the vest pocket until it can be given to a bacteriologist.

Bacteria though still viable may not grow out for some days in infected urine if the patient has been taking a chemotherapeutic drug immediately prior to collection of the specimen. For patients receiving treatment it is important to hold all cultures for 5 to 7 days before reporting them as negative.

With all forms of therapy it is wise to reculture the urine 1 week after the medication has been stopped, in order to make sure that the infection has been eradicated. If no growth is obtained a culture may be taken again after a month or two, should absolute assurance of cure be desired.

Renal tuberculosis should always be suspected in chronic pyuria when repeated urine cultures fail to show any bacterial growth, though other causes of inflammation such as foreign bodies, chemical irritants, and culture-refractory organisms must also be ruled out.

It is a common experience with patients having chronic pyuria or bacteriuria that recurrences after periods of active therapy may be induced by an organism or organisms different than the one originally recovered. In one child with a urinary tract anomaly we encountered six different organisms in as many months. Such observations suggest that recurrences are often new invasions of bacteria. In most chronic childhood infections there is usually some underlying anatomic lesion to trap and retain organisms as they enter from the circulation, regional lymphatics, or urethra.

Since infants with congenital urinary tract obstructions such as a posterior urethral valve are often free from infection when first seen, diagnostic catheterization must be done with complete asepsis or even omitted altogether, in order to avoid the introduction of infectious organisms.

General Principles of Chemotherapy

There is no universal sterilizing agent for urinary tract infections. A sound program of therapy must include (1) locating and correcting anatomic obstructions and foci of infection related to the flow of urine, (2) bacteriologic identification of the responsible microorganism, and (3) utilization of antibiotic sensitivity tests when the organism is one which exhibits strain variability in susceptibility to these substances, in order to select the antibacterial agent or agents which promise to be the most effective (Chap. 76). It is important that the sensitivity tests be carried out with freshly recovered organisms rather than subcultures. Quantitative measurement of the approximate threshold sensitivities of the organism to concentrations of the antibiotics, followed by giving of sufficiently large doses to achieve this threshold value, may sometimes be necessary. With stubborn cases and mixed infections it is often necessary to give several carefully chosen agents concurrently, as, for example, sulfonamides and an antibiotic, or a combination of two or more antibiotics.

Most chemotherapeutic agents are excreted into the urine in concentrations much higher than those present in the blood at the same time and far in excess of what is required to inhibit the growth of susceptible organisms. With the broad-spectrum group, for example, when kidney function is good, the urinary concentration may be 100 times greater than that of the serum. The bactericidal properties are also influenced by the hydrogen ion concentration. Streptomycin is more effective in alkaline urine, whereas penicillin is more potent in acid urine. Neither mandelic acid nor methenamine is effective except in the presence of strong acidity. Except for streptomycin, the antibiotics are readily excreted even when renal function is poor. Recurrent or chronic infections need a urologist's attention, since obstruction or malformation is usually in the background.

In patients with one normal kidney and the other infected, the voided urine may appear free from viable bacteria during therapy but yield positive cultures as soon as the medication is discontinued. As long as the medication is being taken the therapeutic agent excreted by the good kidney kills off within the bladder the bacteria that are coming from the diseased one.

KETONE BODIES

The excretion of acetone, usually with the concomitant presence of acetoacetic and beta-hydroxybutyric acid, is a sign that the metabolism of fats is either imperfect or accelerated (p. 547).

It is advisable to include a test for acetone in every urine analysis made on any child, sick or well. When this is positive, acetoacetic acid should then be looked for to ascertain the severity of the ketosis.

Acetone can be detected by the Lange's sodium nitroprusside test or Wallhauser's test which employs mercuric cyanide and silver nitrate. Acetoacetic (diacetic) acid can be recognized by Gerhard's ferric chloride test. Beta-hydroxybutyric acid reacts with the reagents for acetone and also with Hart's hydrogen peroxide reagent. Instructions for these procedures are described in all good texts on laboratory methods.

The ferric chloride test may respond not alone to acetoacetic acid but also to phenylpyruvic acid and to various coal tar derivatives such as acetylsalicylic acid (aspirin), sodium salicylate, phenacetin, phenazone (antipyrine), and other coal tar drugs. Acetoacetic acid and all drugs except phenacetin give an immediate positive reaction with 10 per cent ferric chloride solution. The dark-brown color due to phenacetin develops slowly and reaches its maximum intensity in 2 or 3 minutes.

It is recommended that an apparently positive test for acetoacetic acid be confirmed. One drop of concentrated nitric acid is mixed with another 4 ml of urine in a test tube. The mixture is boiled for about 2 minutes, cooled thoroughly under the tap, and 2 ml of ferric chloride solution added. If the urine contains acetoacetic acid only, this second test will be negative, since the diacetic acid will be converted to acetone and volatilized away. Should the urine contain a drug, the second test will be still positive though the color may be altered or reduced in intensity.

During starvation states such as malnutrition, vomiting, gastro-enteritis, and postoperative low food intake, the appearance of ketonuria can be taken as indicating that the body is in need of more glucose than is being made available. In the management of such conditions one should endeavor to keep the urine ketone-free at all times. A good working rule to protect against or counteract ketosis is to see that the sick child receives enough sugar each day to supply or exceed his total daily requirement of calories.

Both schools of management of the diabetic child aim to keep the urine free of ketone bodies (p. 369). Excretion of these substances is a sign of incipient or existent diabetic acidosis.

In diabetic ketoacidosis when insulin and extra glucose are suddenly given, or in the ketosis of starvation when glucose is once more made available, the sudden swing of the tissues from ketone to glucose utilization may lead to a transient surplus of ketones in the blood stream and their excretion in great abundance into the urine. Ketonuria in a diabetic patient in the absence of glycosuria is not an indication for further insulin therapy.

LIPIDS

Droplets of doubly refractile lipid are often demonstrable in the urine of nephrotic subjects. These droplets may be free in the sediment or lodged within granular or fatty casts. Similar droplets also appear in chronic nephritis when lipid infiltration of the tubular epithelium has occurred. The double refractility must be searched for by study of the sediment with polarizing lenses attached to the microscope. Normal urine occasionally contains a little lipid, but in kidney disease the droplets are present in much larger numbers and tend to be persistent.

Chemical analysis has shown the urinary lipids in nephrosis and allied syndromes to be a mixture of cholesterol, fatty acids, and phospholipids, all presumably derived from the plasma lipids. These are believed to enter the urine through both glomerular leakage and desquamation of tubular epithelium. The rate of excretion tends to parallel that of the proteinuria and to reflect the degree of kidney damage. Lipids do not escape into the urine when the kidneys are functioning normally, even when the blood lipid level is 10 times the normal.

Small amounts of fat may be found in the urine of patients after severe trauma. Efforts to correlate this observation with the clinical picture of fat embolism have been unsuccessful.

Scuderi's "sizzle" test may be applied to the study of the urine for fat globules. The urine specimen must come from a completely emptied bladder since fat floats on top and is the last to be voided. A platinum loop is introduced into the top layer of the specimen and inserted into a Bunsen flame. Sizzling or popping occurs with urinary fat content of 1:1600 or higher. An alternative procedure is to expose a few drops of top layer urine to fresh concentrated Sudan III stain on a glass slide for at least 5 minutes. Fat globules will be apparent on microscopic examination, but any stained formations under 4 μ in diameter may be artefacts.

ORGANIC ACIDS

Glucuronic and Salicylic Acids

Phenolic and alcoholic substances unite with glucuronic acid within the liver and may be excreted in combination by the kidney. In normal children and in children with inactive rheumatic fever (ages 5 to 13 years), the 24-hour excretion of glucuronic acid was found by Tseng, Elghammer, and Ivy to range from 99 to 361 mg. Slightly higher values were found during active rheumatic fever, tonsillitis, sinusitis, and pharyngitis. The rate of excretion went up when aspirin was taken alone, owing to salicylic acid being excreted as the glucuronide, and subsided when sodium bicarbonate in twice the dosage was added to the aspirin.

Free salicylate can be detected in appreciable amounts in the urine while aspirin or other salicylates are being taken and for 2 to 4 days thereafter. The excretion of salicylic acid in 8 children receiving aspirin was found by the above authors to average 56 per cent of the intake (range 36 to 66 per cent). When twice the amount of sodium bicarbonate was added to the aspirin the excretion of salicylate rose to an average of 70 per cent (range 65 to 82 per cent).

PHENYLPYRUVIC AND RELATED ACIDS

Phenylpyruvic Idiocy (Phenylpyruvic Oligophrenia)

This is a familial and mendelian recessive disease characterized by mental deficiency, neuromuscular disturbances, and overflow of phenylalanine, phenylpyruvic acid, and phenyllactic acid into the urine from high serum content. The serum phenylalanine level, normally 2 to 5 mg per 100 ml, may be between 20 and 60 mg per 100 ml. Metabolic evidence suggests that the normal route of metabolism of phenylalanine is by way of tyrosine, and that the patient with phenylpyruvic idiocy can not convert phenylalanine to tyrosine.

There are no obvious clinical signs which permit one to distinguish this disturbance from many other forms of idiocy. The relation of the metabolic defect to the nervous system involvement has not been elucidated. An unusually high percentage of affected individuals are blond, which may be related to the fact that tyrosine is a metabolic precursor of melanin.

The phenylalanine, phenylpyruvic acid, and phenyllactic acid appear in the urine in the approximate though somewhat variable ratios of 4:2:2. Total excretions become increased when proteins containing an abundance of phenylalanine are fed. They disappear from the urine, along with recession of the serum phenylalanine to normal and some clinical improvement, when a phenylalanine-restricted diet is fed for an extended period of time. Healthy persons receiving average diets do not excrete these substances in detectable amounts.

Of the three substances which appear in the urine, the only one which is easy to test for is phenylpyruvic acid. The test is done by first acidifying about 5 ml of urine if it is alkaline, and then adding about 1 ml of 5 per cent ferric chloride solution. A deep blue-green color which appears within a few moments, and fades away after 5 to 30 minutes, represents a positive reaction. Other colors should be ignored. In our experience the green color can usually be brought out also in neutral or alkaline urine, but initial acidification is helpful. The urine may have a definite aromatic odor. Paper chromatography will demonstrate the abnormal amino aciduria.

The ferric chloride test for phenylpyruvic acid should be an integral step in the study of every infant and child who is mentally retarded. A positive reaction establishes the nature of the condition and makes it unnecessary to carry out more elaborate diagnostic tests.

Prematurity

There is a related but transient metabolic disturbance in the metabolism of tyrosine and phenylalanine in premature infants, prominent when vitamin C is absent from the diet. When such infants were given 5 gm or more of cow's-milk protein per kg body weight per day, Levine, Marples, and Gordon found that L-para-hydroxyphenyllactic and para-hydroxyphenylpyruvic acids were excreted in the urine in quantities of 300 to 500 mg of tyrosine equivalent per kg body weight per 24 hours. The giving of L-ascorbic acid eradicated the defect. With breast-milk or cow's-milk mixtures of reduced protein content, the daily excretion of these substances fell to below 10 mg.

STONES

Pathogenesis

Urinary calculi do not develop spontaneously; their presence is associated either with some local urinary tract disturbance such as stasis or infection or obstruction or with some metabolic fault, usually hereditary. They may be found within the renal pelves, the calcyes, the ureters, the bladder, the urethra, or (rarely) in the prostate or prepuce. Pyuria and hematuria are common associated findings.

Some stones are lamellated or multicrystalline. Others are "pure," being made up almost entirely of a single component. Campbell gives the following order of frequency for the various types of stones seen in the childhood years:

1. Uric acid
2. Urates (ammonium, sodium, potassium)
3. Oxalates (calcium, ammonium, magnesium)
4. Phosphates (calcium, ammonium, magnesium)
5. Carbonates (calcium, ammonium, magnesium)
6. Cystine
7. Xanthine

For proper therapy and prevention of recurrences it is important to subject every stone passed to chemical analysis, in order to determine whether a metabolic fault is present and to have guidance as to the diet and the proper pH at which the urine should be kept in the future.

Stones and crystalluria usually bear little relation to each other. The transient excretion of urates, oxalates, or phosphates does not mean that stones are being deposited in the urinary tract. It is wise, nevertheless, to think of the possibility of a homologous stone when crystalluria of any specific type becomes repeatedly exhibited.

Uric Acid Stones

These, the most common, are related to urinary stasis and infection. They are usually hard and brittle, with a lamellated structure and a yellow or mahogany color as the result of blood pigment absorbed from secondary traumatic hemorrhages. Uric acid itself is not radiopaque, but the contours of these calculi are often roentgenologically evident because of calcium salts incorporated into their substance.

Mention may be made of the needle-shaped masses of uric acid and ammonium urate (uric acid infarcts) which are found often in autopsies of newborn infants within the bladder, collecting ducts, and even the kidney tubules. These are most likely to appear in neutral or alkaline urine and bear no relation to any stone formation that may develop later in life.

Magnesium-Ammonium Phosphate Stones

These customarily develop in the presence of severe chronic urinary infection which makes the urine alkaline. Typically white or grayish yellow, they are soft and crumbly when removed. They may fill a calyx, the entire renal pelvis, or the greater part of the bladder. Their growth is often initiated by a small oxalate or uric acid or some other form of calculus.

Calcium-containing Stones

Primary calcium calculi are usually combined with oxalates, phosphates, or carbonates and form most readily in alkaline or neutral urine. They are radiopaque. Calcium oxalate stones are hard and brownish black, with a spiculated or nodular surface resembling a nutmeg or mulberry. Calcium phosphate stones are small, rounded, lamellated, white or yellow, and radiopaque. Calcium carbonate stones have a consistency that resembles chalk.

Calcium-containing stones may develop whenever there is persistent hypercalciuria, as in hyperparathyroidism, oxalosis, excessive intake of calcium or vitamin D, renal tubular acidosis, chronic pyelonephritis, inability of the renal tubules to form ammonia, or the osteoporosis which accompanies prolonged immobilization. These stones are sometimes found in normal subjects. They have a high recurrence rate, since the disturbance responsible for their presence is usually constitutional and persistent.

Oxalosis is a rare inborn error of metabolism in which oxalic acid is formed excessively, presumably from endogenous sources, and combines with calcium to form inert masses. Calculi of calcium oxalate occur in the urinary passages in association with extensive deposition of calcium oxalate crystals in kidneys, bone marrow, and other internal organs. Crystalluria due to calcium oxalate, not infrequent in otherwise normal children, as a rule does not indicate the existence of a stone.

Cystine Stones

These develop in a minority of those individuals who have a hereditary tendency to excessive urinary excretion of cystine. Usually unilateral, they are small, smooth-surfaced, often multiple, and moderately radiopaque. They are deep yellow or yellow-brown and may slowly become green on exposure to light. They develop only in an acid medium and are soluble in alkali. Microscopically they consist of multiple hexagonal crystals within a yellow organic matrix. The effort has been made to cause them to disappear by keeping the urine strongly alkaline, and some success has been reported with this treatment.

SULFONAMIDES

The direct effect of sulfonamides upon the kidney is not well understood, but there seems no other explanation for the occasional development of temporary oliguria and hematuria with excretion of casts after only one or a few doses of some sulfonamide have been given. More often, however, the obstructive and irritative symptoms seem directly due to the precipitation of sulfonamide deposits anywhere along the excretory tract from collecting tubules to urethra. Hemorrhages follow, and the urine flow becomes obstructed. The factors which facilitate sulfonamide precipitation are (1) low solubility of the drug (whether free or acetylated) at the pH of the urine, (2) high content of the drug in the urinary fluid, and (3) low concentration of concomitant urea, which has solvent properties.

Sulfonamides are excreted in the urine as a mixture of the free and conjugated compounds (glucuronides and N^4-acetylated forms). The relative proportions of the free and conjugated forms are inconstant and variable, even in the same patient, but, in general, about 50 to 60 per cent of sulfanilamide and 25 to 30 per cent of sulfadiazine and sulfathiazole are excreted as conjugates, chiefly in the form of acetyl derivatives.

The solubility of most sulfonamides, including sulfathiazole, sulfapyridine, sulfadiazine, sulfamerazine, sulfamethazine, and their N_4-acetyl derivatives, becomes markedly increased as the pH of the urine is raised to 7.0 or higher. Any patient receiving these sulfonamides in large dosage or for a protracted period should be given liberal amounts of fluids and enough basic substances to keep the urine at or near a pH of 7.5. Hydrogen ion testing paper is helpful for this purpose; with children sick at home the parents can be instructed as to its use. When small dosages are prescribed for but a few days to a child who takes fluids well this precaution is ordinarily not essential.

Another safeguard against crystalluria is to use mixtures of sulfonamides. The triple or quadruple preparations reduce the incidence of crystals in the urine more than the dual mixtures. There are a few molecularly complex sulfonamides, including Gantrisin and Elkosin, which maintain a high urinary solubility within a wide pH range.

Excreted sulfonamides often crystallize within urine specimens which are stored at room or refrigerator temperature for some hours. From the standpoint of urine analysis, therefore, the discovery of crystals does not signify internal crystallization unless the urine is examined when warm and freshly voided or unless erythrocytes are also present in large numbers.

Microscopic hematuria is often induced by sulfonamides, especially sulfathiazole, and need not be viewed with alarm. Nevertheless, every child receiving a sulfonamide in large quantities for more than a few days should have a microscopic urinalysis done daily or every second day. Any marked renal reaction can then be detected in its beginning stages. The urinary output of fluid per day should also be measured, so that the water intake can be raised if the excretion is low.

Gross hematuria or crystalline deposits at the urethral meatus during the period of therapy are signs of crystal deposits within the urinary tract. If either of these findings occurs, one should discontinue the medication, give alkalis to attain the pH of optimal solubility in the urine, and raise to a maximum the ingestion of fluids.

The presence of soluble sulfonamides in urine can be demonstrated by the yellow color which develops when a sulfonamide-containing solution is placed in contact with lignin-containing wood fiber in the presence of an acid. The color results from the interaction of the aniline radical with the lignin. This reaction is produced only by the free sulfonamides, with the acetylated derivatives playing no part. To perform the test, one takes a fragment of newsprint, paper toweling (not rag paper), sawdust, or tongue depressor, and mixes upon it a few drops of 4 per cent hydrochloric acid or other acid with a similar quantity of urine. The distinctive color appears within a few minutes. Pale-yellow hues are given when the concentration is lower than about 75 mg free (unacetylated) sulfonamide per 100 ml of urine. Higher concentrations give a bright-orange color.

There is little need for anxiety concerning calculus formation with a patient receiving sulfonamides so long as the urine is kept sufficiently dilute to yield a yellow rather than an orange color with the wood fiber test and the pH is near that of maximal solubility for the preparation being given.

POISONS

Toxicologic methods are available for testing of urine for ethyl alcohol, bromides, arsenic, mercury, lead, barbiturate derivatives, and similar toxic substances.

Anticonvulsants

Barbiturates, hydantoinates, trimethadione, and related compounds, when taken in excess, can depress the central nervous system and induce a state of coma or semicoma. The diagnosis in these cases is most easily established by obtaining a history of accidental overdosage. If reagents are available, the urine can be tested for these derivatives (Selwyn and Dark).

Lead

Normal urine often contains minute traces of lead. The upper limit of normal for children may be taken as 55 mcg per 24 hours, according to the studies of Byers et al., and outputs of 55 to 80 mcg viewed with suspicion. One must bear in mind that the urinary excretion reflects only the amount of mobile lead in the body, not the total accumulation. Since the content of lead per unit volume of urine varies inversely with the total urinary output, the absolute amount per liter is not of diagnostic value except when excessive. The urine may also contain traces of protein, or sugar, or both. Therapy with the calcium disodium salt of ethylenediaminetetraacetic acid (CaEDTA), whether during the acute stage of intoxication or months afterwards, usually brings about a marked increase in urinary lead output of the magnitude of 1 to 4 mg per 24 hours.

Urine specimens for lead analyses must be collected in paraffined or otherwise lead-free containers which have lead-free covers. A simpler though only presumptive method for detecting lead poisoning is to study the urine for excess coproporphyrin (p. 355).

Copper

Excretion of abnormally large amounts of copper in the urine has been described in hepatolenticular degeneration (Wilson's disease). The output may be increased by administration of BAL. Brain and liver tissue obtained at necropsy of such patients have contained excessive amounts of copper. The concentration of copper in the plasma is low. Patients also excrete an excessive amount of amino acids and dicarboxylic amino acid peptides.

Mercury

Urine analysis for mercury has come into prominence as a result of the belief that many instances of acrodynia or acrocyanosis are idiosyncrasy reactions to ingested mercury (p. 977). Warkany and Hubbard analyzed the urine of 31 children with the acrodynia syndrome for mercury with the di-beta-naphthylthiocarbazone reagent and found detectable amounts in nearly every one. Concentrations of over 50 μgm per liter as determined by this method were deemed indicative of mercury intoxication. Excretion was erratic and continued in some instances for months.

BIBLIOGRAPHY

AMINO ACIDS

Davis, H. A., G. B. Mider, and *J. J. Morton,* Specificity of Paper Partition Chromatography for Analysis of Free Amino Acids in Unhydrolyzed Urine, *Proc. Soc. Exper. Biol. & Med.* 72:553, 1949.

Dent, C. E., The Amino-aciduria in Fanconi Syndrome: Study Making Extensive Use of Techniques Based on Paper Partition Chromatography, *Biochem. J.* 41:240, 1947.

Dunn, M. S., M. N. Camien, S. Shankman, and *H. Block,* Urinary Excretion of Acids by Normal Male and Female Subjects Measured Microbiologically, *Arch. Biochem.* 13:207, 1947.

Harper, H. A., M. Grossman, P. Henderson, and *H. Steinbach,* Renal Amino-Aciduria, *A.M.A. Am. J. Dis. Child.* 84:327, 1952.

Lowe, C. U., M. Terrey, and *E. A. MacLachlan,* Organic-aciduria, Decreased Renal Ammonia Production, Hydrophthalmos and Mental Retardation, *A.M.A. Am. J. Dis. Child.* 83:164, 1952.

Schreier, K., Some Peculiarities of Amino Acid Metabolism in Infancy and Early Childhood, *J. Pediat.* 46:86, 1955.

Spillane, J. D., J. W. Keyser, and *R. A. Parker,* Amino-aciduria and Copper Metabolism in Hepatolenticular Degeneration, *J. Clin. Path.* 5:16, 1952.

Thelander, H. E., and *R. Imagawa,* Amino Aciduria, Congenital Defects, and Mental Retardation, *J. Pediat.* 49:123, 1956.

CYSTINOSIS AND CYSTINURIA

Bickel, H., H. S. Baar, R. Astley, A. A. Douglas, E. Finch, H. Harris, C. C. Harvey, E. M. Hickmans, M. G. Philpott, W. C. Smallwood, J. M. Snellie, and *C. G. Teall,* Cystine Storage Disease with Aminoaciduria and Dwarfism (Lignac-Fanconi Disease), *Acta paediat.* vol. 42, suppl. 90, 1952.

Eberlein, W. R., Aminoaciduria in Childhood: Cystinuria and Cystinosis, *Am. J. M. Sc.* 225:677, 1953.

Ezell, S. D., Cystinuria, *Am. Pract.* 2:748, 1948.

Fanconi, G., and *H. Bickel,* Die Chronische Amino-acidurie, Amino Saurediabetes oder Nephrotisch-glykosrischer Zwergwuchs bei der Glykogenose und der Cystinkrankheit, *Helvet. paediat. acta* 4:359, 1949.

Freudenberg, E., Cystinosis: Cystine Disease (Lignac's Disease) in Children, *Advances Pediat.* 4:265, 1949.

Gatzimos, C. D., D. M. Schulz, and *R. L. Newnum,* Cystinosis (Lignac-Fanconi Disease), *Am. J. Path.* 31:791, 1955.

Israels, S., and *H. J. Suderman,* Cystinosis, *J. Pediat.* 47:73, 1955.

King, F. P., and *E. P. Lochridge,* Cystinosis (Cystine-storage Disease): Report of a Case with Chemical Isolation and Quantitative Determination of Cystine in Lymph Nodes, Spleen and Liver, *A.M.A. Am. J. Dis. Child.* 82:446, 1951.

Lewis, H. B., Cystinuria: A Review of Some Recent Investigations, *Yale J. Biol. & Med.* 4:437, 1931–32.

Sullivan, M. X., A Distinctive Test for Cysteine, *Pub. Health Rep.* 41:1030, 1926.

Williamson, D. A. J., Cystinosis, *Arch. Dis. Childhood* 27:356, 1952.

FREE AMMONIA

Brown, C. P., R. M. Tyson, and *F. H. Wilson,* Dermatitis (Diaper Rash): A Bacteriologic Study of the Diaper Region, *Pennsylvania M. J.* **55:**755, 1952.

Cooke, J. V., Dermatitis of Diaper Region in Infants (Jacquet Dermatitis), *Arch. Dermat. & Syph.* **14:**539, 1926.

———, The Ammoniacal Diaper, Ammonia Dermatitis and Ulceration of the External Urinary Meatus, *Brennemann-McQuarrie Practice Pediat.* vol. 4, chap. 41, 1956.

BACTERIA AND PYURIA

Carroll, G., Chronic Urinary Infections in Infants and Children, *Advances Pediat.* August, 1955, p. 781.

Helmholz, H. F., Practical Points in the Diagnosis and Treatment of Infections of the Urinary Passages in Childhood, *Ann. paediat.* **172:**325, 1949.

Logan, G. B., Urinary Infections in Children, *Proc. Staff Meet. Mayo Clin.* **24:**562, 1949.

Marshall, V. F., A Reconsideration of the Treatment of Urinary Infections, *M. Clin. North America* **34:**525, 1950.

Rhoads, P. S., C. E. Billings, and *V. J. O'Connor,* Antibacterial Management of Urinary Tract Infections, *J.A.M.A.* **148:**165, 1952.

Simons, I., Sterilization of Neurogenic Bladder by Mandelamine (Methenamine Mandelate): Studies in Bladder Function, XIII, *J. Urol.* **64:**586, 1950.

Stansfeld, J. M., and *J. K. G. Webb,* Observations on Pyuria in Children, *Arch. Dis. Childhood* **28:**386, 1953.

Wilhelm, S. F., W. A. Schloss, L. A. Orkin, E. Seligmann, and *M. Wassermann,* Aerobacter Aerogenes Infection of the Urinary Tract: Effective Treatment with Aureomycin, *J.A.M.A.* **141:**837, 1949.

KETONE BODIES

Bridge, E. M., "Epilepsy and Convulsive Disorders in Children," The Blakiston Division, McGraw-Hill Book Company, Inc., New York, 1949.

Heymann, W., (a) Reasons for High Carbohydrate Requirement of Infants and Children, *Am. J. Dis. Child.* **60:** 316, 1940. (b) Metabolism Studies on Age Disposition to Ketosis in Human Beings, *J. Pediat.* **12:**21, 1938. (c) Precipitation of Attacks of Recurrent Acetonemic Vomiting by Means of Ketogenic Diet, *Ohio M. J.* **33:**510, 1937.

Martin, H. E., and *A. N. Wick,* Quantitative Relationships between Blood and Urine Ketone Levels in Diabetic Ketosis, *J. Clin. Invest.* **22:**235, 1943.

Rutherfoord, G. T., Ketonuria in a Child with Cirrhosis of the Liver, *Brit. M. J.* **1:**480, 1949.

Weymuller, C. A., and *O. M. Schloss,* Non-diabetic Ketosis in Children, *Am. J. Dis. Child.* **34:**549, 1927.

Zwarenstein, H., Gerhardt's Test for Aceto-acetic Acid in Urine, *J. Lab. & Clin. Med.* **30:**172, 1945.

LIPIDS

Fishberg, A. M., "Hypertension and Nephritis," 4th ed., Lea & Febiger, Philadelphia, 1939.

Parrish, A. E., and *L. K. Alpert,* Stain for Lipid Bodies in Urinary Sediment, *J.A.M.A.* **152:**1713, 1953.

Quinn, J. R., and *H. J. Zimmerman,* Significance of Oval Fat Bodies in Urinary Sediment, *Am. J. Clin. Path.* **24:**787, 1954.

Scuderi, C. S., Fat Embolism: A Clinical and Experimental Study, *Surg., Gynec. &
Obst.* 72:732, 1941.

PHENYLPYRUVIC AND RELATED ACIDS

Armstrong, M. D., and *F. H. Tyler,* Studies on Phenylketonuria: I. Restricted Phenylalanine Intake in Phenylketonuria. *J. Clin. Invest.* 34:505, 1955.

Bickel, H., J. Gerrard, and *E. M. Hickmans,* Influence of Phenylalanine Intake on
Chemistry and Behavior of a Phenylketonuric Child, *Acta paediat.* 43:64, 1954.

Dann, M., E. Marples, and *S. Z. Levine,* Phenylpyruvic Oligophrenia, Report of a
Case in an Infant with Quantitative Chemical Studies of the Urine, *J. Clin. Invest.* 22:87, 1943.

Horner, F. A., and *C. W. Streamer,* Effect of a Phenylalanine-Restricted Diet on Patients with Phenylketonuria: Clinical Observations in Three Cases, *J.A.M.A.*
161:1628, 1956.

Jervis, G. A., Studies on Phenylpyruvic Oligophrenia: Position of Metabolic Error,
J. Biol. Chem. 169:651, 1947.

Levine, S. Z., Tyrosine and Phenylalanine Metabolism in Infants and the Role of
Vitamin C, *Harvey Lectures* 42:303, 1946–1947.

———, *H. H. Gordon,* and *E. Marples,* A Defect in the Metabolism of Tyrosine
and Phenylalanine in Premature Infants. I. Identification and Assay of Intermediary Products. II. Spontaneous Occurrence and Eradication by Vitamin C, *J.
Clin. Invest.* 20:199, 209, 1941.

Tseng, J. C. S., H. W. Elghammer, and *A. C. Ivy,* Urinary Excretion of Glucuronic
and Salicylic Acids in Normal and Rheumatic Children, *Am. J. Dis. Child.*
79:826, 1950.

Woodruff, C. W., Tyrosine Metabolism in Infantile Scurvy, *J. Lab. & Clin. Med.*
36:640, 1950.

Woolf, L. I., R. Griffiths, and *A. Moncrieff,* Treatment of Phenylketonuria with a Diet
Low in Phenylalanine, *Brit. M. J.* 1:57, 1955.

STONES

Albright, F., W. V. Consolazio, and *F. S. Coombs,* Metabolic Studies and Therapy in
Case of Nephrocalcinosis with Rickets and Dwarfism, *Bull. Johns Hopkins Hosp.*
66:7, 1940.

Brandenberger, E., F. de Quervain, and *H. R. Schinz,* Roentgenographische und
Mikroskopisch-kristalloptische Untersuchungen an Harnsteinen, *Helvet. med. acta*
14:195, 1947.

Burke, E. C., A. H. Baggenstoss, C. A. Owen, Jr., M. H. Power, and *O. W. Lohr,*
Oxalosis, *Pediatrics* 15:383, 1955.

Campbell, M. F., "Pediatric Urology," vol. II, The Macmillan Company, New York,
1937.

Dunn, H. G., Oxalosis: Report of a Case with Review of the Literature, *A.M.A. Am.
J. Dis. Child.* 90:58, 1955.

Engel, W. J., Nephrocalcinosis, *J.A.M.A.* 145:288, 1951.

Israels, S., H. Muth, and *I. Zeavin,* Nephrolithiasis with Renal Tubular Failure,
Am. J. Dis. Child. 78:389, 1949.

Renal Calculi, Transcription of a Panel Meeting, *Bull. New York Acad. Med.* 32:293,
1956.

Rusche, C. F., and *F. R. Morrow,* Calculous Disease in Infants and Children, *Pediat.
Clin. North America* August, 1955, p. 857.

Sendroy, J., Jr., Mineral Metabolism, *Ann. Rev. Biochem.* 14:407, 1945.

Shorr, E., T. P. Almy, M. H. Sloan, H. Taussky, and *V. Toscani,* Relation between the

Urinary Excretion of Citric Acid and Calcium: Its Implications for Urinary Calcium Stone Formation, *Science* 96:587, 1942.

———— and *A. C. Carter,* Aluminum Gels in the Management of Renal Phosphatic Calculi, *J.A.M.A.* 144:1549, 1950.

Thomas, G. J., and *C. O. Tanner,* Urinary Lithiasis in Children, *J. Urol.* 8:171, 1922.

Waller, J. I., and *F. Adney,* Vesical Calculi in Young Female Children, *Am. J. Dis. Child.* 79:684, 1950.

SULFONAMIDES

Fink, H. W., and *C. A. Smith,* Incidence of Reactions to Sulfonamide Drugs in Infants and Children, *J. Pediat.* 28:40, 1946.

Ledbetter, J. H., and *G. E. Cronheim,* The Clinical Use of a Triple Sulfonamide Mixture, *Am. J. M. Sc.* 216:27, 1948.

Lehr, D., and *W. Antopol,* Specific Morphology of Crystals Appearing in the Urine during Administration of Sulfanilamide Derivatives, *Am. J. Clin. Path.* 12:200, 1942.

Northey, E. H., "The Sulfonamides and Allied Compounds," Reinhold Publishing Corporation, New York, 1948.

Rapoport, M., M. I. Rubin, and *A. D. Waltz,* Influence of Sulfanilamide Therapy upon the Course of Acute Glomerulonephritis in Children, *Am. J. M. Sc.* 211:307, 1946.

van Dyke, H. B., The Toxic Effects of Sulfonamides, *Ann. New York Acad. Sc.* 44:477, 1943.

Wolman, I. J., B. Evans, and *S. Lasker,* A Rapid System for Routine Urine Analysis, *Am. J. Clin. Path.* 16:162, 1946.

DRUGS

Selwyn, J. G., and *F. A. Dark,* The Identification of Barbiturate Drugs in Gastric Contents and Urine, *J. Clin. Path.* 3:152, 1950.

LEAD

Byers, R. K., C. A. Maloof, and *M. Cushman,* Urinary Excretion of Lead in Children: Diagnostic Application, *A.M.A. Am. J. Dis. Child.* 87:548, 1954.

Byers, R. K., and *C. A. Maloof,* Edathamil Calcium-Disodium (Versenate) in Treatment of Lead Poisoning in Children, *A.M.A. Am. J. Dis. Child.* 87:559, 1954.

Clark, N. S., Lead Poisoning in Infancy, *Arch. Dis. Childhood* 25:297, 1950.

Johnson, W. S., and *N. E. Whitman,* Coproporphyrinuria as an Index of Lead Absorption, *Arch. Indust. Hyg.* 2:170, 1950.

COPPER

Bearn, A. G., Genetic and Biological Aspects of Wilson's Disease, *Am. J. Med.* 15:442, 1953.

Uzman, L. L., On the Relationship of Urinary Copper Excretion to the Aminoaciduria in Wilson's Disease (Hepatolenticular Degeneration), *Am. J. Med. Sc.* 226:645, 1953.

Zindahl, W. T., I. Hyman, and *W. F. Stafford,* The Effect of Drugs upon the Copper Metabolism in Hepatolenticular Degeneration and in Normal Subjects, *J. Lab. & Clin. Med.* 43:774, 1954.

MERCURY

Holzel, A., and *T. James,* Mercury and Pink Disease, *Lancet* 1:441, 1952.

Warkany, J., and *D. M. Hubbard,* Adverse Mercurial Reactions in the Form of Acrodynia and Related Conditions, *A.M.A. Am. J. Dis. Child.* 81:335, 1951.

CHAPTER 35

Approaches to the Study of Renal Function

When confronted with a child with kidney disturbance it is important to try to (1) ascertain the exact cause, (2) identify the anatomic location of the lesion, and (3) appraise the dysfunction in terms of severity. Diagnosis, treatment, and prognosis depend upon a correlation of the history, the results of laboratory studies, and a good familiarity with the natural histories of the different kidney diseases appearing in childhood.

Many of the newer tests which have been proposed for appraisal of the functional capacity of the kidney are still too controversial or require too elaborate skill and equipment to be applied by the physician in active practice. Those approaches which are generally available can be grouped as follows:

1. Standard tests for study of the urine (Chaps. 28–34)
2. Measurement of the 24-hour urinary output
3. Dilution and concentration tests
4. Addis sediment counts of erythrocytes, leukocytes, and casts
5. Phenolsulfonephthalein excretion
6. Clearance tests for urea and related substances
7. Studies of the chemical composition of the body fluids, especially of blood urea and related substances (Chap. 48)

DAILY VOLUME OF URINE

Valuable insight into the functional status of the kidneys can be obtained from simple measurement of the total 24-hour output of urine. Oliguria or anuria due to kidney damage can take place in shock, trauma, poisonings, dehydration, circulatory failure, severe infections, sulfonamide sensitivity, intestinal obstruction, and a diversity of other conditions. A sudden reduction in output can be the first sign of kidney involvement in a patient ill with some other disease. Conversely, the total daily excretion tends to be above average in the advanced stages of nephritis and related kidney diseases, indicating loss of concentrating power. Polyuria appears also in diabetes mellitus, diabetes insipidus, hypopituitarism, and other diseases affecting the hypothalamus or pituitary gland. The physician should be familiar with the ranges of normal ex-

409

cretion for healthy children of different ages (Chap. 28). A daily chart of fluid intake and output can be of great value in following the progress of seriously ill patients.

DILUTION AND CONCENTRATION TESTS

In many renal diseases the ability to increase or decrease the urinary output or to dilute or concentrate the urine becomes impaired.

Urine Dilution Test

The infant or child, after 6 to 12 hours of fluid restriction, is given 30 to 50 ml of water per kg body weight within 30 to 45 minutes. Urine specimens are then collected every 15 to 30 minutes for the next 4 hours. The peak of the ensuing diuresis should occur in 45 to 120 minutes after the water has been taken. Normally, all or nearly all the ingested water is excreted during the 4 hours, and the specific gravity of at least one urine specimen is 1.004 or below. With infants under 1 month of age the normal rate of excretion will be slower.

Urine Concentration Tests

Homer Smith has suggested that the proximal renal tubule obligatorily absorbs the first 87 per cent of the water coming from the glomerulus, inasmuch as this process goes on isoosmotically. The distal tubule then conserves as much or as little of the remainder as the body requires, up to a total of 99.8 per cent. Here the absorption is of the nature of osmotic work proceeding against the osmotic gradient of the urea, salt, and other unabsorbed constituents. Loss of concentrating power in kidney disease is a sign of defective osmotic function within the distal tubule.

ADDIS CONCENTRATION TEST. This calls for a 24-hour period of fluid deprivation, with collection and testing of the urine during the second 12 hours of this period. The instructions are as follows:

1. The test period begins in the morning, after breakfast. No water, milk, or other liquids may be taken from then until 8 A.M. of the following day. The usual diet is otherwise permitted. The patient should not take more fruit than is customary and no alkaline medication.

2. At approximately 8 P.M. the bladder is emptied and the urine discarded. The exact time of voiding is noted and written down.

3. Every drop of urine passed in the next 12 hours is saved and stored in a refrigerator. The exact times of the starting and ending of the urine collection are noted and written down even though the interval may not be exactly 12 hours.

4. The pooled 12-hour specimen of night urine is brought to the laboratory within the next few hours. It should be kept cold until tested. The Addis sediment count (p. 411) may be performed also, provided a few drops of formalin had been previously placed in the collecting vessel. With young children who may be made uncomfortable by prolonged fluid restriction the preliminary dry interval may be reduced to 8 or 10 hours. A rise in specific gravity to at least

1.026 in children beyond infancy, or above 1.024 in infants, indicates normal concentrating power and no appreciable tubular injury.

In chronic generalized renal disease, as the damage progresses, the urine ultimately achieves the same osmolarity as the glomerular filtrate, with specific gravity fixed at or near 1.010. Neither the concentration nor the dilution tests will any longer evoke significant fluctuations. At this stage the concentration test is not without risk, since any strain placed on the nephrons by the need to excrete a concenrated urine may aggravate permanently the local damage. With nitrogen retention secondary to congestive heart failure a urine concentration response will still be obtained.

MODIFIED MOSENTHAL CONCENTRATION TEST. This measures the physiologic capacity for 24-hour fluctuation in urine specific gravity. Instructions are as follows:

1. Start test at 8 A.M. The usual diet is taken, with liberal amounts of fluid with each meal. No liquids between meals.

2. Collect urine specimens every 2 hours until 8 P.M. Collect one pooled specimen for the period 8 P.M. to 8 A.M.

3. Determine the specific gravity of every specimen.

Normally functioning kidneys will produce urine having a daily swing of at least 10 points (for example, from 1.016 to 1.026) and at least one specimen of 1.025 or higher. Poorly functioning kidneys cannot give so wide a fluctuation, and the highest concentration will not reach 1.025. Other generalizations are the same as with the Addis concentration test.

Inability to exceed a specific gravity of 1.020 can be found in nonnephritic patients with edematous conditions or when the diet is unduly low in protein and sodium chloride. In diabetes insipidus and "water-losing nephritis" the urine is very dilute, and only when clinical dehydration becomes marked will the specific gravity rise from its usual level of under 1.004 up to a range around 1.010.

In acute glomerulonephritis the loss of concentrating power may persist for months after the glomerular filtration rate and the blood urea levels are back to normal. Conversely, at the onset of acute glomerulonephritis and in rapidly accelerating hypertensive disease, the glomerular filtration rate may be much reduced and the blood urea level markedly elevated and yet the concentrating capacity of the kidneys remain apparently unimpaired.

Addis Sediment Count

This, the most widely accepted method for enumerating cells and casts, counts all the erythrocytes, leukocytes, and casts which are passed in a 12-hour period. The specimen is secured as described on page 410. Fluids should not be restricted if there is impaired renal function. The urine should be acid and of high specific gravity; when it is less than 1.010 the red cells and casts may not be preserved.

Wide variations occur in healthy subjects, and no close division can be drawn between normal and abnormal. As Addis pointed out, the test is not strictly quantitative; its chief intent is to express the rates of excretion in terms of approximate magnitude. It is a delicate approach, not needed when microscopy of the urine sediment shows formed elements in excessive numbers. Its chief field of application lies in detecting and following the progress of patients with mild forms of nephritis who exhibit borderline or absent microscopic abnormalities in single specimens of urine.

The upper limits of excretion for a 12-hour period in healthy children under 13 years of age, as compared with adults and expressed in round numbers, have been reported as follows:

Author	No. of children	Casts	Erythrocytes	Epithelial cells and leukocytes
Addis (for adults)		5,000	500,000	1,000,000
Rew and Butler	16	38,000	275,000	850,000 (boys)
				4,000,000 (girls)
Lyttle	74	13,000	600,000	600,000 (boys)
				1,000,000 (girls)
Soto	306	7,300	950,000	3,000,000
Snoke		29,000	800,000	
Boyle et al. (postnephrotic children)	25	18,600	115,000	1,000,000
Giles		10,000	600,000	2,000,000

A good working rule is to take the values of 1,000,000 erythrocytes, 20,000 casts, and 2,000,000 epithelial cells and leukocytes as representing the top upper limits for normality.

These limits are exceeded in kidney diseases, and particularly nephritis. In pyelonephritis and related infective urinary tract lesions there is often a disproportionate increase of urinary white cells over red cells and casts. The Addis approach is more sensitive than the blood urea or phenolsulfonephthalein tests, which often give normal values in the presence of mild or minimal nephritis. During recovery from acute nephritis the abnormal sedimentation rate usually returns to normal before the Addis counts.

During or immediately after acute bacterial infections the urine sedimentary elements are often increased. This is especially noticeable during convalescence from scarlet fever.

PHENOLSULFONEPHTHALEIN (PSP) TESTS

The speed of elimination of this inert dye into the urine is a widely used test for kidney function. Though accurate collections of urine are just as essential as in the urea clearance test, the results are less quantitative.

One- and Two-hour PSP Tests

1. The child first voids several times in order to empty the bladder completely. Catheterization should be done when urinary tract obstruction is suspected, unless there is some contraindication.

2. Slowly inject 6 mg of the sodium salt of PSP intravenously, dissolved in 1 ml of sterile solution as purchased from the manufacturer.

3. Give a liberal intake of fluids. It is advisable for the subject to drink one or more glassfuls of water before and after injection.

4. Collect urine specimens at exactly 1 and 2 hours after the injection. If two urinations are not feasible, procure a single 2-hour specimen.

5. If the PSP cannot be introduced intravenously it may be given intramuscularly. One should allow 10 minutes for absorption before commencing to record the 1- and 2-hour time measurements. The intravenous route is preferred because it eliminates the possibility of delay in absorption.

6. Mix a few drops of 10 per cent sodium hydroxide solution with the urine. Add water to each specimen to bring to a total volume of 1,000 ml. Estimate the percentage of dye excreted by comparing the reddish color of the urine with that of a set of standards.

Fractional PSP Test

The above procedure may be modified in the following particulars:

1. The bladder is first emptied completely by catheterization, and the catheter left in place until the termination of the procedure.

2. Three 20-minute urine specimens are withdrawn in the first hour, and a final specimen at the end of two hours.

Interpretation

Normally about 70 to 80 per cent of the dye will be excreted within 2 hours, with more than 50 per cent within 1 hour. With the fractional test a peak excretion of about 25 per cent is normally observed in the first or second 20-minute specimen.

The rate of excretion is impaired in most forms of nephritis, whether acute or chronic. With chronic nephritis the excretion declines as the disease advances. With liver disease the output may be increased, since a well-functioning liver normally disposes of an appreciable fraction of the dye.

With minor or early impairment of renal function no abnormalities may be revealed. Or the total 2-hour excretion may be normal, with the amount of dye obtained in the first hour no greater than in the second hour. The test may give unreliably low figures if the patient is edematous, oliguric, or in circulatory failure.

CLEARANCES AND RELATED PHYSIOLOGIC TESTS

Sensitive techniques can be applied to the estimation of the efficiency of the discrete excretory operations, in disease states as well as in health. It is now possible to estimate with reasonable accuracy the effective renal plasma flow (RPF) or renal blood flow (RBF), the glomerular filtration rate (GFR), the ratio between GFR and total blood flow through the kidney (the filtration fraction or FF), and the mass of functioning tubular tissue (TM).

These evaluations serve to elucidate in working out the degree of glomerular, tubular, and vascular injury in the respective renal disorders. They are currently not much used in the practical management of individual cases, save in exceptional circumstances, because they are time-consuming and difficult. Their chief merit lies in clarifying problems of pathogenesis and sites of lesions.

The majority of the procedures which have proved most effective are based upon the ability of the kidney to remove or "clear" soluble substances from the blood stream. Such clearance tests fall into three main types, depending on whether they measure (1) glomerular filtration alone, (2) filtration plus tubular excretion, or (3) filtration plus tubular reabsorption. By calculation from proper dosage adjustments, additional deductions can be drawn with respect to circulation rates through glomerular peritubular capillaries.

Renal clearances are conventionally expressed in terms of the minimal volume of plasma which could furnish the quantity of substance excreted in a unit of time. Clearance values are usually reported as the number of milliliters of plasma (or blood) "cleared" per minute. It is customary to relate the values obtained to the surface area of the child as compared with an arbitrary adult surface area of 1.73 square meters.

Clearance of inulin (C_I), mannitol (C_M), and endogenous creatinine (C_{Cr}) are currently deemed the best measures of the GFR. These substances appear to be filtered through the glomeruli and not reabsorbed or excreted through the tubules. The average normal GFR for children beyond infancy, regardless of sex, is about 123 ml per minute per 1.73 square meters of body surface. The average rate for young infants in the postneonatal period is usually 40 to 65 ml per minute and may be even less in small premature infants.

When injected in submaximal amounts to give low plasma concentrations, the clearances of iodopyracet (diodrast; C_D) or of sodium para-aminohippurate (C_{PAH}) are accepted as equivalent to effective renal plasma flow (RPF) since these substances are removed from the arterial blood completely during one passage through the kidneys. The average value for RPF for normal children is approximately 635 ml per minute per 1.73 square meters of body surface; for young postneonatal infants, 20 to 40 per cent of the above. From RPF the effective RBF can be calculated, using a factor based on the venous hematocrit reading.

Maximal excretion of diodrast or sodium para-aminohippurate (PAH), when these substances are given in excess, saturates the mass of functioning tubular tissue. This is the so-called maximal tubular secretory capacity (TM or secretory TM). TM_D refers to diodrast; TM_{PAH} to sodium para-aminohippurate. The average values for TM_{PAH} is about 77 mg per minute per 1.73 square meters of body surface for children and older infants; 12 to 30 mg per minute for postneonatal infants.

The FF measures the proportion of contained water which is removed as the plasma flows through the kidney. FF is calculated from the formula GFR/RPF × 100. It varies with effective filtration pressure provided the glomeruli are intact.

In patients with renal disease one can often demonstrate patterns of altered function which correspond in general with recognized clinical and pathologic changes. In acute nephritis, for example, the picture is essentially one of hampered glomerular filtration. The filtration fraction falls, to return toward normal when healing begins. In chronic nephritis the pattern may be similar until the end stage, when loss of tubular secretory tissue becomes apparent and usually severe. Tubular injury predominates in the toxic nephroses. Normotensive patients suffering from chronic pyelonephritis show a simple loss of function; when hypertension is present some afferent resistance becomes detectable. In advanced renal disease both the plasma flow and the glomerular filtration rate fall and the filtration fraction may rise to normal or above. In congestive heart failure the renal plasma flow and glomerular filtration rates are morbidly reduced, whereas tubular function is normal or perhaps slightly impaired. It is necessary, of course, to be familiar with the techniques, the wide ranges of variation in normal children of various ages, and the limitations which attend the application of these functional measurements to clinical situations.

Clearances measure the work of the kidneys as an organic whole. They cannot distinguish a subtotal loss of function in all nephrons from a complete loss of function in a fractional portion. Repeated clearances may yield essentially identical results even though different groups of nephrons are damaged at the times of the successive tests.

In acute nephritis, serial clearance tests typically show bizarre fluctuations. In chronic kidney disease they measure more effectively the advance or subsidence of the damage. In advanced sickle cell anemia and occasionally in diabetes with normal urine the glomerular filtration rates are reduced.

The reader is referred to the publications cited in the bibliography for theoretical and experimental expositions of clearance measurements, detailed instructions as to performance, and descriptions of the pitfalls and limitations which attend their application. Only the urea clearance test is here discussed in some detail, because it is the oldest and easiest of the clearance tests to carry out and has been subjected to the widest clinical trial.

Urea Clearance

Urea is filtered through the glomeruli very freely and at the same rate as inulin, but unlike the latter, is partially reabsorbed by the tubules in its passage through them.

The urea clearance rises progressively as the urine flow increases from 0.5 to 2 ml per minute per 1.73 square meters of body surface. When the clearance is in this range it is called *standard* (Cs). When the clearance is over 2 ml per minute it is called *maximal* (Cm). Both these expressions of the functional capacity of the kidney to excrete urea from the blood stream tend to be reduced in renal diseases.

When less than 2 ml per minute, the urea clearance may be computed from the formula

$$Cs = \frac{U \times \sqrt{V \times 1.73/SA}}{BUN}$$

When more than 2 ml per minute, the clearance may be

$$Cm = \frac{U \times V \times 1.73/SA}{BUN}$$

U = mg urea N per 100 ml of urine; V = ml urine excreted per minute; BUN = mg urea N per 100 ml of blood; SA = surface area in square meters calculated from height and weight, using the nomogram of Boothby and Sandiford reproduced in most laboratory manuals. With edematous children the ideal weight is used in the calculation.

With a urine output above 2 ml per minute per 1.73 square meters the normal maximal urea clearance averages about 75 ml per minute, with a range of 65 to 85 ml. When the urine flow is below 2 ml per minute the normal standard clearance has a mean of about 55 ml of blood per minute, with a range of 40 to 65 ml.

When measuring urea clearance it is essential to pay precise attention to all details or the results may be in error. Physiologic influences and the protein in the diet affect the figures; a healthy individual may show fluctuations as great as 20 per cent from day to day. The determination is best made when the urine flow is constant.

Because of the wider physiologic variations and the difficulties in procuring urine, the urea clearance is not utilized often for clinical studies in infants under 2 years of age. The clearance rate in children older than 2 years is essentially the same as in adults.

A convenient routine for measuring urea clearance in a child is to start after a light breakfast low in protein. About 250 to 500 ml of water is then taken; the quantity need not be measured. The bladder is emptied and the time noted. Two urine specimens are then collected during the next 2 hours, with the times of voiding being meticulously noted. Incontinent patients must be catheterized for accurate timing. A blood specimen is taken immediately after the second urine collection. Information as to the height, weight, age, and sex of the child is furnished along with the blood and urine specimens. The results are reported in terms of "percentage of normal function."

Clinical conditions in which this test is useful include renal anomalies, acute nephritis, the nephrotic syndrome, and acute nephrotoxic injury. By repeating this determination of kidney function every few months one gains an insight into the course of the disease.

KIDNEY FUNCTION AS RELATED TO AGE

Normal kidney functioning in early infancy differs significantly from that in adult life, having in general a much diminished or "immature" reserve capacity. Renal activity is lowest in premature infants and the neonatal period. Maturation is rapid in the first 6 months, and then proceeds more slowly. In different children the separate functions may mature at disparate rates.

The osmotic pressure of the urine in infancy is low and only rises to adult levels when the serum becomes abnormally concentrated. The osmotic pressure ratio of urine:blood on the basis of surface area in early infancy is nearly always less than 2.0, whereas in adult life it can rise to 3.5 or 4.0.

Some of the clinical phenomena exhibited by younger infants can be ascribed to their comparatively diminished renal function. Such infants have difficulty maintaining a constant internal milieu in states of dehydration, especially when the volume of water available for excretion is small (p. 590). The higher levels of potassium, urea, and uric acid in the blood in the first few days after birth, and the shift of the electrolyte balance in the direction of acidosis, are the results of deficient renal elimination of metabolites. On the other hand, the edema so often seen in newborn premature infants was found by Smith, Yudkin, Minkowski, and Cushman to be governed by unknown, perhaps endocrinal, factors independent of the kidney.

Because their underdeveloped renal function becomes even more handicapped when fluid output is reduced, young infants who are ill should be given water-soluble therapeutic agents such as atropine, phenobarbital, and the antibiotics in restricted dosage. Otherwise the medications may accumulate in the tissue fluids in undesirably high concentrations and give rise to toxic effects.

The comparatively higher levels of serum potassium and chloride and the lower sodium and bicarbonate levels found in the early weeks of life in infants receiving cow's milk likewise reflect low clearance rates. Neonatal tetany may be a consequence of poor excretion of phosphates which are much higher in cow's milk than in breast milk (p. 562). Premature infants receiving concentrated protein milk preparations were shown by Darrow, da Silva, and Stevenson, and also by Hoffman,

Parmalee, and Grossman, to go into severe acidosis with dehydration, loss of weight, and elevated chloride and reduced bicarbonate serum concentrations. This metabolic imbalance was traced to the high content of chloride in the milk preparations widely used at that time.

Since a baby loses a high proportion of ingested water through lungs and skin, a clysis of 0.9 per cent (normal) saline demands a renal excretion of a hypertonic solution of sodium chloride—a task which can be achieved only after the serum becomes grossly abnormal. Edema may develop in newborn and premature infants after such clyses. Parenteral injections of fluid ought not to be of greater tonicity than about 0.2 saline solution, best combined with 4 per cent glucose.

Excretion of contrast agents for intravenous urography, such as iodopyracet (Diodrast), is slow in early infancy. One may have to wait longer for satisfactory filling of the urinary tract when excretory pyelograms are being taken. Not enough dye may be evident in the ureteral passages at any one time to give a satisfactory roentgenogram.

BIBLIOGRAPHY

GENERAL PHENOMENA OF RENAL FUNCTION

Addis, T., Number of Formed Elements in Urinary Sediment of Normal Individuals, *J. Clin. Invest.* 2:409, 1926.

Barnett, H. L., and *F. Sereni,* Kidney Function Tests in Infants and Children, *Pediat. Clin. North Amer.* February, 1955, p. 191.

Brod, J., Acute Diffuse Glomerulonephritis, *Am. J. Med.* 7:317, 1949.

Camara, A. A., A. Reimer, and *L. H. Newburgh,* The Twenty-four Hourly Endogenous Creatinine Clearance as a Clinical Measure of the Functional State of the Kidneys, *J. Lab. & Clin. Med.* 37:743, 1951.

Dubois, D., and *E. F. DuBois,* Clinical Calorimetry. V. Measurement of Surface Area of Man, *Arch. Int. Med.* 15:858, 1915.

Earle, D. P., Jr., Renal Function Tests in the Diagnosis of Glomerular and Tubular Disease, *Bull. New York Acad. Med.* 26:47, 1950.

Etteldorf, J. N., A. H. Tuttle, and *G. W. Clayton,* Renal Function Studies in Pediatrics. I. Renal Hemodynamics in Children with Sickle Cell Anemia, *A.M.A. Am. J. Dis. Child.* 83:185, 1952.

Goldring, W., Clinical Application of Current Tests of Renal Function, *J.A.M.A.* 153:1245, 1953.

"Renal Function in Infants and Children," Report of the Eighth M & R Pediatric Research Conference, 1953, M & R Laboratories, Columbus, 16, Ohio.

Santorius, O. W., Renal Function Tests and Their Physiologic Significance, *New York J. Med.* 52:1777, 1952.

Smith, H. W., W. Goldring, and *H. Chasis,* The Measurement of the Tubular Excretory Mass, Effective Blood Flow and Filtration Rate in the Normal Human Kidney, *J. Clin. Invest.* 17:263, 1938.

Taylor, R. D., J. D. Peirce, and *I. H. Page,* Use of Posterior Pituitary Extract in Tests of Urinary Concentration, *Am. J. M. Sc.* 209:235, 1945.

Weil, W. B., Jr., The Evaluation of Renal Function in Infancy and Childhood, *Am. J. M. Sc.* 229:678, 1955.

UREA CLEARANCE

Emerson, K., and *V. P. Dole,* Diodrast and Inulin Clearances in Nephrotic Children with Supernormal Urea Clearances, *J. Clin. Invest.* 22:447, 1943.

Farr, L. E., Effect of Dietary Protein on Urea Clearance of Children with Nephrosis, *J. Clin. Invest.* 15:703, 1936.

Gordon, H. H., H. E. Harrison, and *H. McNamara,* The Urea Clearance of Young Premature and Full Term Infants, *J. Clin. Invest.* 21:499, 1942.

McIntosh, J. F., E. Moller, and *D. D. Van Slyke,* Studies on Urea Excretion. III. The Influence of Body Size on Urea Output, *J. Clin. Invest.* 6:467, 1928.

Peters, J. P., and *D. D. Van Slyke,* "Quantitative Clinical Chemistry," vol. I, p. 345, vol. II, p. 564, The Williams & Wilkins Company, Baltimore, 1931–1932.

Schoenthal, L., D. Lurie, and *M. Kelly,* Urea Clearance in Normal and in Dehydrated Children, *Am. J. Dis. Child.* 45:41, 1933.

Thomson, J., Urea Clearance in the Immediate Post-natal Period, *Arch. Dis. Childhood* 24:180, 1949.

Van Slyke, D. D., and *V. P. Dole,* The Significance of the Urea Clearance, *J. Clin. Path.* 2:273, 1949.

KIDNEY FUNCTION AS RELATED TO AGE

Barnett, H. L., W. K. Hare, H. McNamara, and *R. S. Hare,* Measurement of Glomerular Filtration Rate in Premature Infants, *J. Clin. Invest.* 27:691, 1948.

———, *H. McNamara, S. Shulta,* and *R. Tompsett,* Renal Clearances of Sodium Penicillin G, Procaine Penicillin G, and Inulin in Infants and Children, *Pediatrics* 3:422, 1949.

——— and *J. Vesterdal,* The Physiologic and Clinical Significance of Immaturity of Kidney Function in Young Infants, *J. Pediat.* 42:99, 1953.

Calcagno, P. L., and *M. I. Rubin,* Effect of Dehydration Produced by Water Deprivation, Diarrhea and Vomiting on Renal Function in Infants, *Pediatrics* 7:328, 1951.

Darrow, D. C., M. M. da Silva, and *S. S. Stevenson,* Production of Acidosis in Premature Infants by Protein Milk, *J. Pediat.* 27:43, 1945.

Dean, R. F., and *R. A. McCance,* Response of New-born Children to Hypertonic Solutions of Sodium Chloride and of Urea, *Nature* 160:904, 1947.

Hoffman, W. S., A. H. Parmalee, and *A. Grossman,* Mechanism of Production of Acidosis in Premature Infants by Protein Milk, *Am. J. Dis. Child.* 75:637, 1948.

McCance, R. A., and *W. F. Young,* The Secretion of Urine by Newborn Infants, *J. Physiol.* 99:265, 1941.

Rubin, M. I., E. Bruck, and *M. Rapoport,* Maturation of Renal Function in Childhood: Clearance Studies, *J. Clin. Invest.* 28:1144, 1949.

Smith, C. A., et al., Adjustment of Electrolytes and Water Following Premature Birth (with Special Reference to Edema), *Pediatrics* 3:34, 1949.

Vesterdal, J., and *F. Tudvad,* Studies on the Kidney Function in Premature and Full-term Infants by Estimation of the Inulin and Paraaminohippurate Clearances, *Acta paediat.* 37:429, 1949.

West, J. R., H. W. Smith, and *H. Chasis,* Glomerular Filtration Rate, Effective Renal Blood Flow, and Maximal Tubular Excretory Capacity in Infancy, *J. Pediat.* 32:10, 1948.

Young, W. F., J. L. Hallum, and *R. A. McCance,* The Secretion of Urine by Premature Infants, *Arch. Dis. Childhood* 16:243, 1941.

———— and *R. A. McCance,* The Secretion of Urine by Dehydrated and Normal Infants, *Arch. Dis. Childhood* 17:65, 1942.

CHAPTER 36

Diseases and Disturbances of the Kidney

Transient disturbances of kidney function may take place in many childhood infections, circulatory failure, surgical shock, states of water and salt imbalance, poisonings of various sorts, polyarteritis nodosa, severe anemia, and many other systemic disturbances. The capacities of the kidney may become affected more permanently in glomerulonephritis, pyelonephritis, interstitial nephritis, the nephrotic syndrome, hydronephrosis, acute renal insufficiency (lower nephron nephrosis), renal tuberculosis, anaphylactoid purpura, and congenital malformations with or without infection.

Injury of the glomerular wall may lead to abnormal escape of proteins or red cells, to diminished permeability with impairment of filtration, or to reduced blood flow to the rest of the nephron. Damage to the tubules may manifest itself as impairment of concentration and dilution, diminished production of ammonia, or disturbances in resorption. Interstitial edema or inflammation can interfere with blood flow and hamper the functioning of both glomeruli and tubules, with scarring and contraction as the end result. Spasm of the arterioles entering the glomeruli reduces the glomerular blood flow. Spasm of the arterioles leaving the glomeruli raises the intraglomerular pressure, increases the rate of filtration, and reduces tubular blood flow. Either kind of spasm may elevate the systemic blood pressure. Severe dehydration increases the osmotic concentration of the blood, thereby retarding glomerular filtration, reducing the volume of filtrate, and hampering the excretory and resorptive functioning of the tubules.

In advanced or terminal chronic glomerulonephritis the renal blood flow, as well as all other functions, becomes greatly restricted. The tubules are usually the most damaged and cannot cope with the glomerular filtrate. This leads to urine of large volume, low specific gravity, low or absent content of ammonia, poorer reabsorption of basic ions, diminished urea clearance with greater urea reabsorption, and retention of many waste products within the body.

With all forms of nephritis the abnormal retention and distribution of water are reflections of disturbances in the relative osmotic concentrations of the electrolytes, protein, and related substances in the intracellular and the extracellular spaces. The total plasma volume is sometimes augmented, sometimes contracted; measurement of this variable is as yet beyond estimation by the routine hospital laboratory. Daily recordings of the body weight and of the intake and output of fluids are important steps in management, whether or not edema is overtly recognizable.

Laboratory observation of the altered equilibria in body chemistry and fluid balances is indispensable for recognition and correction of the disturbances which occur.

EDEMA

In acute glomerulonephritis the inflammatory swelling and proliferation of the glomerular loops slow down the glomerular blood flow and filtration rate. Since tubular function in the milder lesions is impaired little if at all, the sodium and water in the diminished volume of glomerular fluid are reabsorbed by the tubules to an unusual extent and retained in the body. This retention of sodium and water is responsible for most of the edema shown by these patients and is an indication for restriction of sodium intake.

In the nephrotic syndrome the hypoalbuminemia secondary to increased glomerular permeability and massive proteinuria is one major cause of the edema. Swelling of the kidneys and high abdominal pressure from ascites may aggravate the impairment of renal function. A retarded cardiac output will reduce renal blood flow and hamper glomerular filtration even further. Diffuse capillary damage contributes to the seepage of protein-containing fluid into the tissue spaces.

UREMIA

This is a clinical syndrome produced by renal insufficiency. The resulting disturbances of a laboratory nature include an elevation in the blood levels of nonprotein nitrogen, urea, and creatinine, distortions of the various electrolyte equilibria, and abnormal results in renal function tests. Acidosis develops in the late stages and is demonstrable most readily by a low carbon dioxide–combining power of the plasma. The accumulation of metabolites may lead to headache, vomiting, intestinal or pericardial irritation, and in more advanced cases to coma and death. The blood pressure is usually elevated. The term "azotemia" is often applied when laboratory studies show pronounced nitrogen retention in the absence of clinical symptoms.

The retention of urea is not of itself injurious, inasmuch as patients may have high blood urea levels without signs of uremia, and vice versa. The impaired excretion of chlorides, sulfates, and kindred acid waste products contributes to the production of the acidosis.

As the plasma phosphate level rises, that of serum calcium falls. Tetany does not develop often, however, inasmuch as the calcium still in the circulation becomes unusually well ionized in response to the acidosis. The serum potassium may rise sufficiently to depress the heart action or be reduced to dangerously low levels by vomiting, diarrhea, or diuresis. The serum chloride level is typically increased when the food intake is high in sodium chloride or when infusions of saline solution are given. This is related to the fact that the ion ratio of chloride to sodium is 2:3 in the extracellular fluid, but 1:1 in table salt. Hypochloremia, the opposite condition, may be induced by a restricted intake of food chloride; an immoderate loss of body chloride in vomitus, diarrheal stools, diuretic urine, or edema fluid; movement of chloride ions intracellularly; retention of water which dilutes the body fluids; or in response to the piling up of other acid ions such as sulfates, ketone bodies, and lactic acid.

With uremia of obstructive origin, as compared with parenchymal disease, the urine tends to contain less casts, protein, and red cells, but larger numbers of leukocytes which many times are clumped. Obstructive lesions of the outflow tract are best revealed by x-ray and cystoscopy studies.

Not all episodes of uremia are due to renal disease of parenchymal or obstructive origin. Symptomatic derangements of renal function can be brought about by dehydration, shock, hemorrhage, heart failure, or any other disturbance which can raise the osmotic concentration of the blood or lower the blood pressure to levels at which the rate of blood flow to the kidneys is depressed. Permanent damage to the nephrons themselves can follow such extrarenal disturbances when they last more than a few days.

LABORATORY ASPECTS OF SPECIFIC RENAL DISEASES

Renal Glycosuria

Renal glycosuria is believed to be an inherited deficiency in the capacity of the renal tubules to reabsorb glucose. The diagnosis can be suspected from urinary and blood sugar findings (Chaps. 31, 46).

The apparent high renal threshold found in advanced diabetes may be the result of degenerative changes in the renal blood vessels, which interfere with glomerular filtration more than with tubular reabsorption.

Diabetes Insipidus

PITUITARY TYPE. In diabetes insipidus of pituitary origin the affected individual exhibits continuous thirst, a striking output of urine of rarely less than several liters a day, and otherwise normal sugar-free urine of low specific gravity. The disorder may be familial or result from lesions affecting the hypothalamic-posterior pituitary system. The defect lies in impaired water reabsorption by the lower renal tubules as the consequence of a deficiency of the circulating antidiuretic hormone of the pituitary gland. The urine specific gravity cannot be raised above 1.010 by withholding of fluids or by instillation of concentrated saline solution intravenously (p. 767), unless antidiuretic hormone in the form of posterior pituitary substance (Pitressin) is concomitantly given.

NEPHROGENIC TYPE. There is another variety of diabetes insipidus, usually congenital, which appears to result from the kidney being insensitive to the normal control mechanisms of the pituitary. Administration of Pitressin produces no antidiuretic alleviation. The affected patient, often first seen in infancy, tends to have excessive thirst and polyuria and recurring episodes of unexplained fever. When the fluid intake is raised to several liters daily (500 ml per kg of body weight) the patient remains afebrile. The urine specific gravity remains usually at around 1.005 or lower, though it may go as high as 1.010 on infrequent occasions. Affected infants exhibit a steady polyuria of low specific gravity and can become severely dehydrated if fluid is withheld for only 6 to 9 hours. Renal function tests usually give normal results.

The Fanconi Syndrome

This, known also as the Debré-deToni-Fanconi disturbance, consists of a somewhat loose group of rare congenital metabolic disturbances which have in common growth retardation, bone changes (resistant rickets, osteoporosis, osteomalacia), excessive aminoaciduria, glycosuria, hypophosphatemia, and acidosis. Many of the patients, especially in the childhood years, are instances of cystinosis (p. 391). The mechanism of the biochemical changes is (as originally suggested by Fanconi) failure of tubular reabsorption of intermediary metabolites such as glucose, amino and other organic acids, and phosphates. Death is generally by renal failure.

Less consistent phenomena shown by some of the cases have been physical retardation, bouts of dehydration and fever, hypoglycemia an hour or two after glucose ingestion, an increased serum phosphatase level, polyuria, proteinuria, and an acid urine. Cirrhosis of the liver may develop later.

McCune, Mason, and Clarke postulated that glomerular function is normal in these patients (hence no azotemia), but that the ability of the renal tubular epithelium to reabsorb glucose, amino acids, and phosphate from the glomerular filtrate is defective. The records suggest that the Fanconi syndrome is intermediate between hyperphosphatemic renal rickets on the one hand and generalized cystinosis on the other.

Lowering of the serum calcium, when present, is probably a consequence of the unusual output of urinary calcium. Albright and Reifenstein have suggested that the hypercalciuria stimulates a secondary hyperparathyroidism, which in its turn induces a hyperphosphaturia.

Renal Tubular Acidosis

Two distinct clinical syndromes have been described which are apparently the result of primary failure of the renal acidifying mechanisms, located presumably in the distal tubules. Both of these are characterized by low plasma bicarbonate concentrations, hyperchloremia, and the production of a urine either alkaline in reaction or of a higher pH than would be expected with the coexisting degree of acidosis. In both instances there may also be deposition of calcium in the renal tubules and collecting ducts. Intermittent pyuria is not infrequent.

The first type occurs in infants and is characterized by a fairly typical onset at around the age of 6 months with anorexia, failure to gain weight, vomiting, and constipation. Unexplained episodes of fever may occur in which the infant may become severely dehydrated. Apart from the above-mentioned biochemical changes no other abnormalities are usually detected. Treatment with alkalis (sodium citrate, lactate, or bicarbonate) results in striking clinical improvement, but the biochemical changes may be slow in returning to normal. The disease is in most cases self-limited, so that after a few months it is usually possible to discontinue treatment. The renal tubules apparently recover their ability to excrete an acid urine.

The second syndrome occurs in older children and adults. It is not, in the great majority of cases, a continuation of the infantile condition just described. Most of these patients appear to have been healthy during infancy. Apart from the age incidence this type of renal acidosis differs from the first in that most cases exhibit marked skeletal changes. In children these take the form of rickets with osteoporosis, in adults osteomalacia. The bone changes are thought to be due to secondary hyperparathyroidism. The initiating event appears to be the persisting loss of fixed bases (Na, K, Ca, and Mg) into the urine in order to balance the required excretion of metabolic acids. This is followed by a tendency to lowered blood calcium, a secondary hypertrophy of the parathyroid glands, and a consequent increase in the urinary output of phosphorus. As a result of the disturbed blood Ca:P ratio, bone calcification is impaired. The laboratory findings, in addition to the hyperchloremic acidosis and the unduly high urinary pH, are low plasma levels of inorganic phosphorus and potassium, a tendency to raised alkaline phosphatase in the blood, and increased urinary output of phosphorus. Treatment with alkaline mixtures usually results in marked improvement in general health and eventual healing of the bone lesions. Vitamin D is often necessary to increase the absorption of calcium from the bowel, but its use in large doses should not be continued when the acidosis has been corrected because of the risk of hypervitaminosis. The condition is apparently a permanent state. Therapy may have to be continued throughout life.

Acute Tubular Necrosis (Lower Nephron Nephrosis)

This is a syndrome of rapidly progressive renal insufficiency which may follow any of a variety of bodily insults. The predominant features are oliguria or anuria, profound derangements of the fluid acid-base balances, and retention of urinary waste products. Precipitating causes may be severe burns, ingestion of poisons such as mercury or arsenic or potassium bromate, hyperthermia, crushing injuries, prolonged shock, asphyxia neonatorum, protracted major operations, incompatible blood transfusions, massive intravascular hemolysis, or sensitivity to medicaments such as the sulfonamides. The common denominators for these sundry agents seem to be a severe acute vasomotor collapse or extensive destruction of tissue or blood or both. Disintegrating myoglobin seems to be the noxious agent in crush injuries. When sulfonamide sensitivity is responsible there seems to be a block of some of the tubules by crystals along with toxic degeneration of the entire mass of renal tubules.

At the onset there is usually a day to two of shock, with vomiting, hypotension, and urinary frequency. By the second or third day the secretion of urine becomes diminished or absent. Whatever urine is formed is rich in protein, assorted cells, and casts. It is acid in reaction, low in specific gravity, and red in color due to the presence of hemoglobin or its derivatives. Renal failure with azotemia, acidosis, and other disturbances of acid-base balance may follow quickly. Inorganic acids and ketone bodies accumulate in the blood. Hypertension may be slight or moderate. Edema develops unless the fluid intake is kept low. The plasma volume may rise as much as 40 per cent. Venous catheterization studies have shown that the blood flow through the affected kidneys is strikingly decreased.

The kidney begins to function again after 8 to 12 days; if it does not, death may result from uremia or heart failure. Keeping the patient alive by preservation of fluid and electrolytic balance until the return of renal function is the cardinal principle of treatment.

The first sign of resuming kidney activity is the reappearance of urine, usually between 5 and 12 days. The blood pigments disappear from the urine after a few days, but the proteinuria and excretion of casts and leukocytes may continue for several weeks. The soluble nitrogen of the blood may not subside to normal until 3 to 4 weeks after the renal injury began. The rate of urine formation accelerates during the recovery period and can mount to 5,000 ml per day or higher. This diuresis consists of urine which is similar in composition to pure glomerular filtrate. Minerals such as sodium, potassium, and chloride tend to be excreted in abundance, regardless of body needs, and must be replaced if the patient is to be saved. This acute diuretic phase lasts about as long as that of the initial oliguria. There is then an interval in which the diuresis subsides gradually as the tubular function returns to normal.

Acute Nephritis

In the acute nephritis of childhood, the hematuria and proteinuria are ascribed to leakage through the glomerular capillary endothelium. Autopsies of patients who have died early in a severe attack have shown thickening and partial obliteration of the glomerular tufts and only minor morphologic changes in the tubules and blood vessels.

At least 90 per cent of the attacks of acute nephritis seem to be initiated by antecedent infection, usually but not necessarily streptococcic, which takes place 1 to 3 weeks before the edema or hematuria becomes apparent. The renal changes are interpreted as a delayed allergic response, analagous to those seen in association with rheumatic fever and allied infections.

Malaise, hematuria, proteinuria, edema, hypertension, oliguria, and azotemia are obvious manifestations of the disease when moderate or severe. With symptoms which are minimal or mild, however, or when there is a question as to the interpretation of mild proteinuria or microscopic hematuria after an acute infection, the Addis count and the urea clearance tests are the most helpful diagnostic aids.

The urea clearance, if desired, may be redetermined at 2- to 4-week intervals until normal values are obtained. The Addis count, which reverts to normal more slowly, should be repeated at 1- to 3-week intervals until recovery is complete.

A fair number of "outbreaks" of acute nephritis among groups of school children and young adults are on record. Urine studies of the asymptomatic persons within these groups usually uncover additional subclinical cases having microscopic hematuria with or without proteinuria. Nasopharyngeal cultures of both frank and subclinical cases may reveal hemolytic streptococci.

The Nephrotic Syndrome

Generalized edema, hypoproteinemia, massive proteinuria, lipemia, and hypercholesterolemia constitute the characteristics of this disturbance. A low basal metabolic rate is often associated. The course may be acute or chronic with repeated exacerbations and remissions.

The great majority of affected children have either a tubular lesion of unknown cause—the so-called "pure lipid nephrosis"—or pass through a nephrotic stage as a complication of glomerulonephritis. The nephrotic syndrome has at times been induced or simulated by renal vein thrombosis, Tridione intoxication, syphilis of the kidney, renal amyloidosis, congestive heart failure, nutritional hypoproteinemia, acute liver disease, and the end stages of nephritis complicating diabetes (intercapillary glomerulosclerosis). Nose and throat cultures often show pneumococci. Pneumococcic infections such as peritonitis develop with undue frequency.

In all varieties of the syndrome, whatever the cause, the abundant urinary protein is a mixture of serum proteins, with albumins predominant. The great reduction in serum albumin impairs the retention of water in the vascular system and enhances its accumulation in the tissue spaces. This plus abnormally retained amounts of sodium are major factors in the development of edema. Since glomerular filtration appears to be undisturbed in this syndrome, the retention of sodium has been ascribed to its increased reabsorption by the tubules.

The urine tends to have a high specific gravity and be rich in protein, casts, and epithelial cells. Repeated microscopy of the urine may show sporadic showers of erythrocytes when these are not present consistently. The more sensitive Addis counts often bring out a mild increase in red cell excretion which escapes detection in simple examination of the urinary sediment. The proteinuria may be measured quantitatively every few weeks or months to obtain an index of the severity of the disturbance and of the response to the therapy being given. Determinations of urea clearance, once the initial phase is over, give helpful prognostic information; a persistently reduced clearance is an unfavorable sign.

There usually are no changes in the blood count, though leukocytosis or anemia may be induced transiently by a complicating infection. The leukocytosis subsides when the infection is over, though transfusion may be needed to boost the erythrocyte count. The bone marrow shows no special changes. The erythrocyte sedimentation rate is usually elevated and becomes normal in remissions.

In general, normal findings by kidney function studies in children with nephrosis is of good prognostic import, regardless of the prior duration of the syndrome.

Chronic Nephritis

Children who develop chronic nephritis have typically an insidious onset of symptoms unrelated to known antecedent infection. As the disease advances the edema disappears and the patient exhibits fatigue, anemia, gradually increasing acidosis, and terminal azotemia.

From the laboratory standpoint the definitive findings are the continuous but fluctuating urinary excretion of red cells, protein, and casts. The blood urea and other nitrogenous fractions may not be elevated early, but rise as the disease advances. Leukocytosis does not develop. During the phase of generalized edema the serum cholesterol tends to be elevated and the serum proteins depressed, with a reversal of the albumin-globulin ratio. These alterations become rectified later as the patient loses his edema and becomes "dry" and azotemic, though the serum albumin may continue at a depressed value. The proteinuria, which may be less than 0.5 gm total excretion per day in the early stages, may rise to between 4 and 10 gm when the nephrotic syndrome is superimposed or as the disease advances. The casts are predominantly hyaline until the terminal stage and may contain erythrocytes and epithelial cells.

In the early phases the blood urea may be normal in spite of depressed urea clearance, but rises later on. Anemia becomes progressive and refractory when azotemia appears (p. 328). It may be advisable to take several urine cultures on every patient when first seen, in order to rule out chronic pyelonephritis. The urine specific gravity ultimately becomes fixed at or near 1.010, with persistent nocturia and no response to concentration or dilution stimuli.

Polyarteritis (Periarteritis) Nodosa

In more than half the patients with periarteritis nodosa the kidneys and urine may go through phases resembling acute or chronic glomerulonephritis. The urine may contain protein, erythrocytes, leukocytes, and casts, with a lowered specific gravity even when the urine concentration test is done. Urea clearance may be reduced, and the soluble nitrogen of the blood increased. All these signs of functional damage are reflections of periarteriolar or glomerular changes in the kidneys. Sudden hematuria may be the manifestation of an acute infarct within one kidney.

Chronic Pyelonephritis

Chronic infections can be as destructive to the renal parenchyma as are the lesions of chronic glomerulonephritis. Proteinuria, hematuria, cast excretion, edema, nephrotic changes, azotemia, and eventual hypertension and renal failure can be produced. The infections fluctuate in activity, occasionally producing fever and other symptoms for a time, and then subsiding into subclinical latency. The pathologic lesions in the kidney may be focal or diffuse; in either case they involve all types of structures: glomeruli, tubules, blood vessels, and interstitial tissue. If the infection progresses, the kidney architecture becomes gradually replaced by scar formation, with hyalinization of the glomeruli and eventual shrinkage of total size.

Recognition of the bacterial origin of the disorder is imperative. This form of kidney disease, unlike chronic glomerulonephritis, is occasionally amenable to specific therapy by surgery and chemotherapy. The chief differentiations between chronic pyelonephritis and chronic nephritis rest upon the character of the urinary sediment, the fever and other general and local signs of an infectious process, the existence of a urologic obstruction as a rule, and positive results with bacteriologic cultures.

The urinary sediment contains not only erythrocytes and casts, but leukocytes in much higher relative proportion than in chronic nephritis. This is well brought out in the Addis sediment count. The pyuria may be grossly obvious. The proteinuria is as a rule mild, rarely exceeding 1 to 2 gm per 24 hours except when the infectious process is active. Hematuria and cylindruria may be marked during acute flare-ups and absent or nearly so during remissions. The casts are usually granular or may contain epithelial cells and leukocytes.

The hemoglobin level and erythrocyte count may be normal or depressed. A moderate leukocytosis is the rule when the infection is active. The blood proteins are usually normal. The blood urea may be elevated to levels of 30 to 60 mg per 100 ml as a consequence of increased breakdown of tissue proteins from the infection. The urea clearance and glomerular filtration rate are normal or moderately depressed in the milder cases; severely impaired when in the chronic nephritis-like terminal stage.

The urine may or may not show the same bacterium persistently (p. 395). The antibiotic sensitivities should always be determined. Cultures tend to be irregularly positive, with many specimens proving sterile, especially during chemotherapy.

Renal Insufficiency with Bone Decalcification

Chronic renal disease sometimes leads to rickets-like bone changes which are not the true lesions of rickets but a combination of demineralization, softening, and proliferation of osteoid tissue. The bone changes are indistinguishable from osteitis fibrosa generalisata seen in adults with primary hyperparathyroidism, except for epiphysial changes. Once known as "renal rickets," this condition is now referred to more often as "renal osteitis fibrosa generalisata." This syndrome can develop as the end result of chronic nephritis, chronic pyelonephritis, severe bilateral hydronephrosis, congenital hypoplasia of the kidneys, congenital cystic kidneys, and related disorders which interfere with both glomerular and tubular functioning.

The sequence of events, according to Albright and Reifenstein's interpretation, begins with the phosphate retention and chronic acidosis caused by the renal insufficiency. The high phosphorus depresses the serum calcium level. This in turn stimulates the parathyroids to hypertrophy and hypersecretion (p. 573). The bone changes may be caused by the acidosis or by the unusual amount of circulating parathyroid hormone.

In chronic renal disease the serum phosphorus level may rise from a normal of 4 to 5 mg per 100 ml to as much as 6 to 10 mg. The compensatory calcium level may be 6 to 9 mg. The serum bicarbonate can drop as low as half the normal and be near 15 mEq per liter.

Thrombosis of the Renal Veins

This is one of the rarest renal disturbances of children. Massive hemorrhagic infarction of the kidneys may or may not ensue. The lesion is encountered during infancy, as a rule, and is usually preceded by sepsis, gastroenteritis, or some dehydrating disturbance. It may be unilateral or bilateral.

The most prominent presenting symptom is diarrhea with vomiting. Hemoglobinuria is uncommon. More often the urine exhibits only a trace of protein, an occasional red blood cell in the sediment, and an occasional white blood cell. Sometimes, however, oliguria, azotemia, hematuria, pyuria, proteinuria, and cylindruria become apparent.

The possibility of this lesion must always be kept in mind when an infant is ill with dehydration, shock, and diarrhea which are more profound than any evident infection would be expected to cause. In such circumstances the abdomen should be examined repeatedly for palpable kidney masses. Minor abnormalities in the urine should not be cursorily dismissed. Surgical removal of an affected kidney may result in cure.

The nephrotic syndrome usually ensues if the child survives the initial symptoms. In truth, this possibility becomes a probability whenever the nephrotic syndrome is encountered in an infant under 6 months of age, since the "idiopathic" form of this syndrome at this early age is rare.

Mention may be made in this connection of the rare disorder known as familial nephrosis, a congenital disorder which begins in infancy and has been reported a few times.

BIBLIOGRAPHY

KIDNEY FUNCTION IN DISEASE STATES

Barnes, R. W., W. E. Macpherson, R. T. Bergman, G. Hadley, and H. L. Hadley, Classification of Uremia and Differential Diagnosis of Cases, J.A.M.A. 147:1106, 1951.

Bradley, S. E., "The Pathologic Physiology of Uremia in Chronic Bright's Disease," Charles C Thomas, Springfield, Ill., 1948.

――――, G. P. Bradley, C. J. Tyson, J. J. Curry, and W. D. Blake, Renal Function in Renal Diseases, Am. J. Med. 9:766, 1950.

Brod, J., Acute Diffuse Glomerulonephritis, Am. J. Med. 7:317, 1949.

Corcoran, A. C., R. D. Taylor, and I. H. Page, Functional Patterns in Renal Disease, Ann. Int. Med. 28:560, 1948.

Emerson, K., Jr., and V. P. Dole, Diodrast and Inulin Clearances in Nephrotic Children with Supernormal Urea Clearances, J. Clin. Invest. 22:447, 1943.

————, *P. H. Futcher,* and *L. E. Farr,* Relation of High and Low Urea Clearances to Inulin and Creatinine Clearances in Children with Nephrotic Syndrome, *J. Clin. Invest.* 20:361, 1941.

Fanconi, G., Beiträge zur Nierenpathologie, *Acta paediat.* 40:409, 1951.

Rubin, M. I., M. Rapoport, and *E. Bruck,* Renal Function Studies in Acute Glomerulonephritis in Children, *J. Pediat.* 41:823, 1952.

Smith, H. W., "The Kidney: Structure and Function in Health and Disease," Oxford University Press, New York, 1951.

ACUTE RENAL INSUFFICIENCY

Bull, G. M., A. M. Joekes, and *K. G. Lowe,* Renal Function Studies in Acute Tubular Necrosis, *Clin. Sc.* 9:379, 1950.

Jonsson, B., Lower Nephron Nephrosis in Asphyxia Neonatorum, *Acta paediat.* 40:401, 1951.

Kaplan, S. A., and *S. J. Fomon,* Function Recovery Pattern in Acute Renal Failure Following Ingestion of Mercuric Chloride, *A.M.A. Am. J. Dis. Child.* 85:633, 1953.

Riddell, H. I., The Lower Nephron Syndrome in Children, *J. Urol.* 65:513, 1951.

Snapper, I., The Treatment of Acute Renal Insufficiency, *M. Clin. North America* 34:509, 1950.

Warren, S. A., and *W. V. Gross, Jr.,* Clinical Recovery Following Prolonged Anuria in an Infant Two Months of Age: Report of a Case of Potassium Bromate Intoxication, *Pediatrics* 5:954, 1950.

Waugh, D., Acute Nephrosis: The Kidney of Acute Renal Failure, *Am. J. M. Sc.* 226:310, 1953.

DIABETES INSIPIDUS

Blotner, H., "Diabetes Insipidus," Oxford University Press, New York, 1951.

MacDonald, W. B., Congenital Pitressin Resistant Diabetes Insipidus of Renal Origin, *Pediatrics,* 15:298, 1955.

West, J. R., and *J. G. Kramer,* Nephrogenic Diabetes Insipidus, *Pediatrics,* 15:424, 1955.

FAILURE OF TUBULAR FUNCTIONS

Albright, F., and *E. C. Reifenstein, Jr.,* "Parathyroid Glands and Metabolic Bone Disease," The Williams & Wilkins Company, Baltimore, 1948.

Cooke, R. E., and *C. R. Kleeman,* Distal Tubular Dysfunction with Renal Calcification, *Yale J. Biol. & Med.* 23:199, 1950.

Dent, C. E., The Amino-aciduria in Fanconi Syndrome: A Study Making Extensive Use of Techniques Based on Paper Partition Chromatography, *Biochem. J* 41:240, 1947.

Fanconi, G., and *H. Zellweger,* Familiärer Persistierender Phosphatdiabetes mit D-vitamin-resistenter Rachitis, *Acta paediat.* 41:14, 1952.

Israels, S., H. Muth, A. Taber, and *I. Zeavin,* Nephrolithiasis with Renal Tubular Failure, *Am. J. Dis. Child.* 78:389, 1949.

Kelsey, W. M., J. B. Reinhart, and *J. Fishel,* Chronic Acidosis of Renal Origin in Infancy, *Pediatrics* 5:689, 1950.

Latner, A. L., and *E. D. Burnard,* Idiopathic Hyperchloraemic Renal Acidosis of Infants (Nephrocalcinosis Infantum), *Quart. J. Med.* n.s. 19:285, 1950.

Lightwood, R., W. W. Payne, and *J. A. Black,* Infantile Renal Acidosis, *Pediatrics* 12:628, 1953.

Lowe, C. U., M. Terrey, and *E. A. MacLachlan,* Organic-aciduria, Decreased Renal Ammonia Production, Hydrophthalmos, and Mental Retardation: A Clinical Entity, *A.M.A. Am. J. Dis. Child.* 83:164, 1952.

McCune, D. J., H. H. Mason, and *H. T. Clarke,* Late Rickets with Glycosuria and Organic Acid Acidosis (Fanconi Type), *Am. J. Dis. Child.* 58:673, 1939.

Payne, W. W., Renal Tubular Defects in Childhood, *Pediatrics* 17:84, 1956.

Rendle-Short, J., Idiopathic Renal Acidosis in Twins: Alkalosis Resulting from Overdosage of a Citrate Mixture, *Arch. Dis. Childhood* 28:55, 1953.

Stapleton, T., Idiopathic Renal Acidosis in an Infant with Excessive Loss of Bicarbonate in the Urine, *Lancet* 1:683, 1949.

ACUTE AND CHRONIC NEPHRITIS

Dodd, K., Acute Nephritis in Childhood, *Cincinnati J. Med.* 30:8, 1949.

Herbert, H. J., Acute Glomerulonephritis in Childhood: A Study of the Late Prognosis of Twenty-seven Cases, *J. Pediat.* 40:549, 1952.

Jones, D. B., Glomerulonephritis, *Am. J. Path.* 29:33, 1953.

Keith, H. M., Types and Treatment of Nephritis in Children, *M. Clin. North America* 35:1069, 1951.

Rubin, M. I., and *M. Rapoport,* Cardiac Complications of Acute Hemorrhagic Nephritis, *Am. J. Dis. Child,* 55:244, 1938.

—— and ——, Mode of Action of Magnesium Sulfate in Reducing Hypertension of Acute Glomerulonephritis, *Am. J. M. Sc.* 201:734, 1941.

Wedgwood, R. J. P., and *M. H. Klaus,* Anaphylactoid Purpura (Schönlein-Henoch Syndrome: A Long-term Follow-up Study with Special Reference to Renal Involvement), *Pediatrics* 16:196, 1955.

Zuelzer, W. W., S. Charles, R. Kurnetz, W. A. Newton, and *R. Fallon,* Circulatory Diseases of the Kidneys in Infancy and Childhood, *A.M.A. Am. J. Dis. Child.* 81:1, 1951.

THE NEPHROTIC SYNDROME

Barness, L. A., G. H. Moll, and *C. A. Janeway,* Nephrotic Syndrome. I. Natural History of the Disease, *Pediatrics* 5:486, 1950.

Barnett, H. L., C. W. Forman, and *H. D. Lauson,* The Nephrotic Syndrome in Children, *Advances Pediat.* 5:53, 1952.

Bruck, E., M. Rapoport, and *M. I. Rubin,* Renal Functions in the Course of the Nephrotic Syndrome in Children, *J. Clin. Invest.* 33:699, 1954.

Eder, H. A., H. D. Lauson, F. P. Chinard, R. L. Greif, G. C. Cotzias, and *H. D. Van Slyke,* A Study of the Mechanisms of Edema Formation in Patients with the Nephrotic Syndrome, *J. Clin. Invest.* 33:636, 1954.

Eibern, R. M., J. Kleinerman, and *J. C. Cline,* Nephrotic Syndrome in a Neonatal Premature Infant, *J. Pediatrics* 44:195, 1954.

Galan, E., Nephrosis in Children. I. Observations on Eighty-four Patients. II. Clearance and Saturation Tests, *Am. J. Dis. Child.* 77:328, 1949.

Kramer, B., D. D. Casden, H. Goldman, and *S. H. Silverman,* Effect of the Adrenocorticotropic Hormone (ACTH) on Nephrosis in Childhood, *Postgrad. M.* 11:439, 1952.

Metcoff, J., N. Nobuyuki, and *P. Rance,* On the Role of the Kidney during Nephrotic Edema: Potassium Excretion and Sodium Retention, *J. Clin. Invest.* 33:665, 1954.

——, *W. M. Kelsey,* and *C. A. Janeway,* The Nephrotic Syndrome in Children: An Interpretation of its Clinical, Biochemical, and Renal Hemodynamic Features as Variations of a Single Type of Nephron Disease, *J. Clin. Invest.* 30:471, 1951.

Rapoport, M., W. W. McCrory, G. Barbero, H. L. Barnett, C. W. Forman, and *H. McNamara,* Effect of Corticotropin (ACTH) on Children with the Nephrotic Syndrome, *J.A.M.A.* 147:1101, 1951.
Riley, C. M., and *R. A. Davis,* Childhood Nephrosis, *Pediat. Clin. North Amer.* August, 1955, p. 893.
White, J. C., Nephrosis Occurring during Trimethadione Therapy, *J.A.M.A.* 139:376, 1949.

THROMBOSIS OF RENAL VEINS

Angelman, H., E. G. Hall, and *R. Spencer,* The Syndrome of Obstruction of Inferior Vena Cava in Childhood, *Brit. M. J.* 2:752, 1950.
Kobernick, S. D., J. R. Moore, and *F. W. Wiglesworth,* Thrombosis of the Renal Veins with Massive Hemorrhagic Infarction of the Kidneys in Childhood, *Am. J. Path.* 27:435, 1951.
Milburn, C. L., Jr., Hemorrhagic Infarction of the Kidneys in Infants, *J. Pediat.* 41:133, 1952.
Parry, E. W., Unilateral Renal Vein Thrombosis Treated by Nephrectomy and Post-operative Heparin, *Arch. Dis. Childhood* 26:358, 1951.

CHAPTER 37

General Features of the Examination

INDICATIONS FOR EXAMINATION

Examination of the cerebrospinal fluid is an extremely important adjunct to diagnosis and treatment when the existence of disease of the central nervous system or its membraneous coverings is suspected. The lumbar route is the safest and easiest site for the withdrawal of fluid. Cisternal, subarachnoid, and ventricular punctures are employed only when fluid at these sites is expected to be of different character or under different pressure than that in the spinal canal or when fluid cannot be obtained from the lumbar site.

A diagnostic lumbar puncture is important whenever a younger infant displays fever and irritability for which no cause is apparent. Stiff neck, bulging fontanel, and other signs of meningitis sometimes fail to appear in the first day or two of illness, particularly with newborn or premature infants. Convulsions with fever in a child, or a sudden convulsion complicating a systemic illness, should make one suspicious of meningitis or encephalitis as a possibility.

In such situations the "inquiring needle" should be employed at once, to ascertain the existence of meningitis and, if present, to identify the responsible organism. The proper use of antibiotics, sulfonamides, and other therapeutic agents depends on the known susceptibility of the organism. Intrathecal therapy is no longer deemed necessary for therapy of bacterial meningitis except in unusual situations. Hence lumbar puncture is to be viewed as primarily a diagnostic procedure rather than as a route for therapy.

The chief contraindication to diagnostic lumbar puncture is increased intracranial pressure from a space-taking lesion such as a tumor or abscess (p. 439). The eye grounds should always be examined first when this possibility is considered. In the presence of papilledema only a few drops of fluid should be withdrawn.

Every specimen of cerebrospinal fluid should be collected under complete asepsis, with fractional samples distributed through several test tubes. The number of tubes and the quantities placed in each will depend upon the tests to be requested. Traumatic hemorrhage as the direct result of the needle puncture explains the finding of a little fresh blood in the first few drops when those that come later are more clear. For best results the tubes reserved for bacteriology and cell counting should be examined within a few minutes after collection.

There is no evidence that repeated lumbar puncture produces meningeal irritation and resulting pleocytosis or affects adversely a patient with poliomyelitis, virus meningoencephalitis, or bacterial meningitis. When meningitis is a diagnostic possibility, the chance of implanting bacteria in uninfected meninges by the puncture is far less than the risk of overlooking a beginning meningeal infection.

Lumbar Puncture

The performance of a lumbar puncture with an infant or child is in general no different than with an adult, and postpuncture headaches are less bothersome. The fluid flows with more rapidity from the seated posture.

Above infancy, as with adults, the interspace between the third and fourth lumbar vertebrae is the site of choice. With infants under 1 year of age the interspace between the second and third vertebrae is preferable, and with younger prematures that between the first and second. The comparatively shorter length of the spinal cord in relation to the cavity within the vertebral cord is a protection against injury to the cord itself. Since in small or thin infants the distance between skin and subarachnoid space is only about 1 cm, care should be taken not to push the needle too far.

Once the needle point has reached the subarachnoid spaces and the stylet is withdrawn, fluid should drip freely and spontaneously. If no flow occurs the needle should be rotated and 15 to 20 seconds allowed for fluid to emerge before the needle is moved again. Pushing the needle in too far can make it strike the plexus of veins on the anterior aspect of the spinal space and lead to a "bloody tap."

Application of suction by a syringe is ordinarily inadvisable, but with purulent or hemorrhagic exudates is sometimes necessary. A specimen of 1 to 5 ml of fluid can be withdrawn with safety from the newborn and small premature infant, and 5 to 10 ml from the older infant and child, provided the pressure is not increased and no space-occupying intracranial lesion is present. In either of the latter contingencies the brain stem and cerebellum may herniate into the foramen magnum, with catastrophic consequences.

Cisternal Puncture

When doing a cisternal puncture the occipital region and the back of the neck are first shaved. The patient is made to lie down on his side. The head and neck are brought to the edge of the table and held straight or flexed. An antiseptic is applied to the shaved area. The needle used is of the lumbar puncture type, but shorter and with a short bevel. The needle is introduced through the skin in the medial line about 1 cm below the occipital protuberance and advanced in the direction of the nasal bridge until it strikes the bony edge of the occipital crest. The direction is then shifted a little downward and the point advanced further. A characteristic "give" is noted as it penetrates the atlantooccipital ligament and attached dura. The needle should not be forced beyond this point. The stylet is withdrawn. After an adequate amount of fluid has come away the needle is withdrawn and the skin puncture sealed with collodion.

Cisternal puncture is not generally advisable because of the possibility that the needle may be pushed in too far and puncture the medulla or stir up a local tamponading hemorrhage. It is sometimes done in newborn infants when lumbar puncture proves unsuccessful and in conditions associated with opisthotonus in which lumbar or ventricular puncture is not feasible.

Ventricular Puncture

Ventricular punctures are done only when there is a special reason to do so. One may want to study the chemistry or pressure status of the fluid within the ventricle or to replace most of the contained fluid with air for purposes of ventriculography. A dye can be injected when obstructive hydrocephalus is suspected (Blackfan test). In the infancy period when the anterior fontanel is still open, a ventricular puncture is deemed safer than the cisternal approach should lumbar puncture prove unsatisfactory or physically not feasible. Once the anterior fontanel becomes sealed off by growth processes, it becomes necessary to first make burr holes through the skull before going ahead, and a surgeon should be called in for that purpose.

A shortened stylet-containing needle of the lumbar puncture type is best. The scalp is shaved and the skin sterilized. If the fontanel is large the needle is introduced about midway between its lateral angle and the median anteroposterior line of the skull. If the fontanel is small and partly calcified the needle is introduced at or close to the lateral angle. With the patient on his back the needle is directed in the longitudinal line of the body for a distance of 1 to 3 cm, depending on age. If when the stylet is withdrawn no drops of fluid appear, the stylet is reinserted and the needle advanced 0.5 cm. This may have to be done several times. If no fluid is recovered the needle should be withdrawn in a straight line until the point lies just below the fontanel membrane; its angle is then shifted a little to the direction in which the operator thinks the ventricular spaces are situated, and the needle advanced again. When enough fluid is secured the needle is carefully withdrawn and the scalp puncture wound sealed with collodion.

When symptoms suggest a brain tumor, bilateral ventricular punctures may uncover a difference in the character of the fluid in the two ventricles.

PHYSICAL CHARACTERISTICS

The hydrogen ion concentration, specific gravity, viscosity, osmotic pressure, and refractive index of cerebrospinal fluid have been studied intensively by many workers, and the conclusion reached that these determinations are of little aid in the diagnosis of disease states. For this reason, and because appreciable time, skill, and equipment are needed for their measurement, tests for these physical constants are ordinarily not included in the study of specimens received from the sickroom.

The hydrogen ion concentration of cerebrospinal fluid is close to or identical with that of the blood—pH 7.35 to 7.4 under normal conditions. In acidemia and alkalemia the pH shifts parallel to the blood. In purulent meningitis, which is the only disorder with a value significantly different from that of the blood, the pH may drop to 7.2 or 7.3.

The inorganic constituents of normal cerebrospinal fluid are responsible for almost all the specific gravity increment above that of pure water. Sodium chloride and sodium bicarbonate are the two major solutes. The usual specific gravity range in normal fluid from the lumbar area is 1.0060 to 1.0080. A reading below 1.0035 implies that the cerebrospinal fluid is hypotonic in comparison with the tissue fluids—a probability highly unlikely in health—or that the specimen was procured from the ventricles or cisterna magna. In hydrocephalus the specific gravity may fall to less than 1.0040, whereas in uremia and diabetes and purulent meningitis it may approach or even exceed 1.0100. Even higher specific gravities have been encountered in patients with Froin's syndrome due to compression lesions of the upper spinal canal.

COLOR

Normal cerebrospinal fluid is water-clear and colorless. Turbidity may be due to leukocytes or erythrocytes or profuse bacterial growth. Purulent changes are produced by meningeal inflammation. Reddish-pink fluid is the result of bleeding. A yellow tint is given by bilirubin and related pigments and by atabrine. Yellow, orange, or brown xanthochromia is given by resolving hemorrhage or whenever there is an extremely high protein content.

Icterus

The cerebrospinal fluid from newborns often has a yellow tinge and may be bright yellow. This xanthochromia is due to bilirubin derivatives; it rises to a maximum during the second week of life, and then fades gradually. It is more intense when systemic icterus is prominent. In full-term infants the yellow color is usually gone by the end of the first month, but in prematures it may persist up to 2 months or longer.

Beyond the infancy period icteric staining due to bilirubinemia is rare in jaundice states. When the blood urobilinogen is elevated, urobilinogen may escape into the cerebrospinal fluid; readings up to 9 mg per 100 ml have been noted.

Xanthochromia

Yellow to orange-brown xanthochromia due to hemoglobin derivatives derived from erythrocytic breakdown begins to develop within 12 to 24 hours following even minimal intracranial bleeding, whether intracerebral, subarachnoidal, subdural, or related to the dura. The intensity increases as the red cells hemolyze. It reaches a maximum in a few days after the bleeding and begins to recede in 6 to 10 days unless there has been further bleeding. The pigment gives a positive reaction for bilirubin with the van den Bergh test. Once the newborn period is over, therefore, the finding of xanthochromia has great significance when intracranial bleeding is suspected.

To detect minimal xanthochromia, equal amounts of the fluid and distilled water are placed in identical test tubes and compared in daylight by looking directly down into the open ends. Xanthochromic fluid will appear slightly yellow.

PRESSURE

The cerebrospinal fluid pressure in the quiet normal newborn infant is 15 to 80 mm of water; in late infancy and early childhood, 40 to 150 mm; in older children as in adults, 70 to 200 mm. Readings much above these upper limits are indicative of increased intracranial pressure, provided the subject is relaxed physically and emotionally. Struggling makes the measurement of dubious value.

The pressure is usually found elevated in hydrocephalus, meningitis, encephalitis, cerebral edema, hemorrhage, brain tumors, and other lesions which increase the volume of the intracranial contents; and in chronic or subacute meningeal inflammations which can block the absorption of cerebrospinal fluid. When a spinal cord tumor completely obstructs the vertebral canal the first few drops may spurt from the needle at high pressure and then the flow ceases altogether.

During infancy, bulging or tension of the anterior fontanel is a helpful but not infallible indicator of elevated intracranial pressure. Depression of the fontanel portrays a decrease in pressure and is seen almost solely in dehydration.

Meningismus

Meningismus is a state of meningeal and nerve irritability occasionally accompanying acute infections, tetanus, and epileptic and other convulsive disorders. The cerebrospinal fluid pressure may be elevated. Other findings are normal as a rule, except that the protein is often increased to between 50 and 100 mg per 100 ml.

Brain Tumor

In this condition the cerebrospinal fluid pressure is usually elevated. The level of total protein rises in a minority of cases to between 50 and 150 mg per 100 ml. The chloride and sugar show no distinctive changes. The cell count almost never rises except when metastases have spread to the meninges, and then not consistently.

Because of the danger of herniation of the cerebellum and medulla into the foramen magnum, lumbar puncture in questionable cases of brain tumor must be done with great caution and the fluid withdrawn very slowly. After the pressure has been recorded with a manometer of capillary bore, not more than ½ to 1 ml of fluid should be withdrawn for chemical tests. Tumors in the posterior fossa (which comprise four-fifths of the brain tumors of childhood) are especially likely to herniate downward if much fluid is removed. With supratentorial tumors the risk is negligible.

Queckenstedt's Sign

When the vertebral subarachnoid spaces are open, as in the normal individual, compression of the internal jugular veins will dilate the cerebral veins and produce a rapid rise in the monometric reading of cerebrospinal fluid to between 150 and 300 mm of water. When the vertebral canal is blocked, as by a tumor or arachnoiditis in the spinal canal, the spinal fluid pressure as recorded by the manometer does not change on compression of the veins or the rates of rise and later fall may be unusually slow. In lateral sinus thrombosis, pressure on the internal jugular vein on the involved side will evoke no pressure change, whereas pressure on the opposite side will elicit the normal rise.

Testing for Queckenstedt's sign is subject to considerable difficulty, more so in children than in adults. Crying, breath holding, struggling, or any physical resistance on the part of the child can cause the lumbar cerebrospinal fluid pressure to rise regardless of the existence or absence of a block. The point of the needle must be free in the subarachnoid space, away from membrane fragments or nerve fibers which might occlude the lumen. The pressure applied should be enough to block the venous streams without compressing the carotid arteries or interfering with respiration. The operator himself must have some prior experience in the performance of the test, so as to be able to judge the reliability of his observations.

Hydrocephalus

The pressure goes up in hydrocephalus. A needle introduced into the ventricular spaces will have a high reading before fluid is withdrawn. A needle in the lumbar spine will show a high reading if the hydrocephalus is of the communicating type; normal or subnormal if it is noncommunicating. The fluid in hydrocephalus is colorless, unless recent intracerebral hemorrhage or infection has taken place. The cell count, sugar, and chlorides are within normal limits, but the protein content is often slightly increased. When brain tumor is the cause of the hydrocephalus the fluid may be xanthochromic, the protein increased, or the cell count slightly elevated.

Acute Head Injuries

The cerebrospinal fluid pressure may or may not be elevated after accidental injury of the skull or brain tissues. The patient must be completely quiet for elevated readings to be of diagnostic significance. Intracranial hemorrhage can occur without increased pressure or blood being immediately apparent in the spinal fluid.

GLUCOSE

The glucose content of the cerebrospinal fluid normally falls in a wide range between 40 and 90 mg per 100 ml, being about half the blood sugar. The level rises and falls with that of the blood, but after a lag of 1 to 2 hours. With premature and newborn infants the glucose in blood and spinal fluid more nearly approximate each other and may be about equal. In hypoglycemic and fasting states which last more than a few hours the level may drop to as low as 30 mg per 100 ml. If one wants precise information on the permeability of the blood-brain barrier to glucose or on the possible activity of intraspinal glycogenolysis parallel specimens of blood and cerebrospinal fluid should be tested after a 12-hour fast.

At all ages the glucose in the ventricular fluid is 2 to 5 mg per 100 ml higher than in the cisterna magna and 6 to 18 mg higher than in the lumbar region. The remarks which follow on the diagnostic interpretation of changes refer to figures obtained by lumbar puncture.

Diabetes Mellitus

Unusually high glucose may be anticipated in the cerebrospinal fluid in untreated diabetes mellitus. Readings up to 500 mg per 100 ml have been recorded. The fluid may also contain acetone when ketosis is present. We have several times seen the existence of diabetes first recognized by a high cerebrospinal fluid content of sugar in children brought to the hospital for treatment of sudden coma.

Hemorrhage

Blood plasma added to cerebrospinal fluid will destroy the contained glucose within 48 hours. This glycolytic enzymatic activity explains the progressive fall in glucose in stored specimens of normal cerebrospinal fluid which have been contaminated by blood during lumbar puncture. It also explains why blood-tinged ventricular fluid from patients with hydrocephalus may not only be sugar-free but may be able to break down sugar solutions in the laboratory when tested for that property.

Meningitis

Bacterial meningitis or admixture with glycolytic blood plasma is the most usual cause for readings below 30 or 40 mg per 100 ml. Values this low are rare with tumors, abscesses, subdural hematomas, viral and other forms of meningoencephalitis and with "aseptic" meningitis secondary to juxtaposed infection such as lateral sinus thrombosis. The finding of a cerebrospinal fluid sugar level below 30 mg per 100 ml in a child taken suddenly ill with a central nervous system disturbance is presumptive evidence of bacterial meningitis, more likely of pyogenic than of tuberculous origin.

The extent of the depression in glucose level in bacterial meningitis usually reflects the severity of the infection. When therapy is beneficial the level rises again. Readings below 10 or 15 mg per 100 ml call for immediate and energetic treatment. Sometimes, however, the cerebrospinal fluid sugar is found in the normal range in clinically severe meningitis. In untreated tuberculous meningitis the glucose level typically falls early in the disease and rises with recovery.

Rapid Method of Estimation of Glucose in Cerebrospinal Fluid

A simple semiquantitative method is to arrange five small test tubes in a rack, each containing 1 ml of Benedict's quantitative solution. Fresh cerebrospinal fluid in quantities from 0.05 to 0.25 ml (1 to 5 drops) is added to these tubes. The mixtures are placed in a bath of boiling water for exactly 2 minutes, and the sugar reduction read immediately. The threshold for color change is an approximate measure of the concentration of glucose in the fluid.

Amount of cerebrospinal fluid needed to reduce Benedict's solution (green, tan, or red color), ml	Amount of glucose per 100 ml cerebrospinal fluid, mg
0.05	over 50
0.10	40–50
0.15	30–40
0.20	20–30
0.25	10–20

CHLORIDES

The chloride content of cerebrospinal fluid has a wide normal range of from 690 to 760 mg per 100 ml of sodium chloride, or 118 to 133 mEq per liter. The majority of normal specimens fall in the range of 710 to 750 mg (121 to 129 mEq). The level tends to fluctuate parallel with that of the blood. There is a rise when the plasma and tissue fluid chlorides are increased as in renal insufficiency, and a decline when the blood and tissue levels fall as in diarrhea or vomiting.

Meningitis

The chlorides in the cerebrospinal fluid are often reduced slightly in bacterial meningitis, chiefly because of the lowered blood chloride which often accompanies infectious diseases. Tuberculous meningitis tends to evoke an even greater reduction, especially in the late stages when readings below 550 mg per 100 ml (94 mEq per liter) are not uncommon. The values fall steadily as the disease progresses, and rise again if therapy ameliorates the infection.

CALCIUM

The calcium in cerebrospinal fluid normally ranges from 4.5 to 5.5 mg per 100 ml. It may be said to correspond fairly exactly with the diffusible fraction of the serum calcium. Subnormal values are the rule in tetany associated with a low blood calcium.

PROTEIN

Once the neonatal period is over, the content of protein in normal cerebrospinal fluid ranges usually from 15 to 30 mg per 100 ml, with a top upper limit of 45 mg per 100 ml.

Premature infants and newborns under 1 month of age are exceptions to the above rule. Mature newborns may have values up to 200 mg if labor has been prolonged. Samson's mean for the first 2 weeks of life was 60 mg. In Otila's studies of premature infants, one weighing 1,700 gm had 269 mg per 100 ml and another weighing 1,800 gm had 213 mg, both being studied at 14 days of age. Many small premature infants normally have cerebrospinal fluid protein levels of over 100 mg per 100 ml in the first month, and between 50 and 75 mg in the second and third months.

The ventricular fluid normally contains 5 to 15 mg per 100 ml, and that from the cisterna magna about 10 to 20 mg. The slightly higher level in the lumbar region—which obtains in disease states as well as in health—has been attributed to the relative stagnation in this area and the seepage of protein from the perineural and perivascular spaces of the cord.

Disease States

The content of protein in the cerebrospinal fluid goes up in most diseases of the central nervous system and meninges. Values from 50 to 500 mg are found in purulent meningitis, tuberculous meningitis, poliomyelitis, lead poisoning, brain tumor, brain abscess, the encephalitides and nonbacterial meningitides, intracranial and subarachnoid hemorrhage, and cerebral trauma. Values exceeding the 500-mg level are sometimes found with severe meningitis, grossly bloody fluids, spinal cord tumors, and atypical instances of polyneuritis and brain tumor. In all disturbances the level returns progressively to normal as the patient recovers.

Fractionation studies have shown that the cerebrospinal fluid protein consists almost wholly of albumin and globulin in ratios varying from 4:1 to 8:1 (as compared to the 1.5:1 to 2.5:1 ratios obtaining in the serum proteins). Fibrinogen appears in appreciable amounts with pronounced meningeal inflammation as in tuberculous meningitis or when the protein content is high because of other disturbances. Its presence can be shown by the clotted web or pellicle which precipitates when a tube of cerebrospinal fluid stands overnight at refrigerator temperature or when a drop of serum taken from freshly clotted blood is added to the fluid. A pellicle tends to be the rule in active tuberculous meningitis. Fibrinolytic activity by the bacteria or the products of cellular disintegration prevent pellicle formation in purulent meningitis.

An increase in the globulin fraction is the basis of some of the qualitative tests for increase in total protein—the Pandy (10 per cent saturated phenol solution), the K. O. Newman test (5 per cent tannic acid solution), the Ross-Jones test (saturated ammonium sulfate solution), and others. These tests cannot be depended upon to demonstrate increases when the quantitative readings for total protein fall between 10 and 100 mg per 100 ml.

Rapid Method for Estimating Total Protein

A simple turbidimetric method can be set up in ward or office laboratories to provide a quick yet reasonably reliable estimate of the protein content of cerebrospinal fluid when meningitis or encephalitis is suspected. To a measured amount of cerebrospinal fluid—0.5 to 3 ml—is added a triple volume of a precipitant solution, 10 per cent trichloroacetic acid, or 5 per cent sulfosalicylic acid. The mixture is inverted a few times (not shaken violently) and permitted to stand for at least 5 minutes. The cloudiness which develops is compared against the permanent turbidity standards such as those utilized for the estimation of protein in urine. Trichloroacetic acid is preferable to the more widely used sulfosalicylic acid because the turbidity is said to be independent of changes in the albumin-globulin ratio, whereas the turbidity obtained with sulfosalicylic acid can be altered by abnormal ratios of albumin to globulin.

Should the reading in an unknown specimen prove greater than the highest standard, 1 ml of the fluid-precipitant mixture is transferred to another test tube and 9 ml of normal saline solution added. The turbidity reading is then taken and multiplied by 10.

Froin's Syndrome

The so-called loculation syndrome of Froin can appear when the spinal subarachnoid spaces become closed off as the result of a cord tumor, diseased vertebra, epidural abscess or related lesion, or in chronic meningitis after the spinal piarachnoid has become thick and adherent. In Froin's syndrome the fluid is clear or slightly cloudy and with a yellow tint. The withdrawable volume is scanty, and the pressure becomes very low after the first few drops are withdrawn. The protein content may be 100 to 4,000 mg per 100 ml. The spinal fluid glucose may also be high, whereas the chlorides are often unduly low. Spontaneous clotting may take place soon after removal. Fluid with these characteristics is practically pathognomonic of blocking of the downward flow of cerebrospinal fluid through the spinal subarachnoid spaces.

Most spinal cord tumors in the childhood years seem to obstruct the spinal subarachnoid spaces partially rather than completely. Froin's syndrome is then not fully developed. The fluid is clear or slightly turbid, with a normal cell count, chlorides, and sugar, but with protein increased slightly, usually in the range between 40 and 150 mg per 100 ml.

Colloidal Tests

These nonspecific and empirical approaches to demonstrating quantitative disproportions between albumin and globulin in cerebrospinal fluid have their greatest use in the evaluation and management of patients with syphilis. Suspensions of colloidal gold or gum mastic are in widest use. Abnormal but clear cerebrospinal fluid is diluted serially with normal saline to a dilution of 1:64 with gum mastic or to 1:576 or higher with colloidal gold. With maximal precipitation appearing in the first tubes the reaction is described as "first zone," "paretic," or "type D"; in the middle tubes, "middle zone," "syphilitic," or "type B"; in the last tubes, "third zone," "meningitic," or "type C." "Normal" or "type A" fluids may give slight reactions in the mid-zone. Blood-tinged cerebrospinal fluid specimens should not be employed for these tests.

The type D or high first-zone curve is seen often in coccidioidal meningitis, degenerative neurosyphilis, and chronic encephalitis. The type B curve is seen in neurosyphilis, multiple sclerosis, and the recovery phases of acute virus infections. The type C curve is found with exudative inflammation, initial stages of virus infections, subarachnoid block, and hemorrhage. To properly evaluate the results of colloidal tests one must know about the complement-fixation test for syphilis, the spinal fluid cell count, the total protein measurement, and the findings on clinical examination.

Enzymes and Antibodies

A number of enzymes and antibodies are in normal cerebrospinal fluid in negligible amounts. In meningitis and other intracranial diseases the content may increase. During meningitis caused by meningococci, pneumococci, or the Klebsiella it is often feasible to demonstrate type-specific polysaccharide derived from the bacterial capsules. This approach can be of value in identifying the pathogen when prior antimicrobial treatment has prevented bacteriologic isolation of the organism itself. Capsular polysaccharide may persist for some days after the cerebrospinal fluid cultures have become sterile.

CELLS

The leukocytes in the cerebrospinal fluid of normal children are as a rule between 0 and 5 cells per cu mm, though occasionally up to 8 per cu mm. These cells are almost exclusively lymphocytes, with an occasional mononuclear or endothelial cell or migrating neutrophil. Newborn infants, otherwise healthy, may have as many as 15 or even 30 cells during the first 2 weeks. With premature infants this neonatal enhancement may last until the third month.

Pleocytosis

The cerebrospinal fluid cell count goes up in most irritative and inflammatory lesions of the meninges and brain. A pleocytosis of 12 to 20 cells per cu mm is adjudged a minimal increase; 20 to 50 cells slight; 50 to 200 moderate; and 200 to 100,000 or above, great or severe.

Values above 1,000 per cu mm with a predominance of neutrophils are seen most often in acute purulent meningitis, whereas a milder pleocytosis with a majority of lymphocytes and monocytes favors viral or tuberculous meningitis. In the 72 cases of pyogenic meningitis reported by Joffe and Wells, for example, the cell count was between 100 and 1,000 per cu mm in 5 patients; between 1,000 and 10,000 in 54; between 10,000 and 20,000 in 9; and above 20,000 in 2. The 2 patients with initial counts below 100 were instances of meningococcic infection examined during the first few hours of the disease. In only 6 were the lymphocytes in excess of 15 per cent of the total cell count.

Cell Counting

The best way to count the leukocytes in the cerebrospinal fluid is to run the fluid directly into a hemocytometer counting chamber without any added acid or dye. Using the high dry microscopic objective, one enumerates all the leukocytes in the nine fields and multiplies by 10/9. When many red cells are present, it is wise to flush the hemocytometer pipet with glacial acetic acid before drawing up the cerebrospinal fluid. The traces of acid remaining will lyse the red cells and accentuate the contours of the white cells.

The differential cell count may be done on a stained slide made of the sediment after centrifuging or in the counting chamber using a combination staining-diluting solution.

BIBLIOGRAPHY

EXAMINATION AND GENERAL CHARACTERISTICS

Ayer, J. B., and H. C. Solomon, Cerebrospinal Fluid from Different Loci, *Arch. Neurol. & Psychiat.* 14:303, 1925.

Berman, L. B., E. Pastore, and L. W. Lapham, Jaundice and Xanthochromia of the Spinal Fluid, *J. Lab. & Clin. Med.* 44:273, 1954.

Davis, M. R., G. R. Cannefax, and *E. B. Johnwick,* Cerebrospinal Fluid: A Comparative Study of Specimens Taken from the Cisterna Magna and Lumbar Subarachnoid Space, *J. Ven. Dis. Inform.* 32:284, 1951.

Ford, F. R., "Diseases of the Nervous System in Infancy, Childhood and Adolescence," 2d ed. Charles C Thomas, Springfield, Ill., 1944.

Harris, A. H., and *C. Lange,* Routine Examination of Cerebrospinal Fluid, *New York J. Med.* 48:418, 1948.

Levinson, A., "Cerebrospinal Fluid in Health and Disease," 3d ed., The C. V. Mosby Company, St. Louis, 1929.

Lundström, R., and *G. von Reis,* Antistreptolysin Content of Cerebrospinal Fluid, *Am. J. Dis. Child.* 79:438, 1950.

Merritt, H., and *F. Fremont-Smith,* "The Cerebrospinal Fluid," W. B. Saunders Company, Philadelphia, 1937.

Moll, F. C., Examination of Cerebrospinal Fluid, *Pediat. Clin. North Amer.* February, 1955, p. 227.

Otila, E., Studies on the Cerebrospinal Fluid in Premature Infants, *Acta paediat.* vol. 35, suppl. 8, 1948.

Samson, K., Die Liquordiagnostik im Kindesalter, *Ergebn. inn. Med. u. Kinderh.* 41:553, 1931.

Smith, M. J. H., Intrathecal Streptomycin and Cerebrospinal Glucose Estimation, *J. Clin. Path.* 5:199, 1952.

Wikoff, H. L., and *P. Kazdan,* A Critique of Methods for Determination of Protein in Cerebrospinal Fluid, *Am. J. Clin. Path.* 21:1173, 1951.

Wolman, I. J., B. Evans, and *S. Lasker,* Specific Gravity of Cerebrospinal Fluid: Review of Methods and Application of Newer Micromethod in Spinal Anesthesia, *Am. J. Clin. Path.* 16:33, 1946.

FROIN'S SYNDROME AND SPINAL CORD LESIONS

Anderson, F. M., and *M. J. Carson,* Spinal Cord Tumors in Children: A Review of the Subject and Presentation of Twenty-one Cases, *J. Pediat.* 43:190, 1953.

Chambers, W. R., Intraspinal Tumors in Children Resembling Anterior Poliomyelitis, *J. Pediat.* 41:288, 1952.

Ingraham, F. D., Intraspinal Tumors in Infancy and Childhood, *Am. J. Surg.* 29:342, 1938.

CHAPTER 38

Bacterial Meningitis

The meningococcus, the pneumococcus, the influenza bacillus, and the tubercle bacillus are the most common causes of pyogenic meningitis in childhood. Staphylococcus, streptococcus, Pseudomonas, coliform bacilli, Klebsiella, or almost every other microorganism may be encountered. Mixed infections are not infrequent.

The cerebrospinal fluid changes in acute bacterial meningitis are more or less the same regardless of the organism. These changes in general consist of opalescence or cloudiness, increase in pressure and protein and cell count, moderate decline in chlorides, and marked decrease in sugar. The cells rise promptly to between 1,000 and 10,000 per cu mm and may go higher. In the early stages the predominant cell is the neutrophil; as the total count falls, during convalescence, the mononuclears become prominent. The glucose level is nearly always less than 30 mg per 100 ml.

CONGENITAL DERMAL SINUSES

These anomalous skin-lined canals, occurring anywhere along the vertebral column from coccygeal to occipital regions, frequently communicate with the intraspinal spaces through associated defects of the vertebrae and permit entry of bacteria. Coliform organisms are the most common invaders. Every child with meningitis or central nervous system abscess should be examined for the possible presence of one of these sinuses.

IDENTIFICATION OF ORGANISMS

Bacteria in the cerebrospinal fluid are sometimes so numerous as to give rise to a turbid or "ground-glass" appearance during the first hours of illness while the leukocyte count is still below 100 per cu mm. Study of Gram-stained smears of the fluid usually enables the physician to make a provisional morphologic identification. Antecedent chemotherapy often results in negative smear and cultural examinations.

The cerebrospinal fluid should always be cultured when meningitis is suspected. Fluid apparently free from organisms in a direct smear

448

may show recognizable colony growth as early as 12 hours after culturing. The choice of medications will be guided by the nature of the organism and its susceptibility to antibiotics as determined by its usual biologic behavior and the findings on laboratory testing of the recovered strain (p. 932).

Bacteriologic media for recovery of organisms from cerebrospinal fluid are the same as with blood and other body fluids: brain broth and blood agar for routine use, Levinthal's or Fildes' when *Hemophilus influenzae* is suspected, Sabouraud's for possible yeasts, Dubos' or Petrognani's or potato for tuberculosis, etc. The fluid should be placed in several different kinds of media and cultured anaerobically as well as aerobically. One method of taking a culture in suspected meningitis is to permit a little of the fluid to drop directly into the various media directly from the needle during the lumbar puncture.

A blood culture should always be taken prior to therapy. This is frequently positive and furnishes additional material for bacteriologic identification and antibiotic study. Recovery of an organism from the blood stream can be of invaluable assistance should the cerebrospinal fluid culture prove sterile.

When pneumococci, meningococci, or influenza bacilli are recovered the determination of the precise bacterial subtype is of epidemiologic rather than of therapeutic importance. Nevertheless, even though the antibiotics and other chemotherapeutic agents have made it no longer necessary to administer specific immune serum, type identification is desirable when facilities are available.

The organisms which most commonly evade isolation are the influenza bacillus and the meningococcus. Therapy for meningitis of obscure origin should consist of several antimicrobial agents such as penicillin and streptomycin or a broad-spectrum antibiotic and a sulfonamide. Empirical observation of the responses of the infection must then be relied on to govern changes in treatment. When proper therapeutic agents have been selected a striking improvement can be expected within 24 to 48 hours.

PROCEDURE FOR EXAMINATION OF CEREBROSPINAL FLUID WHEN MENINGITIS IS SUSPECTED

Collect the fluid in small sterile test tubes with aseptic technique. Use four tubes (or five if tuberculosis is suspected), distributing as follows:

Tube 1: 1 to 5 ml. Place immediately in bacteriology incubator at 37°C. Examine for bacteria in 12 to 24 hours. Spinal fluid is an excellent culture medium; most of the bacteria which cause meningitis grow well in it.

Tube 2: 1 to 2 ml. Take to laboratory immediately for cell count, before the cells settle out or a coagulum forms. After shaking by hand, a hemocytometer pipet is introduced and a sample withdrawn for cell counting. Do not perform a cell count on a tube which contains visible blood secondary to the trauma of the puncture, for even a trace of bleeding can elevate the apparent cell count above normal limits.

Tube 3: 1 to 5 ml. This should be kept warm in transit by being held in the hand or immersed in tepid water. Centrifuge at 1,000 to 1,500 rpm for 5 minutes, and decant the supernatant. Transfer loopfuls of the sediment to warm blood agar plates and other culture media. Add disks impregnated with selected antibiotics. Prepare two thick air-dried smears of the residual sediment, stain one with aqueous methylene blue for differential counting of leukocytes and demonstration of the shape of the bacteria. Stain the other by the Gram method for provisional identification of the bacteria. Use new glass slides which have been cleaned with chromic acid solution; flame in a Bunsen burner immediately before use.

Tube 4: 2 to 3 ml. Use this for chemical examinations—protein, chloride, sugar, hemoglobin, trytophane, etc. The rapid semiquantitative methods for estimation of protein and glucose may be employed.

Tube 5: Collect at least 5 ml if tuberculous meningitis is suspected and clear or opalescent fluid obtained. Leave test tube undisturbed overnight at 37°C in a bacteriology incubator or in the refrigerator, in order to permit a pellicle to develop. Next day remove the contracted fine fibrin clot (if any) from the center of the tube by a wire loop, spread it over a small section of a new glass slide, and stain for tubercle bacilli with the Ziehl-Neelsen stain. If the clot is not easy to remove, it can be spun down in a centrifuge, cultured on proper media, and then stained. If there is no clot, the fluid should be centrifuged for at least 15 minutes and fluid taken from the lowermost portion for staining.

Should the quantity of collected fluid be too scanty to permit this ideal routine of examination, tubes 1 and 5 may be omitted. The cell count (tube 2) and the search for bacteria (tube 3) can be done from the same tube if the first pipet introduced for withdrawal of fluid for cell counting is bacteriologically sterile.

MENINGOCOCCIC MENINGITIS

As a rule, infection with *Neisseria meningitidis* begins with prodromal symptoms of an upper respiratory tract infection. After one or more days a bacteremia occurs, with a petechial or purpuric or maculopapular rash as a characteristic manifestation. During this phase, blood cultures are usually positive and there is a leukocytosis of 15,000 to 50,000 cells per cu mm with a high percentage of neutrophils which are often immature or vacuolated. Meningitis appears coincidentally or within 1 or 2 days after the onset of the meningococcemia. The organisms are sometimes demonstrable in stained preparations made directly from scrapings of skin hemorrhages.

The organisms are demonstrated more often by direct smear of the cerebrospinal fluid sediment than by growth on culture media. In the smears they appear usually as rounded diplococci, aggregated within the cytoplasm of neutrophils or suspended free in the fluid. For best bacteriologic success the cultures must be made within a few minutes after withdrawal of the fluid, which in the interim is kept warm. Growth is more satisfactory in an atmosphere of 5 to 10 per cent carbon dioxide.

With the aid of serum agglutination, meningococci can be subdivided into groups. The majority of cases of sporadic meningitis are caused by members of group II (p. 804).

Once chemotherapy is started the organisms disappear almost at once from the cerebrospinal fluid, and within a few days the sugar content rises. The protein and cell count return to normal more gradually, and hence are less reliable as indicators of control of the infection.

PNEUMOCOCCIC MENINGITIS

Pneumococci of any type may give rise to meningitis, but types I, III, VI, XI, and XIV are encountered most often. In a typical case the cerebrospinal fluid is under augmented pressure, has a turbid greenish-yellow color, an increased content of protein and cells, and a lowered sugar content. The organisms are extremely abundant in the direct smear unless medications have already been given, and grow out readily in cultures. If the lumbar puncture is done on the first day of illness one may find myriads of organisms free in the turbid cerebrospinal fluid, in association with a cell count which is elevated only moderately. In such situations it is feasible to identify the organisms by demonstration of a quellung reaction when droplets of fluid are mixed with the proper grouping and typing serums.

Most patients with pneumococcic infections have an underlying pneumococcic infection in the throat, nasal sinuses, or lungs.

Penicillin or some other potent antibiotic, given in combination with a sulfonamide, is usually effective therapy. These should be administered as soon as the diagnosis is recognized, since untreated pneumococcic meningitis tends to advance rapidly and cause death within a day or two. Patients in coma or shock when treatment is begun may be given a single initial intrathecal dose of penicillin. Soluble aqueous penicillin should be given in high dosage intravenously at first, followed by as much as 1 million units of penicillin intramuscularly every 2 hours.

STREPTOCOCCIC AND STAPHYLOCOCCIC MENINGITIS

Meningeal infections due to these organisms are as a rule secondary to infections elsewhere in the body. Otitis media with or without mastoiditis, osteomyelitis, pansinusitis, infected wounds or burns, and lobar and bronchopneumonia have all been seen in our experience as precursors to these forms of meningitis. The meninges may be invaded through direct extension as from the temporal bone or frontal sinuses or by bacteremic spread from more distant foci. Therapy is much the same as for pneumococcic meningitis and should be combined with attention to the local lesion when feasible.

INFLUENZA BACILLUS MENINGITIS

Pleomorphic Gram-negative rods or coccobacilli or poorly staining coccoid forms in the direct smear are suggestive of a *Hemophilus influenzae* infection. Culturing on Levinthal or Fildes agar may yield colonies within 12 hours. Blood cultures taken before onset of therapy will yield the organism in more than half the cases.

To identify a suspected organism as *H. influenzae* one may add droplets of fresh cerebrospinal fluid clarified by centrifugation to type-specific diagnostic serums and look for the quellung response. Demonstration of capsular swelling with bacteria from cultures is less satisfactory, since capsules may no longer be evident within 6 hours after first cultivation. Specific antiserums may also be used to detect the specific polysaccharide in cerebrospinal fluid, applying either the direct precipitin reaction or the inhibition of agglutination of erythrocytes previously sensitized with the polysaccharide. The precipitin test alone can be misleading, inasmuch as pneumococcus type IV seems to possess a common antigen with *H. influenzae,* and may give a positive precipitin reaction with antiinfluenzal sera. The strains of *H. influenzae* which give rise to meningitis nearly always are type b, or occasionally type a.

Since different strains of *H. influenzae* differ in their susceptibility to the antibiotics, and since resistance may develop rapidly with any of the antibiotics, it is most important to try to grow the organism from the patient on culture media and to carry out the in vitro tests for sensitivity. Antiserum is difficult to procure, and most cases recover without its use.

MENINGITIS CAUSED BY OTHER GRAM-NEGATIVE BACILLI

Other Gram-negative bacilli such as coliform organisms, Pseudomonas, Klebsiella, Salmonella, or Escherichia found in smears of cerebrospinal fluid may be mistaken at first for *H. influenzae.* Bacteriologic differentiation and antibiotic sensitivity tests should always be made.

These other Gram-negative bacilli are frequent causes of meningitis in premature and debilitated infants. They may act as secondary invaders of an already established meningitis or enter the meninges in the end stages of an overwhelming infection elsewhere. Many cases result from contamination of the meninges by operations on the brain or spinal cord or by invasion through a draining meningomyelocele or similar lesion.

Meningitis caused by *Klebsiella pneumoniae* (Friedländer) tends to have an unusually viscous exudate whose liquefaction may be aided by instillations of streptokinase and streptodornase intrathecally.

TUBERCULOUS MENINGITIS

In tuberculous meningitis the cerebrospinal fluid is typically clear or slightly turbid and under increased pressure. The cell count is usually between 10 and 500 cu mm but may go as high as 1,000 cells. Lymphocytes and other mononuclear cells are as a rule predominant. A high proportion of neutrophils tends to go along with rapid advance of the meningitis. The chloride level falls slowly as the disease advances and rises with recovery. The sugar level drops early and is usually below 35 mg per 100 ml on the initial tap. The protein content varies from 40 to 500 mg in individual cases and goes up as the disease progresses; it is rarely less than 100 mg. The colloidal gold curve may be of any type. The tryptophane test is often positive. A coagulum of clotted fibrin usually forms as the fluid stands, but must not be viewed as pathognomonic.

Demonstration of Organisms

In our hands, the most success in direct demonstration of *Mycobacterium tuberculosis* has been by permitting a weblike pellicle to form in the original test tube, and then centrifuging and staining the coagulum with the Ziehl-Neelsen carbol fuchsin stain. Finding the organisms usually needs 30 to 60 minutes for examination of the slide, scanning each oil-immersion field fully and patiently. They occur singly or in small groups and are far from abundant in the early stages. Failure to demonstrate the mycobacterium is not uncommon, even after extended study with smears, cultures, and guinea pig inoculations.

An alternate method for demonstrating tubercle bacilli is that of Davison, for use with large volumes of cerebrospinal fluid. Samples of 20 to 40 ml of fluid are left to stand at 37°C, in a sterile medicine glass which has a cover slip resting at the bottom. After 24 hours the sediment and any coagulum will have settled upon the cover slip. The excess fluid is carefully sucked off with a medicine dropper. The cover slip with adherent film is removed by forceps, dried in the air, fixed with heat, and stained with carbol fuchsin.

Tryptophane Test

Proteins containing the amino acid tryptophane have been said to appear much more often in the cerebrospinal fluid in tuberculous meningitis than in the pyogenic varieties. A test for this substance is sometimes included in the diagnostic analysis of fluid from suspected cases. The test, however, has not proved of significant reliability. In the study of Toomey, Fulton, and Rea, for example, only 21 of 55 specimens from tuberculous meningitis were positive, whereas 35 of 147 specimens from nontuberculous meningitis were positive. Our own experience is in the same direction.

Positive tryptophane reactions are frequently given by the cerebrospinal fluid of normal premature infants under 1 month of age, and particularly in the first week. This may indicate that the cerebrospinal fluid proteins in premature newborns have a somewhat different amino acid structure than later in life.

Levinson Test

The empirical coagulation test of A. Levinson is sometimes used to follow the progress of treatment in tuberculous meningitis. In this test 1 ml of 2 per cent mercuric chloride solution and 1 ml of 3 per cent sulfosalicylic acid are added to two separate 1-ml samples of cerebrospinal fluid. Flat-bottomed tubes

5 to 6 mm in diameter are used. The contents are mixed by shaking but not centrifuged and left to stand 24 hours at room temperature either corked or stoppered with cotton. The precipitates which settle out are 2 to 3 mm in height normally, but in tuberculous meningitis may exceed 5 mm. That from the mercuric chloride is expected to stand two to five times as high as that from the sulfosalicylic acid and to be gelatinous rather than granular.

Comments on Laboratory Control of Streptomycin Therapy

Miliary tuberculosis may spread to the meninges even while chemotherapy is being given. Since meningitis complicating any form of pulmonary tuberculosis diminishes the chances of recovery materially, and since the therapy of meningitis is much more successful when treatment is begun early, diagnostic lumbar punctures should be performed at periodic intervals in every case of miliary tuberculosis, particularly while the illness keeps the patient apathetic or drowsy.

After recovery from tuberculous meningitis, so long as tuberculosis is active elsewhere, the patient should receive spinal punctures at weekly and later at monthly intervals, in order to detect any recurrence in its beginning stages. If meningeal inflammation becomes evident after an apparently complete remission, the full schedule of therapy should be repeated.

Higher levels of streptomycin in the cerebrospinal fluid are needed for tuberculous meningitis than can be provided by intramuscular therapy alone, especially in the early stages. The number of cases cured by combined intramuscular and intrathecal streptomycin therapy has been much greater than with intramuscular treatment alone. The meningeal barrier seems to become less and less permeable to streptomycin as the inflammation subsides.

Within a few days of starting intrathecal injections of streptomycin the cell count, percentage of neutrophils, and protein content nearly always rise. As the disease subsides the cell count and protein level fall and the sugar content rises more slowly. Streptomycin itself is a reducing agent and may have a minor influence on the readings of cerebrospinal fluid glucose. Intrathecal hemorrhages resulting from puncture trauma may raise the protein and erythrocyte content of the fluid withdrawn, and the glycogenolytic enzymes in the extravasations lower the glucose readings. The chloride levels fluctuate inconstantly and can be depressed by vomiting; they are of little value for prognosis.

Persistence of organisms in the fluid is an unfavorable sign. Unless the organisms are insensitive, or imbedded in a gelatinous exudate or in avascular tuberculomata which resist penetration by streptomycin, they are not recoverable after the first 5 to 10 days if streptomycin therapy is adequate. Distortions in morphology and in staining behavior also become evident. An increase in numbers precedes other alterations in the spinal fluid at the onset of a relapse or of invasion of the meninges during miliary tuberculosis.

Spinal block may complicate repeated instillations of streptomycin into the lumbar spaces. The signs then are those of loculation or Froin's syndrome (p. 444), with fluid of limited quantity, high protein content, and no positive pressure even on bilateral jugular compression. Sometimes the block is only partial, so that the fluid drips from the needle very slowly and at low pressure; such partial obstructions often clear spontaneously within a day or two.

The level of streptomycin in the cerebrospinal fluid after parenteral administration can be of assistance in the recognition of early inflammation of the meninges. In miliary tuberculosis alone the level is usually less than 1 μgm per 100 ml and rarely higher than 3 μgm, whereas at the onset of spread to the meninges it may go to between 5 and 40 μgm before any other cerebrospinal fluid changes are demonstrable.

One cause of late relapse in patients whose meningeal or miliary tuberculosis has improved for a time is the acquiring of streptomycin resistance by the strain of *M. tuberculosis* responsible for the infection. This mutational change can be demonstrated by growing the recovered organisms on media impregnated with the drug in concentration obtaining in the body fluids.

BRAIN ABSCESS

Brain abscess may occur as a complication of general septicemia, paranasal sinusitis, otitis media, bacterial meningitis, or osteomyelitis of the skull. If otitis media precedes, the brain lesion is almost always on the same side as the inflamed ear. The cerebral hemispheres are involved more often than the cerebellum. Multiple foci are not uncommon. Streptococci and pneumococci are the most common causative organisms. The cerebrospinal fluid may or may not show an increased pressure, pleocytosis, or increase in protein. Unless the abscess tract communicates with the leptomeninges the cerebrospinal fluid will be bacteriologically sterile. In well-encapsulated and localized lesions the fluid may not only seem normal, but the peripheral blood may not exhibit any leukocytosis or increase in granulocytes.

Brain abscess is a dreaded and not too uncommon complication of congenital heart disease. Persistent severe headaches with or without lethargy or attacks of vomiting are the early symptoms. Fever, leukocytosis, central nervous system signs, and changes in the cerebrospinal fluid often do not develop until after the abscess has ruptured into the subarachnoid space or the ventricular system. Almost any species of bacteria may be responsible, though often all cultures prove to be sterile.

Patients with intracardiac circulatory shunts appear to be peculiarly susceptible. The pathogenetic mechanism seems to lie in the opportunity for bacteria which constantly enter the blood stream to enter the arterial system through the shunt and thereby reach the brain, instead of being filtered out in the lung capillaries as normally occurs.

ANTIMICROBIAL AGENTS

The individual antibiotics and sulfonamides inhibit or destroy the bacteria causing meningitis in much the same way as they attack these same organisms elsewhere in the body. Therapeutic dosages may have to be unusually high, however, inasmuch as diffusion into the subarachnoid space is not always as efficient as into the other body cavities. In inflammatory diseases of the meninges the meningeal barrier is passed much more readily than in health or in the presence of encephalitis.

Generally, parenteral injections of antibiotics produce higher cerebrospinal fluid levels than can be attained with oral therapy.

The broad-spectrum antibiotics and the sulfonamides can be extremely irritating when injected into the subarachnoid spaces in any appreciable concentration. Sterile meningitis, arachnoid adhesions, convulsions, or central nervous system destruction may follow. Penicillin and streptomycin, on the other hand, are tolerated when injected intrathecally in dilute solutions. Reactions from overdosage consist of meningeal irritation, direct neurotoxic irritation, or depression of the medullary center or cerebral cortex. Injections through the lumbar or intraventricular routes are less likely to excite reactions than those into the cisterna.

All intrathecal instillations of antibiotics should be done with extreme caution and terminated at once if any change appears in physiologic functions or neurologic status. Pleocytosis seems to disappear more rapidly when meningitis is treated with systemic medications alone than when antibiotics are also injected into the cerebrospinal fluid spaces. Upward diffusion of intrathecal medications from the lumbar to the suboccipital spaces seems to be reduced when the protein content of the fluid is high.

Assayable quantities of penicillin in the cerebrospinal fluid of normal subjects are usually not obtainable without a blood concentration of 10 to 30 units per ml for some length of time. After a single massive intravenous injection of aqueous penicillin a cerebrospinal fluid concentration no greater than 0.5 unit per ml will be attained. In contrast, levels of 8 units can be obtained with intramuscular injections of 1 million units of penicillin every 2 hours. When probenecid is given along with penicillin the blood levels become two to five times higher than with penicillin alone, and the cerebrospinal fluid concentrations are doubled.

In normal subjects and those with noninflammatory brain diseases the cerebrospinal fluid concentration after intramuscular administration of 2 gm of streptomycin is usually less than 1 μgm per ml. When meningitis is present, on the other hand, concentrations of approximately 8 to 18 μgm are attained in 2 hours and gradually subside to 1 to 3 μgm at 12 hours. The levels vary with the severity of the infection, diminishing during clinical improvement.

BIBLIOGRAPHY

PYOGENIC MENINGITIS

Alexander, H. E., Guides to Optimal Therapy in Bacterial Meningitis, J.A.M.A. 152:662, 1953.
———, C. Ellis, and G. Leidy, Treatment of Type-specific Hemophilus influenzae Infections in Infancy and Childhood, J. Pediat. 20:673, 1942.

Brainerd, H., Infections of the Central Nervous System: An Approach to Diagnosis, *J. Pediat.* 37:478, 1950.

Goldring, S., and *C. G. Harford,* Effect of Leucocytes and Bacteria on Glucose Content of the Cerebrospinal Fluid in Meningitis, *Proc. Soc. Exper. Biol. & Med.* 75:669, 1950.

Hoyne, A. L., and *H. Herzon,* Streptococcic Viridans Meningitis: A Review of the Literature and Report of Nine Recoveries, *Ann. Int. Med.* 33:879, 1950.

Jackson, W. P. U., A Survey of Recent Development in the Treatment of Pneumococcal Meningitis, *Arch. Dis. Childhood* 25:22, 1950.

Kagan, B. M., J. H. Hess, B. Mirman, and *E. Lundeen,* Meningitis in Premature Infants, *Pediatrics* 4:479, 1949.

Kaufman, B., H. Levy, B. D. Zaleznak, and *A. M. Litvak,* Statistical Analysis of 242 Cases of Meningococcus Meningitis, *J. Pediat.* 38:705, 1951.

Lepper, M. H., N. H. Blatt, P. F. Wehrle, and *H. W. Spies,* Treatment of Bacterial Meningitis of Unusual Etiology and Purulent Meningitis of Unknown Origin, *A.M.A. Am. J. Dis. Child.* 85:295, 1953.

Mount, L. A., Congenital Dermal Sinuses as a Cause of Meningitis, Intraspinal Abscess and Intracranial Abscess, *J.A.M.A.* 139:1263, 1949.

Nemir, R. L., and *J. Israel,* Pneumococcic Meningitis in Infants and Children, *J.A.M.A.* 147:213, 1951.

Neter, E., R. F. Krauss, G. J. Egan, and *T. H. Mason,* Aureomycin Treatment of Meningitis Due to *Bacillus pyocyaneus* and *Bacillus aerogenes, J.A.M.A.* 142:1335, 1950.

Vaden, E. B., E. C. Rice, and *V. Stadnichenko,* Meningitis Due to Simultaneous Double Infections in Children, *J.A.M.A.* 143:1402, 1950.

TUBERCULOUS MENINGITIS

Cairns, H., Neurosurgical Methods in the Treatment of Tuberculosis Meningitis with a Note on Some Unusual Manifestations of the Disease, *Arch. Dis. Childhood* 26:373, 1951.

Cathie, I. A. B., and *J. C. W. MacFarlane,* Adjuvants to Streptomycin in Treating Tuberculous Meningitis in Children, *Lancet* 2:784, 1950.

Committee on Therapy, The Current Status of Isoniazid in the Treatment of Tuberculosis, *Am. Rev. Tuberc.* 67:269, 1953.

Debré, R., et al., "Meningite tuberculeuse et tuberculos miliaire de l'enfant," Masson et Cie, Paris, 1953.

Kendig, E. L., R. Ownby, Jr., G. E. Trevathan, and *L. E. Sutton, Jr.,* The Treatment of Tuberculous Meningitis in Children, *J. Pediat.* 43:532, 1953.

Lincoln, E. M., and *T. W. Kirmse,* The Diagnosis and Treatment of Tuberculous Meningitis in Children, *Am. J. M. Sc.* 219:382, 1950.

Masi, A., and *N. Menabuoni,* Cerebrospinal Fluid Sugar during Tuberculosis Meningitis and Its Relation to the Reducing Power of Streptomycin (La Glicorachia in corso d'meningite tubercolare e suoi rapporti con il potere riducente della streptomicina), *Riv. clin. pediat.* 46:372, 1948.

Rapoport, S., C. D. West, and *W. A. Brodsky,* Salt Losing Conditions: The Renal Defect in Tuberculous Meningitis, *J. Lab. & Clin. Med.* 37:550, 1951.

Stewart, S. M., The Bacteriological Diagnosis of Tuberculous Meningitis, *J. Clin. Path.* 6:241, 1953.

Toomey, J. A., R. P. Fulton, and *F. W. Rea,* Tryptophan Bodies in Tuberculous Meningitis, *J. Pediat.* 14:372, 1939.

Williams, A. L., Pathology of Tuberculous Meningitis, with Particular Reference to Modification in Pathology Following Treatment with Streptomycin, *M. J. Australia* 1:680, 1951.

CHAPTER 39

Viral Meningoencephalitis

Changes in the cerebrospinal fluid are essentially similar in all forms of viral meningoencephalitis. Hence it is not possible to arrive at an etiologic diagnosis solely from the usual tests. Typical fluid is clear and under slightly increased pressure. The cell count usually falls between 50 and 500 per cu mm, though it may be in the normal range or go as high as 2,000 or more. The majority of the cells are lymphocytes or large monocytes. The protein level is usually elevated slightly, in the range from 50 to 200 mg per 100 ml. The glucose and chloride levels are ordinarily normal but may be decreased or increased slightly. Bacteriologic cultures show no growth. The peripheral blood often displays a mild neutrophilic granulocytosis during the first few days. When the clinical differentiation between viral and pyogenic meningitis is uncertain, the findings of monocytosis, normal sugar level, and sterile cultures at the very beginning point to a viral disease, whereas a neutrophilic pleocytosis, low sugar level, and of course a positive culture are more characteristic of a bacterial invasion.

Serologic tests have been perfected for the laboratory identification of most varieties of viral meningoencephalitis (Chap. 73). In lymphocytic choriomeningitis and in mumps the causative virus may be recoverable from the fluid itself. Some comments on the cerebrospinal fluid changes in a few of the more common viral encephalitides are given in the pages which follow.

POLIOMYELITIS

In the early stages of poliomyelitis the cerebrospinal fluid is usually clear but may be mildly opalescent. The pressure may be moderately elevated. The chloride and glucose levels are usually normal but rarely are lowered. The cell count may vary from 5 to 1,000 per cu mm, though most commonly between 50 to 200 cells; it reaches a peak in the first few days and subsides gradually, reaching normal between the second and fifth week. Neutrophils usually pour out in the first few days, amounting to 40 to 90 per cent of all cells; mononuclear cells then become

458

prominent. When symptoms of meningeal irritation are pronounced, the cell count and content of neutrophils are usually high.

In Joffe and Wells' cases the initial protein readings ranged from 12 to 207 mg per 100 ml, with an average of 52.6 mg. In Ford, Eldridge, and Grulee's 31 patients somewhat higher values were shown by those who developed paralysis (geometric mean, 68 mg) than by those who did not (geometric mean, 46 mg).

The protein level rises and falls more slowly than does the pleocytosis and tends to reach a maximum between the tenth and thirty-fifth day. The protein is often still rising after the cell count has returned to normal. It may remain elevated for as long as 3 months after all other cerebrospinal fluid abnormalities have disappeared. Protein values as high as 2,000 mg per 100 ml and a falling cell count after the first week have been described in a few patients with poliomyelitis who exhibited intense radicular pain and sensory disturbances in the affected extremities, simulating the Guillain-Barré syndrome. There are no significant correlations between the protein values, the total cell count, the percentage distribution of cells, the absolute monocyte or neutrophil count, or the levels of chlorides or glucose and the development or character of paralysis.

When a child is first seen several weeks after the onset of an attack of paralysis, the finding of increased protein in the cerebrospinal fluid is suggestive that poliomyelitis was responsible. An elevated cell count should not be expected.

The virology and immunology of poliomyelitis are discussed on pages 887 to 889.

MUMPS

Mumps meningoencephalitis is often unaccompanied by parotitis or other physical evidence that the neurologic disturbance is due to the virus of mumps. Cerebrospinal fluid changes are the same as in other forms of viral encephalitis and may persist for several weeks after clinical recovery is complete. The pressure is increased. A pleocytosis almost always occurs, with the leukocyte count usually in excess of 100 per cu mm and often greater than 1,000. The count tends to reach its high point during the first week of the illness. Lymphocytes usually constitute more than 90 per cent of the cells. The total protein is usually elevated slightly but may rise as high as 250 mg per 100 ml. The sugar and chloride content are as a rule not diminished.

Serologic studies are advisable in suspected cases without other clinically recognizable phenomena such as parotitis. A serum specimen should be taken as soon as possible after the onset of the illness, and another 2 to 4 weeks later for comparison (p. 892). A rise in titer will almost always be demonstrable in the second specimen.

MEASLES

In measles encephalitis the neurologic disturbance begins during or within the first 2 weeks after the eruptive stage. The fluid typically is clear and colorless, with protein content between 35 and 600 mg per 100 ml and glucose and chloride within normal range. The cell count is normal or slightly elevated and rarely exceeds 750 per cu mm. Neutrophils are usually in the minority.

POSTINFECTIOUS ENCEPHALITIS

The cerebrospinal fluid findings in the cerebral complications which may follow some of the viral diseases (p. 890) are similar to what has been described in the foregoing pages as characteristic of the more clearly acknowledged varieties of acute viral meningoencephalitis.

ASEPTIC MENINGITIS

This general term is applied to forms of acute nonbacterial meningitis which are presumptively of viral origin but which cannot be traced to known pathogenic viruses such as those of poliomyelitis, herpes simplex, or lymphocytic choriomeningitis. Some of these may be caused by Coxsackie or ECHO strains (Chap. 73). Patients often exhibit meningeal irritation, nausea or vomiting, pharyngeal injection, vague generalized pains, transitory muscle weakness, or altered tendon reflexes. The cerebrospinal fluid cell count is moderately elevated, usually with a lymphocytic pleocytosis. The protein content is normal or slightly increased. Changes in chlorides and sugar are minimal, if any. These findings may be simulated by some nonviral infections, particularly tuberculosis, leptospirosis, and antibiotic-treated pyogenic meningitis.

BIBLIOGRAPHY

VIRAL MENINGOENCEPHALITIS

Ayres, J. C., and R. F. Feemster, Public-health Aspects of the Virus Encephalitides, New England J. Med. 240:966, 1949.

Donahue, W. L., F. D. Playfair, and L. Whitaker, Mumps Encephalitis, Pathology and Pathogenesis, J. Pediat. 47:395, 1955.

Ford, G. D., F. L. Eldridge, and C. G. Grulee, Jr., Spinal Fluid in Acute Poliomyelitis: Changes in Total Protein and Cell Counts on Serial Study, Am. J. Dis. Child. 79:633, 1950.

Green, W. R., L. K. Sweet, and *R. W. Prichard,* Acute Lymphocytic Choriomeningitis: A Study of Twenty-one Cases, *J. Pediat.* 35:688, 1949.

Hodes, H. L., Common Types of Encephalitis in Children, *New York J. Med.* 50:2277, 1950.

Karzon, D. T., A. L. Barron, M. Winkelstein, Jr., and *S. Cohen,* Isolation of ECHO Virus Type 6 during Outbreak of Seasonal Aseptic Meningitis, *J.A.M.A.* 162:1298, 1956.

Kilham, L., Mumps Meningoencephalitis with and without Parotitis, *Am. J. Dis. Child.* 78:324, 1949.

McLeod, D. L., A. J. Beale, G. A. McNaughton, and *A. J. Rhodes,* Clincal Features of Aseptic Meningitis Caused by Coxsackie-B Virus, *Lancet* 2:701, 1956.

Nicholls, E. E., The Incidence of a Normal Spinal Fluid in Acute Poliomyelitis, *J. Pediat.* 37:894, 1950.

Nilsby, I., Non-bacterial Meningo-encephalitides in Children with Special Reference to Spontaneous, Post-catarrhal and Varicella Meningo-encephalitis, *Acta paediat.* vol. 43, suppl. 95, 1954.

Soto, C. M., and *M. I. Rubin,* An Analysis of One Hundred Cases of Acute Poliomyelitis, *J. Pediat.* 6:343, 1935.

Vasquez, H. J., Encefalitis Postvacunal, *Pediatria de las Americas* 7:373, 1949.

Von Hagen, K. O., and *R. N. Baker,* Infectious Neuronitis: Present Concepts of Etiology and Treatment, *J.A.M.A.* 151:1465, 1953.

CHAPTER 40

Hemorrhages and Effusions

SUBARACHNOID BLEEDING

It is usually possible to make the distinction between blood in cerebro-spinal fluid which has its origin in an early intracranial or subarachnoid hemorrhage and blood due to the immediate trauma of the lumbar puncture (Table 40-1). The clearing of the fluid as it flows and the color of the supernatant after spinning down the red cells immediately after the puncture furnish the most helpful differentiation.

Table 40-1. Criteria for Distinguishing between the Two Main
Causes of Bloody Cerebrospinal Fluid

	Traumatic bleeding from lumbar puncture	Subarachnoid hemorrhage
Pressure	Normal	Often elevated
Color of successive drops	Grow less bloody	Remains uniform or becomes more bloody
Clotting in test tube	Yes, if blood is abundant	Yes, if blood is abundant
Supernatant after immediate centrifuging	Colorless	Xanthochromic if hemorrhage is over 4 hours old; after 1 or 2 days gives positive reaction for bilirubin
Benzidine test of supernatant	Negative	Positive
Microscopic examination	100% crenation of red cells; ° no increase in leukocytes	100% crenation ° or poikilocytosis or anisocytosis of red cells; increased proportion of leukocytes may be present

° Since normal cerebrospinal fluid is slightly more hypotonic than blood plasma with respect to electrolyte content, any red cells which extravasate become crenated within a very few minutes.

In cerebral hemorrhage and chronic subdural or extradural hematoma the cerebrospinal fluid findings vary according to the extent and location of the hemorrhage and its age. Irritation of the meninges may call forth a concomitant leukocytosis and elevation of the protein level. The com-

462

bination of free erythrocytes, xanthochromia, increased pressure, leukocytosis, increase in protein, and decrease in sugars is cogent evidence of an intracranial hemorrhage. With the passage of the days these diverse findings tend to recede at uneven rates, so that after a week or two only some of the changes are still demonstrable. When the bleeding is wholly intracerebral or wholly extradural the erythrocytes may not enter the cerebrospinal fiuid, but faint xanthochromia and a slight elevation of spinal fluid protein develop after a few days.

A number of investigators have reported blood-tinged lumbar puncture fluid in from 10 to 25 per cent of newborn infants. The frequency of this finding seems to have declined in recent years, presumably in consequence of the improved nutrition of mothers and the widespread administration of vitamin K. Conversely, a newborn infant may have cerebrospinal fluid free from demonstrable blood and yet have a massive cerebral hemorrhage as revealed by autopsy soon afterward.

With all intracranial hemorrhages it is of course essential to try to determine the exact cause and site of the bleeding, with a view toward possible surgical repair or correction of a bleeding dyscrasia.

SUBDURAL COLLECTIONS

Hematoma

Hemorrhage into the subdural space is sometimes referable to a head injury, blood vessel anomaly, or constitutional hemorrhagic diathesis. Many of the children who come to medical attention because of an enlarged head or convulsions or other neurologic signs caused by subdural hematoma have no positive history of any probable incitant condition. The diagnosis is best made by needle exploration of the subdural space.

A membrane soon forms about the periphery of the hematoma; this is at first fibrinous, and later fibrous. The contained blood remains liquid and later autolyzes. Further bleeding often occurs from the vessels of the capsule. The content of protein or blood and the degree of xanthochromia in the sac may become intensified in the weeks following the initial injury if the hematoma is not treated. The protein content may range from 100 to 3,000 mg per 100 ml in xanthochromic extravasations, and bloody collections may contain as much as 6,000 mg per 100 ml.

While xanthochromia of the cerebrospinal fluid is always suggestive of a subdural hematoma or effusion, the fluid is often clear and colorless and devoid of changes in composition.

Effusion

An accumulation of protein-rich fluid developing in the subdural space should be suspected whenever a child exhibits signs of increased intracranial pressure after head trauma or pneumoencephalography or during convalescence from acute bacterial meningitis. These accumulations are sometimes bilateral. The fluid obtained by subdural aspiration in these cases may be clear, xanthochromic, blood-tinged, or occasionally bloody. Infants seem most prone to develop this reaction, especially those whose brains are contracted or underdeveloped.

In volume these effusions vary from two to several hundred milliliters. Chemical studies of the contained fluid show an inconstant protein content; usually under 1,000 mg per 100 ml though occasionally 2,000 mg or more. The proportion of albumin to total protein is as a rule higher in the subdural fluid than in the plasma, suggesting that this fluid has leaked from damaged capillary walls. The glucose content is often higher than in the cerebrospinal fluid and may reach 200 mg per 100 ml. Leukocytes and erythrocytes are usually present, in small numbers. Cultures may be sterile, or the organism which caused an antecedent meningitis may grow out.

The lumbar fluid in these patients may be slightly xanthochromic and have a moderate increase in protein. There is usually no pleocytosis, but an elevated leukocyte count may be found exceptionally.

Since subdural collections of fluid will at times yield positive cultures in patients with meningitis when the cerebrospinal fluid seems bacteriologically sterile, it has been suggested that subdural taps be performed for diagnostic purposes when clinical signs and cerebrospinal fluid findings are suggestive of meningitis but organisms are not demonstrable. These fluid accumulations are being found more often since the advent of specific antibacterial chemotherapy; neither trauma, intrathecal injections, nor the degree of purulence of the cerebrospinal fluid has been implicated as an etiologic factor.

Therapeutic aspiration should be done at frequent intervals until fluid is no longer obtainable. If this does not bring about cure, surgical removal of the subdural membrane becomes necessary.

SUBDURAL PUNCTURE

Needling of the subdural space at the lateral angles of the anterior fontanel is a necessary step in detecting subdural hematoma or effusion in infancy. With very young infants the lambdoid suture may similarly be explored. In older children, in whom the fontanels are closed, identification of subdural hematomas requires exploration though bilateral burr holes. This procedure should be referred to a neurosurgeon.

The infant is kept on his back during the puncture, and the skin over the fontanel shaved and sterilized. A small-bored lumbar puncture needle containing a stylet is introduced at the lateral angle of the anterial fontanel. This is advanced cautiously through the scalp and fontanel membrane and dura, in a lateral direction along a line leading to the opposite eye. All sidewise movement of the needle must be avoided. As soon as the dura has been passed the stylet is withdrawn, a glass syringe attached, and negative pressure exerted. If disease is absent, only a few drops of clear fluid under no tension and perhaps containing some noncrenated red cells will be obtained.

Recovery of pink, blood-tinged, or xanthochromic fluid in amounts greater than a few cubic milliliters is abnormal. This fluid sometimes spurts out of the needle, especially when the fused cranial sutures have prevented compensatory expansion of the skull.

If fluid is not immediately obtainable, strong suction should not be exerted, since bits of cortex are easily aspirated. The syringe should be removed, the stylet reinserted, and the needle advanced a little further.

The demonstration in the subdural space of blood-containing or xanthochromic fluid with increased total protein content establishes the diagnosis, particularly when a lumbar tap done simultaneously reveals only minor changes if any. Hemorrhagic fluid obtained by this means will not coagulate unless it consists almost wholly of freshly extravasated blood. Blood-tinged fluid obtained by subdural puncture should always be centrifuged or allowed to stand, in order to inspect for supernatant xanthochromia and to rule out the possibility of any bleeding from the needle.

Samples of the fluid removed during serial aspirations may be placed in sterile corked tubes and kept near the patient. As the days progress the proportions of blood cells and pigment grow less. Cultures should be made of every second or third specimen to make sure that the hematoma sac has not become infected.

THROMBOSIS OF THE DURAL SINUSES

Nonseptic or marantic dural vein thromboses may occur in long-standing debilitating conditions. Their development is related as a rule to sluggish circulation of the blood or to increased viscosity from dehydration or erythrocytosis. Small thrombi usually produce no symptoms or cerebrospinal fluid changes. Larger thrombi lead to congestion, edema, or hemorrhage within the brain, or even massive infarction of some areas. The cerebrospinal fluid may then become xanthochromic or bloody; the protein content and the number of mononuclear cells usually rise.

Septic or suppurative thromboses are nearly always secondary to infections elsewhere in the body. Septic thromboses can originate as marantic thromboses which become infected or as direct extension from a contiguous otitis media or nasal sinusitis. Once established they may give rise to bacteremia, meningitis, brain abscess, or embolic abscesses and infarcts. The most common causative organisms are staphylococci, streptococci, pneumococci, and the influenza bacillus.

BIBLIOGRAPHY

HEMORRHAGES AND EFFUSIONS

Campbell, K., Intracranial Disorders of the New-born Associated with Birth, *M. J. Australia* 2:57, 1948.

Elvidge, A. R., and *I. J. Jackson,* Subdural Hematoma and Effusion in Infants, *Am. J. Dis. Child.* 78:635, 1949.

Gitlin, D., Pathogenesis of Subdural Collections of Fluid, *Pediatrics* 16:345, 1955.

Grant, F. C., and *G. M. Austin,* The Surgical Treatment of Spontaneous and Traumatic Intracerebral Hemorrhage, *Am. J. M. Sc.* 219:237, 1950.

Ingraham, F. D., and *D. D. Matson,* Subdural Hematoma in Infancy, *Advances Pediat.* 4:231, 1949.

Kinley, G., H. D. Riley, Jr., and *C. S. Beck,* Subdural Hematoma, Hygroma and Hydroma in Infants, *J. Pediat.* 38:667, 1951.

Matthews, W. F., and *W. B. Frommeyer, Jr.,* The In Vitro Behavior of Erythrocytes in Human Cerebrospinal Fluid, *J. Lab. & Clin. Med.* 45:508, 1955.

McKay, R. J., F. D. Ingraham, and *D. D. Matson,* Subdural Fluid Complicating Bacterial Meningitis, *J.A.M.A.* 152:387, 1953.

————, *R. A. Morissette, F. D. Ingraham,* and *D. D. Matson,* Collections of Subdural Fluid Complicating Meningitis Due to *Haemophilus influenzae* (Type B), *New England J. Med.* 242:20, 1950.

Smith, H. V., and *B. Crothers,* Subdural Fluid after Pneumoencephalography, *Pediatrics* 5:375, 1950.

Smith, M. H. D., Subdural Lesions in Childhood, with Special Reference to Infectious Processes, *Advances Pediat.* 8:165, 1956.

Toomey, J. A., and H. B. Hutt, Thrombosis of the Dural Sinuses, *Am. J. Dis. Child.* 77:285, 1949.

Williams, J. M., Multiple Subdural Hematomas in an Infant, *Am. J. Dis. Child.* 80:970, 1950.

CHAPTER 41

Miscellaneous Diseases

CRYPTOCOCCOSIS (TORULOSIS)

A severe and chronic form of pyogenic meningitis can be caused by the yeastlike fungus *Cryptococcus neoformans* (known also as *Torula histolytica, C. hominis,* or *Blastomycoides histolytica*). Most patients give a history of respiratory tract infection as an early symptom, and many have subacute roentgen changes in the lungs. The fungus appears to enter the body through the respiratory tract. The liver and spleen also enlarge. In the central nervous system, a chronic meningitis develops with monocytic granulomas about the intracerebral blood vessels. Most affected children are thought to have tuberculous meningitis when first seen, because of the similarity in clinical symptoms and cerebrospinal fluid findings. Affected infants may develop widespread cerebral degeneration, hydrocephalus, and diffuse calcifications which are punctate or confluent and roentgenologically resemble those seen in toxoplasmic encephalitis. It has been possible at times to recover morphologically identical strains from the patient's sputum or urine or from the endocervix of the mother of an infected newborn infant.

The cerebrospinal fluid in cryptococcus meningoencephalitis is under increased pressure and may be clear, turbid, or xanthochromic. The total protein is increased, up to 1,500 mg per 100 ml or even higher. The sugar content tends to be diminished. The cell counts range from 30 to 800, with mononuclear cells predominating. The cryptococci can be identified in the unstained sediment from centrifuged lumbar or ventricular fluid as yeastlike Gram-positive cells, often budding, surrounded by thick capsules. These grow on Sabouraud's and other fungus media, giving colonies of inconstant morphology. Cultures in suspected cases should be kept for a month before being read as negative. Injection of colonies into mice induces a fatal septicemia, with the organisms recoverable from the organs.

GUILLAIN-BARRÉ SYNDROME

The Guillain-Barré syndrome is a term applied to patients who gradually develop polyneuritis with symmetrical flaccid paralysis, loss of tendon reflexes, and preponderance of motor weakness over sensory signs. Complete neurologic recovery is the rule, though orthopedic complications are not uncommon. The spinal fluid protein is elevated, rising to a peak of 50 to 1,000 mg per 100 ml between the first and second month and then subsiding to normal in 1 to 2 months thereafter. The cell count is not elevated, and the glucose, pressure, and chlorides are normal. Xanthochromia is present in a small percentage of cases. The colloidal gold curve is not characteristic.

The diagnosis of Guillain-Barré syndrome is often applied to any disturbance which calls forth most if not all of the above symptoms, and especially the *albumino-cytologic dissociation*. In the opinion of many authorities, however, the term should not be applied when the identity of the disease process which produces this combination of symptoms is known—as, for example, diphtheria, poliomyelitis, diabetes, serum sickness, polyarteritis nodosa, syphilis, lead poisoning, or mustard gas poisoning.

INFANTILE DIARRHEA

A fair proportion of infants ill with diarrhea will be found to have cerebrospinal fluid changes of mild degree if subjected to lumbar puncture. These may be a slight lymphocytic pleocytosis (rarely exceeding 100 cells per cu mm), a mild increase in protein, or both (when the cell count is over 20). The pressure tends to be normal. The sugar level may be elevated or depressed moderately. Bacteriologic cultures are sterile. The changes are most likely to be present when drowsiness, rigidity, or twitching indicate the existence of cerebral irritation.

INFECTIOUS MONONUCLEOSIS

This occasionally involves the nervous system with clinical meningoencephalitis. The cerebrospinal fluid then shows an increased total protein and pleocytosis of lymphocytic nature. In patients with severe infectious mononucleosis but no obvious central nervous system changes, the fluid often reveals a cell count of 15 to 20 lymphocytes and perhaps a minimal increase in protein. Heterophil agglutinins are nearly always in the cerebrospinal fluid when present in the blood.

LEAD ENCEPHALOPATHY

Injury to the nervous system in lead poisoning is more common in childhood than in adult life. Convulsions, vomiting, personality changes, ataxia, nerve palsies, drowsiness, and signs of increased intracranial pressure are common findings. The cerebrospinal fluid typically shows an increase in pressure, a high protein (100 to 1,000 mg per 100 ml), and perhaps a moderate lymphocytosis (10 to 50 cells per cu mm). A pellicle may form when the protein content is high. The sugar and chloride concentrations are not altered except in starvation states. As improvement occurs the increase in the number of cells subsides earlier than the increase of protein.

LEPTOSPIROSIS

Severe acute meningitis can follow leptospiral invasion of the central nervous system after exposure of the mucous membranes or skin to contaminated water, as during swimming. Fever, headache, conjunctival congestion, meningeal irritation, muscular weakness, and transient paralyses are common signs. There is usually no leukocytosis. The cerebrospinal fluid at first may be normal but soon exhibits a pleocytic rise to a count of 50 to 300 cells, mostly lymphocytes. The sugar content usually remains unaffected, but the protein content may increase slightly.

Specific laboratory search for leptospirosis is called for with all cases of "aseptic" or viral meningitis when no other cause can be implicated and a history of contact with potentially infected water or animals can be elicited. Darkfield microscopy of freshly sedimented cerebrospinal fluid during the period of active symptoms usually reveals the parasites. Agglutination tests of the patient's blood during convalescence will show an unusually high titer or a rise in titer with one or more of the leptospiral antigens (p. 861).

SEROUS MENINGITIS FOLLOWING SCARLET FEVER

In children ill with scarlet fever one sometimes encounters transient fever and signs of meningeal irritation 5 to 8 days after the onset of the infection. The cerebrospinal fluid cell count ranges from 30 to 1,000 with 75 to 100 per cent lymphocytes, and the total protein may or may not rise a little, though rarely above 100 mg per 100 ml. The chlorides and dextrose are not affected. The symptoms and spinal fluid changes last about a week.

SYPHILIS

In central nervous system syphilis the severity of the spinal fluid abnormalities depends upon the extent of the meningitis present. The usual findings are an increased pressure, a moderately elevated cell count with a variable percentage of neutrophils, a normal or moderately reduced content of sugar and chlorides, an abnormal colloidal gold reaction, and a positive serologic test for syphilis. Central nervous system syphilis in the childhood age period is almost always on a congenital basis.

The cerebrospinal fluid from a child with congenital syphilis may or may not show a positive reaction with the serologic tests for syphilis when the blood tests are positive. Conversely, instances are sometimes encountered with negative blood reactions despite positive cerebrospinal fluid reactions associated with central nervous system infection.

Rarely, the spinal fluid from a nonsyphilitic patient ill with tuberculous or pyogenic meningitis will give a transiently positive reaction with the test for syphilis. Should this be suspected the quantitative titer of the serologic antibody in the cerebrospinal fluid should be determined quantitatively every 2 weeks. A titer which recedes spontaneously and substantially within a 1- to 2-month period of observation in a child with no clinical indications of syphilis must be adjudged as nonsyphilitic in character. The nonsyphilitic or "false positive" reactions evoked in the blood by some acute infections do not ordinarily induce a similar change in the cerebrospinal fluid.

When true syphilitic involvement of the central nervous system has been established, quantitative estimation of the complement-fixing titer should always be secured. This will serve as a base line for the later evaluation of response to treatment. When the neurosyphilitic infection is treated with penicillin or similar therapy, the cell count subsides to normal in 3 to 6 months, along with a decline or complete disappearance of the complement-fixing antibodies. The colloidal gold reaction takes a year or more to revert to normal and may persist for as long as 4 years or more after all other abnormalities have receded.

TOXOPLASMOSIS

In active infection of the nervous system caused by *Toxoplasma hominis* the protein of the cerebrospinal fluid is increased, there is a pleocytosis of lymphocytes and monocytes, and xanthochromia is frequent. During the beginning phases of the infection these protozoa may be found in the blood, bone marrow, splenic puncture material, cerebrospinal fluid, and possibly sputum.

In subacute toxoplasmosis the foramina of Monro and the aqueduct often becomes blocked by inflammatory exudate. The ventricular spaces then contain fluid of high protein content (1,000 to 2,600 mg per 100 ml), which cannot escape. This high protein content is derived in part from the plasma coming from damaged vascular walls and in part from necrotic brain tissue that has desquamated into the ventricles. The protein level of the subarachnoid fluid is lower, usually between 100 and 600 mg per 100 ml. The organisms may be demonstrable in the sediment of ventricular fluid obtained by aspiration, especially after animal inoculation.

Some of the infants with the congenital form of the disease have had normal-appearing cerebrospinal fluid despite hydrocephalus, chorioretinitis, cerebral calcification, and convulsions.

Another manifestation of toxoplasmosis is the acquired form which usually produces an acute encephalitis along with other visceral manifestations. In this illness, which can occur at any age, the cerebrospinal fluid may undergo a pleocytosis of several hundred cells and an increase in protein. The changes are transient and disappear gradually.

BIBLIOGRAPHY

MISCELLANEOUS DISEASES

Adams, F. H., J. M. Adams, P. Kabler, and M. Cooney, Toxoplasmosis in Children, Pediatrics 2:511, 1948.

DiSpirito, A., Spinal Fluid Findings in Diarrhea: A Clincal Study, Clin. Proc. Children's Hosp. Washington, D. C. 10:220, 1954.

Frenkel, J. K., Pathogenesis, Diagnosis and Treatment of Human Toxoplasmosis, J.A.M.A. 140:369, 1949.

Hallman, N., and H. Tahka, Observations on the Cerebrospinal Fluid in Infantile Diarrhea, Acta paediat. 41:437, 1952.

Mosberg, W. H., Jr., and J. G. Arnold, Jr., Torulosis of the Central Nervous System: Review of Literature and Report of Five Cases, Ann. Int. Med. 32:1153, 1950.

Neuhauser, E. B. D., and A. Tucker, Roentgen Changes Produced by Diffuse Torulosis in Newborn, Am. J. Roentgenol. 59:805, 1948.

Silberstein, J. K., T. C. Bernstein, and T. Stern, Demonstration of Heterophile Antibodies in the Cerebrospinal Fluid from Patients with Infectious Mononucleosis, J. Lab. & Clin. Med. 33:1204, 1948.

Voyles, G. Q., and E. M. Beck, Systemic Infection Due to Torula histolytica (Cryptococcus hominis). I. Report of Four Cases and Review of the Literature, Arch. Int. Med. 77:504, 1946.

CHAPTER 42

Liver Tests

The chief applications of the tests for *liver function* lie in (1) recognition of disease of the liver cells and (2) providing information by serial determinations as to the progress of a patient with liver disease. The correlations between the severity of the liver disorder and the responses to the various tests are not as consistent in children, and especially in infants, as in older patients. Clinical history, physical findings, and experienced judgment are more significant than are the results of liver tests for the making of a diagnosis.

Liver tests are widely used in internal medicine to aid in differentiating so-called extrahepatic obstructive jaundice from hemolytic or hepatocellular jaundice. Most adults with extrahepatic bile duct obstruction give normal responses to the flocculation tests but have elevations in serum alkaline phosphatase and serum total cholesterol and often show depression of the cholesterol ester fraction below 50 per cent. With parenchymal liver disease most adults exhibit abnormal responses in the flocculation tests and are less likely to have disturbances in alkaline phosphatase and cholesterol. This differential diagnostic problem is not common in the childhood years other than in the newborn period when congenital atresia of the bile ducts may be considered; and here the results of these tests are less consistent (Chap. 45).

Because of the multiplicity and diversity of the biochemical activities of the liver, the laboratory appraisal of the efficiency of this organ is peculiarly difficult. The approaches most readily performed with infants and children are the following:

I. Bilirubin metabolism
   A. Urine: bilirubin; urobilinogen (pp. 348–352)
   B. Serum pigments: 1-minute and total serum bilirubin levels; icterus index (pp. 477–478)
   C. Stool: bilirubin; urobilinogen (pp. 702–704)
II. Serum proteins
   A. Fluctuations in total level and fractional composition (pp. 535–541)
   B. Indirect tests for serum protein alterations: cephalin cholesterol flocculation; thymol turbidity and flocculation; zinc turbidity; other flocculation tests (pp. 473–475)

III. Blood enzymes
  A. Alkaline phosphatase (pp. 549–552)
  B. Cholinesterase (pp. 478–479)
  C. Prothrombin (pp. 241–246)
  D. Transaminase (p. 479)
IV. Serum lipids
  A. Total lipids (pp. 517–519)
  B. Total cholesterol (pp. 519–523)
  C. Ratio between free and esterified cholesterol (pp. 523–524)
V. Carbohydrate metabolism
  A. Glucose tolerance tests (pp. 502–507)
  B. Galactose tolerance tests (p. 513)
VI. Excretory and detoxication tests
  A. Bromsulphalein excretion (pp. 475–476)
  B. Hippuric acid synthesis (p. 477)
VII. Needle biopsy of the liver (p. 479)

When interpreting the results given by any of these tests one must bear in mind that other organ systems participate with the liver in practically all the activities listed. Hence abnormal results must be viewed as presumptive rather than as specific for liver damage, to be interpreted in the light of all other findings. As a rule, the more severe the liver damage the greater the percentage of tests that give abnormal results and the higher the abnormalities of the readings. Intercurrent infections or acute metabolic disorders may lead to temporarily abnormal readings in otherwise well children.

SERUM PROTEIN ALTERATIONS

Fractional Analysis

Alterations in the various fractions of the serum proteins are frequent. The albumin or the globulin fraction may rise or fall. The total serum protein level often remains in the normal zone despite disturbances in the individual components. The total tends to be diminished appreciably, and especially the albumin fraction, when parenchymatous destruction is advanced as occurs in advanced cirrhosis or severe viral or toxic hepatitis.

Flocculation Tests

Quantitative or qualitative disturbances in serum protein composition are often demonstrable by diminished stability of standardized colloidal suspensions after addition of a patient's serum. Among such procedures are the cephalin-cholesterol flocculation test, the thymol turbidity and flocculation tests, the colloidal red test, the colloidal gold test, the zinc turbidity test, the Hayem test, the Weltmann test, and the Takata-Ara reaction.

CEPHALIN-CHOLESTEROL FLOCCULATION (CCF) TEST (HANGER'S TEST). The reagent in this test is an emulsion of cephalin from sheep brain combined with cholesterol, usually purchased commercially. In performing the test a sample (0.2 ml) of fasting serum is mixed with the saline-diluted reagent and stored in a dark place at room temperature for 24 hours before being read. Control determinations are run simultaneously on the individual reagents to establish their reliability. The degrees of flocculation are recorded as follows:

Flocculation	Reading	Interpretation
No alteration in opalescence	0	Normal
Slight precipitation, slight clearing of supernatant	+	Normal
Moderate precipitation, moderately clear supernatant	++	Borderline abnormal
Heavy precipitation, almost completely clear supernatant	+++	Abnormal
Heavy precipitation, clear supernatant	++++	Abnormal

Well-defined flocculation (3 or 4 plus) is interpreted as meaning that the plasma protein components are abnormal. Readings of 0 to 2 plus are in the normal range for all infants and children. Abnormal readings are not unusual during the first few days of life, nor in nephrosis and other conditions attended by a low serum albumin level.

THYMOL TURBIDITY (TT) AND THYMOL FLOCCULATION (TF) TESTS. Positive thymol reactions appear to be due to abnormalities in the globulins being released to the blood stream by a damaged liver. The reagent is a barbital buffer solution saturated with thymol.

In performing the tests, 0.1 ml of the patient's serum is mixed with 6 ml of the reagent and a reading taken in 30 minutes. Any turbidity which appears is read photoelectrically or matched in a comparator block against the turbidity of standards similar to those used for estimation of quantitative protein content of urine. Results are expressed in Maclagen turbidity *units*, arbitrarily derived from known concentrations of barium sulfate suspensions. The range for normal subjects, including newborn and premature infants, is 0 to 3 units; 4 units is considered borderline, and 5 units clearly elevated. Rises in liver diseases of childhood rarely exceed 15 units.

The TF test is an addendum to the TT test. After the latter has been read the tube with contained reagents is left for 18 to 24 hours at room temperature, and then observed for flocculation of the particles. Readings are graded from 0 to 4 in the same fashion as for the CCF test. The normal range is 0 to 1 plus. Abnormalities usually run parallel to the TT readings. Lipemic serum in the absence of liver disease may give rise to a positive TT test, but the TF will ordinarily remain negative.

ZINC SULFATE TURBIDITY TEST (KUNKEL). In 1947, Kunkel reported that adding a weak solution of zinc sulfate to serum having an abnormally high content of gamma globulin would produce a turbid precipitate whose optical density would be roughly proportional to the concentration of gamma globulin. The flocculation in such circumstances becomes evident within 4 hours, whereas serum of normal persons does not flocculate for at least 12 hours. This reaction, though positive in all forms of hypergammaglobulinemia, can be useful in following the alterations during the course of infectious hepatitis and in detecting persistence of liver injury after an attack. According to the findings of Harris, the mean reading for newborn infants as the test is customarily performed is approximately 8 units, and lower in premature infants. The readings subside steadily to approximately 4 units at 2 weeks and remain at 1 unit from 3 to 8 months. At 1 year the level rises to 4 units; at 5 years, 6 units; and in adolescence and adult life, 8 to 12 units.

Readings in Disease States

The flocculation tests have their greatest sphere of usefulness in diagnosing and following the course of viral hepatitis and other parenchymal cell disturbances. One or more of the tests will give positive readings in about 80 per cent of patients after the initial stages, independently of the presence of jaundice. Positive readings are not infrequent in acute and chronic infections such as malaria, congenital syphilis, primary atypical pneumonia, infectious mononucleosis, tuberculosis, diphtheria, measles, typhoid fever, streptococcic sore throat, active rheumatic heart disease especially with heart failure or severe dysrhythmia, and also in severe malnutrition with hypoproteinemia.

In viral hepatitis the cephalin cholesterol flocculation tends to become positive earlier than do the thymol tests, whereas during convalescence the latter remain positive longer. When all positive reactivity fades away within a few weeks the prognosis for prompt and full recovery is much more favorable than when any of the reactions remains positive for months.

With infants under 6 months of age, however, the tests may remain negative or borderline despite unequivocal signs of liver involvement. This inconsistency hampers the utilization of these tests in assisting in the differentiation between obstructive and parenchymal liver disease in the severe jaundice of early infancy. The flocculation tests are typically negative in obstructive jaundice unless the liver is involved by complicating cholangitis or related change.

BROMSULPHALEIN (BSP) RETENTION TEST

When Bromsulphalein (phenoltetrabromphthalein sodium sulfate) is injected it is removed rapidly from the blood stream, almost entirely by the action of the liver cells. The rate of excretion of this dye from the blood can be applied to the evaluating of liver function.

Standard Test

The customary dosage is 5 mg per kg body weight in a 0.5 per cent solution, with at least 1 minute being taken for the intravenous injection. At exactly

45 minutes a single blood specimen is drawn from the patient and the concentration of contained dye ascertained. The result is expressed as a percentage, with 10 mg of dye per 100 ml of serum taken arbitrarily as 100 per cent. A child with a normally functioning liver should have less than 5 per cent retention in the blood stream 45 minutes after injection of the test dose. A retention of over 8 to 10 per cent is regarded as abnormal, except in young infants (see below).

Patients with severe parenchymal liver disease productive of jaundice, such as viral hepatitis, liver cirrhosis, and extrahepatic obstructive jaundice, almost always exhibit BSP retention of over 20 per cent at the end of 45 minutes. In most such patients the dye may be detectable in the circulation for 24 hours or more after being injected. Abnormal BSP retention may be encountered also in febrile illnesses, cardiac failure, anemia, and other remote disorders which may induce secondary liver changes.

The BSP retention test is extremely sensitive. It need not be employed when clinical signs or other function tests make it clear that the patient has some liver dysfunction. The particular sphere of application of the BSP test lies in the study of patients with possible liver disease who are free from jaundice. In viral hepatitis the results are usually positive early, before jaundice appears, and during convalescence after the jaundice has gone.

Mollison and Cutbush injected BSP into newborn infants a few hours after birth in a dose of 5 mg per kg body weight, as a 0.5 per cent solution. The content in the circulation was about 20 per cent of the standard in 30 to 40 minutes and disappeared more slowly thereafter. Essentially identical findings, interpreted as immaturity of the excretory function of the liver in the newborn, have been recorded by Yudkin and Gellis. Even at 4 days of age the retention was somewhat greater than adult values.

Percentage Disappearance Rate (PDR)

The liver polygonal cells remove injected BSP at a rate which in normal subjects is more or less constant. When blood samples are tested at regular intervals during the first 30 minutes after injection the findings yield a straight-line curve when plotted against time on semilogarithmic paper. From the slope of the curve is calculated the percentage disappearance rate per minute. In hepatobiliary disturbances abnormal removal patterns (curved lines) are given. Curves obtained by Obrinsky, Danley, and Brauer with premature infants have shown absence of the uniform rate characteristic of normal older children and adults and retention of a larger amount of dye over longer periods than is normal for older children and adults. These changes seem to give evidence of functional hepatic insufficiency.

HIPPURIC ACID SYNTHESIS

Hippuric acid is synthesized in the liver from benzoic acid and glycine. To test this synthesizing function a subject is given sufficient benzoic acid (or sodium benzoate) orally or by vein to elicit the maximum synthesizing capacity of the liver, and the hippuric acid which appears in the urine measured. The excretion of hippuric acid is reported in terms of benzoic acid. If the kidneys are not working well, excretion of synthesized hippuric acid is retarded.

Londe and Probstein recommend an oral test dose of 3 gm of sodium benzoate with children whose ideal weights for height and age are between 20 and 40 kg and of 4 gm when the ideal weights are 40 kg or over. A breakfast of tea and a piece of dry toast is given 1 hour before the sodium benzoate is administered. A small quantity of chocolate syrup sweetened with saccharine may be added to a peppermint-flavored solution of sodium benzoate; this mixture is given cold. Urine specimens are then collected at 1- or 2-hour intervals. In their study, 25 normal children weighing 20 to 40 kg given 3 gm of sodium benzoate excreted 32 to 58 per cent at 2 hours (mean, 46 per cent) and 67 to 88 per cent at 4 hours (mean, 79 per cent). Ten children weighing over 40 kg and given 4 gm of sodium benzoate excreted 41 to 74 per cent in 2 hours (mean, 52 per cent) and 69 to 92 per cent in 4 hours (mean, 82 per cent).

Meneghello and Drinberg deem intravenous injection a more accurate approach for studies with children. The test is made in the morning, breakfast being omitted. A solution of 2 gm of sodium benzoate in 20 ml of distilled water is given intravenously at a very slow rate, so that the entire injection takes approximately 10 minutes. The patient voids just before the test, and a single specimen of urine is collected exactly 1 hour after completion of the injection. Catheterization may occasionally be necessary. Sixteen normal children aged 5 to 11 years excreted 0.93 to 1.65 gm of hippuric acid 1 hour after receiving 2 gm intravenously.

Hippuric acid synthesis is found reduced in most diseases in which parenchymal liver damage is severe, such as viral hepatitis, hepatic cirrhosis, and metastatic malignancy. It is usually normal in obstructive jaundice. Meneghello and Drinberg noted impairment in most or all cases tested of scarlet fever, diphtheria, typhoid fever, lobar pneumonia, and tuberculous meningitis. It has also been found impaired in nephritis, anemia, and after acute infections.

ONE-MINUTE AND TOTAL SERUM BILIRUBIN READINGS

In the performance of the van den Bergh test, when Ehrlich's diazo reagent is added to the serum in the absence of alcohol or other added catalyst, a certain proportion of the contained bilirubin will react with the reagent within the first minute. This is known as the *1-minute* or *direct-reading* fraction. The remaining bilirubin reacts more slowly and may take several hours to show itself fully. This latter fraction, termed the *indirect-reading,* becomes converted much more rapidly when methyl alcohol is added. It was once thought that the 1-minute fraction represents a chemically distinct form of bilirubin which had passed through the liver cells and been regurgitated from the biliary system into the lymphatic and thence into the blood stream. More recent studies, however, indicate that there may not be two types of bilirubin but that the rate of diazotization is conditioned by factors in the serum. The 1-minute level would thus be a selected point on the total conversion curve of bilirubin to azobilirubin.

The range in normal children and postneonatal infants for the 1-minute reading is approximately 0.5 to 0.25 mg per 100 ml; for the total, 0.4 to 1.5 mg per 100 ml. These variations are due as much to technical conditions in the test as to physiologic factors. Values for the neonatal period are discussed in Chap. 44.

The serum bilirubin readings are always elevated, obviously, with any liver lesion sufficient to produce icterus. Less severe hepatic disturbances often produce minor increases in serum level in the absence of visible jaundice.

The differentiation of serum bilirubin into 1-minute and total has been found to be of some clinical value in recognizing icterus of hemolytic origin. The proportion of the 1-minute to the total reading tends to be below 20 per cent in primarily hemolytic jaundice, above 40 per cent in primarily obstructive jaundice, and erratic in hepatocellular diseases.

Bilirubin does not appear in the urine in jaundice of hemolytic origin until the total serum bilirubin level approximates 5 mg per 100 ml. In jaundice of obstructive or hepatocellular origin the pigment is excreted with much lower serum concentrations.

ICTERUS INDEX

The icterus index, or degree of yellowness of the serum when compared with a standard potassium dichromate solution, is nonselective and unreliable as an indicator of jaundice. A yellow color may be given not only by bilirubin itself but by other hemoglobin derivatives, carotene, and various other pigments which may be present. Traces of hemoglobin sufficient to give "abnormal" readings may come from hemolysis during collection or preparation of the specimen.

SERUM CHOLINESTERASE ACTIVITY

The liver appears to be the main site of synthesis of a nonspecific serum enzyme capable of hydrolyzing acetylcholine. The determinations are made by noting the change in pH caused by liberation of acetic acid as acetylcholine is hydrolyzed by cholinesterase.

The serum cholinesterase activity is usually decreased early in liver cell disease such as acute hepatitis and parathion poisoning and returns to normal as the patient convalesces. The activity is usually not distorted in obstructive disorders unless malignancy or malnutrition is present. In hepatic cirrhosis the values tend to parallel the severity of the disease. With most liver diseases, however, this test fails to furnish information beyond that yielded by the other function tests.

TRANSAMINASE (GLUTAMIC OXALACETIC AMINOPHERASE)

This newly described enzyme occurs in appreciable amounts in heart muscle, skeletal muscle, brain, liver, kidney and other tissues, and in the blood serum. Increases in the serum content amounting to two to twenty times normal follow acute myocardial infarctions. Increases of two to twenty times normal have been noted in liver damage caused by toxic or infectious agents. In infectious hepatitis the serum level is said to undergo a rise 1 to 4 weeks before other manifestations of liver injury become detectable by laboratory or clinical approaches.

The serum levels in healthy adults range from 5 to 40 units when measured by standard procedures at 20°C. Values for infants and children in health and disease are currently being explored.

NEEDLE BIOPSY

Needle biopsy can be a most useful adjunct in the diagnostic study of cases of obscure liver disease. Its chief value lies in aiding in the diagnosis of chronic situations in which the organ itself is not shrunken or misplaced. It has proved helpful in making positive (or negative) diagnosis of hepatitis, cirrhosis, glycogen storage disease, xanthomatosis, hemochromatosis, Gaucher's disease, and miscellaneous other conditions. To avoid accidents it is advisable to limit biopsy study to patients whose livers are enlarged and whose prothrombin level and other coagulation studies are within normal limits. The information gained in proper cases is sufficiently valuable to warrant the slight risk taken.

Since most diseases of the liver affect all parts, the small specimens collected by biopsy can be taken as representative of the organ as a whole. With abscesses, cysts, or metastatic tumors, however, positive findings will be secured only if the needle happens to strike a focal lesion.

BIBLIOGRAPHY

LIVER FUNCTION TESTS

Alcalde, J. M. O., Serum Cholinesterase Determination in the Differential Diagnosis of Jaundice, *J. Lab. & Clin. Med.* 36:391, 1950.

Desmond, M. M., H. J. Zimmerman, L. K. Sweet, and *L. J. Thomas,* Thymol Turbidity Values in the Sera of Newborn and Premature Infants and of Mothers at Term, *Pediatrics* 3:49, 1949.

Gellis, S. S., and *D. Y. Hsia*, Liver Function Tests in Infants and Children, *Pediat. Clin. North Amer.* February, 1955, p. 177.

Harris, R. C., Liver Function Tests in Infancy, *Bull. New York Acad. Med.* 28:721, 1952.

Hsia, D. Y., F. H. Allen, Jr., L. K. Diamond, and *S. S. Gellis,* Serum Bilirubin Levels in the Newborn Infant, *J. Pediat.* 42:277, 1953.

———, ———, *S. S. Gellis,* and *L. K. Diamond,* Erythroblastosis Fetalis. VIII. Studies of Serum Bilirubin in Relation to Kernicterus, *New England J. Med.* 247:668, 1952.

Iverson, K., and *F. Raaschou,* Thymol Turbidity Test in Acute Infectious Diseases, *Arch. Int. Med.* 82:251, 1949.

Johnstone, J. M., Bilirubin Values of Cord Blood in Heterospecific Pregnancy, *J. Clin. Path.* 6:215, 1953.

Karmen, A., F. Wróblewski, and *J. S. LaDue,* Transaminase Activity in Human Blood, *J. Clin. Invest.* 34:126, 1955.

Klatskin, G., and *V. A. Drill,* The Significance of the "One-minute" (Prompt Direct Reacting) Bilirubin in Serum, *J. Clin. Invest.* 29:660, 1950.

Kunkel, H. G., Estimation of Alterations of Serum Gamma Globulin by Turbidimetric Technique, *Proc. Soc. Exper. Biol. & Med.* 66:217, 1947.

Londe, S., and *J. G. Probstein,* The Hippuric Acid Liver Function Test in Children, *J. Pediat.* 18:371, 1941.

Maclagan, N. F., N. H. Martin, and *J. B. Lunnon,* The Mechanism and Interrelationships of the Flocculation Tests, *J. Clin. Path.* 5:1, 1952.

Mann, J. D., W. I. Mandel, P. L. Eichman, M. A. Knowlton, and *V. M. Sborov,* Serum Cholinesterase Activity in Liver Disease, *J. Lab. & Clin. Med.* 39:543, 1952.

Meneghello, J., and *M. Drinberg,* Intravenous Hippuric Acid Test of Hepatic Function in Infectious Diseases of Children, *Am. J. Dis. Child.* 66:103, 1943.

Mollison, P. L., and *M. Cutbush,* Bromsulphalein Excretion in the Newborn, *Arch. Dis. Childhood* 24:7, 1949.

Najjar, V. A., The Metabolism of Carbohydrates, Fats and Bile Pigments by the Liver and the Alterations in Hepatic Disease: A Review of Recent Advances, *Pediatrics* 15:444, 1955.

Obrinsky, W., M. L. Denley, and *R. W. Brauer,* Sulfobromophthalein (Bromsulphalein) Sodium Dye Excretion Test, *A.M.A. Am. J. Dis. Child.* 83:401, 1952.

Rapoport, S., Increased Serum Phosphatase and Hyperprothrombinemia in Infectious Hepatitis of Children, *Proc. Soc. Exper. Biol. & Med.* 62:203, 1946.

Sherlock, S., Aspiration Liver Biopsy: Technique and Diagnostic Application, *Lancet* 2:397, 1945.

Vickers, H. E., The Renal Threshold for Bilirubin, *J. Clin. Path.* 3:271, 1950.

Watson, C. J., The Importance of the Fractional Serum Bilirubin Determination in Clinical Medicine, *Ann. Int. Med.* 45:351, 1956.

Wolman, I. J., and *J. D. Farquhar,* The Liver Diseases of Infancy and Childhood: A Brief Summary of Reports and Papers, 1934–1948, *Am. J. M. Sc.* 216:704, 1948.

Yudkin, S., S. S. Gellis, and *F. Lappen,* Liver Function in Newborn Infants with Special Reference to Excretion of Bromsulphalein, *Arch. Dis. Childhood* 24:12, 1949.

Zieve, L., E. Hill, M. Hanson, A. E. Falcone, and *C. J. Watson,* Normal and Abnormal Variations and Clinical Significance of the One-minute and Total Serum Bilirubin Determination, *J. Lab. & Clin. Med.* 38:446, 1951.

CHAPTER 43

Viral Hepatitis

Viral hepatitis has become more prevalent in the civilian population since World War II. What was once known as "catarrhal jaundice" is now viewed as a sproadic form of infectious hepatitis, though occasional instances of such jaundice may be due to bacterial infection traveling up the duodenum and along the biliary ducts into the liver. Leptospirosis (Weil's disease) has a different etiology and epidemiology, runs a more severe course, and displays as a distinctive feature the presence of the spirochete *Leptospira icterohemorrhagica*.

Viral hepatitis without jaundice may be mistaken for almost any other acute infection. Patients without jaundice exhibit the same laboratory signs of liver dysfunction though to a less degree than those with jaundice, but the constitutional disturbances are usually less marked and the serum bilirubin levels less elevated.

Infectious or epidemic hepatitis is caused by a strain of hepatitis virus termed *virus A or IH*. This agent is excreted in the stools of patients and convalescents and is usually spread by direct contact or through contaminated food or water. Just how long the blood and feces of patients in the acute phases of an attack of hepatitis due to virus A remain infective has not been determined. The urine and the nasopharyngeal washings of patients do not seem to contain these agents.

Viral hepatitis A is a common cause of jaundice in infants and children. The ages between 9 months and 25 years appear to be those of maximal susceptibility. The disease is uncommon in individuals over 30, and gamma globulin from pooled plasma of adults has some prophylactic value, suggesting that most older persons acquire immunity.

Serum hepatitis is caused by a different strain, termed *virus B or SH*. This agent is transmitted through injections of infective blood or blood products or the repeated use of syringes or needles which have been inadequately sterilized. It does not appear in the stools in significant amounts but may be carried in the blood of asymptomatic or mildly symptomatic individuals for many years. A number of instances of hepatitis in newborn infants have been recorded, in which the infection seemed to have been acquired transplacentally and was probably due to this B or SH virus.

The incubation period of serum hepatitis ranges from 2 to 6 months, the onset is usually insidious, and the temperature may remain normal during the course of the disease. Infectious hepatitis A tends to be more severe, and its incubation period is 2 to 6 weeks. Otherwise, after the first few days of illness, the two diseases run essentially identical courses.

The viruses which cause hepatitis are too small to be visible under the electron microscope. They are hardy, able to withstand freezing, thawing, and heating up to 56°C for 60 minutes, and will resist most disinfectant solutions. Coagulation, filtration, and chlorination of drinking water to provide total and pure residual chlorine concentration of 1.1 and 0.4 ppm, respectively, as is done in some cities, will inactivate any hepatitis virus present.

The principal hepatic lesions during the early icteric phase include inflammation and necrosis of liver cells with swelling of the Kupffer cells and proliferation of the histiocytes, and periportal infiltration with phagocytes of all sorts. Mild meningoencephalitis may occur. Biliary stasis is prominent in icteric cases.

RELATION OF LABORATORY FINDINGS TO CLINICAL STATUS

An attack of hepatitis typically begins with prodromal symptoms simulating an upper respiratory infection or gastrointestinal upset. Fever and liver enlargement are usually present. Urine studies show the presence of bilirubin several days before jaundice becomes manifest, or even if the patient never becomes icteric.

If jaundice appears it reaches its peak in about 10 days and then subsides more slowly. During this phase the chief clinical findings are icterus and an enlarged tender liver. The urine is dark-colored and rich in bile. The stools are frequent and may be free of bile. The hemoglobin and red cell count may be subnormal. The leukocyte count tends to be between 5,000 and 20,000 cells per cu mm; low counts are usually a reflection of neutrophilopenia. Atypical lymphocytes occur in small numbers in the peripheral blood of most patients.

Readings with the flocculation tests are positive in the majority of patients, though in infants under 6 months of age this finding is less constant. The flocculation disturbances persist for a month or two as a rule, or longer with incomplete healing of the liver lesion.

The serum bilirubin level is elevated in those who have evident jaundice and may be moderately increased in those not jaundiced. Total bilirubin level is usually in the range between 2 and 8 mg per 100 ml. The proportion constituted by the 1-minute-reacting bilirubin is variable, but as a rule is somewhat low (30 to 50 per cent). This bilirubinemia may last from a few days to a few weeks.

The heterophil antibody titer may be slightly elevated, but the antibodies are absorbed on guinea pig kidney and beef cell antigen suspensions (p. 204). The prothrombin time may be prolonged and the serum cholesterol level depressed slightly if cell injury is pronounced. The Bromsulphalein excretion tends to become retarded early in the illness, before jaundice appears. This persists through the illness and may be the last abnormality to subside. The serum alkaline phosphatase level may be elevated or depressed.

VIRAL HEPATITIS IN INFANCY

Viral hepatitis in the first year of life often fails to elicit changes in the "function" tests. Mild cases may exhibit no jaundice, and the total serum bilirubin level may be elevated only slightly if at all. The thymol turbidity response is most often abnormal. Cephalin flocculation is less responsive. The serum alkaline phosphatase is often elevated during the first week and may become subnormal thereafter. The urine urobilinogen output may be increased slightly.

The more severely affected infants will have more overt symptoms. Jaundice may begin as early as the first week or even be evident at birth. The jaundice tends to be progressive at first, continues for some weeks or months, and then subsides spontaneously unless the liver becomes cirrhotic. Fever, watery stools, anorexia, failure to gain weight, poor tissue turgor, and a general appearance of ill health are typical symptoms. At intervals the signs may suggest obstructive jaundice, with pale or completely acholic stools and an enlarged liver and spleen.

In severe cases the urine usually contains bile or urobilinogen or both. The stools may or may not exhibit bile pigment. The total serum bilirubin level tends to be elevated, in the range of 5 to 25 mg per 100 ml. The 1-minute reading is usually elevated also, amounting to 25 to 50 per cent of the total. The serum protein and total cholesterol levels as a rule are not abnormal. The results of liver tests—cephalin flocculation, thymol turbidity and flocculation, and alkaline phosphatase—are abnormal in only a minority of the infants. The zinc turbidity response is frequently elevated. The prothrombin level may be depressed; if so it will rise with vitamin K therapy except in very severe cases. The blood may show a granulocytic leukocytosis, a normochromic anemia, and perhaps a mild reticulocytosis.

Pathology

The liver in biopsy or autopsy specimens exhibits histopathologic changes of the same character as seen in adults with viral hepatitis. The parenchymal cells are swollen or necrotic or otherwise injured and often contain hemosiderin. The interstitial tissue may appear thickened, and the lobular architecture distorted. Infiltrations with leukocytes of diverse varieties are found. The bile canaliculi may be distended with pigment; more often they are not. Usually prominent in infantile cases are giant-sized parenchymal cells, irregular in shape and typically multinucleated. These cells are suggestive but not specifically diagnostic of viral hepatitis since they have been seen in other hepatic disorders of infancy. They have been a prominent feature of the hepatic lesions in a group of young infants reported by Stokes, Wolman, and associates in whom the viral hepatitis seemed to have its origin before the time of birth. The hepatitis B virus was recovered from the blood of one of these infants before death and from the blood of his asymptomatic mother on two occasions.

BIBLIOGRAPHY

VIRAL HEPATITIS

Capps, R. B., A. M. Bennett, E. H. Mills, R. H. Ettinger, M. E. Drake, and J. Stokes, Jr., Infectious Hepatitis in Infants and Small Children, A.M.A. Am. J. Dis. Child. 89:701, 1955.

Cockburn, W. C., J. A. Harrington, R. A. Zeitlin, D. Morris, and E. Camps, Homologous Serum Hepatitis and Measles Prophylaxis: A Report to the Medical Research Council, Brit. M. J. 2:6, 1951.

Craig, J. M., S. S. Gellis, and D. Y.-Y. Hsia, Cirrhosis of the Liver in Infants and Children, A.M.A. Am. J. Dis. Child. 90:299, 1955.

Dible, J. Henry, W. E. Hunt, V. W. Pugh, L. Steingold, and J. H. F. Wood, Foetal and Neonatal Hepatitis and Its Sequelae, J. Path. & Bact. 67:195–206, January, 1954.

Krainin, P., and B. Lapan, Neonatal Hepatitis in Siblings, J.A.M.A. 160:937, 1956.

Lucké, B., (a) Pathology of Fatal Epidemic Hepatitis, Am. J. Path. 20:471, 1944.
(b) Studies on Epidemic Hepatitis and Its Sequelae, Tr. & Stud. Coll. Physicians Philadelphia 16:32, 1948.

Mallory, T. B., Pathology of Endemic Hepatitis, J.A.M.A. 134:655, 1947.

Peace, R., Fatal Hepatitis and Cirrhosis in Infancy, Arch. Path. 61:107, 1956.

Still, W. J. S., Familial Hepatic Cirrhosis, Arch. Dis. Childhood 30:354, 1955.

Stokes, J., Jr., Epidemiology of Viral Hepatitis A, Am. J. Pub. Health 43:1097, 1953.

———, I. J. Wolman, M. C. Blanchard, J. D. Farquhar, and M. E. Drake, Viral Hepatitis in the Newborn, A.M.A. Am. Dis. Child. 82:213, 1951.

CHAPTER 44

Liver Function in the Newborn Period

From the instant of birth the liver of the infant has to assume physiologic activities which are absent or quiescent in intrauterine life. Foodstuffs begin to enter the portal system from the gastrointestinal tract, and the waste bile pigments have to be excreted into the biliary ducts instead of being carried off by the placental vessels. Full adjustment of these added burdens is sometimes not achieved until several days have passed, and especially in infants prematurely born.

CORD BLOOD BILIRUBIN CONCENTRATION

Most newborn infants have a mild hyperbilirubinemia as compared with older infants. In Halbrecht and Brzoza's series of 74 newborn infants, the average total bilirubin in serum of cord blood was 1.41 mg per 100 ml with a range of 0.20 to 4.50 mg per 100 ml. For those under 2,500 gm birth weight the average was 0.95 mg; for those between 2,500 and 3,500 gm, 1.16 mg; and for those above 3,550 gm, 1.34 mg. In the 89 normal newborn infants studied by Hsia, Allen, Diamond, and Gellis, the readings of cord blood for total serum bilirubin averaged 1.9 mg per 100 ml with a range of 0.2 to 5.9 mg. For nine premature infants the average was 1.3 mg and the range 0.0 to 2.9 mg. There were no differences referable to ABO or Rh·Hr incompatibility between mother and infant.

Excretion of the bile pigments before birth appears to be a function of the placenta. This explains Findlay's finding that in 23 newborn infants the bilirubin level in the umbilical artery averaged 14 per cent higher than in the umbilical vein.

ICTERUS NEONATORUM

During the first few days of life the total serum bilirubin levels of all newborn infants tend to pass through a phase of rise and fall, while the 1-minute readings remain undisturbed. The peak is usually reached on the second day. With 24 normal full-term infants followed daily by Hsia, Allen, Diamond, and Gellis, the average reading on the first day was

485

3.7 mg per 100 ml, on the second 6.8 mg, on the third 6.2 mg, and on the fourth 4.7 mg. There was considerable variation, the highest reading being 13.2 mg in one infant on the third day. Of 73 infants followed during the first week by Findlay, Higgins, and Stamier, 34 attained levels greater than 1 mg per 100 ml of serum, and 28 exhibited rises above 2 mg.

In premature infants this period of so-called physiologic hyperbilirubinemia is more pronounced and tends to last longer. With infants of birth weight under 2,250 gm studied by Hsia and associates, the peak of the mean curve occurred on the fourth day with an average of 11.2 mg per 100 ml (range, 0.0 to 27.0 mg). With 27 premature infants studied by Obrinsky and associates, the peak of the mean curve occurred on the fourth day with an average of 7.95 mg (range, 1 to 14 mg). It usually takes 1 to 4 weeks for the elevated plasma bilirubin concentration in premature infants to recede to 1.0 mg per 100 ml or less. In general, the higher the serum level, the longer the bilirubinemia lasts. There is little if any close relation between birth weight and the severity of physiologic bilirubinemia.

The appearance of recognizable jaundice is related somewhat to the height of the plasma level, but there is no critical threshold level. Visible jaundice does not become evident as a rule unless the concentration of bilirubin in serum has reached approximately 4 to 5 mg per 100 ml, and then appears about 1 day later.

Neonatal icterus tends to be much more common, intense, and prolonged in premature than in mature infants. High levels of circulating bilirubin in extremely small or debilitated infants may be associated with injury and pigmentation of areas in the central nervous system and may even lead to death.

Neonatal hyperbilirubinemia seems best explained in terms of sluggishness on the part of the liver of the newborn in adapting itself to excretion of the pigment at the desired physiologic rate. During this adjustment period there is considerable variation in the capacity of the liver to achieve the necessary efficiency in excreting the burden of bilirubin suddenly thrust upon it. There is a pronounced tendency for the fecal excretion of bilirubin to be much lower in jaundiced than in nonjaundiced infants during the first few days of life, but not thereafter. There are wide fluctuations from day to day in the fecal outputs of single infants. The greater height and prolongation of the serum bilirubin levels in infants born prematurely seem referable to functional immaturity of the liver.

The intensity of physiologic hyperbilirubinemia has no correlation with changes in the red cell count in the first few days of life. It is no more severe in normal newborns whose ABO and Rh·Hr red cell antigens are different from those of their mothers than in newborn infants whose groupings are identical, except when there are clinical disturbances related to these blood group antigens.

No differences have been noted in the rates of fall of red cell and hemoglobin levels between jaundiced and nonjaundiced normal newborn infants during the first few weeks of life. In fact, there is little evidence that excessive blood destruction during the first few months causes the "physiologic" drop in red cell and hemoglobin levels. The major mechanism here appears to be a slowdown in the rate of hemopoiesis secondary to the changeover from intrauterine to extrauterine existence. The decline in red cells and hemoglobin is usually less rapid during the first week of life while the bilirubin level is rising; it continues steadily into the third month, long after the hyperbilirubinemia and jaundice have gone.

RESULTS OF OTHER LIVER TESTS DURING THE NEONATAL ADJUSTMENT PERIOD

The cephalin flocculation and thymol turbidity tests in the first week of life give negative results in some infants, weakly positive results in others. The Bromsulphalein retention normally tends to be diminished and is usually between 10 and 20 per cent at 45 minutes. The blood cholesterol content (p. 519) and the plasma proteins (p. 537) are low (see also Chap. 45).

BIBLIOGRAPHY

LIVER FUNCTION IN THE NEWBORN PERIOD

Akerren, Y., Physiological Hyperbilirubinaemia in the Newborn and the Reservoir Function of the Spleen, *Arch. Dis. Childhood* **26**:106, 1951.

Bowman, J. M., The Influence of Blood Group Incompatibility, Sex, Birth Weight, and Birth Order upon Serum Bilirubin Levels in a Newborn Population, *A.M.A. Am. J. Dis. Child.* **92**:482, 1956.

Davidson, L. T., K. K. Merritt, and *A. A. Weech,* Hyperbilirubinemia in the Newborn, *Am. J. Dis. Child.* **61**:985, 1941.

Findlay, L., G. Higgins, and *M. H. Stanier,* Icterus Neonatorum, Its Incidence and Cause, *Arch. Dis. Childhood* **22**:65, 1947.

Halbrecht, L., and *H. Brzoza,* Evaluation of Hepatic Function in Newborn Infants by Means of Chemical Study of Cord Blood, *Am. J. Dis. Child.* **79**:988, 1950.

Hsia, D. Y., F. H. Allen, Jr., L. K. Diamond, and *S. S. Gellis,* Serum Bilirubin Levels in the Newborn Infant, *J. Pediat.* **42**:277, 1953.

Künzer, W., "Über den Blutfarbstoffwechsel gesunder Säulinge und Kinder, Mit besonderer Berücksichtigung der Anämisierungsvorgänge im Verlauf des 1 Trimenons," S. Karger, Basel (Switzerland), 1951.

Larsen, E. H., and *T. K. With,* The Metabolism of Bile Pigments in Infants with Special Regard to Icterus Neonatorum, *Acta paediat.* 31:153, 1943–1944.

Mollison, P. L., Physiological Jaundice of the Newborn: Some New Measurements of the Factors Concerned, *Lancet* 1:513, 1948.

Obrinsky, W., E. L. Allen, and *E. E. Anderson,* Physiologic Hyperbilirubinemia in Premature Infants, *A.M.A. Am. J. Dis. Child.* 87:305, 1954.

Waugh, T. R., F. T. Merchant, and *O. B. Maugham,* Blood Studies on Newborn; Direct and Total Blood Bilirubin; Determinations over 9 Day Period with Special Reference to Icterus Neonatorum, *Am. J. M. Sc.* 199:9, 1940.

Weech, A. A., The Genesis of Physiologic Hyperbilirubinemia, in "Advances in Pediatrics," vol. 2, p. 346, Interscience Publishers, New York, 1947.

CHAPTER 45

Approaches to the Study of Jaundice
and Liver Disease

A good working approach to the elucidation of severe jaundice in an infant or child is to think in terms of whether the disturbance lies primarily in the blood stream or other prehepatic sites, the liver parenchyma itself, or the biliary duct system. This distinction is not always easy to establish. Laboratory evidence of parenchymal cell injury, with or without the poorly defined phenomenon of "inspissation," occurs frequently in both the hemolytic and the obstructive types of disorders. Many patients with liver disease do not have jaundice, and not all patients with jaundice have liver disease. Should the nature of the disturbance still be obscure after clinical observation for some weeks has failed to reveal the true diagnosis or to be attended by spontaneous recovery, surgical exploration or liver aspiration biopsy may be needed.

In infancy particularly, once physiologic icterus and infections such as sepsis or syphilis have been excluded, thorough laboratory study becomes essential. Depending on the clinical indications, one must consider the wisdom of utilizing such exploratory tests as serial serum bilirubin determinations; surveys of the blood of both mother and infant for antibodies secondary to ABO, Rh·Hr, and other possible blood group incompatibilities; checking of the infant's red cells for autoisoagglutinins, increased fragility, and Coombs' test antibodies; duodenal intubation for evidence of absent bile, increased viscosity, or diminished trypsin; analyses of stools and urine. Liver function tests are often of little assistance in the recognition of parenchymal diseases during the first year; one or all tests may yield normal results even when liver damage is advanced.

PRIMARILY HEMOLYTIC DISORDERS

Jaundice in the absence of liver or biliary tract disease is nearly always of hemolytic origin. The typical laboratory findings are (1) hematologic signs of accelerated red cell destruction, (2) a raised total serum bilirubin level with a normal or only slightly elevated 1-minute reading, (3) absence of bilirubin and presence of urobilinogen in the urine, and (4) an abnormally high output of fecal urobilinogen. The results of the tests for flocculation, alkaline phosphatase, Bromsulphalein retention, and plasma protein in "pure" hemolytic cases are ordinarily normal. When the hemolytic disorder is severe, however, it is not uncommon for the hepatic parenchymal cells to be injured by the chronic hypoxia and the heavier burden of augmented hemoglobin destruction. This may be revealed only by a prolonged Bromsulphalein retention, with results of the other tests for parenchymal dysfunction remaining unaltered. In many of the acquired hemolytic disturbances, such as those caused by infections or lead, the same toxic influences which attack the red cells can also injure the liver directly.

Practically all the hemolytic anemias which affect older children may have their onset early in infancy. Any infant with a clearly hemolytic disorder not referable to a blood group antibody transmitted from the mother should be studied with the indicated laboratory tests for septicemia, hereditary spherocytosis, sickle cell disease, autogenous hemolytic mechanisms, and so on. Elevated total serum bilirubin levels, a reticulocytosis, and an increase in urine urobilinogen output are characteristic findings. Signs of disturbed liver function as well as of enhanced red cell destruction may be prominent. A hematologic family survey can be very helpful.

Any jaundice which may occur in hereditary spherocytosis is of fluctuating intensity and may be present for only short periods of time. In active sickle cell anemia the jaundice is typically minimal, with exacerbations only after some "crisis" or when hypersplenism is a complication. In Mediterranean anemia the development of jaundice is a rarity and throws the diagnosis into question except when viral hepatitis is superimposed.

A protracted and excessive rate of blood destruction may be followed after some years by the development of pigment gallstones, which in turn may lead to superimposed biliary tract obstruction. Serum hepatitis may be contracted as a complication of a transfusion. Liver hemosiderosis may develop in children receiving repeated supportive transfusions, but this ordinarily produces no symptoms.

Erythroblastosis Fetalis (see also p. 165)

SERUM BILIRUBIN LEVELS. The pathologically increased rate of red cell destruction is portrayed in the behavior of the serum bilirubin level during the first days after birth. These increases are in the total serum bilirubin; the 1-minute readings are almost never increased. In erythroblastosis fetalis, Hsia and associates found in the cord blood a range of 2.1 to 10.3 mg per 100 ml for total serum bilirubin, with a mean of 5.1 mg. The mean curve for total serum bilirubin attained a maximum of 30 mg per 100 ml by the third day, whereas normal full-term infants attained a maximum of only 7 mg by the second day, and normal premature newborns a maximum of 11 mg by the fourth day. Within a few hours after an exchange transfusion, the elevated levels in erythroblastosis fetalis subside markedly.

OTHER TESTS. Most of the liver tests—cholesterol, alkaline phosphatase, cephalin flocculation, and galactose tolerance—usually give readings in erythroblastosis fetalis which are similar to those exhibited by normal newborns. The cholesterol esterase activity is not much altered. The serum gamma globulin level, as measured by zinc sulfate turbidity, is usually subnormal. The urobilinogen content of the urine may or may not be elevated.

TRANSITORILY PROLONGED JAUNDICE. In about 2 per cent of infants with erythroblastosis fetalis the jaundice, instead of lasting the usual 7 to 10 days, continues for 3 to 8 weeks, and occasionally for as long as a half year. During the period of prolonged jaundice the symptoms and laboratory findings may simulate the pattern resulting from congenital biliary tract obstruction. This complication is sometimes called the "inspissated bile syndrome," though parenchymal cell injury is a more likely cause. An early sign is an unexpected rise in the 1-minute serum bilirubin fraction, commencing on the third or fourth day. The ratio of the 1-minute to the total serum bilirubin reading may rise. The stools remain steadily or intermittently bile-free for several weeks or months, and bile persists in the urine. The serum alkaline phosphatase may mount to 10 to 25 Bodansky units (normal 5 to 12 units). The results of the flocculation tests are as a rule negative. Recovery is spontaneous and complete and the prognosis good. The obstructive syndrome seems more likely to develop when exchange transfusion is not done.

PRIMARILY HEPATOCELLULAR DISORDERS

When the liver cells themselves are affected by an active disease process the expected laboratory findings include (1) an increase in both 1-minute and total serum bilirubin levels, without any consistent ratio between the two, (2) a normal serum alkaline phosphatase level, (3) strongly positive reactions with the flocculation tests, (4) a normal level of total cholesterol but a diminished proportion of cholesterol esters, (5) a somewhat lowered serum albumin level, often with an elevated serum globulin, (6) bile pigments in the urine, with or without bile acids, (7) a normal or low stool output of bile pigments while the jaundice is advancing or continuing, or a high output while the jaundice is subsiding, and (8) unusual Bromsulphalein retention. Urobilinogen may or may not be excreted in the urine in excess.

A diversity of parenchymal diseases can give rise to jaundice in infancy and childhood. Among the possible causes in problem situations are viral hepatitis; necroses or inflammation caused by toxins, drugs, or sepsis; congenital syphilis; cytomegalic inclusion disease; yellow fever; intracellular storage diseases; malnutritional fatty infiltration; circulatory disturbances; infiltrating neoplasms such as dermoids, adenomas, cysts, angiomas, and primary or metastatic sarcoma, teratoma, or even carcinoma; abscesses of bacterial, amebic, syphilitic, tuberculous, or parasitic origin; and assorted forms of nonbiliary cirrhosis including the Laennec type, the infantile cirrhosis seen in India, and that due to circulatory failure. A form of familial jaundice in the newborn has been described (p. 493). The symptoms and laboratory findings in any of these may be highly bizarre.

In many patients the parenchymal disorder is complicated by compression or occlusion of the fine biliary passages. The converse is also true, in that obstructive lesions of any duration tend almost inescapably to cause parenchymal cell injury. Sometimes an intrahepatic neoplasm or abscess will give purely obstructive symptoms by mechanical interference with the flow of bile through the duct system.

Since "physiologic" jaundice does not become apparent until after the second day or later, any icterus which is already apparent at birth must be interpreted as being due to other disturbances. Erythroblastosis fetalis and hemolytic disease due to ABO blood group incompatibility between mother and child are statistically the most frequent.

Viral hepatitis in the newborn, formerly deemed rare, must always be considered in the differential diagnosis of neonatal icterus. More and more cases are being described of newborn infants who experience a jaundice-producing illness which seems best explained as an attack of viral hepatitis. The close proximity to the time of birth, the frequent obtaining of a history of hepatitis in the mother before or during the pregnancy, and the occasional appearance of the same series of symptoms in successive infants are highly suggestive in many instances that the infection was transplacentally transmitted (Chap. 43).

Toxic Hepatopathy

Evidences of derangements in the hepatic intracellular enzyme systems are not uncommon during or immediately after fulminating infections of all kinds, exposure to many drugs and poisons, or severe gastroenteritis or shock or toxemia. Development of liver injury seems to be contingent upon the intensity and duration of the underlying disease. The overt signs in pronounced injury are usually jaundice, fatty involvement of the liver which may enlarge rapidly, and sometimes a lowered prothrombin level leading to hemorrhagic phenomena. Jaundice may be absent even when the serum bilirubin level is raised. Tests of liver function may or may not give abnormal results. Dehydration and potassium deficiency sometimes develop.

Malnutritional Fatty Infiltration

An ill-defined form of fatty liver disease which seems clearly of malnutritional origin occurs in tropical and subtropical areas all over the world. It is known also as malnutritional fatty infiltration, kwashiorkor, malignant malnutrition, polydeficiency disease, m'buaki, syndrome depigmentation-oedème, and infantile pellagra. Its highest prevalence is in infants and young children who may appear well developed and well nourished when first taken ill but who are almost always small for their age. Listlessness is a prominent feature. Jaundice almost never occurs. Occasional survivors of the acute phase develop liver cirrhosis of the Laennec type.

The antecedent history almost always reveals an inadequate diet, with the protein content low. Pathologically the liver cells are distended with fat, usually with one prominent large globule in each cell but sometimes with multiple smaller vacuoles. Mild mononuclear periportal infiltrates are frequent, but no necrosis or fibrosis except in the late stages. The pancreas may show shrinkage of the acinar cells.

Reports of hepatic function tests on these cases are few. Positive flocculation tests and minor rises in total serum bilirubin level have been described. The plasma albumin is low, and the plasma globulin often elevated.

Congenital Familial Nonhemolytic Jaundice with Kernicterus

This descriptive name was applied by Crigler and Najjar to a syndrome presented by 7 patients with a recessively inherited form of nonhemolytic jaundice with brain damage. The only abnormal laboratory findings were pronounced elevation of total serum bilirubin and a delayed excretion of bilirubin given by injection. The concentrations of total serum bilirubin in 6 patients ranged between 10 and 44 mg per 100 ml, with a minimal increase in the 1-minute portion. Very high levels occurred during the newborn period because of the superimposition of physiologic jaundice. Bile thrombi were found in the bile canaliculi in all patients studied pathologically, and a minimal periportal fibrosis in some.

Hypertrophic Steatosis of the Liver

This name was suggested by van Creveld for a poorly understood group of patients whose primary difficulty seems to be excessive accumulation of fat within the cells of the liver. These patients, in association with enlargement of the liver, tend to have retarded growth, hypoglycemia, hyperlipemia, and hypercholesterolemia. There may be a familial incidence. There is no tendency to acetonuria when food is withheld for longer than a few hours—a differentiating feature from glycogen storage disease in which ketosis develops rapidly under like circumstances.

PRIMARILY OBSTRUCTIVE DISORDERS

The positive laboratory findings in purely obstructive disorders form a somewhat characteristic pattern: (1) increase in both 1-minute and total serum bilirubin with the 1-minute reading usually being more than 40 per cent of the total, (2) increased alkaline serum phosphatase, (3) increase in total and esterified cholesterol, (4) presence of bile pigments and bile acids in the urine, (5) an absent or diminished day-by-day output of bilirubin derivatives in the stool, and (6) undue Bromsulphalein retention. The results of the liver tests and of albumin and globulin fractionation are typically undisturbed in the first few months, but later the flocculation tests often become positive and the serum albumin falls as the globulin rises.

Malformation of the Biliary Tract

Biliary tract atresia and related anomalies are the most common causes of complete biliary tract obstruction in early infancy. These infants are not born jaundiced but become so after a few days as the bilirubin begins to be retained within the body. The level of total serum bilirubin tends to rise rapidly in the first few weeks and irregularly thereafter. The usual reading in the first few months is about 12 mg per 100 ml and about 15 to 20 mg by the first birthday. Repeated laboratory studies will show persistent failure of bilirubin to reach the intestinal tract from the liver, except possibly for traces derived from the icteric intestinal mucus.

Some of the accumulating bilirubin seems to be destroyed by internal mechanisms, but much of it is excreted by way of the urinary tract. The urine is heavily loaded with bile pigment at all times. Forcing of fluids is believed by some to promote the urinary output of pigment. Urobilinogen in more than minimal amounts is not found in the urine. The initial meconium may have a green color.

About 80 to 90 per cent of biliary tract anomalies are atresia or absence of one or more segments of extrahepatic passages. Malformation of the intrahepatic network or the development of a choledochus cyst compressing the bile channels from the outside is much less common. The jaundice may not become recognizable until after a few weeks and may be intermittent rather than continuous when there is a choledochus cyst or atresia of only part of the biliary system.

In infants with congenital obstructive disorders the urine contains bile but rarely more than trace amounts of urobilinogen if any. The stools are gray, puttylike, and rich in fat. The quantitative output of fecal urobilinogen is scanty, 1 mg a day or less. The serum alkaline phosphatase is elevated in a minority of the cases, with a range from 5 to 100 units. The prothrombin activity remains unaltered except in very severe cases.

The serum flocculation tests are nearly always negative. Thus during the first 6 months it is not feasible by liver function studies to distinguish reliably between extrahepatic jaundice of obstructive origin and hepatocellular jaundice resulting from parenchymal cell injury.

Infants who survive for more than a year or two usually have retardation in growth. This is attributable to the severe hepatic dysfunction and cirrhosis, with impaired caloric intake secondary to defective absorption of fat-containing foods. The cephalin flocculation results remain negative as a rule, the thymol turbidity becomes erratically increased, and the Bromsulphalein retention impaired. Unless vitamins A, D, and K are fed in water-soluble form, disorders related to poor absorption of fat-soluble vitamins develop, including hypoprothrombinemia, rickets, osteoporosis, or even xerophthalmia. The serum protein levels are normal, with normal albumin-globulin ratios and a normochromic anemia.

The total serum cholesterol and total lipids tend to rise appreciably if the infant survives more than a year. The cholesterol esters tend to be depressed. Eventually there may be frank lipemia. The total lipids may rise to as much as 2,200 mg per 100 ml, the total cholesterol to 200 mg, the free cholesterol to 1,600 mg, and the "neutral fat" to 500 mg. Skin biopsies may show accumulations of foam cells typical of xanthomatous infiltration.

Transitory Obstructivelike Disturbances

Occasional infants in the postneonatal period exhibit a period of obstructive jaundice, usually lasting about 2 months. Sometimes called the "inspissated bile syndrome," this disturbance may be due to erythroblastosis fetalis, viral hepatitis, small or spastic extrahepatic ducts, thick biliary secretions, immaturity of the liver, or toxic injury of the parenchymal cells. The total serum bilirubin level typically rises to 8 to 12 mg per 100 ml. In many of these patients the etiologic diagnosis cannot be made without surgical exploration of the biliary system to exclude anatomic malformations. Intravenous dehydrocholic acid or oral bile salts will sometimes relieve a duct obstruction due to inspissated bile.

Other Obstructive Lesions

Beyond infancy the likelihood of the biliary tract being blocked by a malformation becomes almost negligible, with the exception of a choledochus cyst showing itself late. A diversity of other causes, all extremely unusual, then become suspect—peritoneal adhesions, enlarged hilar nodes, impacted gallstones, neoplastic growths, catarrhal cholangitis, or similar lesions. Obstruction from these acquired causes is more likely to be partial or intermittent, rather than persistent as in the malformational occlusions.

Large space-occupying lesions within the liver such as amebic or echinococcus abscesses may be accompanied by a rise in the serum alkaline phosphatase level and an abnormal retention of Bromsulphalein, with the serum bilirubin level and results of the cephalin flocculation and thymol turbidity tests remaining unaltered.

BIBLIOGRAPHY

PREHEPATIC AND HEPATOCELLULAR DISTURBANCES

Bellin, L. B., and *I. W. Bailit,* Congenital Cirrhosis of the Liver Associated with Infectious Hepatitis of Pregnancy, *J. Pediat.* 40:60, 1952.

Bowden, D. H., and *W. L. Donahue,* Jaundice in the Neonatal Period, *Am. J. M. Sc.* 230:305, 1955.

Craig, J. M., Sequences in the Development of Cirrhosis of the Liver in Cases of Erythroblastosis Fetalis, *A.M.A. Arch. Path.* 49:665, 1950.

Crigler, J. F., Jr., and *V. A. Najjar,* Congenital Familial Nonhemolytic Jaundice with Kernicterus, *Pediatrics* 10:169, 1952.

Dunham, E. C., Septicemia in the Newborn, *Am. J. Dis. Child.* 45:229, 1933.

Gellis, S. S., J. M. Craig, and *D. Y. Hsia,* Prolonged Obstructive Jaundice in Infancy. IV. Neonatal Hepatitis, *A.M.A. Am. J. Dis. Child.* 88:285, 1954.

Harris, R. C., D. H. Andersen, and *R. L. Day,* Obstructive Jaundice in Infants with Normal Biliary Tree, *Pediatrics* 13:293, 1954.

Holzel, A., and *N. Sher,* Familial Jaundice of the Newborn Associated with Hepatosteatosis, *Arch. Dis. Childhood* 27:37, 1952.

Howard, F. H., and *W. A. Meriwether,* Fat Disease of the Liver in Infants on the Isthmus of Panama, *Pediatrics* 10:150, 1952.

Johns, D., Galactosemia: An Unusual Cause of Neonatal Jaundice, *A.M.A. Am. J. Dis. Child.* 85:575, 1953.

Keller, P. D., and *W. L. Nute, Jr.,* Cirrhosis of the Liver in Children: A Clinical and Pathologic Study of Forty Cases, *J. Pediat.* 34:588, 1949.

Sass-Kortzak, A., D. H. Bowden, and *R. J. K. Brown,* Congenital Intrahepatic Biliary Atresia, *Pediatrics* 17:383, 1956.

Schlesinger, B., W. W. Payne, and *E. D. Burnard,* Liver Damage in Gastro-enteritis, *Arch. Dis. Childhood* 24:15, 1949.

van Creveld, S., Diseases of the Liver, Chap. 24 in Fanconi and Wallgren's "Textbook of Paediatrics," ed. by W. R. F. Collis and E. Kawerau, Grune & Stratton, Inc., New York, 1952.

Wróblewski, F., and *J. S. LaDue,* Serum Glutamic Oxalacetic Aminopherase (Transaminase) in Hepatitis, *J.A.M.A.* 160:1130, 1956.

BILIARY TRACT MALFORMATIONS

Dickinson, E. F., F. C. Spencer, Choledochal Cyst, *J. Pediat.* 41:462, 1952.

Gross, H. E., "The Surgery of Infancy and Childhood: Its Principles and Techniques," W. B. Saunders Company, Philadelphia, 1953.

Hsia, D. Y., and *S. S. Gellis,* Prolonged Obstructive Jaundice in Infancy, *A.M.A. Am. J. Dis. Child.* 85:13, 1953.

Kanof, A., E. J. Donovan, and *H. Berner,* Congenital Atresia of the Biliary System, *A.M.A. Am. J. Dis. Child.* 86:780, 1953.

Kiesewetter, W. B., C. E. Koop, and *J. D. Farquhar,* Surgical Jaundice in Infancy, *Pediatrics* 15:149, 1955.

Kirschbaum, J. D., Congenital Absence of the Gallbladder and the Extrahepatic Bile Ducts, *Am. J. Dis. Child.* 47:1080, 1934.

Moschcowitz, E., Morphology and Pathogenesis of Biliary Cirrhosis, *A.M.A. Arch. Path.* 54:259, 1952.

Myers, R. L., A. H. Baggenstoss, G. B. Logan, and *G. A. Hallenbeck,* Congenital Atresia of the Extrahepatic Biliary Tract: A Clinical and Pathologic Study, *Pediatrics* 18:767, 1956.

Schuckmell, N., W. J. Grove, and *A. P. Remenchik,* The Diagnosis of Operable Portal Obstruction in Children, *A.M.A. Am. J. Dis. Child.* 90:692, 1955.

Strauss, A. A., Congenital Atresia of the Bile Ducts, *J. Mt. Sinai Hosp.* 17:552, 1951.

Whitten, W. W., and *G. C. Adie,* Congenital Biliary Atresia, *J. Pediat.* 40:539, 1952.

CHAPTER 46

Blood Glucose

The concentration or level of every chemical constituent of the blood is kept within quantitative physiologic bounds during states of health by the homeostatic mechanisms. Proper interpretation of the report of any blood analysis requires a knowledge of the normal range of spontaneous fluctuation, the extent of variation among normal individuals of the same age and sex in the same environment, and the reliability of the chemical procedure employed.

For most commonly measured substances, good chemistry laboratories give data which are sufficiently precise to be applied clinically to problems presented by patients. It is important to emphasize, nevertheless, that every step in each procedure must be supervised meticulously by the laboratory director. Among other variables he must ascertain the reproducibility of his results, so that the total limits of inherent technical error as well as the scatter of normal readings are known.

In blood chemistry, the samples withdrawn from the peripheral blood stream are as a rule representative of what obtains in the circulation as a whole, though there are certain differences in the portal system and other local areas.

With readily soluble and diffusible substances which are not bound to the serum proteins or subject to the Donnan membrane equilibrium such as glucose, urea, and uric acid the concentrations in the blood reflect the approximate concentrations in the interstitial fluids and lymph. In contrast, substances with large molecules such as proteins and lipids are held within the vascular bed, so that the concentrations measured may differ considerably from those in the interstitial fluids or lymph.

One variable, unconquered practically as yet, is measurement of the blood volume. This is influenced by age, sex, season, climate, illnesses, fluid intake, and other unknown factors and appears to fluctuate markedly throughout day and night. From the concentration of any substance per unit volume of blood or plasma one cannot calculate with accuracy the total amount present within the whole blood stream. Were it possible to measure the blood volume of a patient quickly and accurately at the time a blood sample is withdrawn, one would have a much more satisfying understanding of normal and disturbed physiologic states.

Inability to measure blood volume becomes an especially disturbing handicap in the presence of disturbances of fluid and acid-base equilibria. The levels in the circulating blood give information which is not only inadequate but often misleading. For example, in a dehydrated infant the plasma concentrations of protein, hemoglobin, and mineral ions may seem within or even above the normal range, whereas as soon as the shortage of water is replaced these will fall to markedly subnormal levels. Or, in an edematous child, low levels of sodium, chloride, and hemoglobin may not necessarily denote a total deficiency of these substances. Thus, every deviation from the normal in a blood chemistry report must always be considered in relation to the clinical status and other pertinent data.

The blood glucose concentration is the resultant of an equilibrium regulated by many mechanisms, with the liver playing the leading reservoir role. The chief immediate influences which act to raise the plasma level are intestinal absorption of glucose after meals, breakdown of glycogen in the liver and perhaps other tissues, and gluconegenesis (glucose formation) from fat or amino acids. The chief lowering influences are withdrawal of blood glucose by the tissues, liver, and muscles, lipogenesis, and glycosuria when present.

The glucose of the blood is present both in plasma and red cells, but the intracellular metabolism and lesser water content of the latter result in the glucose content of plasma being slightly higher than that of whole blood.

Insulin lowers the blood glucose level by accelerating the metabolism of glucose within the muscles, while at the same time stimulating hepatic formation of glycogen and decelerating gluconegenesis from noncarbohydrate sources. Acting in the opposite direction, toward glycogenolysis and hyperglycemia, are thyroid hormone, some adrenal cortical steroids, epinephrine, and glucagon from the alpha cells of the islets of Langerhans.

ARTERIOVENOUS DIFFERENCES

The level of glucose is lower in venous than in arterial blood. This difference can vary from 2 to 40 mg per 100 ml in a diabetic within the space of a few hours. The difference is minimal in the fasting state when the muscles are inactive and the blood flowing freely through an open capillary circulation, and maximal shortly after a meal or a large serving of sugar when the skin and muscles are actively withdrawing sugar from the blood stream to store as glycogen.

Blood collected from infants and children for glucose analysis is usually taken from the finger, heel, or ear. Such blood is capillary or arteriolar in origin and possesses the same content of glucose as blood secured by arterial puncture, if the subject is not a newborn infant and the blood is flowing freely. Most blood collections in adults, in contrast, are from the veins, which give readings lower than capillary (arterial) blood.

Venous blood is theoretically preferable for the study of glucose metabolism, as in tolerance tests, because it portrays the utilization of sugar by the tissues as well as by the liver. Practically, however, adequate information can be obtained with capillary (arterial) blood, though the existence of this inconstant differential should always be kept in mind. Capillary blood more accurately reflects the renal threshold to glucose and is preferable in studies for possible renal glycosuria.

NONGLUCOSE REDUCING SUBSTANCES

The circulating plasma contains moderate quantities of reducing substances which are not glucose. Glutathione and ergothionine make up the greatest portion of these, along with creatinine, uric acid, ascorbic acid, and related metabolites. Mucopolysaccharides conjugated with the globulins are present also, though these do not enter into the reactions employed in estimating the glucose of the blood. Jacobs has noted in adults that glucosamine, one of these polysaccharides, has a normal range of about 15 to 25 mg per 100 ml and that the concentration goes up with the blood sugar in uncontrolled diabetes mellitus to levels as high as 90 to 95 mg. The therapeutic injection of streptomycin may be followed by a minor apparent rise in blood glucose which has been ascribed to the reducing activity of the aldehyde groups in this antibiotic.

The Folin-Wu and Hagedorn-Jensen "macro" methods are typical of those which measure all or nearly all the reducing substances. Inasmuch as the nonglucose components of the plasma may vary from 10 to 60 mg per 100 ml, the readings obtained with these methods are higher and less representative of true glucose. The newer methods which use finger tip blood, such as that of Somogyi and Nelson, have minimized the reactivity of the nonglucose constituents to not more than 10 mg per 100 ml. The clinician should ascertain the specificity for glucose of the procedure used in his reference laboratory and the range of "normal" values which can be expected. Since the micro methods are widely used in pediatric practice, the data in the ensuing discussion refer to analyses performed by this approach, with the reducing substances of the blood being almost wholly monosaccharides (glucose).

Blood specimens which are permitted to stand at room temperature for some hours will show a steady disappearance of the contained glucose, as a consequence of the metabolism of the erythrocytes and leukocytes. Hence if delay in analysis is unavoidable, the specimen should be chilled immediately, or fluoride or moniodoacetate added to the collection tube, in order to retard this process. It is best to start the analysis within an hour after collection of the specimen.

NORMAL POSTABSORPTIVE (RESTING) LEVELS

In the normal individual the level of plasma glucose in the resting, fasting, or "postabsorptive" state tends to remain within fairly narrow limits (*normoglycemia*) until the readily mobilized deposits of hepatic glycogen have been exhausted. There is ordinarily enough glycogen in the liver to maintain a balanced level for at least 6 to 12 hours with infants in the first few months of life, and for 12 to 24 hours or longer beyond that age. After the available liver reserves have been exhausted, the plasma level falls (*hypoglycemia*) and the utilization of fats as a body fuel becomes accelerated.

Infancy and Childhood

It is difficult to give a precise set of limits for the normal range of postabsorptive (fasting) blood sugar levels in childhood and infancy. Impressively wide variability is shown by normal children at all ages. Rudesill and Henderson (1941) have tabulated the results of many of the antecedent series of cases, but the source of the blood (arterial or venous) and the procedures in the various studies have been far from identical. In general it may be stated that for normal infants and children the readings during the postabsorptive state with micro methods fall as a rule between 60 and 100 mg per 100 ml. The scatter is greater during infancy than after the second year of life, in accord with the greater lability of most body equilibria during the infancy period.

Newborn Period

At the moment of birth the blood in the umbilical vein (coming from the placenta) contains about 10 per cent more glucose than that in the umbilical artery (coming from the fetus). The blood glucose level declines rapidly in the first 4 hours, and then more slowly to a low point on the first to third day. A gradual rise then begins even when feedings are not given, to continue to the end of the first week.

In a series of 45 newborn infants studied by Hanley, Horn, and Farmer with a modified micro Folin-Wu method, the mean blood glucose value for specimens from the umbilical vein was 111.7 ± 2.9 mg per 100 ml; from the umbilical artery, 96.4 ± 3.1. The mean value for maternal venous blood, taken coincidentally, was 126.8 mg, showing that maternal levels are higher and that the fetus has its own independent capacity for sugar regulation. Blood from the heel or finger of these infants when tested at 1 hour after birth had fallen to a mean of 80.3 ± 3.7 mg; at 6 hours after birth, 77.5 + 1.8 mg (the figures preceded by ± represent the standard error of the mean). No correlation was demonstrable between the birth weight and the extent of the fall, except that premature infants had a mean of 68 mg at 6 hours after birth as compared with 73 mg for those weighing between 2,500 and 4,000 mg and of 82 mg for those with birth weights over 4,000 gm. With a larger group of 130 newborn infants the blood sugar in 22 had dropped below 60 mg per 100 ml at 6 hours. In 3 it was 35, 42, and 46 mg, respectively. No infant gave evidence of shock, twitching, or of later ill health.

Norval, who studied the fasting levels in 33 normal premature infants with a modified Somogyi micromethod, found values from 15 and 117 mg per 100 ml and a mean of 60 mg in the first 2 weeks of life. The mean for the first day was slightly under 45 mg. No signs or symptoms of hypoglycemia were shown by any of the infants. Four other premature infants who died in the first few days had extremely low levels, which were probably secondary to their illnesses.

Clearly the homeostatic mechanisms during the first few days are not wholly effective in keeping the blood glucose at a concentration optimal for tissue metabolism.

GLUCOSE TOLERANCE TESTS

In the normal nondiabetic child the plasma glucose level will frequently rise a few milligrams per 100 ml in the first half hour after a simple meal, to be followed by a slight and transient swing below the original resting value. In children ill with fever or other ailments the rise after a meal may be slightly higher, up to perhaps 30 mg in the first half hour. In children with diabetes mellitus who are not receiving insulin and in a few other conditions such as after a fast or in glycogen storage disease, the rise in level will be much more pronounced. The peak in these conditions will be reached in about 2 hours, with a slow return to the fasting status in 3 to 5 hours.

Much more effective than a meal for testing the capacities of the carbohydrate-regulating mechanisms of the body is to feed or inject a large "loading" dose of glucose after an interval of fasting and note the changes in the blood level or "tolerance" curve over the next few hours. The contour of the curve is determined by the effectiveness of the homeostatic mechanisms of the liver, muscles, and other organs in disposing of the sugar being absorbed, provided the glucose is being absorbed from the gastrointestinal system at a maximal and constant rate. In celiac disease, hypothyroidism, and some intestinal diseases, in which the absorption of glucose may be inefficient, the test dose should be given intravenously.

The determination is best done in the morning, before any energy-containing substance has been eaten and while the patient is at rest and emotionally relaxed. Fever or infection must not be present. The preceding meal should have been a good supper in the case of older children; a late evening or midnight feeding should be given to infants and younger children so that the preliminary fasting period does not exceed 8 to 12 hours.

For several days beforehand the food intake should be adequate and should contain a liberal but not extreme proportion of carbohydrate.

An excessive prior intake of carbohydrate will lead to an unusually low curve, whereas an antecedent interval of starvation or of a high-fat, low-carbohydrate diet will give a high and prolonged curve suggestive of diabetes. When a series of tolerance tests are being made on one child for investigational purposes, it is advisable to allow several days to elapse between the separate determinations so as to have conditions approximately constant with each test.

Oral Tolerance Test

With children older than 2 years a dosage of 1.75 gm of glucose per kg body weight will bring out the desired response. The glucose is best given in 20 per cent solution, after a 12-hour fast, dissolved in water or lemonade. Blood samples are taken at the beginning and at ½-, 1-, 2-, and 3-hour intervals following the taking of the glucose.

The experiments of Livingston and Bridge have indicated that increasing the amount of oral glucose with normal infants will lead to progressively higher responses. Their mean findings may be summarized as follows:

No. of cases	Gm dextrose per kg of body weight	Initial fasting level (mg per 100 ml)	Minutes after glucose			
			30	60	120	180
10	1.0	82	108	115	95	78
10	1.75	86	127	129	100	82
15	3.0	83	142	170	127	85

From these and related observations it seems advisable to give 3 gm of glucose per kg to infants under 2 years of age.

With these oral doses the typical healthy nonstarved nondiabetic infant or child will have a *fasting* blood glucose level between 60 and 100 mg per 100 ml (capillary); a *maximal rise* not higher than 180 mg (capillary) in 30 to 60 minutes; a *return* to the fasting level before 2 or 2½ hours (before 3 hours in infants with a test dose of 3 gm per kg); and a *hypoglycemic counterswing* below the original value of from 10 to 40 mg with a rapid return to the pretest level in the next ½ to 1 hour. Appreciable variations in the curves will be obtained with different subjects, but the same child under standardized conditions will usually give successive curves which are much alike.

With advanced untreated diabetes mellitus the initial or fasting level will be abnormally elevated (usually to between 150 and 400 mg per 100 ml), but with early or mild cases or with children receiving insulin it may fall within normal limits. Conversely, in hypoglycemia due to organic lesions such as severe liver disease or hyperinsulinism due to pancreatic islet adenoma, the initial level may be below 50 or 60 mg, but in functional disturbances of nervous or endocrine origin it is not always found depressed.

The duration of the elevation following a large dose of glucose is of far greater importance than the height of the peak; in fact, the latter is of minor significance. When early diabetes mellitus is being looked for (p. 369), a return to normal before 2 hours will as a rule exclude the diagnosis. In that situation it is usually adequate to take a blood specimen for analysis just before the administration of glucose, and another 2 hours later. A prolonged tolerance will be apparent also in glycogen storage disease, due presumably to the glycogen-loaded liver being unable to metabolize more glucose, but at 6 hours the blood glucose level will be abnormally low. A prolonged curve is often given in the hyperadrenalism of Cushing's syndrome or pheochromocytoma.

When a hypoglycemic disturbance is suspected, it is best to take an initial control blood specimen for glucose determination and to repeat the analyses at $\frac{1}{2}$, 1, 2, 3, 4, and 6 hours (p. 507). Here one is more interested in detecting an unusual speed of return to normal, an unusual drop below the control level, or a prolongation of this beyond the period customarily shown by normal individuals.

A urine specimen should be taken for analysis before the dose of sugar is given, and several others if feasible during the course of the test. Traces of ketones in the first or fasting specimen point to the existence of a state of slight starvation which may invalidate the results. Glycosuria appearing during the test period provides an indication of the renal threshold of the patient. Glycosuria in the presence of a normal glucose tolerance curve may be seen with a low renal threshold, idiopathic pentosuria, lead poisoning, the de Toni-Fanconi syndrome, and other renal tubular disorders (Chap. 31).

If a child is thought to have incipient diabetes mellitus but the diabetes cannot be established by the clinical story or urinary findings, and if the glucose tolerance curve is borderline, the test should be repeated after 1 or 2 weeks of high carbohydrate feeding. The repeat test is better made with venous than with capillary blood. A clear-cut curve of either normal or diabetic character should then be obtained. If the interpretation is still doubtful, the child may be kept under observation for some time with careful clinical and urine examinations and the tolerance test repeated every month or so. However, as discussed on page 369, a long prediabetic period with abnormal elevation of the blood glucose level either fasting or before meals but with no other symptoms is extremely uncommon in childhood.

The same sort of information conveyed by a diabetic type of glucose tolerance curve can often be obtained by testing the blood glucose level about 2 hours after a hearty breakfast containing approximately the test dose of glucose.

Intravenous Tolerance Test

The glucose may be given intravenously when the child refuses to take it by mouth or vomits the test dose or when absorption of glucose from the intestinal tract is sluggish. A satisfactory intravenous test dose is 0.5 gm per kg for an older child, or 1.0 gm per kg for an infant. This is dissolved as a 20 per cent solution in distilled water or physiologic saline and administered over a 3- to 5-minute period. Blood samples are collected when the injection is begun, immediately afterward, and at 15, 30, 60, 90, and 120 minutes thereafter. In normal infants and children the return to the preinjection level will almost always occur within 60 to 90 minutes, whereas in patients with diabetes mellitus the blood level after 2 hours will still be above 100 mg per 100 ml. An unusually steep fall to normal or subnormal values by 30 minutes is indicative of an exceptionally rapid utilization of glucose, as in hyperinsulinism.

Staub-Traugott Effect

If two or more test doses of glucose are given to a fasting subject, the second and later doses induce a lower rise in the blood sugar level than did the first dose. The first hyperglycemia is believed to influence the response to the next dose. Studies by Somersalo have shown that such a response occurs much less consistently in children than in adults; it does not appear when two intravenous tolerance tests are made in succession if the second test is performed after the first curve has returned to normal. The effect has been reported to be absent when a double galactose tolerance test is made.

This phenomenon furnished the rationale for the 1-hour–two-dose glucose tolerance test proposed by Exton and Rose for the detection of subclinical diabetes mellitus. Two large doses of glucose (50 mg each for adults) are taken at 30-minute intervals, and the blood glucose level followed at the time of each ingestion and 30 minutes later. A normal response is said to be one in which the first (fasting) blood level is not elevated; not more than 30-mg difference separates the $\frac{1}{2}$- and 1-hour reading; and the 1-hour reading is less than 160 mg per 100 ml. This two-dose test should have its chief field of usefulness in the detection of subclinical diabetes mellitus. Because of absence of large-scale control studies in infants and children, and the rarity of mild diabetes among children, this test has not been much used in the field of pediatrics.

Tolerance tests have been standardized for levulose and for galactose (p. 513) as measures of hepatic function or of disorders of metabolism specific for these sugars. The liver must be extensively damaged before the tolerance tests begin to show abnormalities, as a rule. Glucose is the monosaccharide most readily absorbed, levulose next, and galactose least. Large amounts of all sugars other than glucose frequently lead to gastrointestinal hypermotility and diarrhealike stools, with only a portion of the sugar being absorbed.

INSULIN SENSITIVITY AND RESISTANCE

In healthy children a single dose of regular insulin evokes an acute moderate fall in blood glucose level, followed by a prompt recovery. An excessively steep fall in blood glucose and unusually slow return are seen in "idiopathic" hypoglycemic conditions, adrenal or pituitary insufficiency, starvation, glycogen storage disease, galactosemia, gastrointestinal disturbances with poor absorption of glucose, and with some organic cerebral lesions. Normal newborn infants may also be hyper-sensitive to insulin in their responses to this test.

When the adrenal glands including the medulla are totally destroyed or when the hepatic stores of glycogen are already depleted, insulin may cause hypoglycemia which cannot be corrected spontaneously (*hypoglycemic unresponsiveness*).

The test for insulin sensitivity can be carried out by giving regular insulin either alone or preferably with some accompanying glucose. Blood samples are withdrawn for glucose analysis just before the injection and at 20, 30, 45, 60, 90, and 120 minutes afterward. When the insulin is given by itself 0.1 unit per kg body weight is injected intravenously or 0.25 unit subcutaneously. Insulin hypersensitivity manifests itself as an abrupt drop in the blood glucose in excess of 30 mg by 1 hour or as abnormal prolongation of the low level. The child should have no food for some hours before this test. Normally the blood sugar exhibits a maximal fall of 20 to 40 mg per 100 ml by 30 minutes and returns to the original fasting level within 120 minutes.

When insulin refractoriness is suspected one may inject $\frac{1}{40}$ unit of crystalline insulin per kg intravenously, calculated on the basis of actual rather than ideal weight. The amount injected can be more accurately controlled by preliminary dilution of the insulin with physiologic salt solution so that 1 ml contains 1 unit. With this smaller dosage the likelihood of an unexpected severe hypoglycemic reaction is minimized and the low blood sugar level is reached in about 30 minutes. Venous blood samples should be withdrawn at 15, 30, and 60 minutes. The reading at 60 minutes will normally be back to the fasting level.

The giving of some glucose along with the insulin protects against the real danger of causing severe hypoglycemic reactions and inhibits the stimulation of other endocrinal mechanisms which act to raise the blood sugar and confuse the pattern of response. It is advisable to perform a standard glucose test first, for control purposes. Five days later the test is repeated with the above dose of regular insulin given 10 minutes after the child has begun to drink a glucose solution in the same dosage as with the glucose tolerance test. The degree of responsiveness to insulin is measured by comparing the 1-hour reading of the two curves. A normal healthy individual will show an approximately flat curve on the second test. In conditions of insulin hypersensitivity, including diabetes with unusual sensitivity to insulin, a hypoglycemic curve will be given. With the opposite phenomenon of "insulin resistance," the glucose tolerance curve will have a contour resembling that of the test without insulin.

Insulin resistance is seen not infrequently in hyperthyroidism, long-standing diabetes mellitus, and other endocrine dysfunctions with over-activity of the physiologic antagonists to insulin. When it appears in severe infections and other febrile states it is ascribed to increased adrenal cortical activity in response to stress. The blood sugar rise shown by some diabetics after insulin is attributed to antibodies acquired against the proteins in insulin preparations or to contaminating glucagon derived presumably from the alpha cells.

EPINEPHRINE TEST

The capacity of the tissues to release glucose can be evaluated by giving an injection of epinephrine and noting the rise in the blood glucose level. In order that the liver glycogen may be in a state of maximum storage and responsiveness, the food intake should be high in carbohydrate for 3 days prior to the test and a glass of orange juice containing added sugar taken the evening before, at bedtime. A satisfactory test dose with older children is 0.01 ml of 1:1,000 solution of epinephrine hydrochloride per kg body weight given subcutaneously or intramuscularly. With infants the dose may be higher: 0.03 ml per kg. The blood glucose is determined before the injection and at 30, 60, 120, and 180 minutes afterward. In a normal child the blood glucose curve thus secured will run more or less parallel to that given by the glucose tolerance test. The maximal rise is reached at or before 60 minutes, and there is a return to normal or nearly normal by 2 hours in older children and by 3 hours in infants. The extent of the rise is more significant than the recovery time; normal children will show an increase of from 30 to 70 mg above the fasting figure. Ten normal infants studied by Livingston and Bridge exhibited responses as follows:

	Blood glucose (mg per 100 ml)
Fasting	80 ± 3
Minutes after injection:	
30	123 ± 4
60	143 ± 5
120	104 ± 8
180	76 ± 2

The maximal rise of blood glucose found was 71, the minimal rise was 40.

Essentially similar results will be given by older children under similar test circumstances.

The outflow of sugar becomes markedly diminished when the liver contains little or no available reserve of glycogen, as in destructive diseases of the liver, starvation states, glycogen storage disease, galactosemia; and in hyperinsulinism as a consequence of the excessively rapid peripheral removal of the carbohydrate released from the liver.

HYPOGLYCEMIA

This term is applied to the disturbed state of carbohydrate regulation in which the blood glucose tends to fall below the normal range during fasting, and also to the collapse syndrome produced by the low glucose level.

Hypoglycemia often has an endocrine origin, as in anterior pituitary insufficiency, hyperinsulinism, severe hypothyroidism, diabetes mellitus when regulation with insulin is difficult, and Addison's disease. An acute infection may precipitate an attack. Glucagon deficiency may play a role in some instances. There is a congenital and presumably hereditary form of the disorder in which hypoglycemic attacks are persistent and disturbing; this disturbance can be alleviated by corticotropin or cortisone or related adrenocortical hormones. Episodes may occur with severe liver disorders such as cirrhosis, advanced hepatitis, phenol or cresol poisoning, galactosemia or glycogen storage disease, and with brain diseases such as encephalitis which involve the hypothalamus.

Infants and young children normally develop hypoglycemia much more readily than do older children and adults. This susceptibility is believed to be related directly to the lesser content of glycogen in the liver in the early years. The liver of the newborn infant normally contains only 2 or 3 gm of glycogen per 100 gm, in contrast to 6 or 8 gm in healthy older children and adults.

Ketosis often develops as an associated phenomenon and may be the first overt indication of the existence of hypoglycemia. Ketosis ordinarily fails to develop in hypoglycemic states of endocrine origin.

Idiopathic Hypoglycemia

The predominant symptoms originate in the central nervous system and are best described as epileptoid; they vary all the way from asthenia and faintness to major convulsive seizures. Episodes occur usually in the early morning, are of short duration, and correct themselves spontaneously even when sugar is not given.

Occasional patients exhibit an abnormal drop in blood sugar with or without the development of symptoms 3 or 4 hours after a meal; these attacks probably represent an extreme degree of postprandial hypoglycemia. A diet low in carbohydrates, according to Holt and Bridge, will prevent episodes in this group.

The diagnosis is made by demonstrating an unusually low blood level for glucose while symptoms are in progress. If spontaneous attacks are infrequent, the attempt may be made to induce an attack by having the patient fast until disturbances become manifest, and then the blood is tested. Should no overt symptoms appear after 24 hours of fasting, a blood specimen should be collected for glucose determination and food given.

The typical glucose tolerance curve exhibits a rise followed by a prolonged drop to an unduly low level. The insulin tolerance test usually gives an insulin-sensitive response; there may be a sharp drop in the blood sugar exceeding 30 mg in 1 hour, or a sustained low level which takes 1 or more hours to return to the control level.

Some hypoglycemia patients respond to fasting by burning less carbohydrate and more fat as the blood sugar fails; others continue to burn carbohydrate, adding greatly to the severity of the hypoglycemia. Information in this regard may be gained by removing carbohydrate from the diet and feeding an adequate caloric intake derived from fat and protein (*carbohydrate-withdrawal test*). Patients able to form sufficient glucose from these other foods—chiefly protein—will sustain their blood sugar level, whereas those unable to do so will exhibit hypoglycemia within 12 to 24 hours.

The relation between blood levels and clinical phenomena is obscure. Some patients may have glucose levels much below 40 mg per 100 ml and even dropping occasionally to 0, without the appearance of symptoms.

Most children with hypoglycemic tendencies are helped by feedings of glucose or sucrose between meals. In advanced disturbances it may be necessary to rouse the child at night for an extra meal. Acute episodes can be arrested almost instantly by feeding orange juice or other form of sugar. Intravenous injections should be given for superimposed coma or convulsions.

Malnutrition

Infants with extreme malnutrition are exceptionally sensitive to hypoglycemia. Fasting levels below 60 mg per 100 ml are not uncommon, but associated symptoms usually do not develop except with precipitating influences such as an infection, severe starvation, or a gastrointestinal disturbance.

Hyperinsulinism

Hypoglycemia is one chief expression of hyperinsulism, being consequent to the excessive combustion of glucose which takes place in these disturbances. Hyperinsulinism may be identified by its intense hypoglycemic tendency, the rapid rate of fall in blood glucose after a normal meal, and the absence of ketosis at the time of hypoglycemia.

Unlike what occurs in adults, the majority of cases of hyperinsulinism in childhood are not due to organic lesions in the pancreas. Nevertheless there is no known preoperative procedure which will differentiate tumor or hyperplasia of the islet beta cells from hypoglycemic disturbances due to undetermined causes.

HYPOGLYCEMIA AND CENTRAL NERVOUS SYSTEM DAMAGE

Since the cells of the central nervous system contain no reserve stores of glycogen, they are extremely susceptible to depression of the circulating glucose. Protracted or recurrent hypoglycemia can result in diffuse brain injury. We have recently seen two such instances of cerebral anoxic damage—one a diabetic child with prolonged insulin shock, the other a child with congenital underdevelopment of the adrenal cortex as revealed by autopsy.

Hypoglycemia can precipitate convulsions in children who have epilepsy. In the management of the epileptic child who also has diabetes mellitus, it is important to so regulate the diet and insulin that the diurnal cycle never falls to the hypoglycemic level.

The electroencephalogram during hypoglycemia can be indistinguishable from that of epilepsy. Accordingly, no child with both diabetes mellitus and convulsions should be subjected to an encephalogram without the blood glucose being determined at the time of the readings. If the glucose level is within normal limits, any brain wave irregularities signify some other disturbance.

BLOOD GLUCOSE IN DIABETES MELLITUS

When a child first becomes ill with diabetes mellitus the prodromal symptoms usually last only a few weeks. The younger the age, the briefer this preliminary period. One almost never sees the protracted "prediabetic" disturbances shown by adults or the mild form of the disease controllable without insulin.

Parents often ignore the early symptoms of polydipsia, polyuria, loss of strength, and changes in disposition. Glycosuria, ketonuria, ketosis, and hyperglycemia are usually well advanced by the time the child comes to medical attention. On looking over 11 consecutive case histories of children hospitalized for beginning diabetes, the initial blood glucose levels before any insulin was received ranged from 200 to 480 mg per 100 ml. The fasting level did not necessarily reflect the severity of the diabetes.

In diabetic children under treatment with insulin and diet, the blood glucose is labile and difficult to regulate. During the night sleeping period the blood sugar mounts rapidly, unless a late dose of standard insulin or a substantial dose of slower-acting insulin has been given, and tends to be the highest in the morning. Moderate doses of insulin may then bring about sharp and abrupt hypoglycemia from a high hyperglycemic level previously. Soskin ascribes this so-called insulin sensitivity of the diabetic child to the high efficiency of liver function at this age. Determinations of the blood glucose levels before breakfast and at selected periods during the day help in working out the requirements of the various forms of insulin in children ill enough to require hospitalization.

It is not ordinarily necessary to carry out a glucose tolerance curve with a child who has the history and urine and blood findings typical of diabetes. The peculiar usefulness of the tolerance curve with respect to diabetes lies in ruling out the disease or in detecting the mild beginning case.

DIABETIC COMA

The child in diabetic coma is dehydrated, acidotic and in shock, with air hunger, drowsiness, vomiting, hypotension, soft eyeballs, a flushed dry skin, and acetone-smelling breath. The urine is rich in glucose, acetone, and diacetic acid, and the blood displays a raised glucose content and low carbon dioxide–combining power. Differentiation must be made from insulin overdosages when the child is a known diabetic under treatment. In the latter condition ketosis and dehydration are usually absent. When the differentiation is not immediately apparent one can administer some glucose solution orally or by vein. This therapy will correct an insulin hypoglycemia without aggravating a ketonemic hyperglycemic coma.

Insulin shock due to the effect of slow-acting insulin may give profound unconsciousness rather than convulsions. Unless the urine being excreted at the time of examination is known to contain sugar, this possibility in the diabetic patient who is unconscious should be disproved before a diagnosis of coma is made and more insulin given. Other causes of severe acidosis and deep rapid breathing must also be excluded, such as uremia, salicylate poisoning, severe infection, poisoning, cerebral hemorrhage, meningitis, or encephalitis.

The management of a child in diabetic coma calls for multiple corrections—of the dehydration, the ketosis, the mineral deficits, and the faulty carbohydrate metabolism. For best regulation of therapy it is important to determine the blood levels of glucose, CO_2-combining power, chlorides, and potassium if possible, both before beginning treatment and every 4 to 6 hours thereafter. The urine should be tested at 2-hour intervals for sugar and ketone bodies, by catheterization if necessary. The patient who does not improve satisfactorily should be reexamined carefully for signs of an occult infection or other undiscovered complication.

NEWBORN INFANTS OF DIABETIC MOTHERS

Infants born to diabetic mothers tend to have a greater average birth weight than those born to normal mothers. They have unduly high morbidity and mortality rates in both the late intrauterine and the neonatal periods. Listlessness, pallor, cyanotic spells, convulsions, muscular twitchings, circulatory failure, or erythroblastemia appears not infrequently in the first few days and may be fatal. At autopsy these infants may exhibit enlargement of the visceral organs and excessive hemopoiesis in the liver.

The blood glucose level is usually unduly high in such infants at the time of birth and falls to the moderate or marked hypoglycemic range in the first or second day. Only exceptionally, however, do infants exhibit clinical symptoms suggestive of hypoglycemia. Liberal feedings of glucose when disturbances are present usually fail to produce any immediate improvement, suggesting that the hypoglycemia bears no direct relation to the symptoms.

GLYCOGEN STORAGE DISEASE (VON GIERKE)

The systemic form of this congenital disturbance is characterized by the accumulation of excessive quantities of glycogen in the liver, kidneys, skeletal muscles, or heart, along with physical retardation of growth. Lipemia is a frequent concomitant. The severity and chief focus of the disturbance seem to vary somewhat from patient to patient. The urine may contain acetone, but usually not diacetic acid, and is free of sugar. The fasting blood glucose level tends to be a little low (around 50 to 60 mg per 100 ml). The glucose tolerance curve is described on page 504. Since patients are not able to mobilize glucose quickly from the glycogen in the liver, they go into marked hypoglycemia after 6 to 12 hours without food or when an acute infection is contracted. Their hypoglycemic response to the insulin tolerance test may be normal, or so violent as to be fatal. The blood glucose rise with the epinephrine test is negligible.

CELIAC DISEASE

The fasting blood glucose levels in children ill with the celiac syndrome have approximately the same range as in normal children. With the oral glucose tolerance test most of the curves secured will show no elevation at all or a slight rise to perhaps 20 mg per 100 ml above fasting level. Some may even have a period of actual fall of 10 to 35 mg. This low tolerance curve is customarily explained as being due to a lag in gastrointestinal absorption, but Emery's studies suggest that the body tissues may have an unusual avidity for glucose. With the intravenous insulin tolerance test Emery found the immediate fall of blood glucose to be normal, but the return to original level often protracted. Oral glucose restored the blood level when it was low after insulin. Epinephrine alone produced a rise in blood sugar which was lower and more sluggish than normal. The carbohydrate metabolism in these children thus appears to correspond with the carbohydrate metabolism found in other marasmic states.

GALACTOSEMIA

This rare and congenital inability to metabolize galactose efficiently is characterized clinically by undernutrition, galactosuria, galactosemia, and enlargement of the liver, with severe icterus in the neonatal period as a common complication. The capacity of the liver to convert and to store galactose seems impaired but not completely lost. The urinary excretion of galactose may range from 15 to 50 per cent of the intake and seems to improve after several years provided the patient survives. The galactosuria, galactosemia, and other symptoms can be eliminated by removing milk from the diet of the patient. These same symptoms can be made to recur by feeding the patient lactose and galactose once more.

The urine in these patients persistently contains enough galactose to give a 1 to 4 plus reaction with the reagents for sugar testing so long as galactose or lactose is in the diet. It usually also contains small amounts of protein but never any acetone or diacetic acid. The galactosuria and proteinuria disappear within 1 to 2 days after the feedings of these sugars are discontinued.

The fasting blood sugar level in untreated cases is typically between 150 and 300 mg per 100 ml. On fractional analysis, usually made with yeast, only part of the blood sugar proves to be fermentable glucose. The nonfermentable portion (presumably galactose) constitutes 25 to 75 per cent of the total, depending upon the character of the preceding meal.

The cerebrospinal fluid also contains galactose, in approximately the same concentration as the blood, showing that this sugar is readily diffusible into other body fluids and tissues.

In the oral galactose tolerance test, usually made by feeding 1.75 gm of galactose per kg body weight, the content of this sugar in the blood rises steeply to a peak level between 200 and 300 mg per 100 ml at 1 to 2 hours, and then subsides so slowly as not to reach the fasting level until another 4 to 6 hours. The peak is slightly higher and more prolonged when the subject is taking milk than when on a milk-free diet, but the contour remains the same. A normal child given the same test will show a peak between 50 and 75 mg in the first hour and exhibit complete removal of the galactose by 1 to 1½ hours. During the period of galactose elevation the blood glucose level in these patients becomes depressed, suggesting the existence of a reciprocally antagonistic competition between galactose and glucose within the enzyme systems of the liver. Hypoglycemic symptoms are not seen even when the blood glucose falls to negligible levels after the test administration of large amounts of galactose.

In the intravenous galactose tolerance test, made by injecting 0.5 gm of galactose per kg intravenously, the level of blood galactose remains high for several hours, and then subsides slowly as in the oral test. With normal individuals, in contrast, the galactose usually is gone by 1 hour. Tests of this sort with galactose may aggravate the symptoms.

The glucose tolerance test, whether oral or intravenous, gives a normal or flat curve, indicative of efficient utilization of glucose, provided correction is made for the galactose also present in the blood. During this test the blood galactose level may drop a little. Injection of epinephrine produces a moderate rise in the blood glucose and total blood sugar and a slight fall in the blood galactose.

BIBLIOGRAPHY

METHODOLOGY AND GENERAL FEATURES

Altschule, M. D., and *E. P. Siegel,* Inadequacy of the Glycemic Reaction to Epinephrine as a Measure of Hepatic Glycogen, *Am. J. M. Sc.* 222:50, 1951.

Bongiovanni, A. M., Use of the Glucose Tolerance Test in Pediatric Practice, *Quart. Rev. Pediat.* 10:23, 1955.

Hamwi, G. J., and *E. von Haam,* The Differential Diagnosis of Hyperglycemic States by Laboratory Methods, *Am. J. Clin. Path.* 21:701, 1951.

Jacobs, H. R., The Bound Glucosamine of Serum Mucoid in Diabetes Mellitus: Fluctuations Observed under the Influence of Insulin, *J. Lab. & Clin. Med.* 34:116, 1949.

Lowe, C. U., and *C. D. May,* Metabolic Studies in Patients with Intolerance to Complex Carbohydrates, *A.M.A. Am. J. Dis. Child.* 81:81, 1951.

Mosenthal, H. O., Evaluation of Blood Sugar Tests: Significance of the Nonglucose Reducing Substances and the Arteriovenous Blood Sugar Difference, *Quart. Bull. Northwestern Univ. M. School* 20:99, 1946.

Najjar, V. A., The Physiology and Disorders of Carbohydrate Metabolism, *J. Pediat.* 41:804, 1952.

Somersalo, O., Staub Effect in Children: Studies of the Blood Sugar Regulation by Means of Double and Triple Glucose Tolerance Tests, *Acta paediat.* suppl. 78, 1950.

Somogyi, M., Reducing Sugars and Non-sugars in Human Blood, *J. Biol. Chem.* 75:33, 1927.

Soskin, S., Use and Abuse of the Dextrose Tolerance Test, *Postgrad. Med.* 10:108, 1951.

Stadie, W. C., The Problem of the Action of Insulin, *Am. J. M. Sc.* 229:233, 1955.

Stettin, D., Jr., Metabolic Effects of Insulin, *Bull. New York Acad. Med.* 29:466, 1953.

Waters, E. T., Review of Studies on Blood Sugar, *Bull. New York Acad. Med.* 25:32, 1949.

FASTING VALUES IN INFANTS AND CHILDREN

Cornblath, M., E. Y. Levin, and *H. H. Gordon,* Studies of Carbohydrate Metabolism in the Newborn, 1. Capillary-venous Differences in Blood Sugar in Normal Newborn Infants, *Pediatrics,* 18:167, 1956.

Desmond, M. M., Observations Related to Neonatal Hypoglycemia, *J. Pediat.* 43:253, 1953.

Gittelman, I. F., and *J. B. Pincus,* Blood Sugar and Citric Acid Levels in Newborn Infants, *Pediatrics* 9:38, 1952.

Norval, M. A., Blood Sugar Values in Premature Infants, *J. Pediat.* 36:177, 1950.

———, *R. L. J. Kennedy,* and *J. Berkson,* Blood Sugar in Newborn Infants, *J. Pediat.* 34:342, 1949.

Rudesill, C. L., and *R. A. Henderson,* Normal Blood Sugar Values in Children, *Am. J. Dis. Child.* 61:108, 1941.

HYPOGLYCEMIA

Aballi, A. J., Disturbances of Carbohydrate Metabolism in Infantile Malnutrition, *Rev. cubana pediat.* 22:509, 1950.

Conn, J. W., and *H. S. Seltzer*, Spontaneous Hypoglycemia, *Am. J. Med.* **19**:460, 1955.

Fabrykant, M., and *B. I. Ashe*, Significance of Arterial Blood Sugar in Spontaneous Hypoglycemia, *Am. J. M. Sc.* **221**:61, 1951.

Greenlee, R. G., R. R. White, and *C. Phillips*, Chronic Hypoglycemia in an Infant Treated by Subtotal Pancreatectomy, *J.A.M.A.* **149**:272, 1952.

Holt, L. E., Jr., and *E. M. Bridge*, Hypoglycemia in Early Life, *Nebraska M. J.* **30**:45, 1949.

Livingston, L., and *E. M. Bridge*, Tests of Carbohydrate Metabolism in Infants, *J.A.M.A.* **119**:117, 1942.

McQuarrie, I., Idiopathic Spontaneously Occurring Hypoglycemia in Infants, *A.M.A. Am. J. Dis. Child.* **87**:399, 1954.

Roxburgh, R. C., Islet-cell Adenoma of the Pancreas in a Child Aged Seven Years, *Lancet* **1**:1057, 1954.

Schwartz, O., M. G. Goldner, J. Rosenblum, and *J. Avin*, Neonatal Hypoglycemia: Report of a Course of Unusual Duration, *Pediatrics* **16**:658, 1955.

Talbot, N. B., J. D. Crawford, and *C. C. Bailey*, Use of Mesoxalyl Urea (Alloxan) in Treatment of an Infant with Convulsions Due to Idiopathic Hypoglycemia, *Pediatrics* **1**:337, 1948.

INFANTS OF DIABETIC MOTHERS

Gilbert, J. A. L., The Association of Maternal Obesity, Large Babies and Diabetes, *Brit. M. J.* **1**:702, 1949.

Hanley, B. J., P. Horn, and *A. Farmer*, Comparative Blood Sugar Studies in the Parturient Woman and the Newborn Infant, *Am. J. Obst. & Gynec.* **46**:502, 1943.

Komrower, G. M., Blood Sugar Levels in Babies Born of Diabetic Mothers, *Arch. Dis. Childhood* **29**:28, 1954.

Miller, H. C., and *R. A. Ross*, Relation of Hypoglycemia to the Symptoms Observed in Infants of Diabetic Mothers: Report of Six Cases, *J. Pediat.* **16**:473, 1940.

Reis, R. A., E. J. DeCosta, and *M. D. Allweiss*, The Management of the Pregnant Diabetic Woman and Her Newborn Infant, *Am. J. Obst. & Gynec.* **60**:1023, 1950.

MISCELLANEOUS

Behrer, M. R., D. Goldring, and *A. F. Hartmann*, The Treatment of Diabetic Acidosis: Comparison of Treatment Regimes With and Without Parenteral Potassium, *J. Pediat.* **49**:141, 1956.

Cori, G. T., and *C. F. Cori*, Glucose-6-phosphatase of the Liver in Glycogen Storage Disease, *J. Biol. Chem.* **199** (part 2):661, 1952.

―――― and *J. L. Schulman*, Glycogen Storage Disease of the Liver. Eleven Enzymic Studies, *Pediatrics* **14**:646, 1954.

Danowski, T. S., "Diabetes Mellitus with Emphasis on Children and Young Adults," The Williams & Wilkins Company, Baltimore, 1957.

Emery, J. L., Carbohydrate Metabolism in the Coeliac Syndrome, *Arch. Dis. Childhood* **22**:41, 1947.

Guest, G. M., Diabetes Mellitus in Early Infancy, Treated without Dietary Restrictions, *Acta paediat.* **38**:196, 1949.

Hartmann, A. F., Pathologic Physiology in Some Disturbances of Carbohydrate Metabolism, *J. Pediat.* **47**:537, 1955.

Landing, B. H., and *R. Bangle, Jr.*, Glycogen Storage Disease. I. Familial Cardiac Glycogen Storage Disease: Report of Two Cases and Discussion of Relation to

Other Forms of Abnormal Glycogen Deposition, *Bull. Internat. Assoc. M. Museums* 31:84, 1950.

Schulman, J. L., and P. Saturen, Glycogen Storage Disease of the Liver. I. Clinical Studies during the Early Neonatal Period, *Pediatrics* 14:632, 1954.

Sheldon, W., and A. MacMahon, Studies in Coeliac Disease: Glucose Absorption, *Arch. Dis. Childhood* 26:446, 1951.

Sprague, R. G., and M. H. Power, Electrolyte Metabolism in Diabetic Acidosis, *J.A.M.A.* 151:970, 1953.

Stephens, J. W., and H. F. Root, Treatment of Diabetic Coma, *Postgrad. Med.* 13:164, 1953.

Van Creveld, S., Glycogen Disease, *Medicine* 18:1, 1939.

GALACTOSEMIA

Bray, P. T., R. J. Isaac, and A. G. Watkins, Galactosaemia, *Arch. Dis. Childhood* 27:341, 1951.

Hartmann, A. F., M. D. Grunwaldt, M. D. Edgar, and D. H. James, Blood Galactose in Infants and Children, *J. Pediat.* 43:1, 1953.

CHAPTER 47

Plasma Lipids

The prominent lipids of plasma are in four classes: neutral fats, free cholesterol, esterified cholesterol, and phospholipids. Collectively these are often referred to as total lipids. Except for the cholesterol, each contains some fatty acids in its molecular structure. The total of plasma fatty acids can be ascertained by measurement after hydrolysis of the plasma lipids.

The fasting levels of each of the four fractions, of the total lipids, and of the total plasma fatty acids differ widely among normal children but remain more or less constant for any single child. Accordingly, the best standard of reference for a suspected alteration in lipid constituents is a previous determination on the same individual, if available, or a reading made after the clinical disturbance has been corrected.

The discussions which follow are based on results of selected published studies. They illustrate both the poorly defined limits for normality and the significant deviations which occur in diseases which alter the normal concentrations. It will be noted that determinations of the total of serum lipids and the various major components are of practical utility in only a limited number of conditions, and then are best applied to appraising the results of therapy.

TOTAL PLASMA LIPIDS

Once the neonatal period is over, the mean fasting values for total plasma lipids undergo no systematic trend of change during childhood. There are no major sex or race differences. Representative data for normal children are listed in Table 47-1. The total increases whenever the concentration of any fractional component increases, unless some other fraction is coincidentally depressed.

The increase after a usual meal amounts to 20 to 50 per cent, contingent in height and duration on the fat content of the meal. With a high intake of butter or cream this may be 50 to 100 per cent above the preprandial reading. The rise is chiefly in the phospholipid and neutral fat components and subsides to normal in 6 to 10 hours. Because of this

517

alimentary response, all determinations of total blood lipids are best conducted with specimens collected in the morning, before breakfast is taken. Elevations are found in ketotic states.

Table 47-1. Total Plasma Lipids in Normal Children, as Reported by Various Authors (*Mg per 100 ml*)

Author	No. of children	Age distribution	Range of readings	Mean	Standard deviation
Erickson	16	5–9 years		454	±73
Thomas	24	6–14 years	480–755	620	
Radwin	54	2 months–16 years		614	±103
Hansen	22	0–2 years	326–662	519	±79.5
Hansen	28	2–15 years	415–720	558	±95.4
Boyd	29	Newborn infants	97–367	198	±80

In poorly controlled diabetes mellitus there is usually an elevation of all components—free and combined cholesterol, neutral fat, and phospholipids—and especially in the neutral fat. Lipemia of the magnitude of 1,000 or 2,000 mg per 100 ml is not uncommon. It is not known why these rises are seen only in some diabetic children. The later development of juvenile arteriosclerosis is assumed to be related to these high levels. In most children with well-regulated diabetes the lipid concentrations are within normal limits or the cholesterol fraction may be slightly elevated.

In 17 children with untreated hypothyroidism, Radwin and associates found a rise in total lipids in every instance. Readings ranged from 854 to 1,531 mg per 100 ml, with a mean of 1,104 mg. No consistent relation was seen between extent of the elevation and severity of the hypothyroidism. The values dropped to a mean of 601 mg per 100 ml after some weeks of therapy with thyroid preparations and returned to former levels within 10 weeks after discontinuance of therapy.

In the nephrotic syndrome and in glycogen storage disease the total lipid levels are almost always elevated. There is augmentation of all the constituent fractions. Neutral fat is usually the most increased. Marked fluctuations occur, with maximum rises during severest clinical activity. Readings up to 5,000 mg per 100 ml may be seen. There is no parallelism between the total or fractional blood lipid levels and those of total serum protein or total globulin.

Idiopathic Familial Hyperlipemia

This is a rare congenital error of metabolism, often associated with hepatosplenomegaly. The blood serum typically appears milky, because of a high total lipid content, which is usually between 3,000 and 9,000 mg per 100 ml in florid cases. The increase is largely in neutral fat, though the cholesterol and other lipid constituents are elevated also.

Other features of laboratory interest are huge vacuolated reticulo-endothelial cells in the bone marrow and in xanthomatous skin lesions. Family surveys occasionally discover parents or siblings with milder and asymptomatic forms of the disorder.

This form of lipemia may be differentiated from the lipemia of the nephrotic syndrome by the absence of hypoproteinemia, edema, and urinary changes and from the lipemia of glycogen storage disease by the absence of ketosis and hypoglycemic episodes.

NEUTRAL FAT

There is no simple method for the direct measurement of neutral fat (fatty acid esters of glycerol, esterified fatty acids) in plasma. Readings are made by determining the quantity of total fatty acids and then subtracting the fatty acids estimated to be in the phospholipids and cholesterol esters.

In 16 normal children aged 5 to 9 years reported by Erickson and associates, the mean value for plasma neutral fat was 100 mg per 100 ml. In Thomas' 24 children the range was 40 to 305 mg per 100 ml, with a mean of 120 ml. In 29 newborn infants described by Boyd one sample of plasma contained none, whereas the highest had a reading of 283 mg per 100 ml; the mean was 90 ± 50 mg per 100 ml. Postprandially the serum neutral fat attains a peak increase of 10 to 50 mg per 100 ml in 3 to 6 hours, and then subsides slowly.

In eight nephrotic children repeatedly studied by Thomas and associates readings above 300 mg per 100 ml were secured almost consistently. Many of the values were above 1,000 mg per 100 ml; one was as high as 3,150 mg. In diabetes mellitus not carefully regulated, the levels are often very high, 500 to 2,000 mg per 100 ml. In a patient with glycogen storage disease Thomas noted fluctuations between 1,785 and 5,420 mg per 100 ml. Elevations may occur also in severe liver disturbances and in familial hyperlipemia.

Hirsch and associates have suggested the feeding of cream containing 36 per cent butterfat as a test for evaluating pancreatic function in children suspected of having cystic fibrosis of the pancreas. With doses of 4 gm of cream fat per kg body weight, normal children exhibited an increase in blood esterified fatty acids of 56 to 211 per cent in 3 to 6 hours. Children with cystic fibrosis, on the other hand, had little or no postprandial rise.

TOTAL CHOLESTEROL

The levels in normal children and in infants above 2 months of age fall in approximately the same range as those of adults. Representative values are listed in Table 47-2. Values at birth are low, but a rise begins immediately. By the fourth day many infants have attained serum levels

Table 47-2. Plasma Cholesterol Values in Normal Children, as Reported by Various Authors

Authors	No. of observations	Age distribution	Total cholesterol (mg/100 ml)		Free cholesterol (mg/100 ml)		Cholesterol esters (mg/100 ml)	
			Range of readings	Mean	Range of readings	Mean	Range of readings	Mean
Hodges et al.	417	2 months–13 years	82–180	206 ± 38	17–46	35	109–235	183
Erickson et al.	16	6–14 years	130–275	143	40–140	70	75–255	140
Thomas	24	2 months–12 years		210				
Offenkrantz and Karshan	325	2 months–16 years	107–299	184 ± 38		51 ± 10		
Radwin et al.	54	0–2 years		193 ± 28	24–79	47 ± 10		
Hansen	22	2–15 years		176 ± 32				
Hansen	28	2–13 years		199 ± 26				
Bruch	89	(obese)	108–301	200 ± 38				
Boyd	29	Newborn	17–86	34 ± 15	6–29	14 ± 7	0–57	20 ± 12
Sperry		Newborn	50–70					
Sperry	71	4–25 days	71–190	133 ± 25	25–61	46	36–126	86
Whitelaw	9	Newborn	51–96	71				

deemed normal for adults, and by 1 to 2 months of age nearly all are at the adult level.

In Whitelaw's series of premature newborn infants the mean of 71 mg was of the same order of magnitude as in full-term newborn infants. The absolute levels and partition of serum cholesterol did not vary with degree of prematurity. The cholesterol levels of mother and infant bore no relationship to each other.

Unlike the phospholipids and neutral fats, the cholesterol components of the blood remain more or less constant throughout the day. Ordinary meals are not followed by a rise in plasma level, though a large test dose of a sterol-containing fat may induce an elevation of about 10 per cent of the initial value for a few hours. Eczema induces no abnormalities, according to Hansen. In the 89 obese children studied by Bruch, the total cholesterol bore no relation to the basal metabolic rate and was not affected by thyroid medication or its interruption.

Hypercholesterolemia

The level of total cholesterol tends to be elevated in the nephrotic syndrome, hypothyroidism, diabetes mellitus, glycogen storage disease, some forms of liver disease, and some forms of xanthomatosis. It frequently rises during therapy with cortisone or corticotropin, receding when these hormones are withdrawn; it is often elevated in Cushing's syndrome.

In children with the nephrotic syndrome the levels for total cholesterol range usually from 200 to 1,000 mg per 100 ml but may be higher or lower.

In hypothyroid children over 1 or 2 years of age the serum cholesterol is usually above 280 mg per 100 ml and may go to 600 mg or more. The total and fractional lipids and the plasma carotene are also increased, and carotenemia may be recognizable clinically. Wilkins and Fleischmann have pointed out that after thyroid medication has been discontinued in a hypothyroid child, the serum cholesterol level mounts within 6 to 12 months to much higher levels. Since this does not take place in children who are not hypothyroid, the long-range curve for serum cholesterol during and after a period of thyroid therapy can be used as a diagnostic test in questionable cases.

When an infant is being surveyed for causes of idiocy, the determination of blood cholesterol as an index of possible hypothyroidism is not very helpful. The hypercholesterolemia characteristic of hypothyroidism does not usually become apparent until after the first or second year of age. The protein-bound iodine determination is a much more satisfactory indicator for this purpose.

The hypothyroidism of pituitary origin is commonly not associated with high serum cholesterol. The failure to rise may be related to the usually poor nutrition of these individuals.

In most children with liver disease the total cholesterol and the various lipid fractions exhibit no recognized changes. Hypercholesterolemia sometimes appears with congenital biliary tract obstruction, or occasionally with hepatitis or cirrhosis in which jaundice due to intrahepatic obstruction is prominent. This increase may involve both the free and the esterified cholesterol, particularly the former. With severe liver injury the total cholesterol may be depressed, especially in the esterified portion.

In diabetes mellitus the total serum cholesterol is often elevated. The cholesterol partition ratio is customarily within normal limits.

In six diabetic children described by Thomas, for example, the level was between 185 and 300 mg per 100 ml. In their follow-up study of young adults whose diabetes had begun in childhood Jackson and associates found a mean total serum cholesterol of 401.8 ± 138 (standard deviation) mg per 100 ml in 6 whose regulatory control had been consistently poor, and of 233.6 ± 52 in 21 whose control had been consistently good. The incidence of hypertension, proteinuria, and fundal arteriosclerosis was higher in the group which had been poorly regulated.

Mention may be made of so-called Mauriac's syndrome encountered in children whose diabetes mellitus is poorly regulated. This is characterized by enlargement of the liver, retardation of growth, hyperglycemia, glycosuria, and hypercholesterolemia with levels above 500 mg per 100 ml. The disturbance is reversible and can be cleared in a few months by regulation of the insulin and dietary requirements.

In glycogen storage disease the blood cholesterol may show a marked augmentation and the neutral fat and other lipid constituents are also increased. Values of over 2,000 mg per 100 ml for cholesterol alone have been reported.

Attention is being directed to an asymptomatic condition known as hereditary hypercholesterolemia. This seems to be most prevalent (an estimated 5 per cent of adults) in the Jewish population group. The only criterion thus far available for its recognition is that some members of a family have a total serum cholesterol level (Sperry-Schoenheimer method) above 280 mg per 100 ml in the absence of other known cause.

Dermatologists find the determination of serum cholesterol and other lipids helpful in studying xanthomatous disorders with lipid deposits in the skin. The levels are not elevated with simple skin xanthomas of the xanthoma disseminatum group or with xanthomas associated with eosinophilic granulomas and the Hand-Schüller-Christian syndrome. On the other hand, elevations are encountered in xanthoma tuberosum, poorly regulated diabetes mellitus, and the chronic disorders already discussed.

Hypocholesterolemia

The level of total serum cholesterol falls rather consistently in the low normal or subnormal range (below 150 mg per 100 ml) in malnutrition, acute and chronic infections, severe parenchymal liver diseases, hyperthyroidism, and severe forms of anemia. The feeding of a cholesterol-free diet for a prolonged period may lower the blood cholesterol to some extent; moderate restrictions of dietary cholesterol have little effect upon the level.

RELATION OF ESTER CHOLESTEROL TO FREE
CHOLESTEROL (CHOLESTEROL PARTITION)

In normal children the uncombined cholesterol may range from 25 to 150 mg per 100 ml, with an average of approximately 75 mg. The combined cholesterol, i.e., combined with fatty acids, or esterified, varies widely from about 70 to about 250 mg per 100 ml (Table 47-2). In the young infant both readings are lower.

After the neonatal period the proportion between the two forms of cholesterol in states of health normally remains within narrow limits. The quantitative relationships can be expressed as the ratio of the ester to the free form, or the reverse, or as the percentage of the total cholesterol which is constituted by either one of these forms. Expressed generally, 65 to 75 per cent of the cholesterol in the child's plasma is combined or ester cholesterol, and the remaining 25 to 35 per cent is free cholesterol.

In Sperry's series of young infants the ratio of ester to total cholesterol ranged from 0.7 to 2.6, equivalent to between 41 and 72 per cent; in every infant 2 weeks of age and over the ratio was higher than 2.0. Physiologic icterus seemed to exert no effect on this ratio or on the level of total cholesterol. Deviations in the proportion of the two forms are not uncommon in disease states. The ratio of combined to free cholesterol was found by Hodges, Sperry, and Andersen to average 2.15 ± 0.36 in 78 children with malnutrition; 2.32 ± 0.26 in 38 children with severe anemia of various kinds; 1.94 ± 0.35 in 14 children with infection not complicated by loss of weight; 0.64 ± 0.38 in 15 children with congenital atresia of the bile ducts. In 10 patients with acute catarrhal jaundice the ratio fell to low levels during the acute stage and promptly returned toward normal with fall of temperature and clearing of clinical icterus. In 11 patients with nonobstructive liver cirrhosis (Laennec type) there was no significant fall below normal except when infection was superimposed.

In the nephrotic syndrome and in hypothyroidism, even though both the ester cholesterol and the free cholesterol are elevated, the ratio between these substances is ordinarily not altered. In 89 children with obesity Bruch found a normal ratio of 2.6 ± 0.24.

Comparison of the free and esterified forms in the serum is sometimes used as a liver test in the differential diagnosis of jaundice, since the esterified fraction tends to be diminished in many forms of liver disease. The ratio may be said to be altered significantly when the cholesterol ester fraction is less than 50 per cent of the total cholesterol.

Cholesterol and Arteriosclerosis

Cholesterol metabolism seems to be somehow linked to human arteriosclerosis, but the evidence is fragmentary and controversial. Extensive atheromatous deposits tend to form prematurely in disease in which the serum lipids are much increased, as in uncontrolled diabetes mellitus, hypothyroidism, the nephrotic syndrome, and the hyperlipemic xanthomatoses. Normal individuals whose cholesterol levels are in the higher ranges are thought to be more prone to the later development of arteriosclerosis.

Though the habitual intake of cholesterol bears no significant correlation to the fasting serum cholesterol level, complete elimination of cholesterol from the diet for several weeks will bring about a moderate decline in the serum level. Such diets are essentially fat-free as well, and there are some data which imply that fat is just as important as cholesterol in maintaining the level of serum cholesterol. The relation between dietary cholesterol and serum levels is most complex, inasmuch as the liver and other organs are capable of synthesizing cholesterol and apparently do so regularly; tissue synthesis may become accelerated when cholesterol is not being ingested.

PLASMA PHOSPHOLIPIDS

This class comprises the lecithins, cephalins, sphingomyelins, and cerebrosides. Their approximate total can be calculated by multiplying the inorganic phosphate found in the hydrolyzed lipid extract by the factor 26.

In Stearns and Warweg's series of normal children of all ages the serum phospholipids (expressed as *lipid phosphorus*) averaged 5.3 mg per 100 ml in the newborn period, rose rapidly in early infancy, and more slowly during late infancy. They reached a maximum of 9.6 mg at 2 years, then fell to 8.6 mg by the fourth year, and remained at this level throughout childhood and early adolescence. The range for total phospholipids was between 9 and 14 mg per 100 ml of whole blood; the mean was near 10.5 mg in the first few months, and 12 mg thereafter. The individual values had a wide range of variation.

Adlersberg, Schaefer, et al. found mean serum phospholipid levels of approximately 227 mg per 100 ml for boys aged 3 to 17. For girls the means were 262 mg at ages 3 through 7; 242 mg at ages 8 through 12; and 236 mg at ages 13 through 17.

The serum phospholipid level often rises to approximately double the normal in diabetes mellitus, the nephrotic syndrome, and untreated hypothyroidism, and occasionally in many other diseases.

SERUM LIPOPROTEINS

The major portion of the blood lipids is combined with large protein molecules (*lipoproteins*) and thereby becomes miscible with plasma. These lipoprotein macromolecules as they occur in human serum have been studied by Gofman and associates by measuring their rates of movement (S_f, Svedberg units of flotation) in an ultracentrifugal field.

The following classes have been identified: (1) Those with migration values greater than 75 S_f units. These increase following fat-containing meals and hence represent part of acute alimentary lipemia. Chylomicrons are included in this fraction. (2) Those with migration values between 30 and 70 S_f units. These constitute the major fraction of acute alimentary lipemia and fluctuate widely in relation to meals. (3) Those with migration values between 10 and 20 S_f units. Having molecular weights in the neighborhood of 3 million, these are said to be in abnormally high concentrations in the blood of adults with atherosclerosis or diseases associated with atherosclerosis (old myocardial infarction, diabetes mellitus, the nephrotic syndrome, hypothyroidism, coronary artery insufficiency). When the daily intake of dietary cholesterol is restricted to 200 mg or less and the dietary fat to 50 gm or less for 4 weeks or longer, the concentration of these molecules in adult patients becomes lowered. (4) Those with migration values between 3 and 10 S_f units. These contain cholesterol, phospholipid, and protein. They carry a major fraction of the serum cholesterol, in concentrations differing among individuals but at essentially constant levels in the same individual. They do not appear to be related to atherosclerosis.

Kempe, Silver, Smyth, Gofman, and Jones have reported on the levels of lipoproteins of the S_f 10–20 class in 147 children from birth to 15 years of age. The distributions of values for both sexes were approximately identical. In 26 boys and 20 girls aged 7 to 20 years with diabetes mellitus the serum levels of the S_f 10–20 class were higher than in normal boys and girls of the same age. No close correlation was found between the serum levels, the diabetic phenomena, the serum cholesterol levels, or the dietary intake of fat.

Rosenthal and associates found exceptionally high concentrations of serum lipoproteins in a child with progeria.

CHYLOMICRON COUNTS

By enumerating the emulsified particles of fat in the serum at half-hour intervals for 3 or 4 hours after a fatty meal, one obtains a curve of *chylomicron count* which is presumably the reflection of the rate of intestinal absorption of the unhydrolyzed fat particles.

In the procedure introduced by Frazer and Stewart a specimen of blood is first taken from the finger tip in the morning, after an overnight fast. A test meal of fat is then given. This may consist of heavy cream, in amounts of

30 ml per kg body weight, with a maximum of 120 ml. No other foods or liquids are given until the studies are over. Capillary blood specimens are then taken at hourly intervals for 3 to 5 hours. These are centrifuged, and the serum studied on a glass slide with a darkfield microscope, counts being made of the numbers of particles of visible fat in a single horizontal plane of an oil-immersion field or a standardized fraction thereof. The centrifuging is sometimes omitted. The rise and fall in the curve after a fatty meal—the *chylomicrograph*—should take about 5 hours. Meals composed of fat-free or essentially fat-free foods do not give rise to chylomicronemia, and the serum remains clear and free of large particles.

For example, in healthy children studied by Sheldon and MacMahon the chylomicron curves began to rise in the first hour and reached a maximum averaging 53 particles per field in 2 to 3 hours. In children with untreated true celiac disease the curves were much flatter, exhibiting a maximum rise at about 3 hours but with an average of only 20 particles per field. This suggests that particulate fat absorption is defective in the florid phase of true celiac disease. Similar impairment of absorption in cystic fibrosis of the pancreas has been reported by Elghammer, Reichert, and Philipsborn.

A more precise though more involved technique for measuring fat particles in serum is the nephelometric method of Moreton. This utilizes an intense parallel beam of light passed through a small glass cell. At right angles to the beam, and carefully shielded from it, is a sensitive photoelectric cell which measures only the light scattered by the particulate matter in the serum (the Tyndall effect). The intensity of this light will be proportional both to the number and the size of the chylomicrons.

BIBLIOGRAPHY

NORMAL BLOOD AND PLASMA LIPIDS

Adlersberg, D., L. E. Schaefer, A. G. Steinberg, and *C. I. Wang,* Age, Sex, Serum Lipids and Coronary Atherosclerosis, *J.A.M.A.* 162:619, 1956.

Boyd, E. M., Lipid Composition of Blood in New-born Infants, *Am. J. Dis. Child.* 52:1319, 1936.

Bruch, H., Obesity in Childhood: II. Physical Growth and Development of Obese Children, *Am. J. Dis. Child.* 58:1001, 1939.

Erickson, B. N., H. J. Sonders, M. L. Shepherd, D. M. Teague, and *H. H. Williams,* Relation between Cerebroside and Neutral Fat Contents of Blood Plasma, Erythrocytes and Stroma, *Proc. Soc. Exper. Biol. & Med.* 45:153, 1940.

———, *H. H. Williams, F. C. Hummel,* and *I. G. Macy,* The Lipid and Mineral Distribution in the Serum and Erythrocytes of Normal Children, *J. Biol. Chem.* 118:15, 1937.

Gofman, J. W., H. B. Jones, F. T. Lindgren, T. P. Lyon, H. A. Elliott, and *B. Strisower,* Blood Lipids and Human Atherosclerosis, *Circulation* 2:161, 1950.

Hodges, R. G., W. M. Sperry, and *D. H. Andersen,* Serum Cholesterol Values for Infants and Children, *Am. J. Dis. Child.* 65:858, 1943.

Kempe, C. H., H. K. Silver, F. S. Smyth, J. W. Gofman, and *H. B. Jones,* The Lipoproteins of Serum in Infancy and Childhood. I. Lipoproteins in Normal Children, *J. Pediat.* 40:11, 1952.

Man, E. B., and *J. P. Peters,* Variations of Serum Lipids with Age, *J. Lab. & Clin. Med.* 41:738, 1953.

Offenkrantz, F. M., and *M. Karshan,* Serum Cholesterol Values for Children, *Am. J. Dis. Child.* 52:784, 1936.

Peters, J. P., and *D. D. Van Slyke,* "Quantitative Clinical Chemistry," vol. I, "Interpretations," The Williams & Wilkins Company, Baltimore, 1931.

Sperry, W. M., Cholesterol of the Blood Plasma in the Neonatal Period, *Am. J. Dis. Child.* 51:84, 1936.

Stark, V. J. M., The Blood Cholesterol Content in Childhood, *Arch. Dis. Childhood* 15:255, 1940.

Stearns, G., and *E. Warweg,* Studies of Phosphorus of Blood. I. The Partition of Phosphorus in Whole Blood and Serum: The Serum Calcium and Plasma Phosphatase from Birth to Maturity, *J. Biol. Chem.* 102:749, 1933.

Thomas, E. M., Total and Fractional Blood Lipid Levels in Diseases of Childhood, *Am. J. Dis. Child.* 74:563, 1947.

CHYLOMICRON COUNTS

Elghammer, W. R., J. M. Reichert, and *H. F. Philipsborn,* Postprandial Lipemic Response in Infants and Children, *Pediatrics* 5:621, 1950.

Fourman, L. P. R., The Chylomicron Count in Normal Subjects and Patients with Sprue, *Tr. Roy. Soc. Trop. Med. & Hyg.* 41:537, 1948.

Frailing, J. M., and *C. I. Owen,* Chylomicrons of Blood: A Resume of Literature and a Recommended Counting Procedure, *Am. J. Clin. Path.* 21:508, 1951.

Frazer, A. C., and *H. C. Stewart,* The Interpretation of the Normal Chylomicrograph, *J. Physiol.* 95:23P, 1939.

Moreton, J. R., Chylomicronemia, Fat Tolerance and Atherosclerosis, *J. Lab. & Clin. Med.* 35:373, 1950.

Sheldon, W., and *A. MacMahon,* Studies in Coeliac Disease: Fat Absorption, *Arch. Dis. Childhood* 24:245, 1949.

Zinn, W. J., and *G. C. Griffith,* A Study of Serum Fat Globules in Atherosclerotic and Non-atherosclerotic Male Subjects, *Am. J. M. Sc.* 220:597, 1950.

IDIOPATHIC FAMILIAL HYPERLIPEMIA

Bruton, O. C., and *A. J. Kanter,* Idiopathic Familial Hyperlipemia, *A.M.A. Am. J. Dis. Child.* 82:153, 1951.

Gaskins, A. L., R. B. Scott, and *A. D. Kessler,* Report of Three Cases of Idiopathic Familial Hyperlipemia: Use of ACTH and Cortisone, *Pediatrics* 11:480, 1953.

Holt, L. E., Jr., F. X. Aylward, and *H. G. Timbres,* Idiopathic Familial Lipemia, *Bull. Johns Hopkins Hosp.* 64:279, 1939.

PLASMA LIPIDS IN DISEASE STATES

Adlersberg, D., L. E. Schaefer, and *S. R. Drachman,* The Incidence of Hereditary Hypercholesteremia, *J. Lab. & Clin. Med.* 39:237, 1952.

Bridge, E. M., and *L. E. Holt, Jr.,* Glycogen Storage Disease: Observations on the Pathologic Physiology of Two Cases of the Hepatic Form of the Disease, *J. Pediat.* 27:299, 1945.

Carr, J. H., C. H. Kempe, H. K. Silver, F. S. Smyth, J. W. Gofman, and *H. B. Jones,*

The Lipoproteins of Serum in Infancy and Childhood. II. Lipoprotein Levels in Juvenile Diabetes Mellitus, *J. Pediat.* 40:19, 1952.

De Rodriguez, M. L. S., Sindromo de Mauriac en niños diabeticos, *Arch. pediat. Uruguay* 20:587, 1949.

Hansen, A. E., Serum Lipids in Eczema and in Other Pathologic Conditions, *Am. J. Dis. Child.* 53:933, 1937.

Harslöf, E., Idiopathic Familial Hyperlipemia Attended with Hepato-splenomegaly, *Acta med. scandinav.* 130:140, 1948.

Hirsch, E. F., L. Carbonaro, A. D. Biggs, and F. L. Phillips, Postprandial Hypolipemia of Pancreatic Fibrocystic Disease: A Diagnostic Test, *A.M.A. Am. J. Dis. Child.* 86:721, 1953.

Jackson, R. L., R. C. Hardin, G. L. Walker, A. B. Hendricks, and H. G. Kelly, Degenerative Changes in Young Diabetic Patients in Relationship to Level of Control, *Pediatrics* 5:959, 1950.

Radwin, L. S., J. P. Michelson, J. Melnick, and S. Gottfried, Blood Lipid Partition in Hypothyroidism of Childhood, *Am. J. Dis. Child.* 60:1120, 1940.

Rosenthal, I. M., I. P. Bronstein, F. D. Dallenbach, S. Pruzansky, and A. K. Rosenwald, Progeria: Report of a Case with Cephalometric Roentgenograms and Abnormally High Concentrations of Lipoproteins in the Serum, *Pediatrics* 18:565, 1956.

Schick, B., and W. M. Sperry, Essential Xanthomatosis: Fifteen Years' Observation on a Case Occurring in a Family with Hypercholesteremia, *Am. J. Dis. Child.* 77:164, 1949.

Stoesser, A. V., and I. McQuarrie, Influence of Acute Infection and Artificial Fever on the Plasma Lipids, *Am. J. Dis. Child.* 49:658, 1935.

Thannhauser, S. J., Serum Lipids and Their Value in Diagnosis, *New England J. Med.* 237:546, 1947.

Thomas, E. M., A. H. Rosenblum, H. B. Lander, and R. Fisher, Relationships between Blood Lipid and Blood Protein Levels, in the Nephrotic Syndrome, *A.M.A. Am. J. Dis. Child.* 81:207, 1951.

van Creveld, S., Glycogen Disease, *Medicine* 18:1, 1939.

Whitelaw, M. J., The Serum Cholesterol Level of the Prematurely Born Infant and Its Mother, *J. Clin. Invest.* 27:260, 1948.

Wilkins, L., and W. Fleischmann, Hypothyroidism in Childhood. III. The Effect of Withdrawal of Thyroid Therapy upon the Serum Cholesterol: Relationship of Cholesterol, Basal Metabolic Rate, Weight and Clinical Symptoms, *J. Clin. Endocrinol.* 1:91, 1941.

———, ———, and W. Block, Hypothyroidism in Childhood. I. The Basal Metabolic Rate, Serum Cholesterol and Urinary Creatine before Treatment. II. Sensitivity to Thyroid Medication as Measured by the Serum Cholesterol and the Creatine Excretion, *J. Clin. Endocrinol.* 1:3; 1:14; 1941.

Wilkinson, C. F., Jr., Essential Familial Hypercholesterolemia: Cutaneous, Metabolic and Hereditary Aspects, *Bull. New York Acad. Med.* 26:670, 1950.

CHAPTER 48

Nonprotein Nitrogenous Constituents

TOTAL NONPROTEIN NITROGEN (NPN)

This is a heterogeneous mixture of soluble nitrogen-containing compounds, with urea constituting about half the total in normal subjects. Uric acid, creatinine, creatine, and amino acids are present in lesser degree, and ammonia, nitrates, polypeptides, purines, glutathione, and miscellaneous other substances in trace amounts.

Total NPN is measured usually by the Folin-Wu method, after prior precipitation of the serum proteins with sodium tungstate and sulfuric acid. For whole blood the normal for NPN through infancy and childhood ranges from 20 to 40 mg per 100 ml and is usually below 30 mg. For serum the normal varies from 10 to 30 mg per 100 mg and is usually below 20 mg.

At the moment of birth the concentrations of total nonprotein nitrogen and its major components are essentially the same in both mother and fetus. This indicates free diffusion of these substances across the placenta. In the neonatal period the averages are a little higher.

When renal excretion of nitrogenous substances is impaired (*azotemia*), values between 40 and 300 mg per 100 ml will be encountered. Up to 90 per cent of this increment in total NPN may be due to urea retention. Peters and Van Slyke give the formula NPN = 10 + 1.07 × urea N to describe the approximate relationship between urea and the nonurea nonprotein nitrogenous constituents in both normal conditions and states of disease.

UREA NITROGEN

Urea is the chief end product of protein catabolism. It is formed in the liver from arginine, glutamine, and perhaps other circulating amides. Being highly soluble, it permeates uniformly both the water-containing spaces and the interior of the tissue cells. Excretion is almost entirely through the kidney. Trace amounts occur in the perspiration and other body secretions, but not much is lost by these routes except when perspiration is marked. Urea will act as a diuretic agent in the normal subject

529

when food or tissue proteins are being catabolized rapidly or when the intake of urea itself is excessive.

The blood urea level reflects the intake and breakdown of protein and the efficiency of the kidneys. A meal rich in protein will evoke a transitory rise except when a large volume of water is taken concurrently; in the latter event there may even be a postprandial drop as a reflection of the diuretic influence of the water. To eliminate the influence of recent meals the best time to secure a blood sample is in the morning before breakfast, while the patient is in the resting or so-called postabsorptive phase.

Normal Concentrations

Blood urea levels are customarily expressed in terms of the nitrogen content, in order to permit comparison with the nonprotein nitrogen. Each molecule of urea, with molecular weight of 60, contains two atoms of nitrogen, with atomic weight 14. Hence urea concentration can be calculated from urea nitrogen concentrations by multiplying the latter by 60/28, or 2.14.

In normal infants and children the fasting blood urea nitrogen concentration ranges usually from 8 to 22 mg per 100 ml, with a mean of about 12 mg. The higher levels are found in those who habitually take a high protein diet and small amounts of fluid.

The neonatal rise is a consequence of the active endogenous protein metabolism and the comparatively low intake and output of fluid. In a series of infants studied by McCance and Widdowson, the average urea N rose from 18.9 mg per 100 ml at birth to 29.1 mg on the third day of life, subsided to 19.7 mg on the sixth day, and became stable by the eighth or ninth day.

Rothe-Meyer observed lower blood levels during the first 2 weeks of life among breast-fed prematurely born infants than among those receiving cow's-milk formulas, though readings up to 40 mg per 100 ml were shown by individual members of each group. By 4 weeks of age the levels in nearly all the breast-fed infants had subsided to between 5 and 15 mg per 100 ml, whereas in the bottle-fed infants the levels were still between 20 and 40 mg, or even higher.

In premature infants the blood concentration of urea is usually in direct proportion to the protein intake. Barnett has demonstrated that the fasting levels in such infants can be made to rise from below 5 to over 40 mg per 100 ml by raising the protein intake progressively from 1 to 9 gm per kg body weight per day.

Retention up to 60 mg per 100 ml of blood or more may be induced in younger infants free from disease or dehydration by feeding a high intake of protein. This azotemia may be accompanied by slight proteinuria and cylindruria. Similar responses may occur when an infant with the celiac syndrome is given casein hydrolysate or a high protein diet. These urinary phenomena along with the blood nitrogen retention may simulate mild nephritis, but the changes revert quickly to normal when the high protein or amino acid intake is reduced.

Abnormal Increases

The blood urea N level is elevated whenever sufficient acute or chronic parenchymal damage has occurred in the kidney to seriously impair the excretory functions. The more advanced the lesions the higher the level of accumulated urea, generally speaking. The nitrogen content of the food and the rate of endogenous protein metabolism are contributory influences. Readings up to 500 mg per 100 ml or even higher have been seen in extremely ill children with severe renal disease. Retention of urea, however, is not responsible for the toxic symptoms exhibited by the "uremic" patient (p. 422).

Diseases of the kidney which may transiently or permanently elevate the blood urea include acute and chronic renal diseases, bichloride of mercury and other poisonings, acute hemoglobinuria, and neoplastic infiltration of the kidneys. With exceptionally low systolic blood pressure, as in circulatory failure due to heart disease, the sluggish glomerular filtration rate may permit the urea in the filtrate to be reabsorbed almost entirely by the tubules. The blood urea is often elevated in diabetic acidosis, oxalosis, cerebral hemorrhage, acute hyperparathyroidism, severe diarrhea, intestinal obstruction, endocrinal disorders with either hypo- or hyperactivity of the adrenal cortex (e.g., Addison's disease, adrenocorticism), massive hemorrhages into the gastrointestinal tract, and the oliguria which sometimes follows major surgical operations; also in severe febrile infections, when protein catabolism is accelerated and not enough fluids are being taken to sustain a liberal output of urine.

Doxiadis analyzed the case histories of 47 sick infants under 1 year of age who had blood urea levels between 50 and 500 mg per 100 ml. The common etiologic factor seemed to be dehydration. In general, higher urea levels were associated with greater rises in hematocrit and falls in body weight, but exceptions were many. Those infants who died despite rehydration and correction of the azotemia had no renal lesions at autopsy, whereas those whose blood urea levels remained elevated after relief of the dehydration exhibited degenerative changes in the renal tubular epithelium. Doxiadis concluded that a blood urea level which continues to mount after relief of rehydration is a sign of an organic renal lesion and carries a poor prognosis.

Readings often reach 50 to 200 mg per 100 ml in children dying from infection or any debilitating disease. Dehydration, hypotension, anoxia, increased destruction of tissue proteins, toxic substances from necrotic or infected tissues, and degeneration in the renal tubular epithelium are participant causes. That the urine specific gravity is often low in such illnesses indicates that the urea retention is more than a response to simple dehydration.

Subsidence of an elevated blood urea level, whatever the character of the renal lesion, usually means an improvement in renal function. In chronic nephritis, however, the loss of concentrating power and consequent polyuria may pull down the level of blood urea while the patient's clinical condition is actually growing worse.

Unusually Low Concentrations

Subnormal values for blood urea may be found in starvation states with a low rate of nitrogen catabolism, in untreated diabetes insipidus due to washing out of urea, and in acute diseases of the liver which are severe enough to impair urea-producing capacity.

URIC ACID

The uric acid of the blood and urine comes in part from endogenous breakdown of the proteins of the tissues and in part from the proteins of the food. Uric acid is the final product of the catabolism of the nucleic acids, the nucleotides, and the purine bases adenine and guanine. Some may perhaps be derived from the pyrimidine bases thymine and cytosine.

Not all the uric acid leaves the body by way of the urine; an indeterminate portion is destroyed by the body, and some is excreted in the bile. As brought out in the review of Peters and Van Slyke, the entire story of uric acid metabolism remains peculiarly obscure despite a half century of intensive work devoted to it. The uric acid levels in whole blood of healthy children usually fall between 0.6 and 3.2 mg per 100 ml, with an average in the neighborhood of 2.0 mg.

Abnormal Increases

The blood uric acid may become transitorily elevated during the course of acute infections. In chronic retention of nitrogenous end products due to renal disease the level is usually elevated also, but with no direct relation to the extent of retention of other nitrogenous products or to the severity of any uremic symptoms present. The blood nitrogen level is often elevated in advanced leukemia, as an accompaniment of the accelerated production and metabolism of the leukocytes. Renal insufficiency from precipitated urates in the tubules may follow the sudden dissolution of myriads of leukemic cells when chemotherapy is first given.

Gout is the most specific of the diseases with a high blood uric acid concentration. The blood levels in untreated gout usually range between 3 and 16 mg per 100 ml. Solid urates may be deposited in the tissues. The degree of hyperuricemia bears no obvious relation to the severity of the disease or to the frequency of exacerbations. Some patients with gout have blood uric acid levels within the normal range. The disease is almost never seen in infancy, but appears occasionally in early childhood when there is a strong hereditary history. At least 2 per cent of adult patients put the date of their initial symptoms at some time in their second decade.

Gout which has its first symptoms during childhood or adolescence usually displays a rapid progression of symptoms and leads to pronounced disability. In many such instances the nature of the disorder is not suspected until the deformities have become advanced. Surveys in patients' families frequently uncover asymptomatic individuals with abnormally high blood uric acid levels. These individuals are deemed to be either potential cases or genetic carriers of the trait with the capacity to transmit it to their offspring.

CREATININE

This, the internal anhydride of creatine or methylguanidine-acetic acid, is produced by the muscles. It normally occurs in the blood of normal children in a range between 0.5 and 3.0 mg per 100 ml and is usually approximately 1.5 mg or less. In chronic renal disease the level may rise to 4 or 5 mg per 100 ml or higher. It is elevated more often in chronic nephritis than in acute nephritis or in the nonrenal conditions which sometimes induce a rise in blood urea.

The chief clinical interest in creatinine lies in its urinary excretion. The excretion of the small quantities of creatinine normally present in blood seems to be entirely by way of the glomeruli. Furthermore, when the kidneys are normal the amount excreted per 24 hours can be used as an index of endogenous protein metabolism.

The so-called endogenous creatinine clearance is a renal function test based on the rate of excretion of metabolically produced creatinine by the kidneys and is conducted according to the same quantitative principles as the urea clearance test. After correction for differences in body surface area the rate of creatinine clearance as computed from studies of blood and urine is about the same in normal children of all ages. In early life and in malnutritional states this clearance is reduced. The values for endogenous creatinine clearance are usually parallel to those obtained with inulin clearance tests on the same subjects.

OTHER NITROGENOUS PRODUCTS

The normal serum level of amino acids is about 6 to 7 mg per 100 ml and has been said to double or even triple in malnutrition. Creatine concentration is usually less than 0.6 mg per 100 ml.

BIBLIOGRAPHY

NONPROTEIN NITROGEN

Barnett, H. L., and *J. Vesterdal,* The Physiologic and Clinical Significance of Immaturity of Kidney Function in Young Infants, *J. Pediat.* 42:99, 1953.

Bernstein, S. S., Gout in Early Life, *J. Mt. Sinai Hosp.* 14:747, 1947.

Doxiadis, S. A., Azotaemia in Infancy, *Arch. Dis. Childhood* 23:50, 1948.

Hoffman, W. S., Metabolism of Uric Acid and Its Relation to Gout, *J.A.M.A.* 154:213, 1954.

McCance, R. A., and *E. M. Widdowson,* Blood-Urea in the First Nine Days of Life, *Lancet* 1:787, 1947.

Peters, J. P., and *D. D. Van Slyke,* "Quantitative Clinical Chemistry," vol. 1, "Interpretations," The Williams & Wilkins Company, Baltimore, 1931.

Roscoe, M. H., The Estimation of Creatinine in Serum, *J. Clin. Path.* 6:201, 1953.

Rothe-Meyer, A., High Protein Nutrition in Prematures, *Acta paediat.* suppl. 77, p. 109, 1949.

CHAPTER 49

Plasma Proteins

The plasma proteins form a complex interdissolved mixture made up of many individual components. Those which have been separated out or are of known clinical significance include fibrinogen; several fractions of albumin and globulin; several complement components; enzyme precursors (prothrombin, plasminogen); enzymes (thrombin, plasmin, amylase, lipase, peptidase, esterase, alkaline phosphatase); and portions which carry lipid fractions, vitamins, hormones, and minerals.

Acting collectively the plasma proteins are largely responsible for maintaining the colloid osmotic pressure of the blood and the distribution of water between blood and tissues. The albumin, with its lower molecular weight and higher net negative charge at the pH of blood, is much more important than the globulin or fibrinogen for this activity.

Many empirically developed laboratory tests are based upon alterations in the fractional composition of the plasma. Elevation of the sedimentation rate is referable in part to an increase in fibrinogen or globulin. A positive thymol turbidity reaction depends upon elevated globulins and lipids, which precipitate a globulin-thymol-lipid complex. The colloidal gold test is influenced by the globulin content and its relationship to albumin. Cephalin cholesterol flocculation is due primarily to depressive alteration in the albumin fraction.

METHODOLOGY

A variety of methods are used to study the total plasma proteins and their respective fractions. The more important are chemical precipitation, Tiselius electrophoresis, ultracentrifugation, immunochemical study, and amino acid analysis.

Whenever data on plasma protein fractions are given, the method employed should be stated and the nomenclature should conform to that customary with that method. With precipitation approaches the nature and concentration of the precipitant should be made known. Values differ with techniques. Comparisons of values under standardized conditions are more important than absolute figures.

Circulatory stagnation at the time of collection of blood samples for protein

535

studies may result in transfer of water from the vessels into the tissues. Nordmann found, for example, that when two blood samples were collected from the same arm, one before a tourniquet was applied and the other after it had been in place for 6 minutes, the rapidly increasing hemoconcentration could raise total serum protein from 7.3 to 9.5 gm per 100 ml. Blood specimens for this analysis should be taken from the vein as soon as the tourniquet is applied.

Specific Gravity Measurement

A linear relation exists between plasma specific gravity and its total protein content. Measurements are easy once the apparatus has been installed and the technique mastered. This approach is useful for nutritional surveys and for following the course of patients being treated for shock, dehydration, or edema. Results are clinically adequate when the individual protein fractions do not deviate much from the normal.

Chemical Precipitation

That portion of plasma protein which remains in solution after half saturation with ammonium sulfate or 22 per cent sodium sulfate has been defined in the past as albumin, and the precipitated portion as globulin. Globulin has been subdivided further by selective solubility into moieties which have been known as euglobulin, pseudoglobulin I and II, and fibrinogen. With the development of electrophoresis, however, these classical distinctions have been generally abandoned in favor of the nomenclature of Tiselius based upon electrochemical properties. This revision of interpretations is based in part on observations which show the precipitated fractions to be impure heterogeneous mixtures. Pseudoglobulin has been found to consist of 85 per cent alpha globulin and 15 per cent gamma globulin, whereas euglobulin is chiefly beta and gamma globulins.

Tiselius Electrophoresis

This is the most illuminating of the methods for determining protein fractions. The accuracy of the results secured is especially appealing to the investigator, but the complexity of the apparatus unfortunately places its application beyond the reach of the average hospital laboratory except for reference purposes.

Electrophoretic readings appear as a series of waves, with each crest or peak due to a different group of proteins. The areas under each peak represent the concentration of the respective fractions. Results are customarily expressed in terms of percentages or absolute values. Six definite boundaries usually are observed, which in the order of their mobilities at pH 8.6 are as follows: albumin, alpha$_1$ and alpha$_2$ globulins, beta globulin (also seen as two fractions under certain conditions), fibrinogen, and gamma globulin. Leutscher claims to have separated human albumin at pH 4.0 into two components: alpha (67 per cent) and beta (33 per cent) albumin, both of which show some alterations in disease states. Fibrinogen is present in plasma; absent in serum obtained from clotted blood.

Comparison of the precipitation methods with electrophoresis, as was done by Martin and Morris, indicates that the results with 22 per cent sodium sulfate, sodium sulfite, or magnesium sulfate are markedly at variance from the electrophoretic values, whereas fairly close agreement is given by precipitation with methyl alcohol or 26 per cent sodium sulfate.

Paper Electrophoresis

Comparatively simple devices are now available for differentiating the serum proteins by placing a small amount of serum on a strip of filter paper which has been moistened with a buffer solution and passing a weak current of electricity through for some hours. After the electrophoresis the separated protein components on the filter paper are stained with a dye such as bromphenol blue. One may then measure the pattern of absorbed dye on the filter paper by photometric methods or cut the strip segments containing the various fractions and analyze each segment for its quantitative content of protein by micro-Kjeldahl analysis.

NORMAL VALUES

The concentrations of the individual plasma proteins do not fluctuate appreciably from day to day. Values are lowest with newborn and premature infants; rise slowly through the first year of life. Above this age significant differences are usually not found and the values in general are in the same range as with adults (Table 49-1).

Table 49-1. Plasma Protein Concentrations from Birth to Maturity *
(*Gm per 100 ml*)

	Total protein	Albumin	Total globulin	Gamma globulin
Premature infants				
Average	5.5	3.7	1.8	0.7
Range	4.0–6.0	2.5–4.5	1.2–2.0	0.5–0.9
Full-term newborn infants				
Average	6.4	3.4	3.1	0.8
Range	5.0–7.1	2.5–5.0	1.2–4.0	0.7–0.9
1–3 months				
Average	6.6	3.8	2.5	0.3
Range	4.7–7.4	3.0–4.2	1.0–3.3	0.1–0.5
3–12 months				
Average	6.8	3.9	2.6	0.8
Range	5.0–7.5	2.7–5.0	2.0–3.8	0.4–1.2
1–15 years				
Average	7.4	4.0	3.1	0.9
Range	6.5–8.6	3.2–5.0	2.0–4.4	0.6–1.2

* Plasma fibrinogen averages 0.28 gm per 100 ml (range 0.22 to 0.32) at all ages.

The albumin fraction rises steadily and attains the adult range by the end of the first year, whereas the globulin may not reach there for several years. Fibrinogen exhibits little alteration with age, being close to the adult level at the moment of birth. The total *serum* protein does not include this fibrinogen content, whereas that of total *plasma* protein does. Since the fibrinogen is usually less than 0.3 gm per 100 ml, plasma and serum values correspond closely and may be used interchangeably for clinical purposes. The standard precipitation methods, which measure the globulins as a group, are not able to detect the absence of gamma globulin.

In individual infants there is no close correlation between the plasma components and the birth weights or later body weights except that, in general, the more mature infants tend to exhibit higher values. During the first few months many infants will show erratic fluctuations if determinations are repeated weekly. The levels in premature infants tend to be lower in the ones who are less mature.

In the representative study by Beach and associates no significant differences were found between the values for males and females, between white and Negro boys, or between determinations made near the beginning and end of 6 weeks in a health camp. Their study dealt with total serum protein determinations in 390 well Michigan children, determined by the specific gravity method. The means for all subgroups fell within the narrow range of 6.7 to 7.2 gm per 100 ml, with an average of 7.0 gm per 100 ml. All but 5 of the children showed levels between 6.0 and 8.6 gm per 100 ml. Those below 7 years of age had slightly lower values. As in other nutritional surveys, it was not possible to correlate slight diminutions in the readings with recognized signs of undernutrition.

From their analytic studies with paper electrophoresis, Oberman and associates concluded that mean values for albumin are 50 to 60 per cent of total serum proteins at all childhood ages.

ALTERATIONS IN DISEASE STATES

Illnesses have to be severe or protracted before the total or major fractions of the plasma proteins become grossly altered. Increases or decreases of any of the fractions occur, but almost never in a pattern that is pathognomonic of a specific disease.

Acute fluid loss from diarrhea, vomiting, burns, ketosis, hyperpyrexia, and heat exhaustion can quickly raise the concentrations of all components. As the dehydration is corrected the values return to normal.

Augmentation of the albumin level is seen only when there is acute fluid loss with transitory hemoconcentration. Hypoalbuminemia, on the other hand, occurs often; it is an almost regular feature of severe rheumatic fever or other protracted infections, the nephrotic syndrome, severe nephritis, extensive burns, pronounced liver disorders, and diseases associated with severe malnutrition.

Just as the plasma albumin almost never increases, the total of plasma globulin almost never falls. Hyperglobulinemia is seen with fair regularity in nephrosis, Still's disease, cirrhosis of the liver, acute hepatitis, protracted febrile infections, sarcoidosis, lupus erythematosus, Addison's disease, and miscellaneous chronic infections and reticuloendothelial disturbances. Electrophoretic analyses show that the globulin increases in these diseases are due to diverse and often strikingly different alterations among the $alpha_1$, $alpha_2$, beta, and gamma globulins (which themselves are far from chemically homogeneous). The gamma globulin seems to be related to antibody formation, for this fraction frequently increases after infections and remains elevated for several weeks or months.

Cryoglobulins are globulin fractions which precipitate spontaneously when the serum is chilled and redissolve when it is warmed again. Cryoglobulins are uncommon; they have been described in serum sickness, rheumatoid arthritis, multiple myeloma, and chronic lymphocytic leukemia. When present in quantity they are associated with Reynaud's phenomenon of hypersensitivity to cold, in which the immersion of a patient's fingers in water at 4°C for 5 minutes produces pallor locally and livid cyanosis of the rest of the hand, the other hand, and often of both feet.

ALBUMIN-GLOBULIN (A/G) RATIO

Normally the ratio of plasma albumin to globulin is approximately 2:1 or 3:21. When changes occur in disease the albumin level usually falls and the globulin level rises. As a result the calculated A/G ratio approaches 1:1 or even becomes reversed. Under such circumstances the determination of total protein, without partition studies, may fail to demonstrate the alterations which have taken place. It is not possible to deduce from a change in the A/G ratio whether one component is elevated or depressed. Should both components move in the same direction the ratio remains unchanged. The actual concentrations of albumin and globulin per unit volume are much more meaningful than their numerical relation.

RELATION OF PLASMA PROTEIN LEVEL TO EDEMA

Clinically recognizable edema may appear when the total plasma proteins drop below about 5.0 gm or the albumin fraction below 3.0 gm per 100 ml. These threshold values are indefinite and variable, for the development of edema may be influenced by many other factors— capillary permeability, capillary blood pressure, lymph flow, nutritional status, salt and water retention, tissue tension, and percentage composition of the plasma proteins themselves. Edema may not develop with a low plasma albumin if the globulin fractions are in great excess.

In congestive heart failure all levels drop a little, probably in reflection of the increased blood volume. When there is a clinical differentiation to be made between the edema of uncomplicated heart failure and the edema of renal insufficiency, the finding of a total protein level above 5.5 gm or of albumin above 3.0 gm indicates that the edema is probably of cardiac origin.

LIVER DISEASES

The liver plays an important part in the production of serum albumin, and the synthesis is deficient when the parenchymal cells are damaged. The usual finding is a fall in serum albumin, accompanied by a corresponding rise in the serum globulins. In infectious hepatitis the serum albumin usually returns to normal by the end of the first month, whereas the rise in globulins may persist for several months longer. The giving of plasma or concentrated serum albumin intravenously to patients with cirrhosis and ascites may raise the serum albumin temporarily, with loss of edema and increased urinary output. The plasma proteins are often low in poorly controlled diabetes mellitus, probably because of poor liver function.

THE NEPHROTIC SYNDROME

The total protein falls markedly in nephrotic states, in large measure as the result of the severe persistent proteinuria. The albumin content as determined by precipitation is usually below 2 gm and may be down to 0.3 gm per 100 ml. Even such low values are falsely high, since electrophoretic study of precipitated albumin reveals some alpha and beta globulin trapped within the albumin. A rise in globulin, and usually in fibrinogen also, is sometimes sufficient to raise the figure for total protein to near normal, obscuring the low albumin level. There is no evidence that a high protein intake stimulates blood protein synthesis.

Concentrates of serum albumin, if injected daily over long periods to patients with nephrosis, sometimes produce a moderate rise in albumin and a decrease in globulin; these changes are not permanent. The urinary output of albumin goes up markedly while such injections are being given.

MALNUTRITION

In starvation and other states of protein depletion the total blood volume shrinks before the plasma level drops. In nutritional surveys, readings have to be at least 1.0 gm below the mean before one can feel safe in making any positive statement, inasmuch as the standard deviations for the so-called normal standards are approximately ±0.7 gm.

Many patients with moderate malnutrition exhibit a slight rise in the albumin component after the dietary deficiencies have been corrected;

but the initial value cannot be taken as lowered until viewed in retrospect.

Only when malnutrition is well advanced does a drop in plasma proteins become demonstrable, and then usually in the albumin portion. Of the emaciated Italian children studied by Gollan at the end of World War II, most had an unusually low concentration of albumin with a slight increase in globulin; they were presumably salt-depleted as well, for edema did not develop until intravenous fluids were given.

The malnourished child with extreme hypoproteinemia may have such generalized edema and ascites as to superficially mimic the nephrotic syndrome. The urine, however, will be essentially normal except perhaps for a mild proteinuria. A high-protein high-calorie diet with vitamin supplements and a period of bed rest will quickly remedy the symptoms.

INFECTIONS

The alpha globulin and the fibrinogen often rise during acute infections. Later on, during convalescence, the gamma globulin fraction which contains antibodies may become moderately augmented. In active tuberculosis and active rheumatic fever the gamma globulin and alpha$_2$ globulin are elevated early; the albumin fraction tends to fall, so that the level of total protein remains essentially constant. A few children have been described with recurrent or persistent bacterial infections in whom the increases of serum gamma globulin have amounted to as much as 2 to 4 gm per 100 ml (normal range, 0.6 to 0.9 gm). In these cases the total proteins have also been at a high level, from 7 to 8.5 gm.

C-REACTIVE PROTEIN (CRP)

A protein fraction which reacts with the somatic C polysaccharide of pneumococci appears in the blood within 1 or 2 days after the onset of many inflammatory diseases. Illnesses in which this protein has been detected include pneumonia, osteomyelitis, endocarditis, empyema, myocardial infarction, widespread malignant diseases, and following typhoid vaccination. It is not found in healthy normal individuals. Its presence can be detected and measured semiquantitatively by means of a specific antiserum prepared from rabbits.

The CRP precipitin test often but not invariably becomes positive early in active rheumatic fever. It becomes negative during convalescence, often weeks or months before the rapid sedimentation rate disappears. During hormonal treatment of rheumatic fever the CRP disappears within 2 to 4 weeks and may return if the suppressive agent is discontinued before the acute attack has run its full course. When congestive failure complicates active carditis the CRP precipitin test tends to remain positive, unlike the sedimentation rate which may transitorily revert to normal. The current impression is that in patients with chronic or questionable carditis a negative reading with this test does not exclude the existence of rheumatic activity, whereas persistent positives are indicative of inflammatory activity provided other possible causes of inflammation can be excluded.

SERUM MUCOPROTEINS

These carbohydrate-rich complexes of alpha globulin are measured by analyzing the blood serum filtrate for the mucoproteins which remain after the major serum proteins are precipitated with perchloric acid. Serum levels in adults and normal children are typically between 1.9 and 4.5 mg per 100 ml (expressed as milligram percentage of mucoprotein tyrosine) and show no significant variation with age. Elevations to between 3.5 and 20 mg per 100 ml are usual in active rheumatic fever. These increases become apparent during the acute phase of the disease and subside with clinical quiescence. The rise is proportional to the severity of the rheumatic fever and fluctuates parallel to the clinical symptoms, fever, and changes in the erythrocyte sedimentation rate. Patients with chorea minor unaccompanied by other signs have normal or only slightly elevated levels. Elevations have been noted also in generalized malignancy, rheumatoid arthritis, and some bacterial and viral infections. Subnormal values are customary in the nephrotic syndrome.

When patients with active rheumatic fever are treated with hormones and the overt symptoms of the disease subside, the sedimentation rate may return temporarily to normal but the decline in serum mucoproteins may be only partial. The serum mucoprotein level is depressed in most adult cases of viral hepatitis and portal cirrhosis but not in those with obstructive biliary tract lesions.

CONGENITAL HYPOPROTEINEMIA

Defective production of both plasma albumin and plasma globulin but not of plasma fibrinogen of apparently congenital origin has been recorded. The chief and usually the only manifestation is mild continual edema. There are no indications that the proteins are being destroyed at an excessive rate. High-protein diets or infusions of plasma or blood have no permanent effect on this form of hypoproteinemia.

FAMILIAL IDIOPATHIC DYSPROTEINEMIA

This syndrome was described by Homburger and Petermann. The syndrome is characterized by hypoproteinemia and abnormalities in the plasma electrophoretic patterns. In the adult one also finds peripheral vascular changes (ulcers of the legs in the men, low oscillometric indices in the women) and edema. Some of the cases have had malformations of the thoracic cage and of the occipital hair.

HYPOGAMMAGLOBULINEMIA

That fraction of plasma proteins comprised by the gamma globulins contains nearly all the circulating antibodies as well as some unstudied proteins. After early infancy the normal concentration is 0.6 to 1.2 gm per 100 ml, representing 10 to 15 per cent of the total plasma proteins (Table 49-1).

At the time of birth all, or nearly all, the gamma globulin found in the circulation appears to be derived from the mother, by passive transfer across the placenta. The level at birth is normally in the range of 0.7 to 0.9 gm per 100 ml. This declines gradually until 1 to 3 months of age when the level is lowest, usually 0.1 to 0.5 gm per 100 ml. Active synthesis begins at about the third month. This "physiologic" hypogammaglobulinemia as a rule is so brief that no difficulties occur. Rarely it persists for several months and may be associated with recurrent severe infections. Caution is advisable when seeking to establish the existence of a persistent deficiency until after the first 6 months.

Children with nephrosis and pronounced loss of urinary proteins often have serum gamma globulin levels as low as 0.2 gm per 100 ml. This may contribute to the poor resistance to bacterial infections in this disease.

A rare disturbance, poorly understood, is one in which a deficiency of gamma globulin occurs in association with hypoproteinemia and edema. This may be long-lasting or transitory.

CONGENITAL AGAMMAGLOBULINEMIA

This term denotes a hereditary deficiency of gamma globulin in the presence of normal concentrations of all other plasma protein constituents. Practically all the instances reported to date have been males. There is a pronounced familial incidence, with a genetic pattern which appears to be recessive and sex-linked.

Unusual susceptibility to severe bacterial infections has been prominent, with recurrences of pneumonia, meningitis, or other septic illnesses as common expressions. Symptoms usually begin during the first year of life, and most of the patients could not survive infancy in the absence of chemotherapy. Early recognition of the disturbance is essential if one is to commence prophylactic supportive therapy before permanent and irreversible tissue injury occurs. To most viral infections the immune responses seem relatively normal. The usual leukocytic response is not impaired. The most frequent bacterial invaders appear to be pneumococci, staphylococci, influenza bacilli, streptococci, and meningococci. It has been suggested that sudden deaths in infants from acute respiratory infections, which are most frequent at the ages of 2 to 3 months, may be referable in part to the low serum gamma globulin which exists normally in this age period.

With electrophoretic analysis the plasma of these patients seems to be completely devoid of gamma globulin. However, this method often fails to detect concentrations below 0.2 gm per 100 ml. With the more sensitive immunochemical approach some patients show trace amounts, usually between 5 and 20 mg per 100 ml. Intravenous or intramuscular injections of gamma globulin concentrates are followed by the appearance of this protein fraction in the blood plasma in moderate amounts, with gradual fading away over the ensuing few weeks at a normal or slowed rate. Intramuscular injections of 0.1 to 0.15 gm (0.6 to 1.0 ml) per kg once a month are of considerable prophylactic benefit against fresh bacterial infections. Antibiotics are more effective in controlling infections already developed. On histologic study these children show few or no plasma cells in their tissues.

The adult form of agammaglobulinemia is somewhat similar in clinical manifestations, but symptoms do not begin until late childhood and there is no sex selectivity. The plasma level may be between 0 and 100 mg per 100 ml.

There have been reports of a few infants who suffer recurrent severe infections even though their circulating gamma globulin is above normal.

A preliminary laboratory approach is to test the serum for isohemagglutinins. These antibodies are absent in congenital agammaglobulinemia, provided the patient is in blood group O, A, or B; they are, of course, naturally lacking in subjects of blood group AB.

Gitlin has described an original quantitative immunochemical procedure which is said to be more reliable for diagnosis than electrophoresis. Horse antiserum against human gamma globulin is incorporated in agar and placed in a long thin test tube left at room temperature for 18 to 24 hours; sterile conditions are not observed. The presence of a band of precipitate in the agar indicates the presence of gamma globulin in the patient's serum. The distance the precipitation band has migrated away from the interface between agar and patient's serum reflects the content of gamma globulin.

BIBLIOGRAPHY

METHODS AND NORMAL VALUES

Beach, E. F., A. P. Harrison, M. Lesher, M. Kaucher, C. Roderuck, W. Lameck, and E. R. Moyer, Nutritional Status of Children. V. Blood Serum-Protein, J. Am. Dietet. A. 24:405, 1948.

Bongiovanni, A. M., and I. J. Wolman, Plasma Protein Fractionation in Pediatrics: A Review of its Present Status, Am. J. M. Sc. 218:700, 1949.

Kagan, B. M., and J. R. Stern, Blood Protein Measurements in Diagnosis of Disease, Ped. Clinics North America, p. 265, February, 1955.

Kempe, C. H., H. K. Silver, F. S. Smyth, J. W. Gofman, and *H. B. Jones*, The Lipoproteins of Serum in Infancy and Childhood. I. Lipoproteins in Normal Children, *J. Pediat.* 40:11, 1952.

Knapp, E. L., and *J. I. Routh*, Electrophoretic Studies of Plasma Proteins in Normal Children, *Pediatrics* 4:508, 1949.

Luetscher, J. A., Jr., Electrophoretic Analysis of Plasma and Urinary Proteins, *J. Clin. Invest.* 19:313, 1940.

Marrack, J. R., and *H. Hoch*, Serum Proteins: A Review, *J. Clin. Path* 2:161, 1949.

Martin, N. H., and *R. Morris*, The Albumin/Globulin Ratio: A Technical Study, *J. Clin. Path.* 2:64, 1949.

Nordmann, J., On an Important Source of Error in Determinations of Serum Proteins, *Presse méd.* 55:830, 1947.

Oberman, J. W., K. O. Gregory, F. G. Burke, S. Ross, and *E. C. Rice*, Electrophoretic Analysis of Serum Proteins in Infants and Children. I. Normal Values from Birth to Adolescence, *New England J. Med.* 255:743, 1956.

Rapoport, M., M. I. Rubin, and *D. Chaffee*, Fractionation of Serum and Plasma Proteins by Salt Precipitation in Infants and Children, *J. Clin. Invest.* 22:487, 1943.

PREMATURE AND NEWBORN INFANTS

Desmond, M. M., and *L. K. Sweet*, Relation of Plasma Proteins to Birth Weight, Multiple Births and Edema in the Newborn, *Pediatrics* 4:484, 1949.

Longsworth, L. G., R. M. Curtis, and *R. H. Pembroke, Jr.*, Electrophoretic Analysis of Maternal and Fetal Plasma and Sera, *J. Clin. Invest.* 24:46, 1945.

McMurray, L., J. H. Roe, and *L. K. Sweet*, Plasma Protein Studies on Normal Newborn and Premature Infants. I. Plasma Protein Values for Normal Full Term and Normal Premature Infants. II. Use of Concentrated Normal Human Serum Albumin in Treatment of Premature Infants, *Am. J. Dis. Child.* 75:265, 1948.

Norton, P. M., H. Kunz, and *E. L. Pratt*, Electrophoretic Analysis of Serum Proteins in Premature Infants, *Pediatrics* 10:527, 1952.

Saito, M., I. F. Gittleman, J. B. Pincus, and *A. E. Sobel*, Plasma Protein Patterns in Premature Infants of Varying Weights on the First Day of Life, *Pediatrics* 17:657, 1956.

DISEASE STATES

Fischer, M. A., P. A. Steinman, A. M. Carpenter, and *M. L. Menten*, Qualitative and Quantitative Changes in the Plasma Proteins of Lipoid Nephrosis Demonstrated by Electrophoresis, *J. Lab. & Clin. Med.* 37:894, 1951.

Fisher, B., Recent Contributions of Electrophoresis to Clinical Pathology, *Am. J. Clin. Path.* 23:246, 1953.

Gollan, F., Blood and Extracellular Fluid Studies in Chronic Malnutrition in Infancy, *J. Clin. Invest.* 27:352 1948.

Hertzog, F. V., Edema Associated with Temporary Idiopathic Hypoproteinemia, *J. Pediat.* 36:641, 1950.

Homburger, F., and *M. L. Petermann*, Studies on Hypoproteinemia: Familial Idiopathic Dysproteinemia, *Blood* 4:1085, 1949.

Jonsson, B. J., and *V. Lagercrantz*, Severe Hypoproteinemia, Probably Caused by Hepatic Damage, *Acta paediat.* 39:165, 1950.

Klenerman, P., Nutritional Edema: A Survey of Cases at the King Edward Hospital, Durban, *South African M. J.* 24:891, 1950.

Levin, B. M., H. Kaufman, and *J. de la Huerga*, Gamma Globulin Studies in Tuberculosis in Children, *A.M.A. Am. J. Dis. Child.* 83:26, 1952.

Luetscher, J. A., Jr., A. D. Hall, and *V. L. Kremer*, Treatment of Nephrosis with Concentrated Human Serum Albumin. I. Effects on the Proteins of Body Fluids, *J. Clin. Invest.* 28:700, 1949.

Routh, J. I., E. L. Knapp, and *C. K. Kobayashi,* Electrophoretic Studies of Plasma and Urinary Proteins in Children with Lipoid Nephrosis, *J. Pediat.* 33:688, 1948.

Steigman, A. J., Normal Distribution of Serum Protein Levels in Acute Poliomyelitis Patients, *J. Lab. & Clin. Med.* 39:757, 1952.

Sterling, K., The Serum Proteins in Infectious Mononucleosis, Electrophoretic Studies, *J. Clin. Invest.* 28:1057, 1949.

Wilson, M. G., and *R. Lubschez,* Immunologic and Biochemical Studies in Infants and Children with Special Reference to Rheumatic Fever. VI. Electrophoretic Patterns of Blood Plasma and Serum in Rheumatic Children, *Pediatrics* 2:577, 1948.

Wungaarden, J. B., J. D. Crawford, H. R. Chamberlin, and *W. F. Lever,* Idiopathic Hypoproteinemia: Report of a Case of Transient Edema, Depression of Plasma Albumin and Gamma Globulin and Eosinophilia, *Pediatrics* 9:729, 1952.

C-REACTIVE PROTEIN; MUCOPROTEINS

C-Reactive Protein, Editorial, *Lancet* 1:350, 1954.

Good, R. A., V. C. Kelley, T. A. Good, and *D. Glick,* Mucolytic Enzyme Systems. XX. Comparison of Mucoprotein and Hyaluronidase Inhibitor Concentrations in Maternal and Infant Serum, *Pediatrics* 12:575, 1953.

Kelley, V. C., F. H. Adams, and *R. A. Good,* Serum Mucoproteins in Patients with Rheumatic Fever, *Pediatrics* 12:607, 1953.

Jackson, R. L., H. G. Kelly, E. K. Smith, P. Wang, and *J. I. Routh,* Electrophoretic Analyses of Plasma or Serum Proteins of Rheumatic Fever Patients in Relation to Stages of Disease, *A.M.A. Am. J. Dis. Child.* 86:403, 1953.

Roantree, R. J., and *L. A. Rantz,* Clinical Experience with the C-Reactive Protein Test, *A.M.A. Arch. Int. Med.* 96:674, 1955.

Stollerman, G. H., S. Glick, D. J. Patel, I. Hirschfeld, and *J. H. Rusoff,* Determination of C-reactive Protein in Serum As a Guide to the Treatment and Management of Rheumatic Fever, *Am. J. Med.* 15:645, 1953.

GAMMA GLOBULIN

Bruton, O. C., Agammaglobulinemia, *Pediatrics* 9:722, 1952.

————, *L. Apt, D. Gitlin,* and *C. A. Janeway,* Absence of Serum Gamma Globulin, *Pediatrics* 9:722, 1952.

Gitlin, D., Paper 3 in W. H. Cole (ed.), "Serological Approaches to Studies of Protein Structures and Metabolism," Rutgers University Press, New Brunswick, N.J., 1954.

————, Low Resistance to Infection: Relationship to Abnormalities in Gamma Globulin, *Bull. New York Acad. Med.* 31:359, 1955.

Hayles, A. B., G. B. Stickler, and *B. F. McKenzie,* Decrease in Serum Gamma Globulin (Agammaglobulinemia): Report of 3 Cases, *Pediatrics* 14:449, 1954.

Janeway, C. A., J. Craig, M. Davidson, W. Downey, D. Gitlin, and *J. Sullivan,* Hypergammaglobulinemia Associated with Severe Recurrent and Chronic Nonspecific Infection (abstract) in *Trans. Am. Pediat. Soc., A.M.A. Am. J. Dis. Child.* 88:388, 1954.

Orlandini, T. O., A. Sass-Kortsak, and *J. H. Ebbs,* Serum Gamma Globulins in Normal Infants, *Pediatrics* 16:575, 1955.

Schick, B., and *J. W. Greenbaum,* Edema with Hypoproteinemia Due to Congenital Defect in Protein Formation, *J. Pediat.* 27:241, 1945.

Spain, D. M., V. A. Bradess, and *I. J. Greenblatt,* Possible Factor in Sudden and Unexpected Death during Infancy, *J.A.M.A.* 156:246, 1954.

CHAPTER 50

Miscellaneous Organic Constituents

BLOOD KETONES

Ketosis with ketonuria is more common in children than in adults, and carbohydrate impoverishment plays a role in its production. The liver is the main site for formation of the three principal metabolic ketones—acetone, acetoacetic acid (diacetic acid), and beta-hydroxybutyric acid. The physiologic mechanisms which govern an excessive production of ketone bodies are not understood wholly, but it seems clear that ketosis is usually associated with a depleted glycogen reserve within the liver. When this occurs the fat metabolism accelerates but fatty acid breakdown seems to be incomplete, with resulting stimulation of ketogenesis and the piling up in the blood and tissue fluids of these substances. Any disturbance which increases the metabolic need of the tissues for carbohydrates (e.g., fever) or which decreases the availability of carbohydrate for storage in the liver (e.g., uncontrolled diabetes mellitus, ketogenic diet, starvation) or which damages the liver itself (e.g., cirrhosis, glycogen disease, many poisonings) seems to favor ketogenesis and the establishment of ketonemia. Hence the need for a liberal intake of sugar-containing substances, at night as well as during the day if necessary, for any child who is ill with an infection or liver disease or whose food intake has been reduced because of gastrointestinal disturbance or a surgical operation.

In general, the younger the child the greater the susceptibility to ketosis, with the exception of very early infancy (Heymann). A ketogenic diet is sometimes given deliberately by the physician as a form of treatment in epilepsy. With children above age 7 years the ketotic state is best induced by an initial period of complete starvation lasting 3 to 5 days. A diet having a ratio of 4 or 4.5 gm of fat to 1 gm of carbohydrate plus protein (the *ketogenic-antiketogenic ratio*) is then begun. With younger children, who go into ketosis more easily, one can start with a dietary ratio of 1:1, and then increase this ratio to 2:1, 3:1, and 4:1 in successive steps every 4 to 7 days. Either regimen will induce and maintain ketosis for as long as it is continued. In the past the ketogenic regimen was occasionally used as a means of sterilizing the urine in urinary tract infection, but this therapeutic application generally has been abandoned since the antibiotics have become available.

The acute ketosis induced by infections is typically accompanied by anorexia, nausea, and even vomiting as the disturbance continues. Inability to take food aggravates the starvation and deepens the ketosis, thereby giving rise to a circular progression of disturbances, which often cannot be broken until glucose in large amounts is given by some parenteral route.

The accumulating acetoacetic and beta-hydroxybutyric acids combine with some of the base of the blood and tissue fluids to diminish the alkali reserve of the body. The urinary excretion of these acid ketone substances is accompanied by an increased output of sodium and other basic ions, thereby producing an acidosis as well. With ketogenic diet therapy this acidosis gradually disappears after about 2 weeks, though the ketosis persists.

Ketosis is also accompanied at the beginning by the excretion of large amounts of water as well as sodium, indicating a depletion of the extracellular fluid compartment. A shift of potassium from the intracellular to the extracellular compartment also takes place, and this may have serious constitutional effects in the severe acidosis and ketosis which can be a part of diabetic coma (p. 510). In renal failure the urinary excretion of the ketone bodies is impaired.

Under ordinary normal circumstances, ketone bodies are present in the circulating blood in trace amounts. In mild ketosis this rises to between 2 and 10 mg per 100 ml, expressed as beta-hydroxybutyric acid. In moderate to severe ketosis the levels may vary from 10 to 20 mg in infections and gastroenteritis, up to 100 to 150 mg per 100 ml in diabetic acidosis.

The relation between the blood and urine ketones is complex, as shown by the studies by Martin and Wick with diabetic adults. The urinary output is comparatively low—less than 100 mg per hour—when the blood level is below 20 mg per 100 ml and the ketone which is excreted is largely acetone. As the blood ketone level rises above this value the urinary output per hour increases markedly in disproportionate amounts. The relative proportions of the three ketone bodies within the urine is far from consistent or constant, even in the same patient in successive phases of his illness.

These observations with respect to renal excretion are reflected in the familiar finding that in mild ketosis the very sensitive nitroprusside reaction for acetone becomes positive while the ferric chloride (Gerhardt) reaction for acetoacetic acid remains negative. With more severe ketosis the latter also becomes positive.

The blood ketone level is a more sensitive indicator of an accelerated fat catabolism than is the appearance of ketone bodies in the urine. When blood ketones are only moderately increased and the renal function good, the renal tubules reabsorb the ketone bodies completely and the voided urine is free of these substances. Also, when renal function is very poor, the ketonuria may be minimal because of poor excretion by the kidney. A child with fever and dehydration may have an indisputable odor of acetone in the breath and yet have urine which tests negatively for acetone.

BLOOD PHOSPHATASES

The phosphatases are a family of intracellular and circulating enzymes which break down organic phosphates of all sorts including the phospholipids, phosphoproteins, and phosphorylated carbohydrates. Three types of phosphomonesterases, referred to more simply as phosphatases, are the varieties ordinarily contained in the blood stream, in concentrations which may become increased or decreased in certain disease states. These, with their pH optima, are alkaline phosphatase, pH 9.0 to 10.0; acid phosphatase, pH 4.5 to 5.0; and red cell phosphatase, pH 5.3.

Test Procedures. A number of simple organic phosphates are employed as substrates for clinical testing, each under differently standardized conditions. The Bodansky method measures the liberation of inorganic phosphates from beta-glycerophosphate. One Bodansky unit is that amount of enzyme in 100 ml of plasma which will liberate 1 mg of phosphorus (as the phosphate ion) during the first hour of incubation. With the Kay or Jenner-Kay method, one unit represents the liberation of 1 mg of phosphorus from an excess of disodium beta-glycerophosphate at pH 8.8 in 3 hours at 37.5°C. The King-Armstrong method uses disodium phenylphosphate as substrate and measures the phenol liberated in 30 minutes under the conditions of the test. One Jenner-Kay or King-Armstrong unit is approximately equivalent to two Bodansky units. To avoid the venipuncture demanded by the above methods, Bessey, Lowry, and Brock have developed a micromethod for finger tip blood which employs para-nitrophenyl phosphate as the substrate and expresses the results in nitrophenol units. One nitrophenol unit is approximately equivalent to 1.8 Bodansky units.

Because of this diversity of methods it is important to know which procedure is employed by the laboratory whose services are being utilized and what the limits of normality are, not only for that particular procedure but for the individual laboratory as well.

Red Cell Acid Phosphatase

The acid phosphatase in human erythrocytes has a strong activity in the range between pH 4.8 and pH 6.1, with an optimum at about pH 5.3. With phenylphosphate as substrate, King and Armstrong found the values in normal persons to be from 200 to 400 units per 100 ml with an average of 340 units. Behrendt's averages for the acid red cell phosphatase was between 94.4 and 305.3 Bodansky units, with an average of 159.1

units. It is stated that the level is a little higher in the newborn than later. Measurement of this enzyme has no clinical pertinence at present.

Serum Acid Phosphatase

A minimal amount of acid phosphatase can ordinarily be demonstrated in the serum of every child, regardless of age or sex. The level is almost never enhanced except in carcinoma of the prostate with extension of metastasis, so that the determination has little application during childhood.

Large quantities of acid phosphatase are present in adult semen. Riisfeldt has applied this knowledge to the medicolegal problem of rape. Recovery of large amounts of acid phosphatase from dried spots on clothing is presumptive evidence when an accusation of rape has been made.

Serum Alkaline Phosphatase

This enzyme is believed to be formed mainly in the bones, transported by the blood stream, and excreted by the liver into the bile. Its level in the plasma tends to remain more or less constant from day to day, unaffected by meals or incidental occurrences. The elevations which occur in many bone and liver diseases are believed to represent either a continuously greater output of the enzyme from the site of origin or some block in the normal pathway of excretion. The diminutions observed in scurvy, hypothyroidism, and a few other miscellaneous conditions are ascribed to decreased rates of formation.

Alkaline phosphatase is excreted to variable extent in both feces and urine. A normal adult excretes an average of 23 units of alkaline phosphatase (Bodansky method) per dry weight of feces; this is presumably derived from the bile, succus entericus, and other sources. The urinary content is scanty and irregular with no relation to age or sex.

NORMAL VALUES IN CHILDHOOD. Bodansky and Jaffe, using the Bodansky method, found the average for 27 children to be 7.3 units per 100 ml, with values ranging from 3.1 to 13.1. Readings from 10 to 13 units were common between 10 and 15 years. In 300 other children hospitalized for a variety of clinical conditions (excluding anemia, malnutrition, jaundice, and known diseases of bone) the spread was approximately the same, from 5 to 14 units, with an average of about 7.5 units. Similarly, with 70 healthy children between 2 and 10 years of age, Talbot and associates found values from 4.5 to 12 Bodansky units, with an average of 7.2 units. Essentially similar values have been found by most workers and are generally accepted as normal. There are no differences due to age and sex between 1 and 10 years. The range for adults is lower, 2 to 4 units.

At puberty the serum alkaline phosphatase often doubles in value. The rise begins and ceases earlier in girls than in boys; with the latter it may persist through the seventeenth year.

The test for serum alkaline phosphatase seems to have its greatest usefulness in corroborating clinical impressions based on other findings. Serial determinations can serve as an indicator of response to therapy or progress of an illness.

RICKETS AND OTHER BONE DISEASES. The serum alkaline phosphatase is often elevated in disturbances of the bones which are accompanied by overactivity of the osteoblasts. Such rises may be found in infantile rickets, hyperparathyroidism, late osteogenic or refractory rickets, osteogenic sarcoma, osteomalacia, osteosclerosis fragilis (marble bones), epiphyseal dysgenesis, infantile cortical hyperostosis, malignant infiltrations, and polyostotic fibrous dysplasia. Slight rises have been occasionally noted in renal rickets. Essentially normal findings are obtained in most patients with skeletal abnormalities, arthritis, treated osteomyelitis, and calcinosis universalis. An increase or decrease cannot be interpreted as being diagnostic or even indicative of any one disturbance, in the absence of other pertinent information regarding the patient.

There is pronounced parallelism between the activity of rickets and the level of phosphatase, though the individual variations often seem out of proportion to the severity of the disease. This is brought out by the study of Klasmer, who found the mean value in 55 children between 6 months and $2\frac{1}{2}$ years of age with active rickets to be almost always above 20 units. Fourteen children with increased alkaline phosphatase (mean, 16.8 units) at the first examination but dubious clinical signs of rickets subsequently exhibited obvious rickets.

The phosphatase activity of the serum remains high so long as the rickets is active. Decline to normal values coincides fairly well with clinical recovery, whereas a rise often antedates the first clinical symptoms. The rise in alkaline phosphatase has proved much more reliable as a sign of rickets than have changes in serum calcium or phosphorus.

Klasmer found that the average for 925 children rose 1.5 units in the winter. This suggests a mild lack of vitamin D during the winter. Most of the studies on the incidence of rickets have not always differentiated between active rickets and healed rickets, which may account for some of the discordances among the published reports. Stearns and Warweg followed the levels of three children aged 3 to 12 years with late rickets. The values for plasma phosphatase were elevated at first and decreased slowly with vitamin D therapy, though they were still above normal when roentgenologic healing was complete.

MALNUTRITION. The determination of alkaline phosphatase is frequently included in nutritional surveys to serve as a rough indicator of the extent of vitamin D deficiency in a given population. To determine the reliability of this approach Harrison and associates studied the range and frequency distribution of serum alkaline phosphatase in a total of 377 healthy American boys and girls of various ages. The figures showed wide divergences, with no evidence that moderately elevated or depressed values were in any sense abnormal. Thus because of the breadth of the zone of normal variation, single readings cannot be interpreted accurately without full knowledge of the history and status of the patient.

HYPOPHOSPHATASIA. A number of ill children have been described who exhibited poor bone calcification, dwarfing, reduced serum alkaline phosphatase activity, elevation of serum calcium in some instances, and almost absent alkaline phosphatase in the bones and other tissues after death when looked for. The low to absent enzyme in blood and tissues is believed to be the primary pathogenetic defect.

SCURVY. The alkaline phosphatase level falls in active scurvy. In 18 scorbutic infants reported by Schwachman the average serum level on admission to the hospital was 3.2 Bodansky units, with a range of 1.1 to 4.9 units. After 1 to 4 weeks of treatment the levels had risen to 8 to 19 units.

HYPOTHYROIDISM. The alkaline phosphatase determination is a useful index of thyroid function in children, provided other diseases which may cause a lowering are excluded. In a group of infants and children with cretinism and juvenile hypothyroidism, Talbot and associates found the levels prior to thyroid therapy to be below 4.5 Bodansky units per 100 ml. During replacement treatment the level rose to normal or nearly normal in every patient and fell again when the dosage of thyroid was reduced or discontinued. Low levels were not observed in diseases which might be confused with juvenile hypothyroidism or cretinism other than some instances of idiopathic dwarfism.

LIVER DISEASE. In children with infectious hepatitis the alkaline phosphatase is often elevated in the early stages. In infectious mononucleosis it is also usually elevated, as a manifestation presumably of altered liver function.

The level may or may not be increased in congenital atresia of the bile ducts. This rise is less consistent than the elevation which is more or less regularly observed in adult patients with jaundice due to complete obstruction of the common bile duct. Hepatitis in adults may or may not evoke an increase.

MISCELLANEOUS. The alkaline phosphatase may be depressed in Mediterranean anemia, obscure bone disease, severe malnutrition, progeria, and in the postacidotic states of infantile diarrhea. Of 11 children with celiac and celiac-like disease studied by Yieh and Wissler, 7 had subnormal values, 1 with a reading of 2.2 units; one child with uremic vomiting gave a reading of only 2.4 units. In glycogen storage disease, there may be a slight change in either direction.

BIBLIOGRAPHY

BLOOD KETONES

Debré, R., P. Royer, and *H. Lestradet,* Metabolic Significance of Nervous Symptoms due to Attacks of Vomiting with Ketosis in Children, *J. Pediat.* 48:409, 1956.

Dumm, R. M., and *R. A. Shipley,* A Simple Estimation of Blood Ketones in Diabetic Acidosis, *J. Lab. & Clin. Med.* 31:1162, 1946.

Fisher, P., The Role of the Ketone Bodies in the Etiology of Diabetic Coma, *Am. J. M. Sc.* 221:384, 1951.

Heymann, W., Metabolism Studies on Age Disposition to Ketosis in Human Beings, *J. Pediat.* 12:21, 1938.

Martin, H. E., and *A. N. Wick,* Quantitative Relationships between Blood and Urine Ketone Levels in Diabetic Ketosis, *J. Clin. Invest.* 22:235, 1943.

Sherry, S., Current Concepts of Diabetes, *Bull. New York Acad. Med.* 29:202, 1953.

Warming-Larsen, A., and *E. O. Errebo-Knudsen,* Peroral Glucose Treatment of Acute Diarrhoea in Infants, *Acta paediat.* 77:184, 1949.

PHOSPHATASES

Adamson, J. S., et al., Medical Survey of Nutrition in Newfoundland, *Canad. M. A. J.* 52:227, 1945.

Behrendt, H., Phosphatases in Blood of Man: Values in Whole Blood, Plasma, Cytolysates and Erythrocytic Suspensions, *Am. J. Clin. Path.* 19:167, 1949.

Bessey, O. A., O. H. Lowry, and *M. J. Brock,* A Method for the Rapid Determination of Alkaline Phosphatase with Five Cubic Millimeters of Serum, *J. Biol. Chem.* 164:321, 1946.

Bodansky, A., Phosphatase Studies; Determination of Serum Phosphatase; Factors Influencing Accuracy of Determination, *J. Biol. Chem.* 101:93, 1933.

—— and *H. L. Jaffe,* (a) Phosphatase Studies: Serum Phosphatase in Diseases of Bone; Interpretation and Significance, *Arch. Int. Med.* 54:88, 1934. (b) Phosphatase Studies: Serum Phosphatase as Criterion of Severity and Rate of Healing of Rickets, *Am. J. Dis. Child.* 48:1268, 1934.

Clark, L. C., Jr., and *E. Beck,* Plasma "Alkaline" Phosphatase Activity. I. Normative Data for Growing Children, *J. Pediat.* 36:335, 1950.

Drabkin, D. L., Hyperglycemia, Glycosuria and Dephosphorylation: The Role of Phosphatases, *Proc. Am. Diabetes A.* 8:3, 1948.

Harrison, A. P., C. Roderuck, M. Lesher, M. Kaucher, E. Z. Moyer, W. Lameck, and *E. F. Beach,* Nutritional Status of Children: Blood Serum Alkaline Phosphatase, *J. Am. Dietet. A.* 24:503, 1948.

Josefsson, E., (a) On the Plasma Phosphatase Titer in Rickets with Particular Reference to the Shock Treatment, *Ann. paediat.* 157:169, 1941. (b) On the Values for Plasma Phosphatase and Blood Phosphorus in Healthy Children Born at Term and in Premature Children, *Ann. paediat.* 157:193, 1941.

Klasmer, R., Serum Phosphatase Activity and Clinical Rickets in Children in Jerusalem, *Am. J. Dis. Child.* 67:348, 1944.

Lanman, J. T., Hypophosphatasia: A Newly Recognized Disease, *J. Pediat.* 47:509, 1955.

Lorch, I. J., Alkaline Phosphatase and the Mechanism of Ossification, *J. Bone & Joint Surg.* 31B:94, 1949.

McKerrow, J. R., E. Lau, and *E. W. McHenry,* Serum Phosphatase Values of School Children, *Canad. J. Pub. Health* 41:322, 1950.

Payne, **W. W.**, Plasma Phosphatase in Jaundice in Children, *Proc. Roy. Soc. Med.* **32:**1265, 1939.

Rapoport, **S.**, Increased Serum Phosphatase and "Hyperprothrombinemia" in Infectious Hepatitis of Children, *Proc. Soc. Exper. Biol. & Med.* **62:**203, 1946.

Riisfeldt, **O.**, Acid Phosphatases Employed as a New Method of Demonstrating Seminal Spots in Forensic Medicine, *Acta path. microbiol. scandinav.* suppl. 58, 1946.

Schwachman, **H.**, Serum Phosphatase in Infantile Scurvy, *J. Pediat.* **19:**38, 1941.

Stearns, **G.**, and **E. Warweg**, I. The Partition of Phosphorus in Whole Blood and Serum: The Serum Calcium and Plasma Phosphatase from Birth to Maturity, *J. Biol. Chem.* **102:**749, 1933.

—— and ——, Studies of Phosphorus of Blood. III. The Phosphorus Partition in Whole Blood and in Serum and the Serum Calcium and Plasma Phosphatase during Healing of Late Rickets, *Am. J. Dis. Child.* **49:**79, 1935.

Talbot, **N. B., A. M. Butler, E. L. Pratt, E. A. MacLachlan,** and **J. Tannheimer,** Progeria, Clinical, Metabolic and Pathologic Studies on a Patient, *Am. J. Dis. Child.* **69:**267, 1947.

——, **G. Hoeffel, H. Schwachman,** and **E. L. Tuohy,** Serum Phosphatase as an Aid in the Diagnosis of Cretinism and Juvenile Hypothyroidism, *Am. J. Dis. Child.* **62:**273, 1941.

Vermehren, **E.**, (*a*) Variationen im Phosphatasegehalt des Plasmas im Anschluss an die verschiedenen Lebensalter, *Acta med. scandinav.* **100:**244, 1939. (*b*) Von den Jahreszeitenabhängige Variationen im Phosphataseinhalt des Plasmas normaler Kinder, *Acta med. scandinav.* **100:**267, 1939.

Wolman, **I. J.**, and **A. N. Evans**, The Phosphatases in Relation to Clinical Pediatrics, *Am. J. M. Sc.* **217:**690, 1949.

Yieh and **H. Wissler,** Ueber Serumphosphatase, *Ann. paediat.* **152:**348, 1938.

CHAPTER 51

Iron

The iron in foodstuffs, largely in the ferric state, is ionized and reduced during transit through the acid environment of the stomach. Absorption, probably solely as ferrous (Fe^{++}) ions, occurs chiefly through the upper small intestine, at a rate regulated by the epithelial cells of the mucosa to meet body needs. Ascorbic acid and other reducing substances in the stomach and duodenum seem to increase the nutritional availability of food iron. Ferrous compounds given by mouth for therapy of anemic states are absorbed more efficiently than are ferric compounds. Overdosage of iron, as when young children ingest a goodly number of ferrous sulfate tablets, has produced acute collapse ending in death.

The total of normal body iron varies from approximately 40 to 60 mg per kg, regardless of age. After infancy, hemoglobin accounts for approximately 55 to 70 per cent of the body iron, ferritin, and hemosiderin stores in liver; spleen and marrow 20 per cent; and muscle myohemoglobin 10 to 20 per cent. The remainder occurs chiefly in the cytochrome and other cellular enzyme systems and in the beta globulin fraction of plasma protein.

Ferritin, a water-soluble protein of molecular weight 400,000, normally constitutes about two-thirds of the reserve iron stores; each molecule contains approximately 17 to 23 per cent iron which is not demonstrable with the usual staining reagents. Hemosiderin, a chemically similar water-insoluble protein, constitutes the remaining third of the reserve stores; it may hold as much as 35 per cent iron in the form of large visible and stainable granules of iron hydroxide. The amount of iron in these reservoirs, which are in dynamic equilibrium with each other, can increase enormously in hemosiderotic states.

IRON TRANSPORT

Iron, after absorption from the intestine, is taken directly into the blood stream and oxidized to the ferric (Fe^{+++}) form. In the plasma it combines almost exclusively with a specific fraction of beta globulin known as siderophilin or transferrin. This iron-binding fraction constitutes approximately 3 per cent of all the serum proteins, or 0.24 gm per 100 ml of serum; 100 ml of plasma contains enough to combine with 300 to 420 μgm of iron, but 100 per cent "saturation" is seen only when there

555

is a surplus of iron in the body. The usual degree of saturation is 30 to 50 per cent in normal subjects, and 10 to 20 per cent in iron deficiency. The unsaturated portion is termed the *serum iron-binding capacity*. The unsaturated and saturated fractions constitute together the *total iron-binding capacity* (TIBC).

IRON KINETICS

Once within the body, iron is used over and over again. Healthy men probably assimilate less than one milligram daily from food, and excrete equivalent traces in urine, stool, and sweat. With women, the loss of iron-containing blood during menstruation averages an additional 0.5 to 1 mg per day over a 28-day menstrual cycle (Moore). During pregnancy the amount transferred transplacentally to the fetus averages 1 to 2 mg daily. Hence women, who eat less than men, are more prone to develop iron deficiency when the diet is inadequate or intestinal absorption poor.

The total balance of iron within the body is controlled exclusively by the absorption mechanisms. There is no effective physiologic mechanism for the elimination of any surplus which may accumulate from pathologically rapid absorption or the receiving of unusual amounts parenterally by injection or transfusion. Here the child has one advantage over the adult; if an excess has accumulated and the source of the excess removed, the growth of the body gradually consumes the surplus and restores normal equilibrium.

Movement of iron within the body is rapid. Studies of adults with radioactive iron have indicated that half of the serum iron content is removed and replaced every 90 minutes. This turnover is largely related to the destruction and production of hemoglobin.

The continual reuse of iron in the hemoglobin cycle is illustrated strikingly in the observations of Smith, Cherry, and associates with infants whose mothers had been transfused during pregnancy with erythrocytes tagged with radioactive iron (Fe^{55}). Considerable radioactive iron was present in the blood of the infants at birth. This persisted through infancy. At 2 years, about 90 per cent of the transplacentally received radioactive iron was still detectable within hemoglobin.

When single tracer doses of radioactive iron (Fe^{55} and Fe^{59}) are given intravenously, "tagged" erythrocytes begin to appear in the circulation within 24 hours. This indicates that the injected iron begins to be incorporated almost immediately into hemoglobin. It takes 2 to 3 weeks for the radioactivity of circulating red cells to rise to a plateau. The slope of the curve portrays the rate of erythropoiesis. A rapidly rising high curve is seen in iron depletion or when red cell destruction is abnormal. A low flat curve is seen when iron is in excess as in hemosiderosis, and with the anemic disorders in which storage iron is not greatly altered but erythropoiesis is sluggish as in myelophthisis, cachexia, and infection.

NUTRITIONAL REQUIREMENTS OF IRON

The older view that infants are born with appreciable stores of iron has been disproved by the more recent studies of McCance and Widdowson, Sturgeon, and others. Nearly all of the iron at birth is in the hemoglobin; storage iron represents only about one-twelfth of the total in the body. The additional iron required for growth must accordingly come from dietary or medicinal sources.

During the first 2 or 3 months of life there is little absorption of utilizable iron from the gastrointestinal tract. Growth of the body and dilution of its iron content results in a state of "physiologic anemia" for a few months (Chap. 2). In fact, the status of the blood hemoglobin level throughout infancy is conditioned in large measure by the quantity of the hemoglobin present in the body at the time of birth. Important influences are the duration of gestation, the rates of intrauterine hemopoiesis and postnatal growth, and the volume of umbilical cord blood permitted to drain into the infant during the delivery.

Healthy adults who take a representative American diet ingest an average of 12 to 15 mg of food iron daily. Of this, approximately 10 per cent is absorbed. Assimilation may be higher when the body is deficient in iron, and especially when the dietary content of ascorbic acid is high.

Similar studies of iron metabolism in infants and children are still inadequate. It is known that prematurely born infants regularly develop lower hemoglobin levels than full-term infants, despite liberal supplementation of the diet with oral iron. Even well nourished and well fed full-term infants are prone to exhibit levels of hemoglobin and serum iron which are lower in the first few months than later on.

The Food and Nutrition Board of the National Research Council (1953) has recommended the following dietary allowances of iron for infants and children per day:

Age	Mg of iron	Age	Mg of iron
Under 1 year	6	10–12 years	12
1–3 years	7	Over 12 years	15
4–6 years	8	(Adult males and	
7–9 years	10	nonpregnant	
		females)	12

These values are for food iron; medicinal ferrous iron may be assimilated at a better rate than the estimated 10 per cent of food iron. The recommended intakes appear to be adequate to meet the maintenance and growth needs of most healthy infants and children. Available evidence indicates, however, that during periods of rapid growth in some infants the dietary iron content and the rate of gastrointestinal absorption may not be fully adequate to meet optimally the enlarging blood volume and the anabolic needs of other iron-utilizing tissues. This is the reason for not relying on dietary iron exclusively and for giving supplemental oral or parenteral medication to correct an obvious iron deficiency state in an infant or child. Supplementation of the diet with a ferrous salt should be continued for several months after the hemoglobin level of the blood has returned to normal, in order to establish a reserve of this metal in the metabolic pool.

A transfusion of 100 ml of blood bank blood will provide approximately 35 mg of iron. The new iron-dextran preparations for intramuscular administration contain 50 mg of elemental iron per ml.

PLASMA IRON LEVELS

The concentration of iron in the circulating plasma must be viewed as being in physiologic equilibrium with (1) what is being absorbed from the gastrointestinal tract, (2) what is being released by destruction of erythrocytes, and (3) what is being removed for utilization by the bone marrow and other body structures. Hence it is not surprising that plasma iron levels fluctuate considerably during the course of a single day and have a wide range of normal variation from person to person.

In 27 girls aged 13 to 16 years Schlapoff, Johnston, and Boroughs found afternoon values ranging from 39 to 127 μgm per 100 ml with a mean of 77 μgm. Determinations made in the mornings had a mean value 23 μgm higher. In 130 normal adults studied by Fowler and Barer the plasma iron levels ranged from 20 to 265 μgm per 100 ml. Values were slightly lower in women than in men. There was no significant difference between subjects with achlorhydria and those with normal gastric acidity. With normal ranges so wide one must be conservative in ascribing significance to single random readings.

In 51 normal children aged 5 days to 12 years, Smith, Schulman, and Morganthau found the serum iron content to range from 34 to 250 μgm per 100 ml. The TIBC of these sera ranged from 103 to 551 μgm. The percentage saturation of the latter varied from 10 to 100 per cent.

Generally speaking, the serum iron level is high in the newborn period (60 to 140 μgm), falls to a low point by 4 months (30 to 80 μgm), and then rises slowly to the usual childhood range (50 to 150 μgm). The TIBC of the serum, however, is low in the newborn period (100 to 250 μgm) and then rises in the first year to the more or less constant level of childhood (200 to 500 μgm). The percentage saturation of the TIBC averages about 75 per cent in the newborn period, about 12 per cent at 4 months, and then rises slowly to about 20 per cent in young children and 30 to 50 per cent in older children (Table 51-1). There is wide normal variation, so that individual readings as much as 20 per cent above or below these average figures may still be normal. Many of the generalizations based on levels of serum iron and serum iron-binding capacity in healthy and disease states are based on trends shown by large series of cases.

A very sharp fall in serum iron was reported by Vahlquist to take place in the first day of life, with an average reading of 159.8 μgm per 100 ml at birth and of 51.5 μgm at 24 hours. This may be a reflection of the abrupt stoppage of transfer of iron from placenta to fetus at the time of delivery.

The plasma (or serum) level of iron is depressed when the dietary supply is inadequate or when an excessive amount of blood has been lost as in hemorrhage. The level is low also in many infections, especially

Table 51-1. Mean Iron and Iron-binding Capacity of Serum in Normal Children at Various Ages *

Age group	Serum iron (μgm/100 ml)	TIBC of serum (μgm/100 ml)	Per cent saturation of iron-binding protein of serum
5–8 days	147.9	261.8	65.0
1–6 months	132.4	411.7	32.2
6–12 months	105.7	428.6	25.0
1–2 years	94.9	414.1	22.2
2–6 years	116.0	395.4	28.1
6–12 years	126.9	340.3	37.9

* Adapted from Smith, Schulman, and Morgenthau, Iron Metabolism in Infants and Children, *Advances Pediat.* 5:195, 1952.

of the chronic variety, as a consequence in part of a greater need for iron by the tissue cells in those disturbances. The TIBC falls concomitantly, so that the percentage saturation remains about the same. With recovery from infection these both return to normal.

In 15 infants and young children with iron-deficiency anemia studied by Smith and associates, the serum iron was low, ranging from 31 to 76 μgm, with a mean of 49 μgm. The TIBC was markedly elevated, 330 to 660 μgm with a mean of 507 μgm. The percentage saturation varied from 3.7 to 17.6 per cent. There was no correlation between the iron values or percentage saturation with the blood hemoglobin or hematocrit of these patients.

When iron medication is given to patients with iron-deficiency anemia the plasma content reaches a peak from 30 to 70 per cent above the initial level in about 6 hours after the dose is taken.

The iron level and the percentage saturation of the iron-binding protein are both high in hereditary spherocytosis, sickle cell anemia, and Mediterranean anemia. In the active forms of these disorders the serum iron readings may rise to 300 or even 400 μgm per 100 ml.

In patients receiving multiple transfusions the serum iron content and the TIBC tend to be identical. The latter may be lower than normal. Smith's values for both factors in 10 children with severe Cooley's anemia ranged from 141 to 273 μgm per 100 ml, with a mean of 203 μgm.

IRON STORAGE DISEASES

Hemochromatosis of the "classic" type, with finely granular liver cirrhosis, pancreatic fibrosis, testicular atrophy, and rich deposits of hemosiderin in the viscera, is limited almost exclusively to late adult life.

A somewhat similar condition has been seen at times in children with long-standing anemia. It is not clear whether the organ changes are induced by the chronic hypoxia of the tissues or are the end results of the administration of medicinal iron or of transfusions. Analyses of postmortem tissues from some of the cases have revealed a greater content of iron than can be accounted for by the treatment. One pathogenetic factor may be that in anemia the absorption of food iron from the intestinal tract becomes abnormally enhanced.

Hemosiderosis is the term applied when iron accumulates within the body after transfusions of blood or intravenous injections of iron. Liver cirrhosis and other tissue lesions of hemochromatosis do not develop. It is debatable whether hemosiderotic deposits are directly injurious to the tissues, inasmuch as this is a physiologic storage substance.

BIBLIOGRAPHY

IRON

Cartwright, G. W., C. M. Huguley, Jr., H. Ashenbrucker, J. Fay, and M. M. Wintrobe, Studies on Free Erythrocyte Protoporphyrin, Plasma Iron and Plasma Copper in Normal and Anemic Subjects, *Blood* 3:501, 1948.

Darby, W. J., Iron and Copper, *J.A.M.A.* 142:1288, 1950.

Feuillen, Y. M., and A. Lambrechts, Iron Metabolism in Infants. III. The Influence of Vitamin C on the Absorption of Iron, *Acta paediat.* 43:188, 1954.

Finch, C. A., J. G. Gibson II, W. C. Peacock, and R. G. Fluharty, Iron Metabolism: Utilization of Intravenous Radioactive Iron, *Blood* 4:905, 1949.

————, M. Hegsted, T. D. Kinney, E. D. Thomas, C. E. Rath, D. Haskins, S. Finch, and R. G. Fluharty, Iron Metabolism: The Pathophysiology of Iron Storage, *Blood* 5:983, 1950.

Food and Nutrition Board, "Recommended Daily Allowances, Revised 1953," Publication 302, National Academy of Sciences, National Research Council, Washington, D.C., 1953.

Fowler, W. M., and A. P. Barer, Plasma Iron: Normal Values; Response Following Medication, *Am. J. M. Sc.* 223:633, 1952.

Gorten, M. K., and *J. E. Bradley,* The Treatment of Nutritional Anemia in Infancy and Childhood with Oral Iron and Ascorbic Acid, *J. Pediat.* 45:11, 1954.

Granick, S., Iron Metabolism, *Bull. New York Acad. Med.* 30:81, 1954.

Hoppe, T. O., G. M. A. Marcelli, and *M. L. Tainter,* A Review of the Toxicity of Iron Compounds, *Am. J. M. Sc.* 230:558, 1955.

Josephs, H. W., Iron Metabolism and the Hypochromic Anemia of Infancy, *Medicine* 32:125, 1953.

Kleckner, M. S., Jr., A. H. Baggenstoss, and *J. F. Weir,* Iron-storage Diseases, *Am. J. Clin. Path.* 25:915, 1955.

McCance, R. A., and *E. M. Widdowson,* Metabolism of Iron during Suckling, *J. Physiol.* 112:450, 1951.

Metabolism and Function of Iron. "Report of the 19th Ross Pediatric Research Conference," Ross Laboratories, Columbus, Ohio, 1956.

Moore, C. V., and *R. Dubach,* Metabolism and Requirements of Iron in the Human, *J.A.M.A.* 162:197, 1956.

Oettinger, L., Jr., W. B. Mills, and *P. F. Hahn,* Iron Absorption in Premature and Full-term Infants, *J. Pediat.* 45:302, 1954.

Reissmann, K. R., T. J. Coleman, B. S. Budai, and *L. R. Moriarty,* Acute Intestinal Iron Intoxication. I. Iron Absorption, Serum Iron and Autopsy Findings, *Blood* 10:35, 1955.

Schlaphoff, D., F. A. Johnston, and *E. D. Boroughs,* Serum Iron Levels of Adolescent Girls and the Dirunal Variation of Serum Iron and Hemoglobin, *Arch. Biochem.* 28:165, 1950.

Schulman, I., Commentary—Iron Metabolism, *Pediat.* 18:299, 1956.

Smith, C. A., R. B. Cherry, C. J. Maletskos, J. G. Gibson II, C. C. Roby, W. L. Caton, and *D. E Reid,* Persistence and Utilization of Maternal Iron for Blood Formation during Infancy, *J. Clin. Invest.* 34:1391, 1955.

Smith, C. H., I. Schulman, and *J. E. Morganthau,* Iron Metabolism in Infants and Children, *Advances Pediat.* 5:195, 1952.

———, *T. R. C. Sisson, W. H. Floyd, Jr.,* and *S. Siegal,* Serum Iron and Iron-binding Capacity of the Serum in Children with Severe Mediterranean (Cooley's) Anemia, *Pediatrics* 5:799, 1950.

Sturgeon, P., Studies of Iron Requirements in Infants and Children. I. Normal Values for Serum Iron, Copper and Free Erythrocyte Protoporphyrin, *Pediatrics* 13:107, 1954.

———, Iron Metabolism: A Review with Special Consideration of Iron Requirements during Normal Infancy, *Pediatrics* 18:267, 1956.

Vahlquist, B., Das Serumeisen, *Acta paediat.* vol. 28, suppl. 5, 1941.

Vannotti, A., and *A. Delachaux,* "Iron Metabolism and Its Clinical Significance," Grune & Stratton, Inc., New York, 1949.

CHAPTER 52

Phosphorus, Calcium, and the Parathyroids

Calcium and phosphorus are best considered together, for the reason that almost every disease which disturbs the serum concentration of one of these minerals affects the other, directly or secondarily. Alternations in the metabolism of calcium or phosphorus occur principally in conditions related to malnutrition, vitamin D, acid-base disequilibria, the steatorrheic disorders, parathyroid disturbances, some bone diseases, some kidney diseases, pseudohyperparathyroidism, and immobilization osteoporosis.

PHOSPHORUS METABOLISM

Phosphorus occurs in many more foods than does calcium. Being a constituent of all nucleic acids and phospholipids and of most proteins, it is found in all organic foodstuffs which contain cells or cellular residues such as meat, vegetables, cereals, milk, and bone ash. The inorganic phosphorus content of breast milk averages about 0.02 gm per 100 ml; of cow's milk, about 0.09 gm per 100 ml; of goat's milk, about 0.08 gm per 100 ml.

The phosphorus intake of a child should be at least equal to that of calcium. A good diet which meets the requirements of calcium and protein will in general meet the phosphorus requirement as well.

The phosphorus of foods is ordinarily well absorbed, in the form of phosphates or organic combinations. The calcium-phosphorus (Ca:P) ratio or ion product of the diet is important in this connection. Both of these minerals seem best absorbed when the value of this ratio, in terms of milligrams, falls between 2:1 and 1:1. The usual child's diet which contains milk gives values within this range. An otherwise normal diet with a standard intake of vitamin D can be made rachitogenic by adding a large excess of either calcium or phosphorus.

Any surplus of ingested phosphorus above the needs of the bones and tissue cells is excreted chiefly by the kidneys, with a small proportion finding its way into the feces. When the serum phosphorus falls below

562

about 3 mg per 100 ml, the excretion of urinary phosphorus (urinary phosphate) practically ceases.

Blood Chemistry

In whole blood the phosphorus occurs in (1) organic phosphate esters extractable by acids, (2) insoluble phospholipids unextractable by acids (p. 524), (3) dissolved acide-soluble inorganic phosphates, and (4) free nucleotides in trace amounts.

ACID-SOLUBLE ESTER COMPOUNDS. Hexose mono- and diphosphates, triosephosphates, adenylic acid, adenosinetriphosphate, phosphopyruvic acid, diphosphoglyceric acid, cocarboxylase, and many other essential acid-soluble phosphorus-containing substances occur largely within the blood cells; the serum content is usually, though not necessarily, negligible. Wide differences occur in the total concentrations of these in blood of normal individuals. Analyses by Stearns and Warweg showed mean totals of 30 mg of ester phosphorus per 100 ml of whole blood at birth, a fall to the 20-mg level at 3 months of age, a rise to 25 mg at 1 year, and then a gradual subsidence to 23 mg at age 15 years. These fluctuations are in part a reflection of alterations in red cell corpuscular volume with age.

With rises in the urinary excretion of phosphates, the concentration of these substances in the blood usually becomes diminished. Such changes have been described in malnutritional rickets, hyperparathyroidism, and acidotic states when renal function is unimpaired. If the plasma content increases, as in hypochloremia or nephritic acidosis, that of intracellular phosphates goes up also.

INORGANIC PHOSPHATE. The inorganic phosphorus of the blood is acid-soluble and is carried wholly or almost wholly by the plasma in the form of phosphate ions. Measurements are performed preferably with serum rather than with plasma or whole blood. Serum should be separated from erythrocytes within the first hour after clotting, the earlier the better, in order to avoid a falsely high reading from products of the cells.

In normal children above the age of 1 year the fasting values for serum inorganic phosphorus are usually in the zone of 5.0 to 6.0 mg per 100 ml. In Macy's group of normal children aged 5 to 12 years the average was 5.6 mg per 100 ml. In Stearns and Warweg's series the mean declined gradually from 5.5 mg at 1 year to 5.0 mg at 12 years. During adolescence this falls to the 3- to 4-mg level obtaining in normal adults.

In infancy the normal range is 4 to 7 mg per 100 ml. Levels are said to be a little lower in winter than in summer. Prematurely born infants may exhibit slightly higher values for the first 6 months, in the range from 5 to 8.5 mg per 100 ml.

The taking of a large amount of carbohydrate as in a tolerance test, or the depression of the blood glucose level by an injection of insulin or epinephrine, brings about a fall in serum phosphorus of 1.0 to 1.5 mg per 100 ml, which lasts for several hours. The increased carbohydrate utilization in the tissues temporarily draws off some phosphate ions for the phosphorylation reactions.

Ingestion of calcium may be followed by a slight and transient rise in the blood phosphorus, whereas injection of a magnesium salt induces a significant fall. A slight rise to 6 or 7 mg per 100 ml may be noted during the healing of fractures.

There is a strong propensity for the calcium and phosphorus of the serum to bear a reciprocal relationship to each other. Disturbances which bring about a drop in serum calcium tend to evoke a phosphorus rise, and the reverse.

CALCIUM METABOLISM

The average older child on a good diet ingests 800 to 1,200 mg of calcium daily. Of this from 15 to 30 per cent is retained for maintenance and growth of bone and other tissues. Some 8 to 15 per cent is eliminated in the urine. The balance is excreted in the feces. The excretion of calcium can be increased above the normal limits by the giving of mineral acids or acid salts such as ammonium chloride, by a ketogenic diet, and by diets with an acid residue.

An infant who is nonrachitic and on a good feeding schedule ordinarily takes in between 100 and 200 mg of calcium per kg body weight per day. His calcium retention (i.e., the difference between the intake and the total of urinary and fecal losses) is of the magnitude of 30 to 60 mg per kg daily. The rachitic infant retains a lesser amount; values from −22 to +61 mg per kg were found by Barnes, Munks, and Kaucher in 30 such infants, with a mean of +20.4 mg. The giving of vitamin D to these infants improved the retention.

Milk

The intake of calcium comes largely from milk and milk products. The only other foods in the childhood dietary with an appreciable content of calcium are those artificially enriched, such as the baby cereals with bone meal added or white bread made with milk. The average child will receive enough calcium if milk is taken in the equivalent of 1 qt a day.

In the balance study of a normal 12-year old boy conducted by Macy, the calcium intake over a 55-day period averaged 912 mg per day. Of this, 590 mg came from milk, 113 mg from cheese, and 62 mg from bread (which was enriched with added milk solids). The remaining 147 mg represented small contributions from a diversity of foods.

Milk's content of calcium is far from constant. Analyses conducted by the Canadian Council on Nutrition on hundreds of samples of cow's milk showed that 95 per cent contained between 108 and 165 mg calcium per 100 ml. The mean was 124 mg per 100 ml, equivalent to 1,170 mg, or 1.17 gm, per qt. Calcium is highest in Jersey milk and lowest in Holstein, being inversely proportional to the water content. The content in milk from goats of the four common breeds was found by Holmes et al. to vary from 112 to 164 mg per 100 gm of milk, with an average of 137 mg. Breast milk averages approximately 33 mg per 100 ml.

Serum Chemistry

Serum or heparinized or defibrinated plasma is best for blood calcium estimation; oxalate and citrate react with calcium and are undesirable. Whole blood gives greater variation and yields less reproducible results, presumably because there is practically no calcium in the erythrocytes and the total corpuscular volume varies from patient to patient.

About half of the serum calcium (45 to 55 per cent) is extractable by diffusion through artificial membranes. This "diffusible fraction" is presumed capable of passing through capillary walls and cell membranes. The remainder is "nondiffusible" and bound to the plasma proteins, chiefly the albumin. Approximately 1 mg per 100 ml of the diffusible fraction and all of the nondiffusible calcium is not ionized. The diffusible and nondiffusible fractions may vary independently of each other. McLean and Hastings have constructed a chart from which it is possible to calculate the approximate concentration of ionized calcium if the values for total serum calcium and serum protein are known.

Clinical disorders characterized by hypercalcemia or hypocalcemia are ordinarily discussed in terms of abnormalities in the level of total serum calcium. Disturbances in the ratio between diffusible and nondiffusible calcium, or in the degree of ionization of the diffusible calcium, are undoubtedly of significance, but technical difficulties make it impossible for most laboratories to carry out analyses with respect to these fractions. Alterations in the relative proportions of these may explain why one patient may have a significant disturbance of calcium metabolism despite a normal value for total serum calcium, as in mild hyperparathyroidism, or why another may be tetany-free despite a strikingly low value, as in nephrosis. Related to these mechanisms is the frequent finding of mild hypercalcemia (12 to 14 mg per 100 ml) in diseases in which the carbon dioxide content of the blood is increased, as in cyanotic congenital heart disease, chronic circulatory failure, and emphysematous conditions.

NORMAL VALUES. In normal children the serum calcium level is almost always between 9.6 and 11.6 mg per 100 ml (4.8 and 5.8 mEq per liter). Macy found a mean of 10.4 mg per 100 ml for children 5 to 12 years of age. Infants in the first few months of life, while receiving prophylactic vitamin D, may have levels up to 12 mg per 100 ml.

In the absence of hypoproteinemia, levels of serum calcium between 9 and 10 mg per 100 ml can be adjudged as being in the borderline low zone and those below 9 mg as clearly subnormal. Conversely, readings above 12 mg may be interpreted as unusually high.

During the first week or two of life the calcium and phosphorus levels tend to undergo poorly understood fluctuations. These occasionally become manifest clinically as tetany of the newborn (p. 572).

Calcium Salt Therapy

The absorbability of any calcium salt taken by mouth is dependent upon its solubility, which becomes much higher when the pH is acid. Calcium compounds are best given in water or with acid fruit juices before meals, since milk and meals call out the pancreatic and intestinal secretions which are alkaline. Vitamin D and lactose also promote absorption.

For sustained oral therapy of hypocalcemia, calcium chloride is deemed superior to calcium lactate or calcium gluconate. Part of this difference may lie in the calcium content, which is 30 per cent in the chloride, 17 per cent in the lactate, and only 9 per cent in the gluconate. The effectiveness of calcium chloride in correcting the disturbances of tetany seems to be enhanced by its internal acidifying action. When rickets is present it is ordinarily not possible to raise the blood calcium level to normal with calcium salts unless a liberal amount of vitamin D is also given.

Calcium compounds when given by intramuscular injection sometimes cause local necrosis and sterile abscesses. This approach to therapy should be avoided.

Indirect Transfusions

About 0.4 gm of soluble sodium citrate per 100 ml of blood or 50 ml of plasma is present in stored citrated blood for transfusions (p. 139). When introduced intravenously this citrate may neutralize temporarily some of the circulating calcium and inhibit its physiologic activity. With the customary transfusion the liver destroys the citrate with sufficient rapidity to prevent the development of symptoms of hypocalcemia. With exchange transfusions in the newborn period, however, when as much as 500 ml of citrated blood may be introduced within 1 to 2 hours into a small newborn baby, tremors, irritability, and other signs of tetany may appear. An electrocardiogram may show electrical evidences of somatic skeletal muscle tremors, not discernible clinically. Hence the need for adding some calcium gluconate solution at intervals during exchange transfusions. Too much calcium in this circumstance may cause bradycardia or even sudden stoppage of the heart.

Calcium salts for intravenous use should never be mixed with citrated plasma or blood prior to transfusions, even in highest dilutions, else clotting will follow.

VITAMIN D

A closely related group of sterol derivatives differ among themselves in antirachitic activity and in capacity to produce toxic symptoms. D_2 or D_3, or a mixture of these two, constitute the active principles in most of the commercial preparations available for the prophylaxis and treatment of rickets and appear to have approximately equal antirachitic potency for human beings. Cod liver oil contains a preponderance of D_3. Viosterol is a nonproprietary name for commercial preparations of irradiated ergosterol; it consists of approximately 50 per cent calciferol (D_2), with nonactive lumisterol and tachysterol accounting for the remainder.

One international unit of vitamin D represents the vitamin D activity of an international standard solution of calciferol, equal to 0.025 μgm of the crystalline vitamin. There are 350 or more units in each teaspoonful of cod liver oil, 400 units in each quart of milk fortified with vitamin D, and 400,000 units in 1 mg of D_2 or D_3. Dosages of 400 to 1,000 units daily are adequate for the prevention of rickets and infantile tetany if started within the first month of life and provide a margin of safety in case of illness or temporary neglect. Once rickets is established the dose of vitamin D required for cure becomes appreciably larger.

Infantile Rickets

Rickets on a nutritional basis is a deficiency disease which tends to subside spontaneously after the first year of life. The pathogenesis is complex, being participated in by five major variables: calcium, phosphorus, vitamin D, rapidity of bone growth, and the congeries of unknown factors which constitute individual susceptibility. Among the conducive circumstances are (1) an inadequate dietary content of calcium or phosphorus or of vitamin D (less than 100 units daily, more or less), (2) an altered Ca:P dietary ratio, which can be either unusually high or unusually low, or (3) faulty absorption of ingested calcium or phosphorus or vitamin D due to steatorrhea or related disturbance, especially when the rate of bone growth is excessively rapid as in the first months of life. It may be estimated that rickets of some degree would develop in the majority of infants in northern North America during the winter months if milk with its rich content of calcium and phosphorus were not the staple food at this age and if additional vitamin D were not supplied.

BLOOD CHANGES. The concentration of phosphorus in the serum of the rachitic child is almost always subnormal. When the disturbance is at all advanced the phosphorus may fall below 3 mg per 100 ml and may be as low as 1 mg. The serum concentration of calcium, in contrast, may or may not be depressed. The serum alkaline phosphatase level is regularly elevated. During recovery from rickets, or when the treatment is inadequate, the serum phosphorus may rise transitorily to unusually high levels (6 to 8 mg per 100 ml).

Rapidly growing premature infants frequently exhibit minimal rickets without tetany despite receiving relatively large amounts of vitamin D. The existence of the disturbance is recognizable by roentgen study of the bones, a moderate rise in serum phosphatase, and histologic findings in the bones should death occur. The serum calcium and phosphorus levels in these infants are typically within the high normal ranges. The bone changes in these premature infants appear to result from production of cartilage and bone matrix faster than the deposition of the inorganic mineral aggregates.

Human milk with its approximate content of 0.04 gm per 100 ml for calcium and 0.02 gm for phosphorus has a Ca:P ratio of approximately 2:1. This ratio appears to be much more favorable for normal bone growth than the 1.3:1 ratio of cow's milk—0.124 gm per 100 ml for calcium and 0.09 gm for phosphorus—even though the latter has a much higher content of these minerals. Where vitamin D is not given during the winter months, artificially fed infants in temperate climates are much more prone to develop severe rickets than those who are breast fed.

Evaporated milk and many proprietory milk preparations designed for infant feeding have phosphate-containing stabilizers added during the processing. This may alter the ratio even more unfavorably, to become approximately 1:1.

VITAMIN D THERAPY. Vitamin D promotes absorption of calcium and phosphorus through the intestinal wall, assists the kidney in reducing the loss of phosphorus into the urine, and acts favorably and directly upon the metabolic processes within bone tissue itself. When a child with rickets is given vitamin D in therapeutic amounts, or is exposed to ultraviolet rays, the serum phosphorus level rises, and the serum calcium also if depressed. The bone lesions commence to heal, the muscle tone improves, and the serum alkaline phosphatase reverts slowly to normal. Balance studies will show an increased retention of both calcium and phosphorus.

Osteomalacia (Adult Rickets)

In this disease, metabolic and bony changes differ little from those of infantile rickets, except that the older age of the patients results in absent or minimal disturbances of calcification at the growing epiphyseal ends of the bones. There is an abundance or even an excess of osteoid matrix, but the concentrations of serum calcium or phosphorus or both seem to be too low for normal precipitation of calcium salts to take place.

CAUSES. Osteomalacia has multiple incitants. Nutritional osteomalacia due solely to an insufficient intake of vitamin D and mineral-containing foods is not seen in this country or Europe in children beyond infancy.

In fact, nutritional hypocalcemia is so rare that nutritional surveys of most populations do not include determinations of the calcium content of the blood, except perhaps among infants. The alkaline serum phosphatase is a much more sensitive indicator of the occurrence of vitamin D or calcium deficiency in children (p. 551).

Osteomalacic and rachitic changes may develop during the course of cystic fibrosis of the pancreas, celiac disease, and related diseases associated with steatorrhea unless ample vitamin D is given in water-miscible rather than fat-soluble form. Osteomalacia may also be seen in renal acidosis with the compensatory hypercalciuria secondary to inability of the tubules to produce ammonia; in the Fanconi syndrome of tubular malfunction; and in the idiopathic hypercalciuria which sometimes seems to be associated with urinary tract infections. Osteomalacia appearing in kidney diseases is often referred to as "renal rickets." Osteomalacia may develop in hyperparathyroidism with osteitis fibrosa generalisata following removal of a parathyroid tumor.

RESISTANT RICKETS. This form of osteomalacia is produced by endogenous resistance of the tissues to a normal intake of vitamin D. The architectural changes in the shafts of the bones are the same as in rickets caused by insufficient vitamin D intake. The condition appears to be of hereditary origin. The serum phosphorus level is almost always subnormal and appears responsible for the bone lesions. Physiologic studies in some cases have demonstrated defective phosphorus reabsorption within the renal tubules.

Cure, or at least repression of the bone changes, can be achieved by daily dosages of 50,000 to 100,000 units of vitamin D or higher, coupled with an optimal diet and careful nutritional supervision of the patient. Vitamin D_2 and vitamin D_3 seem equally effective. When these are discontinued the rickets becomes active again, except that spontaneous improvement sometimes occurs at puberty. The hypophosphatemia may persist despite large doses of vitamin D daily continued for years.

During treatment with the large amounts of vitamin D needed for therapy the urine should be tested every week or so with Sulkowitch reagent for excessive calcium output and with the microscope for signs of calcium casts. Either finding calls for discontinuance or reduction of the dosage of vitamin D for a week or two. An abnormally high blood level of either calcium or soluble nitrogen is a warning of vitamin D excess. Hyperplasia of the parathyroid glands seems to occur regularly. Osteotomy for bowed legs has been followed by dangerous hypercalcemia, consequent to immobilization and decalcification of the bones.

Idiopathic Hypercalcemia of Infancy

This is a syndrome in which normally developing infants begin to exhibit vomiting, anorexia, constipation, hypotonia, dehydration, and failure to gain weight. The usual recognizable onset is between the ages of 2 and 9 months, though occasional infants seem to have the disturbance from birth. Blood chemistry studies reveal hypercalcemia and soluble nitrogen retention. The serum calcium level is typically between 12 and 17 mg per 100 ml, and the blood urea level between 30 and 90 mg per 100 ml. The serum alkaline phosphatase is sometimes slightly elevated, and the serum inorganic phosphorus within the normal range. The pH of the urine is variable, and proteinuria is absent. Most of the clinical phenomena can be attributed to the hypercalcemia. Under therapy with a feeding regime low in calcium and free from vitamin D the disturbance subsides gradually and growth begins again. The serum urea level returns to normal more slowly than the serum calcium. Milk in adequate amounts may then be given again, but with no added vitamin D. It has been suggested that the origin of the disturbance in these infants is an abnormal transitory hypersensitivity to vitamin D.

Hypervitaminosis D

Toxic effects from commercial vitamin D preparations may be due to other contaminating sterols rather than to the calcemic-producing principles D_2 or D_3. Symptoms usually do not appear until after daily doses of 50,000 units or higher have been taken for several weeks. With the preparations currently on the market the zone of safety between the antirachitic and the toxic dosages is extremely broad.

None of the disturbances seen in patients receiving large doses of vitamin D can be viewed as pathognomonic or specific, except for unusual amounts of calcium in the blood and urine. Symptoms suggestive of hypervitaminosis D, in patients receiving this substance in abundance, include anorexia, pallor, lassitude, thirst, gastrointestinal discomfort, weight loss, fever, anemia, and leukocytosis. Hypertension and convulsions may occur. The urine becomes profuse and of low specific gravity; it contains traces of protein, excessive calcium, occasional casts, or erythrocytes.

The serum calcium can range from 11 to 25 mg per 100 ml; this increase is believed to be chiefly in the ionized portion. The blood phosphorus may be low, normal, or slightly elevated. The zones of provisional calcification in the long bones become dense. Calcium deposits appear erratically and unpredictably, in the kidney tubules, walls of the arteries, or around the joints. The blood urea becomes elevated, and the urea clearance is depressed. Uremia may ensue if the kidneys are badly damaged. Demineralization of the skeleton may follow; if the cause is not recognized still more vitamin D or some ultraviolet therapy may be given.

Treatment consists of discontinuance of the vitamin D and administration of extremely large amounts of fluid by mouth. If the kidneys show signs of damage suggestive of calcinosis, the diet should be kept low in milk and other calcium-containing foods and the same precautions instituted as for other kinds of chronic nephritis.

Most of the symptoms are reversible if the intoxication is recognized early. The blood chemistry changes revert to normal after several weeks. The erythrocyte sedimentation rate may remain increased for a much longer period. A marked eosinophilia may become evident at the onset of the recovery stage.

HYPOCALCEMIA AND TETANY

The serum calcium level tends to be low in a diversity of disorders, including hypoparathyroidism, pseudohypoparathyroidism, privational rickets, osteomalacia due to vitamin D deficiency, and nephrosis and chronic nephritis. Hypocalcemia may occur also in the newborn period, in malnutritional states associated with starvational or liver diseases which have low serum proteins, and in the steatorrheic disturbances of celiac disease, cystic fibrosis of the pancreas, and sprue. Tetany as a complication of the hypocalcemia may occur in any of these, except when the drop in calcium is solely in the nondiffusible fraction bound to low serum proteins, as in nephrosis.

The physiologic relationship between calcium metabolism and tetany is still far from clear, but the demonstration of hypocalcemia is a requisite to the diagnosis of hypocalcemic tetany. Nevertheless the influences which depress the level of serum calcium should be separated from the mechanisms which precipitate the signs and symptoms of tetany in hypocalcemia.

There is no fixed threshold level of total serum calcium for evoking the symptoms of tetany, though these may develop whenever the serum calcium falls below 9 mg per 100 ml. The overt manifestations of tetany in rachitic infants are not referable to the severity of the rickets but to the low serum calcium level. Many infants with a low serum calcium do not exhibit signs of tetany until an attack of gastroenteritis or a respiratory tract or other acute infection supervenes.

Acidosis of the body fluids acts to inhibit the appearance of clinical tetany, whereas alkalosis facilitates its development. Hence the importance of giving acid-producing calcium chloride along with dihydrotachysterol or vitamin D when treating a patient with hypoparathyroidism and hypocalcemia.

ALKALOTIC TETANY

Alkalosis can produce tetany as readily as can hypocalcemia, even though alkalosis does not alter the total serum concentration of calcium or the urinary calcium output. Tetany-inducing alkalosis in childhood is usually induced through one of three mechanisms: (1) hyperventilation of central nervous system origin, as for example in emotional excitement or salicylate poisoning, (2) excessive vomiting, as in congenital hypertrophic pyloric stenosis or upper intestinal obstruction, or (3) ingestion of large amounts of alkali such as sodium bicarbonate or sodium citrate, especially when renal function is poor because of dehydration or other causes.

TETANY, HYPOCALCEMIA, AND HYPERPHOSPHATEMIA IN THE NEWBORN PERIOD

The frequent concurrence of hypocalcemia, hyperphosphatemia, and tetany in newborn infants is suggestive of a common pathogenesis, but this has not been clearly established. The prompt alleviation of symptoms and signs attributed to tetany after calcium has been given is often empirically accepted as a demonstration of an underlying hypocalcemia, even when hypocalcemia has not been looked for as the cause of the symptoms. Calcium can act as a nerve sedative and relieve neuromuscular irritability in conditions other than tetany.

Normally during the first few days of life the serum calcium level falls transitorily and the serum phosphorus tends to rise.

These changes are well exemplified in the data of Gittelman and Pincus, from a group of artificially fed newborn infants in Brooklyn, N.Y. For the first 24 hours these infants received glucose solution only; they were then given an evaporated milk formula fortified with vitamin D. Approximately 20 per cent had serum calcium levels below 9 mg per 100 ml in the first day, approximately 40 per cent on the second day, and approximately 50 per cent at some time between ages 3 and 15 days.

Serum phosphorus changes were in the reverse direction. Serum levels were less than 7 mg per 100 ml in more than 90 per cent of those tested in the first day and exceeded 7.4 mg per 100 ml in nearly 80 per cent between 3 and 15 days. The alkaline phosphatase level ranged between 2.6 and 13.6 Bodansky units.

Bakwin was the first to demonstrate that administration of phosphate solutions to newborn infants encouraged the development of hypocalcemia and to suggest that cow's milk with its lower Ca:P ratio and higher total phosphorus concentration may be a causative significance in neonatal tetany.

McCrory, Forman, McNamara, and Barnett have reported that newborn infants whose endogenous levels of serum phosphate are or have been elevated (with decreased levels of serum calcium) display a diminished capacity for renal excretion of phosphate. It is possible that the feeding of cow's-milk mixtures calls for a higher level of activity by the parathyroids than does breast milk. Animal experiments indicate that the parathyroids hypertrophy when the dietary Ca:P ratio is low, as in cow's milk.

Suggestive confirmation lies in the observation of Gardner and associates and of Kaplan that the parathyroids of eight autopsied newborn infants fed cow's milk had "idiopathic hypertrophy," whereas those from seven breast-fed newborn infants were "normal."

Thus diverse influences seem able to affect the levels of serum calcium and phosphorus and the development of tetany during the newborn period. Illnesses affecting the acid-base equilibria—vomiting with hypochloremic alkalosis, hyperventilation with respiratory alkalosis, postacidotic imbalances, and toxemia from acute infections—can cause tetany at any age and are occasionally operative during the newborn period. Cerebral hemorrhage, erythroblastosis fetalis, prematurity, and presence of maternal diabetes or prediabetes may also be accompanied by hypocalcemia with or without tetany.

Clinical and roentgenologic signs of rickets are ordinarily not found in newborn infants, and the serum alkaline phosphatase is not elevated. On the other hand, histologic irregularities characteristic of rickets were demonstrated by Ranström and von Sydow in 57 per cent of a series of newborn Swedish infants dying during the first day of life. Likewise Follis, Jackson, Eliot, and Park uncovered histologic rickets in 21 per cent of 90 infant autopsies during the first month of life. In many similar infants personally studied these histologic changes were minimal and of only brief duration, portraying perhaps only a disturbance in bone growth during the terminal illness.

KIDNEY DISEASES

Hyperphosphatemia

One of the cardinal signs of renal functional insufficiency is an increase in the level of serum phosphorus. This increase becomes evident whether the kidney disease is accompanied by acute or chronic nephritis, hydronephrosis, pyelonephritis, or destruction of the kidneys by tumor. Hyperphosphatemia may be said to be present when the level mounts above 8 mg per 100 ml; it has been found as high as 40 mg in some cases. As the uremia improves, the hyperphosphatemia subsides.

Hypocalcemia

Being intimately bound to the serum proteins, the total calcium level usually becomes diminished in the hypoproteinuria which accompanies the nephrotic syndrome. Since the diffusible fraction of the calcium is not altered, tetany is exceptional, though sometimes occurring just before death. The same phenomenon of hypocalcemia with hypoproteinemia takes place in kala-azar, because of the low serum albumin.

In kidney diseases severe enough to produce uremia, impairment of the capacity of the renal tubules to make acid-neutralizing ammonia promotes a compensatory loss of urinary calcium and depletes the calcium reserves. The hyperphosphatemia from retained phosphates not only acts to depress the serum calcium but may also inhibit the extent of its ionization despite the acidosis these patients show. If the excretion of endogenous phosphates shifts to the intestine, absorption of dietary calcium may be hindered by the local formation of insoluble calcium phosphate. Osteomalacic bone changes (so-called "renal rickets") may follow if these interacting phenomena persist for more than a few weeks. It is sometimes advisable to give calcium as part of the corrective therapy for the acidosis of chronic nephritis to protect against a fall in blood calcium and development of tetany.

Magnesium therapy of the hypertension in nephritis calls for caution if the blood calcium is already low, since the antagonism of this ion to calcium may lead to severe hypocalcemic complications.

HYPERPARATHYROIDISM

The parathyroid hormone, according to Albright and Reifenstein, acts directly upon the electrolyte equilibria of the body fluids, and bone changes, when they occur, are secondary to the chemical changes. The sequence of events with excessive stimulation of the body tissues by parathyroid hormone is believed to be somewhat as follows. The parathyroid hormone makes the phosphate dissolved in body fluids more readily excretable by the kidney, with a resulting decrease in the serum phosphorus level. Resorption of calcium phosphate salts from the bones becomes thereby stimulated. An elevated serum calcium level results. This stimulates hypercalciuria, which in turn tends to cause undersaturation of the body fluids; so that unless there is a liberal supply of calcium from the gastrointestinal tract the bones have to supply the deficit. As the bones decalcify they respond to stresses and strains by laying down of osteoid tissue, which also drains off calcium and phosphorus.

Hyperparathyroidism in the childhood years may develop (1) as a manifestation of adenoma or otherwise unexplainable "primary" hyperplasia of the parathyroid glands, or (2) as a "secondary" or compensatory complication in chronic renal disease, malnutritional osteomalacia, or hypocalcemia due to other causes. Surgery is the most satisfactory approach to primary hyperparathyroidism but is contraindicated in the secondary forms; hence the importance of ruling out primary renal disease and of establishing the origin of the disturbance in all cases. With a primary adenoma, removal of too much parathyroid tissue may be followed by transient hypoparathyroid tetany or persistent residual hypoparathyroidism.

The characteristic laboratory findings in uncomplicated hyperparathyroidism consist of a low serum phosphorus (2 to 4 mg per 100 ml or lower), a high serum calcium (12 to 18 mg per 100 ml), a high urinary output of both calcium and phosphorus, and an elevation of serum alkaline phosphatase if the skeletal changes are marked and active. Anemia may also ensue.

The level of ionized serum calcium can be calculated from the values for total calcium and total protein by reference to the chart of McLean and Hastings. The ionized fraction may be elevated when that for total serum calcium is normal, in consequence of an accompanying hypoproteinemia.

Demonstration of a high urinary calcium output while on a low calcium neutral ash diet is a confirming sign. A total excretion over 100 mg per 24 hours by an infant or young child, over 150 mg by an older child, and over 200 mg by an adolescent may be deemed abnormally high. The urinary calcium may be low, contrary to the usual rule, if there is secondary renal damage. A low serum phosphorus is helpful diagnostically, though hypophosphatemia may be masked by phosphate retention in renal failure.

Calcium phosphate and calcium oxalate stones may accumulate in the urinary passages, or calcium may become deposited within the tubules. The skeletal lesions are inconstant and variable, consisting of ill-defined skeletal pains, epulis formation, multiple giant cell tumors, or generalized decalcification of the bones with tendency to fracture (osteitis fibrosa generalisata). Differentiation must be made from hypervitaminosis D, multiple myeloma, and sarcoidosis of bone, any of which can also give elevated serum calcium. In the milder forms of hyperparathyroidism there may be no obvious change in either the bones or the urologic tract.

HYPOPARATHYROIDISM

Symptoms consist of increased neuromuscular irritability, attacks of tetany which may simulate generalized convulsions, softening of the bones, hypoplasia of the teeth, and a tendency to cataracts. Laboratory studies reveal the serum calcium low, the phosphorus high, the alkaline phosphatase normal or low, and the urinary content of calcium and phosphorus both diminished as a rule. Stubborn moniliasis due to *Candida albicans* not infrequently develops on the oral or intestinal mucosa or the nails.

PHOSPHORUS EXCRETION TEST. A helpful diagnostic procedure for distinguishing true hypoparathyroidism from the fundamentally different syndrome of "pseudohypoparathyroidism" is the phosphorus excretion test, perhaps better known as the Ellsworth-Howard test. Older children and adolescents are given 2 ml (200 USP units) of parathyroid extract intravenously while fasting. The phosphorus content of the urine is determined hourly for 3 hours before the injection and 3 to 5 hours afterward. A normal individual or one with true hypoparathyroid hypocalcemia will be stimulated by the parathyroid hormone to increase the rate of urinary phosphorus excretion from the usual 10 to 20 mg per hour up to between 60 to 120 mg per hour. Contrariwise, the hypocalcemic patient with pseudohypoparathyroidism, being refractory to parathyroid hormone, will demonstrate no rise in phosphorus output under this stimulation. The potency of the parathyroid hormone preparation used should always be checked by performing the test on a normal individual of suitable size and age.

With younger children this test may have to be modified because of the difficulty of obtaining hourly specimens of urine from a young child. Proportionately smaller doses of parathyroid hormone are needed, and the urine specimens pooled. Or one may substitute the procedure employed by Collins-Williams with his 6-year-old patient. While a uniformly low phosphorus diet was being given, three consecutive 24-hour collections of urine were taken, the first being the control. Parathyroid extract was injected, 50 units every 12 hours for four injections, commencing at the beginning of the second 24 hours. The urinary output of inorganic phosphorus, which had been 250 mg in the first 24 hours, rose to 548 and 397 mg in the second and third periods. A rise of this magnitude is interpreted as normal.

Treatment of hypoparathyroidism consists of giving large doses of either soluble vitamin D or dihydrotachysterol (AT-10), along with oral calcium salts and a diet high in protein, low in fat, and low in phosphorus. The urinary calcium excretion as estimated by the Sulkowitch test is a helpful guide to the dosages needed (p. 360).

PSEUDOHYPOPARATHYROIDISM

This condition, known also as the Seabright bantam syndrome, was first described by Albright, Burnett, Smith, and Parson in 1942. Affected patients exhibit the signs and symptoms of clinical tetany: convulsions, carpopedal spasm, laryngeal stridor, and positive Chvostek and Trousseau signs. The bodily configuration is distinctive, as a consequence of early closure of the epiphyses: short stature, sturdy build, rounded features, and irregularities in length of the metacarpals and metatarsals. There are soft-tissue calcifications, reduced serum calcium, and elevated serum phosphorus. Parathyroid extract in the phosphorus excretion test fails to raise the serum calcium or the rate of excretion of phosphorus in the urine, as occurs in normal individuals and patients with true hypoparathyroidism. The giving of dihydrotachysterol or vitamin D results in improvement, but much more slowly than in true hypoparathyroidism.

IMMOBILIZATION OSTEOPOROSIS

Osteoporosis is a form of bone demineralization in which the matrix becomes resorbed without osteoid proliferation taking place. Such bone changes can be seen in sudden protracted immobilization and also in scurvy, severe malnutrition, Cushing's syndrome, and the milder forms of osteogenesis imperfecta. The serum calcium and phosphorus do not necessarily show alterations, and the alkaline serum phosphatase remains normal or low.

In normal nongrowing bony tissue an approximately equal balance prevails between the opposing processes of mineral deposition and mineral removal. Fractures or severe paralysis which abruptly immobilize a previously active individual may be followed by an unusual release of calcium and phosphorus into the body fluids. Hypercalcemia may ensue, or even renal injury if the kidney is unable to excrete the calcium as rapidly as liberated. The urinary excretion of calcium mounts to a maximum at about a month after the beginning of the prolonged immobilization and may continue until motion of the limbs is regained. Roentgenograms may fail to detect the demineralization in its early stages.

BIBLIOGRAPHY

PHOSPHORUS AND CALCIUM METABOLISM

Burnett, C. H., R. R. Commons, F. Albright, and *J. E. Howard,* Hypercalcemia without Hypercalcuria or Hypophosphatemia, Calcinosis and Renal Insufficiency, *New England J. Med.* 240:787, 1949.

Calcium and Phosphorus Metabolism in Man and Animals with Special Reference to Pregnancy and Lactation (Symposium), *Ann. New York Acad. Sci.* vol. 64, art. 3, p. 279, 1956.

Calcium and Phosphorus Metabolism: Report of the Fourth M & R Pediatric Research Conference, Feb. 15, 1952, M & R Laboratories, Columbus 16, Ohio.

Cantarow, A., "Calcium Metabolism and Calcium Therapy," Lea & Febiger, Philadelphia, 1933.

Clark, N. S., Familial Renal Insufficiency, *Arch. Dis. Childhood* 26:351, 1951.

Dodd, K., H. Graubarth, and *S. Rapoport,* Hypercalcemia, Nephropathy and Encephalopathy Following Immobilization: Case Report, *Pediatrics* 6:124, 1950.

Guest, G. M., and *S. Rapoport,* Organic Acid-soluble Phosphorus Compounds of the Blood, *Physiol. Rev.* 21:410, 1941.

Holmes, A. D., J. W. Kuzmeski, H. G. Lindquist, and *H. B. Rodman,* Goat's Milk as a Source of Bonebuilding Minerals for Infant Feeding, *Am. J. Dis. Child.* 71:647, 1946.

Kinsman, G., D. Sheldon, E. Jensen, M. Bernds, J. Outhouse, and *H. H. Mitchell,* Utilization of the Calcium of Milk by Pre-school Children, *J. Nutrition* 17:429, 1939.

Macy, I. G., "Nutrition and Chemical Growth in Childhood," vol. I, "Evaluation," Charles C Thomas, Springfield, Ill., 1942.

McLean, F. C., and *A. B. Hastings,* Clinical Estimation and Significance of Calcium-ion Concentration in the Blood, *Am. J. M. Sc.* 189:601, 1935.

Mills, R., H. Breiter, E. Kempster, B. McKey, M. Pickens, and *J. Outhouse,* The Influence of Lactose on Calcium Retention in Children, *J. Nutrition* 20:467, 1940.

Robinson, C. H., I. Hlynka, F. A. Herman, and *J. W. McArthur,* Calcium Content of Fluid Milk, *Canad. J. Pub. Health* 38:236, 1947.

Shohl, A. T., "Mineral Metabolism," Reinhold Publishing Corporation, New York, 1939.

Stearns, G., and *E. Warweg*, Studies of Phosphorus of Blood. I. The Partition of Phosphorus in Whole Blood and Serum: The Serum Calcium and Plasma Phosphatase from Birth to Maturity, *J. Biol. Chem.* **102**:749, 1933.

HYPOCALCEMIA AND TETANY

Bruck, E., Hypocalcemia: Suggestions for Treatment, *Quart. Rev. Pediat.* **4**:221, 1949.
Calamari, A., Apoplessia delle paratiroidi in lattante con sindrome tetanica, *Riv. clin. pediat.* **46**:19, 1948.
Dodd, K., Hypocalcemic States, *Pediatrics* **2**:737, 1948.
Rapoport, S., K. Dodd, M. Clark, and *I. Syllm*, Postacidotic State of Infantile Diarrhea; Symptoms and Chemical Data; Postacidotic Hypocalcemic and Associated Decreases in Levels of Potassium, Phosphorus and Phosphatase in the Plasma, *Am. J. Dis. Child.* **73**:391, 1947.

NEWBORN PERIOD

Bakwin, H., Tetany in Newborn Infants: Relation to Physiologic Hypoparathyroidism, *J. Pediat.* **14**:1, 1939.
Bruck, E., and *D. H. Weintraub*, Serum Calcium and Phosphorus in Premature and Full-term Infants: A Longitudinal Study in the First Three Weeks of Life, *A.M.A., Am. J. Dis. Child.* **90**:653, 1955.
Dodd, K., and *S. Rapoport*, Hypocalcemia in the Neonatal Period: A Clinical Study, *Am. J. Dis. Child.* **78**:537, 1949.
Gardner, L. I., Tetany and Parathyroid Hyperplasia in the Newborn Infant: Influence of Dietary Phosphate Load, *Pediatrics* **9**:534, 1952.
———, *E. A. MacLachlan, W. Pick, M. L. Terry*, and *A. M. Butler*, Etiologic Factors in Tetany of Newly Born Infants, *Pediatrics* **5**:228, 1950.
Gleich, M., S. Smoller, and *B. E. Scott*, Calcium and Phosphorus Studies in Negro Premature Infants, *J. Pediat.* **39**:677, 1951.
Kaplan, E., Parathyroid Gland in Infancy, *Arch. Path.* **34**:1042, 1942.
McCrory, W. W., C. W. Forman, H. McNamara, and *H. L. Barnett*, Renal Excretion of Inorganic Phosphate in Newborn Infants, *J. Clin. Invest.* **31**:357, 1952.
Pincus, J. B., and *I. F. Gittleman*, Mean Serum Calcium and Phosphorus Levels in Infants Fed Formulas Containing and Not Containing Vitamin D during the First Weeks of Life, *A.M.A. Am. J. Dis. Child.* **84**:773, 1952.
———, ———, *A. E. Sobel*, and *E. Schmerzler*, Effects of Vitamin D on the Serum Calcium and Phosphorus Levels in Infants during the First Week of Life, *Pediatrics* **13**:178, 1954.
Ranström, S., and *G. von Sydow*, Rickets in Newborn Infants: Clinical and Histologic Study, *Pediatrics* **4**:406, 1949.
Wolman, I. J., Hypocalcemia and Tetany in the Newborn, *Quart. Rev. Pediat.* **5**:271, 1950.

HYPERCALCEMIA, VITAMIN D, AND BONE DISTURBANCES

Anning, S. T., J. Dawson, D. E. Dolby, and *J. T. Ingram*, The Toxic Effects of Calciferol, *Quart. J. Med.* **17**:203, 1948.
Barnes, D. J., B. Munks, and *M. Kaucher*, Effect of Vitamin D from Cod-liver Oil and Tuna-liver Oil upon Serum Phosphatase Concentrations in Rachitic Infants, *J. Pediat.* **24**:159, 1944.
Copeland, M. M., Bone Diseases with Osteoporotic or Malacic Changes, *South. Surgeon* **16**:677, 1950.
Creery, R. D. G., and *D. W. Neill*, Idiopathic Hypercalcemia in Infants with Failure to Thrive, *Lancet* **2**:110, 1954.

Eliot, M. M., and *E. A. Park,* in Brennemann-McQuarrie, "Practice of Pediatrics" chap. 36, W. F. Prior Co., Hagerstown, Md., 1957.

Engleson, G., Refractory Rickets, *Acta paediat.* **38**:135, 1949.

Fanconi, G., and *E. Chastonay,* Die D-Hypervitaminose im Säuglingsalter, *Helvet. paediat. acta* **5**:5, 1950.

Follis, R. H., Jr., D. A. Jackson, M. M. Eliot, and *E. A. Park,* Prevalence of Rickets in Children between Two and Fourteen Years of Age, *Am. J. Dis. Child.* **66**:1, 1943.

——, *E. A. Park,* and *D. Jackson,* The Prevalence of Rickets at Autopsy during the First Two Years of Age, *Bull. Johns Hopkins Hosp.* **91**:480, 1952.

——, ——, and ——, The Relationship of Vitamin D Administration to the Prevalence of Rickets Observed at Autopsy during the First Two Years of Life, *Bull. Johns Hopkins Hosp.* **92**:426, 1953.

Freeman, S., and *I. Dunsky,* Resistant Rickets, *Am. J. Dis. Child.* **79**:409, 1950.

Harrison, H. E., Mechanisms of Action of Vitamin D, *Pediatrics* **14**:285, 1954.

—— and *H. C. Harrison,* Further Studies of the Effects of Citrate Feeding on the Calcium, Phosphorus and Citrate Metabolism of Rachitic Infants, *J. Pediat.* **41**:756, 1952.

Jeans, P. C., Vitamin D., *J.A.M.A.* **143**:177, 1950.

McCune, D. J., Refractory Rickets, *Am. J. Dis. Child.* **77**:112, 1949.

Pedersen, H. E., and *H. R. McCarroll,* Vitamin-resistant Rickets, *J. Bone & Joint Surg.* **33A**:203, 1951.

Ross, S. G., Vitamin D Intoxication in Infancy: A Report of Four Cases, *J. Pediat.* **41**:815, 1952.

Shohl, A. T., and *A. M. Butler,* Citrates in the Treatment of Infantile Rickets, *New England J. Med.* **220**:515, 1939.

Wiederhold, R. A., and *M. Gonzalez R.,* Rickets in Out-patient Practice. (El Raquitismo en la practica del consultorio externo), *Arch. venezol. de puericult. y pediat.* **16**:25, 1953.

PARATHYROIDS AND THEIR DISTURBANCES

Albright, F., and *E. C. Reifenstein, Jr.,* "The Parathyroid Glands and Metabolic Bone Disease: Selected Studies," The Williams & Wilkins Company, Baltimore, 1948.

Bakwin, H., W. F. Gorman, and *S. R. Ziegra,* Pseudohypoparathyroid Tetany, *J. Pediat.* **36**:567, 1950.

Burnett, C. H., P. H. Smith, and *W. Parson,* Pseudo-Hypoparathyroidism—An Example of "Seabright-Bantam Syndrome," *Endocrinology* **30**:922, 1942.

Collins-Williams, C., Idiopathic Hypoparathyroidism with Papilledema in a Boy Six Years of Age: Report of a Case Associated with Moniliasis and the Celiac Syndrome and a Brief Review of the Literature, *Pediatrics* **5**:998, 1950.

Ellsworth, R., and *J. E. Howard,* Studies on the Physiology of the Parathyroid Glands: Some Responses of Normal Human Kidneys and Blood to Intravenous Parathyroid Extract, *Bull. Johns Hopkins Hosp.* **55**:296, 1934.

Lowe, C. U., A. J. Ellinger, W. S. Wright, and *H. M. Stauffer,* Pseudohypoparathyroidism (the Seabright Bantam Syndrome), *J. Pediat.* **36**:1, 1950.

McLean, F. C., Activated Sterols in the Treatment of Parathyroid Insufficiency, *J.A.M.A.* **117**:609, 1941.

Philips, R. N., Primary Diffuse Parathyroid Hyperplasia in an Infant of Four Months, *Pediatrics* **2**:428, 1948.

Snapper, I., Parathyroid Hormone and Mineral Metabolism, *Bull. New York Acad. Med.* **29**:612, 1953.

Waife, S. O., Parathyrotoxicosis: The Syndrome of Acute Hyperparathyroidism, *Am. J. M. Sc.* **218**:624, 1949.

CHAPTER 53

Plasma Potassium

DISTRIBUTION WITHIN THE BODY

Most of the potassium of the body is held within the tissue cells. Plasma and other extracellular fluids contain only 2 to 5 per cent of the total. According to Shohl, the body of the prematurely born infant of 7 months contains approximately 2.1 gm; of the newborn infant, 5.1 gm; and of the average adult, 160 gm. In the adult the muscles contain approximately 110 gm; blood cells, 8 gm; skeleton, 6 gm; skin, 4 gm; brain, 4 gm; intestines, 5 gm; liver, 3 gm; interstitial fluid, 2.5 gm; lungs, 1.5 gm; and blood plasma, 0.3 gm. The remainder is distributed in lesser amounts in the body fluids and other organs. One hundred grams of fresh muscle contains approximately 365 mg of potassium.

The atomic weight of potassium is 39.1, and its valence is 1. Hence a liter of solution with 39.1 mg of dissolved potassium will contain 1 mEq. One liter of intracellular fluid typically contains 155 mEq of potassium, in contrast to the 5 mEq of potassium in a liter of plasma. The gastric secretion can contain as much as 40 mEq of potassium per liter, and the intestinal secretions about 10 mEq per liter. These secretions are reabsorbed normally in the large intestine but may be lost from the body during vomiting or diarrhea. Normal urine contains 20 to 60 mEq per liter, and vomitus 8 to 20 mEq per liter.

AVERAGE DAILY INTAKE

Since all vegetable and animal cells contain potassium, the everyday human diet, whether omnivorous or vegetarian, is inescapably rich in this element. Milk contains approximately 35 mEq per liter; meat broth, approximately 25 mEq per liter; commercial meat juice concentrates approximately 1,200 mEq per liter. Of the 0.75 gm per 100 ml of mineral ash in cow's milk, 15 to 25 per cent of the positive ions is potassium. The potassium intake of the typical adult is 75 to 130 mEq, or 3 to 5 gm per day. That of the child is proportionately less.

INTERNAL HOMEOSTATIC MECHANISMS

Potassium is filtered through the glomeruli, reabsorbed by the proximal tubules, and perhaps excreted by the distal tubules. Normally, about 80 to 85 per cent of ingested potassium is eliminated in the urine. Urinary excretion goes up whenever the levels of serum potassium or serum bicarbonate are elevated, or whenever a diuresis has been induced by any cause.

In Addison's disease the excretion of this ion is depressed, with a resultant accumulation in the interstitial spaces and the interior of the cells. Conversely, in hyperadrenalism and during prolonged administration of corticotropin or adrenal cortical hormones, extraordinary amounts are lost in the urine.

Actually, the movement of potassium into and out of body cells is far more complex than the above generalizations concerning kidney and adrenal cortex would indicate. Potassium moves out of the fibers during muscle contraction and returns during relaxation. Oral ingestion of a large amount leads to a transient rise in tissue stores, followed in a few hours by a return to normal when renal excretion begins. Water retention in edema may lower the plasma level by dilution even when the body content is far from depleted. Both glycogen and protein formation retain potassium, whereas breakdown of these nutrients liberates this element. Hence it enters the body cells during cellular anabolism as after the administration of testosterone, or insulin and glucose, and leaves during catabolism. Excessive withdrawal of potassium from the body cells may be associated with movement of sodium intracellularly.

The plasma concentration of potassium may need to fluctuate only 1 or 2 mEq above or below normal limits for electrocardiographic changes or disturbances in cardiac rhythm to become evident. Conduction of nerve impulses in both the voluntary and involuntary nervous systems is altered by either high or low concentrations. The skeletal muscles become weak when their content is lowered.

The concentration of potassium in the plasma resembles somewhat that in the interstitial fluids. Measurement per unit volume, however, does not indicate whether the total volumes of these fluids are excessive, normal, or diminished. A total deficit of potassium may be masked by a state of dehydration which may keep the concentration in the body fluids close to normal.

In disease states in which the normal equilibria between intracellular and extracellular potassium may shift, the extracellular concentration of potassium may be low for many hours before clinical signs of cellular depletion appear. Contrariwise, when potassium is being administered therapeutically for hypopotassemia, several days are needed for the content in the tissues to be restored to normal. The serum level may be normal or high at the time the intracellular content is depleted.

One cannot use postmortem chemistry studies to reconstruct possible disturbances. The potassium levels in plasma and cerebrospinal fluid go up immediately after death as the result of autolysis of cells.

NORMAL LEVELS

Red cells contain considerable potassium which diffuses out quickly or is released by hemolysis unless the blood sample is handled with proper care. When collecting a venipuncture specimen for testing, one should draw the blood with a sterile syringe and needle, add anticoagulant at once, and separate the plasma completely from the cells within a few hours by rapid centrifuging. Should the supernatant fluid show more than the faintest trace of hemolysis, the specimen should be discarded and another one taken. The concentrations of potassium in venous and arterial (capillary) blood do not differ appreciably from each other.

Until the flame photometer was applied to this problem, the older chemical methods of estimating potassium in plasma were slow, requiring many hours for their performance. Use of the flame photometer with an internal standard is the most rapid and accurate approach. With it, the range for normal plasma extends from 4.0 to 5.8 mEq per liter, regardless of age. During the first 10 days of life, however, readings up to 6 and 7 mEq per liter are not uncommon. This postnatal rise reaches a peak at the third to fifth day and is usually over by the tenth day, but in premature infants may not subside until the fifteenth or twentieth day. In cerebrospinal fluid the normal spread of potassium is from 2.2 to 3.0 mEq per liter.

CARDIAC RESPONSES

In the absence of a flame photometer the electrocardiogram is the quickest approach to detecting aberrations in potassium level. Electrocardiographic disturbances appear when the plasma level rises above 6 or 7 mEq per liter or falls to 3 mEq per liter or less. The chemistry changes and the intensity of the electrocardiographic changes are not always strictly parallel.

Hyperpotassemia is potentially much more dangerous than is hypopotassemia, because of toxic myocardial depression and the possibility of heart block and ventricular arrest at levels above 10 mEq per liter.

A peaked T wave is the first sign of hyperpotassemia. As retention progresses the R and P waves diminish in height and the S wave increases. The RST segment then becomes depressed. The QRS complex may coincidentally lengthen. With extreme potassium retention an intraventricular or other block may develop and the rhythm become irregular. These changes are best detected with precordial leads.

Hypopotassemia lowers, inverts, or notches the T waves, depresses the RST segment, and lengthens the QT interval. U waves often appear. When potassium is given, the cardiac changes subside within a few minutes, but the skeletal muscle strength may not return for several hours.

HYPERPOTASSEMIA (HYPERKALEMIA)

Pathogenesis

Since healthy kidneys eliminate any reasonable excess, the piling up of potassium within the body is less frequent than its deficiency. An older child can ingest as much as 10 gm of potassium chloride a day with no long-lasting rise in plasma level.

Hyperpotassemia may be said to exist when the plasma level is above 5.8 mEq per liter. This state may be brought about by a diversity of disturbances: increased tissue catabolism; poor renal function caused by anatomic disease, toxemia, or dehydration; massive hemolytic reactions; too rapid intravenous administration of potassium, especially in renal or cardiac disease; adrenocortical insufficiency as in Addison's disease; transfer of intracellular potassium to the extracellular fluids as in dehydration; impairment of the uptake of potassium by the cells as in anoxia. The intracellular content of potassium may be simultaneously high (adrenocortical deficiency, renal failure) or low (infantile diarrhea, postoperative states, diabetic acidosis).

When hyperpotassemia is due to advanced dehydration or the shock syndrome, the serum sodium level is usually subnormal and the plasma volume reduced. In such cases, and particularly when the electrolyte loss has exceeded the water loss, normal or hypertonic saline solution should be a major component of therapy. Restoration of the plasma volume corrects the circulatory impairment and the low blood pressure. This reestablishes kidney function and permits the excretion of the excess potassium. One must be certain, however, before giving saline solution, that the sodium depletion is not consequent to a shift of sodium from extracellular to intracellular areas (p. 596). In this circumstance the giving of additional sodium may decrease the hyperpotassemia temporarily by dilution, but at the same time favor the further movement of sodium into and potassium out of the cells.

Hyperpotassemia occurs exceptionally in acute glomerulonephritis, in all forms of chronic nephritis including pyelonephritis and polycystic disease, and occasionally in the nephrotic syndrome. With the complete renal shutdown of mercury poisoning or the uremia which follows accidental ligation of the ureters, the body content of potassium rises quickly to inordinately high levels and can be the precipitating cause of death. Potassium intoxication may occur even when the blood urea level is elevated only minimally.

Every patient with renal or cardiac disease who has a low urine volume should be watched closely for signs of potassium intoxication. Symptoms and signs are vague and inconsistent. Numbness, weakness, or paresthesias may be complained of in the hands or feet. The heart rate slows without changes in blood pressure or signs of circulatory failure. Flaccid paralysis, pallor, peripheral vascular collapse, cardiac dilatation, or mental confusion may develop. If the accumulation continues, the slowed heart may stop in diastole.

Management

General approaches to the prevention and correction of hyperpotassemia include (1) a very low potassium intake (no milk, meat, fruit juices, vegetables, or potassium-containing medications or parenteral fluids), (2) a diet high in carbohydrates, fats, and calories, in order to minimize protein breakdown, (3) augmentation of the urinary output by administration of proper solutions, (4) digitalization if the heart is failing, (5) minimizing of tissue catabolism by restriction of physical activity, and (6) if thought necessary, a high intake of glucose in concentrated form (25 to 100 gm a day), along with insulin (10 to 30 units), in order to promote glycogen deposition. When anuria or oliguria are not present, sodium chloride and water may be fed in liberal quantities to reduce the potassium level by dilution. In advanced renal hyperpotassemia an ammonium cation-exchange resin may be given by mouth or enema two to four times daily (p. 626) or, where facilities are available, intestinal or peritoneal lavage or "artificial kidney" dialysis.

Careful laboratory control is essential during therapy of the hyperpotassemic patient with anuria. One should determine frequently the serum levels not only of potassium but of sodium, chloride, carbon dioxide, calcium, phosphorus, and the plasma pH.

HYPOPOTASSEMIA (HYPOKALEMIA)

Pathogenesis

A low serum potassium level may be observed in a wide variety of conditions. It often follows parenteral alimentation with potassium-free solutions of patients with dehydration following diarrhea or vomiting, gastric or intestinal drainage, or diabetic ketosis. As already mentioned, cellular breakdown occurs during these disturbances, releasing potassium which is then excreted. As the patient is rehydrated, some potassium returns to the cells, the extracellular space is expanded, and the circulating potassium decreases. Hypopotassemia can also complicate postoperative states, familial periodic paralysis, bulbar poliomyelitis with inability to swallow, adrenal cortex hyperactivity, and treatment with corticotropin, cortisone, or related hormones. The biochemical mechanism may be deficient intake, excessive loss through the gastrointestinal tract or sweat, or metabolic withdrawal of potassium from the cells to the extracellular spaces and thence to the urine. Urinary excretion continues for a time whether the intake is adequate or not, for the renal mechanisms respond slowly and inadequately to the body's need for conservation of potassium.

Diabetic Acidosis

Potassium deficiency is frequent in diabetic acidosis. The most important factor in its production is movement of the ion from the cells to the plasma to the urine as a consequence of dehydration and breakdown of tissue. Phosphate is usually lost simultaneously as well. If potassium-free parenteral solutions and insulin are given to combat the hyperglycemia and ketosis, the fluid-correcting effect of the added fluid and the need for potassium with glucose in intracellular anabolism may lower the potassium level rapidly. The serum concentration may be 4 mEq per liter at the time of hospitalization and less than 2 mEq per liter within 3 to 18 hours after this therapy is begun. The posttherapy decline may give rise to complicating symptoms of myocardial depression and muscular paralysis, at a time when satisfactory progress toward recovery would otherwise be anticipated. Hence it is important in diabetic acidosis to administer potassium salts early, as soon as the renal function is restored.

The diabetic child in profound acidosis and coma may present an especially difficult problem in potassium therapy because of the anuria and diarrhea which so complicate this situation. Frequently repeated laboratory controls are most essential.

Infantile Diarrhea

Infants with diarrhea, dehydration, and acidosis lose potassium and other electrolytes in stools, urine, and vomitus, in amounts proportional to the severity and duration of symptoms. The content of potassium in the muscles may be reduced by as much as 30 per cent, and in the body as a whole by as much as 20 to 25 per cent. The blood potassium level is not a good indicator of the extent of body loss, since normal readings may be given even when the total body deficit is marked. Therapy with potassium salts restores the intracellular potassium and releases sodium to the extracellular fluids.

Potassium deficiency, when not already present in persistent severe diarrhea, may be induced by therapy consisting essentially of solutions of glucose, sodium chloride, and sodium bicarbonate. Hence potassium should be added to these solutions whenever infantile diarrhea is severe enough to interfere with the oral absorption of potassium-containing fluids or foods.

Persistent Vomiting

After continuous gastric drainage or persistent vomiting from pyloric stenosis or other forms of intestinal obstruction, the serum potassium level may fall to as low as 1.5 mEq per liter. There is usually an attendant metabolic alkalosis with a low serum chloride and a secondarily elevated serum bicarbonate (p. 612). The alkalosis as a rule is proportional in severity to the hypotassemia. Therapy of the alkalosis with potassium-free fluids may lower further the serum potassium level. The kidneys appear to have difficulty in excreting bicarbonate in the presence of hypopotassemia, and the urine may remain acid in the presence of alkalosis.

Postoperative States

Every infant or child who has been subjected to major surgery may develop potassium deficiency as a consequence of (1) an antecedent deficit of potassium, (2) unusual loss of potassium in the urine as the result of stress, (3) delay in resuming a normal intake by mouth, or (4) absence of this ion in the supporting parenteral solutions.

Poliomyelitis

With bulbar lesions, the inability to swallow coupled with breakdown of body proteins during the early stages may be attended by loss of large quantities of potassium (along with nitrogen) into the urine, so that the serum potassium level falls significantly. Hence when supporting the nutrition of such patients parenterally the injected fluid should contain potassium salts as well as other nutrients. Current advice is to introduce 0.15 gm (approximately 4 mEq) of potassium chloride per kg body weight each day for the first day or two and 0.1 gm daily thereafter. Once the patient is able to take food by mouth the parenteral potassium becomes no longer necessary. Restoring the plasma level to normal will remove flaccidity from hypopotassemia but will not benefit paralysis from the disease.

Sometimes in unusually severe cases of poliomyelitis the blood level of potassium goes up. This seems to be due to a shift of potassium from the cells to the extracellular fluid, due to tissue destruction, dehydration, and metabolic acidosis, and is aggravated by low renal blood flow and poor urine formation.

Renal Hypopotassemia

Exceptionally in a patient with nephritis or renal failure the excretion of potassium will continue unimpaired or even be abnormally augmented and may eventuate in potassium depletion. The serum potassium level may fall to 1.5 to 3.0 mEq per liter even though the patient ingests a good diet. Satisfactory retention may not be achieved until the daily intake is raised to many times the normal.

Since hyperpotassemia rather than hypopotassemia is the rule in renal disease, however, the blind administration of potassium to correct a possible deficit is most unwise. The same caution applies in all other situations in which renal excretion may be transitorily impaired, such as acute dehydrative states or in the first 24 hours after a major operation.

Excessive urinary loss of potassium is unusual in the nephrotic syndrome. During corticotropin or cortisone therapy, however, the level of serum potassium may fall significantly, especially in those patients who develop diarrhea. Serum levels less than 3.0 mEq per liter may be attained. To avoid hypopotassemia during such hormone therapy it is important to administer a therapeutic supplement of 3 to 5 mEq per kg body weight of potassium each day during and for a few days afterward.

Familial Periodic Paralysis

This is a rare hereditary syndrome in which susceptible patients suffer from intermittent flaccid paralysis of the muscles and extremities. The deep tendon reflexes become lost, and the muscles do not respond properly to galvanic stimulation.

In affected individuals attacks can be induced by fatigue, chilling, overeating, epinephrine, insulin, or glucose in large amounts and can be terminated by giving a potassium salt. It has been hypothesized that extreme activity of the intermediate carbohydrate metabolism within the liver lowers the potassium content of the muscle cells in susceptible individuals below the threshold for proper tonal function.

Studies of childhood cases have shown serum potassium levels below 3.7 mEq per liter during attacks and 4.5 to 5.5 mEq per liter when asymptomatic. A less sustained fall in serum phosphorus occurs coincidentally. Balance studies demonstrate that this drop in serum potassium is due to a shift of potassium from plasma and other extracellular fluids into the interior of the cells. No unusual urinary excretion takes place.

Management of Hypopotassemia

There is no simple formula by which an internal potassium deficit can be calculated. The following general principles are helpful guides to therapy, but treatment must always be individualized.

Potassium deficiency practically always is a component of a generalized disequilibrium, with the acid-base balance and other biochemical mechanisms of the body being disturbed simultaneously. Correction of the potassium deficiency cannot therefore be undertaken as an isolated procedure, except in familial periodic paralysis. One must restore simultaneously the imbalances in water, sodium, chloride, phosphate, glucose, ketone bodies, and other ionizable and non-ionizable solutes. Body weight, respiratory movements, urinary volume, and chemical studies of the blood and urine become important guides. If the shock state is present, whole blood or plasma should be administered to prevent further changes in this direction.

The concentration of potassium in the plasma is approximately the same as in the interstitial fluid, so that one is the measure of the other. When the therapy of dehydration is first begun the concentration of potassium in the blood may be found normal or slightly elevated because of diminished blood volume, even while the deficit in the body as a whole is marked. In this circumstance it is best to start with an intravenous injection of physiologic saline solution containing glucose in order to counteract shock, improve the circulation, and stimulate renal function. Potassium-containing fluids may then be given subcutaneously or intravenously as soon as the peripheral vascular tone is restored and the kidneys are active. Further comments on the use of potassium in parenteral fluid therapy will be found on page 627.

BIBLIOGRAPHY

POTASSIUM

Almaden, P. J., Temperance in Potassium Therapy, *Am. J. Clin. Path.* 22:622, 1952.

Barnett, H. L., and *H. McNamara*, Electrolyte Balances in a Male Infant with Adrenocortical Insufficiency and Virilism: The Effect of Desoxycorticosterone Acetate and Salt Therapy with Special Reference to Potassium, *J. Clin. Invest.* 28:1498, 1949.

Berry, R. E., L. V. Iob, and *K. N. Campbell*, Potassium Metabolism in the Immediate Postoperative Period, *Alexander Blain Hosp. Bull.* 8:34, 1949.

Bower, A. G., F. M. Morgan, and *A. L. Chaney*, Nitrogen and Potassium Metabolism: The Reaction Pattern in Poliomyelitis, *Am. J. M. Sc.* 223:532, 1952.

Brown, H., G. O. Tanner, and *H. H. Hecht*, The Effects of Potassium Salts in Subjects with Heart Disease, *J. Lab. & Clin. Med.* 37:506, 1951.

Butler, A. M., N. B. Talbot, C. H. Burnett, J. B. Stanbury, and *E. A. MacLachlan*, Metabolic Studies in Diabetic Coma, *Tr. A. Am. Physicians* 60:102, 1947.

Cardelle, G., R. M. Jimenez, and *M. G. Vazquez*, Diarrea de Verano. II. Trastornos en el metabolismo del potasio en el curso de las diarreas graves del lactante, *Rev. cubana pediat.* 24:3, 1952.

Currens, J. H., and *J. D. Crawford*, The Electrocardiogram and Disturbances of Potassium Metabolism, *New England J. Med.* 243:843, 1950.

Danowski, T. S., and *J. R. Elkinton*, Exchanges of Potassium Related to Organs and Systems, *Pharmacol. Rev.* 3:42, 1951.

Darrow, D. C., Body-Fluid Physiology: The Role of Potassium in Clinical Disturbances of Body Water and Electrolyte, *New England J. Med.* 242:978, 1014, 1950.

———, Physiological Basis of Potassium Therapy, *J.A.M.A.* 162:1310, 1956.

———, *E. L. Pratt, J. Flett, Jr., A. H. Gamble*, and *H. F. Wiese*, Disturbances of Water and Electrolytes in Infantile Diarrhea, *Pediatrics* 3:129, 1949.

Earle, D. P., H. Bakwin, and *D. Hirsch*, The Plasma Potassium Level in the Newborn, *Proc. Soc. Exper. Biol. & Med.* 76:756, 1951.

Elkinton, J. R., J. K. Clark, R. D. Squires, L. W. Bluemile, Jr., and *A. P. Crosley, Jr.*,

Treatment of Potassium Retention in Anuria with Cation Exchange Resin, *Am. J. M. Sc.* **220**:547, 1950.

——, *R. Tarail,* and *J. P. Peters,* Transfers of Potassium in Renal Insufficiency, *J. Clin. Invest.* **28**:378, 1948.

Engel, F. L., S. P. Martin, and *H. Taylor,* On the Relation of Potassium to the Neurological Manifestations of Hypocalcemic Tetany, *Bull. Johns Hopkins Hosp.* **84**:285, 1949.

Fox, C. L., and *L. B. Slobody,* Tissue Changes in the Nephrotic Syndrome: Demonstration of Potassium Depletion, *Pediatrics* **7**:186, 1951.

Fourman, P., Ability of the Normal Kidney to Conserve Potassium, *Lancet* **262**:1042, 1952.

Gardner, L. I., N. B. Talbot, C. D. Cook, H. Berman, and *C. Uribe,* The Effect of Potassium Deficiency on Carbohydrate Metabolism, *J. Lab. & Clin. Med.* **35**:592, 1950.

Gass, H., M. Cherkasky, and *N. Savitsky,* Potassium and Periodic Paralysis: A Metabolic Study and Physiological Considerations, *Medicine* **27**:105, 1948.

Greenman, L., F. M. Mateer, R. C. Gow, J. H. Peters, and *T. S. Danowski,* Some Observations on the Development of Hypokaliemia during Therapy of Diabetic Acidosis in Juvenile and Young Adult Subjects, *J. Clin. Invest.* **28**:409, 1949.

Lans, H. S., I. F. Stein, R. J. Becker, A. L. Hoyne, and *K. A. Meyer,* Potassium Deficiency in Bulbar Poliomyelitis, *J.A.M.A.* **146**:1017, 1951.

Lowe, C. U., M. Rourke, E. MacLachlan, and *A. M. Butler,* Use of Parenteral Potassium Therapy in Surgical Patients: Its Role in Preventing Chloride Loss, *Pediatrics* **6**:183, 1950.

Martin, H. E., T. B. Reynolds, E. N. Snyder, C. J. Berne, R. E. Homann, Jr., H. A. Edmondson, N. Blatherwick, I. Fields, M. Wertman, and *L. Westover,* Etiology and Treatment of Serum Potassium Deficits, *J.A.M.A.* **147**:24, 1951.

Mateer, F. M., L. Greenman, A. C. Austin, J. H. Peters, H. Mermelstein, F. Weigand, and *T. S. Danowski,* The Use of Potassium Chloride in the Pre-operative Treatment of Pyloric Stenosis in Infants, *Am. J. M. Sc.* **221**:21, 1951.

Mudge, G. H., Potassium Imbalance, *Bull. New York Acad. Med.* **29**:846, 1953.

Nadler, C. S., Recent Advances in Potassium Metabolism, *Am. J. M. Sc.* **226**:88, 1953.

Oliver, C. P., M. Ziegler, and *I. McQuarrie,* Hereditary Periodic Paralysis in a Family Showing Varied Manifestations, *Am. J. Dis. Child.* **68**:308, 1944.

Sarnoff, S. J., J. L. Whittenberger, and *J. E. Affeldt,* Hypoventilation Syndrome in Bulbar Poliomyelitis, *J.A.M.A.* **147**:30, 1951.

Schwartz, R., E. J. Tomsovic, and *I. L. Schwartz,* Hyperpotassemia and Body Water Distribution in an Anuric Child, *Pediatrics* **7**:516, 1951.

Schwartz, W. B., Potassium and the Kidney, *New England J. Med.* **253**:601, 1955.

Sherry, S., L. W. Eichna, and *D. P. Earle, Jr.,* The Low Potassium Syndrome in Chronic Nephritis, *J. Clin. Invest.* **27**:556, 1948.

Shohl, A. T., "Mineral Metabolism," Reinhold Publishing Corporation, New York, 1939.

Stephens, J. W., and *H. F. Root,* Treatment of Diabetic Coma, *Postgrad. Med.* **13**:164, 1953.

Wallace, W. M., and *F. C. Moll,* Balance and Electrocardiographic Studies in a Child with Potassium Deficiency, *Pediatrics* **4**:287, 1949.

CHAPTER 54

Body Water and Electrolytes

NORMAL WATER METABOLISM

Water, the most abundant of the body ingredients, is a major constituent of the contents of the vascular, subarachnoid, and synovial spaces. It is held loosely in the connective tissue and intercellular spaces and is united intimately with the proteins and other molecular substances found intracellularly and interstitially.

The equilibria between water in the blood stream, tissue interstices, and intracellular protoplasm are difficult to separate from the distribution of electrolytes and plasma and tissue proteins. The selective permeability of membranes, the osmotic pressure of the proteins, the differences in ion content between protoplasm and interstitial fluid, the excretory activities of the kidney, the movement of water into areas of greater osmotic tonicity—all participate in the maintenance of a stable water metabolism.

The very rapid intermediary metabolism can be followed by tracing the movement through the body of water containing deuterium or tritium. A 98 per cent equilibrium with the extravascular body fluids is achieved within an hour after water containing either of these two isotopes of hydrogen is injected into the blood stream. The volumes of water which move in and out of the blood stream per minute seem to be considerably greater than the amount in the blood stream itself. The average time that a molecule of water remains in the body between ingestion and excretion is about 10 days, as noted in experiments with normal adults.

Water Intake and Output

The body receives water from liquids that one drinks, the fluid contained in foods, and food materials as they are catabolized. The quantities of water which are formed when 100 gm of the principal food types are consumed within the body are protein, 39 gm; fat, 107 gm; carbohydrate, 56 gm.

For a normal 7-kg infant in a temperate climate the total daily intake of water from all sources (fluids drunk, food eaten, and water of oxidation) averages 700 ml, or approximately one-tenth the body weight. For a comparable adult the intake averages 2,000 to 2,500 ml or approximately one-thirtieth of the body weight.

Water leaves the body (1) through the pulmonary alveoli and the skin surface by "insensible" evaporation, (2) through the kidneys, (3) through frank sweating, and (4) through the bowel (negligible except in vomiting or diarrhea). The water lost by the average adult each day may amount to as much as 1 to 2 liters in urine, 0.5 to 1 liter by evaporation from the lungs, 0 to several liters in sweat, and 50 to 100 ml in feces. For infants under 1 year of age the average daily loss is approximately 40 to 80 ml per kg in urine, 40 ml per kg in evaporation, 0 to 100 ml per kg in sweat, and 0 to 20 ml per kg in feces. In general, 42 ml of water is lost from the lungs for each 100 calories of heat produced.

The irreducible water losses, according to Gamble, amount to about 1,400 ml a day in the 70-kg adult and about 300 ml a day in the 7-kg infant. Proportionately, therefore, the starving and thirsting adult loses only 2 per cent of his body weight per day, but the infant nearly 5 per cent. Death from water deprivation in the infant can be expected in half the time needed for its occurrence in the adult.

The average healthy normal infant, in an environment in which sweating is not marked, will have enough water for all metabolic and excretory requirements if 140 to 150 ml per kg body weight is provided. Sweating, diarrhea, or other unusual losses may increase the need for water beyond these limits. The greater requirements of the infant, as compared with the older child or adult, are the consequence of (1) the larger surface area in proportion to body mass resulting in a greater rate of heat loss and insensible perspiration, and (2) the functional immaturity of the kidney which, when coupled with the relatively greater abundance of end products of tissue catabolism, necessitates comparatively larger minimal volumes of urine.

When the balances of intake and output of water and electrolytes are measured accurately in metabolic experiments, considerable oscillation of the retention and excretion of these components is found to take place from day to day and week to week. These normal physiologic phenomena are responsible for the lack of absolute constancy in body-weight curves when weighings are conducted daily under conditions comparable with respect to meals and elimination.

During a 24-hour period the typical normal adult secretes into his gastrointestinal system as much as 1.5 liters of saliva, 2.5 liters of gastric juice, 1 liter of pancreatic juice, 3 liters of succus entericus, and 0.5 liter of bile— a total of 8.5 liters. These secretions pour out in waves which attain their maxima soon after meals. After a heavy meal the needs for water may reduce significantly the blood volume and the interstitial fluid compartment. Within the colon these fluids are practically completely reabsorbed, except when there is diarrhea, vomiting, or a draining intestinal fistula. Loss of water in these latter conditions is accompanied by loss of electrolytes, the ionic composition depending upon site of the loss and nature of the disturbance. In gastroenteritis of moderate degree the daily stool volume may amount to approximately 35 ml per kg per day; in severe disturbances to as much as 70 ml per kg per day.

About 80 per cent of the water which is filtered through the glomeruli must be reabsorbed in order to enable the contained solutes such as sodium, chloride bicarbonate, glucose, and amino acids to be drawn back through the tubular epithelium. Most of the remaining 20 per cent of the glomerular filtrate is reabsorbed also, varying with need. In the healthy adult, approximately 1,175 liters of water a day is filtered through the glomeruli, and all but 1 or 2 liters reabsorbed in the tubules.

Water losses from the lungs and skin increase during hot weather. As much as 60 or 70 ml of water per kg body weight per day may be lost through sweat alone, in addition to the insensible water loss from the skin and lungs. Daily losses may be estimated at about 25 to 50 mM (millimols) for sodium and chloride and 15 mM for potassium.

Total Body Water

Data regarding the precise water content of the body as a whole are meager. Figures ranging from 65 to 80 per cent of body weight have been secured by desiccation analyses of the bodies of newborn infants. Values of about 75 per cent body weight for three newborn infants were obtained by Flexner and associates with the deuterium oxide method. Readings of from 70 to 83 per cent of body weight were obtained by Friis-Hansen and associates in premature and newborn infants; there was a gradual decline during the first 6 months of life with both the deuterium oxide and the antipyrine methods. Between 6 months and 11 years, the values varied between 53 and 63 per cent, uncorrelated with age and sex. Studies by Katcher and associates of 10 normal infants 6 weeks to 8 months of age, using deuterium oxide, gave values for total body water ranging from 55 to 71 per cent with a mean of 62 per cent. Variations in individuals of the same age or body surface area are probably due largely to differences in fat content.

Friis-Hansen and associates give the following empirical formulas for calculation of total body water in children weighing up to 20 kg or having body surface areas up to 1 square meter:

$$\text{Total body water, liters} = (0.55 \times \text{wt., kg}) + 0.51 \ (\text{S.D.} \pm 7.4\%)$$

Total body water, liters
$$= (\text{surface area, square meters} \times 15.05) - 0.71 \ (\text{S.D.} \pm 7.1\%)$$

With adults the body water has been found to be 40 to 72 per cent of total body weight. The more obese the subject, the lower his water content. The widely cited value of 70 per cent holds only for the exceptionally lean individual. The body fat content can be estimated from the reading for specific gravity of the whole body.

Concept of Compartments

Despite the continuous to-and-fro movement of individual molecules of water across the enormous aggregate surface area of the tissue cells, the water in the body as a whole can be presented as being partly intracellular and partly extracellular. The so-called "intracellular compartment" refers to the water contained in the aggregate protoplasm of all the cells. The so-called "extracellular compartment" refers to the contents of the interstitial spaces, the blood and lymph vessels, the cerebrospinal fluid spaces, and so forth. The application of this concept to experimental physiologic data has been productive of great advances in the development of corrective treatment for states of fluid and electrolyte imbalance.

The concentrations of mineral ions in the fluids of the connective tissues and other interstitial areas vary with location and age, and rise and fall parallel with alterations in the respective plasma concentrations. For practical purposes, when calculations on the amounts and kinds of salts needed for therapeutic purposes are being made, the electrolytic composition of the blood plasma is usually taken as representative of that of the interstitial fluid throughout the body.

Measurement

The volumes of these subdivisions can be approximated by injecting measured amounts of test substances into the blood stream and then determining the extent of the dilution. Certain dyes, such as Evans blue, combine with the plasma proteins and for a limited time remain confined to the intravascular spaces. Other soluble substances, such as thiocyanate, inulin, sucrose, and radioactive sodium (Na^{24}), diffuse promptly through the entire extracellular compartment and a little more slowly through the cerebrospinal fluid, but do not enter the cells in quantity until many hours have passed. Another group of soluble substances, including urea, thiourea, antipyrine, and especially deuterium oxide (heavy water), because they distribute themselves rapidly through all parts of the body, are employed as indicators of the total amount of free water. By simultaneously measuring plasma volume and total extracellular water and subtracting one from the other, the volume of the "interstitial space" can be estimated. Similarly, by subtracting total extracellular water from total body water, the volume of intracellular water can be estimated.

Results secured with parallel methods are not always in close agreement. Confusing variation occurs in the rates of diffusion, equilibration, excretion, and catabolism. Totals obtained by such means are best viewed as approximate rather than absolute values. With serial determinations of a patient by any one method, however, one can attempt to follow the water shifts and thereby estimate the changes in compartment size. Statistical assessments of alterations with age in normal growing subjects are presumably valid also.

Sodium Thiocyanate (NaSCN) Space (Extracellular Fluid)

When sodium thiocyanate (NaSCN) was injected into normal infants and children by Ely and Sutow, the "thiocyanate space" was found to average 39 per cent of the body weight during the first 6 months of life, 33 per cent at 6 to 12 months, 32 per cent at 1 to 2 years, 30 per cent at 3 to 5 years, and 29 per cent at 5 to 15 years. These values may be compared with reported figures of 20 to 25 per cent for adults secured with the same method. Correlations with the data of Friis-Hansen and associates suggest that during the first half year of life the fall in total body water with age occurs principally in the extracellular compartment.

Plasma Volume

Ely and Sutow's readings for plasma volume with Evans blue dye (T-1824) in 13 infants under 1 year of age ranged from 32 to 66 ml per kg body weight, with a mean of 50 ml. In 50 children up to 10 years of age the range was 29 to 84 ml per kg, with a mean of slightly under 50 ml. No sex differences were noted. Katcher and associates, using the Evans blue method, found a mean in 10 normal infants 6 weeks to 10 months of age of 58 ml per kg, with a standard deviation of ±7 ml. Russell reported a mean of 48 ml in 64 children weighing 10 to 30 kg.

Thus the round number of 50 ml per kg may be used as an average for estimating plasma volume in infants and young children. The adult average is about 45 ml per kg.

Blood Volume

Total blood volume can be estimated from the hematocrit reading and from the value for plasma volume obtained by the dye method. Ely and Sutow calculated the blood volumes in their infants under 1 year of age as 55 to 116 ml per kg body weight, with a mean of 80 ml. The blood volumes in their 50 infants and children up to 10 years of age ranged from 46 to 140 ml per kg, with a mean of slightly over 80 ml.

Mollison has pointed out that a corrective factor of 0.83 should be introduced into such calculations. This factor is the product of 0.95×0.87, 0.95 being the correction for trapped plasma in the hematocrit tube and 0.87 the relation of the proportion of red cells in the body as a whole to the proportion in venous blood. The more precise formula is, therefore,

$$\text{Blood volume} = \text{plasma volume} \times \frac{100}{100 - (\text{hematocrit} \times 0.83)}$$

Introduction of this corrective factor brings the above-quoted average blood volume for Ely and Sutow's children to approximately 75 ml per kg body weight, which is in the same range as figures submitted by other workers.

When calculating deficits for fluid therapy in infants and young children, the value of 7.5 per cent of body weight may be taken as the average normal for the amount of whole blood in the body. Of this, roughly 70 per cent is plasma and 30 per cent is red cells, in the absence of anemia or erythrocytosis. In the newborn period the total blood volume may be closer to 8.0 per cent, chiefly because of a higher red cell count.

Magnitude of Compartments as Related to Age

Wide variations have been found in the estimated volumes of interstitial fluid and plasma in the same normal individual on successive days, and even wider differences in random observations of groups of individuals of the same approximate age and body size. In the premature infant the interstitial fluid seems to average 40 to 50 per cent of the total body weight; in the full-term newborn 30 to 40 per cent. At all ages, the intravascular fluid (plasma) represents about 5 per cent of the body weight, or approximately 50 ml per kg. Estimates for the intracellular water, which is less labile, vary from 25 to 40 per cent of the body weight throughout childhood. The volume of interstitial fluid is thus proportionately greater (and the concentration of solids perhaps slightly lower) in early infancy as compared with adult ages. These differences decline rapidly during late infancy and more slowly throughout childhood.

In disturbances involving water and electrolytes the volume of the interstitial fluid fluctuates most markedly, that of the intravascular plasma somewhat less so, and that of the cells themselves least.

THE PLASMA CATIONS

Total cations in extracellular fluid average about 155 mEq per liter in infancy and childhood. Of this, approximately 142 mEq, or 92 per cent, is sodium; 5 mEq, or 3 per cent, is potassium; 5 mEq is calcium; and 3 mEq, or 2 per cent, is magnesium. This compares with the estimated 155 mEq of potassium, 14 mEq of sodium, and 26 mEq of magnesium in intracellular fluid.

Until a few years ago, when one wanted to analyze the plasma chemically for the basic ions it was customary to test for them together under the category of "total base." This determination was within the scope of the better-equipped hospital laboratories but took at least a day to carry out. The more recent popularization of flame photometry has made it possible to secure accurate estimations of sodium and potassium within an hour. Since sodium is the most abundant single ion, knowledge of its concentration can be very helpful in evaluating both the total cation concentration and the osmotic status of the full electrolyte equilibrium.

Sodium

PHYSIOLOGY. The sources of dietary sodium are few. Unsalted vegetables are low in sodium, and meats and most other foods contain but small amounts. Fish is a richer source. Cow's milk averages about 50 mg per 100 gm. Most of the sodium ingested by older children and adults derives from sodium chloride added to foods, either in processing or at the table. Breads, butter, oleomargarine, and processed cheeses contain from 0.15 to 1.5 per cent sodium.

Sodium is excreted chiefly in the urine. When the intake of sodium is stopped, the urinary output diminishes gradually and ceases within a few days. The amounts lost through perspiration or gastrointestinal contents are ordinarily not very great but may mount significantly as the result of sweating, vomiting, diarrhea, or intestinal fistula.

The total content of sodium in bodies of young infants seems to vary from 60 to 90 mEq per kg body weight, with an average of 75 mEq. Beyond infancy the proportional content declines gradually in curvilinear fashion with increasing age, until adult values of approximately 42 mEq per kg are reached.

In plasma and interstitial fluid, sodium is the most abundant ion and is responsible for almost half of the total osmotic force exerted by the extracellular electrolytes. Not much sodium is found inside the body cells except for bone, which contains about 20 per cent of the total content of body sodium, mostly in a non-ionized structurally bound form. When in excess, sodium ion is pharmacologically inert except that a large intake may promote the accumulation of fluid. According to present knowledge, the principal clinical disturbances referable to sodium are related to acid-base equilibrium and the distribution of water.

The urinary excretion of sodium seems to be controlled in part by the adrenal cortical hormones. The glomerulosa zone is believed to decrease when intake and output of sodium are high and enlarge when reverse conditions obtain. Hormones from the other endocrine glands also affect sodium metabolism; for example, deprivation of thyroid substance diverts sodium into myxedematous tissues. The need for sodium is increased in adrenal cortical insufficiency (p. 744).

The ionized intracellular sodium is about 7 mEq per kg at all ages. Sodium may move from the extracellular to the intracellular fluid and back in electrolyte disturbances, to balance variations in extracellular bicarbonate. Intracellular accumulation may take place during dehydration, shock, or tissue anoxia, at the same time as potassium is migrating out into the extracellular environment.

Sodium can be driven into the cells by giving large quantities of sodium without furnishing an equivalent amount of chloride or potassium simultaneously. When Gamble and associates fed 80 mM of sodium bicarbonate over an 8-day period to an 8-kg infant, a total of 79 mM was retained in the body. Of this, only 23 mM appeared to lie extracellularly, whereas 56 mM was taken up by the cells.

The normal plasma concentration of sodium tends to range from 134 to 154 mEq per liter, regardless of age. The usual or median level is 143 mEq. Practically all is ionized. Maintenance of this constant level with varying intakes of water and sodium is effected by adjustments in renal excretion. Efficiency of the kidneys in conserving the salt supplies of the body may become impaired in (1) various kidney diseases, (2) Addison's disease and related forms of adrenal cortical insufficiency, (3) some intracranial lesions, tuberculous meningitis, advanced pulmonary tuberculosis, and, occasionally, in other disorders. The extreme limits of variation for plasma sodium compatible with life have been said to be 105 and 170 mEq per liter.

HYPONATREMIA. Sodium may be lost in excess of an equivalent amount of water during therapy with fluids of low sodium content or the absence of good renal or adrenocortical functions (water intoxication, p. 617). The corresponding phenomenon occurs when patients with diarrhea or vomiting are given large amounts of water or plain glucose solution by mouth or proctoclysis, instead of normal or slightly hypotonic saline solutions.

Administration of large volumes of glucose solution parenterally can induce a wave of hypotonicity in the body fluid reservoirs (p. 622).

When the extravascular fluids become hypotonic with respect to sodium, osmotic pressure pulls water into the cells. This reduces the volumes of the interstitial and the intravascular compartments. The result is a form of prostration resembling shock, in which circulatory efficiency is impaired, blood pressure reduced, and the cardiac output diminished. This form of sodium depletion is sometimes a factor in the dehydration which accompanies diarrhea, diabetic acidosis, extensive burns, and the loss of fluids through vomiting or gastrointestinal fistulas (p. 619). Similarly, children with communicating hydrocephalus which has been treated surgically by anastomosis of a renal pelvis to the subarachnoid space may do well for many months until a sudden infection or illness, by curtailing the food intake or evoking diarrhea, exhausts the low salt reserves.

The shocklike state of sodium depletion can be corrected by giving sodium, preferably in hypertonic saline solution, unless protracted delay has resulted in extreme intracellular changes. In such circumstance, whole blood or plasma should be administered with or before the saline solution.

Intravenous therapy for patients with hyponatremia should consist of a 3 per cent hypertonic saline solution. Each 10 ml of this contains enough sodium to take care of its own water content and raise the sodium content of 1 liter of extracellular fluid by about 3.5 mEq.

Associated disturbances of the anions while sodium is being lost can result in a low plasma content of bicarbonate or chloride or both. When chloride is deficient as well as sodium the restorative therapy should be saline solutions; when carbonic acid is low the indication is for the use of solutions of sodium bicarbonate or lactate (Chap. 56).

Estimation of the deficit of sodium from that of chloride or bicarbonate or their total has certain limitations. When acidosis is present, chloride and bicarbonate can vary independently of each other. A high content of organic acids as in diabetic acidosis may depress the concentrations of both chloride and bicarbonate, while that of sodium remains normal.

HYPERNATREMIA. The extracellular concentration of sodium may become elevated to levels above the top normal of 155 mEq per liter in fluid and electrolyte imbalances in which water deficit exceeds sodium deficit. These conditions are discussed under Hyperelectrolytemic Dehydration (p. 620).

Other Cations

The pathologic physiology of potassium is discussed in Chap. 53 and of calcium in Chap. 52.

MAGNESIUM. One of the less abundant minerals, magnesium occurs in the blood plasma in a concentration of about 2 mEq per liter. The usual daily intake of an older child on a regular diet, according to Macy, is 250 to 600 mg a day. From 35 to 60 per cent of this is absorbed. Of the amount absorbed, 10 to 30 per cent is retained in the body. The rest is lost in the feces and urine. Important dietary sources of magnesium are nuts, cocoa, wheat, corn, oatmeal, beans, and peas. About 70 per cent of the magnesium in the body is in the bones.

Magnesium appears to follow the same physiologic pathways as phosphorus within the body and seems related to carbohydrate and fat metabolism. Intravenous injections of magnesium salts promote the urinary excretion of calcium; other pharmacologic phenomena also indicate an antagonism between these two elements.

Magnesium deficiency in childhood as an entity is almost unknown. In experimental animals the signs of deficiency are hyperirritability, convulsions, renal lesions, tachycardia, vasodilatation, and changes in the teeth and bones. It is probable that the magnesium ion participates in some poorly understood manner in the clinical manifestations of tetany during hypocalcemic disturbances.

THE PLASMA ANIONS

Bicarbonate with an average of 27 mEq per liter and chloride with an average of 103 mEq per liter are the principal anions of the blood plasma. The other constituent ions which make up this moiety of normal plasma are, per liter, organic acids 6 mEq, phosphate 2 mEq, sulfate 1 mEq, and the plasma proteins which at pH 7.4 ionize to about 16 mEq.

Chloride

Chloride, the most abundant extracellular anion, plays an important role in the maintenance of total osmotic pressure and acid-base balance.

Whether this ion occurs in more than trace amounts elsewhere than in the extracellular fluid and the gastric mucosa is still a subject of controversy. Some evidence suggests that appreciable intracellular quantities may be found in the connective tissue, testis, and lung.

Chloride is widely distributed through all foods and tends to be ingested in excess. Its excretion is largely through urine and sweat. When the intake and body content begin to be depleted the urinary output ceases within a day or two as a conserving measure.

The total quantity of chloride ions in the body as a whole is about 30 mEq per kg body weight. In the blood plasma and the interstitial fluid the concentrations tend to be essentially the same. The range of normal variation of plasma chloride levels in infants is 100 to 110 mEq per liter, with the usual reading near 105 mEq per liter. In adults the usual concentration of the chlorides in the extracellular fluids is usually approximately 103 mEq per liter.

HYPERCHLOREMIA. Increases in plasma chloride are encountered (1) in acute dehydrative and hyperelectrolytemic states, in which reduced intake or loss of water hampers the renal mechanisms which carry off electrolytes, (2) when the exchange of water remains normal or only slightly reduced but unusual amounts of chloride are being supplied to the body, (3) when renal excretion of chloride is impaired, as in severe nephritis, after surgical operations, and in congestive circulatory failure, or (4) in alkalosis produced by chronic hyperventilation as in salicylate poisoning, where a compensatory rise in chloride replaces the diminished bicarbonate level and sustains the normal pH of the plasma.

HYPOCHLOREMIA. Decreases in plasma chloride may occur in the same conditions which decrease the sodium level, but the relative losses of these two ions do not necessarily run parallel. A moderate fall in the plasma level of chloride is accompanied by no prominent disturbance except dehydration. Pronounced depletion results in impaired digestion, poor water retention, muscle cramps, hyperexcitability, and even convulsions.

Loss of fluids and electrolytes is frequent in intestinal obstruction and diarrheal disorders. Pancreatic juice, bile, jejunal and ileal secretions, and diarrheal discharges ordinarily contain more sodium than chloride; whereas gastric fluid lost through vomiting or drainage tends to contain proportionately much more chloride. Chloride may shift from the plasma to tissues and red cells concomitantly. Hypochloremia which may result evokes a retention of carbon dioxide and a trend to alkalosis. The kidney then excretes increased quantities of sodium to correct the alkalosis. Dehydration, hemoconcentration, and loss of fixed base follow. Weakness and muscle cramps may be prominent symptoms. A 2 per cent solution of ammonium chloride is sometimes given intravenously as part of the therapy, but is almost never necessary.

Extracellular fluids maintain their isotonicity during chloride loss by an increase in bicarbonate or organic acids or both. A fall in chloride concentration from the usual level of 95 to 110 mEq per liter down to 70 or even 60 mEq does not produce any specific group of symptoms, in the way that hypopotassemia produces cardiac weakness or hypocalcemia results in tetany. Nevertheless, muscular twitching and muscular and intestinal cramps are frequent in such patients and are alleviated by the therapeutic administration of chlorides. This is the reason for giving extra sodium chloride in the form of enteric-coated salt tablets or salty broth to laborers or febrile patients who sweat profusely.

In prolonged inanition the chloride level may fall to near 70 mEq per liter, compensated in part by an increase in bicarbonate; the sodium level also falls. In severe acute febrile illnesses such as pneumonia, both the chloride and sodium levels in the serum may decrease because of the inanition, diminished intake of salt, and retention of water in the extracellular spaces. Typical plasma readings in severe febrile illnesses are 90 mEq per liter for chloride and 130 mEq for sodium.

In nephritic diseases and the nephrotic syndrome the serum chloride level often remains in the normal range despite marked changes in other components. Vomiting or marked retention of phosphate, sulfate, and other inorganic acids may bring about a diminution. With adrenal cortical insufficiency the serum chlorides may fall to 80 or 90 mEq per liter, coincident with the depression of the sodium level.

Plasma Bicarbonate

CARRIAGE OF CO_2 IN THE BLOOD. Carbon dioxide when first liberated by the catabolic processes of the tissue cells is believed to pass through the interstitial fluid into the blood as a gas dissolved in water. Once in the blood the greater part of this gas diffuses promptly into the red cells. Here some of it combines with hemoglobin, while the rest is converted into carbonic acid through the catalytic activity of the red cell enzyme carbonic anhydrase. Much of this newly formed carbonic acid is ionized instantly to yield hydrogen ions and bicarbonate ions. The bulk of the bicarbonate ions then diffuse out of the red cells into the plasma to balance ionically with the basic ions there present. The entire cycle of reactions is reversed in the pulmonary capillaries as the blood gives off CO_2 and takes up oxygen. Chloride ions "shift" into the red cells as the bicarbonate ions move out.

A representative sample of normal adult whole blood, according to Henderson, may contain 21.53 mM of CO_2 per liter in the arterial state and 23.21 mM in the venous state. The amount of CO_2 transported from the tissues to the lungs for excretion thus is about 1.68 mM per liter.

BUFFER ACTION OF CO_2 AND BICARBONATE. When the ratio of free CO_2 to combined CO_2 (bicarbonate) in the plasma is 1:20 the pH of the plasma is maintained at 7.4. Any disturbance in either the pulmonary excretion of CO_2 or the level of circulating bicarbonate would force the plasma pH in either an acidic or basic direction, were not these influences counterbalanced to some extent by other physiologic mechanisms (see discussion of acidosis and alkalosis, Chap. 55).

In the acid-base equilibrium of the plasma, the bicarbonate anion in healthy children averages approximately 26 mEq per liter. The corresponding amount of basic ion is known as "alkali reserve" or "available base," since it will neutralize any metabolic excess of anions (e.g., lactic acid, ketone acids) or any abnormal absorbed anions (e.g., salicylic acid).

CO_2 CAPACITY AND CONTENT. The CO_2 capacity, known also as "CO_2-combining power," is a fairly reliable indication of the alkali reserve. The determination is done on freshly separated plasma (or serum).

The CO_2 capacity in children is usually near 58 ml or "volumes" CO_2 per 100 ml. To convert to milliequivalents per liter this value is multiplied by the factor 0.45, giving 26 mEq per liter. The normal range is 45 to 70 ml per 100 ml, corresponding to 20 to 31 mEq per liter. Readings below 40 ml are found in metabolic acidosis and respiratory alkalosis; above 75 ml, in respiratory acidosis and metabolic alkalosis (Chap. 55). The plasma pH is usually reduced when values are less than 30 ml or elevated when higher than 85 ml per 100 ml.

The plasma CO_2 "content," measured on blood or plasma collected anaerobically, is a technically difficult but most direct approach to determining the existence of a CO_2 deficit or excess. When combined with a plasma pH determination done simultaneously, exact information concerning the acid-base equilibrium is given.

BIBLIOGRAPHY

BODY WATER AND ELECTROLYTES

Adolph, E. F., The Metabolism and Distribution of Water in Body and Tissues, *Physiol. Rev.* 13:336, 1933.

Cheek, D. B., Observations on Total Body Chloride in Children, *Pediatrics* 14:5, 1954.

Elliot, H. C., Jr., and *H. L. Holley,* Serum Sodium and Potassium Values in Four Hundred Normal Human Subjects, Determined by the Beckman Flame Photometer, *Am. J. Clin. Path.* 21:831, 1951.

Ely, R. S., and *W. W. Sutow,* Growth of Thiocyanate Space in Infancy and Childhood, *Pediatrics* 10:115, 1952.

Evans Blue: Accepted for Admission to New and Nonofficial Remedies, *J.A.M.A.* 150:1486, 1952.

Fellers, F. X., H. L. Barnett, K. Hare, and *H. McNamara,* Change in Thiocyanate and Sodium Spaces during Growth, *Pediatrics* 3:622, 1949.

Flexner, L. B., W. S. Wilde, N. K. Proctor, D. B. Cowie, G. J. Vosburgh, and *L. M. Hellman,* Estimation of Extracellular and Total Body Water in the Newborn Human Infant with Radioactive Sodium and Deuterium Oxide, *J. Pediat.* 30:413, 1947.

Flink, E. B., Magnesium Syndrome in Man, *J.A.M.A.* 160:1406, 1956.

Forbes, G. B., Chemical Growth in Infancy and Childhood, *J. Pediat.* 41:202, 1952.

——— and *A. Perley,* Estimation of Total Body Sodium by Isotopic Dilution. I. Studies on Young Adults, *J. Clin. Invest.* 30:558, 1951. II. Studies on Infants and Children: An Example of a Constant Differential Growth Ratio, *ibid.* 30:566, 1951.

Friis-Hansen, B. J., M. Holiday, T. Stapleton, and *W. M. Wallace,* Total Body Water in Children, *Pediatrics* 7:321, 1951.

Gamble, J. L., Companionship of Water and Electrolytes in the Organization of Body Fluids, *Lane M. Lect., Stanford Univ. Publ. M. Sc.* vol. 5, no. 1, 1951.

Gaunt, R., J. H. Birnie, and *W. J. Eversole,* Adrenal Cortex and Water Metabolism, *Physiol. Rev.* 29:281, 1949.

Gottfried, S. P., M. Bogin, and *N. V. Levycky,* Blood and Electrolyte Studies on Normal Newborn Full-term Babies, *A.M.A. Am. J. Dis. Child.* 87:543, 1954.

Graham, B. D., J. L. Wilson, M. U. Tsao, M. L. Baumann, and *S. Brown,* Development of Neonatal Electrolyte Hemeostasis, *Pediatrics* 8:68, 1951.

Hardy, J. D., and *D. L. Drabkin,* Measurement of Body Water, Techniques and Practical Implications, *J.A.M.A.* 149:1113, 1952.

Heller, H., The Water Metabolism of Newborn Infants and Animals, *Arch. Dis. Childhood* 26:195, 1951.

Henderson, L. J., "Blood," Yale University Press, New Haven, Conn., 1928.

Iob, V., and *W. W. Swanson,* Mineral Growth of Human Fetus, *Am. J. Dis. Child.* 47:302, 1934.

Kaltreider, N. L., G. R. Meneely, J. R. Allen, and *W. F. Bale,* Determination of the Volume of Extracellular Fluid of the Body with Radioactive Sodium, *J. Exper. Med.* 74:569, 1941.

Katcher, A. L., M. F. Levitt, A. Y. Sweet, and *H. L. Hodes,* Studies of Body-water Distribution in Normal Infants and in Infants during Dehydration and Subsequent Recovery, *A.M.A. Am. J. Dis. Child.* 84:744, 1952.

Levine, S. Z., Respiratory Metabolism in Infancy and Childhood: Daily Water Exchange of Normal Infants, *Am. J. Dis. Child.* 56:83, 1938.

Levitt, M. F., and *M. Gaudino,* Measurements of Body Water Compartments, *Am. J. Med.* 9:208, 1950.

Mollison, P. L., "Blood Transfusion in Clinical Medicine," Charles C Thomas, Springfield, Ill., 1951.

Nyham, W. L., and *R. E. Cooke,* Symptomatic Hyponatremia in Acute Infections of the Central Nervous System, *Pediatrics,* 18:604, 1956.

Overman, R. R., J. N. Etteldorf, A. C. Bass, and *G. B. Horn,* Plasma and Erythrocyte Chemistry of the Normal Infant from Birth to Two Years of Age, *Pediatrics* 7:565, 1951.

Perley, A., G. B. Forbes, and *M. M. Pennoyer,* Determination of Sodium[24] "Space" in Infants, Children and Adults, *J. Pediat.* 38:299, 1951.

Pinson, E. A., Water Exchanges and Barriers as Studied by the Use of Hydrogen Isotopes, *Physiol. Rev.* 32:123, 1952.

Reardon, H. S., B. D. Graham, J. L. Wilson, M. L. Baumann, M. U. Tsao, and *M. Murayama,* Studies of Acid-Base Equilibrium in Premature Infants, *Pediatrics* 6:753, 1950.

Russell, S. J. M., Blood Volume Studies in Healthy Children, *Arch. Dis. Childhood* 24:88, 1949.

Smith, C. A., S. Yudkin, W. Young, A. Minkowski, and *M. Cushman,* Adjustment of Electrolytes and Water Following Premature Birth (with Special Reference to Edema), *Pediatrics* 3:34, 1949.

Wallace, W. M., Chemical Composition, Physiology and Pathology of Intracellular Fluid, *Pediatrics* 9:141, 1952.

Widdowson, E. M., R. A. McCance, and *C. M. Spray,* The Chemical Composition of the Human Body, *Clin. Sc.* 10:113, 1951.

────── and *C. M. Spray,* Chemical Development in Utero, *Arch. Dis. Childhood* 26:205, 1951.

CHAPTER 55

Osmotic and Acid-Base Equilibria

During health the totals and relative proportions of the individual mineral ions within the body compartments are kept more or less constant by delicately responsive homeostatic mechanisms. In disease states the major chemical equilibria may become disturbed in three directions which are amenable to laboratory investigation. These are (1) the total osmotic pressure which is related to the total amount of contained solutes, whether electrolytes or nonelectrolytes, (2) the hydrogen-ion concentration or electrochemical balance between the totals of the acidic and basic ions, and (3) the distribution of the acidic and basic ions. These are all integrated and are best considered together.

The equilibria of all body fluids with respect to osmotic pressure, total electrolytes, and ionic balance are continuously making adjustments to new substances being absorbed from the gastrointestinal tract or liberated by tissue metabolism, to changes in the internal environment from water and carbon dioxide being lost through the lungs, and to water, electrolytes, and other products being excreted through kidneys and skin. Water, mineral ions, and smaller nonelectrolytes undergo a lively interchange between the plasma, interstitial spaces, and cell interiors. The larger molecules of proteins and similar substances, which are in dissimilar concentrations on opposite sides of cell membranes, exert their influence through the Donnan equilibrium. Sudden demands on the electrolytes of the extracellular and intracellular fluids are defended by the large reserves and by the corrective capacities of the kidneys and lungs. Distortions of the internal ionic environment occur only when losses of water and electrolytes are large, as with severe diarrhea or vomiting or deprivation of water or when greater quantities are taken in than the excretory mechanisms can handle.

OSMOTIC PRESSURE

The osmotic pressure of a solution is directly proportional to the total number of dissolved chemical particles per unit volume of solvent. Neither molecular weight nor valence is of significance in this regard.

604

The osmotic pressure of a molar solution of a nonelectrolyte such as sugar or urea is the same as that of 1 equivalent of a univalent ion and is termed the osmol. An identical osmotic pressure of 1 osmol or 1,000 milliosmols (mOsm) per liter of distilled water will be exerted by 23 gm of Na^+ of atomic weight 23, by 40 gm of Ca^{++} of atomic weight 40, by 180 gm or 1 mol of glucose of molecular weight 180, and by 200 kg or 1 mol of a globulin whose molecular weight is 200,000. The so-called "osmolar concentration" of a body fluid, usually expressed in milliosmols, is established by the sum of the concentrations of the various ions and of the undissociated molecules.

The osmotic constancy of the various body compartments is protected by shifts of ions or water and by the selective excretory activity of the kidneys. The renal responses seem to be governed by the sensitivity of the hypothalamus and posterior pituitary to the osmotic pressure of the blood. When the latter rises slightly either as the result of water loss or solute increase, enough posterior lobe hormone is liberated to stimulate the distal tubular epithelium and enhance the reabsorption of water.

The total osmotic pressure of a solution can be measured by any one of four approaches: (1) depression of freezing point, (2) lowering of vapor pressure, (3) elevation of boiling point, or (4) direct estimation of osmotic pressure itself. Of these, the most practical for use with body fluids is freezing-point depression. Normal serum shows a freezing point depression of about 0.56°C. This is equivalent to an osmolar concentration of approximately 302 mOsm. The contributions of the major serum constituents are electrolytes 290 mOsm (96 per cent), glucose plus urea 10 mOsm, and other nonelectrolytes 2 mOsm.

TOTAL ELECTROLYTES

The electrolyte constituents of normal plasma are in balance at a pH of 7.4. They consist of Na^+, K^+, Ca^{++}, and Mg^{++}; and HCO_3^-, Cl^-, $H_2PO_4^-$, SO_4^{--}, organic acids, and partially ionized protein. Their concentrations in the blood plasma of healthy children are given in Table 55-1.

Table 55-1. Electrolyte Composition of Normal Plasma
(*In milliequivalents per liter*)

Cations	Range	Average	Anions	Range	Average
Na^+	134–154	143	Cl^-	100–110	103
K^+	4.0–5.5	5	HCO_3^-	20–31	27
Ca^{++}	4.8–5.8	5	$H_2PO_4^-$	2.6–3.2	2
Mg^{++}	1.9–2.3	2	SO_4^{--}	0.6–1.2	1
Total		155	Organic acids		6
			Anion equivalent of plasma proteins		16
			Total		155

With elements or radicals which form monovalent ions the equivalent weights are the same as the atomic or radicular weights. With elements or radicals which form bivalent ions the equivalent weights are one-half the atomic or radicular weights. The distribution of these in body fluids is most conveniently presented as milliequivalents per liter. A milliequivalent is 1/1,000 equivalent. To convert from milligrams per 100 ml to milliequivalents per liter, one first divides the number of milligrams by the atomic or radicular weight and multiplies by the valence; the result is then multiplied by 10 (Table 55-2).

Some workers report the results of analyses of body fluids in terms of millimol concentrations. A millimol (mM) is 1/1,000 mol. A mol is the molecular weight expressed in grams. A molar solution contains 1 mol of solute in a measured volume of solution, usually 1 liter. Since 1 mM of a divalent ion forms 2 mEq, and of a trivalent ion 3 mEq, it is preferable to compare the concentrations of ions in solution in terms of milliequivalents.

Table 55-2. Factors for Converting Milligrams per 100 ml
to Milliequivalents per Liter

Ion	Atomic or radicular weight	Valence	Factor by which mg per 100 ml is multiplied to convert to mEq per liter
Sodium (Na+)	23	1	0.435
Potassium (K+)	39	1	0.256
Calcium (Ca++)	40	2	0.5
Magnesium (Mg++)	24.3	2	0.823
Chloride (Cl−)	35.5	1	0.282

To convert CO_2 (volumes per 100 ml "as bicarbonate") to milliequivalents per liter, multiply by 0.45.

To convert protein (grams per 100 ml) at pH 7.4 to milliequivalents of base effect per liter, multiply by 0.0243.

IONIC BALANCE

When the constituents of human plasma are scrutinized in terms of their concentrations in milliequivalents per liter, numerous relationships become apparent: The total concentration of cations is essentially equal to the total concentration of anions. Sodium, constituting about 92 per cent of the total base, is by far the most abundant of the cations and therefore the most important from the standpoint of electrolyte balance. Chloride represents about 66 per cent of total acid. The other prominent anion, HCO_3^-, appears to be the most labile of all the electrolytes in the metabolic stream. The plasma proteins, not found in the interstitial fluid, are charged negatively and are balanced by an equal amount of base. The plasma pH is 7.4 rather than 7.0 since the bicarbonate and protein radicals are weak acids, whereas all the cations are strong bases.

Of the acid ions, the concentration of HCO_3^-, which is the most labile, ordinarily balances the amount of base in excess of that required to match the other acid ions. The Cl^-, HPO_4^{--}, and SO_4^{--} anions and all the cations are exclusively under renal control except when perspiration is occurring. The plasma protein concentration is maintained largely by the liver. The organic acids, produced by tissue cells, may be metabolized and destroyed by other tissue cells or be excreted by the kidneys when in excess. The relative proportions of Cl^- and HCO_3^- are mutually compensatory; the absolute concentration of each is less constant physiologically than that of sodium. The potassium, even though quantitatively in minor amount, must be present within physiologic limits, or else the sodium distribution becomes distorted.

In healthy children the bicarbonate content usually falls within 5 mEq of the sodium content, and the chloride within 15 mEq.

RENAL REGULATION

In addition to being the outlets for nitrogenous waste products, healthy kidneys selectively excrete water and individual ions in order to maintain the integrity of the body fluids and cells. In response to alkalosis the urine becomes rich in sodium and bicarbonates, is free of ammonium, and is alkaline in reaction. In response to acidosis it becomes free of bicarbonate, rich in ammonium, and acid in reaction.

Influences from the adrenal can alter the urine composition. A circulating excess of the adrenal cortical hormones may act on the tubular epithelium to promote unusual reabsorption of sodium and enhance the loss of potassium. The reverse, as in Addison's disease, leads to increased loss of sodium and retention of potassium.

Water

For efficient functioning the kidneys must receive a water supply adequate for the solute load. The older child instinctively takes in more than enough water for this purpose. The infant, on the other hand, has a proportionately greater need and must depend on water given by another individual. During the first months of life, when the kidneys are still functionally immature, it is important that the milk mixture given be at least as dilute as unmodified cow's milk, or else that water be given supplementarily. Additional water must be supplied whenever the extrarenal water loss is increased by sweating or diarrhea. It has been found experimentally that small infants in a protected environment can cope with feedings as concentrated as 2 parts of evaporated milk and 1 part of water and no additional fluid, but that this high renal solute load reduces dangerously the margin of safety against dehydration. The very early feeding of solid foods has been criticized as throwing a burden upon the neonatal excretory mechanisms.

Bicarbonate

The normal glomerular filtrate contains bicarbonate in essentially the same concentration as plasma, namely 23 to 33 mEq per liter. The total amount of bicarbonate delivered to the renal tubules each day constitutes about five times the amount of bicarbonate in the body at any one time. Normally, however, only 1 or 2 mEq of bicarbonate is lost into the urine each day, because the filtered bicarbonate ion is reabsorbed by the tubules with great efficiency. However, if an excess of base is taken into the body as sodium bicarbonate or lactate or as a diet with an alkaline ash residue, bicarbonate ions make their appearance in the urine in combination with the surplus base. Dissolved CO_2 itself is not secreted by the kidney but is transferred to the urine in the same concentration as in the plasma.

The renal threshold for bicarbonate excretion is a plasma concentration of 25 to 27 mEq per liter. A change in urinary pH from 7.0 to 7.4 is accompanied by a doubling of the urine bicarbonate. A further rise from pH 7.4 to 7.8 more than doubles it again.

When the plasma concentration is less than 25 mEq per liter, no bicarbonate is excreted into the urine. An exception to this generalization occurs during hyperventilation, when, despite a lowered plasma bicarbonate concentration, sufficient bicarbonate continues to be excreted along with base to render the urine alkaline. Another exception occurs when a high plasma bicarbonate level corrects for a lowered chloride level. In the hypochloremia that may attend prolonged vomiting, the compensatory elevation in bicarbonate can lead to alkalosis and even to tetany, and yet the urine will remain acid and contain almost no bicarbonate as long as the chloride level remains subnormal.

Organic Acids

Radicals of organic acids, such as the ketone bodies, are weakly acidic substances which can be excreted directly into the urine. The free hydrogen ions which accompany these acids are elaborated within the renal tubules, presumably through the action of the carbonic anhydrase in the renal epithelial cells. In the ketosis of unregulated diabetes mellitus the body is flooded with a far greater load of organic acids than the renal tubules can excrete.

Other Ions

Phosphoric acid circulates in the plasma almost entirely as the divalent phosphate. This can be converted and excreted directly by the kidney as monovalent phosphate. Hence phosphate can be eliminated with the loss of only one-half the base which balances it in plasma. In contrast, the chloride and sulfate radicals which are strong acids must be excreted in combination with mineral cations or neutralizing ammonium ions elaborated by the tubular epithelial cells. The acidosis of chronic nephritis results in part from the inadequacy of these ion-exchange and ammonium-producing mechanisms. The body cations are drained away by the need to balance the acids being excreted. In addition, the excretion of sulfate and phosphate ions is impaired as the result of both glomerular and tubular damage. These mineral acids accumulate in the body fluids and reduce the plasma concentration of bicarbonate.

RESPIRATORY REGULATION

The plasma CO_2 system, though quantitatively the least important of the buffers of the blood, is more than a passive indicator of fluctuations in the electrolyte equilibrium. The slightest change tends to disturb the ratio between blood H_2CO_3 and HCO_3^-. The respiratory mechanisms, highly sensitive to variations in this bicarbonate system, immediately correct by adjusting the CO_2 concentration in the residual air of the lungs. The pulmonary response to an increase in fixed plasma acids consists of enlarging the air spaces, thereby reducing the CO_2 concentration in the expired air by dilution. This enlargement, achieved by deeper rapid breathing, becomes recognizable clinically as acidiotic or Kussmaul breathing and is practically pathognomonic of plasma bicarbonate reduction. Conversely, when the plasma bicarbonate concentration rises above normal the respirations become shallow and slower. The quieter respiratory movements, characteristic of alkalosis, reduce the residual air space and increase its CO_2 tension.

Respiratory adjustments to changes in plasma CO_2 begin to act immediately. Renal responses to changes in electrolyte balance are much slower and require the excretion of water along with the excess of anions or cations. Hence the CO_2 system may be regarded as the front line for defending acid-base stability. It counteracts disturbances as soon as they begin, both by virtue of the immediate responsiveness of the respiratory exchanges and by the intimate relation of the bicarbonate buffer system to the other physiologic buffer systems of hemoglobin and phosphate.

ACIDOSIS AND ALKALOSIS

These conditions are distortions in the equilibrium of the acidic and basic ions, as reflected in the hydrogen-ion status (pH) of the blood. Should the pH be lowered the blood becomes acidic or acidotic; should the pH rise, the blood becomes basic or alkalotic. According to this definition, a blood specimen with a high CO_2 content has an alkali excess but is not alkalotic until the pH is increased. Conversely, a low CO_2 content or alkali deficit is not acidotic until the pH becomes reduced.

In clinical usage the term *acidosis* is often mistakenly applied whenever the plasma CO_2 is reduced below normal, and *alkalosis* when this is above normal, regardless of whether the deviation is sufficient to overcome the sustaining buffers and shift the pH of the blood to a measurable extent. With this nomenclature, such disturbances are referred to as "compensated" as long as the ratio between the concentration of H_2CO_3 and HCO_3^- is unaffected and the pH remains at 7.4.

The plasma pH is best determined on arterial blood. In practice, the minor difference between arterial and venous blood is usually neglected. The temperature gradient makes any pH reading on blood about 0.1 unit higher at room temperature than at 37°C.

Acidosis and alkalosis can be subclassified as (1) of metabolic origin when the bicarbonate content of the plasma is reduced primarily because of disorders in the mineral ion or buffer salt content of the blood, or (2) of respiratory origin when breathing difficulties are responsible for the changed bicarbonate content. The metabolic varieties are the more common in pediatric practice and develop more slowly.

The distinctions between these various disturbances *when the total base remains unaltered* can be epitomized as follows:

	Blood HCO_3^-	Total of other blood anions	Blood pH °	Urine reaction
Metabolic acidosis	Low	High	Low	Acid
Respiratory acidosis	High	Low	Low	Variable
Metabolic alkalosis	High	Low	High	Alkaline
Respiratory alkalosis	Low	High	High	Variable

° Deviations in pH occur only when acidosis or alkalosis is marked and uncompensated.

Acidosis and alkalosis of respiratory origin can usually be diagnosed or at least be reasonably suspected from the clinical story. The usual problem is to determine whether a disturbance in breathing is due to nervous system stimulation or is the result of an internal metabolic disturbance. Knowing solely the plasma CO_2 content in a patient with an acid-base deviation is often inadequate for either diagnosis or treatment. This information should be combined with an accurate pH measurement whenever feasible.

In all forms of acidosis and alkalosis the sums of the anion and cation milliequivalents may be depressed, normal, or elevated. The plasma bicarbonate level is the key variable.

Metabolic Acidosis

In this disturbance the acid-base equilibrium of the plasma is distorted in the direction of a low bicarbonate level as the consequence either of a relative increase in one or more of the "fixed" acids of the blood—

chlorides, phosphates, sulfates, organic acids—or of a relative decrease in the concentration of total cations. When the hydrogen-ion concentration is undisturbed the metabolic acidosis is said to be "compensated"; when shifted to a pH below 7.35, "uncompensated." A superimposed poor pulmonary elimination of CO_2 can result in the simultaneous occurrence of both metabolic acidosis and respiratory acidosis. Conversely, a complicating hyperventilation can add respiratory alkalosis to an initial metabolic acidosis.

The causes of metabolic acidosis in infancy and childhood are diverse and usually multiple: (1) Beta-hydroxybutric, acetoacetic, and related intermediary ketonic products of fat metabolism accumulating in the body will displace the bicarbonate ions and usually to a lesser extent, the chloride ions as well. Such excessive production of organic acids (ketosis) can take place in starvation, untreated diabetes mellitus, von Gierke's glycogen storage disease, and the dehydrative intoxication of acute febrile infections. (2) Excessive amounts of phosphate, sulfate, lactic acid, and other acid products of protein catabolism are liberated into the body fluids in fever or whenever protein catabolism is accelerated. Dehydration by impairing renal function favors the retention of these waste acids and, secondarily, aggravates the development of acidosis initiated by other causes. Lactic acid tends to accumulate in excessive quantities in patients with shock and in ill premature infants. (3) During nephritis and other kidney diseases of any severity, the phosphate may rise to 6 to 8 mEq per liter (normal 2 mEq) and the sulfates to a lesser extent (normal 1 mEq). Some urinary loss of base as a consequence of depressed ammonia production may take place. In chronic renal insufficiency of long standing these disturbances become more pronounced and intricate (p. 428). (4) Gastroenteritis and related diarrheal disorders and intestinal tract fistulas can lead to significant outpouring of basic and bicarbonate ions in the lost intestinal fluids. (5) Ingestion of acid-producing substances such as ammonium chloride tends to depress the plasma bicarbonate level by raising its chloride content. Such an acidosis has been described in premature and newly born infants being fed protein milk high in chlorides (p. 417).

Prolonged metabolic acidosis may bring about other electrolyte changes of clinical significance. Potassium and calcium, instead of being absorbed efficiently by the renal tubules as occurs normally, may be lost in the urine in excessive amounts. The potassium depletion can lead to muscle hypotonicity or cardiac disturbances in extreme cases. In oliguric states, on the other hand, excess potassium may be retained and lead to hyperpotassemia. The depletion of calcium would be conducive to tetany were it not that an acid blood pH favors the ionization of the remaining calcium and thereby corrects for the lowered total level. However, should the acidosis be treated with large doses of sodium bicarbonate or lactate, its correction may precipitate an attack of tetany (postacidotic tetany). A continuing urinary calcium loss may initiate a series of physiologic disturbances ending in structural bone lesions (p. 568).

Metabolic Alkalosis

The plasma bicarbonate can become comparatively elevated as a metabolic consequence of (1) a chloride deficit from pronounced vomiting, extreme chloride loss in the stools in some diarrheas, or urinary depletion of chloride in excess of sodium during mercurial diuresis; (2) excessive ingestion of compounds of sodium with organic acids, such as sodium bicarbonate; or (3) a primary deficit of potassium accompanied by movement of sodium into the cells. The plasma bicarbonate readings may rise to 35 to 50 mEq per liter. With pronounced changes the pH of the blood may go as high as pH 7.65.

Metabolic alkalosis must be differentiated from the more frequent respiratory alkalosis in which the plasma CO_2 level is unduly low. Its most frequent cause in infancy is gastrointestinal tract obstruction with vomiting as in congenital hypertrophic pyloric stenosis, volvulus, intussusception, and upper intestinal tract anomalies. Lost gastric juice usually contains more chloride than sodium and also some potassium. Excessive drainage of the stomach or even the duodenum by suction devices will sometimes drain away more acid gastric juice than alkaline intestinal fluid. Along with the muscular weaknesses and other symptoms of hypopotassemia, the loss of potassium in the vomitus is followed by increase of intracellular sodium.

Recovery from metabolic alkalosis begins when the cause is removed and the normal balance restored by the giving of a sodium salt such as sodium chloride. If the kidneys are functioning efficiently, the sodium will be conserved and the surplus chloride excreted in the urine. Hypopotassemia when present must be corrected also for this to proceed efficiently.

An unusual form of alkalosis is sometimes seen in patients with cardiac failure who are being treated with mercurial diuretics and whose edema becomes refractory to the mercurials. Biochemical studies of the plasma of such patients show the sodium level to be normal, the potassium normal or low, the bicarbonate usually elevated, and the chloride low. Corrective therapy of this so-called hypochloremic alkalosis consists in discontinuing mercurial diuretics for some days and administering ammonium chloride orally or intravenously or hydrochloric acid orally.

Respiratory Alkalosis

This is evoked primarily by an increase in rate and depth of the respiratory movements. Such hyperventilation can be induced by voluntary or emotional stimuli, fever, bronchopneumonia, exposure to high external temperatures, congenital heart disease, encephalitis or meningitis, salicylate poisoning, anoxic anoxemia as the result of exposure to high altitudes or reduced atmospheric oxygen tension, and other influences which act upon the respiratory center. Breathing in excess of physiologic requirements leads to an unusual loss of CO_2 through the lungs and reduces the free CO_2 content of the plasma. So long as the base which had been combined with $HCO_3{}^-$ is balanced by compensatory mechanisms, the $H\cdot HCO_3:B\cdot HCO_3$ ratio will stay at 1:20 and the blood pH will remain undisturbed. When the surplus of base is not longer corrected, a rise in plasma pH and uncompensated alkalosis will ensue. The surplus of base may be neutralized in part by a rise in the plasma content of chlorides and organic acids. If subclinical alkalosis is already present, clinical symptoms can be made to appear by a few minutes of hyperventilation.

In infants ill with infection and hyperpyrexia, nitrogenous waste products may accumulate from excessive respiratory loss of water, facilitated by diminished fluid intake and immaturity of renal function. Respiratory alkalosis in such infants may be distorted by a superimposed metabolic acidosis.

A syndrome of respiratory alkalosis induced reflexly by psychogenic hyperventilation is not uncommon in excitable older children confronted with acute situations which evoke emotional stress. Dizziness, malaise, peripheral numbness, and shortness of breath become evident as the pH of the blood rises above 7.45. Carpopedal spasm and other signs of enhanced excitability of the peripheral sensory nerves may follow the poorer ionization of calcium as the blood becomes alkalotic. Studies of the total blood calcium will show no abnormalities. The diagnosis of a propensity to emotional hyperventilation can be verified by asking such a child to breathe deeply and rapidly. Typical distress ensues in 5 to 10 minutes. The pH of the venous blood if determined before and after the period of voluntary hyperventilation will show a rise, sometimes to as high as 7.6.

Good therapy for such acute tetany is for the patient to hold his breath or to breathe in and out of a closed paper or plastic bag. Inhalations of carbon dioxide in 10 to 15 per cent concentration along with oxygen will usually give immediate relief. Administration of sodium solution parenterally or ammonium chloride by mouth (0.5 to 1 gm every 4 hours for an older child) may be helpful.

Respiratory Acidosis

The plasma CO_2 and bicarbonate concentrations can become elevated through various disturbances in the respiratory mechanisms: (1) an abnormally high CO_2 content in the inhaled air; (2) hampered excretion of CO_2 across the alveolar membranes or through the respiratory passages as a consequence of pulmonary edema, exudate, fibrosis, atelectasis, infiltrations, or of spasm, foreign body, or mucus plugs in the larynx, trachea, or bronchi; (3) poor vascular transport of CO_2 from the tissues to the lungs because of shock, circulatory failure, anoxia, congenital heart disease, or pulmonary artery occlusions; or (4) depression of respiratory movements as the results of opiate or barbiturate poisoning, cerebral immaturity, or nervous system lesions. Mechanism 2 is the most common. Since oxygen is less soluble than carbon dioxide, any diffusion difficulty due to respiratory tract lesion will produce anoxemia before the carbon dioxide mounts. Placing such a patient in an oxygen tent favors the penetration of oxygen through the alveoli.

Respiratory acidosis is often complicated by accumulation of endogenous organic acids and other electrolyte distortions. The ensuing biochemical findings can be very confusing and require astute clinical judgment for their correct interpretation.

The increase in blood carbon dioxide which accompanies these disorders tends to raise the $H \cdot HCO_3 : B \cdot HCO_3$ ratio and cause the pH to become more acid. After a few hours, if the fluid intake is adequate, the renal tubules start to selectively excrete chloride in excess of sodium. As the urine becomes acid the plasma chloride falls and the released base combines with the excess carbonic acid. The plasma bicarbonate level may rise to as high as 40 to 50 mEq per liter as the ratio of the buffer system returns to 1:20. With a scanty fluid intake or impaired renal function the plasma pH may fall to 7.0 or even lower ("uncompensated respiratory acidosis") and the bicarbonate level does not rise. The urinary output of potassium usually becomes high in this situation. Chloride-containing therapeutic fluids such as saline or Ringer's solution are contraindicated in respiratory acidosis.

If the cause of the respiratory acidosis is alleviated suddenly, as when a tracheotomy is done for laryngeal obstruction, the accumulated carbon dioxide may leave the blood with such speed that uncompensated base remains in the blood in excess. Transitory alkalosis and even tetany may then follow.

The presence of respiratory acidosis can be surmised from the underlying disturbance. Its demonstration requires the finding of high levels of plasma CO_2 or an acid shift in the plasma pH in advanced disturbances. Breathing is shallow and slow when the respiratory tract is open, but may be rapid and labored when obstructed.

The hypoventilation which attends central nervous system lesions seems to result from loss of responsiveness by the respiratory center to changes in the partial pressure of arterial carbon dioxide. The respiratory rate may fall to as low as four per minute. Efficiency of ventilation varies from hour to hour, with corresponding fluctuations in the carbon dioxide content of the blood. To demonstrate a lowered plasma pH the blood specimen must be taken without disturbing the patient, since excitement may increase the breathing sufficiently to produce transitorily normal blood gas values. In the study of such cases it has been suggested that a needle and syringe with a three-way stopcock attachment be left in an artery for at least 5 minutes before the blood is drawn. The therapeutic attack should be directed against the underlying cause. The first repair solutions should be chloride-free. Administration of oxygen in severe asphyxia is not advised by some authorities, since this may diminish the reflex stimulation to the respiratory center from the carotid and aortic bodies. Artificial respiratory aid of some kind is recommended instead, until a period of adequate ventilation has restored the sensitivity of the respiratory center.

BIBLIOGRAPHY

MAINTENANCE OF OSMOTIC AND ELECTROLYTE EQUILIBRIA

Baskin, J. L., H. M. Keith, and *B. H. Scribner,* Water Metabolism in Water Intoxication: Review of Basic Concepts, *A.M.A. Am. J. Dis. Child.* 83:618, 1952.

Bischoff, H. W., and *E. F. Fantazier,* The Role of the Donnan Membrane Equilibrium in the Production of Edema, *Clin. Proc. Child. Hosp.* 4:128, 1948.

Bland, J. H., Role of the Kidneys in Regulation of Fluid and Electrolyte Balance, *Am. J. Clin. Path.* 23:1070, 1953.

Farnsworth, E. B., Electrolyte Partition in Patients with Edema of Various Origins, Sodium and Chloride, *Am. J. Med.* 4:338, 1948.

Ferraro, A., The Reaction of the Brain Tissue to Intravenous Injection of Hypotonic Solutions, *J. Nerv. & Ment. Dis.* 71:129, 1930.

Gamble, J. L., "Chemical Anatomy, Physiology and Pathology of Extracellular Fluid: A Lecture Syllabus," 2d ed., Harvard University Press, Cambridge, Mass., 1952.

Gillespie, J. B., The Hyperventilation Syndrome in Childhood: Report of Two Cases, *Arch. Pediat.* 71:197, 1954.

Johnstone, D. E., and *E. Bruck,* Respiratory Acidosis in Children with Cerebral Pulmonary and Cardiovascular Disorders, *Am. J. Dis. Child.* 80:578, 1950.

Marriott, H. L., "Water and Salt Depletion," Charles C Thomas, Springfield, Ill., 1950.

McQuarrie, I., and *D. B. Peeler,* The Effects of Sustained Pituitary Antidiuresis and Forced Water Drinking in Epileptic Children: A Diagnostic and Etiologic Study, *J. Clin. Invest.* 10:915, 1931.

Pitts, R. F., Acid-Base Regulation by the Kidneys, *Am. J. Med.* 9:356, 1950.

Sarnoff, S. J., J. L. Whittenberger, and *J. E. Affeldt,* The Hypoventilation Syndrome in Bulbar Poliomyelitis, *J.A.M.A.* 147:30, 1951.

Shohl, A T., "Mineral Metabolism," Reinhold Publishing Corporation, New York, 1939.

Singer, R. B., A New Diagram for the Vizualization and Interpretation of Acid-Base Changes, *Am. J. M. Sc.* 221:199, 1951.

——— and *A. B. Hastings,* An Improved Clinical Method for the Estimation of Disturbances of the Acid-Base Balance of Human Blood, *Medicine* 27:223, 1948.

Spector, S., and *C. F. McKhann,* Respiratory Acidosis and Alkalosis in Children, *J Pediat.* 32:227, 1948.

Weisberg, H. F., Respiratory Factors in Disturbance of Acid-Base Balance, *Am. J. Clin. Path.* 23:1082, 1953.

CHAPTER 56

Disturbances in Body Water

and Electrolytes: General Principles

of Management

Infants and children of the same age exhibit appreciable differences with respect to water and salt content of fat, muscle, and other tissues, volume of circulating blood, mineral density of bone, and other physiologic entities which relate to the metabolism of the healthy body. Furthermore, even the same child during the course of the day undergoes poorly understood spontaneous minor fluctuations in the volume and chemical composition of the various fluid compartments and of tissues rich in water. For these reasons the problem of management of any disturbance of fluid balance must be highly individualized. Nevertheless, as with all other diseases, there are certain general features and principles which must be understood if therapy is to be administered intelligently.

When estimating losses or retention of water or salts in patients with water and electrolyte disturbances, the clinical history, objective signs and symptoms, breathing patterns, changes in body weight, daily fluid intakes and outputs, and serial findings in urine and blood plasma must all be taken into consideration. Such studies permit the physician to recognize shock, ketosis, dehydration, edema, acidosis, alkalosis, hypo- or hyperpotassemia, and related derangements. The full pattern of the disturbances determines the proper composition and sequence of repair solutions.

Present knowledge makes it feasible to sustain an acutely ill infant or child by parenteral feeding of water, electrolytes, calories, proteins, amino acids, fats, and vitamins. A good fluid therapy program endeavors to provide (1) the daily maintenance needs (Table 56-1), (2) extra amounts if the metabolic rate is elevated or if losses are continuing, and (3) replacements for any accumulated deficits of water, sodium, chloride, potassium, protein, or even phosphate. Appropriate consideration must always be given to therapy of the patient's diseases—diarrhea, adrenal

616

insufficiency, diabetes mellitus, the nephrotic syndrome, renal failure, or whatever. Poorly chosen therapeutic measures can aggravate the shortages or imbalances.

Biochemical studies should be as comprehensive as reasonable judgment and laboratory facilities will permit, but entire reliance should not be placed on these alone. One should think physiologically in terms of the total body water, the individual electrolytes in their relations to the body compartments, the functional activity of the kidneys and lungs, maintenance requirements, deficits, calorie needs, and the efficiency of the body metabolism. It must be remembered that absolute deviations in the concentrations of pertinent substances per unit volume of blood or plasma represent only a fraction of the alterations in the total body stores.

Table 56–1. Approximate Daily Maintenance Allowances for
Infants and Children at Rest *

Age	Calories per kg	Protein (gm per kg)	Water (ml per kg)	Chloride (mEq per kg)	Sodium (mEq per kg)	Potassium (mEq per kg)
First week	60	2.0	100	0.9	0.9	1.0
Up to 6 months	55	2.0	150	0.8	0.8	1.0
6 months–1 year	50	2.0	135	0.8	0.8	1.0
1–6 years	30	1.0	100–125	0.7	0.7	0.9
7–12 years	30	0.6	75	0.6	0.6	0.8
Adolescence	25	0.6	50	0.5	0.5	0.6

* Divide values by slightly more than one-half to express them in units per pound. The physician should learn to compute needs for parenteral fluids in both the metric and avoirdupois systems since few American hospitals weigh infants and children on scales calibrated in the metric system.

A high urinary specific gravity generally represents a constitutional need for conservation of water. However, this response may be inhibited when renal function is poor or hypoelectrolytemia is present. The urinary pH usually, but not necessarily, reflects the existence of acidosis or alkalosis. Quantitative studies of the electrolytes contained in random urine specimens are of some significance, but the 24-hour outputs and the findings with the usual tests are much more helpful.

OVERHYDRATION

Overhydration may be subclassified in terms of whether the retention is predominantly that of water alone (*water intoxication*) or of electrolytes as well (*edema*).

Water Intoxication

Flooding of the organism with large amounts of water renders the extracellular fluids abruptly hypotonic. Salts are drained from the body cells at the same time as water is pulled into them by osmotic pressure. The first symptoms of cellular dysfunction appear in the central nervous system, usually before the blood and interstitial fluid volumes expand sufficiently to cause recognizable tissue swelling. Early symptoms are nervousness, salivation, and vomiting, followed in severe cases by disorientation, muscular twitchings, stupor, or even convulsions.

Rapidity of osmotic pressure decrease is a major factor in production of symptoms. A sudden drop in total cation level to 130 mEq per liter of plasma in an individual who was healthy up to this time is more likely to evoke clinical manifestations than a gradual fall to 120 mEq in a patient with a chronic illness.

The principal childhood situation in which water intoxication may develop is after the administration of large amounts of glucose solution parenterally or of water by protoclysis. It occurs rarely as a complication of renal or adrenal insufficiency.

Stopping the administration of water and giving a 2 to 3 per cent hypertonic solution of sodium chloride intravenously is effective counter-treatment. Salt reverses the osmotic gradient and relieves the cells of some of their excess water. Only enough of the hypertonic solution should be given to alleviate the symptoms, since more may overload the circulation and cause circulatory failure.

Edema

Undue retention of electrolytes is accompanied by retention of a proportional amount of water. The body fluids remain normotonic or perhaps very slightly hypertonic despite their greatly augmented volume. Such accumulations may occur in congestive circulatory failure, the nephrotic syndrome, severe liver disease, trichinosis, severe infectious diseases, nephritis, malignant malnutrition, adrenal cortical hyperplasia, or following therapy with corticotropin or adrenal cortical hormones. In all these conditions, large amounts of sodium-containing foods or medicaments aggravate the retention and increase the edema. Unless osmotic changes are superimposed, however, the tissue cells as a rule suffer no injury.

The mechanisms behind the development of edema represent a mixture of influences derived from the heart, kidney, liver, capillary bed, serum albumin level, intraabdominal pressure, circulating antidiuretic substances, lymphatic drainage, tissue inflammatory reactions, and other factors. Minimal degrees of generalized edema are detectable only by increases in body weight. More pronounced accumulation of fluid and electrolytes leads to visible pitting and swelling of the subcutaneous and other tissues and accumulations within the body cavities. Extreme retentions may result in pulmonary edema or circulatory failure. This is in contrast to retention of water alone, where water pulled osmotically into the cells produces symptoms of intoxication before the extracellular compartment can become visibly distended.

DEHYDRATION

Water deficiency tends to occur in all serious childhood illnesses which are attended by reduced fluid intake, fever, hyperventilation, sweating, vomiting, or diarrhea. Acidosis, ketosis, or alkalosis is often superimposed. Clinical signs become apparent when the water shortage exceeds 5 per cent of the body weight.

Observing the daily changes in weight and the totals of fluid intake and output is a crude but helpful means of following the progress of a disturbed water balance. Laboratory signs of value for demonstration of acute dehydration are those referable to hemoconcentration—elevations in hemoglobin, hematocrit, serum protein, and red cell count. Furthermore, since kidney function tends to be depressed, particularly in infants, the values for blood urea or nonprotein nitrogen in the absence of organic renal disease are good indicators of the severity of the dehydration as affecting the functional status of the kidneys. In pronounced dehydration the urea or nonprotein nitrogen content of the serum may rise to 100 mg per 100 ml or higher. Declining values in serial determinations usually denote restoration of circulatory and renal function, whereas an increase implies inadequate treatment or specific renal disease. The specific gravity of the urine may be high. The plasma electrolytes may be increased in total concentration, but the components are more likely to be distorted by associated disturbances in the acid-base equilibria.

Salicylates, sulfonamides, and many other drugs will be retained when renal function is poor and may attain toxic levels if given to a dehydrated child in customary dosages. Salicylates are especially dangerous in dehydration because of their propensity to stimulate the respiratory rate and thereby aggravate water loss through the lungs.

Hypoelectrolytemic Dehydration

This term is applied when both electrolytes and water are lost from the body but with the electrolytes relatively more depleted. In this condition, when acute, the plasma concentrations of sodium and chloride and other ions tend to become subnormal while the plasma proteins and the hematocrit reading remain undisturbed or even increase. Oliguria develops, and the blood urea and nonprotein nitrogen levels soon rise.

In the dehydration of gastrointestinal disorders the reserves of both water and electrolytes become depleted, the comparative proportions being contingent upon volume and composition of the food and fluid intake and losses through vomiting, diarrhea, and insensible and sensible perspiration. In some diseases—e.g., pneumonia, peritonitis, pulmonary tuberculosis, tuberculous meningitis, severe liver damage—plasma concentrations of sodium and chloride tend to persist at subnormal levels.

An early physiologic change in hypoelectrolytemic dehydration is shrinkage of the interstitial compartment. The plasma volume is less reduced because of the osmotic activity of the plasma proteins. The osmotic pressure inside the cells of the organs, now relatively higher, attracts additional water into the cell interiors. This diminishes further the volume of the interstitial fluid. Pallor, dry skin, weakness, prostration, low blood pressure, and circulatory failure become manifest. The syndrome is sometimes called medical shock; it responds to therapy with isotonic solutions of electrolytes, but the results are more satisfactory when blood or plasma accompanies the electrolyte solutions. Sometimes, in the late stages of such dehydration, the loss of water into the cells may bring about a rise in plasma electrolyte concentration, even while the total interstitial fluid content remains much diminished.

Hyperelectrolytemic Dehydration

A primary increase in the electrolytes in the plasma and interstitial fluid can be brought about by prolonged restriction of water or of water and food, by injections of urea or of hypertonic salt solutions to induce diuresis, by limitation of fluid intake to electrolyte-rich solutions, or by an inadequate water intake in the presence of acute severe diarrhea, febrile illnesses, diabetes insipidus, or hyposthenuric forms of chronic nephritis. It may be brought about by the therapeutic administration of hypertonic solutions of sodium, or of normal or hypotonic solutions followed by subsequent losses of water without salt, or after giving normal saline solution to premature and newborn infants whose renal concentrating power is still imperfect (p. 417). Contributory factors may be fever, hot dry environments, convulsions, physical activities which promote the expenditure of energy, or inadequate renal functions. Some of these mechanisms seem a major component in the difficulties exhibited by castaways on a raft who have only sea water to drink or by premature infants kept in a hot bed or incubator without extra moisture being added to the atmosphere. Once hyperelectrolytemia becomes established the ensuing loss of appetite and inadequate food intake enhance the destruction of body protein and the liberation of additional endogenous salts. Other situations in which sodium seems to accumulate but concerning which knowledge is incomplete include some of the phenomena exhibited in hypertensive and vascular diseases, hypopotassemia, adrenocortical insufficiency, diabetic acidosis, and renal, intracranial, and hepatic disorders.

Characteristic clinical findings are fever, lethargy, and dehydration of the tissues with puttylike consistency of the skin. Symptoms may resemble those of shock, but with circulatory collapse less prominent than in hypotonic dehydration. The increase of plasma electrolytes is chiefly in sodium and chloride; the potassium and bicarbonate components are subject to other variations. The levels of retained ions can rise as high as 180 or 190 mEq per liter for sodium and 145 to 155 mEq per liter for chlorides. The serum nonprotein nitrogen level tends to rise to between 40 and 120 mg per 100 ml and may go even higher. The disturbance is sometimes complicated by hyperpnea of uncertain origin; this promotes excessive water loss from the lungs and tends toward respiratory alkalosis.

The hyperelectrolytemia together with the increase in nitrogenous end products leads to osmotic hypertonicity of the interstitial fluids and plasma. This withdraws water from the body cells. Irritation or injury of the brain cells may be prominent, leading to convulsions or even lethal respiratory paralysis.

Water in Therapy

Enough water should be given to meet the daily requirements and to restore the amount in deficit.

Water loss is usually more pronounced than electrolyte loss in febrile states and can be corrected by 5 per cent glucose in distilled water or hypotonic saline.

The dehydrated patient who cannot take or retain fluids by mouth must perforce receive the fluid parenterally. Whether the intravenous, subcutaneous, intramuscular, or intraosseous route is chosen depends on the accessibility of veins, the skill of the attending physician, and the availability of nursing supervision. Hyaluronidase is sometimes added to subcutaneous or intramuscular fluids as an accelerator, but only when absorption would otherwise be undesirably slow; too rapid absorption may overload the circulation.

When calculating the fluid needs of an ill infant, if the skin is inelastic it is reasonable to assume that the true body weight has been reduced by approximately 10 per cent. A 10 per cent weight drop represents extreme dehydration in an older child but only moderate dehydration during the first year. Infants who lose more than 15 per cent of their total body weight during a severely dehydrating illness are likely to be in shock, and the physiologic changes may be irreversible.

Water losses can be corrected and the maintenance needs met, with most ill infants and children, by the total water intakes shown in Table 56-2 (see also Table 56-1). Exceeding the maximums may overload the circulation except when extreme water loss is continuing. For an infant being kept in an atmosphere of high humidity the recommended water intake should be reduced by one-third.

Exceptionally a very young or premature infant may not do well until as much as 150 ml per lb per day, or even more, is given. Such infants must be managed with meticulous supervision, and their need for such a high amount established by gradual increments.

Table 56-2. Approximate Daily Water Requirements during Parenteral
Fluid Therapy *
(*In milliliters per pound body weight*)

Body weight (lb)	1st day	2d day	3d, 4th, 5th days, etc.
Under 15	100	75	60–75
15–25	75	50–75	Same as 2d day
25–40	60	40–60	Same as 2d day
Over 40	30–40	Same as 1st day	Same as 1st day

* Multiply the volumes cited by 2 if it is desired to express them as requirements per kilogram body weight.

The rate of administration of fluids should be so adjusted as to take about 48 hours to relieve any water deficit while satisfying simultaneously the maintenance needs. If the kidneys are inactive an infusion of approximately one-third of the daily fluid requirement within 2 to 4 hours helps to reestablish this function. When shock is present an initial transfusion of whole blood or plasma is advisable; this will also facilitate the absorption of any aqueous solution injected subcutaneously.

Glucose

Glucose solutions restore renal activity, help to meet caloric requirements, and counteract dehydration and ketosis. However, once dehydration is corrected a small amount of electrolyte should be added to the glucose solution, since the production of urine of very low specific gravity is a strain on the kidneys.

A 5 per cent glucose solution is isotonic with plasma and is the strength usually given intravenously. Solutions more concentrated than 10 per cent irritate the lumens of the veins and cannot be kept up for a long time; should they extravasate they may cause tissue necrosis. Infusions of glucose alone, when given subcutaneously or intraperitoneally, are likely to remain at the sites of injection for several hours and pull electrolytes into them before absorption begins.

It has been established that glucose when given intravenously cannot be metabolized to serve immediate caloric needs more rapidly than 10 to 12 gm an hour in an adult or about 2 gm an hour in an infant. Any surplus is lost in the urine or converted into glycogen or fat. Hence only about 70 per cent of the minimal caloric maintenance needs per 24 hours can be met by parenteral glucose.

Fructose (levulose) may be substituted for glucose in intravenous solutions. It disappears from the blood more promptly, does not produce as high hyperglycemic levels, and is not lost in the urine in significant amounts even when infused in fairly high concentration. Apparently the liver converts fructose into glycogen more rapidly than glucose.

Dextran

This high molecular weight polymer of glucose may be injected intravenously in isotonic sodium chloride solution to expand temporarily a decreased effective blood volume in shock states. Its activity lasts for some hours, until it is excreted in the urine or catabolized within the body. Dextran is less satisfactory than plasma; the dosages advised are the same as for plasma.

Blood and Plasma

Elements of the shock syndrome, even though inconspicuous, are nearly always present in dehydration from any cause. For this reason the amelioration of dehydration is usually aided by the intravenous administration of plasma, whole blood, or concentrated serum albumin solution. Whole blood is preferable after hemorrhage or in the presence of anemia.

Dehydrated infants in mild shock from a gastrointestinal disturbance with diarrhea or vomiting usually recover quickly after a single transfusion of whole blood or plasma, followed by infusions of electrolytes and glucose if necessary and a gradually increasing rate of feeding. Several transfusions may be needed with illnesses which are more severe or have a propensity to relapse. The first transfusion should amount to 10 to 15 ml per lb of body weight. The initial portion of this is run in rapidly, and the remainder more slowly. The rate of administration may vary from 30 ml per hour with marasmic infants, up to 90 ml per hour with older infants when the shock is extreme. Enough should be given to support hydration.

Whole blood and plasma contain globulins which may be of some specific therapeutic value in acute infections, but today the physician relies on antibiotics and other chemotherapeutic agents for this effect.

In critical cases of depletion the proteins in transfused plasma may serve for immediate protein replacement. For parenteral feeding of protein, however, infusions of plasma are more costly than an amino acid mixture and furnish only about 6 gm per 100 ml. Furthermore, 10 to 30 ml of citrate solution is contained in each 100 ml of plasma preserved with ACD solution (p. 139). This is equivalent to approximately 0.5 gm of sodium citrate and may be deleterious in hypocalcemia, hyponatremia, and related disorders.

Electrolytes in Therapy

Enough information should be secured with respect to both anions and cations to permit an estimation of the major electrolyte disequilibria

(Chap. 55). The presence of hypo- or hyperelectrolytemia can be evaluated from the level of sodium, or less clearly from the sum of bicarbonate plus chloride when ketosis is absent.

Distortions of the bicarbonate level should be considered in relation to the respiratory movements in order to adjudge the efficiency of gaseous exchange within the lungs and should be correlated with plasma pH whenever salicylism is suspected. The serum bicarbonate level does not indicate accurately the actual deficit of sodium and potassium and other cations within the body as a whole. Nevertheless the apparent plasma deficit is often used as a guide to the number of milliequivalents of base needed for its correction.

The potassium reading shows whether its concentration is abnormal, but fails to indicate the state of the body reserves. As a rule, an elevation in potassium is found more often in acidosis, and a depression in alkalosis. The hematocrit, red cell count, and hemoglobin and plasma protein levels are so dependent upon other factors that they cannot be used as indicators of hemoconcentration except when their pre-illness levels are known to have been normal.

The normal maintenance 24-hour requirement of sodium chloride totals 0.25 to 0.5 gm for infants below 1 month of age; 0.5 to 1 gm for infants up to 6 months; 1.5 to 2 gm for those up to 2 years; 3 to 4 gm for older children and adolescents. A 10-lb infant would thus need about 125 ml of physiologic saline (0.85 per cent) solution if this were given in full strength; an older child would need about 350 ml. Larger amounts may be required to replace deficits.

One liter of physiologic saline solution (0.85 per cent) contains 145 mEq each of sodium and of chloride. This represents very little more sodium than the 143 mEq per liter representative of the extracellular body fluids, and considerably more chloride than the approximately 103 mEq per liter in these fluids. This excess of chloride over sodium is a benefit in the treatment of the hypochloremic alkalosis which attends the dehydration from gastric vomiting, but a disadvantage in most forms of metabolic acidosis. After the interstitial fluid volume has been restored, unless the kidneys are able to excrete the surplus chloride as rapidly as it is infused, the plasma chloride level and the acidosis become augmented and the bicarbonate level depressed further. In the absence of enough potassium (p. 587) the plasma level of chloride may rise above normal, with depression of the bicarbonate to the alkalotic zone. If there is a deficit of calcium, the therapeutic raising of a low potassium level may evoke the symptoms of tetany unless the calcium disturbance is simultaneously corrected.

The giving of greater quantities of normal saline solution to non-acidotic ill infants or children whose renal excretory power is poor may result in fluid retention and strain on the circulation, but with no other toxic results. Premature and newborn infants seem exceptionally prone to develop retention edema; their intake of normal saline is best kept below a total of 25 ml and their total fluid intake below 200 ml per day, except when appreciable deficits of either salt or water have been incurred.

When giving saline solution intravenously for acidotic or hyperelectrolytemic disturbances it is best to begin with a hypotonic solution since isotonic solutions tend to induce a temporary further dehydration. A suitable preparation could be a mixture of one-third physiologic saline and two-thirds 5 per cent glucose solution. When sixth-molar ($M/6$) sodium lactate solution is required, this too may be mixed with 5 per cent or 10 per cent solution of glucose in water. When parenteral fluids are going to be continued for more than a single injection, it is important to begin by computing the total amounts and kinds needed, considering not only the maintenance requirement but replacement of losses.

Treatment solutions (Table 56-3) which approximate interstitial fluid composition more closely than does sodium chloride solution include (1) plasma itself, (2) Hartmann's lactated Ringer's solution, and (3) mixtures of 2 or 3 parts of normal saline solution with 1 part of $M/6$ sodium lactate solution. In acidosis, 2 ml $M/6$ sodium lactate or 1.5 per cent sodium bicarbonate solution per lb body weight will raise the plasma bicarbonate level by about 1 mEq per liter. When a reading of the plasma carbon dioxide cannot be secured but metabolic acidosis seems evident clinically, one may assume that the bicarbonate level has fallen 5 mEq per liter. $M/6$ sodium lactate or 1.5 per cent sodium bicarbonate solution in amounts of 20 ml per kg (10 ml per lb) may then be included in the fluid therapy program.

Table 56-3. Composition of Electrolyte Solutions Used in Parenteral Fluid Therapy
(In milliequivalents per liter)

	Na+	K+	Ca++	Cl−	Lactate−
Normal (0.9%) saline	154			154	
½ Strength normal saline	77			77	
M/6 sodium lactate	167				167
⅔ Normal saline; ⅓ M/6 sodium lactate	158			103	55
Ringer's solution	146	4	5.4	155	
Hartmann's Ringer lactate	128	4	3.6	110	
Darrow's solution	121	35		103	53
Glucose solutions	0	0	0	0	0

In dehydration with hyperelectrolytemia the corrective fluids, whether given by mouth or parenterally, should be sufficiently hypotonic to provide enough water to reduce the excessive electrolyte concentrations and to permit the kidneys to carry off metabolic end products. Normal saline solution contains little free water beyond that needed to maintain the osmolarity of its contained solutes; this is a disadvantage when one is trying to administer water to replace a deficit or take care of insensible water losses and other physiologic needs. Administration of isotonic sodium chloride solution at the initiation of therapy when kidney function is submaximal may lower the level of nitrogenous substances in the blood without alleviating the hyperelectrolytemia, or even aggravate the latter. Similar criticism may be directed against an initial infusion of plasma (except perhaps the salt-poor type). In the absence of renal disease the height of the blood nonprotein nitrogen level is a good indication for a therapeutic solution free from salt. For this condition an intravenous infusion of 5 per cent glucose solution is ordinarily the best to employ first, since 10 per cent glucose solution may transitorily increase the tissue fluid hypertonicity. Sodium bicarbonate or lactate solution may be added if acidosis is a complication, or a dilute calcium solution if hypocalcemia is present or suspected. When recovery has progressed to the point where diuresis begins, saline-containing solutions become necessary. Correction of the water deficit often brings out electrolyte deficits hitherto hidden, with the result that symptoms due to hypocalcemia or hypopotassemia may then supervene. Hyperelectrolytemic dehydration sometimes injures the renal tubules, so that for a time afterward there may be poor tubular reabsorption and undue loss of essential mineral ions.

With any new patient needing parenteral fluid therapy in whom the status of the kidney function is unknown, it is best to administer first an infusion of 5 per cent glucose in order to stimulate urine flow.

Fecal excretion of sodium can be increased in the edema associated with chronic congestive circulatory failure, cirrhosis of the liver, renal disease, or the nephrotic syndrome by giving a mixture of ion-exchange carbacrylic or carboxylic acid resins by mouth. These give up their hydrogen ions in exchange for cations. Sodium, being the most abundant cation of the gastrointestinal contents, is the chief one to be removed by the resin. To prevent depletion of potassium, an appreciable fraction of the resin mixture is usually already combined with this ion, provided urinary function is adequate to protect the subject from hyperpotassemia. A small amount of a polyamine methylene or anion-exchange resin is often included in order to remove some of the chloride and other intestinal anions. If these resins succeed in reducing the edema, the various blood electrolyte levels should be followed by laboratory tests in order to avoid the secondary development of distortions in carbon dioxide, chloride, calcium, potassium, and sodium metabolism from continued use of this form of therapy. Additional causative factors such as hypoproteinemia should be looked for when resins under suitable circumstances fail to reduce edema.

Potassium

When potassium is needed therapeutically the serum level does not return permanently to normal until after the intracellular deficit has been corrected (Chap. 53). A typical deficit is 10 mEq (391 mg) per kg body weight. A depleted infant weighing 5 kg would require a total restorative amount of 50 mEq. This is about 2 gm of potassium or 4 gm of potassium chloride (1 gm = 13.4 mEq K^+). The potassium should not be given until after renal function has been established by prior fluid therapy. Approximately one-third or one-fourth of the total deficit (2 to 3 mEq per kg) may be given each day, with an additional 1 mEq per kg to meet the daily needs. Less than 2 mEq per kg is unlikely to repair the deficit.

Intravenous solutions for therapy of hypopotassemia must be given slowly and in relatively dilute form, to avoid toxic effects on the heart muscle. This is especially important when the urine flow has been depressed. With older children a good rule for intravenous administration is at a rate not exceeding 15 mEq per hour. After a deficit has been rectified the infusion of 1 to 2 mEq per kg per day, depending on circumstances, should maintain the serum potassium satisfactorily until oral feedings are established.

For prophylaxis of potassium deficits one may give a solution of potassium chloride containing 1 to 2 gm per liter intravenously or subcutaneously without local reactions. For oral use a 1 per cent solution of potassium chloride is satisfactory and may be fed by gavage.

As replacement therapy in infantile diarrhea Darrow and associates have recommended a premixed solution containing 4 gm NaCl, 2.7 gm KCl, and 52 ml of molar sodium lactate per liter. This solution is best injected subcutaneously without dilution. Four or more hours should be taken for giving the calculated daily dose. In the first 24 hours of treatment 80 ml per kg is sufficient for replacement of the deficit of water and electrolyte. Thereafter, 20 to 50 ml per kg per day is adequate. It is essential that losses of water in the urine, stools, lungs, and skin be compensated for by sufficient electrolyte-free water. Stool loss may amount to as much as 80 ml per kg per day and sweat in hot weather may be 100 ml per kg per day. Adequate renal function requires 25 to 50 ml of urine per kg per day. Hence, in addition to the fluids containing potassium, the water requirement during the first 24 hours of treatment is 125 to 200 ml per kg. After the first day the total fluid requirement can usually be met by 150 ml per kg per day, including the solution containing electrolyte, which should not be more than one-third of the total. Solutions with adequate amounts of potassium will restore the serum bicarbonate level to normal in 1 or 2 days without additional bicarbonate or lactate, even when diarrhea is very severe. Larger doses can raise the serum bicarbonate to normal more rapidly but involve the risk of producing alkalosis or lowering the level of serum calcium.

Butler has recommended a phosphate-containing therapeutic solution for intravenous rather than subcutaneous injection. This contains about 30 mEq of sodium, 22 mEq of chloride, 20 mEq of lactate, 15 mEq of potassium, and 5 mM of phosphate per liter in 5 or 10 per cent glucose. The content of electrolytes is adequate if the volume is sufficient to meet the water requirement. The presence of phosphate is helpful in diabetic coma and perhaps so in diarrhea.

Most infants with diarrhea do not require prolonged administration of parenteral fluid. Even those severely ill can usually take fluid by mouth after 12 to 24 hours of parenteral therapy. Darrow and associates have diluted their potassium-containing solution with 2 parts of 5 per cent glucose in water and offered 150 ml per kg per day by mouth. The efficacy of the carrot-soup therapy used widely in Europe is probably due to the approximate 40 mEq content of potassium per liter, along with some sodium, chloride, and phosphate. When a well-rounded diet is taken, its content of potassium will correct even a marked deficit within a few days.

In older children a solution with a higher content of potassium and no sodium is preferred usually, especially for postoperative situations and for patients with heart disease. A concentrated solution containing 10, 20, or even 30 per cent of potassium chloride in distilled water can be added to other solutions before they are given intravenously. An isotonic solution of potassium chloride, which contains 11.4 gm (154 mEq) per liter, is likely to cause painful venospasm when introduced directly. A 5 per cent glucose solution containing 2 to 4 gm of potassium chloride per liter is safe if given over a 3- to 4-hour period and may be repeated after a few hours if the kidneys are functioning properly. Once the deficit is corrected this solution may be infused once daily.

Cautious supervision is necessary for all patients receiving parenteral potassium. The blood potassium level or electrocardiographic status should be determined every day or two. Hyperpotassemia calls for an immediate cessation of therapy, whereas hypopotassemia indicates that the corrective measures should be continued.

There seems to be a relation between potassium and the overt manifestations of hypocalcemic tetany. Clinical studies have shown that the symptoms of hypocalcemic tetany will subside in the presence of hypopotassemia, to recur after the level of serum potassium has been raised.

THERAPEUTIC EXAMPLES

Numerous systems have been proposed for calculating the amount of any ion needed to correct a deficiency or distortion of that ion in the extracellular fluid. The following type of approach may be utilized when fluid loss has been acute.

Example 1. A 6-month-old infant weighed 16 lb at the onset of acute diarrhea and shock. He now weighs 14 lb and has a plasma sodium level of 133 mEq per liter. How much saline solution is needed to restore the sodium content to normal in the extracellular fluid?

Calculations

a. To convert pounds to kilograms divide the infant's weight by 2.2:

Normal weight: 16/2.2 = 7.3 kg
Present weight: 14/2.2 = 6.4 kg
Acute weight loss (presumably water loss): 7.3 − 6.4 = 0.9 kg

It is assumed in situations such as this that the extracellular and intracellular water stores have been depleted about equally.

b. The value for extracellular fluid at this age is approximately 20 per cent of 7.3 kg, or 1.46 liters. However, 0.9 liter of water has been lost, of which approximately 0.45 liter comes from the extracellular fluid. Hence the estimated value of the extracellular fluid at hospitalization is 1.46 − 0.45, or about 1.0 liter. The amount of sodium needed to raise the concentration to normal is 1.0 × (143 − 133) = 10 mEq.

c. Sodium is needed also to provide a concentration of 143 mEq per liter in the 0.45 liter of interstitial fluid which must be replaced.

0.45 × 143 = 64 mEq   64 mEq + 10 mEq = 74 mEq Na needed

Inasmuch as the illness is very acute the change in sodium content in the intracellular fluids is comparatively negligible and may be ignored.

d. Since normal physiologic saline solution (0.85%) contains 145 mEq of sodium per liter, the quantity needed to replace a deficit of 74 mEq is approximately 500 ml. If half-strength saline solution in 5 per cent glucose is to be administered, 1,000 ml is required.

Example 2. A 1-year-old infant weighing 20 lb (9.1 kg) is hospitalized because of acute volvulus. The plasma chemistry levels are not disturbed. Continuous gastric suction is maintained after operation and 250 ml of gastric juice recovered in 24 hours. Parenteral fluids must be given for some days—what kind and how much?

Calculations

a. Maintenance requirements per 24 hours:

Water: 135 ml per kg × 9.1 = 1,230 ml
Sodium: 0.8 mEq per kg × 9.1 = 7.3 mEq
Chloride: 0.8 mEq per kg × 9.1 = 7.3 mEq
Potassium: 1.0 mEq per kg × 9.1 = 9.1 mEq

b. Depletion through gastric suction per 24 hours:

Water: 250 ml
Sodium: 0.25 × 60 mEq per liter = 15.0 mEq
Chloride: 0.25 × 90 mEq per liter = 22.5 mEq
Potassium: 0.25 × 10 mEq per liter = 2.5 mEq

c. Total daily requirements $(a + b)$:

Water: 1,230 + 250 = 1,480 ml
Sodium: 7.3+ 15 = 22.3 mEq
Chloride: 7.3 + 22.5 = 29.8 mEq
Potassium: 9.1 + 2.5 = 11.6 mEq
Calories: 50 per kg × 9.1 = 455 cal
Protein: 2 gm per kg × 9.1 = 18.2 gm

d. Prescription for parenteral fluids per 24 hours:

Solution	Amount (ml)	Cal per ml	Total cal	Na (mEq)	Cl (mEq)	K (mEq)	Protein
5% protein hydrolysate with 5% glucose	360	0.4	144				18.0
5% glucose in normal saline	150	0.2	30	22	22		
5% glucose with 0.2% KCl	400	0.2	80		11	11	
5% glucose alone	600	0.2	120				
Total	1,510	1.0	374	22	33	11	18.0

Example 3. An 8-month-old infant with diarrhea and dehydration weighed 8 kg before an acute illness and weighs 7 kg today. His plasma bicarbonate level is 17 mEq per liter. Sodium and chloride levels are within normal limits. How much fluid and alkaline salts are needed to repair the dehydration and metabolic acidosis (ignoring the needs for potassium and for transfusion of whole blood or plasma)?

Calculations

a. Replacement of the lost interstitial fluid. This amounts to 50% of 1 kg, or 0.5 liter. The sodium needed is 0.5 ×143 = 71 mEq. This is contained in approximately 500 ml of normal saline solution and should be given with 5 per cent glucose added. The missing chloride will be simultaneously restored.

b. Specific treatment to correct the acidosis: 27 − 17 = 10 mEq bicarbonate per liter to be replaced. 4 ml of $M/6$ sodium lactate or of 1.5% sodium bicarbonate solution per kg body weight will raise the plasma bicarbonate level 1 mEq per liter. 4 × 10 × 8 = 320 ml. This may be given intravenously and subcutaneously in 5% glucose solution.

c. Repair of water deficit: Water required to restore weight deficit of 1 kg = 1,000 ml. In addition, 125 ml of water is required to maintain hydration for 24 hours at this age (8 × 125 = 1,000 ml). Total requirement, 2,000 ml.

2,000 − (320 + 500) = 1,180 ml of 5% glucose solution to be administered in addition to solutions a and b. The 2,000-ml total with its 5% glucose content will furnish 100 gm of glucose, equivalent to 400 calories.

Note: The above solutions should be given over the first 36 hours. If kidney function is reestablished early and the infant begins to take fluids by mouth, the full program may be curtailed.

Example 4. An 8-year-old child weighing 60 lb (27.3 kg) is unable to produce appreciable amounts of red cells because of leukemic infiltration of the bone marrow. His hemoglobin level at the time of hospitalization is 7.0 gm per 100 ml. How much transfused blood is needed in order to raise this level to optimal (13 gm per 100 ml)?

Calculations

a. Normal blood volume is approximately 7.5% of body weight.

$$7.5\% \times 27.3 = 2.05 \text{ liters, or } 2,050 \text{ ml}$$

b. Deficit is 13 − 7 or 6 gm hemoglobin per 100 ml.

$$2,050/100 \times 6 = 123 \text{ gm total hemoglobin deficit}$$

c. Since 1 ml of "sedimented red cells" supplies approximately 0.24 gm of hemoglobin, the child needs 123/0.24 or 513 ml of sedimented red cells. This can be given with safety as two 250-ml transfusions on successive days. If whole citrated blood is used, the total volume required will be twice as great, best given as three 350-ml transfusions.

Other Nutrients

The daily amino acid requirement estimated to cover average nitrogen loss under basal conditions is 1.5 mg per kg for young infants, 1 mg for older infants, and 0.6 mg for children and adults. The commercial amino acid mixtures prepared for intravenous use are given in concentrations under 4 per cent, or as specified by the manufacturer. Ascorbic acid, along with thiamine, riboflavin, niacinamide, and other elements of the vitamin B complex should be added to nutrient repair solutions if parenteral feeding is kept up for more than a day or two. Since most of these vitamins are unstable in an alkaline environment, they should not be added to solutions containing bicarbonate or lactate.

BIBLIOGRAPHY

DISTURBANCES IN BODY WATER AND ELECTROLYTES

Black, D. A. K., "Sodium Metabolism in Health and Disease," Charles C Thomas, Springfield, Ill., 1952.

Blecha, E., Low Sodium Diets, Am. J. Nursing 51:464, 1951.

Bower, A. G., J. S. Chudnoff, and A. L. Chaney, Bio-chemical Alterations in Acute Human Poliomyelitis: Electrolyte Patterns and Trends, California Med. 73:406, 1950.

Cole, S. L., Tap Water Sodium in the Low Salt Diet, J.A.M.A. 140:19, 1949.

Danowski, T. S., Newer Concepts of the Role of Sodium in Disease, Am. J. Med. 10:468, 1951.

———, Fundamental Features of Metabolism of Sodium and Potassium, Am. J. Clin. Path. 23:1095, 1953.

Darrow, D. C., The Importance of Deficit of Sodium and Chloride in Dehydration, J. Pediat. 13:670, 1938.

Elkinton, J. R., A. W. Winkler, and T. S. Danowski, Transfers of Cell Sodium and Potassium in Experimental and Clinical Conditions, J. Clin. Invest. 27:74, 1948.

Hiatt, R. B., The Pathologic Physiology of Congenital Megacolon, *Ann. Surg.* 133:313, 1951.

Leiter, L., The Role of Sodium Chloride in the Mechanism and Treatment of Congestive Heart Failure, *Bull. New York Acad. Med.* 24:702, 1948.

————, *R. E. Weston,* and *J. Grossman,* The Low Sodium Syndrome: Its Origins and Varieties, *Bull. New York Acad. Med.* 46:833, 1953.

Macguire, W. B., Jr., Risk of Uremia Due to Sodium Depletion, *J.A.M.A.* 137:1377, 1948.

Musselman, M. M., Management of Water and Electrolyte Problems in Surgery, *Am. J. Clin. Path.* 23:1121, 1953.

Overman, R. R., Sodium, Potassium and Chloride Alterations in Disease, *Physiol. Rev.* 31:285, 1951.

Peters, J. P., Diagnostic Significance of Electrolyte Disturbances, *Bull. New York Acad. Med.* 25:749, 1949.

Rapoport, S., Hyperosmolarity and Hyperelectrolytemia in Pathologic Conditions of Childhood, *Am. J. Dis. Child.* 74:682, 1947.

————, The Role of Overventilation in Diseases of Infancy, *Ann. paediat.* 176:12, 1951.

Sawyer, W. H., and *C. Solez,* Salt-losing Nephritis Simulating Adrenocortical Insufficiency, *New England J. Med.* 240:210, 1949.

Whittinghill, J. A., W. H. Danielson, A. Robinson, and *L. E. Holt, Jr.,* Diarrhea with Hyperelectrolytemia and Post-acidotic Collapse, *Bull. Children's Hosp. Denver, Colo.* 2:57, 1950.

GENERAL PRINCIPLES OF MANAGEMENT

Barness, L. A., and *P. Gyorgy,* Errors in Fluid Therapy for Children, *Postgrad. Med.* 17:302, 1955.

Butler, A. M., and *N. B. Talbot,* Parenteral-fluid Therapy. II. The Estimation of Losses Incident to Starvation and Dehydration with Acidosis or Alkalosis and the Provision of Repair Therapy, *New England J. Med.* 231:621, 1944.

Cooke, R. E., Contributions of the Laboratory to the Practical Management of Disorders of Body Water and Electrolyte, *Pediatrics* 16:555, 1955.

Council on Pharmacy and Chemistry of the A.M.A., Carbacrylamine Resins, *J.A.M.A.* 151:210, 1953.

Danowski, T. S., A. W. Winkler, and *J. R. Elkinton,* Biochemical and Hemodynamic Changes Following the Subcutaneous Injection of Glucose Solution, *J. Clin. Invest.* 26:887, 1947.

Darrow, D. C., Therapeutic Measures Promoting Recovery from the Physiologic Disturbances of Infantile Diarrhea, *Pediatrics* 9:519, 1952.

———— and *E. L. Pratt,* Fluid Therapy: Relation to Tissue Composition and the Expenditure of Water and Electrolyte, *J.A.M.A.* 143:432, 1950.

———— and ————, Fluid Therapy: Relation to Tissue Composition and the Expenditure of Water and Electrolyte, *J.A.M.A.* 143:365, 1950.

Finberg, L., and *H. E. Harrison,* Hypernatremia in Infants: An Evaluation of the Clinical and Biochemical Findings Accompanying This State, *Pediatrics* 16:1, 1955.

Forbes, G. B., and *J. A. Erganian,* Parenteral Administration of Ammonium Chloride for Alkalosis of Congenital Hypertrophic Pyloric Stenosis: A Preliminary Report, *Am. J. Dis. Child.* 72:649, 1946.

Hill, F. S., "Practical Fluid Therapy in Pediatrics," W. B. Saunders Co., Philadelphia, 1954.

Hoffman, W. S., Theoretical and Practical Considerations in Correcting Fluid and Electrolyte Losses: A Résumé, *Am. J. Clin. Path.* 23:1142, 1953.

Koop, C. E., and *R. W. P. Mellish*, Some Aspects of Nutrition in Pediatric Surgical Patients, *Am. J. Clin. Nutrition* 3:487, 1955.

Lowe, C. U., T. S. Danowski, and *R. Ebert*, Symposium on Parenteral Fluid Therapy in Pediatrics, *Pediatrics* 15:488, 1955.

Marriott, H. L., "Water and Salt Depletion," American Lectures in Physiology, Charles C Thomas, Springfield, Ill., 1950.

Nickerson, D. A., Role of Pathologist in Management of Patients with Fluid and Electrolyte Disturbances, *Am. J. Clin. Path.* 23:1061, 1953.

Schechter, A. J., M. K. Cory, A. L. Carpentier, and *D. C. Darrow*, Changes in the Composition of Fluids Injected into the Peritoneal Cavity, *Am. J. Dis. Child.* 46:1015, 1933.

Schroeder, H. A., and *H. M. Perry, Jr.*, Disturbances of the Internal Environment and Their Correction, *Am. J. Clin. Path.* 23:1100, 1953.

Snyder, C. H., Practical Scheme for Fluid and Electrolyte Therapy in Children, *J.A.M.A.* 158:1004, 1955.

Talbot, N. B., G. A. Kerrigan, J. D. Crawford, W. Cochran, and *M. Terry*, Application of Homeostatic Principles to the Practice of Parenteral Fluid Therapy, *New England J. Med.* 252:856, 1955.

Wallace, W. M., Quantitative Requirements of the Infant and Child for Water and Electrolyte under Varying Conditions, *Am. J. Clin. Path.* 23:1133, 1953.

CHAPTER 57

Fluid and Electrolyte Disturbances in Specific Disorders

CHRONIC NEPHRITIS

Every patient with nephritis presents an individualized set of derangements and requires a program of management tempered for his own needs. Complicating problems of pathogenesis and treatment are the general tendency for all functioning parts of the kidney to be affected no matter what the nature of the renal disease. The biochemical disturbances which appear are the end results of the interplay of vascular lesions, impaired glomerular filtration, and deranged tubular activities. Altered body metabolism, gastrointestinal dysfunctions, impairment of appetite, or enfeebled gaseous exchange through the lungs as a consequence of edema may hamper further the already disturbed economy of water and electrolytes.

The more advanced the renal destruction and the more curtailed the renal homeostatic mechanisms, the more meticulous must be the selection and administration of drugs, diet, and therapeutic fluids (Chap. 36). For intelligent management of patients the physician must have a clear understanding of renal physiology and the assistance of a reliable chemistry laboratory.

CHRONIC RENAL ACIDOSIS

Poor tubular reabsorption of bicarbonate can result in an alkaline urine rich in bicarbonate, a low plasma bicarbonate level, and a compensatory elevation of plasma chloride. Characteristic blood findings are a plasma bicarbonate level of about 20 mEq per liter, a plasma chloride level of about 115 mEq per liter, and a sodium level of about 135 mEq per liter. The urine has a pH near that of the blood, its specific gravity is about 1.010, and its ammonia content is diminished.

Chronic hyperchloremic acidosis of this type with bony changes has been seen in chronic pyelonephritis of infants and young children, along

634

with the bony changes of osteomalacia or "renal rickets." It sometimes complicates diabetes insipidus. It may develop when there is an undue excretion of organic acids, a tubular dysfunction of ammonia production or hydrogen-ion exchange, tubular damage secondary to toxins, or acute infections. There is a bizarre syndrome becoming apparent soon after birth, in which dysfunction and roentgenologically visible nephrocalcinosis of the distal tubules is accompanied by hyperpnea, polyuria, dehydration, and hyperchloremic acidosis (p. 425).

CONGESTIVE CIRCULATORY FAILURE

One of the principal manifestations of pure congestive circulatory failure is the retention of salt and water. Elevated pressure in the capillary bed, hypoalbuminemia, and altered renal hemodynamics are important pathogenetic factors. Any coincident or secondary renal lesion makes the pathogenesis of the edema and the management of the patient even more complex; for example, preexisting renal disease may lead to a "salt-losing" syndrome.

Physiologic studies have shown that in congestive failure the diminished cardiac output slows the renal plasma flow and the glomerular filtration rate and enhances the tubular resorption of sodium. The renal retention of sodium may be aided by an unusual output of the salt-and-water adrenal hormones. Sodium is often absent from the urine. The osmotic activity of the retained sodium retards the excretion of water into the urine.

Occasional patients with cardiac decompensation exhibit low blood sodium levels. Here a specific disturbance of water balance not wholly dependent on retention of salt is believed to be operating.

The electrolyte disturbances in congestive heart failure may be aggravated by other factors. Diffuse pulmonary disease, if it impairs the respiratory exchange of gases, may first produce a respiratory acidosis from carbon dioxide retention. This can change to a metabolic alkalosis after the kidneys have excreted an unusual amount of chloride as compensation. With other patients who hyperventilate, as occurs not infrequently in heart failure, the plasma CO_2 falls, the pH of the blood rises, the kidneys excrete sodium and bicarbonate in excess but retain chloride, and respiratory alkalosis ensues.

When patients with congestive failure are treated by drastic restriction of fluid intake, the blood may become hypertonic and urea as well as sodium is retained. Heart failure in this circumstance may remain refractory to treatment until a liberal intake of water has been restored.

Digitalis by raising cardiac output facilitates the renal excretion of sodium, chloride, and water. Concomitant oxygen therapy sometimes depresses the respiratory center, leading to a decrease in ventilation and a rise in the CO_2 of the blood.

The therapeutic administration of ammonium chloride in adequate amounts to cardiac patients raises the chloride concentration of the plasma and the edema fluid. The urinary output of chlorides mounts also, depleting the sodium and also the potassium and calcium. The plasma volume then decreases, with hemoconcentration as shown by a rise in the hematocrit and plasma protein levels. It takes about 4 days for the kidneys to develop sufficient ammonia production to inhibit this further loss of fixed base. Should the production of ammonia be impaired by renal disease the excessive loss of base into the urine may continue, resulting in chloride retention and even "chloride acidosis."

Mercurials tend to increase the excretion of chloride in excess of that of sodium. Such a regimen may lead to hypochloremic alkalosis. Diuresis ceases when the plasma chloride level falls below 86 mEq per liter. The patient may then become prostrated, and the nonprotein nitrogen level rise precipitously. The addition of ammonium chloride prevents the hypochloremic alkalosis. Should the bicarbonate become depleted during the alkalosis with secondary excretion of sodium, dehydration will follow. Although the patient is in alkalosis the urine becomes acid ("paradoxical aciduria").

Low-sodium Therapy

Most patients with edema of circulatory origin are helped by a restricted sodium intake, except those who because of renal disease continue to lose sodium into the urine. The usual daily diet of an older child contains 2,000 to 4,000 mg of sodium, corresponding to 1 to 2 level teaspoons of salt. This intake can be cut in half by eliminating obviously salty foods and not adding salt to meals at the table. If it is desired to restrict the intake further, one should give low-sodium milk, eliminate salt, soda, and baking powder from foods, and avoid meat juices, broths, gravies, fish, oleomargarine, salted butter, and all other foods of high sodium content. The desired range for diets low in sodium is 50 to 100 mg per day, depending on the age of the child and extent of restriction desired.

Drinking water from public water supplies varies considerably in sodium content and can be as high as 200 ppm (20 mg per 100 ml). Use of water softeners in hospital buildings may raise the sodium content a little. When sodium intake is being rigidly controlled, therefore, one must have information regarding the tap water. Distilled water or spring water low in sodium may have to be given.

Care must always be taken, whenever a patient is receiving a low sodium intake, to avoid inducing a "low-salt syndrome" or sodium-depletion state. Early signs are lethargy, mental confusion, nausea, low urine output, and a high nonprotein nitrogen content in the blood. The giving of sodium chloride causes improvement promptly. Frequent estimations of blood sodium levels are integral parts of the management of all patients being deprived of sodium.

Since the sodium ion in food and drinking water is accompanied by the chloride ion in approximately equivalent amounts, a crude office aid in control of a patient on a low-sodium diet is to test the urine for chloride. The test can be performed by the patient at home.

Procedure

Solution *A:* 10 per cent solution of potassium chromate.

Solution *B:* 0.74 per cent solution of silver nitrate (stored in a dark-glass bottle).

To 10 drops of the early-morning urine specimen add 1 drop of solution *A.* Shake well. Add solution *B,* counting the drops until the urine becomes a permanent light brown or brick-red color. Each drop of solution *B* represents approximately 250 mg of sodium chloride or 100 mg of sodium per liter. If the diet is low in chloride and sodium, not more than 8 drops will be required. Misleading results will be obtained if nonchloride sodium salts such as sodium bicarbonate are being taken, or halide salts such as bromides or potassium chloride, an important constituent of salt substitutes.

CYSTIC FIBROSIS OF THE PANCREAS

In this disorder the chloride concentration of the sweat varies from 80 to 220 mEq per liter, in contrast to the usual 1 to 110 mEq range of normal individuals. A comparable amount of sodium and traces of potassium accompany the chloride. The total volume of sweat is not abnormal.

Collection and chemical analysis of sweat for its content of salt is useful in differentiating cystic fibrosis of the pancreas from other chronic disorders of the digestive tract or lungs and from familial dysautonomia. It is helpful also in uncovering subclinical forms of cystic fibrosis.

Sweat Test

The skin of a limb or most of the body is first washed with soap and water, rinsed thoroughly, and dried. This is then wrapped in a plastic sheet. The environment is then made hot by covering the part with an excess of blankets or placing it under a blanketed cradle holding a 100-watt light bulb. A small infant may be placed in an air-controlled incubator set at 95°F with 100 per cent humidity. The sweat is aspirated directly from the sheet and the skin by means of a glass syringe. A sample of 2 to 20 ml of sweat may be thus collected.

An alternative method for procuring a sample of sweat is to apply a piece of dry gauze to body surface, sealed under a larger piece of plastic cloth. The gauze is weighed before and after being applied, and its contents extracted with a measured amount of water.

Schwachman and Gahm have described a procedure whereby a finger or hand or foot is pressed lightly upon an agar test medium containing silver nitrate and potassium chromate. When the chloride content of the sweat is excessive a pronounced whitish-yellow discoloration appears immediately. When the content is normal the imprint is barely detectable. Since newborn infants do not sweat perceptibly, this approach cannot be used diagnostically to recognize meconium ileus.

The exceptionally high content of salt in the sweat in this disease, perhaps along with an undue propensity to perspiration, makes affected children unusually likely to develop subnormal levels of serum sodium and chloride during hot weather. Hypoelectrolytemic symptoms and dehydration may result. Isotonic sodium chloride solution in large amounts should be administered intravenously as rapidly as possible for this type of heat prostration. Prophylaxis consists of giving goodly amounts of salt and water daily to such children during the summer months.

DIABETIC ACIDOSIS

Electrolyte Disturbances

Derangements can vary enormously in diabetic acidosis, depending on duration of the disturbance and speed of development, age of the child, functional reserves of kidney and liver, character of the respirations, and extent of vomiting, diarrhea, sweating, and infection. In general, the younger the child the more rapid the onset of ketosis and coma.

Accumulation of ketone bodies depresses the plasma concentrations of bicarbonate and chloride anions, which are excreted largely in the urine. Being acid, they carry off large quantities of neutralizing base and deplete the reserve of cations. The polyuria induced by the excessive output of salts, ketone bodies, and glucose promotes dehydration, which in turn impairs the renal production of ammonia and aggravates further the loss of body base. Protein catabolism, accelerated as long as the diabetes remains uncontrolled, raises the level of nitrogenous products in both plasma and urine. The blood proteins may be partially consumed, but lowered levels may not become apparent until after the disturbed fluid and electrolyte equilibria have been repaired. The hypoproteinemia which then appears may be sufficiently marked to cause edema.

The water loss results in shrinkage of interstitial fluid volume and blood volume. The osmotic tonicity of the plasma increases as the process advances. The end result may be a shocklike syndrome with peripheral vascular collapse, low blood pressure, oliguria or anuria, and sometimes even the uremic syndrome. If vomiting supervenes, the available supplies of fluids and electrolytes, chiefly chlorides and potassium, are reduced further. Various important intracellular components, especially potassium, magnesium, and phosphate, can become depleted.

The plasma levels of sodium, potassium, chloride, bicarbonate, phosphate, and other ions can undergo bizarre distortions. The values represent the concentrations of the respective substances in terms of unit volumes of blood plasma; they do not describe the contractions of the various body fluid compartments or the imbalances inside the cells. The magnesium and phosphate are usually depressed also, but cannot be measured readily. The presence of acetone is detectable in the urine and circulating blood. The plasma levels of glucose, cholesterol, fat, and non-protein nitrogen are above normal.

The plasma bicarbonate is usually markedly depressed and may be lower than 1.5 mEq per liter. The pH reading of the plasma if coincidentally determined may fall between 7.2 and 6.9. Failure of the usual acidotic hypoventilation in marked shock can further augment the CO_2 loss and aggravate the decline in plasma pH. The blowing off of CO_2 in the expired air may persist after the initiation of therapy and result in a respiratory alkalosis superimposed upon a metabolic acidosis. Treatment of diabetic acidosis with intravenous solutions of sodium lactate or sodium bicarbonate can elevate the bicarbonate value toward normal, but the concomitant base added may displace the serum pH to the alkaline side for a time.

Comments on Therapy

Treatment must be adjusted to the deficits of the individual patient and carried out with careful laboratory control. Butler has recommended that the first infusion be a hypotonic solution consisting of 550 ml of pyrogen-free distilled water plus 400 ml of isotonic saline plus 40 ml molar sodium lactate. This furnishes 100 mEq of Na^+ per liter, 60 mEq of Cl^-, 45 mEq of lactate, and water to correct the immediate dehydration and induce urine flow. Insulin is given in large doses, commencing as soon as the patient is seen.

If the patient is in shock with dehydration and anuria, the blood volume may be first restored by a rapid infusion of plasma or fresh whole blood.

As recovery progresses, the various ions in deficit are replaced after kidney function has been restored. Butler's hypotonic solution containing electrolytes and glucose may be given. One liter of this contains 75 gm of glucose and 45 mEq of Na^+, 30 of Cl^-, 30 of K^+, 5 of Mg^{++}, and 16 of PO_4^{--}.

Gastric lavage with isotonic saline or sodium bicarbonate solution may be performed when the patient is first seen, if there has been extensive vomiting or evidence of gastric dilatation, and several hundred milliliters of the lavage solution may be left within the stomach. Antimicrobial therapy is needed for any infection present. Fluids and food should be taken by mouth as soon as the patient is able. Bacteriologic cultures of the urine are advisable.

The hematocrit, hemoglobin, and red cell levels are good indicators of the extent of hemoconcentration and the progress of recovery. Repeated urine analyses for specific gravity, sugar, ketone bodies, pH, protein, casts, and other characteristics aid in following recovery. The severity of the ketonuria is a rough indicator of the intensity of the ketosis, though many patients with high blood ketone levels may excrete only scanty amounts into the urine. Urine with a liberal content of chloride, especially when alkaline, indicates that the kidneys are excreting coincidentally a relative excess of basic ions. Return of the urine to an acid pH indicates that this loss is ceasing.

Serial determinations of the blood sugar level guide the administration of insulin and glucose. The blood nonprotein nitrogen level is a good indicator of renal function. Electrocardiograms may be utilized to detect abnormalities in the potassium level.

EKIRI

This serious disease of Japanese children in the age group 2 to 6 years, prevalent in the summer season, has been characterized by diarrhea, high fever, vomiting, hyperventilation, convulsions, and tetany as the chief symptoms. In most children this illness is usually bacillary dysentery complicated by tetany (Dodd, Buddingh, and Rapoport). The plasma CO_2 content is usually diminished to levels between 12 and 21 mEq per liter, the nonprotein nitrogen between 60 and 90 mg per 100 ml, and the serum calcium below 9 mg per 100 ml. In most of the cases the plasma pH remains within normal limits. These plasma changes suggest that much of the disturbance is an expression of primary respiratory alkalosis from hyperventilation induced by the infection, with a complicating secondary metabolic acidosis perhaps due in part to lactic acid accumulation. The tetany is ascribed to an underlying hypocalcemia from a low prior intake of milk and other calcium-containing foods.

INFANTILE GASTROENTERITIS

The more severe gastrointestinal disturbances of infancy, and especially in the first year of life, often induce serious disturbances in internal biochemical equilibria. Vomiting and diarrhea, when combined with fever, infection, sweating, and a reduced fluid and food intake, can seriously deplete the body stores of water and electrolytes and bring about ketotic changes within but a few hours. Infants with diarrhea who become sufficiently ill and dehydrated to require hospitalization are nearly always in shock and have a concomitant metabolic acidosis. Poor tissue turgor, Kussmaul breathing, hypotension, oliguria, and other physical indications of dehydration and acidosis are usually present.

The electrolyte content of diarrheal stools varies greatly from case to case, and from stool to stool in the same case. Water lost in the stools generally exceeds 200 ml per day, even in small infants, and may exceed 500 ml per day in cholera-like illnesses. Typical daily losses in severe infantile diarrhea, noted by Darrow, Pratt, and associates, are 250 gm of water, 16 mM of sodium, 11 mM of chloride, and 8 mM of potassium. The amounts of sodium and potassium lost are almost always greater than those of chloride. However, there is a rare anomaly of intestinal absorption in which watery stools are passed which contain more chloride than sodium, so that the infant remains in continual metabolic alkalosis.

The character of the plasma electrolyte pattern is determined by the intensity and duration of the illness and the extent of depletion of water as compared with electrolytes. The younger the infant, the more extreme are the deviations likely to be. In the more severe cases the electrolyte changes are usually those of metabolic acidosis. The plasma may be hypertonic or hypotonic with respect to the total ionic content. The plasma sodium level in a series of reported cases has ranged from 115 to 165 mEq per liter (normal, 134 to 154 mEq) but is usually moderately below the lower limits for normal infants of similar ages. The plasma potassium level is usually reduced, more so in older infants; the range may be from 1.0 to 7.5 mEq per liter (normal, 3.5 to 5.5 mEq). The potassium level and the severity of the acidosis show no clear correlation. The plasma calcium level usually does not deviate from the normal range, at least before treatment is begun. The plasma chloride level tends to be mildly or moderately depressed; it usually falls between 80 and 115 mEq per liter (normal, 100 to 110 mEq). The changes of chloride often parallel those of sodium.

The plasma bicarbonate level is often significantly depressed. The usual range is 3 to 25 mEq per liter (normal, 20 to 31 mEq). The clinical severity of the gastroenteritis tends to be correlated more closely with the drop in plasma bicarbonate than with that of any other plasma electrolyte.

The levels of hemoglobin, erythrocytes, hematocrit, and plasma protein are usually elevated, portraying a shrinkage in blood volume. The blood nonprotein nitrogen level is as a rule elevated also and may be as much as 100 mg per 100 ml or more (normal, 25 to 40 mg). The centrifuged red cells in infants with dehydration due to gastroenteritis show questionably slight elevations in sodium content, normal values for chloride, and slight diminutions in potassium; these changes reflect dimly the much greater ones in the muscle cells which are the great reservoir of body electrolytes, and notably potassium.

Metabolic balance studies, carried out by Darrow, Pratt, and associates, demonstrated that the major quantitative deficits in infantile diarrhea are in water, sodium, potassium, and chloride. The average retentions during recovery in 8 infants with moderate to severe diarrhea were, per kilogram body weight, 125 ml water, 9.2 mM (or mEq) chloride, 9.5 mM sodium, and 10 mM potassium. The deficit in extracellular fluids averaged about 100 ml per kg. Thus the losses of extracellular water and salts are about one-fourth of the usual normal content. The deficit of potassium may be equivalent to about one-seventh of the total intracellular sodium. Loss of potassium and shift of sodium are greatest in the sickest patients, especially those with prolonged diarrhea, and may be minimal in brief illnesses.

Solutions to replace deficits of water and electrolyte in diarrhea should contain potassium as well as sodium and chloride. When restorative therapy consists of sodium and water alone, as when solutions of sodium lactate or bicarbonate are given, more sodium moves into the cells even though the plasma bicarbonate concentration may be raised to an alkalotic level. This aggravates the clinical signs of potassium deficiency so long as the diarrhea persists and food cannot be absorbed. The alterations in the electrocardiogram so consistently seen in hypopotassemia have been described in diarrheal infants with normal serum potassium levels but extremely low plasma bicarbonate.

It is commonly advised to withhold milk feedings during vomiting or severe diarrhea, and then resume them in gradual increments. Parenteral fluids high in sugar content but low in electrolyte tonicity are given first, up to a total fluid intake of 200 to 300 ml per kg of body weight. Transfusions with blood or plasma are also desirable. After the first day the fluid intake may be reduced to 150 ml per kg and need not be given parenterally if tolerated by mouth. The restoring of milk should be regulated by the symptoms; return of diarrhea or vomiting suggests that the milk is being increased too rapidly.

Rarely one encounters infants whose diarrhea recurs every time milk is given, even after fasting for 4 or 5 days. These infants seem to have an allergy or a sensitivity to milk, which in some may antedate the gastroenteritis and in others seems to have been acquired during the illness. Milk substitutes made from glucose–amino acid–fat mixtures, soybean preparations, and formulas based on homogenized meat are useful. Veal and beef should be avoided; these are antigenically related to cow's-milk protein and occasionally prove irritating.

OPERATIVE PROBLEMS

Most children undergoing simple elective operations such as tonsillectomy or herniorrhaphy require no parenteral fluid therapy except when oral fluids are refused for several days because of emotional trauma or some unforeseen reaction. With more severe operations a single clysis on the day of surgery may be required to prevent dehydration or starvation secondary to anesthesia. With patients already dehydrated or in shock, and especially if the operation involves the gastrointestinal tract, parenteral fluid and electrolytes may be needed for several days both before and afterward to replace deficits and meet the daily maintenance requirements until a sufficient intake can be taken orally. Transfusions of whole blood or plasma support the patient during the operation and afterward.

The water and electrolyte content of the parenteral fluids given should be based on the total of insensible water loss, kidney and stool losses, and any losses during operation or by drainage. Steady vomiting or the liberal suctioning off of gastric fluid result typically in a predominantly chloride deficit. If bile or pancreatic or intestinal fluids are drained away the loss of sodium and other bases tends to exceed that of chloride.

The most difficult problems are presented by newborn infants, often premature, with a gastrointestinal or other anomaly. The attendant vomiting, starvation, distention, and shock, acting in combination with the normal neonatal difficulties, result in involved patterns of dehydration, malnutrition, ketosis, acid-base imbalances, and hypopotassemia. If these continue for some days it is often impossible to save the infant even after the anatomic defects have been corrected.

PREFERENTIAL CHLORIDE RETENTION FROM IMMATURE RENAL FUNCTION

Kidneys which are functioning efficiently are well able to cope with unusual loads of sodium chloride. When the chloride is taken free in an acid medium, or accompanied by an organic ammonium ion, the excretory burden is more difficult. Many of the patients subjected to bilateral ureterosigmoidostomy have hyperchloremia and compensated mild acidosis, consequent to mucosal absorption of chloride from the acid urine flowing into the colon and rectum.

In prematurely and immaturely born infants, a high content of chloride and other mineral ions in cow's-milk feeding mixtures may burden the kidneys. Electrolyte-rich feeding formulas made from protein milk powder containing 5.7 mEq of chloride and 2.0 mEq of sodium per 100 calories were found by Darrow, Da Silva, and Stevenson, and also by Hoffman, Parmalee, and Grossman, to produce within 3 days a profound acidosis with elevated plasma chloride, greatly reduced plasma bicarbonate, loss of weight, and intracellular dehydration. Balance studies showed these changes to be due to retention of chloride in excess of sodium. There were no consistent alterations in the concentrations of serum potassium, nitrogen, calcium, or phosphate. Full-term newborn infants given the same milk mixtures exhibited the same sequence of changes but to a lesser degree. Their slightly more mature renal function seemed to permit a more concentrated urine output and a greater conservation of sodium and excretion of chloride (p. 417).

Electrolyte balance studies of premature infants being raised on formulas consisting of evaporated cow's milk diluted with an equal quantity of distilled water and added carbohydrate have shown an elevation in serum chloride levels (average 110 mEq per liter) and a drop in bicarbonate levels (average 18 mEq per liter).

Breast milk with its lower content of salts provides a much wider physiologic margin for the immature kidney than does cow's milk. Typical figures on the content per 100 calories, presented by Darrow, Da Silva, and Stevenson, are as follows:

	Protein (gm)	Fat (gm)	Carbo-hydrate (gm)	Cl (mM*)	Na (mM*)	K (mM*)	P (mM*)	Ca (mM*)
Human	1.84	5.2	11.0	1.5	0.7	1.8	0.7	1.3
Cow	4.2	5.3	7.2	5.0	4.0	6.0	4.4	4.6
Half-skimmed cow's milk with added carbohydrate	3.4	2.2	16.0	3.0	2.4	4.6	3.3	3.4

* For monovalent ions, millimols and milliequivalents are identical. For divalent ions, 1 mM yields 2 mEq when ionized.

SALICYLATE INTOXICATION

Acetylsalicylic acid (aspirin) or sodium salicylate can be prescribed safely for children in the low dosage of 0.04 gm per kg body weight per day (¼ grain per lb per day). When somewhat larger doses are given, such as 0.07 to 0.30 gm per kg per day, many of the patients will exhibit mild symptoms of salicylism in the form of lassitude, anorexia, tinnitus, or even hyperpnea. With greater intakes, or in occasional sensitive individuals given the above doses, the more profound disturbance known as salicylate intoxication may be produced with dehydration, vomiting, stupor, cyanosis, or convulsions. Increased rate and depth of breathing is a nearly constant feature at all stages. Vomiting, which may be persistent, will aggravate the electrolyte losses and interfere with the ingestion of carbohydrates.

Salicylates in large doses stimulate the respiratory center centrally. The ensuing hyperventilation leads to an undue excretion of CO_2 from the lungs, followed by a fall in the plasma CO_2 content. The bicarbonate reading in patients receiving moderate doses of salicylates often drops to less than 20 mEq per liter from pretreatment levels of 25 to 32 mEq and may fall below 15 mEq. There is, however, only a slight rise in the pH of the blood.

The extent of the depression of the plasma bicarbonate level in children receiving salicylates is proportional roughly to the total daily dosage. This is much more than can be explained by accumulation of the salicylate anion in the plasma, since with a large intake the salicylate level is only of the magnitude of 2 to 4 mEq per liter and subsides within a few hours after the ingestion is discontinued.

Homeostatic correction of the alkalosis induced by the respiratory loss of CO_2 is achieved by (1) rise in the plasma chloride from about 103 to about 120 mEq per liter, (2) excretion of bicarbonate into the urine which becomes alkaline, (3) a less pronounced and less consistent decline in the plasma sodium level amounting to 4 to 10 mEq per liter. These latter changes are effected by the kidney. If symptoms of tetany develop and pH studies show the blood to be alkaline, inhalations of CO_2 gas may give relief.

This compensated respiratory alkalosis is soon complicated by ketosis and metabolic acidosis. The ketosis is brought about in part by the infection for which the salicylate is being given therapeutically and in part by a toxic action of the salicylate ion itself on the liver and other organs with depletion of the glycogen reserves. A lowered plasma sodium level may contribute to the difficulties. The reaction of the urine changes to acid, and acetone becomes demonstrable. The pH of the blood shifts to acid and may fall to 7.30, 7.20, or even lower. The hyperventilation enhances also the loss of water through the lungs and thereby aggravates any tendency to dehydration and poor renal function which may already be present.

Mild salicylism is best treated by withdrawal of the drug and the giving of a liberal intake of fluids and sugar. Therapy of severe prostration and intoxication consists of (1) vigorous specific treatment of the underlying infection, (2) infusion of sodium lactate in the form of $M/6$ or stronger solutions to correct the acidosis, (3) administration of glucose, both in the venoclysis and by mouth if tolerated, in order to counteract the ketosis and the presumed injury to the liver, and (4) control of other untoward symptoms by symptomatic measures such as hydrotherapy for hyperpyrexia, sedation for convulsions, or oxygen for cyanosis or collapse. The sudden onset of prostration after ingestion of many aspirin tablets by a young child should be treated immediately with an intravenous injection of 1.4 per cent sodium bicarbonate in a 5 per cent glucose solution.

When a child accidentally ingests methyl salicylate, or one of many other hepatotoxic poisons, the signs and symptoms of extreme metabolic acidosis with a low blood pH develop promptly, along with hyperpnea and other disturbances similar to those described above. Signs of liver injury are also prominent. The stomach should be washed out if ingestion is recent, or a cathartic given if the child is seen too late for lavage to be useful. An intravenous injection of sodium bicarbonate is here preferable to one of sodium lactate which may not be metabolized promptly. Prothrombin deficiency if it appears in salicylism is corrected by vitamin K administration in large doses.

The urine of patients taking salicylates reacts with ferric chloride solution to yield a color resembling that of diacetic acid. A slightly positive reaction with Benedict's test solution for glucose may also be obtained. This combination of responses in salicylate intoxication may lead to the erroneous diagnosis of diabetic acidosis. Differentiation of the ferric chloride reaction is made by boiling the urine. The color produced by salicylates will not change, whereas that due to diacetic acid will disappear because the latter is volatile. Other tests for acetone and diacetic acid will also be negative. The glucose-like substance will not be fermented by yeast. The ferric chloride test may be applied to the examination of serum or cerebrospinal fluid in suspected cases.

EDEMA IN LIVER DISEASE

The pathogenesis of the edema which develops in patients with severe liver disease is still a mystery. Numerous mechanisms have been proposed, but none are fully accepted. Hypoalbuminemia or increased venous pressure may be contributory. Representative blood chemistry levels in advanced liver disease are sodium, 133 mEq per liter; chloride, 95 mEq; calcium, 4.2 mEq; potassium, 3 mEq; and phosphorus, 1.2 mEq. The fact that ascites is a not infrequent complication of severe liver diseases suggests that local disturbances in or about the liver may play a part. The ascitic fluid contains sodium, chloride, and other solutes in approximately the same proportions and osmotic tonicity as the interstitial fluid.

SHOCK

Tissue anoxia is a prime component of shock. Even though the oxygen content of the arterial blood is usually normal, the slowing of the circulation results in peripheral anoxemia and leads to an unusually low content of oxygen in the venous blood. The brain is highly susceptible to such anoxia, but the immediate survival of the patient is more contingent upon the degree of injury to the kidney and liver. Kidneys when subjected to prolonged anoxia may undergo distal tubular damage and give rise to the syndrome of toxic nephritis, once known as lower nephron nephrosis. The irreversible stage of shock with paralysis of the capillaries and fall in blood pressure has been ascribed to inability of the liver to destroy a vasopressor substance (ferritin).

From the clinical manifestations one can estimate with fair accuracy the contraction of blood volume. Clinical signs of shock are *mild* when the blood volume is reduced 15 to 20 per cent, *moderate* when 20 to 30 per cent is lost, and *severe* when 30 to 50 per cent is lost. Infusions of small amounts of blood, plasma, or a plasma substitute may cause a transitory improvement and a temporary rise in blood pressure, but the full volume of intravascular and interstitial fluid lost must be replaced for good recovery. A vigorous program of oral and parenteral fluid therapy is thus advisable. For the immediate therapy of mass casualties in major disasters the oral administration of a solution of sodium bicarbonate in hypotonic sodium chloride has been proposed.

The physiologic abnormalities in the shock syndrome are loss of blood volume, depression of metabolism, stagnation in the peripheral circulation, metabolic acidosis with a high blood lactic acid level, and decline in the oxygen content of venous blood. There may be hyperglycemia in the early acute phase, changing to hypoglycemia as the condition progresses. In so-called traumatic shock the fluid moves from the blood stream into the injured tissues, whereas in the hemorrhagic form a significant quantity of the blood itself is lost directly. Pallor, vasoconstriction, sweating, and vertigo appear when the total volume of circulating blood is reduced by 15 per cent or more. The systolic blood pressure may go up at the beginning and not decline until after 25 per cent of the circulating blood volume has been lost.

Traumatized tissues tend to swell as the consequence of local extravasation of fluid, which may be relatively enormous. The capillary permeability, however, is not generally increased. The infiltrating fluid contains chloride, sugar, nonprotein nitrogen, and total protein in approximately the same concentrations as in the plasma. The cells in the traumatized areas lose some potassium and take up excess sodium and water. This extensive focal edema can be so great as to dehydrate the remainder of the body. When the edema begins to be absorbed several days later, the circulatory mechanisms may have difficulty in coping with the sudden return of the water and electrolytes.

Depletion by natural routes aggravates the fluid loss in shock. The insensible respiratory loss continues and may be increased by hyperventilation which is a part of the reaction. There is usually some vomiting and diarrhea. Sweating is usually marked. Production of urine, on the other hand, is markedly diminished as the consequence of altered renal circulation. This blocks the renal regulation of plasma electrolyte levels.

Signs of metabolic acidosis often develop rapidly. These comprise an increase in the plasma levels of phosphate, chloride, and organic acids, particularly lactate; a compensatory fall in the bicarbonate level which is augmented by increased volume and depth of respirations; a fall in the pH of arterial blood to as low as pH 7.1 in severe shock; and relatively little change in the plasma levels of sodium, potassium, and calcium at first. Terminally the plasma potassium may be elevated.

Generally speaking, the hemoglobin and hematocrit readings go up in burns, crush wounds, or other injuries which bring about a transudation of plasma. The readings tend to be low after a direct hemorrhage or in traumatic lesions which have hemorrhage as a prominent feature, whether the loss of blood be external or into an injured site. Movement of interstitial fluid into the circulation after a hemorrhage may reduce the hematocrit readings, to be followed perhaps by another rise if death draws near.

STARVATION

Infants and children who subsist on grossly defective diets exhibit inconstant disturbances in the functions approachable by familiar laboratory tests. Analysis of their intakes usually reveals deficiencies in calories, animal proteins, calcium and other minerals, and assorted vitamins. The blood hemoglobin and red cell concentrations may not show much apparent lowering unless dietary iron is deficient though the total blood volume and the total amount of circulating hemoglobin may be decreased. Plasma concentrations of sodium and chloride may be reduced slightly. Blood nonprotein nitrogen levels remain within normal limits. The extracellular fluid volume as estimated indirectly may be either reduced or elevated. The total protein level tends to be diminished when the malnutrition is extreme, with a reduction in albumin and an increase in globulin. Such patients may not be edematous, but become so very rapidly when fluids are given intravenously. Starvation may advance to a stage from which recovery is impossible; failure of absorption from the gastrointestinal tract is believed to be an important mechanism here. Transfusions may be of some benefit.

Edema usually appears in kwashiorkor (p. 493). Affected children are usually 1 to 5 years of age. Associated features are retardation of growth, changes in the skin and hair, diarrhea, and morphologic changes in the liver and pancreas. Electrolyte studies indicate overhydration of both the extracellular tissues and the cells. There may be slight lowering of the plasma levels for sodium and chloride but no significant change in potassium. Many of the children do not have much depression of their plasma proteins. When there is a low protein level there may be cachexia rather than edema. Some of the children appear superficially to be in good nutrition with liberal deposits of body fat. Damage to the liver, often irreversible and resulting from inadequate intake of protein and calories, appears to be a major intermediate mechanism. Increased capillary permeability, intestinal parasitism, and respiratory tract or other infections can be contributory factors. The poorer the antecedent diet, the less pronounced these infections have to be to precipitate acute symptoms.

Recovery from starvation under feeding therapy may take many weeks. The total plasma protein content returns quickly to normal levels, with the gamma globulin fraction unusually high and the albumin fraction somewhat subnormal.

TUBERCULOUS MENINGITIS

Through mechanisms which are still obscure, patients with florid tuberculous meningitis tend to have lowered levels of plasma sodium and chloride, elevated or normal levels for plasma bicarbonate, and normal levels of potassium, urea nitrogen, and total protein. The serum calcium and serum phosphorus may be in the low normal range. Determinations with Evans blue, thiocyanate, and antipyrine as indices of plasma volume, extracellular fluid volume, and total body water, respectively, have been made in several such patients with low serum sodium and have not uncovered significant alterations in the size of these compartments. Typical plasma values are 125 mEq per liter of sodium and 92 mEq of chloride. These changes may not be alleviated by a good intake of liquid food or infusions of sodium chloride. When the tuberculous meningitis subsides under treatment, these levels return to normal.

During the period of active meningitis the glomerular function is essentially undisturbed, but tubular regulation of sodium and chloride becomes impaired. Excretion of both sodium and chloride into the urine is excessive. Responses to test loads of electrolytes are not as efficient as in the normal child.

BIBLIOGRAPHY

CONGESTIVE CIRCULATORY FAILURE

Baumann, D. P., Electrolyte Disturbances in Congestive Heart Failure, *Am. J. Clin. Path.* **22**:616, 1952.

Bryant, J. M., V. Iob, G. L. Phillips, and *E. E. Blecha,* Estimation of Urinary Sodium: A Simple Test for Patients on Low Sodium Diets, *J.A.M.A.* **140**:670, 1949.

Mokotoff, R., G. Ross, and *L. Leiter,* Renal Plasma Flow and Sodium Reabsorption and Excretion in Congestive Heart Failure, *J. Clin. Invest.* **27**:1, 1948.

Stapleton, J. F., and *W. P. Harvey,* Hypochloremic Alkalosis Induced by Mercurial Diuretics in Congestive Heart Failure, *A.M.A. Arch. Int. Med.* **90**:425, 1952.

Talso, P. J., N. Spofford, and *M. Blaw,* The Metabolism of Water and Electrolytes in Congestive Heart Failure. I. The Electrolyte and Water Content of Normal Human Skeletal Muscle, *J. Lab. & Clin. Med.* **41**:281, 1953.

CYSTIC FIBROSIS OF THE PANCREAS

Barbero, G. J., J. MacGavran, and *I. C. Kim,* A Simplified Technique for the Sweat Test in the Diagnosis of Cystic Fibrosis of the Pancreas, *Pediatrics* **18**:189, 1956.

Di Sant'Agnese, P. A., R. C. Darling, G. A. Perera, and *E. Shea,* Abnormal Electrolyte Composition of Sweat in Cystic Fibrosis of the Pancreas, *Pediatrics* **12**:549, 1953.

Schwachman, H., and *H. Leubner,* Mucoviscidosis, *Advances Pediat.* **7**:249, 1955.

———— and *N. Gahm,* Studies in Cystic Fibrosis of the Pancreas: A Simple Test for the Detection of Excessive Chloride on the Skin, *New England J. Med.* **255**:999, 1956.

DIABETIC ACIDOSIS

Darrow, D. C., and *E. L. Pratt,* Retention of Water and Electrolyte during Recovery in a Patient with Diabetic Acidosis, *J. Pediat.* **41**:688, 1952.

Sprague, R. G., and *M. H. Power,* Electrolyte Metabolism in Diabetic Acidosis, *J.A.M.A.* **151**:970, 1953.

INFANTILE GASTROENTERITIS

Calcagno, P. L., and *M. I. Rubin,* Effect of Dehydration Produced by Water Deprivation, Diarrhea and Vomiting on Renal Function in Infants, *Pediatrics* **7**:328, 1951.

Cheek, D. B., Changes in Total Chloride and Acid-Base Balance in Gastroenteritis Following Treatment with Large and Small Loads of Sodium Chloride, *Pediatrics* **17**:839, 1956.

Darrow, D. C., E. L. Pratt, J. Flett, Jr., A. H. Gamble, and *H. F. Wiese,* Disturbances of Water and Electrolytes in Infantile Diarrhea, *Pediatrics* **3**:129, 1949.

Etteldorf, J. N., F. S. Hill, A. H. Tuttle, D. Pinheiro, A. C. Bass, and *R. R. Overman,* Alterations in Blood Chemistry Caused by Diarrhea during Infancy as Determined by Direct Analysis of Plasma and Erythrocytes, *Pediatrics* **10**:694, 1952.

Friedman, A., Experiences in Two Hundred Eighty-nine Cases of Infantile Diarrhea in a Nutritionally Deficient Group of Infants, *A.M.A. Am. J. Dis. Child.* **85**:675, 1953.

Mann, N. M., S. Ross, and *W. H. Patterson,* Gastro-enteritis in Infancy: An Account of 286 Cases Treated in a General Paediatric Hospital, *Arch. Dis. Childhood* **27**:457, 1952.

Tarail, R., L. W. Bass, and *A. S. Runco,* The Frequency and Nature of Hypertonicity of the Body Fluids in Infantile Diarrhea, *A.M.A. Am. J. Dis. Child.* 86:658, 1954.

SHOCK

Danowski, T. S., A. W. Winkler, and *J. R. Elkinton,* The Treatment of Shock Due to Salt Depletion: Comparison of the Hemodynamic Effects of Isotonic Saline, of Hypertonic Saline, and of Isotonic Glucose Solutions, *J. Clin. Invest.* 25:130, 1946.

Frank, H. A., Present Day Concepts of Shock, *New England J. Med.* 249:445, 1953.

Randall, H. T., The Shifts of Fluid and Electrolyte in Shock, *Ann. New York Acad. Med.* 55:412, 1952.

STARVATION

Gollan, F., Blood and Extracellular Fluid Studies in Chronic Malnutrition in Infancy, *J. Clin. Invest.* 27:352, 1948.

Gómez, F., R. Ramos Galván, J. Cravioto, and *S. Frenk,* Malnutrition in Infancy and Childhood, with Special Reference to Kwashiorkor, *Advances Pediat.* 7:131, 1955.

Venkatchalam, P. S., S. G. Srikantia, and *C. Gopalan,* Nutritional Oedema in Children, *Indian J. Pediat.* 19:165, 1952.

TUBERCULOUS MENINGITIS

Harrison, H. E., L. Finberg, and *E. Fleishman,* Disturbances of Ionic Equilibrium of Intracellular and Extracellular Electrolytes in Patients with Tuberculous Meningitis, *J. Clin. Invest.* 31:300, 1952.

Rapoport, S., C. D. West, and *W. A. Brodsky,* Salt Losing Conditions: The Renal Defect in Tuberculous Meningitis, *J. Lab. & Clin. Med.* 37:550, 1951.

SALICYLATE INTOXICATION

Harvie, F. H., and *R. B. Singer,* Salicylate Poisoning, *A.M.A. Am. J. Dis. Child.* 89:149, 1955.

Riley, H. D., Jr., and *L. Worley,* Salicylate Intoxication, *Pediatrics,* 18:578, 1956.

Singer, R. B., The Acid-Base Disturbance in Salicylate Intoxication, *Medicine* 33:1, 1954.

Wallace, W. M., The Use of Salicylates in Pediatrics, *Quart. Rev. Pediat.* 9:135, 1954.

MISCELLANEOUS

Cheek, D. B., Pink Disease (Infantile Acrodynia): A Physiological Approach (An Evaluation of Adrenal Function and the Importance of Water and Electrolyte Metabolism), *J. Pediat.* 42:239, 1953.

Dodd, K., G. J. Buddingh, and *S. Rapoport,* The Etiology of Ekiri, A Highly Fatal Disease of Japanese Children, *Pediatrics* 3:9, 1949.

Lightwood, R., W. W. Payne, and *J. A. Black,* Infantile Renal Acidosis, *Pediatrics* 12:628, 1953.

Lockwood, J. S., and *H. T. Randall,* The Place of Electrolyte Studies in Surgical Patients, *Bull. New York Acad. Med.* 25:228, 1949.

Spector, S., and *V. V. Startzman,* Respiratory Acidosis and Alkalosis in Infants with Acute Pulmonary Infections, *Am. Pract.* 3:744, 1949.

CHAPTER 58

Vitamins and Their Blood Levels

DETECTION OF SUBCLINICAL VITAMIN-DEFICIENCY STATES

When a partial or occult vitamin deficiency is suspected, the physician tends to turn to assessment of pertinent biochemical variables. Retrospective surveys of dietary intake in minor disturbances may be highly misleading, and physiologic phenomena such as cardiovascular or ophthalmologic responses are subject to too many extraneous influences. As has been emphasized by Thomson and Duncan, specific deficiencies referable to inadequate food intakes are ordinarily not recognizable before the appearance of physical signs; the early manifestations of malnutrition are nonspecific.

Regrettably, most of the analytic methods for detection of the hypovitaminoses are too complicated for evaluation of individual patients. Of those few that are available, such as measurements of serum calcium, iron, vitamin A, or the water-soluble vitamins, either the physiologic interrelations are far from simple or chemical changes do not appear until signs and symptoms are pronounced. For example, the urinary excretion of a water-soluble vitamin may relate more or less directly to the current intake but does not necessarily portray the quantitative status of that vitamin inside the tissue cells. If the intake is low on the day of the test, the output may be low, whether the tissue stores are adequate or depleted. Blood levels usually give unsatisfactory information regarding tissue reserves, and normal individual differences in blood concentrations are extremely wide. Determining the intracellular concentration of vitamins by direct analysis of biopsy specimens is impractical. Circulating leukocytes are sometimes analyzed for vitamin C concentration, on the thesis that their content of this vitamin is representative of the body tissues generally.

The total mass of body tissues is conceived to be "saturated" with an essential nutrient when further amounts cannot be stored. "Unsaturation" may be tested for by giving a large or "loading" dose of the nutrient and noting the changes which take place in the blood and urine. Rises in blood levels or urinary signs of undue retention are taken to signify that

651

the body stores are in a depleted state. Deviations from this rule are numerous. For example, the giving of a large test dose of a nutrient after a prolonged period of deprivation may raise the blood and urine levels in the absence of adequate tissue utilization or reversal of the physiologic disturbance. Excessive tissue breakdown from starvation or other causes in a depleted patient may lead to the excretion of nutrients or their derivatives in amounts compatible with a state of saturation. Certain diseases may give rise to blood chemistry changes resembling those produced by faulty food intake. The chemical methods of analysis which measure thiamine alone give much lower values than those based on yeast fermentation which determine also the pyrimidines which are metabolic derivatives of thiamine.

The vitamin-deficiency states which are at least potentially subject to evaluation by laboratory approaches without too highly complicated procedures include deficiencies of thiamine, riboflavin, and niacin in the B complex, vitamin A, vitamin C, vitamin E, and vitamin K (Chap. 22).

THIAMINE

Thiamine (vitamin B_1) plays an active role within most if not all of the body cells. It appears to be a coenzyme catalyst in the metabolism of carbohydrate, and particularly in the breakdown of pyruvic acid. Mild states of deficiency may be encountered in starvation, gastrointestinal disorders, diabetes mellitus, alcoholism, hyperthyroidism, and polyneuritis of various types. Beri-beri is a manifestation of extreme deficiency.

Among the approaches which have been suggested for detection of subclinical nutritional deficiency with respect to thiamine are 24-hour urinary excretion; 4-hour urinary output after a large test dose; direct measurement of thiamine in whole blood, leukocytes, erythrocytes, or muscle tissue; cocarboxylase level of whole blood; and determination of either blood pyruvic acid content or the ratio of pyruvate to lactate. A recently proposed carbohydrate metabolism index (CMI) is calculated from the blood concentrations of glucose, pyruvic acid, and lactic acid; in thiamine deficiency the CMI index becomes unusually high after glucose is given and mild exercise taken.

The urinary excretion of thiamine drops considerably in deficiency states, but there is no close correlation between the extent of the deficiency and the quantity excreted. A daily output of less than 100 μgm per day (determined by chemical assay) has been suggested as indicative of a deficiency in adults. The range for thiamine in the whole blood of children on a good diet, according to studies of Waisman and associates with a modified thiochrome method, is approximately 5 to 17 μgm per 100 ml, with the average at about 10 μgm per 100 ml.

The recommended dietary allowance of thiamine is approximately 0.5 mg per 1,000 calories of intake per day. Holt and associates, by employing the "point of minimal excretion technique," have noted that an intake of 0.2 mg a day seems to meet the presumed basal excretion of thiamine.

RIBOFLAVIN (VITAMIN B₂)

This vitamin is an important constituent of the intracellular oxidation-reduction and other enzyme systems. Since milk which is a rich source is widely used in the United States, deficiency states in infants and children are almost never seen here. It is possible also that riboflavin is synthesized by the bacteria of the colon. Presumptive physical signs of deficiency are corneal vascularization, seborrhea, glossitis, chelosis, angular fissures, and general weakness. Biologic and fluorometric procedures are available for assay of body fluids.

The urinary excretion is related both to the dietary intake and the body size. In the average adult the daily output remains negligible unless the daily intake exceeds 1.1 mg. Loading urinary tests are frequently used for appraisal of possible riboflavin subnutrition; disagreement attends the size of dose to be given and the interpretation of the response.

The riboflavin content of whole blood is approximately 50 μgm per 100 ml. This may or may not be diminished in deficiency states. The recommended dietary allowances range from 0.6 mg daily for infants up to 2.5 mg for adolescent boys and 2.0 for adolescent girls.

NIACIN

The intracellular metabolism of niacin is bound up with that of protein and particularly tryptophane, since this amino acid is a precursor of niacin. The appraisal of nutritional status with respect to niacin by analytic methods is involved and far from satisfactory. The excretory products consist chiefly of N^1-methyl derivatives—not accurately measurable by routine methods—along with niacinamide, nicotinic acid, nicotinuric acid, and other derivatives. The allowances recommended for niacin have been set empirically at ten times those for thiamine.

VITAMIN B₆

Three closely related chemical substances comprise this vitamin: pyridoxine, pyridoxal, and pyridoxamine. It is now clear that a deficiency in vitamin B_6 can occur in infants under special circumstances and give rise to a syndrome of hyperirritability and convulsive seizures. Simple laboratory tests are not available for recognition of the deficiency state. An elevated level of protein in the cerebrospinal fluid, of the magnitude of 50 to 100 mg per 100 ml, is not uncommon in infants with deficiency severe enough to induce convulsions. Their serum calcium and phosphorus levels fall in the normal range, and anemia is not apparent.

The data of Coursin and others indicate that human milk contains approximately 100 μgm and fresh cow's milk approximately 500 μgm per liter. Current processes of commercial evaporation reduce the concentration of this vitamin moderately: higher temperatures (above 247°F) or more protracted heat treatment are dangerously destructive.

Present information, admittedly incomplete, suggests that 100 μgm daily is an adequate daily intake for infants, whereas 50 μgm daily is insufficient. For normal adults an intake of 2 mg (2,000 μgm) seems to meet the nutritional requirements very satisfactorily.

VITAMIN A

Much remains to be learned about the role of this unsaturated cyclic alcohol in the body economy, but from the fact that it circulates continually in all well-nourished individuals one must infer that it is needed metabolically. Prolonged shortages results in keratinization of the ciliated epithelium in the internal organs, with secondary susceptibility to local bacterial invasion. Xerophthalmia and cessation of growth are signs of extreme deficiency. Vitamin A enters into the formation of rhodopsin, the visual pigment. Psychologic tests for evaluating the adaptability of individuals to light are available, but complicating subjective factors make these appraisals subject to much question.

Vitamin A concentrations may be expressed as *international units* or as micrograms. One international unit is equivalent to 0.34 μgm of the alcohol. The recommended allowances increase from 1,500 IU daily for infants up to 5,000 IU daily for adolescent boys and girls.

Good dietary sources of vitamin A are butter, egg yolk, fortified margarine, fish-liver oils, and the milk of cows and humans. Many vegetables are rich in carotene and in provitamin A, which is converted to the vitamin itself in the liver after absorption. The liver serves also as a reservoir for the maintenance of the plasma level and will slowly destroy excessive amounts when taken.

The oily concentrates of vitamin A as a rule have refined fish-liver oil as the vehicle or menstruum. The water-soluble dispersions contain vitamin A combined chemically with either an alcohol or fatty acids, suspended in propylene glycol or glycerin or some similar medium with the aid of solubilizer agents; the extremely fine diameter of the individual particles promotes their direct absorption through the intestinal mucosa without the aid of lipase.

Normal Serum Levels

The mean values in groups of Michigan children 2 to 8 years old studied by Robinson and associates with the Bessey and Lowry microchemical technique ranged from 30 to 42 μgm per 100 ml. Individual readings varied from 0 to 140 μgm. Most well-fed healthy infants and children have serum levels above 40 μgm, which is the same as the adult levels.

On the first day of life the values are ordinarily 20 to 30 μgm per 100 ml. Lewis found a sharp drop during the first 48 hours, with a return to normal by the fourth day.

In single individuals the serum vitamin A content tends to remain at an approximately constant level. An enormous intake is needed to raise the fasting level permanently.

Hypovitaminosis A

A low serum level (less than 20 μgm per 100 ml) may be due to a low intake, to scanty reserve stores, or to some disease which interferes with vitamin A metabolism. Clinical signs of avitaminosis A do not become manifest until after the blood level has remained subnormal for several months.

Children with the celiac syndrome tend to have subnormal serum levels except when supplementary vitamin A is given in large amounts, preferably in the water-soluble form. Unless this precaution is taken the tissue changes of vitamin A deficiency may ultimately become manifest.

Hypervitaminosis A

Ingestion of excessive amounts of vitamin A by infants and children can lead to anorexia, loss of weight, pallor, weakness, fretfulness, hepatomegaly, low-grade fever, tender swelling of the limbs, and dry lips and skin. The alkaline phosphatase and total lipids of the serum may be moderately elevated. A mild anemia may be present. The blood sedimentation rate is sometimes increased. Roentgenologically one may find bone thickenings and hyperostoses in the ribs, clavicles, or long bones. When a patient exhibits these phenomena one usually can elicit a history of excessive intake of vitamin A over many months, such as a concentrate taken by the teaspoonful rather than by the drop, perhaps with a high intake of butter or fortified oleomargarine as well.

Serum levels in chronic hypervitaminosis A range from 100 to 800 μgm per 100 ml. Data are not available as to the length of time the levels must remain elevated before symptoms begin. Once the excessive ingestion is stopped, several weeks are required for return to normal.

The rarity of hypervitaminosis A despite the possibilities for overdosage inherent in the wide use of the concentrates suggests that individual susceptibility is a contributory factor.

Vitamin A Tolerance Test

Fat-soluble preparations of vitamin A may be used diagnostically for study of patients suspected of having defective intestinal absorption of fat.

After a 24-hour period in which no vitamin A concentrates are taken, the fasting serum level of vitamin A is determined. A test dose of 5,000 or 10,000

USP units of oily vitamin A per kg of body weight is given, and serial readings taken at 3-, 5-, and 8-hour intervals thereafter. Additional readings are advisable at 12 or 24 hours if absorption is expected to be slow. A regular diet may be taken during the test period except that foods rich in vitamin A are omitted. It is important for each laboratory to establish its own set of normal curves for a uniform test dose.

With normal children having good fat absorption the serum vitamin A reaches a maximum in 3 to 5 hours after the test dose is taken and returns to the initial fasting value within 8 hours. The peak usually falls between 300 and 450 μgm per 100 ml (1,000 to 1,500 units). In children with the celiac syndrome the test dose of oil brings a rise of only a few units above the initial fasting level, and this itself will be abnormally low if the disturbance has not been treated previously.

Children with cystic fibrosis of the pancreas can absorb appreciable amounts of the water-soluble forms of vitamin A, whether ester or alcohol, whereas children with true celiac disease usually cannot. For example, a child with pancreatic fibrosis and a fasting serum level of 10 μgm per 100 ml of vitamin A may exhibit a moderate rise in the vitamin A tolerance test, whereas the same dose in oil will be followed by practically no rise. In contrast, a child with true celiac disease and a low fasting serum level will exhibit little change with either preparation. The giving of pancreatin along with vitamin A in oil will induce a marked rise in serum vitamin A in cystic fibrosis of the pancreas, but not in true celiac disease (Gibbs).

In newborn and young infants the absorption of large doses of vitamin A in oil is less efficient than that of aqueous dispersions, as shown by tolerance tests.

Vitamin A Metabolism

Popper and associates have reported that the ester form of vitamin A is transported from the intestine to the liver to be stored there as such. After release from the liver, however, the alcohol form normally represents about 80 per cent of the total plasma vitamin A. The rise in total serum vitamin A which follows the ingestion of a large test dose, whether in an oily menstruum or an aqueous dispersion, is confined entirely to the ester fraction.

The serum vitamin A level ordinarily does not fall (1) unless some disease interferes with regulatory hepatic mechanisms or (2) unless the hepatic reserves become exhausted after weeks or months of insufficient absorption of vitamin A and its precursor carotene, as in prolonged severe starvation or steatorrhea. Since low levels are not uncommon in liver diseases and tend to fluctuate with the severity of the disturbance, serial determinations can be indicators of hepatic function.

Moderate depression of the fasting level occurs during most febrile illness such as upper respiratory tract infections, pneumonia, and exacerbations of rheumatic fever. In progressive and ultimately fatal infections the levels may be unusually low, despite an ample content in the liver at autopsy. Fever induced by physical means may depress the level for 12 hours or longer.

CAROTENE

The carotenes or carotenoids are red, yellow, and orange hydrocarbon pigments which occur in vegetables, fruits, flowers, and egg yolks. These pigments are referred to collectively as carotene. Carrots, squash, and oranges are rich sources. Most green vegetables, and especially spinach and kale, also contain carotene, though the color is masked by the chlorophyll and other pigments present.

Carotene is the metabolic precursor of vitamin A. Its conversion to vitamin A is believed to take place in the intestinal wall and in the liver and may be impaired in liver disease. Absorption of carotene from the human intestine is facilitated by diets high in fat and diminished or absent in liver or bile duct diseases in which bile is not liberated into the intestine. Within the liver the transformation of carotene into vitamin A appears to be effected by the enzyme carotenase and is accelerated by thyroxin.

Normal Levels

Serum levels are far from uniform and drop rapidly when the diet is carotene-free for as brief a period as 1 week. The usual range for fasting serum carotene during childhood is 60 to 180 μgm per 100 ml as a rule, but may extend from 50 to 300 μgm. The level in the infant at birth is usually about 25 μgm per 100 ml.

Carotenemia (Hypercarotenemia)

Excessively high blood levels of serum carotene, when continuing for some weeks, will impart a golden-yellow color to the skin. Such "carotenosis" or xanthosis cutis, the external manifestation of carotenemia, is not uncommon in some infants who have a high intake of carrots, squash, and other vegetables; an individual peculiarity has been hypothesized. The pigment is deposited most abundantly where the epithelial keratinization is thickest, as in the palms and soles and along the margins of the alae nasae. Carotenemia sometimes appears in hypothyroidism, the nephrotic syndrome, and other disturbances associated with hyperlipemia.

Serum levels up to 800 μgm per 100 ml have been encountered during carotenemia. A transitory mild increase in serum lipids may be associated. The serum level of vitamin A is not elevated. When carotene-rich foods are removed from the diet the yellow staining of the skin subsides over a period of weeks but the serum levels may take 6 months or more to revert to normal. No symptoms of illness are known to be associated with unusually high serum levels. The propensity to carotenemia in otherwise well infants tends to disappear during childhood.

ASCORBIC ACID (VITAMIN C)

Vitamin C is a water-soluble and easily oxidized dietary essential which occurs in significant amounts in raw milk, raw fruits, raw vegetables, citrus fruits, and tomatoes. It enters into many intracellular reactions, is an important constituent of the adrenal cortex, and is essential to the proper formation and maintenance of supporting tissues of mesenchymal origin (connective tissue, bone, dentin, cartilage). Since it is not synthesized or stored by any of the tissues it must be provided regularly by the food intake. Diets low in ascorbic acid and folic acid or the citrovorum factor result in a megaloblastic type of anemia.

The body need for ascorbic acid is proportional to body mass. Exercise, febrile illnesses, and all other conditions which enhance tissue metabolism increase the requirements. The recommended intakes range from 30 mg daily for infants up to 80 mg daily for adolescent girls and 90 to 100 mg daily for adolescent boys. Nutritional surveys in all parts of the world have indicated that in most populations the mean intakes of ascorbic acid do not meet these recommendations.

Premature infants require a more liberal supply (approximately 100 mg a day). Otherwise their internal metabolism of phenylalanine and tyrosine is imperfect and intermediary products are lost in the urine.

Generally speaking, when a child's dietary intake of ascorbic acid is below 20 mg a day the fasting plasma level will vary from 0 to 0.2 mg per 100 ml; with a 30- to 50-mg daily intake, 0.2 to 0.6 mg per 100 ml; with a 60- to 100-mg intake, 0.5 to 0.8 mg per 100 ml; with more than 100 mg, up to 1.5 mg per 100 ml. Plasma contents above 1.5 mg per 100 ml are exceptional, inasmuch as ascorbic acid is excreted into the urine by a threshold mechanism at this level.

Infants with the bleeding gums, bone rarefaction, and subperiosteal hemorrhages of frank scurvy typically have plasma levels between 0 and 0.3 per 100 mg. When ascorbic acid in large quantities is given to such infants there is usually a lag of several days before the serum content exhibits any appreciable rise. This is interpreted as signifying that the tissues are in a state of "unsaturation." Only after the deficit has been met does the blood level begin to go up.

Individuals without frank scurvy but on an inadequate diet tend to have low plasma ascorbic acid. For example, in a survey of 868 poorly nourished residents of Newfoundland carried out by Adamson and associates in 1945, the level was less than 0.2 mg per 100 ml in 28 per cent and less than 0.4 mg in 59 per cent.

Controversy still attends the importance of the ascorbic acid level in the fasting plasma as an indicator of nutritional status. Day-to-day readings on single individuals on a fixed intake may show fluctuations of 0.2 to 0.4 mg per 100 ml. Hence a single plasma determination is less accurate as a measure of the state of vitamin C storage than are several repeated determinations.

In depletion states the leukocytes and platelets retain appreciable ascorbic acid for a considerable time after the vitamin has disappeared from the plasma. Lowry, Bessey, and associates found that serum levels of 0.4 mg per 100 ml or higher were associated with concentrations in the leukocytes of more than 20 mg per 100 ml, whereas levels under 0.3 mg were associated with leukocyte concentrations of less than 20 mg.

The urine ordinarily contains little or no ascorbic acid except when the plasma contains well above 1.0 mg per 100 ml or when large amounts of the vitamin are being taken in single doses. The ascorbic acid content of cord blood ranges from 0.6 to 2.2 mg per 100 ml, whereas mothers' blood at the time of birth contains only one-half to two-thirds of this amount. This suggests that prenatal physiologic processes require greater tissue saturation of the vitamin than in extrauterine existence. The blood levels in the first days of life fall to the same range as in older infants, and considerable ascorbic acid appears in the urine.

A number of "loading" tests have been proposed for evaluating the ascorbic acid needs and state of deficiency if present. A single large dose is given and measurements made of the changes which follow in the blood or urine content within a fixed period of time. The standards for evaluation are constructed from the responses of normal individuals. Details and dosages vary with the individual procedures.

VITAMIN E

Three separate but closely related fat-soluble groups of substances—the alpha, beta, and gamma tocopherols—possess similar biologic activities and are referred to collectively as *vitamin E.*

The requirements of the human being for vitamin E are unknown. Large doses can be administered without production of any major symptoms.

The tocopherols have marked antioxidant activity. Vitamin A and carotene, readily oxidized in the presence of unsaturated fats, seem to derive some protection within the body from the tocopherols. In experiments with dystrophic animal muscle tissue the respiratory reactions can be markedly altered by the addition of vitamin E.

The serum tocopherol level in the normal adult is approximately 1 mg per 100 ml. Newborn infants on the first or second day, before receiving any supplementary tocopherol through feedings, have serum levels which may vary from 0.02 to 0.6 mg per 100 mg but are usually between 0.1 and 0.4 mg per 100 ml. There are wide variations in both term and premature infants regardless of birth weight. The serum tocopherols in breast-fed infants increase much more rapidly than in bottle-fed infants and reach a mean value of approximately 1.5 mg per 100 ml by the end of the first week. Breast milk is richer in tocopherol than cow's milk.

Rose and Gyorgy noted that newborn infants' red blood cells are more readily hemolyzed by H_2O_2 than red blood cells of older infants or of any other age group. Vitamin E will prevent this phenomenon when added in vitro to blood or to washed blood cells (suspended in saline solution) or when given to the newborn infant by mouth.

Filer and associates reported that when oral doses of tocopherol or of tocopherol esters are given in doses of 20 mg per kg of body weight, and serum tocopherol (vitamin E) levels determined every 3 hours over a 12-hour period, the resulting data when plotted yield a "tolerance curve" with a maximum at 9 hours. Premature infants were found to absorb vitamin E as well as full-term infants, in contrast to their diminished ability to utilize vitamin A and fats.

BIBLIOGRAPHY

NUTRITION

Bourne, G. H., and G. W. Kidder (eds.), "Biochemistry and Physiology of Nutrition," vols. 1 and 2, Academic Press, Inc., New York, 1953.

Clements, F. W., "Infant Nutrition: Its Physiological Basis," John Wright, Bristol (England), 1949.

Elvehjem, C. A., Mineral Nutrition: The Role of Trace Elements, Food Technol. 8:531, 1954.

Nutrition Surveys: Their Techniques and Value, Bull. Nat. Res. Council 117, Washington, D.C., May, 1949.

Pollack, H., and S. L. Halpern, Therapeutic Nutrition, Nat. Acad. Sc., Nat. Res. Council, Publ. 234, 1952.

"Present Knowledge in Nutrition," The Nutrition Foundation, Inc., New York, 1953.

Recommended Dietary Allowances: A Report of the Food and Nutrition Board, Nat. Acad. Sc., Nat. Res. Council, Publ. 302, rev. 1953.

Spies, T. D., Recent Advances in Diagnosis and Treatment of Deficiency Diseases, J.A.M.A. 145:66, 1951.

Thomson, A. M., and D. L. Duncan, The Diagnosis of Malnutrition in Man, Nutrition Abstr. & Rev. 24:1, 1954.

Waisman, H. A., J. B. Richmond, and S. J. Williams, Vitamin Requirements in Adolescence, J. Pediat. 37:922, 1950.

VITAMIN B COMPLEX

Benson, R. A., C. M. Witzberger, and L. B. Slobody, An Evaluation of Blood and Urinary Thiamine Determinations in Vitamin B₁ Sub-nutrition, J. Pediat. 23:437, 1943.

Coryell, M. N., M. M. Rutledge, M. C. Drummond, F. Meyer, F. Mead, and *E. F. Beach,* Nutritional Status of Children. XIV. Urinary Excretions of Thiamine and Riboflavin, *J. Am. Dietet. A.* **26**:979, 1950.

Holt, L. E., Jr., and *V. A. Najjar,* A Simple Method for the Laboratory Diagnosis of Subclinical Deficiencies of Thiamin, Riboflavin and Nicotinic Acid, *Bull. Johns Hopkins Hosp.* **70**:329, 1942.

Waisman, H. A., T. S. Cho, J. B. Richmond, and *S. J. Williams,* Blood Level of Thiamine in Normal Children, *A.M.A. Am. J. Dis. Child.* **82**:535, 1951.

VITAMIN B₆

Coursin, D. B., Vitamin B₆ (Pyridoxine) in Milk, *Quart. Rev. Pediat.* **10**:2, 1955.

Filer, L. J., Jr. (ed.), Vitamin B₆ in Human Nutrition: Report of the Tenth M & R Pediatric Research Conference, M & R Laboratories, Columbus 16, Ohio, 1954.

Hunt, A. D., Jr., J. Stokes, Jr., W. W. McCrory, and *H. H. Stroud,* Pyridoxine Dependency: Report of a Case of Intractable Convulsions in an Infant Controlled by Pyridoxine, *Pediatrics* **13**:140–145, 1954.

Snyderman, S. E., L. E. Holt, Jr., R. Carretero, and *K. Jacobs,* Pyridoxine Deficiency in the Human Infant, *J. Clin. Nutrition* **1**:200, 1953.

Vilter, R. W., J. F. Mueller, H. S. Glazer, T. Jarrold, J. Abraham, C. Thompson, and *V. R. Hawkins,* The Effect of Vitamin B₆ Deficiency Induced by Desoxypyridoxine in Human Beings, *J. Lab. & Clin. Med.* **42**:335, 1953.

VITAMIN A AND CAROTENE

Adlersberg, D., S. Kann, A. P. Maurer, K. Newerly, W. Winternitz, and *H. Sobotka,* Studies on Serum Carotene in Man, *Am. J. Digest. Dis.* **16**:333, 1949.

Caffey, J., Chronic Poisoning Due to Excess of Vitamin A: Description of the Clinical and Roentgen Manifestations in Seven Infants and Young Children, *Am. J. Roentgenol.* **65**:12, 1951.

Castellanos, A., Disturbances of Carotene Metabolism in Childhood (Perturbaciones del metabolismo de las carotinas en el niño), *Rev. cubana pediat.* **20**:377, 1948.

Gibbs, G. E., Effect of Pancreatin on Plasma Vitamin A Curves in the Celiac Syndrome, *Pediatrics* **6**:593, 1950.

Josephs, H. W., Hypervitaminosis A and Carotenemia, *Am. J. Dis. Child.* **67**:33, 1944.

——, The Carotenemia of Hypothyroidism, *J. Pediat.* **41**:784, 1952.

Kagan, B. M., D. A. Jordan, and *P. S. Gerald,* Absorption of Aqueous Dispersions of Vitamin A Alcohol and Vitamin A Ester in Normal Children, *J. Nutrition* **40**:275, 1950.

Lewis, J. M., O. Bodansky, J. Birmingham, and *S. Q. Cohlan,* Comparative Absorption, Excretion and Storage of Oily and Aqueous Preparations of Vitamin A, *J. Pediat.* **31**:496, 1947.

——, ——, and *L. M. Shapiro,* Regulation of Level of Vitamin A in Blood of Newborn Infants, *Am. J. Dis. Child.* **66**:503, 1943.

——, *S. Q. Cohlan,* and *A. Messina,* Further Observations on the Absorption of Vitamin A: Influence of the Particle Size of the Vehicle on the Absorption of Vitamin A, *Pediatrics* **5**:425, 1950.

May, C. D., and *C. U. Lowe,* The Absorption of Orally Administered Emulsified Lipid in Normal Children and in Children with Steatorrhea, *J. Clin. Invest.* **27**:226, 1948.

McCoord, A. B., C. P. Katsampes, C. G. Lavender, F. J. Martin, R. A. Ulstrom, R. H. Tully, III, and *A. J. Keenan,* The Absorption of Oily and Aqueous Preparations of Ester and Alcohol Vitamin A by Normal Children and Children with Various Diseases, *Pediatrics* **2**:652, 1948.

Popper, H., F. Steigmann, A. Dubin, H. A. Dyniewicz, and *F. P. Hesser,* Significance of Vitamin A Alcohol and Ester Partitioning under Normal and Pathologic Circumstances, *Proc. Soc. Exper. Biol. & Med.* 68:676, 1948.

Robinson, A., M. Lesher, A. P. Harrison, E. Z. Moyer, M. C. Gresock, and C. Saunders, Nutritional Status of Children. VI. Blood Serum Vitamin A and Carotenoids, *J. Am. Dietetic A.* 24:410, 1948.

Ryersbach, G. C., J. Hanelin, and R. J. Joplin, Vitamin A Intoxication, *New England J. Med.* 246:978, 1952.

Sobel, A. E., L. Besman, and B. Kramer, Vitamin A Absorption in the Newborn, *Am. J. Dis. Child.* 77:576, 1949.

Wang, P., H. L. Glass, L. Goldenberg, G. Stearns, H. G. Kelly, and R. L. Jackson, Serum Vitamin A and Carotene Levels in Children with Rheumatic Fever, *A.M.A. Am. J. Dis. Child.* 87:659, 1954.

Wyatt, T. C., C. A. Carabello, and M. E. Fletcher, Hypervitaminosis A: Report of a Case, *J.A.M.A.* 144:304, 1950.

ASCORBIC ACID

Adamson, J. D., N. Jolliffe, H. D. Kruse, O. H. Lowry, P. E. Moore, B. S. Platt, W. H. Selrell, J. W. Tice, F. F. Tisdall, R. M. Wilder, and P. C. Zamecnik, Medical Survey of Nutrition in Newfoundland, *Canad. M. A. J.* 52:227, 1945.

Cooperstock, M., E. Morse, E. Z. Moyer, and I. G. Macy, Nutritional Status of Children. IV. Nutritional Conditioning in a Health Camp, *J. Am. Dietet. A.* 24:205, 1948.

Follis, R. H., Jr., E. A. Park, and D. Jackson, The Prevalence of Scurvy at Autopsy during the First Two Years of Age, *Bull. Johns Hopkins Hosp.* 87:569, 1950.

Hamil, B. M., B. Munks, E. Z. Moyer, M. Kaucher, and H. H. Williams, Vitamin C in the Blood and Urine of the Newborn and in the Cord and Maternal Blood, *Am. J. Dis. Child.* 74:417, 1947.

Hollinger, M. E., and R. B. Attaya, Comparison of the Ascorbic Acid Content of Plasma and of Whole Blood as Criteria of Nutritional Status, *J. Nutrition* 37:203, 1949.

Kajdi, L., J. Light, and C. Kajdi, Test for Determination of Vitamin C Storage: Vitamin C Index, *J. Pediat.* 15:197, 1939.

Lowry, O. H., O. A. Bessey, M. J. Brock, and J. A. Lopez, Interrelationship of Dietary, Serum, White Blood Cell and Total Body Ascorbic Acid, *J. Biol. Chem.* 166:111, 1946.

Meiklejohn, A. P., "The Physiology and Biochemistry of Ascorbic Acid in Vitamins and Hormones: Advances in Research and Applications," Academic Press, Inc., New York, 1953.

Moyer, E. Z., A. P. Harrison, M. Lesher, and O. N. Miller, Nutritional Status of Children. III. Blood Serum Vitamin C, *J. Am. Dietet. A.* 24:199, 1948.

Storvick, C. A., M. L. Fincke, J. P. Quinn, and B. L. Davey, A Study of Ascorbic Acid Metabolism of Adolescent Children, *J. Nutrition* 33:529, 1947.

Vitamin C Content of Commercially Canned Tomato Juice and Other Fruit Juices as Determined by Chemical Titration: A Report of the Council on Foods, *J.A.M.A.* 110:650, 1938.

VITAMIN E

Butt, H. R., Fat-soluble Vitamins A, E, and K, *J.A.M.A.* 143:236, 1950.

Filer, L. J., Jr., S. W. Wright, M. P. Manning, and K. E. Mason, Absorption of ω-Tocopherol and Tocopherol Esters by Infants and Children, *Pediatrics* 8:328, 1951.

Moyer, W. T., Vitamin E Levels in Term and Premature Newborn Infants, *Pediatrics* 6:893, 1950.

Rose, C. S., and *P. Gyorgy,* Specificity of Hemolytic Reaction in Vitamin E-deficient Erythrocytes, *Am. J. Physiol.* 168:414, 1952.

Wright, S. W., L. J. Filer, Jr., and *K. E. Mason,* Vitamin E Blood Levels in Premature and Full Term Infants, *Pediatrics* 7:386, 1951.

CHAPTER 59

Stomach

The known major constituents of digestive importance in the child's gastric juice are hydrochloric acid and pepsin. Enzymes other than pepsin participate to a lesser extent in the breakdown of foods: cathepsin, gelatinase, Brücke-pepsin, lipase, lipokinase, and an amylase-accelerating factor. The concentration or degree of activity of any of these after ingestion of a regular meal can be estimated only by inference, since measurements are not feasible.

VOLUME OF RESTING (BASAL) SECRETION

The child's stomach in the resting state, between meals, is contracted and empty except for a small gas bubble and some resting or basal secretion. The latter is a mixture of saliva, gastric mucosal secretion, and regurgitated duodenal juice. In 695 of such specimens aspirated by the author from 59 children aged 3 to 14 years, the resting or basal volumes ranged from 0.4 to 80 ml. Of these, 83 per cent were between 0.1 and 10 ml; the mean was 8.8 ml with a standard deviation of ±8.2. The older children tended to have larger volumes, but there were no sex differences. Serial studies showed that the mean rates of accumulation of this resting fluid were 0.1 to 3 ml per minute, with a mean of 0.84 ml and a standard deviation of ±0.42. The pH ranged from 0.9 to 7.7; in most instances it was between pH 3.0 and 7.0. Bile was identified by its color in 159 of the specimens. This high incidence suggests that reverse peristalsis from duodenum to stomach is common and normal during childhood. In the bile-tinged samples the hydrogen-ion concentration was higher than pH 7.0 in only 11, below pH 3.0 in 80, and below pH 2.0 in 72. This shows that regurgitated duodenal fluid may impart a yellow tint to the gastric contents, but the quantity is ordinarily not enough to neutralize the gastric acidity.

The possibility that asphyxial disturbances in newborn infants may be aggravated by an excessive quantity of gastric fluid has been explored by Gellis, White, and Pfeffer. The average volume of gastric contents in 25 infants of diabetic mothers delivered by cesarean section was 20 ml, in 12 control infants delivered by cesarean section 14 ml. With 15 infants from nondiabetic mothers delivered by low forceps the average was only 2 ml. Prompt aspirations of the gastric fluid from infants delivered by cesarean section seemed to reduce neonatal asphyxia.

664

HYDROCHLORIC ACID

The studies of Hollander have indicated that the gastric hydrochloric acid is secreted by the mucosa at a more or less constant high concentration under both normal and pathologic circumstances, regardless of the rate of secretion. It is estimated that the concentration of hydrochloric acid in the pure parietal secretion is 165 to 170 mg per liter. This figure becomes, when expressed in more familiar terms, 0.6 per cent HCl, with a pH value of 0.87; 100 ml will be neutralized by about 165 ml of 0.1 N alkali, equal numerically to 165 "clinical units" or milliequivalents per liter.

Secondary mechanisms are constantly active to neutralize and dilute acidity strength to the lower potency customarily found in the normal stomach. Among these acidity-reducing mechanisms are saliva, gastric mucus and watery secretions, and regurgitated duodenal fluid.

Single specimens of gastric juice, as withdrawn during fasting, exhibit wide and inconstant hour-to-hour fluctuations. Fever and emotional factors may depress secretion.

Of the 695 resting specimens cited earlier, 197 or 35.3 per cent were negative for free hydrochloric acid. Individual readings for the positive specimens ranged from 4 to 100 mEq per liter. The mean was 28.1 mEq, with a standard deviation of ±17.9. The range for total acidity was 4 to 126 mEq per liter, with a mean of 38.2 mEq and a standard deviation of ±21.6. There was no close correlation with pH. These wide variations in the resting or fasting gastric juice of essentially normal children and the high percentage of hydrochloric acid-free specimens emphasize the necessity for using a stimulant such as histamine for testing the acid secretory capacity.

Free and Total Acidity

Töpfer's quantitative procedure is widely used for the titration of gastric hydrochloric acid. Ten milliliters of filtered gastric juice is mixed with 3 or 4 drops of dimethylaminoazobenzol (0.5 per cent alcoholic solution) and 3 or 4 drops of phenolphthalein (1 per cent alcoholic solution) in a porcelain dish. $N/10$ NaOH is then added drop by drop from a buret until the last trace of red color disappears. The number of milliliters which produce this first color change in 100 ml of gastric juice is the measure of *free acidity*, or hydrogen ions not linked to the buffer substances. Titration is then continued further until the red tint of phenolphthalein appears and reaches a maximum. The number of milliliters or units which produce the second color change, or *total acidity*, is a measure of both free acid and the entire buffer capacity to the end point of phenolphthalein. Subtraction of the free acidity from the total acidity gives the *combined acidity*, or buffer capacity. These values are now expressed in milliequivalents (mEq) per liter; numerically the number of units per 100 ml and milliequivalents per liter are identical and transposable.

Several criticisms of Töpfer's method are pertinent. Gastric juice is a buffered mixture of assorted secretions. Titration to the full yellow color of dimethylaminoazobenzol corresponds to a pH value of 4.0 to 5.0, whereas the end point for free HCl actually falls at pH 2.8. Most of the phosphates and acid proteins in the gastric secretion become neutralized in the pH range 3 to 3.8 and hence are included in the free acidity. Moreover, the red color of phenolphthalein marks a pH of 8 to 10, which is much more alkaline than the blood serum from which the acid digestive juice was derived.

Histamine Stimulation

Histamine not only evokes the most nearly maximal secretory response, it permits measurement of approximately pure secretions instead of the mixture of juice, food, saliva, and perhaps regurgitated intestinal juices which enter the stomach after a test meal. Toxic side effects are uncommon and not serious. Urecholine as a gastric stimulant produces excessive salivary secretion and may induce toxic systemic reactions.

The response to histamine in children, as in adults, is contingent upon the amount given. The optimal dose for children of all ages appears to be 0.01 mg of active histamine per kg body weight. The dose should be calculated in terms of the amount of histamine base contained in the preparation being given; e.g., histamine dihydrochloride is 60 per cent histamine base whereas histamine acid phosphate consists of but 36 per cent of active substance.

Procedure. 1. The test is best performed in the morning. The child receives no food for 12 hours prior to the test but may have water in reasonable quantities.

2. The equipment, already prepared and autoclaved on a tray, consists of a size no. 14 flexible catheter, or smaller for younger children, 24 inches long; a glass-tipped 10-ml syringe; a curved kidney basin; a medicine glass containing water; lubricant; a rubber apron and bib; glass test tubes or centrifuge tubes; and labels to mark the specimens.

3. If the child is old enough to understand, the procedure is explained to him in advance, and every effort is made to secure his cooperation. Restraint may otherwise be needed, but excitement must be avoided.

4. The child remains seated if possible. The rubber apron and bib are put on.

5. The tube is lubricated with jelly or glycerin.

6. The distance from the crown to the xyphoid process is measured, and a corresponding line marked on the tube with ink, to indicate how far it should be inserted.

7. The tube is introduced through one nostril while the patient makes swallowing movements. If it cannot be passed through the nose, the mouth is used.

8. When the lower end of the tube is thought to be in the stomach, its upper end is inverted in a medicine glass filled with water. No bubbles should appear. If bubbles stream continuously, the tube is withdrawn, reinserted, and retested. The tube is then fastened by a clamp to the patient's shirt. If the tube accidentally enters the trachea the patient will cough and gag and cyanosis may appear.

9. The syringe is attached to the end of the tube, and the intragastric air drawn off. The gastric contents are then gently aspirated by suction until no more can be obtained; this is saved and labeled Resting secretion.

10. Histamine is then injected subcutaneously, approximately 0.01 mg of active histamine per kg body weight.

11. The gastric fluid is again drawn off as fully as possible at 15, 30, and 45 minutes after the injection. Each specimen is placed in a separate large tube, labeled, and sent for analysis. Yellow specimens whose color is suggestive of contamination with regurgitated duodenal juice are not titrated; these are infrequent.

12. After the 45-minute collection (or after an added 60-minute collection if the 15-minute specimen was scanty) the tube is withdrawn and the test terminated.

NORMAL VALUES AFTER HISTAMINE. With children, as with adults, the range of variation among individuals of the same age and state of health is extremely wide. The range of spread which has been encountered in healthy American children after approximately 0.01 mg histamine base per kg body weight is indicated in Table 59-1.

Table 59-1. Ranges of Response of the Child's Stomach to Histamine at Various Ages

Age	Secretory rate (ml per minute)	Free acidity (mEq per 100 ml)	Total acidity (mEq per 100 ml)	pH
Prematures	0.12–0.15	0	0–8	3.0–7.0
Newborns	0.20–0.45	0–20	15–40	2.5–7.0
2 weeks–6 months	0.25–1.10	0–60	5–70	1.5–3.4
7–12 months	0.40–1.50	12–80	25–105	1.5–2.2
1–2 years	0.70–1.80	15–95	26–106	1.2–2.0
2–5 years	0.50–2.20	29–90	38–102	1.4–2.0
5–10 years	0.10–3.30	53–113	61–145	1.4–2.0
10–15 years	2.70–3.60	49–115	61–128	1.4–2.0

The secretory rate can be calculated by dividing the total number of milliliters secreted after the initial emptying by the number of minutes required for the collection.

The acid of the gastric juice appears to be secreted at a constant rate when the electrolyte composition of the blood is normal, whether the individual be normal or ill. Variations in observed gastric acidity are reflections of differences between the relative amounts of gastric juice and such neutralizing substances as food, swallowed saliva, mucus from the pyloric antrum, and regurgitated alkaline duodenal juice. The increased concentration of free gastric hydrochloric acid found in ulcer patients is thus a manifestation of an increased rate of secretion rather than of an increase in the acid concentration of the gastric juice itself.

As indicated by the above data, healthy infants and children are usually able to secrete an abundance of free hydrochloric acid.

Other Stimulants

When other stimulants are employed the procedure is the same as with histamine stimulation, except as indicated below. Normal responses are of slightly lower magnitude than those obtained with histamine.

EWALD-TYPE TEST MEAL. Two arrowroot crackers are given to children up to age 4 years, four to children from 4 to 8 years, and six to children above 8 years. Give 200 to 400 ml of water with the crackers or immediately afterward. One hour after starting to feed the crackers, a tube is passed and the gastric contents aspirated as completely as possible.

ALCOHOL STIMULATION. A stomach tube is passed, and the resting secretion withdrawn. An aqueous solution of 7 per cent alcohol is then introduced through a funnel by gravity. The dose is 25 ml for children under 5 years of age; 50 ml for children 5 years and over. The secretions are then withdrawn at 15 minutes, 30 minutes, and 45 minutes. The specimens may be pooled or tested separately.

Achlorhydria

Complete anacidity after histamine stimulation is occasionally discovered as a random finding in otherwise asymptomatic adults and may be familial. More often, in adults it is deemed a precursor or concomitant of pernicious anemia or cancer of the stomach. Persistent histamine-resistant anacidity in childhood is rare. Transitory absence of acid is seen in some of the megaloblastic anemias of nutritional origin.

Hypochlorhydria

A tendency to a diminished response to histamine is not uncommon in children with chronic ailments such as asthma, rheumatic fever, the celiac sydrome, and anemia. The deficiency tends to clear as the underlying conditions are corrected. Normal variability is so great, however, that the diagnosis of hypochlorhydria or complete anacidity should not be made until after at least two separate determinations made while the child is not acutely ill or disturbed emotionally.

In pyloric stenosis the gastric secretion prior to the onset of symptoms is normal in quantity and acidity. As soon as stasis and vomiting begin, the free and total acidities become increased. Few analyses of gastric fluids have been recorded in children with gastric or duodenal ulcers, but hyperchlorhydria may be expected, just as with adults.

Apart from chronic ailments and ulcers, therefore, there are almost no known disorders of childhood in which either anacidity, hypoacidity, or hyperacidity occur regularly and consistently enough to be of service in diagnosis.

Newborn Period

Unexpectedly high acid values are often present in the immediate postnatal period.

Griswold and Shohl's tests of 25 normal newborns showed a pH range from 1.7 to 4.4 (numerical average 2.6) in the fasting secretion. Miller found the resting gastric acidity to be highest on the first or second day of life and to subside to a negligibly low level by the seventh day. The resting volume during this period as a rule is less than 3 ml.

PEPSIN

The principal proteolytic factor in gastric juice is pepsin. This shows wide differences in concentration in the resting state.

In our study of 695 childhood specimens the readings (Helmer-Fouts method) ranged from 0.00 to 18.5 mg of pepsin per ml, with a mean of 3.9 mg and a standard deviation of ± 3.2. The correlations between pepsin, acid content, and pH indicated that in the fasting child the secretion of pepsin is closely associated with that of hydrochloric acid.

Pepsin is inactive unless the environmental medium is strongly acid, below pH 4.0. The optimum pH with casein as substrate is slightly under pH 2.0. Regurgitated duodenal juice can neutralize secreted acid and destroy its accompanying enzyme.

Dozens of techniques are available for the measurement of peptic strength of gastric juice. For the average physician's office or clinical laboratory the simple methods based upon milk-clotting power are reasonably accurate and easy to work with. The powerful milk-clotting enzyme known as rennin which occurs in the calf and the kid but not in the adult cow or mature goat seems to be absent from the human stomach.

CATHEPSIN

Intragastric digestion of milk has been reported at pH values of 5.0 and 6.0, whereas proteolysis by pepsin cannot occur when the surrounding medium is at a pH above 4.0. This phenomenon has been explained by Freudenberg and Buchs in terms of the occurrence of another proteolytic enzyme, cathepsin, within the child's gastric juice. Two other proteinases of minor if any significance which have also been demonstrated are (1) gelatinase and (2) a protein-free preparation of noncrystallizable material known as Brücke-pepsin.

AMYLASE-ACCELERATING ACTION

Davison noted that the addition of infant gastric contents to fresh hog pancreas extracted in saline solution increased the starch-liquefying activity of the latter nearly eightfold. Swallowing of saliva may explain the presence of amylase in the stomach.

LIPASE

A weak lipolytic activity appears to be constantly present through infancy and childhood, even in unfed newborns. The optimum range for this enzymatic action is pH 4.0 to 5.0. Its occurrence explains the distinctive odor of butyric acid when vomiting occurs after milk or any other food containing butterfat has been taken. There is uncertainty as to whether this lipase comes from the gastric mucosa or from duodenal regurgitation.

Milk Lipase

Both breast milk and cow's milk contain lipase which is thermolabile. Cow's-milk lipase becomes destroyed during pasteurization or boiling. Since breast milk ordinarily receives no heat treatment in advance of being fed, its lipase appears to play a significant role in the digestive breakdown of milk fats. The optimal hydrogen-ion concentration for this milk enzyme lies between pH 7.0 and 8.0; its activity is reduced to one-tenth at pH 5.0. Regurgitation studies have shown that with young infants receiving breast milk, which is normally slightly alkaline, the acidity of the gastric contents following nursing does not fall to pH 6.0 until 30 minutes and to pH 5.5 until nearly 2 hours.

LIPOKINASE

Breast milk when left standing at room temperature for some hours does not exhibit spontaneous changes, yet when mixed with gastric juice will become rancid immediately. Freudenberg has been able to extract a thermolabile lipase-activating agent from the gastric wall of some species of animals and to demonstrate the presence of this same agent in human gastric fluid, during infancy as well as throughout life. This lipokinase activates the fat-splitting enzyme which in normal breast milk occurs in the inactive or prolipase precursor state.

ERYTHROCYTE MATURATION FACTOR

An "intrinsic" hemopoietic factor is elaborated by the gastric and duodenal mucosa. This combines with the extrinsic factor, now believed to be vitamin B_{12}, to produce a nutrient principle essential for normal red cell maturation. The pernicious anemia syndrome, seen in adults who have an irreversible atrophy of the stomach wall and deficiency of the intrinsic factor, is almost never seen in childhood (p. 48).

GASTRIC DIGESTION OF MILK

In a series of original studies carried out with 59 children aged 3 to 14 years, the fasting gastric secretions were withdrawn through an indwelling catheter at 10-minute intervals for 50 minutes. A glassful (240 ml) of milk was then swallowed while the catheter remained in place. Samples of the gastric contents were then aspirated every 10 minutes until the stomach had become empty. Wide individual variations in the fasting gastric secretion were found, epitomized as follows:

	Range	Mean	Standard deviation
Volume (ml)	0.4–80	8.7	±8.2
Rate of formation (ml per minute)	0.1–3.0	0.84	±0.42
Hydrogen-ion concentration (pH)	0.9–7.7	3.27	±2.01
Free acidity when present (mEq per liter)	0–100	28.1	±17.9
Combined acidity (mEq per liter)	4–40	19.6	±6.2
Total acidity (mEq per liter)	4–126	38.2	±21.6
Pepsin, Helmer-Fouts method (mg per ml)	0–18.5	3.89	±3.19

Bile was present in one-fourth of the specimens.

Pepsin and hydrochloric acid seemed to be secreted in more or less parallel fashion. There was indirect evidence that cathepsin was being secreted as well. The buffer capacity of this amount of milk neutralized the gastric contents almost completely, even when it had contained a comparatively large amount of strong acid. The observed coagulation times for the ingested milk ranged from 8 to 52 minutes, with a mean of 19.7 minutes. Gastric emptying times ranged from 25 to 170 minutes, with a mean of 118.5 minutes. No measurable differences could be demonstrated in the responses to "soft-curd" homogenized milk as compared with more "hard-curd" plain pasteurized milk. The mean pH did not fall below 4.7 until after 30 minutes, failed to go below 3.3 until nearly an hour, and never fully attained the low pH values necessary for maximal activation of pepsin. Since evacuation of milk into the duodenum begins a few moments after drinking, there is not much opportunity for the gastric digestant principles to act. The child's stomach seems to serve largely as a reservoir. The intestinal tract beyond the pylorus carries the main burden of the digestive breakdown of milk.

During infancy the circumstances are even more unfavorable for pepsin action. The intragastric pH is usually above 5.0, and food remains in the stomach for an even briefer period. Breast milk, despite its lower buffer capacity, tends to evoke a weaker secretory response than that produced by cow's milk.

PEPTIC ULCER

Chronic duodenal and gastric ulcers are uncommon in infancy and childhood. Symptoms are vague and indefinite, as a rule. The lesion is usually not suspected until an ominous complication such as hemorrhage or perforation supervenes. Recurrent pain in the upper abdomen, symptoms of partial pyloric obstruction, or stools which are intermittently tarry or which contain occult blood call for a careful roentgen study of the gastrointestinal tract for signs of ulceration or of any related lesions.

Acute mucosal lesions may develop in the stomach, duodenum, or esophagus during the course of profound toxemia (e.g., burns, septicemia) or of illnesses affecting the brain stem (e.g., encephalitis, tumors, bulbar poliomyelitis).

BLOOD IN VOMITUS

The spontaneous vomiting of blood in a massive hematemesis is rare in childhood; when it occurs one must study the patient for peptic ulcer, for a blood dyscrasia with impairment of coagulation, for esophageal varices secondary to liver cirrhosis, for esophageal hiatal hernia, and for related lesions. Blood-tinged fluid secured by gastric aspiration is best ascribed to mechanical trauma associated with passage of the tube, unless other more positive evidence of intragastric hemorrhage is available. Vomiting of "coffee-ground" gastric fluid is indicative of a bloody ooze from the mucosa and is seen in hemorrhagic states, gastritis, uremia, anoxemia, and terminally from any cause.

TUBERCLE BACILLI IN GASTRIC WASHINGS

Aspiration of the fasting gastric contents for *Mycobacterium tuberculosis* is a means of procuring sputum for examination from children too young or too uncooperative to expectorate and can supplement direct sputum examinations in suspected cases when sputum examinations have been repeatedly negative. Children under 6 or 7 years of age usually swallow sputum instead of expectorating. The gastric contents should be collected as sterilely as possible.

Technique of Aspiration for Tubercle Bacilli

1. The test is done in the early morning. The child should receive no food or drink since the evening before, or with young infants, after 2 A.M. If the child vomits as the tube is being introduced, the vomitus is collected and saved.

2. The gastric contents are removed by suction after the tube has been inserted. Should no fluid be obtained, 5 to 10 ml of water is run in and withdrawn 2 to 3 minutes later. The recovered aspirate contains flecks of mucus; if milk or other foods are present the test should be discontinued since these substances make it impossible to perform proper bacteriologic studies. All the material aspirated is sent to the laboratory. The upper end of the tube is then clamped off with the fingers and gently withdrawn.

3. The specimen is labeled "gastric contents, resting secretion," with patient's name, ward, date, etc. Specimens which cannot be cultured immediately are stored in a refrigerator.

4. The equipment is thoroughly washed with soapy water, autoclaved, and prepared for the next using.

5. In the laboratory the gastric contents and lavage fluids are mixed with warm 5 per cent sodium or potassium hydroxide solution to disintegrate the mucus and are centrifuged. The sediment is then neutralized with dilute hydrochloric acid, recentrifuged, washed with normal salt solution, smeared and cultured or injected into guinea pigs if deemed necessary.

6. Experience has shown that a single negative specimen is not adequate for ruling out the diagnosis. The examination should be repeated three to five

times in suspicious cases, at intervals of 1 to 7 days. Since M. *tuberculosis* tends to lose its viability when left in contact with the digestive enzymes from the saliva and gastric juice, even at room temperature, it is best to study each lavage specimen individually, as soon after collection as possible. Three or more such specimens may be pooled for guinea pig inoculation, but each should be neutralized and washed when collected and then preserved in the refrigerator.

Clinical Interpretations

Smear or culture of the sediment from gastric washings frequently reveals acid-fast organisms which are not M. *tuberculosis*. These so-called saprophytic acid-fast bacilli are believed to enter the stomach from previously ingested raw fruits and vegetables. Some of the strains seem to be derived from the dust in the laboratory air or on the equipment. In growth characteristics the colonies are often golden, round, smooth, and glistening, rather than the typical whitish or pale-buff, rough, dry crumblike colonies of the tubercle bacillus. When there are doubts about pathogenicity, atypical strains may in inoculated into guinea pigs since they produce no disease in these animals. The cultural method alone is considered reliable by most workers for the recognition of tubercle bacilli when the stained appearances and colony structure are characteristic.

BIBLIOGRAPHY

STOMACH

Buchs, S., and *E. Freudenberg*, Die Rolle des Kathepsins bei der Eiweissverdauung, *Ergebn. inn. Med. u. Kinderh.* 2:544, 1951.

Davison, W. C., The Amylase-Accelerating Action of Gastric Contents, *Am. J. Dis. Child.* 63:728, 1942.

Dragstedt, L. R., H. A. Oberhelman, Jr., and *E. R. Woodward*, Physiology of Gastric Secretion and Its Relation to the Ulcer Problem, *J.A.M.A.* 147:1615, 1951.

Freudenberg, E., "Physiologie und Pathologie der Verdauung in Säuglingsalter," Julius Springer, Berlin, 1929.

Gellis, S. S., P. White, and *W. Pfeffer*, Gastric Suction: A Proposed Additional Technic for the Prevention of Asphyxia in Infants Delivered by Cesarean Section, *New England J. Med.* 240:533, 1949.

Griswold, C., and *A. T. Shohl*, Gastric Digestion in Newborn Infants, *Am. J. Dis. Child.* 30:541, 1925.

Helmer, O. M., and *P. J. Fouts*, Gastric Analysis Methods, *Am. J. Clin. Path.* (*Tech. Suppl.*) 7:41, 1937.

Hollander, F., The Chemistry and Mechanics of Hydrochloric Acid Formation in the Stomach, *Gastroenterology* 1:401, 1943.

Ingram, M. D., Jr., Gastric Ulcer in Childhood, *Am. J. Roentgenol.* 64:765, 1950.

Jones, J. A., B. Margolis, and *T. Potterfield,* The Gastric Response of Normal Children to Urecholine, *J. Pediat.* **40**:456, 1952.

Lichtenberg, H. H., Untersuchungen zur Verdauungsphysiologie des Säuglings. XVI. Zur Kenntnis der Magenlipase, *Ztschr. Kinderh.* **54**:732, 1933.

Miller, R. A., Observations on Gastric Acidity during the First Month of Life, *Arch. Dis. Childhood* **16**:22, 1941.

——, Gastric Acidity during the First Year of Life, *Arch. Dis. Childhood* **17**:198, 1942.

Northrop, J. H., Isolation and Properties of Pepsin and Trypsin, *Harvey Lect.* **30**:229, 1934–1935.

Plummer, G. W., and *S. J. Stabins,* Bleeding Duodenal Ulcer in Infancy: A Surgical Problem, *J. Pediat.* **37**:899, 1950.

Wolman, I. J., Gastric Digestive Secretions in Infancy and Childhood: A Review, *Am. J. M. Sc.* **206**:770, 1943.

——, Gastric Phase of Milk Digestion in Childhood: A Study of the Fasting Secretions and of the Physiologic Responses to "Hard Curd" (Pasteurized) and "Soft Curd" (Homogenized) Milks, *Am. J. Dis. Child.* **71**:394, 1946.

CHAPTER 60

Duodenum, Gallbladder, Pancreas, and Small Intestine

DUODENAL SECRETIONS

The intraduodenal fluid is a pool or composite of secretions forming simultaneously (1) from Brunner's glands and the duodenal mucous membrane, (2) from the pancreas (amylase, lipase, trypsin) and (3) from the liver, gallbladder, and bile ducts (bile, mucus). In addition (4) fluid containing gastric or salivary enzymes and hydrochloric acid trickles in intermittently from the pyloric antrum. The relative amounts from these separate sources at any one time depend upon a diversity of mechanisms, constitutional as well as local, with autonomic and hormonal influences exerting major control.

Specimens collected from a fasting child by duodenal intubation usually contain little bile and are composed chiefly of pancreatic fluid. If contaminated with gastric juice they contain gray floccules and are paler, more acid, and of greater volume.

The external secretion of the duodenal mucous membrane is not abundant and seems to contain only two major enzymes: enterokinase and amylase. The mucosal amylase is weak as compared with pancreatic amylase and therefore not of much significance. The enterokinase appears to be a powerful activant as it enters the intestine.

Since the pancreatic component is the greatest in volume and the most potent in enzymes, the findings in aspirated duodenal fluid during the so-called "interdigestive period," when the stomach is empty, are taken as representative of the secretion of the pancreas. Because of the possible flow of some of the duodenal contents into the jejunum during a collection period and probable contamination with material derived from the stomach or saliva, results of analyses must be regarded as only semiquantitative.

Rate of Production

The usual volumes range from 1 to 5 ml per hour in healthy infants under 2 months, up to 5 to 50 ml per hour in older children. The rate of formation is not affected appreciably by crying or excitement. Older children tend to produce more potent secretions at faster rates than do infants. Individual differences are prominent. There is no decrease in malnutrition, and an occasional increase in celiac disease. In cystic fibrosis of the pancreas the rate of formation is much diminished and the consistency highly viscid.

Excitation of pancreatic flow can be effected by humoral, neural, or pharmacologic mechanisms. Stimulation with intravenous secretin produces a large volume of duodenal juice rich in bicarbonate but poor in enzymes. Parasympathetic (vagal) stimulation or Urecholine and similar cholinergic drugs evoke thicker juice poor in bicarbonate but rich in enzymes. Secretin sometimes causes systemic reactions in infants and children and is not often employed.

Hydrogen-ion Concentration

The intraduodenal hydrogen-ion concentration of the fasting healthy infant and child is usually between pH 6.5 and 7.5. In acute gastroenteritis of infancy the pH has been found between 4.5 and 6.2.

Evidently the duodenal secretion when "pure" is neutral or slightly alkaline, but when "contaminated" with gastric contents becomes acidic. The exact pH status seems of minor clinical importance, even though the pancreatic enzymes have their optima for activity at neutrality or on the basic side. Food and gastric secretions pass quickly to the jejunum, where the succus entericus there elaborated mixes with and determines the pH of the material which comes in from the duodenum.

Viscosity

Duodenal fluid is normally thin and watery. In nephrosis the viscosity is moderately increased and the proportion of mucus increased. In true celiac disease it is normal.

A pronounced increase in viscosity is the rule in cystic fibrosis of the pancreas and in jaundice due to liver disease in young infants. In pancreatic fibrosis the fluid is sometimes too viscid to flow through a viscosimeter. It will adhere to a glass rod or to the side of a test tube and flow very slowly. When biliary tract obstruction is responsible for the liver disease the viscosity returns to normal after the obstruction is relieved.

Enzymes

Amylase, trypsin, and lipase, the chief enzymes of duodenal juice, come largely if not almost entirely from the pancreas. In normal children, any stimulus which provokes the appearance of any one of these enzymes ordinarily calls forth its two companions simultaneously in strict parallelism. This is true following excitation by pilocarpine or inhibition by atropine.

Transitory dissociation of the enzymatic triad is present occasionally in nutritional disturbances or after severe infections (p. 692). Lipase hyposecretion is sometimes encountered in the first few months of life, and amylase deficiency in true celiac disease (p. 691).

Study of aspirated duodenal fluid for enzymatic abnormalities is a cardinal approach to differentiation of the entities which together make up the celiac syndrome (Chap. 61). The results of enzymatic analyses are best expressed as comparisons with control results obtained in the same laboratory.

AMYLASE. Amylases are carbohydrates which attack starches and glycogen. Pancreatic extracts can digest raw starch from corn, wheat, and potato, whereas salivary amylase must be placed with cooked starches before its enzymatic activity begins. Davison noted that admixture with gastric juices increased the amylolytic power of some duodenal fluids as much as eightfold, and others have noted acceleration of enzymatic starch hydrolysis by addition of bile.

Amylase activity is normally low in the neonate and premature infant and increases gradually with growth into childhood. Because of the lesser activity per unit volume and the total lower output of secretions, the young infant does not digest starch as efficiently as when older. In gastrointestinal diseases the secretion of amylase may be diminished.

LIPASE. The pancreatic secretion is a highly potent hydrolytic agent for neutral fats which are triglycerides of fatty acids, but is weak or ineffective with esters of organic acids with alcohols or carbohydrates. Hence the term lipase rather than esterase is applied.

During digestion the triglyceride fats are first emulsified by the bile and then split by the lipase. The fatty acids so liberated promptly go into a water-soluble freely diffusible combination with bile salts and are absorbed by the intestinal mucosa in this complex form.

Most of the recent work on pancreatic lipase in children utilizes a titrative method for assaying lipolytic activity. A standardized alkali solution measures the fatty acids liberated in vitro within a standard period of time (usually 1 hour) from a standardized oil emulsion. Lipolytic potency of the duodenal contents is then expressed as the number of milliliters of alkali solution required to neutralize the free fatty acids which form, or more indirectly in terms of calculated Willstätter "units."

Wide variations normally occur in infants and children of all ages, with no gradations in lipase activity associated directly with age. Lipase is typically absent in cystic fibrosis of the pancreas, but undisturbed in idiopathic celiac disease. Low values occur at times in other disease conditions, such as atresia of the common bile duct; absent or very low lipase of itself is not pathognomonic of pancreatic fibrosis.

TRYPSIN. The breakdown of proteins and protein products by enzymes in aqueous solution is a most complex set of processes with innumerable subsidiary equilibrium reactions acting one upon another. Coenzymes, cosubstrates, and acid and basic ions all participate in multiple component reactions which go on simultaneously. It is customary to refer to the sum of the protein-digestant principles in pancreatic juice as *trypsin,* and that is the meaning of the term as usually employed for clinical purposes. More precisely, however, these proteases can be subdivided into proteinases and polypeptidases. The differentiation is based upon the power of proteinases to dissolve amino acid linkages anywhere within the protein molecules, whereas peptidases are more limited and can break off single amino acids only from one or the other end of the peptide chain. Studies with experimental animals indicate that most of the proteolytic behavior of pancreatic juice is due to proteinases; the peptidases seem weak and few in number.

The proteinases of the pancreas are secreted in a precursor or zymogen form, in the same way as the pepsin of the stomach first appears as pepsinogen. Freshly secreted pancreatic juice will exhibit no proteolytic activity until after coming in contact either with acid or with enterokinase of the small intestine.

A diversity of methods is available for measuring the activity of trypsin-containing preparations. The general approaches include measurement of increases in amino groups, COOH groups, nonprotein nitrogen or residual protein nitrogen in the substrate; changes in viscosity of protein solutions or in milk-clotting power; or liberation of tyrosine from hemoglobin. The widely used Fermi method modified by Andersen and Early is based upon the property of gelatin to no longer solidify at refrigerator temperature after being enzymatically hydrolyzed beyond a certain point. When serial dilutions of duodenal fluid are incubated with a standard amount of melted gelatin solution and then placed in a refrigerator, the extent of liquefaction indicates the approximate proteolytic activity of the fluid.

The variation in the trypsin activity of fasting secretion among normal individuals is wide, with no significant trend in relation to age. In cystic fibrosis of the pancreas the trypsin is usually completely absent. Occasional infants with this disorder may exhibit a minor degree of activity, which tends to fade away with the passage of months. In idiopathic celiac disease, nephrosis, marasmus, and bile duct obstruction, the trypsin activity may be normal or decreased. In bile duct obstruction the diminution is attributed to the absence of bile, which is a pancreatogogue.

Premature infants have unimpaired secretion of pancreatic trypsin. With 16 small premature infants Madey and Dancis found that gelatin was liquefied by

0.01 ml of duodenal juice and that 12 of the 16 showed activity with 0.005 ml. Such findings and observations of weight gain indicate that there is no need to "predigest" protein foods for premature infants.

TECHNIQUE FOR DUODENAL INTUBATION
AND STUDY OF DUODENAL FLUID [1]

Debility may be a contraindication, depending on its degree, especially in small infants. The procedure may be long and exhausting for the patient unless due restraint is exercised. The long period without food or water may be tolerated poorly, especially in the summer for patients with pancreatic disease. A maximum of 2 hours should seldom be exceeded.

1. Administer nothing by mouth after midnight except water which is allowed freely up to 1 hour before the test.
2. Preliminary mild sedation is often worthwhile for patients over 2 years.
3. Proper restraint if necessary. Older children may give better cooperation if allowed some freedom after the tube is in place.
4. Two tongue blades taped together may be placed between the teeth if necessary to avoid biting the tube.
5. A properly instructed assistant is needed to keep the patient's head straight, to keep the tube in the mid-line (which reduces the chance of regurgitating it), and to prevent movement of the tube after it is in place.

Contamination of the duodenal juice by gastric contents is probably undesirable, especially with respect to amylase determinations. A double-lumened tube is most convenient, with two sets of holes 2½ to 5 in. apart so the distal set can be in the duodenum and the proximal holes in the stomach. An Abbott-Rawson tube can be used with the distal segment appropriately shortened; a Miller-Abbott tube can be altered by removal of the balloon and adding holes where needed; or two Levine tubes, nos. 10 and 12, can be tied together so the opening of the smaller one will lie in the stomach when the other one is in the duodenum. A smooth metal tip in the distal opening (slightly thicker than the tube) facilitates passage through the pylorus and is easily visualized fluoroscopically. Passage through the mouth is less distressing than nasally and makes manipulation of the tube easier.

The patient lies supine with the head in the mid-line. Pass the tube to the stomach and check the position by fluoroscope. If it turns to the left, pull back to the cardia, turn the patient on the right side, and try again. Manual pressure through the abdominal wall may occasionally be helpful. If the tube curls or kinks, pull back and readvance slowly, about 2 or 3 minutes for 3 in. of tube. Once the tip is in the pyloric antrum, it can usually be forced slowly and gently into the duodenum. The terminal opening should lie well into the duodenum, and the proximal one in the stomach. Testing the aspirated juice with Nitrazine paper will help to confirm the positions. The procedure is

[1] Technique of J. Albright Jones, M.D., from "Pediatric Methods and Standards," University of Pennsylvania, School of Medicine, Department of Pediatrics, 1954. Reproduced by permission.

usually easy, but it may require much patience and perseverance of both physician and patient. When in position without excess slack in the stomach, mark the tube at the lips with a piece of tape so further swallowing of the tube can be avoided. Empty the stomach thoroughly and keep it empty by continuous or intermittent suction on the shorter tube. Discard the first milliliter of duodenal juice which appears. Collect at least 3 ml by gentle suction with a syringe. If the tube becomes plugged, it can be cleared by injection of a few cubic centimeters of air. Suction is more effective if gentle. The character of the juice must be checked frequently with Nitrazine paper to avoid contamination with gastric juice or saliva; it should be strongly alkaline. Transfer the juice to a tube set in ice and send it *as soon as collected* to the laboratory. The study must be scheduled in advance with the laboratory to ensure prompt handling of the specimen. If the enzyme studies cannot be carried out at once, the juice must be frozen and stored promptly. A small amount (about 0.5 ml kept warm) can be subjected to immediate microscopic study if desired; unsuspected giardiasis may be found.

A second specimen of juice is sometimes collected after pancreatic stimulation with Urecholine 1 to 5 mg subcutaneously or with secretin 1 clinical unit intravenously, but these agents have not added much to the study method. Either one may produce undesirable reactions. The proper dose of Urecholine is difficult to estimate, and atropine should be kept at hand to counteract possible side effects.

Warning: Use the fluoroscope sparingly. Learn to see enough with a short exposure. Fluoroscopic tubes vary in the amount of radiation delivered. Probably exposure should not be more than a total of 5 minutes per week from the average tube, the less the better.

GALLBLADDER

Bile

The chemical composition of the bile in healthy children appears to be much the same as in the normal adult. Reported analyses indicate that in infancy a random specimen of bile will contain (in round numbers) water, 93 per cent; mucin, 1.5 per cent; sodium glycocholic acid, 2 per cent; sodium taurocholic acid, 1 per cent; cholesterol and other lipids, 2 per cent; mineral salts, 0.5 per cent. Great fluctuations occur in the proportion of these various constituents, in specimens secured by gallbladder drainage as well as with fistula fluid. During and after an interval of active hepatic secretion the composition of the gallbladder bile approaches that coming directly from the liver. During stasis the relative content of solids increases as a consequence of resorption of water and salts by the gallbladder wall. Agents such as bile salts themselves, which stimulate secretion by the liver, are called choleretics, whereas magnesium sulfate and fatty meals which cause emptying of the gallbladder are cholagogues. Anticholeretics and anticholagogues, chiefly pharmacologic substances, exert the opposite effects.

Duodenal Drainage for Bile Examination

The test is carried out in the morning before breakfast. A thin metal-tipped flexible tube, about 3 ml in diameter, is introduced into the stomach and the gastric contents aspirated. The child is then placed on the right side, preferably under the fluoroscope, and the tube is advanced slowly. When the tip has entered the duodenum, yellow fluid can be aspirated which is neutral or weakly alkaline in reaction. An injection of 5 to 20 ml of a warmed 25 per cent solution of magnesium sulfate solution is then given, the quantity being contingent upon the age of the child.

Three "types" of bile ordinarily appear in succession: A bile, golden yellow, supposedly coming from the common duct; B bile, much darker, more viscous, and more abundant, supposedly from the gallbladder; and C bile, clear, light yellow, and of low specific gravity, supposedly freshly secreted by the liver. Often, however, these appearances are inconstant and variable. The color depends upon the content of bilirubin. Infants with congenital atresia of the bile ducts have colorless duodenal fluid even after cholagogues. With other forms of infantile jaundice the administration of cholagogues may or may not evoke the appearance of bile.

Partial or intermittent biliary tract occlusion can lead to diminished output of bile. Faint yellow staining of the duodenal secretions may be noted even when occlusion is complete, the color being produced by the icteric secretions from the mucosa of duodenum and stomach.

More than trace amounts of bile pigment in the duodenal aspirate of jaundiced infants rules out complete atresia of the bile passages, especially when the Pettenkofer test for bile acids is also positive.

With infants who are fed milk while the tube is in place, the bilirubin coloring of the duodenal secretions begins to fade at about 15 minutes after the feeding is begun. It usually disappears in another 15 minutes and returns 1 to 1½ hours afterward.

Cholecystitis

Cholecystitis is uncommon but not unheard of in children. It may be due to bacterial invasion or to giardial infestation. It is looked for by microscopic examination of uncentrifuged unstained fluid from all three bile fractions. Inflammatory changes in the bile may consist of excessive mucus, floccules, segmented leukocytes, cholesterol crystals, or the presence of *Giardia lamblia* or *Trichomonas hominis*. These are usually present in the A and B fractions. Changes in the C bile are suggestive of cholangitis. Bacteriologic cultures may be made if the tube and all collecting equipment had been autoclaved previously and the collections made with sterile precautions. Except when Giardia are present, repeated drainages by cholagogues may bring the bile back to normal with concomitant relief or amelioration of symptoms.

Cholelithiasis

Most children with cholelithiasis—which is also rare in this age period—have some obvious predisposing factor. This may be a congenital anomaly of the biliary system, an extrabiliary tract disturbance which blocks the flow of bile, or a chronic hemolytic disorder. Infection may or may not be associated. These patients tend to have recurrent episodes of pain in the abdomen, usually on the right side, which are aggravated by a fatty meal. X-rays may demonstrate calcified densities in the gallbladder region. Bilirubin stones are the most frequent.

PANCREATIC DISORDERS

Diseases of the pancreas other than cystic fibrosis (p. 687) or transient depression of function (p. 692) are conspicuously exceptional during childhood. Carcinoma and pancreatitis caused by impacted gallstones are almost never seen. In acute pancreatitis due to spasm at the ampulla of Vater with retrograde flow of the bile into the duct, pain and other symptoms are referable to the upper abdomen; positive laboratory findings include an elevated amylase in the blood serum and the urine. In chronic pancreatitis the prominent symptoms are abdominal pain and distention, irregularly large stools, and weight loss. Ascites, hepatomegaly, splenomegaly, or hyperlipemia have been seen in some cases, and the serum amylase level may be elevated. Fibrotic changes and dysontogenetic pancreatic cysts do not give rise to the celiac syndrome unless the entire gland is severely involved; glycosuria may then develop, probably as a result of injury to the islet cells.

SMALL INTESTINE

Succus Entericus

Not many studies have been carried out on physiologic conditions within the jejunum and ileum, either in the fasting state or during the digestion of foods. Available information indicates that the contents of these segments of the intestine are clear and yellow-green during fasting, cloudy and light yellow when foods are being digested. The hydrogen-ion concentration is usually between pH 6.0 and 8.0. Lipases, amylases, and proteases are present, derived both from the intestinal wall itself and from the topographically higher duodenum, pancreas, stomach, and salivary apparatus.

The duodenum tends to be bacteriologically sterile during health, but enterococci and other bacteria may be found in the jejunum and ileum, particularly the latter. Lactobacilli are common in the terminal ileum of breast-fed infants, but not with those receiving cow's milk.

That the quantities of intestinal enzymes may vary considerably from individual to individual is suggested by the wide variations in digestive capacity which are seen in cystic fibrosis of the pancreas. In this disease the pancreatic secretions for practical purposes may be said to be absent; the differences in stool composition and nutritional status of patients may be attributed at least partially to differences in the enzyme productivity of the small intestine.

Meckel's Diverticulum

This embryonic structure often has patches of heterotopic gastric mucosa in its walls. Secondary ulcers, the source of intestinal hemorrhages (p. 705), often develop near the junction of the diverticulum with the intestinal lumen. To search for such an ulcer a duodenal intubation tube may be advanced slowly under fluoroscopic control through the small intestine in order to avoid traumatic bleeding. Small samples of succus entericus are aspirated at successive levels and tested for pH status and gross or microscopic blood. The pH, which in the jejunum and ileum is normally between 6.0 and 8.0, may drop suddenly to 5.0 or lower when an ulcer is reached, and free erythrocytes may make their appearance. An opaque barium suspension may then be introduced through the tube, and roentgenograms made of the local contours. Care must be taken to avoid mechanical trauma to the nasopharyngeal mucous membrane while the tube is being passed, since bleeding from this region can confuse the results.

BIBLIOGRAPHY

DUODENUM, PANCREAS, GALLBLADDER, AND SMALL INTESTINE

Andersen, D. H., and *M. V. Early,* Method of Assaying Trypsin Suitable for Routine Use in Diagnosis of Congenital Pancreatic Deficiency, *Am. J. Dis. Child.* 63:891, 1942.

Anfanger, H., M. H. Bass, R. Heavenrich, and *J. J. Bookman,* Pancreatic Achylia and Glycosuria Due to Cystic Disease of the Pancreas in a 9 Year Old Child, *J. Pediat.* 35:151, 1949.

Davis, M. L., and *W. M. Kelsey,* Chronic Pancreatitis in Childhood, *A.M.A. Am. J. Dis. Child.* 81:687, 1951.

Guilbert, P. W., and *I. J. Wolman,* The Importance of Trypsin in Infancy and Childhood, I, *Am. J. M. Sc.* 226:688, 1953.

Hamilton, H. B., C. O. Rich, and *J. D. Bisgard,* Cholecystitis and Cholelithiasis of Childhood, *J.A.M.A.* 103:829, 1934.

Jaeger, H. W., Acute Pancreatitis in Children (Pancreatitis aguda hemorragica en el niño), *Rev. chilena pediat.* 14:18, 1943.

James, R., Chronic Pancreatitis in Childhood, *Arch. Dis. Childhood* 27:364, 1952.

Jones, J. A., Studies on Pancreatic Enzymes: A Comparison of Fasting Duodenal Juice before and after Gastric Aspiration, *J. Pediat.* 49:672, 1956.

Lynch, K. M., Pancreatitis: An Analysis of Types and Causes, *Ann. Int. Med.* 14:628, 1940.

Madey, S., and *J. Dancis,* Proteolytic Enzymes of the Premature Infant with Special Reference to his Ability to Digest Unsplit Protein Food, *Pediatrics* 4:177, 1949.

Patterson, P., A Study of the Duodenal Fluid in Infants with Jaundice, *A.M.A. Am. J. Dis. Child.* 83:415, 1952.

Philipsborn, H. F., G. Lawrence, S. Gibson, and *H. Greengard,* An Analysis of the Duodenal Drainage in the Steatorrheas, *J. Pediat.* 26:107, 1945.

Poulsen, H. M., Familial Lipaemia: A New Form of Lipoidosis Showing Increase in Neutral Fats Combined with Attacks of Acute Pancreatitis, *Acta med. scandinav.* 138:413, 1950.

Shapiro, D. J., F. J. Dzurik, and *E. W. Gerrish,* Obstruction of Duodenum in the Newborn Infant Due to Annular Pancreas, *Pediatrics* 9:764, 1952.

Snyder, W. H., Jr., L. Chaffin, and *L. Oettinger,* Cholelithiasis and Perforation of the Gallbladder in an Infant with Recovery, *J.A.M.A.* 149:1645, 1952.

Thomas, J. E., Physiology of the External Secretion of the Pancreas, *Tr. New York Acad. Sc.* ser. II, 14:310, 1952.

Ulin, A. W., J. L. Nosal, and *W. L. Martin,* Cholecystitis in Childhood, *J.A.M.A.* 147:1443, 1951.

Wolman, I. J., The Intra-duodenal Secretions in Childhood, *Am. J. M. Sc.* 209:788, 1945.

CHAPTER 61

Celiac Syndrome

DEFINITION

The celiac syndrome is a reaction syndrome rather than a clinical entity. Regardless of the causative mechanism, in established cases the prominent features include poor absorption of foodstuffs and especially fats or starches, an increased volume of feces often but not necessarily associated with diarrhea or gross steatorrhea, a distended abdomen, and malnutritional complications. In mild or early cases these symptoms may be minor and go unrecognized.

The digestive difficulties of the celiac syndrome can be brought about by a diversity of disorders—cystic fibrosis of the pancreas, "idiopathic" or "true" celiac disease with intolerance to starches or fats or both, "idiopathic" infantile steatorrhea, subacute pancreatitis (rare in childhood), prolonged therapy with oral antibiotics, chronic incomplete intestinal obstruction, severe giardiasis or other chronic enteric infections, intestinal tuberculosis, nontropical sprue, marked gastrointestinal allergy, especially to wheat gluten, congenital megacolon, lipid storage diseases, starvation, or mental retardation with poor feeding and failure to grow. Since prognosis and general management vary with the pathogenesis, it is essential with every patient to try to identify the exact nature of the disorder. The possibility of this symptom complex should be thought of whenever there is persistent colic or diarrhea refractory to the usual therapy, malnutrition despite accessibility to a well-balanced diet, meconium ileus, or a chronic or recurrent nontuberculous lung lesion even in the absence of digestive symptoms.

Nutritional deficiencies, usually multiple, tend to complicate the severe or poorly managed cases of the celiac syndrome. Hypoproteinemia is not uncommon. Hypocalcemia, tetany, or osteoporosis may develop secondary to trapping of dietary calcium by the unabsorbed fatty acids. Hypoprothrombinemia and hemorrhagic tendencies may indicate poor absorption of vitamin K. Deficiencies attributable to poor absorption of vitamins A, D, B complex, or even C may be observed.

685

ABSORPTION OF FAT

A fatty or steatorrheic stool is typical of most forms of the celiac syndrome. Fecal loss of fat may also be increased in congenital bile duct obstruction, in chronic abdominal lymphatic obstruction, and in sprue.

In order to interpret excessive loss of fat in the stools it is essential to have an understanding of the processes of normal fat digestion. This has been divided into three phases (Frazer): (1) intraintestinal emulsification and hydrolysis, (2) passage through the intestinal cells, (3) distribution within the body.

In the intraintestinal phase the food fat, ingested chiefly as triglycerides, first becomes emulsified into submicroscopic particles less than 0.5 μ in diameter. The dispersion mechanism is in the upper intestine, where the essential components are the bile salts from the liver and the fatty acids and monoglycerides derived from the food itself after lipolysis by the pancreatic enzyme. The dispersed food fat is broken down—to great extent if not completely—by the enzymatic hydrolysis, resulting in the liberation of fatty acids, soaps, and glycerine. The effective enzymes are the lipases, which come chiefly from the pancreas but also from the succus entericus. The prolipase normally present in breast milk becomes activated within the stomach and aids in the hydrolysis of breast-milk fat. The long-chained triglycerides such as tributyrin appear to be emulsified chiefly in the lower intestine where the intestinal pH is more alkaline and the pancreatic lipase more active.

In the intestinal wall phase the water-soluble fatty acids are believed to diffuse into the mucosal cells in soluble form, possibly as soaps, whereas the split fats and water-insoluble glycerides are transported directly through the cells as intact globules if dispersed colloidally to a size of less than 0.5 μ in diameter. Choline seems to facilitate both routes of transport. Phospholipids derived from the intestinal cells are believed to alter the interfacial film structure and keep undissolved fat particles finely dispersed after entry into the blood.

Complex dietary fats throw more of a burden on the intestine than do the more soluble short-chained fatty acids in all patients with impaired fat digestion. The dispersion phase seems to be defective in biliary tract obstruction, liver disease with no excretion of bile salts, and cystic fibrosis of the pancreas. This may be corrected therapeutically in part by homogenization of the fat before ingestion or by the addition to the diet of surface-active emulsifying or "solubilizing" agents such as polyoxyethylene sorbitan monooleate (Tween 80). Absorption rather than dispersion would seem to be at fault in most patients with sprue, true celiac disease, gastrocolic fistula, and related disorders. Stool examination shows that the fecal fat is emulsified and much of it is hydrolyzed.

Transitory lipemia normally follows a fatty meal; if it does not, the absorption of emulsified fat particles is usually defective. The chylomicron curve (p. 525) represents a laboratory means for observing this process.

In the distributive phase within the body, the hydrolyzed dissolved fatty acids are routed chiefly through the portal vein system and carried to the liver; unhydrolyzed triglycerides and other lipids reach the general circulation directly by way of the lacteal lymphatic channels.

CYSTIC FIBROSIS OF THE PANCREAS

This entity within the celiac syndrome comprises those cases which have fibrocystic changes in the pancreas and a propensity to chronic lung infections, of familial character. The pancreatic secretions are scanty, viscid, and deficient in all enzymes. Abnormal secretions and morphologic changes homologous to those in the pancreas may occur also in the gastrointestinal mucosa, sweat glands, salivary glands, and other secretory tissues. The stools are steatorrheic and bulky, rich in unabsorbed nutrients, and lacking in proteolytic enzymes (Table 61-1). Appetite is excellent, but growth is retarded. Excessive amounts of electrolytes are found in the sweat (p. 637). The glucose tolerance curve is usually flat. The plasma glycine, vitamin A absorption, and chylomicron curves are subnormal.

Table 61-1. Differential Laboratory Features between Idiopathic Celiac Disease and Cystic Fibrosis of the Pancreas

	Idiopathic celiac disease	*Cystic fibrosis of the pancreas*
Salivary amylase	Normal	Normal
Gastric fluid		
Rate of secretion	Low	Normal
Hydrochloric acid	Usually low	Normal
Pepsin	Low	Normal
Duodenal fluid		
Viscosity	Normal	Increased
Rate of secretion	Normal	Decreased
Trypsin	Normal	None or very low
Amylase	Low or none	None or very low
Lipase	Normal	None or very low
Serum protein (over 6 months of age)	Often low	Normal
Oral glucose tolerance curve	Usually flat	Usually normal
Plasma–vitamin A level	Usually normal	Usually low
Plasma-carotene level	Low	Low
Vitamin A tolerance curve with vitamin A ester	Usually poor	Normal or poor
Trypsin in stool	Present	Absent
Excess fat in stool (after treatment)	Absent	Present

The name "mucoviscidosis" has been proposed to bring out the concept of a general disease. The severity and refractoriness of the pulmonary changes are the most important factors in determining the course and prognosis of the patient under treatment.

Pancreatic fibrosis typically becomes apparent in early infancy. Occasionally the symptoms are apparent at birth as meconium ileus. Conversely, the existence of the condition may not be recognized until the late childhood years.

Gibbs and others have reported several instances of "partial" pancreatic fibrosis, confirmed by autopsy, in which trace amounts of pancreatic enzymes were in the duodenal aspirates and vitamin A absorption curves fell in the low normal range.

The anatomic changes as revealed by autopsy become progressively more advanced with increasing age. The newborn infant usually shows a full complement of acini and ducts, moderately distended with mucus and enveloped by an only slightly thickened fibrous stroma. At this stage the pancreatic secretion may still show traces of enzymatic activity even though its consistency is highly viscid. After the first few months the tissue destruction, cellular infiltration, and fibrous replacement become progressively more prominent and the enzymes are no longer demonstrable. Rarely in either early or late infancy the stools may become so puttylike as actually to obstruct the intestinal lumen.

Mild degrees of dilatation of the pancreatic acini, inspissation of secretion, and flattening of the duct epithelial cells are occasionally found at autopsy in children dying of uremia or sepsis who had had no prior digestive difficulties. The gap is wide between these comparatively slight alterations and the enormously dilated ducts and glands filled with eosinophilic matter and enveloped by fibrous proliferation which constitute the morphologic lesions of true pancreatic cystic fibrosis.

Duodenal Enzymes

Absence of trypsin and increase in viscosity are the most typical abnormalities of the duodenal fluid (Chap. 60). Traces of lipase or amylase are occasionally demonstrable.

Caution must always be applied when interpreting duodenal amylase readings. Low concentrations are found normally in infants in the first months of life. Positive readings in older children with pancreatic fibrosis may be due to salivary amylase which has passed through the stomach without being inactivated. Conversely, when the pancreatic fluid is scanty and weak as occurs typically in pancreatic fibrosis but may at times be induced by other disorders, gastric acid may overbalance the neutrality or alkalinity of the duodenal secretions and, by destroying trace amounts of any enzyme there contained, make a partial pancreatic deficiency appear complete.

Gastrointestinal Features

The most prominent digestive disturbance is the frequent passage of large stools rich in undigested food residues. The odor has been described by di Sant'Agnese and Andersen as being "like stale marigolds." In breast-fed infants the lipase in the human milk along with the traces from the stomach may induce active lipolysis, so that the stools though more abundant may appear normal in color and consistency. With feedings of unskimmed cow's milk the stools are not only large and bulky; 20 to 80 per cent of their total dry weight is undigested fat, giving them a greasy or oily appearance. Later in life the stools may be pale, fatty, mushy, semiliquid, foul-smelling, or frothy, varying with the contents of the diet.

It is suggested that the pediatrician personally inspect one of the patient's stools. Parents are often unaware of abnormal characteristics and may fail to supply necessary information.

The stool fat output becomes diminished when the fat intake is curtailed. Unusual amounts of dietary fat increase the excretion not only of fat but of protein and ash as well. Enteric-coated pancreatin taken by mouth in large amounts may reduce the fecal fat content and total bulk of the feces and improve the absorption of vitamin A. Nutrition becomes adequate only when the diet contains all nutrients in exceptionally large amounts.

Vitamin A deficiency, hypoprothrombinemia, or even osteoporotic undercalcification of the bones may develop unless the poor absorption of the fat-soluble vitamins is compensated for by intakes much higher than normal, in a water-miscible vehicle.

Respiratory Tract

Bronchopulmonary involvement parallels the process in the pancreas and is an integral manifestation of the disease. The respiratory tract symptoms typically begin before 3 months of age though sometimes much later. The bronchial and tracheal glands extrude viscid mucus which accumulates in the air passages. Secondary infection usually supervenes and becomes chronic. *Staphylococcus aureus, Proteus,* or *Pseudomonas aeruginosa* are the usual invading organisms. These are often recoverable from the nose and throat during life and from the lungs in fatal cases. The characteristic lesion at autopsy is that of severe obstructive emphysema and atelectasis, with tenacious mucopurulent or (rarely) mucoid exudate in all air passages. Usually associated is some combination of chronic bronchopneumonia, bronchiolectasis, bronchiectasis, and parenchymal abscesses. However, an occasional patient may experience only minor or minimal lung symptoms for many years, even though pancreatic enzymes are completely absent.

Meconium Ileus

In severely affected infants the meconium may be so inspissated and tightly packed as to block the intestinal lumen, usually in the ileum (p. 710). Fibrosis and calcification in the wall, or even complete obliteration of the lumen, may be associated. The intestine may rupture and give rise to peritonitis, either before or after birth. The diagnosis can be suspected if abdominal roentgenography shows scattered calcified specks. Stenosis or volvulus of the small intestine with obstruction of the lumen may produce similar inspissated meconium. If the disturbance is not due to pancreatic disease, there will be no further difficulty after the obstruction is relieved. If pancreatic fibrosis is responsible, those who survive will later exhibit the absent duodenal enzymes and the other characteristic signs and symptoms.

Glycine Absorption Test

The plasma glycine urine after the feeding of gelatin with its high glycine content has been proposed by Christensen and Schwachman as a diagnostic procedure for the detection of pancreatic fibrosis. This is based on the principle that liberation of amino acids from ingested protein is retarded when pancreatic enzymes are inadequate. Patients with good pancreatic trypsin activity exhibit increases in blood glycine to more than 2.5 times the fasting value, whereas those with no significant enzyme activity do not. This test is more cumbersome than duodenal intubation and of no greater diagnostic value.

Stool Gelatinase Test. See page 707.

Sweat Electrolyte Test. See page 637.

IDIOPATHIC OR TRUE CELIAC DISEASE

This diagnosis is applied to children who, without demonstrable parasitic or anatomic cause, have chronic or recurrent diarrhea and are unable fully to digest fat-containing diets normal for their age. Untreated cases exhibit diarrhea, abdominal distention, poor weight gain, underdeveloped flabby musculature, and retardation of growth. The fundamental defect seems to be that of faulty absorption through the intestinal wall. The disease is often familial; in some families there are other individuals with diabetes mellitus. Symptoms usually develop within the first 2 years. The onset is later in breast-fed infants than in those given cow's-milk formulas. Vomiting rather than diarrhea may be the prominent symptom, should the disturbance first become apparent at 1 or 2 months of age. Multiple nutritional deficiencies may become superimposed if proper therapy is not given. Most of the overt manifestations are remediable by diet. Once treatment is begun and recovery initiated, a prolonged maintenance phase ensues which lasts 1 to many years. Therapy is gradually relaxed as improvement advances.

In many patients, gluten in the diet seems related to the digestive defect. Rapid improvement is often exhibited after wheat and rye are removed from the diet. More often, taking away cow's milk for a time seems to be beneficial.

Pathologic Physiology

In idiopathic celiac disease both trypsin and lipase occur in the duodenal fluid in normal amounts, provided the determinations are made when the patient is not acutely ill or marantic. This is a critical differentiation from cystic fibrosis of the pancreas, in which these enzymes are absent or nearly so. Pancreatic amylase is almost always reduced or even absent, according to Andersen, and may not rise for many years after the symptoms appear to have cleared under dietary therapy.

Much of the flatulence and diarrhea during infancy and early childhood seems attributable to digestive intolerance to starch. Excessive quantities of starch granules can be demonstrated by microscopic examination of a fresh stool in smears stained with Lugol's solution, provided that starch-containing foods are being taken in normal or unusual amounts (p. 697). Symptomatic relief, often complete, attends the change to a low starch diet. Balance studies have shown that both starch and dextrins lower the capacity of the intestine to absorb fats.

Most children with celiac disease also have microscopically or chemically demonstrable steatorrhea while on a normal diet, whether or not diarrhea or grossly fatty stools are evident. Gross steatorrhea when present tends to fade away a few months after therapy is begun. Impaired digestion of fat is often still demonstrable in children over 4 years of age, whether treated or not, whereas intolerance to dietary starch becomes much less prominent after this age.

The serum protein level is usually low when malnutrition is prominent and in extreme situations may be accompanied by edema. This tendency to hypoproteinemia recedes with a change to a high protein diet and clinical recovery. The hypoproteinemia cannot be explained on the basis of nitrogen loss in the feces, which is usually not above normal.

Additional phenomena commonly present in florid untreated cases are gastric hypoacidity; subnormal serum carotene levels; anemia of nutritional character; intestinal hyper- or hypomotility and hyper- or hypotonicity in the roentgenograms; flat glucose tolerance and vitamin A absorption curves; hypoprothrombinemia secondary to poor vitamin K absorption; low chylomicron curve; and osteoporosis despite normal levels of serum calcium and phosphorus and the absence of rickets (Table 61-1). Many children seem to have associated food allergies. Emotional disturbances or acute infection may aggravate the symptoms temporarily.

INFANTILE STEATORRHEA

Infants are seen not infrequently who for their first few months exhibit digestive difficulties, persistent diarrhea, and failure to gain weight. The development of these symptoms may be preceded by an attack of gastroenteritis. The stools contain excess fat, especially when a normal milk mixture is fed. Duodenal enzyme studies often reveal diminished concentrations of trypsin and lipase. Amylase, it will be remembered, is usually low in the duodenal secretions during the first few months of life, so that no conclusions can be drawn from the level of this enzyme.

This disturbance tends to clear spontaneously after the age of 6 months, after which the duodenal enzymes are found at normal levels. The customary treatment consists primarily of feeding of fat-free milk mixtures and removal of fat-containing foods from the diet. Attacks of watery diarrhea and sudden dehydration may be precipitated by an intercurrent upper respiratory infection or a dietary deviation.

PANCREATIC INSUFFICIENCY

Disturbances of the pancreas other than cystic fibrosis are oddities in pediatrics, at least to a degree which is clinically recognizable. One almost never encounters in childhood the acute edema or inflammation of the pancreas leading to the combination of upper abdominal symptoms, obstruction of the ducts, steatorrhea, diminution in duodenal enzymes, and elevation of serum amylase—the "acute pancreatitis" of the internist.

Transitory Depression of Function

Pancreatic function will sometimes become transitorily disturbed in dehydration, in states of ill health, and in infectious diseases. Decrease or absence of one or more pancreatic enzymes may be demonstrable by duodenal intubation even when overt signs of altered pancreatic function are missing. Lipase seems to be the enzyme most commonly depressed. Hyperglycemia, glycosuria, and even acetonuria may appear if the islets of Langerhans are also involved. This toxic depression of pancreatic function, if prolonged, may eventuate rarely in steatorrhea, malnutrition, or the full celiac syndrome. Early diagnosis and therapy are essential for prompt recovery. Therapy consists of the same regimen as with idiopathic celiac disease, along with large doses of pancreatic preparations orally. These measures are relaxed gradually as the patient improves.

Occasionally children with the celiac syndrome may have a selective and permanent deficiency of only one or two of the pancreatic enzymes. Thus the duodenal fluid of an undernourished 13-year-old boy described by Lowe and May had diminished trypsin, lipase within normal range, but no amylase activity at all. The number of reported cases of this type has not been great enough to permit the validation of clinical entities corresponding to different deficiencies. We have seen similar cases.

In 32 children ill with scarlet fever Véghelyi found all three pancreatic enzymes diminished in 14, both trypsin and lipase in 6, trypsin alone in 1, and lipase alone in 5. The lipase was quantitatively the most depressed. All returned to normal by the fourth week. In only two children did clinical symptoms point to inflammation of the pancreas.

McDougall encountered partial and transient supression of duodenal trypsin, lipase, and amylase in four children ill from various causes. In three of these, when the studies were repeated after health was regained, the content of enzymes had returned to normal. A fourth child died without the enzyme studies having been repeated. A fifth child with complete suppression of enzyme activity while ill with a respiratory infection had appreciable return of enzyme activity coincident with clinical recovery.

In the nephrotic syndrome, according to Carpenter and Menten who studied 10 cases, the trypsin and amylase of the duodenal juice are usually reduced in potency. Both the duodenal and gastric secretions are rich in mucus and small in quantity.

In mumps the serum amylase level frequently goes up, but this rise is likely to be due to overflow from the parotids rather than from the pancreas. Symptoms attributable to the pancreas are almost never seen during mumps in children.

Chronic Depression of Function

Among 165 children who had or were suspected of having chronic intestinal disease or fibrocystic disease of the pancreas, McDougall found 25 with suppression of duodenal lipase in conjunction with normal trypsin and amylase. Eighteen other severely malnourished children, mostly infants, exhibited normal duodenal enzyme activity, contrary to the common belief that malnutrition suppresses pancreatic function.

BIBLIOGRAPHY

CYSTIC FIBROSIS OF THE PANCREAS

Baker, H. M., Jr., and S. B. Silverman, Meconium Ileus, Am. J. Dis. Child. 80:803, 1950.

Bodian, M., "Fibrocystic Disease of the Pancreas," Grune & Stratton, Inc., New York, 1953.

Boesen, I., Fat Resorption in Congenital Cystic Fibrosis of the Pancreas in a Child Aged 6 Months, Acta paediat. 37:309, 1949.

Christensen, H. N., and H. Schwachman, Determination of the Plasma Glycine after Gelatin Feeding as a Diagnostic Procedure for Pancreatic Fibrosis, J. Clin. Invest. 28:319, 1949.

Di Sant'Agnese, P. A., Fibrocystic Disease of the Pancreas with Normal or Partial Pancreatic Function, Pediatrics 15:683, 1955.

Gibbs, G. E., W. L. Bostwick, and P. M. Smith, Incomplete Pancreatic Deficiency in Cystic Fibrosis of the Pancreas, J. Pediat. 37:320, 1950.

Goodman, H. O., and S. C. Reed, Heredity of Fibrosis of the Pancreas, Possible Mutation Rate of the Gene, Am. J. Human Genet. 4:59, 1952.

Johnstone, D. E., and E. Neter, Studies on the Laboratory Diagnosis of Cystic Fibrosis of the Pancreas, Pediatrics 7:483, 1951.

Jones, J. A., Congenital Fibrocystic Disease of the Pancreas, Pennsylvania Med. J. 56:559, 1953.

May, C. D., "Cystic Fibrosis of the Pancreas in Infants and Children," Charles C Thomas, Springfield, Ill., 1954.

Richmond, R. C., and *H. Schwachman,* Studies of Fibrocystic Disease of the Pancreas (Mucoviscidosis): Chymotrypsin Activity of Duodenal Fluid, *Pediatrics* 16:207, 1955.

Schwachman, H., H. Luebner, and *P. Catzel,* Mucoviscidosis, *Advances Pediat.* 7:249, 1955.

————, *P. R. Patterson,* and *S. Farber,* Significance of Altered Viscosity of Duodenal Content in Pancreatic Fibrosis (Mucoviscidosis), *Am. J. Dis. Child.* 80:864, 1950.

————, ————, and *J. Laguna,* Studies in Pancreatic Fibrosis: A Simple Diagnostic Gelatin Film Test for Stool Trypsin, *Pediatrics* 4:222, 1949.

Webster, R., and *H. Williams,* Hepatic Cirrhosis Associated with Fibrocystic Disease of the Pancreas: Clinical and Pathological Reports of Five Patients, *Arch. Dis. Childhood* 28:343, 1953.

Wolman, I. J., Cystic Fibrosis of the Pancreas, *Am. J. M. Sc.* 203:900, 1942.

Zuelzer, W. W., and *W. A. Newton, Jr.,* The Pathogenesis of Fibrocystic Disease of the Pancreas: A Study of 36 Cases with Special Reference to the Pulmonary Lesions, *Pediatrics* 4:53, 1949.

APPROACHES TO STUDY OF THE CELIAC SYNDROME

Anfanger, H., and *R. M. Heavenrich,* Amino Acid Tolerance Tests in Children, *Am. J. Dis. Child.* 77:425, 1949.

Chung, A. W., S. Morales, S. E. Snyderman, J. M. Lewis, and *L. E. Holt, Jr.,* Studies in Steatorrhea: Effect of the Level of Dietary Fat upon the Absorption of Fat and Other Foodstuffs in Idiopathic Celiac Disease and Cystic Fibrosis of the Pancreas, *Pediatrics* 7:491, 1951.

Frazer, A. C., Aetiology of Steatorrhoea, *Brit. M. J.* 2:641, 1947.

Gibbs, G. E., Secretin Tests with Bilumen Gastroduodenal Drainage in Infants and Children, *Pediatrics* 5:941, 1950.

Lelong, M., J. Colin, and *C. Polonovski,* Les Stéatorrhées infantiles: Leur caractérisation, *Arch. franç. pédiat.* 10:561, 1953.

Nothman, M. M., The Value of Functional Tests for the Diagnosis of Diseases of the Pancreas, *Ann. Int. Med.* 34:1358, 1951.

Véghelyi, P. V., Pancreatic Enzymes: Normal Output and Comparison of Different Methods of Assay, *Pediatrics* 3:749, 1949.

CELIAC DISEASE

Andersen, D. H., Celiac Syndrome. VI. The Relationship of Celiac Disease, Starch Intolerance, and Steatorrhea, *J. Pediat.* 30:564, 1947.

———— and *P. A. Di Sant'Agnese,* Idiopathic Celiac Disease. I. Mode of Onset and Diagnosis, *Pediatrics* 11:207, 1953.

Dicke, W. K., H. A. Weijers, and *J. H. van de Kamer,* Coeliac Disease. II. The Presence in Wheat of a Factor Having a Deleterious Effect in Cases of Coeliac Disease, *Acta paediat.* 42:34, 1953.

Di Sant'Agnese, P. A., Idiopathic Celiac Disease. II. Course and Prognosis, *Pediatrics* 11:224, 1953.

Emery, J. L., Carbohydrate Metabolism in the Coeliac Syndrome, *Arch. Dis. Childhood* 22:41, 1947.

Gibbs, G. E., Effect of Pancreatin on Plasma Vitamin A Curves in the Celiac Syndrome, *Pediatrics* 6:593, 1950.

Sheldon, W., and *A. MacMahon,* Studies in Coeliac Disease: Fat Absorption, *Arch. Dis. Childhood* 24:245, 1949.

Weijers, H. A., and J. H. van de Kamer, Coeliac Disease. III. Excretion of Unsaturated and Saturated Fatty Acids by Patients with Coeliac Disease, Acta paediat. 42:97, 1953.

MISCELLANEOUS

Carpenter, A. M., and M. L. Menten, Studies on Nephrosis: Quantitative Changes in Enzymes of the Gastroduodenal Fluids, Am. J. Clin. Path. 20:619, 1950.

Chaptel, J., C. Benezech, D. Brunel, R. Jean, and E. de Marmier, Syndrome coeliaque du nourrisson et lambliase intestinale: Etude métabolique, Arch. franç pédiat. 9:148, 1952.

Davis, M. L., and W. M. Kelsey, Chronic Pancreatitis in Childhood, A.M.A. Am. J. Dis. Child. 81:687, 1951.

Garaguso, P., and R. Labourdette, Tratamiento de la giardiasis en la infancia, Prensa pediat. 4:77, 1953.

Hinden, E., Meconium Ileus with No Pancreatic Abnormality, Arch. Dis. Childhood 25:99, 1950.

James, T., Chronic Pancreatitis in Childhood, Arch. Dis. Childhood 27:364, 1952.

Lowe, C. U., and C. D. May, Selective Pancreatic Deficiency: Absent Amylase. Diminished Trypsin, and Normal Lipase, A.M.A. Am. J. Dis. Child. 82:459. 1951.

Madey, S., and J. Dancis, Proteolytic Enzymes of the Premature Infant with Special Reference to His Ability to Digest Unsplit Protein Food, Pediatrics 4:177, 1949.

McDougall, C., Clinical Evaluation of Abnormal Enzyme Content in the Pancreatic Juice of Children, Pediatrics 5:114, 1950.

Merliss, R. R., and A. Hoffman, Steatorrhea Following the Use of Antibiotics, New England J. Med. 245:328, 1951.

Mithoefer, J., Pseudocyst of Pancreas in Childhood, Pediatrics 8:534, 1951.

Véghelyi, P. V., Giardiasis, Am. J. Dis. Child. 59:793, 1940.

————, Secondary Pancreatitis, Am. J. Dis. Child. 74:45, 1947.

————, Pancreatic Function in Scarlet Fever, Pediatrics 4:94, 1949; correction 4:824, 1949.

CHAPTER 62

Colon: Stools

INTESTINAL MOTILITY IN INFANCY AND CHILDHOOD

In the small intestine the mixture of food and gastrointestinal secretions is highly dilute. Most of the water is reabsorbed within the colon, leaving a semisolid pasty food residue for evacuation. Factors which contribute to the rate of laxation are length of the intestine, rapidity of movements, efficiency of water absorption, irritant food materials, quantity and consistency of fecal residues, and inflammatory and other stimuli acting on the intestinal walls.

Personal studies of more than 1,000 infants receiving a variety of cow's-milk mixtures gave the following mean values for laxation rate per day:

Age (months)	Laxation rate	Age (months)	Laxation rate	Age (months)	Laxation rate
1 *	2.67	5	2.28	9	1.97
2	2.63	6	2.27	10	1.82
3	2.41	7	2.29	11	1.75
4	2.37	8	2.02	12	1.72

* Infants aged 3 and 4 weeks only.

The usual period required for food to pass through the entire alimentary tract, as measured with carmine markers, has been found to range from 9 to 20 hours in the first year of life, 10 to 24 hours in the second year, and 20 to 48 hours in the older child and adult. These differences in total passage time between infants and adults can be ascribed chiefly to longer retention in the colon after infancy.

COMPOSITION OF STOOLS

Water and Solids

The stools of normal children exhibit wide variations in composition. With 18 normal children aged 4 to 12 years studied by Macy, the wet weight of the stools ranged from 77 to 117 gm per day, the dry weight from 15 to 21 gm. The fecal content of water averaged 74 to 84 per cent and was not related to the water intake.

With 11 normal infants aged 2 to 6 months Andersen observed the wet

696

weight of 24-hour stools to range from 6.6 to 37.0 gm, average 17.2 gm. The dry weight ranged from 2.0 to 5.7 gm and averaged 4.1 gm. With 11 children 2 to 6 years of age the average wet weight was 25.7 gm and the range 6.6 to 48.5 gm; the average dry weight was 6.6 gm and the range 2.0 to 12.9 gm. Fat constituted about 22 per cent (average) of the dry weight of the stools of younger infants, 17.6 per cent of those aged 6 to 12 months, and 14 per cent of children aged 1 to 6 years.

Nitrogen

The fecal content of nitrogen is derived from cellular debris, mucosal secretions, undigested food residue, and bacterial products. The normal child excretes a little over 1 gm of nitrogen per day in the stools as measured by the Kjeldahl procedure; of this about one-half is due to bacteria and one-fourth to protein. Nitrogen excretion is practically uninfluenced by the amount of protein ingested but can be made to increase by a diet high in unabsorbable residue. Studies of amino acid excretion by Ross with paper chromatography have indicated that in the stools of breast-fed infants the amino acids are free and abundant, whereas in stools from infants receiving cow's milk the amino acids tend to be combined with each other or other substances. This may be the result of differences in intestinal flora.

Electrolyte Content

In seven children 8 to 12 years of age studied by Macy, the average total excretion of Zn was 10.5 mg and of Fe 8.7 mg. Ca, Mg, Na, and K together constituted about 7 per cent of the total weight of the fecal solids, and P, Cl, and S another 3 per cent.

Particles

On microscopy a fresh normal stool diluted with saline solution appears to consist chiefly of bacterial bodies, debris, and undigested food fragments. Leukocytes, yeast cells, erythrocytes, and fatty acid crystals may also be seen. Eosinophils and Charcot-Leyden crystals may appear in ulcerative colitis, intestinal parasitism, and allergic gastroenteritis.

Muscle fragments and elastic and connective tissue fibers become abundant when the meat intake is excessive or protein digestion poor. Muscle fragments are cylindrical or oval; even when partly digested they retain the distinctive property of taking a red color when a weak eosin solution is added. Elastic tissue fibers branch and anastamose, whereas connective tissue fibers appear as colorless pale-yellow mats; both varieties become more distinct when glacial acetic acid is added to the wet preparation.

STARCHES

About 20 per cent of the intake of the higher vegetable carbohydrates and starches is excreted more or less intact into the stools, usually in undigested vegetable cells.

Starch granules when not digested take on a blue or blue-black color if iodine is added to the stool specimen; when partly digested they appear red. The clinical significance is much greater when they occur free than when in intact vegetable cells. They appear in unusual amounts in young infants given feedings of granule-containing cereals, since digestive efficiency for starch is normally incompletely developed in the first 6 months of life. Dusting powder from the perianal skin may be a source of starch found in the stools in infants.

Stool Test for Starch Digestion

The child should have a liberal intake of potato, bread, and farina or some similar breakfast cereal for 1 or 2 days, and the stool should then be examined for starch granules.

The so-called precooked infant cereals are not satisfactory for this test. The manufacturing process reduces the contained starch to amorphous particles, which are difficult to recognize even when excreted abundantly.

PROCEDURE. Add a small particle of fresh feces to a large drop of water or normal saline solution on a glass slide and mix thoroughly with a wooden applicator. Stir in 1 or 2 drops of Lugol's solution (resublimed iron 5 gm; potassium iodide, CP, 10 gm; distilled water 100 ml). Cover with a cover glass pressed down. Examine with both low and high power of microscope after a few minutes.

The quantity of organized granules present is noted (amorphous starch is difficult to recognize with certainty). The granules often occur in intracellular and extracellular clumps. The report is described as follows: *None* (less than 1 per low-power field); *scanty* (1 to 5 per low-power field); *moderate numbers* (6 to 20 per field); *abundant* (over 20 per field).

FECAL FATS

More than half of the lipid in any normal stool is fatty acids and soaps, and the remainder is a mixture of unsaponifiable sterols and free neutral fats. Most of this lipid seems to be derived from the intestinal mucosa since even in starvation or with a fat-free intake the stool will contain fat—0.5 to 3.0 gm a day in an adult. For example, in Macy's 18 children above 4 years of age the daily excretion of stool lipids averaged 2.3 gm, well under 10 per cent of the total fat intake. The output of unassimilated fat rises when the intake of fats, especially those with high melting points, becomes excessive.

Because successive stools from the same individual can exhibit wide variation of fat content even with a constant intake, balance studies will have little validity unless based on a pooled specimen from at least a 3-day period and preferably longer.

In infancy the percentage of fat in the stool is greater than in older children. The infants studied by Holt and associates excreted an average of about 45 per cent of the amount ingested during the first month, and about 33 per cent in the sixth month. Breast milk yielded about 1 gm of combined fats (soaps) in the stool each day, whereas butterfat gave approximately twice that excretion. In Andersen's studies the stool fat of infants receiving an evaporated-milk mixture averaged 0.8 gm a day (range 0.3 to 1.3 gm); of children up to 6 years of age, 1 gm a day (range, 0.3 to 1.8 gm).

In premature infants both the splitting and absorption of fat are highly variable and much less efficient. In Söderhjelm's study of 17 premature infants receiving cow's-milk mixtures about 60 per cent of the milk fat was retained whether the milk was boiled, pasteurized, or homogenized. With 12 other infants receiving breast milk the absorption varied from 78 to 99.7 per cent, with no differences elicited by prior boiling of the milk.

Breast-milk fat seems to be absorbed more efficiently than the butterfat of cow's milk, presumably because of its higher content of unsaturated and short-chained fatty acids. Olive oil resembles breast-milk fat in this respect, as do many other vegetable fats such as those from the palm, cocoanut, soybean, and peanut; hence the rationale for employing these in modified milk mixtures developed for infant feeding.

Steatorrhea and Celiac Syndrome

In most of the disorders comprised in the celiac syndrome, and particularly during the advanced stages, the amount of fat lost in the stool is greater than normal. Current opinion holds that the absolute amount of fat excreted is not as significant physiologically as is the amount relative to that which is ingested. When facilities are available the quantities of fat both ingested and excreted within a reasonable period are measured quantitatively and the results appraised according to the following ratio:

$$\frac{\text{Gm fat ingested} - \text{gm fat excreted}}{\text{gm fat ingested}} \times 100$$
$$= \text{coefficient of absorption (expressed in \%)}$$

In states of health, after the first few months of life, over 90 per cent of the intake is ordinarily well absorbed. In true celiac disease the coefficient of absorption is generally between 60 and 90 per cent. Exact values depend largely upon the quantity and quality of the dietary fat and the severity of symptoms at the time of the test. In cystic fibrosis of the pancreas the coefficient of absorption can range from 20 to 80 per cent on diets with a normal content of fat.

Increasing the intake of fatty foods when fat digestion is not at top efficiency is accompanied usually by an absolute augmentation of absorption. Conversely, with a diet practically devoid of fat the stool will still contain detectable amounts because of the endogenous excretion.

Simple Stool Test for Fat Digestion

Direct microscopic examination of random fecal material, when performed and interpreted properly, can yield most valuable information regarding the efficiency of fat digestion. Quantitative chemical analysis of stools for fat, even though newer techniques have reduced the number of manipulations considerably, is still too elaborate for routine use and has the disadvantage also of requiring at least a total 3-day specimen. It is important, however, when planning a stool study of a child with suspected steatorrhea to give whole milk and an appreciable amount of fatty foods for 1 or 2 days beforehand. When the capacity to utilize fats is extremely defective, the complete removal of all fats from the diet including a change to fat-free milk will result in stools containing only a normal amount of fat.

PROCEDURE. Place one large drop (1 to 2 mm in diameter) of 36% acetic acid on a glass slide. Add a small particle of fresh feces with a wooden applicator and mix thoroughly. Stir in a few drops of Sudan III or scarlet red solution (dye 1 gm; 70% alcohol 250 ml; acetone 250 ml). Cover with cover glass pressed down. Heat slide gently over a low flame until bubbles appear. Examine with low- and high-power magnifications of microscope before and after heating.

The proportion of fat is estimated from the number and size of the stained particles. Neutral fat appears as rounded globules. These are yellow (Sudan III), deep orange-red or scarlet-red and melt when the slide is warmed; on cooling their margins become more sharply defined. In the cooled preparation the fatty acids crystallize as amorphous flakes or sheaves of long straight or short curved needles which stain faintly if at all. Soaps (chiefly calcium salts of the fatty acids) occur as short plump coarse crystals or yellowish round or irregular opaque masses that do not melt or take the stain. Cod-liver oil, mineral oil, or castor oil give droplets which may be confused with those of neutral fat but stain less deeply.

Fatty acid crystals and soaps are found almost always when fat globules are in abundance, regardless of the presence or absence of pancreatic disease. The percentage of split fat tends to be higher in true celiac disease than in pancreatic fibrosis.

Reports may be expressed as follows: *Normal content* (no more than 4 or 5 droplets and fatty acid crystals per low-power field); *moderate increase* (6 to 50); *marked increase* (too many to count).

BACTERIA

About 50 per cent of the usual fecal specimen consists of living and dead bacteria of many kinds. Counts of colonies on culture plates do not portray accurately the relative frequency of the various species within the body since the rates of growth of individual bacteria on artificial media are far from the same. Microscopy of stained smears would seem a more direct approach to the comparative appraisal of Gram-positive and Gram-negative organisms, but most dead Gram-positive intestinal bacteria stain Gram-negatively in fecal smears.

When breast milk is fed exclusively the stool organisms seem to be at least 90 per cent *Lactobacillus acidophilus* and *Bacillus bifidus* (these may be variant forms of the same Gram-positive species). With cow's-milk mixtures the Gram-positive and Gram-negative organisms seem about equal, with no one organism dominant. Lactobacilli are scanty or not evident, and the stool flora seem to consist largely of coliform organisms, nonhemolytic streptococci and other micrococci, clostridia, bacteroides, and yeast.

The higher ratio of lactose to protein in breast milk is believed to favor the growth of lactose fermenters and thereby produce enough acidity in the intestinal environment to suppress the growth of coliform strains. With cow's-milk feedings the longer-chained amino acid polymers which reach the colon seem to encourage the coliform flora.

Coliform organisms become established in all newborn infants during the first days of life, but are soon supplanted by lactobacilli when breast milk is given. In gastroenteritis there seems to be a marked shift toward a wholly Gram-negative intestinal flora.

The hydrogen-ion concentration of the stool tends to have a pH range 4.5 to 6.5 in breast-fed infants and 5.0 to 8.5 in those artificially fed. Stools with values lower than pH 6 tend to have an "acid" odor, higher than pH 7 a "fecal" odor.

The most important use of stool bacteriology in clinical practice is to search for pathogenic microorganisms when infectious gastroenteritis is suspected. Most bacterial enteric infections are caused by strains of Shigella or Salmonella. Streptococcus, Staphylococcus, Proteus, Pseudomonas, colon bacillus, or paracolon or Klebsiella organisms sometimes seem responsible. These usually have to be sought for with selective techniques which inhibit the growth of the nonpathogens. Tuberculous enteritis is rare in this country. Some epidemics of gastroenteritis seem to have a viral origin.

Another application of stool bacteriology is to control the effectiveness of reduction of fecal bacteria prior to intestinal surgery by antibacterial drugs. Streptomycin, the broad-spectrum antibiotics, polymyxin B, and nonabsorbable sulfonamides are employed for this purpose, singly or in combination, given orally.

After the first 1 or 2 days of oral antibacterial therapy the susceptible strains no longer multiply. The stools may be unusually bulky for the first few days and then tend to become small and constipated. That the bacteria are inhibited rather than killed can be demonstrated by culturing serial dilutions of the stools. As the antibacterial therapy continues for more than a few days the resistant organisms—Proteus and

Pseudomonas bacilli, yeasts, fecal streptococci and other micrococci, and Aerobacter at times—begin to proliferate in large numbers. The yeast *Candida albicans* often proliferates excessively during such therapy and may give rise to proctitis, stomatitis, or vaginitis (p. 931). Or a resistant staphylococcus may stir up a serious enteritis and diarrhea (p. 821).

The urobilinogen content of the feces and urine declines rapidly during oral antibacterial therapy, while the bilirubin mounts reciprocally. Quantitative studies of urobilinogen excretion have no reliability at these times (p. 348).

Many fecal strains of Pseudomonas, Proteus, and other stool bacteria have the biologic property of liquefying gelatin. Their presence in large numbers may lead to weakly positive film tests in the absence of pancreatic trypsin (p. 708).

FECAL BILE PIGMENTS

The color of the stool is due largely to bile pigment derivatives. Pigments from food residues (e.g., milk, spinach, beets, carrots, squash, chocolate, cocoa) and unabsorbed drugs (e.g., iron, bismuth, calomel) will sometimes influence the color.

Intermediary Metabolism

Bilirubin is excreted by the liver as sodium bilirubinate. This does not undergo any chemical alteration in the gallbladder or small intestine. Once the large intestine is reached, however, decomposition by bacteria begins. By way of the intermediary pigments *mesobilirubin* and *mesobilirubinogen* the sodium bilirubinate becomes converted into the almost colorless *stercobilinogen* or *fecal urobilinogen*. In the terminal colon or after passage of the stool the fecal urobilinogen becomes oxidized by the intestinal bacteria to orange-yellow *urobilin* (known also as *stercobilin*).

The content of urobilinogen and related pigments in the stool can be measured with a fair degree of quantitative accuracy by means of the Ehrlich aldehyde reagent.

The intestinal mucosa and portal vein system absorb a significant moiety of the urobilinogenic substances formed in the colon, thereby initiating the so-called enterohepatic-renal circulation of urobilinogen. On reaching the liver the absorbed urobilinogen is filtered out by the parenchymal cells, where some is metabolized and the rest reexcreted into the bile. Most healthy infants and children, unlike adults, rarely have urobilinogenuria. The normal urinary output is well under 1 mg a day; it ceases altogether when absorption of urobilinogen from the colon is diminished, and also in severe hypochromic anemia with its reduced production and destruction of erythrocytes. Conversely, urinary urobilinogen becomes comparatively abundant when hemodestruction is excessive or when hepatic function is inadequate (p. 348).

In the first few days of life, until the intestinal flora is well established, the stool pigment consists almost entirely of bilirubin. Fecal urobilinogen begins to make its appearance in appreciable amounts at about the third day in infants given cow's-milk mixtures, but not until the second week or even later in breast-fed infants.

The fecal conversion of bilirubin to urobilinogen seems to proceed much more slowly when the predominating fecal organisms are the Gram-positive lactobacilli, as in breast-fed infants or in older children given large amounts of carbohydrates with acidophilus milk; or when the Gram-negative intestinal flora are inhibited by antibiotics or nonabsorbable sulfonamides given orally.

The study by Tat, Greenwalt, and Dameshek on 30 normal newborn infants gave the following daily outputs for fecal bilirubin: first to fifth day, 1 to 23 mg, average 8.6 mg; sixth to tenth days, 0 to 16 mg, average 5.7 mg; tenth to fifteenth days, 0.3 to 12.4 mg, average 5.3 mg. The fecal urobilinogen in this interval was minimal, up to 0.7 mg per day.

Bilirubin disappears from the stools between the third and twelfth months after undergoing wide day-to-day fluctuations. Its daily excretion during this period rarely exceeds 15 mg a day. The stool urobilinogen in most normal infants is usually between 3 and 5 mg per day, but occasionally may be as high as 20 mg.

The fecal urobilinogen output rises with age. The average output per day for normal children 1 to 5 years of age is about 10 mg; for those 6 to 10 years of age, about 25 mg; for adolescents 11 to 15 years of age, about 45 mg. For adults the accepted range is 40 to 230 mg.

Obstructive Disorders

The stool is practically free of urobilinogen and bilirubin in complete obstruction of the bile passages, and often in severe cirrhosis of the liver or viral hepatitis. Trace amounts may appear when the blood bilirubin is high as the consequence of desquamation of icteric mucus and cells from the intestinal mucosa.

Hemodestructive Disorders

When blood destruction is unusually rapid, as in erythroblastosis fetalis, hereditary spherocytosis, active sickle cell anemia, and other hemolytic anemias, the output of fecal bile pigments rises to many times the normal. The day-to-day excretion is irregular even when the patient's blood picture and clinical signs are comparatively stable.

With three infants having erythroblastosis fetalis, total outputs of 19.4 to 109 mg per day of stool pigments were noted by Tat and associates. With five infants having assorted hemodestructive disorders Mills and Mason found a mean daily output of 15 mg (range 0.07 to 37 mg). With 15 children aged 1 to 14 years the mean was 188, with a range from 72 to 1,400 mg. Daily excretions up to 2,000 mg per day are not unusual during hemolytic episodes. When carrying out studies on such patients, one may encounter misleadingly low values if antibiotics which inhibit bacterial conversion of bilirubin to urobilinogen are being administered concurrently.

THE HEMOLYTIC INDEX. The output of bile pigments reflects the absolute rate of hemoglobin destruction, which in turn is proportional to the quantity of circulating hemoglobin in the body and indirectly to blood volume. This relationship is portrayed in the so-called hemolytic index:

$$\frac{\text{Total daily excretion of urobilinogen and bilirubin (mg)} \times 100}{\text{total circulating hemoglobin (gm)}}$$

$$= \text{hemolytic index}$$

The total circulating hemoglobin is calculated from the blood volume (estimated from body weight—see p. 594) and the grams of hemoglobin per 100 ml of blood.

The hemolytic index permits one to compare the rates of erythrocyte destruction in individuals of different ages, body weights, and blood volumes or in the same individual under varying conditions. For example, a 24-hour pigment excretion totaling 50 mg in a child may signify excessive red cell destruction when the blood hemoglobin level is only 4 mg per 100 mg, but may be within normal limits when the level is 12 mg. The index is useful also for evaluating possible benefits from any specific therapy, by contrasting the rates of excretion before and after such therapy.

MELENA

Blood in the stools in childhood can have its origin anywhere in the gastrointestinal tract from lips to anus. The quantity necessary to impart a black tarry or red appearance (melena) ranges from 3 to 10 ml in the infant to between 50 and 100 ml in the mature adult. In nursing infants the source of the melena may be a mother's cracked and bleeding nipple. With lesser degrees of gastrointestinal bleeding it becomes necessary to employ chemical tests for the recognition of occult blood in stools with a normal appearance. Blood originating in the stomach will still react with the diagnostic reagents except when in minimal amounts. In the newborn period the stools often give positive reactions, as the result presumably of capillary oozing from the intestinal mucosa.

Melena may be simulated by the gray-black color given to the stools by iron or bismuth medication or the deep red color which attends the liberal ingestion of beets. Most normal stools become black on the surface after exposure to the air for several hours, but will be found to retain the normal yellow-brown in the interior.

A positive finding of blood in the stools, especially if persistent, calls for a thorough survey of the patient by sigmoidoscopy, gastrointestinal radiography, and study of the efficiency of the blood coagulation mechanisms.

Repeated stool studies for occult blood are advisable with every patient who has persistent anemia of the iron-deficiency type without obvious cause. We recall such an anemic child in whom a positive stool test led to the discovery that he sucked vigorously every night on a chronic fissure in one finger. In anaphylactoid purpura, occult blood in the stools is found in one-third of the cases.

Recognition of Source of Bleeding

When the bleeding site is at or near the anus, as a rectal fissure, polyp, hemorrhoid, inserted foreign body, or recurrent sigmoid intussusception, bright or dark-red streaks adhere to the outside of or are coarsely blended with the stool. When the site is in the large intestine or when small intestinal bleeding is profuse, the stool will be bright red. With minor small intestinal bleeding or lesions in the duodenum or higher the stool becomes a uniform tarry black if the blood content is abundant.

A Meckel's diverticulum with an ulceration secondary to ectopic gastric mucosa will often reveal itself by the painless sudden passage of a stool which is largely blood. The appearance may be brick red or bright red when the bleeding is profuse. When this condition is suspected, a digital rectal examination will usually withdraw feces with the brick-red color which is almost diagnostic. Occasionally a child may become pale and listless or even collapse before the hemorrhage is apparent. Chronic anemia can result from persistent mild oozing. Soon after the onset of acute intussusception or volvulus the stools may consist of fecal matter intermingled with bloody mucus.

Polyps, hemangiomas, bowel duplications, systemic diseases, and recurrent intussusceptions are more prone to cause recurrent small hemorrhages. In blood dyscrasias the bleeding or clotting or prothrombin times are apt to be prolonged and hematologic abnormalities or hemorrhages elsewhere may guide one to the correct explanation for the blood loss. The possibility of food allergy or of liver disease must be considered in the differential diagnosis.

In bacterial gastroenteritis or ulcerative colitis with erosions or ulcers of the colon mucosa, flecks of blood and pus are passed with fair consistency. Typical stools are watery, unformed, green, increased in number, and contain incompletely digested food particles. The mucus content is usually in excess.

Ulcers, varices, or more uncommon lesions of the esophagus, stomach, or duodenum are often accompanied by vomiting of black "coffee-ground" material or frank blood. Vomiting is ordinarily not seen with bleeding lesions below the ligament of Treitz except when there is complete intestinal obstruction with fecal vomiting or an ulcer near the stoma of a gastroenterostomy. Esophagoscopy or roentgen study of the esophagus is in order when local varices are suspected.

The sudden passage of a large blood-containing stool which appears to originate in the upper gastrointestinal tract should initiate a train of studies to ascertain the cause of bleeding. It must always be remembered that lesions can be multiple and that an obvious hemorrhoid or rectal fissure is not necessarily the major source of the bleeding. Severe liver disease should be suspected when a gastrointestinal hemorrhage is associated with defective coagulation in a child who is not a hemophiliac or has no other detectable blood disturbance.

Tests for Blood in Feces

The approved procedures are based on color reactions with the heme portion of the hemoglobin or its breakdown products. All tests must be made exactly as directed.

Positive reactions with the highly sensitive benzidine or its derivative orthotolidine are given not only by extravasated blood itself but also by the peroxidase of leukocytes, any meat or fish particles still containing blood pigments, and at times even by the red cells which diapedese through the mucosa during lively intestinal peristalsis. A positive reading with these reagents is therefore not deemed significant unless the patient is free from colitis and has had no meat or fish for at least 3 days preceding the test. When blood dilutions are added to stool in vitro, clear-cut positive reactions in 60 seconds will be given by orthotolidine to blood in 1:100,000 dilution, by benzidine to 1:20,000 dilution; and by gum guaiac to 1:5,000 dilution. Prior exposure of the blood to digestive enzymes reduces these sensitivities considerably. The benzidine and guaiac tests do not give positive reactions when ferrous medications are being taken, but orthotolidine may do so.

Gum guaiac is the least sensitive of the reagents mentioned and therefore the most satisfactory. It does not react with meat residues or most medications, and hence preliminary preparation of the patient is not necessary. Normal subjects on an unrestricted diet show faintly positive reactions to guaiac after the ingestion of 2 to 3 ml of blood.

A negative chemical reaction for blood does not necessarily exclude a bleeding lesion when other evidence favors its presence. Digested blood which no longer reacts with specific reagents may be detectable by spectroscopic examination of a stool extract for the absorption bands of porphyrin.

CHEMICAL TESTS FOR OCCULT BLOOD. 1. Smear a little fecal matter on clean filter paper with a tongue depressor or a gloved finger after rectal examination.

2. If using benzidine dihydrochloride, add 3 to 4 drops of a 1 per cent solution. [This is made by dissolving 1 mg of purified benzidine dihydro-

chloride (Merck) in 20 ml of glacial acetic acid, and then mixing with 30 ml of distilled water and 50 ml of 95 per cent ethyl alcohol. The solution will keep for many months at room temperature if stored in a brown bottle.] A color reaction varying from light green (trace) to dark blue (large amount) will appear in 1 to 5 minutes if the stool contains blood.

3. If using gum guaiac, add in succession 2 drops each of (1) saturated 95 per cent alcoholic solution of gum guaiac (will keep for at least a month), (2) glacial acetic acid, and (3) fresh hydrogen peroxide kept refrigerated in a brown bottle. A faint-blue color developing within a few minutes indicates a trace amount of blood, whereas an immediate deep blue represents an abundant amount. A faint green without any blue component or any other delayed color change can be due to iron or other substances and may be disregarded.

4. One should check a doubtful reaction to benzidine dihydrochloride with gum guaiac, and vice versa, bearing in mind that the former reagent is much more sensitive. With trace amounts of blood the benzidine test may be positive and the guaiac test negative; this finding must raise doubt as to the clinical significance of the positive benzidine reaction and is best ignored unless there is gastrointestinal disease or other hemorrhagic phenomena.

5. It is wise always to carry out two control tests: (1) a "blank" or "negative" control using the reagents on the filter paper preferably with some normal stool added, and (2) a "positive" control with a dilute aqueous solution of blood.

Melena in the Newborn

Apt introduced blood into the stomachs of newborn infants and found that at least 35 ml of blood was usually required to give the meconium a bloody appearance. In contrast, with infants a few days old whose meconium had already been evacuated, only 10 ml was sufficient. Guaiac tests with stools from 35 normal newborn infants were all negative.

Apt and Downey have proposed a simple approach based on the presence or absence of fetal hemoglobin (p. 108), to differentiate maternal from infant blood in a grossly bloody stool. One milliliter of a 1 per cent solution of sodium hydroxide is added to 5 ml of a centrifuged suspension of stool. After 2 minutes, if the blood comes from the baby and contains alkali-resistant fetal hemoglobin, the supernatant will retain a distinct pink tint. If the hemoglobin in the stool is of maternal origin, as from a bleeding nipple, the supernatant will turn yellow-brown within 2 minutes. This alkali denaturation test is not reliable if the stool is tarry rather than bloody.

GELATINASE (TRYPSIN; PROTEASE)

Enzymes derived from the gastrointestinal mucosa occur in normal stools in inconstant amounts. A comparatively simple screening test for pancreatic fibrosis is based on the absence from the stools of proteolytic gelatinase, one manifestation of pancreatic tryptic activity.

Test for Gelatinase (Trypsin)

1. Mix serially 1 ml of fresh unconstipated feces with sterile water or saline solution to make 1:1, 1:10, and 1:100 suspensions.

2. Place separate large drops (approximately 0.1 ml) of each dilution well mixed on a 3 × 8 cm strip of unfixed gelatin x-ray or photographic film. The sensitivity of the film to weak trypsin solutions should be established by control studies. The film edges may be stapled to cardboard to prevent curling. The back of the film at the spots where the test material is to be placed may be scraped to make the readings easier.

3. As control, prepare similar stool suspensions from a normal infant or use a standard weak trypsin solution.

4. Incubate the films at 37°C for 1 hour or (less preferably) at warm room temperature for 1½ to 2 hours, covered by an inverted flat glass dish to prevent drying.

5. Wash the film surfaces with a cold stream of water. Gentle rubbing may help to dislodge loosened gelatin. With incomplete gelatin liquefaction the gelatin may appear opaque but not wash off or appear transparent.

6. Complete clearing of the film areas is designated as 4 plus; intermediate degrees are 3 plus, 2 plus, and 1 plus. If the suspensions have dried during the incubation the test should be repeated.

7. No pancreatic preparations should be given for at least 3 days prior. Enzymes from melon or pineapple in the diet or from contaminating urine may give positive stool reactions. Sanitary precautions should be employed when dealing with stools from cases of suspected enteric infections.

The positive gelatin film reaction can be a helpful adjunct in ruling out the presence of pancreatic fibrosis. Occasional infants with pancreatic fibrosis have a diminished rather than absent pancreatic production of gelatinase, and their stools may give a weakly positive reaction. Constipation or obstipation may give rise to negative results in older children whose pancreatic secretions are normal, through destruction of the enzyme by intestinal bacteria. When slow movement of feces is responsible the giving of a laxative will make such stools become positive; with pancreatic fibrosis they remain negative.

Large numbers of gelatin-liquefying strains of Proteus, Pseudomonas, or other coliform bacteria in the intestines or stools are capable of giving rise to weakly positive film reactions. A positive reaction in the 1:100 suspension is strong evidence for good pancreatic function, since few fecal organisms can produce enough enzyme to liquefy gelatin in that dilution. When, however, the test is positive in only the 1:10 dilution the following differential steps have been suggested: (1) The fecal specimen should be studied bacteriologically for the presence of gelatin-liquefying bacteria. (2) A suspension of twice the minimal concentration of the stool specimen which yields a clearly positive gelatin film test may be mixed with equal amounts of a solution containing 2 mg per liter of soybean trypsin inhibitor, and the test repeated. Complete inhibition of gelatin liquefaction by trypsin inhibitor is indicative of human trypsin rather than bacterial enzymes.

In doubtful situations there is no substitute for duodenal drainage and study of the enzymatic content of the aspirated fluid. Film tests can be carried out with duodenal fluid if more accurate methods of chemical analysis are not available or if immediate information is desired.

ULCERATIVE COLITIS

In the active phases of this disease the stools, which number 2 to 20 per day, are typically liquid or semisolid and contain mucus, pus, and blood cells. Clots indicative of hemorrhage are sometimes seen and may be abundant. With active inflammation in the rectal region the exterior of the stool may be streaked with blood-stained mucus. Microscopic study may reveal an excess of fat, starches, or meat particles to signify poor food digestion.

The hemoglobin level of the blood falls in proportion to the severity of the intestinal involvement and the associated malnutrition if any. Changes in the leukocyte count and sedimentation rate are less consistent. Entozoa, enterococci, and other nonhemolytic Gram-positive short-chained cocci may dominate the flora; hemolytic *Escherichia coli* or streptococci may also be found in abundance. Examinations for Salmonella, Shigella, *Endamoeba histolytica,* and related pathogens are negative. *Endamoeba coli* seems to thrive in the blood-containing fluid stools of this disease, but it is doubtful whether this parasite contributes to the anatomic lesions in the intestine.

Lysozyme

This mucolytic enzyme, normally present in small amounts in gastric and intestinal secretions and tears, saliva, cartilage, and urine, occurs in unusually high titer in the wet stools of patients with active ulcerative colitis. Fecal lysozyme is measured by a viscosimetric method, using a mucopolysaccharide substrate prepared from *Micrococcus lysodeikticus.* In the active phases of the disease the lysozyme content of the stools can vary from 40 to 500 units per gm (normal, 0 to 5 units). States of emotional tension evoke transiently higher titers. In patients in the chronic inactive phase the range may be from 10 to 25 units. During remissions the titer may subside to normal. The lysozyme rise appears to be secondary to the tissue responses and is not significant in pathogenesis. There is no significant increase in acute gastroenteritis or in most other diseases of the colon. In clinical remissions induced by corticotropin or cortisone, the fall in titer of fecal lysozyme becomes striking within 1 to 3 weeks.

MECONIUM

The meconium in the gastrointestinal tract at birth has been estimated to vary from 60 to 200 gm and to have a water content of about 70 per cent. It contains proteolytic enzyme, little ash or lipid, and no protein. The color is thought to be due to bile pigment derivatives. The greater part of normal meconium is a mucopolysaccharide which is related chemically to the blood-group substances. Buchanan and Rapoport found the saliva and meconium of secretor infants of blood group A, B, or AB to react with specific blood group sera in the same manner as their erythrocytes.

In meconium ileus the consistency is exceptionally viscid. It contains much protein, little carbohydrate, and no proteolytic enzyme. When emulsified in water, permitted to stand for a few hours, and then filtered, the filtrate will yield a heavy precipitate with trichloracetic acid. In contrast, the filtrate of normal meconium yields almost no precipitate (Schwachman, Pryles, and Gross).

Meconium is sterile at birth, except at times when there has been early rupture of the membranes.

Cornified epithelial cells are normally evident in abundance. Desquamated from the fetal skin into the amniotic fluid, these are swallowed by the baby in utero and pass through the gastrointestinal tract undigested. They can be demonstrated by Emery's modification of Farber's technique, described below. With intestinal atresia these cells are absent, or present in very small numbers. Normal meconium sometimes contains very little cornified epithelium. When a newborn infant is being studied for congenital intestinal atresia, helpful information can be obtained by study of the meconium for cornified epithelial cells.

Demonstration of Cornified Epithelial Cells

To avoid false results from contact with the perianal skin, the meconium is taken from the interior of a passed stool or collected by a swab passed through a short rubber tube inserted in the rectum. Rub the material on a glass slide. Place the slide in a flat dish containing ether to dissolve the fat. Dry in air. Stain for 2 minutes with Masson's ponceau-acid fuchsin. Decolorize for 15 minutes in 1 per cent phosphomolybdic acid. Counterstain for 15 minutes in 2 per cent light green. Wash in water, blot, dry, and mount in either glycerin or balsam. Cornified cells stain red, and the background stains green.

EOSINOPHILIA

Gastrointestinal symptoms produced by food allergy in infants and growing children are chiefly colic or diarrhea or sometimes vomiting. The stools may be rich in mucus and often contain demonstrable eosinophils. Fluid stools containing flecks of pus or blood may be exhibited by young infants who are sensitive to cow's milk. Eosinophils are absent or sparse in normal stools and in those from bacillary or amebic dysentery, cystic fibrosis of the pancreas, and nonallergic diarrhea.

Test for Stool Eosinophils

Fresh-stool material is necessary, procured if desired by insertion of a gloved finger into the rectum. The surface is inspected for bits of mucus or pus; these are picked up with an applicator or fine forceps and placed unstained on a glass slide. If microscopy under a coverslip shows the presence of leukocytes, a smear is prepared and stained. Study under the oil-immersion lens quickly reveals the presence or absence of eosinophils.

Nance suggests that the smear be heated briefly over a flame, flooded while still hot with Wright's stain, and diluted immediately with water or buffer solution. When the surface becomes greenish and opaque the stain is washed off and the slide dried. Rosenblum advises that the slide remain unheated and be permitted to dry in the air. The May-Grünwald stain is applied for 30 seconds, an equal quantity of distilled water added, and the mixture washed off after 30 seconds.

Eosinophils from the stools often appear distorted or ruptured, with granules which seem over- or understained. If the color is too light for positive identification, the slide may be restained.

Some patients with gastrointestinal allergy excrete an excess of starch or fat in the stools, as demonstrable by special stains, and exhibit symptoms which simulate closely true celiac disease. Conversely, some patients with true celiac disease have gastrointestinal allergy as a complication. Allergic bronchitis along with gastrointestinal allergy can give rise to a clinical picture suggestive of pancreatic fibrosis, but stool or duodenal studies will show normal production of trypsin.

Planned manipulation of the diet is the best approach to establishing the existence of food allergy. When the offending foods are removed by elimination diets the stools revert promptly to normal and the eosinophils disappear. Blood eosinophilia is an inconstant and unreliable indicator of gastrointestinal allergy, and skin tests are of little practical value.

ACUTE GASTROENTERITIS

Infectious inflammation of the intestinal wall resulting in diarrhea can be produced by Salmonella, Shigella, Pseudomonas, Klebsiella, enterococci, hemolytic or nonhemolytic streptococci, staphylococci, pathogenic strains of *Esch. coli*, paracolon or coliform bacilli, or even a virus or protozoan.

Except when the invading organism is exceptionally invasive or toxicogenic, the profound constitutional derangements which may accompany an attack of infantile gastroenteritis are usually associated with some contributory factor such as malnutrition, chronic digestive disease, a "parenteral" infection elsewhere in the body, or a major anomaly of some vital organ. Success in elucidating the precipitating and contributory causes is directly proportional to the thoroughness of the clinical survey and the laboratory diagnostic workup.

"Virus" Diarrhea ("Intestinal Flu")

Some epidemics of diarrhea or vomiting appear to be caused by an as yet unknown virus or family of viruses. The outbreaks are usually recognized in institutions such as schools, camps, barracks, and hospitals. The typical illness is acute and mild and lasts 12 to 48 hours. Symptoms consist of anorexia, nausea, diarrhea, dizziness, malaise, and abdominal discomfort or cramps. About one-third of the patients exhibit vomiting. The incubation period appears to be about 2 days.

Epidemic Diarrhea of the Newborn

This term is applied somewhat loosely to institutional outbreaks of gastroenteritis among infants. Sometimes the outbreak can be traced to a bacterial agent such as a pathogenic strain of *Esch. coli* (p. 790) or rarely to a virus, but equally often the studies of the stools and other body discharges prove to be negative.

The predominant findings in the affected infants are usually constitutional. Dehydration tends to develop rapidly, with concentration of the formed and chemical constituents of the blood and a propensity to the development of metabolic acidosis. The stools are usually but not invariably diarrheic; they are profuse, yellow, and watery and contain a little mucus but not pus or blood. Fever and leukocytosis as a rule are not seen in the absence of dehydration.

Cultures should be taken of the stools, throats, and skin lesions of affected infants and all other patients and institutional employees with whom there has been contact. Regardless of whether a pathogenic bacterium is recoverable, a survey of the nursery will usually uncover one or more violations of sanitary principles. The operation of the milk-preparation room should also be investigated, and cultures made of the formulas and nipples. All supplies and solutions should be checked for sterility. The procedure of scrubbing the hands should be reviewed. As a precautionary measure, hospitals and nurseries are advised to autoclave all bottles which contain infants' feeding after the nipples have been attached and covered (*terminal sterilization*). Visitors should not handle ill babies or their clothing or feeding equipment.

BIBLIOGRAPHY

INTESTINAL MOTILITY

Brackett, A. S., Diarrhea in the Otherwise Healthy Infant, *Yale J. Biol. & Med.* **22**:429, 1950.

Hatfield, M. A., R. A. Simpson, and *R. L. Jackson,* A Study of the Comparative Response of Young Infants to Human Milk and to Various Types of Cow's Milk Formulas, *J. Pediat.* 44:32, 1954.

Nyhan, W. L., Stool Frequency of Normal Infants in First Week of Life, *Pediatrics* 10:414, 1952.

Wolman, I. J., Major Motility Patterns of the Child's Digestive Tract: A Review, *Am. J. M. Sc.* 207:782, 1944.

—— and *S. Borowsky,* Influence of Minor Dietary Changes on Frequency of Infants' Stools: Study of the Effect of Varying the Content of Lactose, Milk Fat and Thiamine, *Am. J. Dis. Child.* 65:827, 1943.

STOOL COMPOSITION

Albanese, A. A., V. I. Danis, N. Lein, and *E. M. Smetak,* Biochemistry of the Metabolic Fecal Protein Nitrogen, *J. Biol. Chem.* 176:1189, 1948.

Andersen, D. H., Celiac Syndrome. I. Determination of Fat in Feces; Reliability of Two Chemical Methods and of Microscopic Estimate; Excretion of Feces and of Fecal Fat in Normal Children, *Am. J. Dis. Child.* 69:141, 1945.

Culver, P. J., and *R. H. Ham,* in T. H. Ham (ed.), "A Syllabus of Laboratory Examinations in Clinical Diagnosis," Unit 19, Harvard University Press, Cambridge, Mass. 1950.

Holt, L. E., Jr., H. C. Tidwell, C. M. Kirk, D. M. Cross, and *S. Neale,* Studies in Fat Metabolism: I. Fat Absorption in Normal Infants, *J. Pediat.* 6:427, 1935.

Lewis, G. T., and *H. C. Partin,* Fecal Fat on an Essentially Fat-free Diet, *J. Lab. & Clin. Med.* 44:91, 1954.

Macy, I. G., "Nutrition and Chemical Growth in Childhood," vol. I, "Evaluation," Charles C Thomas, Springfield, Ill., 1942.

Ross, C. A. C., Amino-acids in the Faeces of Breast-fed and Bottle-fed Infants: Preliminary Communication, *Lancet* 1:716, 1950.

——, Direct Microscopical Examination of Faeces in Infants, *Brit. Med. J.* 1:465, 1950.

Söderhjelm, L., Fat Absorption Studies in Children: Influence of Heat Treatment on Milk on Fat Retention by Premature Infants, *Acta paediat.* 41:207, 1952.

STOOL FLORA

Bierman, H. R., and *E. Jawetz,* The Effect of Prolonged Administration of Antibiotics on the Human Fecal Flora, *J. Lab. & Clin. Med.* 37:394, 1951.

Brown, R. L., The Gastrointestinal Tract and Stool Following Aureomycin Therapy, *Antibiotics & Chemother.* 2:5, 1952.

Cook, G. T., and *R. Knox,* Bacteriological Examination of Faeces, *J. Path. & Bact.* 61:353, 1949.

Frisell, E., Studies on *Bacterium bifidum* in Healthy Infants, *Acta paediat.* vol. 40, suppl. 80, 1951.

Gerstley, J. R., E. Penruddocke, and *G. Lawrence,* Beta-Lactose: A Study of Its Effect upon the Flora of the Infant's Stool, *Arch. Pediat.* 52:552, 1935.

Johansson, K. R., and *W. B. Sarles,* Some Considerations of the Biological Importance of Intestinal Microorganisms, *Bacteriol. Rev.* 13:25, 1949.

Hughes, J. D., Antibiotics and Chemotherapeutic Agents in Diseases of the Gastrointestinal Tract, *J.A.M.A.* 150:1456, 1952.

Metzger, W. I., L. T. Wright, R. F. Morton, J. C. DiLorenzo, and *M. Marmell,* Contents of the Colon of Man, *Antibiotics & Chemother.* 2:91, 1952.

Olsen, E., "Studies on the Intestinal Flora of Infants," E. Munksgaard, Copenhagen, 1949.

Riddell, M. I., A Review of the Literature on Preoperative Prophylaxis of the Bowel with Antibacterial Agents, *Am. J. M. Sc.* 223:301, 1952.

Stahl, C., and *E. Olsen,* Gram-negative Staining of Gram-positive Intestinal Bacteria with Particular Reference to Examinations of Faeces in Infants, *Acta paediat.* 39:471, 1950.

Williams, N. B., R. F. Norris, and *P. Gyorgy,* Antigenic and Cultural Relationships of *Lactobacillus Bifidus* and *Lactobacillus Parabifidus, J. Infect. Dis.* 92:121, 1953.

STOOL PIGMENTS

Brereton, H. G., and *S. P. Lucia,* Quantitative Method for Determination of Urobilinogen in Stool and of Urobilinogen and Bilirubin in Urine, *Am. J. Clin. Path.* 18:887, 1948.

Hollan, O. R., The Site of Formation of Urobilinogen in the Intact Human Gastrointestinal Tract, *Gastroenterol.* 16:418, 1950.

Kaplan, E., and *S. R. Lewis,* The Effect of Human Plasma Transfusions on the Fecal Urobilinogen Excretion in Sickle Cell Anemia, *Blood* 4:947, 1949.

Mills, S. D., and *H. L. Mason,* Values for Fecal Urobilinogen in Childhood, *A.M.A. Am. J. Dis. Child.* 84:322, 1952.

Sborov, V. M., A. R. Jay, and *C. J. Watson,* The Effect of Aureomycin on Urobilinogen Formation and Fecal Flora, *J. Lab. & Clin. Med.* 37:52, 1951.

Schwartz, S., V. Sborov, and *C. J. Watson,* Studies of Urobilinogen. IV. The Quantitative Determination of Urobilinogen by Means of the Evelyn Photoelectric Colorimeter, *Am. J. Clin. Path.* 14:598, 1944.

Tat, R. J., T. J. Greenwalt, and *W. Dameshek,* Output of Bile Pigment by Newborn Infants and by Older Infants and Children, *Am. J. Dis. Child.* 65:558, 1943.

BLOOD IN STOOLS

Apt, L., Melena Neonatorum: An Experimental Study of the Effect of the Oral Administration of Blood on the Stools, *J. Pediat.* 47:1, 1955.

—— and *W. S. Downey,* "Melena" Neonatorum: The Swallowed-Blood Syndrome; A Simple Test for the Differentiation of Adult and Fetal Hemoglobin in Bloody Stools, *J. Pediat.* 47:6, 1955.

Berman, E. J., A. Schneider, and *W. J. Potts,* Importance of Gastric Mucosa in Meckel's Diverticulum, *J.A.M.A.* 56:6, 1954.

Bonar, B. E., Blood in the Stools of the New-born, *Am. J. Dis. Child.* 51:255, 1936.

Brayton, D., and *W. J. Norris,* Gastrointestinal Hemorrhage in Infancy and Childhood, *J.A.M.A.* 150:668, 1952.

Gettler, A. O., and *S. Kaye,* The Phenolphthalin Test for the Detection of "Occult" Blood, *Am. J. Clin. Path., Tech. Sec.* 7:77, 1943.

Hoerr, S. O., W. R. Bliss, and *J. Kauffman,* Clinical Evaluation of Various Tests for Occult Blood in Feces, *J.A.M.A.* 141:1213, 1949.

Kiesewetter, W. B., R. Cancelmo, and *C. E. Koop,* Rectal Bleeding in Infants and Children, *J. Pediat.* 47:660, 1955.

Levin, M. B., and *J. Y. C. Watt,* A Simple Benzidine Test for Occult Blood in Feces, *Rev. Gastroenterol.* 16:650, 1949.

Neilson, R., Jr., and *J. H. Black,* Massive Bleeding from Duodenal Ulcer in Infancy Treated by Gastrectomy, *Pediatrics* 15:433, 1955.

Peranio, A., and *M. Bruger,* The Detection of Occult Blood in Feces Including Observations on the Ingestion of Iron and Whole Blood, *J. Lab. & Clin. Med.* 38:433, 1951.

Rider, J. A., and *F. J. Owens,* Evaluation of an Orthotolidine Test (Fecatest) for Determination of Occult Blood, *J.A.M.A.* 156:31, 1954.

Rozenfeld, I. H., and *J. R. McGrath,* Melena in the Newborn Infant, *J. Pediat.* 40:180, 1952.

Schwartz, S. O., and C. S. Vil, Benzidine-negative Stools during Iron Therapy, *J. Lab. & Clin. Med.* 32:181, 1947.

Thompson, H. L., and D. W. McGuffin, Melena: A Study of Underlying Causes, *J.A.M.A.* 141:1208, 1949.

Zamcheck, N., T. C. Chalmers, M. Ritvo, and M. P. Osborne, Early Diagnosis in Massive Gastrointestinal Hemorrhage, *J.A.M.A.* 148:504, 1952.

STOOL ENZYMES

Gaffney, P. C., Source of Error in Test for Stool Trypsin, *Pediatrics* 8:82, 1951.

Grace, W. J., P. H. Seton, S. Wolf, and H. G. Wolff, Studies of the Human Colon. I. Variations in Concentration of Lysozyme with Life Situation and Emotional State, *Am. J. M. Sc.* 217:241, 1949.

Johnstone, D. E., and E. Neter, Studies on the Laboratory Diagnosis of Cystic Fibrosis of the Pancreas: Positive Gelatin Film Tests Due to Gelatin-liquefying Bacteria in Feces and Duodenal Juice, *Pediatrics* 7:483, 1951.

Meyer, K., and E. Hahnel, The Estimation of Lysozyme by a Viscosimetric Method, *J. Biol. Chem.* 163:723, 1946.

Schwachman, H., P. R. Patterson, and J. Laguna, Studies in Pancreatic Fibrosis: A Simple Diagnostic Gelatin Film Test for Stool Trypsin, *Pediatrics* 4:222, 1949.

ULCERATIVE AND ALLERGIC COLITIS

Lagercrantz, R., Ulcerative Colitis in Children, *Acta paediat.* suppl. 75, p. 89, 1949.

Nance, F. D., Stool Eosinophilia in Gastrointestinal Allergy of Infancy, *J. Pediat.* 33:313, 1948.

Rosenblum, A. H., and P. Rosenblum, Gastrointestinal Allergy in Infancy, *Pediatrics* 9:311, 1952.

Rothman, P. E., Diarrhea of Allergic Origin: A Review, *A.M.A. Am. J. Dis. Child.* 86:201, 1953.

Turell, R., Pediatric Proctology: Review with Comment, *Am. J. Dis. Child.* 79:510, 1950.

MECONIUM

Buchanan, D. J., and S. Rapoport, Chemical Comparison of Normal Meconium and Meconium from a Patient with Meconium Ileus, *Pediatrics* 9:304, 1952.

Emery, J. L., The Tryptic Activity and Presence of Cornified Squames in Meconium as a Diagnostic Aid in Congenital Intestinal Obstruction, *Arch. Dis. Childhood* 27:67, 1952.

Schwachman, H., C. V. Pryles, and R. E. Gross, Meconium Ileus: A Clinical Study of Twenty Surviving Patients, *A.M.A. Am. J. Dis. Child.* 91:223, 1956.

Snyder, M. L., Bacterial Flora of Meconium Specimens Collected from 64 Infants within 4 Hours after Delivery, *J. Pediat.* 9:624, 1936.

ACUTE INFECTIOUS GASTROENTERITIS

Abramson, H., Acute Diarrheal Disorders of Newborn Infants, Differential Diagnosis, *Am. J. Dis. Child.* 79:698, 1950.

Colgan, M. T., The Bacterial Flora of the Intestinal Tract: Changes in Diarrheal Disease and Following Antimicrobial Therapy, *J. Pediat.* 49:214, 1956.

Dodd, K., Virus Diarrhea, *Advances Pediat.* 2:298, 1947.

Epidemic and Endemic Diarrheal Diseases of the Infant, *Ann. New York Acad. Sci.* vol. 66, art. 1, p. 3, 1956.

Hodes, H. L., The Etiology of Infantile Diarrhea, *Advances Pediat.* 8:13, 1956.

Hunter, C. A., and P. R. Ensign, An Epidemic of Diarrhea in a New-born Nursery Caused by *Pseudomonas Aeruginosa*, *Am. J. Pub. Health* 37:1166, 1947.

Ingalls, T. H., and S. A. Britten, Epidemic Diarrhea in a School for Boys, J.A.M.A. 146:710, 1951.

Levinson, J. D., and W. B. Raycraft, A Study of Three Hundred Cases of Diarrhea in Infants and Children during the Summer and Fall of 1948, J. Pediat. 36:316, 1950.

Scott, J. P., and J. G. Kety, Experiences with Epidemic Diarrhea of the Newborn, J. Pediat. 33:573, 1948.

Scott, R. B., G. P. Brown, and A. D. Kessler, Diarrhea of the Newborn: Report of Epidemic and Results of Treatment with Streptomycin, A.M.A. Am. J. Dis. Child. 83:192, 1952.

Smith, M. H. D., C. G. Loosli, and M. H. Ritter, Outbreak of Aerobacter Infections on Infants' Wards, Pediatrics 7:550, 1951.

CHAPTER 63

Intestinal Parasites

CLASSIFICATION

The intestinal parasites most often encountered in children in North America can be divided into three great divisions: (1) the single-celled protozoa, (2) the roundworms, and (3) the tapeworms. Infestation with any of these parasites is more often subclinical and unsuspected than overt and symptom-producing. But despite this comparative latency, the physician should test for intestinal parasites whenever their presence is suspected, and institute treatment and measures of control if any are found, in order to protect public health and relieve the child from a possibly debilitating handicap. Since routes of contagion such as contact with fecal-contaminated fomites or spread through dust are common to more than one species of parasite, infestations are often multiple.

1. Intestinal Protozoa

AMEBAE	CILIATES	FLAGELLATES
Endamoeba coli	Balantidium coli	Trichomonas hominis
Endolimax nana		Chilomastix mesnili
Iodamoeba butschlii		Enteromonas hominis
Endamoeba histolytica		Giardia lamblia

2. Roundworms (Nemathelminthes)

Those of most concern fall in the zoologic class of Nematoda. These possess an intestinal tract and a body cavity not lined with epithelium and lack a proboscis.

NEMATODES

Pinworm (*Enterobius vermicularis*)
Ascaris (*Ascaris lumbricoides*)
Hookworm (*Necator americanus, Ancylostoma duodenale, A. braziliense*)
Whipworm (*Trichocephalus trichiurus*)
Strongyloides (*Strongyloides stercoralis*)
Trichina (*Trichinella spiralis*)

3. Flatworms (Platyhelminthes)

These are usually bilaterally symmetrical and lack a body cavity; their digestive system when present usually has no oval opening. Those of pediatric interest belong to two groups: tapeworms, or Cestoda; and flukes, or Trematoda.

TAPEWORMS

	Adult host	Intermediate host
Taenia saginata (beef tapeworm)	Man only	Cattle
Taenia solium (pork tapeworm)	Man only	Hog (man)
Diphyllobothrium latum (fish tapeworm)	1. Man	1. Cyclops and Diaptomus
	2. Dog	2. Fresh-water fish
Hymenolepis nana (dwarf tapeworm)	Man, rat, mouse	None
Hymenolepis diminuta	Rat, mouse, man	Fleas
Dipylidium caninum (dog tapeworm)	Dog, cat, man	Fleas

Flukes, or trematodes, have been practically unknown in the United States in the past. The immigration of inhabitants of the Caribbean islands and the return of servicemen's families from Asia, Africa, and the Orient have made it necessary to consider the possibility of infestation in all such individuals with suspicious symptoms.

FLUKES

Blood flukes (*Schistosoma haematobium, S. mansoni, S. Japonicum*)
Liver flukes (*Clonorchis sinensis, Opisthorchis felineus, Fasciola hepatica*)
Intestinal flukes (*Heterophyes heterophyes, Metagonimus yokogawai, Fasciolopsis buski*)
Lung fluke (*Paragonimus westermani*)

DIAGNOSTIC APPROACHES

Clinical manifestations alone are never sufficient to enable one to establish the diagnosis of intestinal parasitism without aid from the laboratory except when worms migrate out from some portal of the body. The two principal methods for recognition of intestinal parasites are (1) examination of stool specimens and (2) microscopy of scrapings from the perianal region. Serologic approaches and skin tests are being energetically investigated but as a rule are not yet satisfactory for specific diagnostic purposes in individual patients. Blood eosinophilia is a frequent but far from essential concomitant.

With many of the parasites, though not with Enterobius or the tapeworms, the number of cysts or ova in the stools is a rough index of the intensity of the infestation. Recognition of light infestations requires concentration techniques, whereas liberal numbers of cysts or ova in a simple wet smear of stool usually indicate moderate to heavy parasitism. Most laboratories have mastered and use one or more of the numerous available concentration techniques, among which may be named the Faust zinc flotation method, the Lane direct centrifugal flotation, the Willis brine flotation, the Ritchie formalin-ether sedimentation method, and others. For quantitative approximation of the fecal content of cysts and ova one may mention the Stoll dilution method and Beaver's direct egg-count technique.

Soft mushy stools are more satisfactory for direct examination than those that are hard and constipated or liquid and diarrheic. Liquid petrolatum or castor oil confuse the readings of the tests.

The reported prevalence of single or multiple infestations with intestinal parasites varies with the climate, the hygienic habits of the community, and the thoroughness of the diagnostic studies. In common experience the screening of members of a community by a single stool examination will detect only 50 per cent or less of those who are infested. The percentage of total positives rises with each repetition of the examination.

At least one out of every two American children carry one or more protozoa, usually asymptomatically. The most common of these are *Endamoeba coli, Giardia lamblia,* and *Endolimox nana.* Of the worm species, *Enterobius vermicularis* is by far the most prevalent. Amebiasis and hookworm diseases are rare in the northern part of the United States.

INTESTINAL PROTOZOA

Endamoeba coli

Endamoeba coli, 15 to 50 μ in diameter, is a common inhabitant of the large intestine of man, found most often in and near the cecum. Its chief importance lies in having to be differentiated from *Endamoeba histolytica.* Not uncommonly the two species occur together. *Endamoeba coli* can be differentiated by shorter pseudopodia, more sluggish motility, absence of ingested erythrocytes, and slightly larger cysts which contain irregular chromatoid bodies and 1 to 8 or 16 nuclei with thick uneven nuclear membrane and eccentric large karyosome.

Endamoeba coli as a rule is a harmless saprophyte. We have, however, seen a number of children with obscure upper abdominal complaints, suggestive of duodenitis or even of a mild celiac syndrome, in whom duodenal intubation recovered fluid which seemed normal in all respects except for containing *E. coli* in moderate numbers. Antiamebic therapy was followed by prompt return of appetite and disappearance of all other symptoms.

Endolimax nana

Endolimax nana is another common nonpathogenic ameba which must be differentiated from *Endamoeba histolytica*. Its trophozoite form, 6 to 15 μ in diameter, is about half the size of *Endamoeba histolytica* or *Endamoeba coli*. It does not ingest human erythrocytes. The cysts are the size of those of *Endamoeba histolytica* and also contain one to four nuclei. They are pale green instead of greenish yellow, the nuclear membranes are indistinct, the karyosomes lie on or near the nuclear membranes and may appear broken into several masses, and cytoplasmic chromatoid bodies are not present.

Endamoeba histolytica

Infection with *Endamoeba histolytica* typically begins insidiously, with abdominal discomfort, diarrhea, nausea, flatulence, and lassitude. Many cases do not progress beyond this stage. The bowel movements, usually increased, may contain mucus and be spotted with blood or appear as an "explosive" combination of semiformed stool material and abundant gas. Diarrhea may alternate with constipation. Spontaneous remissions can occur, but with the apparently well individual carrying the parasite for months or even years. Or the clinical course may be fulminating, with a bloody diarrhea followed by lymphatic invasion to the liver and other organs.

The ulcers in the colon result from amebic invasion and cytolysis, combined with secondary invasion of the tissues by enterococci, clostridia, and similar bacteria. Proper antibiotic therapy reduces the symptoms by inhibiting these associated invaders.

Every child with chronic diarrhea should be studied for amebiasis, especially when bloody mucus occurs in the stools. The absolute diagnosis of amebiasis rests upon detection of the parasites by adequate stool examination.

RECOGNITION OF AMEBAE. *Endamoeba histolytica* has a two-stage life cycle—the motile trophozoite stage and the nonmotile cyst stage. The mature trophozoites, 15 to 60 μ in diameter, are found within the wall of the large intestine and in extensions elsewhere. Their cytoplasm is finely granular and may contain ingested red cells. Amebae are actively motile in fresh warm stool specimens and are killed by drying or low temperatures. They can be demonstrated in the stools only when the patient has bowel symptoms with diarrhea. In the absence of diarrhea the active amebae are not seen except in liquid stools passed after a cathartic.

The cysts are smaller, measuring 4 to 20 μ in diameter, and may remain viable for days. Usually spherical, they have a refractile hyalinelike outer membrane and one to four nuclei. They are excreted in asymptomatic disturbances and following subsidence of active symptoms. They must be distinguished from the cysts of *E. coli, E. nana,* and *Iodamoeba butschlii* and from free macrophages. It has been estimated that patients with acute symptoms may excrete as many as 15 million cysts daily.

It is these cysts, excreted in the feces, which are responsible for the spread from host to host. They are not injured by freezing or by chlorine in concentrations far above those usually employed in water purification and can remain viable in water for a month or longer. In temperate zones they seem to be spread most often by infected food handlers. Uncooked food mixed with polluted water or fertilized by human excreta is another major route of contagion. House flies, cockroaches, and rats may sometimes transmit the cysts. Contaminated drinking water can be made safe by boiling or by removal of the cysts through coagulation or sand-bed filtration.

Cysts, like active amebae, are not uniformly mixed with the feces and are most abundant on the stool surface and in blood or mucus. Charcot-Leyden crystals frequently accompany them. They should be sought for both in unstained preparations and in slides stained with iodine solution. The stools need not be fresh. Concentration techniques are often successful when direct search has failed to show any cysts.

Since trophozoites and cysts may be passed only intermittently, it is helpful in problem cases to examine as many as five or six stool specimens, separated by intervals of several days. In cases of florid diarrhea, at least three loose stools should be examined, on three successive days, before the diagnosis of amebiasis is excluded.

RECTAL INSPECTION. Rectosigmoidoscopy is indicated in the management of recurrent bloody diarrhea when the diagnosis of amebiasis is suspected but cannot be made by stool examination. Its purpose is twofold: to search for evidences of inflammation or ulceration and to procure mucosal scrapings or fresh specimens of feces or mucus for immediate microscopic examination. Proctoscopes of adult size have proved highly satisfactory with children. By serial inspections of the lesions one is better able to follow the progress of the lesions with patients receiving amebicidal drugs. Material obtained by sigmoidoscopy should be collected with a glass tube rather than on a cotton swab, since organisms may adhere to the latter and not be transferred to the glass slide. Detection of parasites by proctoscopy material has not been as successful statistically in detecting mild cases or carriers as study of several stools including a purgation specimen.

COMPLEMENT-FIXATION TEST. A complement-fixation test is available for serum antibodies against *E. histolytica.* The antigen, derived from cultures, is of doubtful specificity; positive reactions occur occasionally in the absence of demonstrable amebiasis. Conversely, the serum response is not universally positive in active infections. The antibody tends to disappear from the circulation after adequate therapy. The serologic approach is sometimes used to corroborate the suspicion of an extracolonic amebic lesion such as hepatic abscess when stool examinations are negative.

Balantidium coli

Rare in temperate climates, this is the largest of the intestinal protozoa. In trophozoite form it appears as a large ovoidal motile ciliate 40 to 100 or even 200 μ in length and 45 to 65 μ in diameter. It lives in the mucosa of the large intestine where exceptionally it will produce ulceration and intestinal irritation. The cysts, more rounded, are 45 to 65 μ in diameter.

This ciliate has been found in pigs, sheep, fowl, turtles, cockroaches, primates, and other species. Close contact with pigs has been noted in 50 per cent of the reported cases of clinical balantidiasis.

Trichomonas hominis (Tr. intestinalis)

This small pear-shaped saprophyte has three to five anterior flagella and a long undulating membrane with another free flagellum at the end. It may inhabit almost any portion of the small or large intestine but is most abundant in the cecum. There is no known cyst stage. Motile forms are not ordinarily found in the stool of carriers except during diarrhea or after a purgative. A related variety (Tr. vaginalis) may cause vaginitis in young girls.

Chilomastix mesnili

The motile trophozoite forms of this nonpathogenic intestinal flagellate are ordinarily excreted only when the stools are liquid and rapidly passed. The cysts, on the other hand, are common in formed stools, where they appear as rounded bodies about 7 μ in diameter displaying a small blunt projection at the smaller end.

Enteromonas hominis

This rare protozoan saprophyte possesses three anterior and one posterior flagellum and gives rise to oval cysts 6 to 8 μ in length.

Giardia lamblia

This may infest the duodenum and upper jejunum in myriad numbers and give rise to duodenitis, cholecystitis, the celiac syndrome, or even ulcerative ileitis or colitis. Infection is acquired by ingestion of cyst-contaminated food.

The adult trophozoite is pear-shaped, with a sucking disk, two nuclei, a pear-shaped tail, and four pairs of flagellae; the length ranges from 10 to 20 μ. In fresh wet unstained preparations of infected duodenal fluid the parasites are actively motile, with jerky dancing movements. Only encysted or dead and disintegrating forms are excreted in the stools except during acute diarrhea. The cysts are oval and 8 to 12 μ in length, with smooth well-defined walls which appear refractile and double-outlined. Several paired nuclei, short fibrils, and a V-shaped group of rods may be recognized after staining.

Duodenal drainage will frequently demonstrate the presence of parasites when the stools are negative. Conversely, when the stools contain cysts, the motile forms will often be found in the duodenal fluid if looked for specifically.

The most common complaints in heavy giardial infestations are abdominal pain, anorexia, slow weight gain, nausea, and sometimes diarrhea. Many of Maris and Bushong's 86 infested children had an eosinophilia up to 24 per cent in the differential white blood count. Most of the cases in this series were satisfactorily treated by 3 days of Atabrine, in dosages from 45 mg twice a day for those 2 to 4 years old, up to 90 mg three times daily for those 9 years old and upward.

ROUNDWORMS

Enterobius vermicularis

Known also as the pinworm, seatworm, or oxyurid, this is the most common intestinal nematode in the United States. It inhabits the cecum, the appendix, and the contiguous regions of the ileum and ascending colon. The male worms, 2 to 5 mm in length, do not live as long as the females and are seen less commonly. They die within the intestine, presumably soon after copulation, and are passed in the feces.

To deposit her ova the mature female, 8 to 13 mm in length, migrates out of the rectum at a time when the host is asleep or inactive. After laying an estimated 11,000 ova in or near the anus, she then dies. Within 6 hours thereafter the ova have matured and become infectious, and may reinvade the rectum. They can be spread by the hands, toys and bed linen, and are light enough to float in air currents. In infested homes they have been recovered from the upper walls and ceiling. Ova ordinarily are not present in the stools except as the result of surface adsorption during defecation. A superimposed diarrhea or the giving of a high enema may throw out the worms in large numbers.

Man is the only known reservoir host. Every new worm comes from an ovum deposited outside the body. These may be carried to the mouth by the fingers and swallowed, or the larvae may hatch on the perianal skin and migrate back into the intestine through the anus. Since the life cycle of the individual worm is 2 months or less, the infestation would be self-limited were reinfection not the rule.

ENTEROBIASIS. Enterobiasis seems to occur more often in whites than Negroes, and in temperate rather than tropical climates. The infestation tends to subside spontaneously during adolescence, especially in males. The prevalence rates seem to be highest during the school ages. When one child in a household is infected, the rest are usually also. The number of worms in the intestine at any time shows great individual variation and may range from a dozen to several thousand. The majority of patients have only a few migrating worms nightly at the perianal region. Local itching is the most common symptom, along with restlessness, scratching, and insomnia. The importance of pinworms in appendicitis is questionable, though in excised specimens they often are found within the lumen or partially imbedded in the mucosa. Pinworms may enter the vagina or even the female peritoneal cavity to produce disturbances. Swabs of the vulva are occasionally positive for ova.

Current therapy is generally with piperazine salts. Parents and siblings should all be treated at the same time. Children's fingernails should be kept clean and short, and the perianal region should be washed with soap and water every morning. The walls, furniture, and floors of the house must be simultaneously scrubbed or cleaned daily with a vacuum cleaner. Otherwise the untreated individuals or the ova in the environment may initiate the reinfestation of the entire household.

Household dogs and cats can spread ova from person to person in a family. This has been demonstrated by Pryor, who advises standing the suspected animal on a sheet of waxed paper and brushing his fur. The debris is then accumulated by folding the paper, and adhesive tape preparations made for microscopic examinations.

STUDY OF THE PERIANAL SKIN. The diagnosis of enterobiasis is made most easily by smearing or scraping the perianal region and examining the material thus secured for microscopic ova. This examination is best made in the early morning. The buttocks and perineum should not be washed or wiped on arising nor medicated ointments applied the night before. Ova or larvae of other worms (Ascaris, Taenia, Trichocephalus, Necator) are sometimes encountered by this approach, since they may adhere to the perianal skin during passage of an infected stool.

THE ADHESIVE SWAB. To search for ova a short strip of cellulose adhesive tape is placed sticky side out over the end of a tongue depressor or test tube or finger and pressed and rolled against the anal folds. The yield of ova is highest at the edge of the anal canal. The sticky side of the adhesive strip is then spread on a glass slide over a drop of water, oil, or toluol. Toluol dissolves the adhesive material on the tape and is a good cleansing agent. Neither a cover slip or staining is necessary. The undersurface of the strip is then scrutinized with the low power of the microscope. Such slides may be kept for many days when mounted with oil or water; toluol will lyse ova after 3 or 4 days.

If the adhesive is to be forwarded elsewhere for examination, it should be folded in the middle with the smooth side out. In the laboratory, if quick microscopy of the unfolded tape shows no ova immediately apparent, the tape should be unfolded and spread on a slide.

Recovery of one or two ova is as significant diagnostically as a much larger number. Air bubbles or other artefacts simulating pinworm eggs may be seen in the preparations, but these contain no larvae. As many as 3,000 ova may be picked up on a single adhesive strip and yet come from only a few ovipositing females.

The migration of mature worms often exhibits cyclic fluctuations. There may be weeks during which no ova are deposited, followed by an interval in which the perineum is showered nightly. Hence, before a child can be adjudged free of the infestation, perianal examinations must be consistently negative for weeks or months. Reappearance of ova on the skin within 2 to 3 months after the last day of treatment may be interpreted as a relapse, whereas ova reappearing after that time presumably signify a fresh infestation.

Ascaris lumbricoides

The large roundworm stays chiefly within the intestine, though its migratory habits can lead to serious complications in other organ systems. The diagnosis of infestation is made by demonstration of the ova in the stools or finding the adult worm at some body orifice.

ASCARIASIS. Diarrhea, anorexia, malnutrition, anemia, or abdominal pains are signs of heavy infestation. There may be no symptoms if the worms are few. Eosinophilia is not seen often; its presence or absence is no indication of the number of parasites. The x-ray may show increased bronchovascular markings caused by larval invasion; when associated with eosinophilia and ascariasis this represents one variety of Loeffler's syndrome. The parasites may enter the biliary, hepatic, or pancreatic ducts and produce local obstruction or infection. Perforation of the large or small intestine can discharge the worms into the peritoneal cavity. Intestinal obstruction due to masses of ascaris demands immediate surgical evacuation. Ascariasis is a possible cause of abdominal symptoms whenever recurrent vomiting is associated. Sanitary disposal of all stools is mandatory to prevent spread.

Laboratory Diagnosis. The female worms discharge ova continuously; a single worm can emit enough ova each day to make every stool examination positive. In general, however, the more abundant the excretion of ova the more severe the infestation. The ova, elliptical and 40 to 100 μ in length, are yellow-brown and smoothly encapsulated when fertilized, or irregular and nodular when unfertilized. In suspected cases they should be searched for first in a direct smear of a stool and are usually demonstrable when infestation is present. A concentration technique may demonstrate ova when direct examination has been unsuccessful (p. 731). Should only male or immature female worms be present, as may happen, ova are not excreted. When treatment is given on clinical suspicion alone, the appearance in the stool of one or more dead worms after the administration of the drug confirms the diagnosis. A skin test antigen is available, but a positive reaction means only that the individual has become sensitized; the infestation may no longer be present.

Stool examinations should be repeated after every course of treatment to make sure that all the worms have been eliminated. The therapeutic agents currently employed, including piperazine, may not eradicate larvae from the circulation or lungs. Patients who have migratory larvae should have monthly stool examinations for at least 3 months after the course of therapy, to make sure that mature forms have not again become implanted in the intestine.

Hookworms

Of the three recognized species of hookworm—*Necator americanus, Ancylostoma duodenale,* and *A. braziliense*—Necator is the one widely prevalent in the United States, occurring almost exclusively in the South.

Hookworms tend to inhabit the middle segment of the small intestine, where they anchor themselves to the mucosa with two pairs of teeth. Each worm sucks out an estimated 1 ml of blood each day and may liberate a hemolytic toxin which is systemically absorbed. Each female discharges several thousand ova each day.

When an infected stool is deposited in shaded muddy soil the ova develop first into the so-called rhabditoid larvae and then into the filarial form which is infective for humans. These latter penetrate the skin between the toes and are carried by the blood to the lungs. In the lungs they are coughed up and swallowed. Once in the intestine they grow and mature and attach themselves to the mucosa to start the cycle again. Sanitary disposal of feces is thus the essential public-health measure for blocking the spread.

ANCYLOSTOMIASIS (UNCINARIASIS). Hookworm disease is more disturbing in children than in adults, and the carrier state is seen less often. There is flatulence and transitory abdominal pain; in the more severe and chronic infestations these may be associated with low fever, vasomotor disturbances, malnutrition, or retardation of growth. A hypochromic anemia develops ultimately, especially with Ancylostoma infections; this is microcytic at first, but may become macrocytic later. Eosinophilia, leukocytosis, or monocytosis may accompany the anemia. The larvae of *A. braziliense* can migrate through the skin to produce the serpiginous lesions of "creeping eruption" or "larva migrans."

LABORATORY DIAGNOSIS. This is best made by finding the ova in the stools. Mature worms are rarely found under ordinary circumstances. The ova are elliptical, measure about 60 μ in length, and have thin hyaline shells through which the embryos can be seen. In freshly passed stools these are usually at the two- to eight-cell stage of segmentation, but in older or constipated stools they may be further matured. Ova counts on the direct smear reflect the severity of the infestation. Stool concentration techniques may be needed with light infestations. Cultural methods are available by which larvae may be grown and isolated for identification.

Adult worms usually appear in the feces during drug treatment. They can be demonstrated by stirring the fresh stool in a tall container with a large volume of water or half-normal saline solution. After the suspension has settled, the supernatant fluid is decanted off and discarded; this is repeated several times. Parasites if present can then be seen by inspecting the sediment in a shallow glass dish against a black background or by straining it through a fine sieve. This form of direct stool study is helpful in establishing the diagnosis in cases subjected to therapy on suspicion alone.

Trichocephalus trichiuris

The whipworm lives mainly in the cecum and appendix. The mature worm measures 30 to 50 mm in length, with the anterior three-fifths being delicate and narrow and the posterior two-fifths broader and fleshy. The ova, which are discharged in the stools in large numbers, measure about 50 μ in length and have pluglike projections at each end. Mild infestations are usually asymptomatic; more severe ones can lead to appendiceal irritation, undernutrition, anemia, chronic diarrhea, and other symptoms. Heavy infestations in which the worms extend from their usual habitat, the cecum, into the entire bowel, including sigmoid and rectum, occur most often in the age period 2 to 4 years. The intestinal irritation can then be as severe as in amebiasis of the colon, with severe diarrhea and even prolapse of the rectum. Eosinophilia is frequent in the early stages; unusual in chronic infestations.

The number of ova in the stool smear is proportional to the intensity of the infestation and the severity of the symptoms. In advanced cases the stools contain many eosinophils and Charcot-Leyden crystals.

Strongyloides stercoralis

Threadworm infestation is moderately prevalent among children in subtropical areas. The parasite occurs most abundantly in the duodenum and jejunum but may be in any portion of the gastrointestinal tract. The male is about 1 mm in length, the female about 2 mm. The complex life cycle is like that of the hookworm, though the host can become reinfected by filarial forms which mature in the intestinal tract and burrow into the anal skin or rectal mucosa. The ova resemble those of the hookworm but tend to mature within the bowel. Stools are more likely to contain some motile rhabditoid or filariform larvae than unhatched unembryonated eggs. Common symptoms in severe infestations are nausea, diarrhea, weakness, recurrent urticarial eruptions, and rectal prolapse. Eosinophilia is usually present and marked; monocytosis appears in the more chronic cases. Anemia is not produced inasmuch as this parasite, unlike the hookworm, does not ingest blood.

Duodenal intubation will occasionally reveal the worms when stool examinations are repeatedly negative; the reverse is also true. Sigmoidoscopy may discover the pale worms attached to the mucosa by their imbedded slender portions.

Trichinella spiralis

Clinically recognizable infections with *Trichinella spiralis* are comparatively uncommon, even though Trichina larvae have been found in the diaphragmatic muscles of over 15 per cent of adults examined at autopsy. Human infections originate nearly always from the meat of hogs which contains encysted viable larvae. These larvae, released from their capsules by the digestive juices, burrow into the intestinal villi, where they mate about 2 days after ingestion. During this period the patient may display signs of gastrointestinal irritation, but stool studies will throw no light on the cause of the disturbance. The male then dies, whereas the female grows and after about 5 days begins to deposit successive groups of larvae into the capillaries and lymph spaces over the next 4 or 5 days. It has been estimated that up to 1,000 larvae may be released by each female. The new larvae circulate through the blood stream of the host and lodge in every organ. Only in striated muscles, however, do they survive and become encysted; elsewhere they degenerate and give rise to local inflammatory responses.

Constitutional disturbances of fever, chills, muscle pains, malaise, weakness, or focal edema may be prominent during this stage of general dissemination of larvae. Skin rashes, cardiac signs, or encephalitic or meningitic phenomena may appear if these organs are heavily involved. Larvae have occasionally been found in the cerebrospinal fluid sediment.

Leukocytosis is usually apparent during the second and third weeks of the illness. Eosinophilia is present almost invariably, with these cells ranging from 10 to 90 per cent of all leukocytes. There is, however, little positive correlation between the intensity of the eosinophilia and the severity of the clinical manifestations. The plasma albumin level may be depressed. The red cell sedimentation test is usually not altered appreciably.

The laboratory tests which are diagnostically applicable typically do not become positive until after the second or third week. One may use the intradermal test with Bachman trichinella antigen, read like the tuberculin test, or specific precipitin, flocculation, and complement-fixation reactions. Muscle biopsy will reveal characteristically degenerating muscle fibers and invading larvae; these can be taken most conveniently and with the greatest likelihood of success from near the tendinous attachments of the deltoid or gastrocnemius muscles. The intradermal test remains positive as a rule for about 3 years, and the serologic tests for 6 to 18 months.

TAPEWORMS

Suspicion of tapeworm infestation is often aroused by digestive difficulties, abdominal pains, and loss of weight, usually with nervousness, anemia, and eosinophilia or by the discovery of a chain of proglottid segments in the stools. *Taenia solium* sometimes forms encysted lesions in the skin, muscle, or brain which are known as *cysticerci*.

LABORATORY DIAGNOSIS. With all the tapeworms the diagnosis is best made by the recovery of either ova or proglottid segments in the stools. Ova are excreted abundantly in the stools, but those from all species of Taenia are so similar that identification cannot be achieved by this means alone. Ova often adhere to the perianal surfaces during defecation and may be detected with the adhesive-tape method (p. 724).

Proglottids are best identified by pressing a freshly discharged segment between two glass slides and scrutinizing the internal structure with a hand lens against a bright light. The pork tapeworm *T. solium* possesses 7 to 13 main lateral arms of the uterus on each side of each proglottid, in contrast to the beef tapeworm, *T. saginata*, which has 15 to 20. The proglottids of *T. saginata* may be actively motile in fresh specimens. The fish tapeworm, *Diphyllobothrium latum*, which belongs to a different genus, has easily identifiable ova and proglottids.

During treatment and for a few days thereafter all stools should be saved and passed through a fine sieve, about 20 meshes to the inch, in a thorough search for the head or scolex. Should the scolex fail to come away with the proglottid segments the probability is that the body of the worm will regenerate. Stool studies should be repeated in 2 or 3 months. If ova or segments are not found in several examinations the patient may be adjudged as cured.

STOOL EXAMINATIONS FOR PARASITES

Spontaneous evacuations are preferable to material obtained by enemas or cathartics, though the latter may be needed to recover worm segments when taeniasis is suspected. Stool specimens collected at home should be submitted as promptly as possible, in sterile glass jars or clean paper containers. There should be no contamination with urine. The entire evacuation is brought to the examiner to select the portions most suitable for study and to scrutinize for mucus or blood which might not be present in a small sample. Warm specimens must be examined within a few minutes in order to detect living protozoa.

Gross Examination

Spontaneously passed stools are preferable for detection of cysts and ova, since the number per unit of stool volume is much higher in a formed than in a postcathartic liquid stool. The latter is preferable for recovery of adult worms or the segments or proglottids of tapeworms. When ova alone are to be searched for, stool specimens may be several days old; a representative sample weighing a few grams is ample. The color and consistency are noted, and the surface inspected for blood, pus, mucus, nematodes, foreign bodies, or segments of taenia.

To search for worms buried in the substance, the greater part of the stool is placed in the topmost of a pile of progressively finer sieves, with the lowermost having a mesh of 60 holes to the inch. The sieves are then placed under a cold-water spigot and the water stream allowed to play on the stool until it disintegrates. As the particles wash through, any worms or worm segments are caught and become evident.

Adult worms possess distinctive morphologic features which permit their ready identification. Young stages may present more difficulty. The observer should be on the alert for mixed infections and also for worms not ordinarily associated with human infestations such as *Toxocara cati,* the ascarid of cats, or *T. canis,* the ascarid of dogs (p. 197). Descriptions of adult worms and ova and larvae and of concentration techniques for their recovery from feces can be found in textbooks on parasitology or laboratory methods.

Direct Microscopy

Each gram of stool, it has been estimated, must contain over 1,000 ova for direct smears to detect their presence regularly. Hence, except with the tapeworms which give off ova in unusual abundance, the finding of many ova or cysts in a direct smear is an indicator of a moderate or heavy infestation rather than of a carrier or subclinical state.

Ova and cysts tend to be distributed uniformly throughout an infected stool, so that any random fragment is representative. Live amebae and schistosome ova, on the other hand, are more likely to be found in specks of mucus or of blood.

When searching for live protozoa, a mucus-containing fragment of feces is emulsified in normal saline solution and mounted on a clean glass slide under a cover glass. At least three such preparations should be scrutinized microscopically before the presence of parasites can be excluded. Even one larva or ovum establishes the diagnosis. Additional slides may be stained, for study, with iodine solution or with neutral red. Cultures for amebae can be made if desired.

Many laboratories spread slides with stool material and immerse them while still wet in Schaudinn's fluid or some other fixative. These are then stored for later staining with one of the hematoxylin methods. Slides so fixed can be prepared in the physician's office and brought or mailed to a reliable laboratory. This approach to the demonstration of amebae furnishes a permanent record for filing purposes.

The ova of most human parasitic worms have diameters between 40 and 80 μ and can be detected with the low power of the microscope. *Balantidium coli,* the largest of the intestinal protozoa, has a similar diameter and its cysts are only slightly smaller. Active forms of the other intestinal protozoa, on the other hand, are generally 10 to 25 μ in diameter, and their cysts are 7 to 15 μ; these are best searched for with the high power, preferably with a warm stage. It is practically impossible to find motile protozoa in the first week after a roentgen study with barium or while a patient is receiving bismuth medication or mineral oil or other oily cathartic.

Concentration Procedures

When direct miscroscopic examinations of the wet smear are negative, one next resorts to concentration methods. For demonstrating small numbers of ova and cysts these are much more effective. Motile trophozoites cannot survive the procedure. The techniques in widest use are zinc sulfate flotation and formalin-ether sedimentation.

BIBLIOGRAPHY

LABORATORY DIAGNOSIS OF INTESTINAL PARASITES

Bittner, G., Detection of Parasites in Human Excretions, *J. Lab. & Clin. Med.* 35:121, 1950.

Craig, C. F., and *E. C. Faust*, "Clinical Parasitology," 5th ed., Lea & Febiger, Philadelphia, 1951.

Headlee, W. H., Intestinal Parasite Infections among In-patients of the Indiana University Medical Center Hospitals, *Am. J. Trop. Med.* 22:341, 1942.

Simmons, J. S., and *C. J. Gentzkow*, "Medical and Public Health Laboratory Methods," Lea & Febiger, Philadelphia, 1955.

INTESTINAL PROTOZOA

Arean, V. M., and *E. Koppisch*, Balantidiasis: A Review and Report of Cases, *Am. J. Path.* 32:1089, 1956.

Brooke, M. M., and *M. Goldman*, Polyvinyl Alcohol-fixative as Preservative and Adhesive for Protozoa in Dysenteric Stools and Other Liquid Materials, *J. Lab. & Clin. Med.* 34:1554, 1949.

Dolkart, R. E., *B. Halpern*, and *J. Cullen*, The Diagnosis of Amebiasis, the Role of the Complement-fixation Test, and the Incidence of the Disease in the Chicago Area, *J. Lab. & Clin. Med.* 38:804, 1951.

Maris, E. P., and *S. Bushong*, The Diagnosis of *Giardia intestinalis* Infestation by Means of Intestinal Intubation: The Treatment with Atabrine and Follow-up Studies of 68 Cases, *Pennsylvania M.J.*, 45:724, 1942.

Sapero, J. J., *D. K. Lawless*, and *C. P. A. Strome*, An Improved Iodine-staining Technique for Routine Laboratory Diagnosis of Intestinal Protozoa, *Science* 114:550, 1951.

Swartzelder, C., Laboratory Diagnosis of Amebiasis, *Am. J. Clin. Path.* 22:379, 1952.

Taylor, J. A., and *W. A. Riddell*, Entozoa of Children in Two Regina Institutions, *Canad. J. Pub. Health* 41:471, 1950.

WORMS

Avery, J. L., Treatment of Enterobiasis with One Dose of Promethazine Hydrochloride, *J.A.M.A.* 161:681, 1956.

Beaver, P. C., Methods of Pinworm Diagnosis, *Am. J. Trop. Med.* 29:577, 1949.

————, The Detection and Identification of Some Common Nematode Parasites of Man, *Am. J. Clin. Path.* 22:481, 1952.

Brown, H. W., K-F. Chan, and *K. L. Hussey,* Treatment of Enterobiasis and Ascariasis with Piperazine, *J.A.M.A.* **161:**515, 1956.

Hood, M., Laboratory Diagnosis of Platyhelminthiasis, *Am. J. Clin. Path.* **22:**396, 1952.

Jenkins, M. Q., and *M. W. Beach,* Intestinal Obstruction Due to Ascariasis: Report of Thirty-one Cases, *Pediatrics* **13:**419, 1954.

Jung, R. C., and *P. C. Beaver,* Clinical Observations on *Trichocephalus trichiuris* (Whipworm) Infestation in Children, *Pediatrics* **8:**548, 1951.

Markey, R. L., An Anal Swab Method for Detection of *Enterobius vermicularis, Am. J. Clin. Path.* **20:**493, 1950.

Pryor, H. B., Oxyuris Vermicularis: The Most Prevalent Parasite Encountered in the Practice of Pediatrics, *J. Pediat.* **46:**262, 1955.

Sadun, E. H., and *D. M. Melvin,* The Probability of Detecting Infections with *Enterobius vermicularis* by Successive Examinations, *J. Pediat.* **48:**438, 1956.

TRICHINOSIS

Freeman, L. C., F. J. Brady, A. D. Kessler, and *R. B. Scott,* Observations on Trichinosis: Report of a Community Outbreak, *A.M.A. Am. J. Dis. Child.* **89:**194, 1955.

Most, H., and *M. M. Abeles,* Trichiniasis Involving the Nervous System: Clinical and Neuropathologic Review, with Report of 2 Cases, *Arch. Neurol. & Psychiat.* **37:**589, 1937.

Roett, C. J. E., L. C. Freeman, and *R. B. Scott,* Incidence of "Subclinical" Trichinosis in Children: Observations Based on Reaction to Intradermal Test with Trichinella Antigen, *A.M.A. Am. J. Dis. Child.* **87:**464, 1954.

Rosen, E., Cortisone Treatment of Trichinosis, *Am. J. M. Sc.* **223:**16, 1952.

Wright, W. H., K. B. Kerr, and *L. Jacobs,* Studies on Trichinosis: Summary of Findings of *Trichinella spiralis* in Random Sampling and Other Samplings of Population of United States, *Pub. Health Rep.* **58:**1293, 1943.

CHAPTER 64

Thyroid

Any increase or diminution in the hormone elaborated and released by the thyroid gland results in derangements of tissue functions elsewhere in the body. The degree of activity of this gland is related to the regulatory control of thyrotropin (TSH, thyroid-stimulating hormone) of the anterior pituitary and related also to the amount of iodine made available by the circulation.

The polygonal epithelioid cells of the thyroid gland usually line the follicles or acini as a single layer. The lumens of the follicles are filled with hormone-containing eosinophilic material known as *colloid*. The iodine-containing hormones produced by the gland consist principally of thyroxin and triiodothyronine; most of the former is combined with a serum protein.

Metabolically, the iodine of food normally is absorbed into the circulation as inorganic iodine. Some of the iodide may be excreted by the kidney, but much of it is withdrawn from the blood stream ("trapped") by the thyroid gland. The acinar cells oxidize the iodide enzymatically to iodine and then build up thyroxin through the intermediate stages of monoiodotyrosine and diiodotyrosine.

APPRAISAL OF THYROID FUNCTION

When the history or physical examination of a patient suggests the existence of a thyroid disorder, laboratory studies should be resorted to in order to validate the diagnosis, rule out disturbances of other organs which may be affecting thyroid activity, and obtain measurable indexes to serve as guides during therapy. The most used test procedures are (1) basal metabolic rate, (2) serum protein-bound iodine concentration, and (3) studies with radioactive iodine.

Any of these approaches can serve for following the progress of a patient once the diagnosis has been established. In the early phases of a diagnostic study it is advisable to substantiate the interpretations by performing at least two of the tests. The basal metabolic reading is not reliable with patients with cardiac disorders, with children who are unable or unwilling to cooperate, or with any individual whose physical habitus is markedly deviant from the normal range. Readings within normal limits in serum protein-bound iodine and radioactive iodine studies practically always rule out thyroid disease.

Other less direct approaches to the efficiency of thyroid function which may be utilized in selected situations include (4) determinations of the serum levels of cholesterol, alkaline phosphatase, lipids, or carotene, (5) the creatine tolerance response, (6) estimation of thyrotropin concentration of blood or urine, (7) roentgen estimation of bone age and roentgenography for the epiphyseal dysgenesis found in hypothyroidism.

Basal Metabolic Rate (BMR)

Basal metabolism is the term applied to the total heat production by the body while in absolute rest. Since direct calorimetric measurement of the total heat output is very difficult technically, recourse is had to so-called indirect calorimetry. This is based on the established principle that oxygen consumption under standardized controlled conditions runs parallel to heat production and can be determined by measuring the amount of oxygen consumed by the patient in a given unit of time (corrected to 0°C and 760 mm Hg barometric pressure). The devices in widest use are of the closed-circuit type, which have the subject breathe oxygen through a tightly fitting face mask. The amount of oxygen consumed in an arbitrary interval of time, when multiplied by an arithmetical factor, converts the reading into the total number of calories produced during that interval. From this can be calculated the expected total caloric output in 24 hours were the child to remain in a basal status.

To eliminate variables due to digestion, physical activities, increased body temperature, and specific dynamic action of foods, the oxygen consumption is measured at least 12 hours after a meal while the digestive processes are quiescent and the subject is relaxed. This reading is deemed a measure of the vegetative functions alone. Ideally the subject should be asleep, since the rate is a little lower than when awake, but the value in the resting awake state is taken as the definite datum by common consent. A 1-hour rest period should precede the test. Since the first readings may be enhanced as a consequence of emotional and other causes, one or more preliminary rehearsals are often advisable, especially with apprehensive children.

STANDARDS. Emission of basal heat and the consumption of oxygen are proportional to total body size. Hence a corrective factor of reference must be introduced when one individual is compared with another or when changes are being looked for in the same individual with a weight change between successive readings. In healthy adults an excellent factor of reference is body surface area. In the childhood years the oxygen consumption and basal heat output may be referred to body surface area, weight, height, or combinations of these. Age before puberty has been found to be of negligible importance.

The tabulated sets of so-called normal data used most widely are those of F. B. Talbot (height, weight); Benedict (height); Dreyer (height); Boothby-Sandiford (surface area); Vogelius (weight-height ratio); Lewis, Duval, and Iliff (weight, height, surface area). With well-proportioned children the calculated basal metabolism rates as derived from any of these sets of standards run more or less parallel. With obese, thin, dwarfed or overtall children whose measurements deviate appreciably from those of the normal children utilized in preparing these standards, the rates derived from the different approaches may not conform one with another.

When calculating a child's basal metabolic rate from standard tables, one should first appraise the body size by referring to one of the accepted tables for height and weight as related to age. If the weight is near the average for height, the reading derived from oxygen consumption can be compared with the corresponding figure for a normal child of the same weight and sex. The difference between the observed and the expected reading, computed as plus or minus per cent, is the expression of the basal metabolism. However, should the child's weight deviate markedly from the average, or should physical inspection reveal abnormal body proportions, it is better to refer to the table for height.

Because of the many pertinent considerations which attend the clinical use of basal metabolism readings of children, the formal report from the laboratory should state—in addition to the final computed percentage—the child's physical measurements, the average weight of a child of the same sex, age, and height as given by an authoritative source which should be named, the measured rate of oxygen consumption, the source of the standard used for reference, and a statement as to the child's cooperation during the test.

INFANCY AND CHILDHOOD. Readings with an infant may be made while at rest in a special boxlike respiratory chamber covering the entire body or his head alone. Reference standards for infants are those of Benedict and Talbot, Levine and Marples, Clagett and Hathaway, Benjamin and Weech, and Karlberg. The energy metabolism has been found to be about 15 per cent lower in the first week of life than later. There are no sex differences. Individual infants exhibit day-to-day variations up to 15 per cent in their resting metabolism, especially during the early months of life. Differences up to 20 per cent have been found with healthy infants of the same weight, height, and age.

The basal metabolism (caloric output per square meter of body surface per hour) diminishes gradually during the age period 10 to 16 years for both boys and girls. The basal metabolism for boys is higher than for girls of comparable age.

A deviation of ±15 per cent from the mean will take in approximately 95 per cent of normal children. A deviation of ±20 per cent from the mean value is necessary to comprise 98 per cent. With the surface-area standards the results of tests of obese children having no signs of hypothyroidism may be as low as −25 to −40 per cent. Parallel difficulties attend the recognition of increased basal metabolism in excitable or overthin children suspected of being hyperthyroid.

A fall in basal oxygen consumption takes place in the year prior to the onset of menstruation.

ABNORMAL STATES. When interpreting a basal metabolic reading one should bear in mind that deviations from the normal average do not occur in thyroid disturbances alone. Nutritional reserves, antecedent diet, rate of growth, and hormones from other endocrine glands can affect the metabolism. The rate tends to be elevated by fever, emotional disturbance, lymphoma, leukemia, cardiac failure, and some forms of hyperpituitarism; and to be depressed by hypoadrenalism, starvation, the nephrotic syndrome, intracranial tumors, and hypopituitarism.

In pronounced hypothyroidism the basal metabolic readings are typically at least 25 per cent below the standards; in pronounced hyperthyroidism, at least 25 per cent above. In borderline thyroid dysfunctions the readings are often in the normal range. Even when the conduct of the test has been satisfactory, selection of a proper standard for comparison becomes difficult. If the hypothyroid child is dwarfed, inadequate standards are available; if he is obese the low oxygen consumption of adipose tissue gives rise to abnormally low figures when referred to surface-area standards.

Despite these limitations, serial determinations can be useful in following the response to therapy of a child with a thyroid disturbance. The necessary cooperation as a rule cannot be secured until the patient is at least 7 years of age, or higher if mentally defective.

Protein-bound Iodine Level in Serum (PBI)

The great proportion of the iodine in the plasma or serum is in the form of thyroxin (tetraiodothyronine), which circulates combined with serum protein. Small amounts are in related substances, or free as inorganic iodine. The latter occurs ordinarily in concentrations of the magnitude of 1 μgm per 100 ml, but may be raised if iodine-containing substances have been ingested recently. The protein-bound iodine concentration, on the other hand, usually parallels that of circulating thyroid hormone.

The accuracy of the determination when reliably done is one part per million. The blood specimen may be drawn at any time of day without relation to meals, fever, physical activity, nervous tension, diet, or any of the other variables which distort the basal metabolic rate. The quantities of iodine measured are so minute that a high degree of technical skill is necessary.

Falsely high readings will be encountered for weeks after iodine-containing compounds have been given for urinary tract excretory studies, or for months after diagnostic cholecystography or bronchography.

Whenever the diagnostic study of a patient requires both a protein-bound iodine determination and a procedure using an iodide, the former should always be done first.

NORMAL VALUES. During the first week of life the usual range for the protein-bound iodine of serum is 8 to 14 μgm per 100 ml, with the average at 11 to 12 μgm per 100 ml. In the large series reported by Danowski and associates the extremes spread from 6.5 to 15.4 μgm. Unduly high contents at this age period were ascribed presumptively to passive transfer from maternal blood.

The mean curve falls gradually in the neonatal period, and then remains constant from the third month until the end of the first year. The average for this period was found by Danowski in a study of 110 Pittsburgh infants to be 6.3 ± 1.0 μgm. With healthy children the same authors found a mean of 4.7 ± 0.8 μgm per 100 ml, with no trend of change in relation to age. The 3d to 97th percentile range was 3.2 to 7.0 μgm; the 20th to 80th percentile, 4.0 to 6.0 μgm. Readings were slightly higher in early adolescence.

THYROID DISEASES. In childhood hyperthyroidism the levels typically range from 9 to 25 μgm per 100 ml, whereas in hypothyroidism they are less than 4 or even 3 μgm. When therapy is begun for either form of dysfunction the readings for protein-bound iodine return to normal more rapidly than does the basal metabolic rate. Low values may be found also in hypoproteinemia and following radiation injury of the gland.

Radioactive Iodine (Radioiodine, I¹³¹)

The metabolism of iodine can be followed quantitatively by observing the progress through the body of an oral dose of radioactive iodine (I¹³¹). Numerous phases of the cycle may be measured, such as the curve of the rise and fall of plasma radioactivity after a test dose or the rate of uptake of radioactive iodine by the thyroid gland itself or the excretion in the urine, as determined within a convenient number of hours. All such measurements of radioactivity are carried out with shielded mechanical assemblies containing Geiger-Müller counters. When urinary excretion is being measured, the results may be distorted if renal function is abnormal.

In hypothyroid states the metabolic cycle of radioactive iodine proceeds more slowly than normal, in hyperthyroid states more rapidly. The percentage of aberrant results in euthyroid (normal) individuals is much lower than with the basal metabolic rate. In borderline disturbances the readings do not always deviate sufficiently from the normal range to lead to reliable conclusions. Some well-differentiated thyroid tumors will accumulate radioactive iodine.

Perhaps the most frequent method of utilizing I¹³¹ is to give an oral dose of sodium radioiodine of known potency (usually from 10 to 50 microcuries) and measure the uptake by means of a counter placed over the thyroid 24 to 48 hours later. In Oliner's representative study of children of all ages, the normal 24-hour uptakes ranged from 17 to 50 per cent with a mean of 31.1 ± 7.63. The 48-hour readings were in the same range. In hyperthyroidism the uptakes were over 70 per cent; in hypothyroidism, below 15 per cent. Absorption in any patient can be depressed temporarily by prior ingestion of antithyroid drugs, thyroid substance, or stable iodine in any form.

Studies with radioactive iodine can be applied only by laboratories having radiation subdepartments. There is also the fear, thus far unsubstantiated, that even with the most cautious dosage the retention of this radioactive material may later result in some other serious thyroid disorder, or even in some mutational changes within the ova of the ovary.

HYPOTHYROIDISM

In childhood this is most often an expression of a congenital or primary defect of the gland (athyreosis, cretinism). Hypothyroidism due to hypoiodinism (endemic goiter) has largely disappeared from this country as the consequence of direct fortification of table salt and other foods with iodine in geographic areas where this element is otherwise lacking. A rare variety is that in which the thyroid can take up iodine but is unable to synthesize thyroxin from it; I^{131} uptakes are normal in these cases.

Cyanates, perchlorates, thiourea, para-aminosalicylic acid, resorcinol, perhaps cobalt, and a number of other drugs sometimes become goitrogenic by interfering with the initial organic binding of iodine or a later step in hormone synthesis. Iodine itself, absorbed over a long period (often in a medicament), will sometimes paradoxically induce a nontoxic goiter. Exceptionally the iodinated hormones in the circulation may seem pharmacologically inert even though measurable in the total serum PBI.

Rarer causes of acquired or secondary hypothyroidism (juvenile hypothyroidism) are thyroiditis, operative removal, and unknown influences. Minimal degrees of secondary hypothyroidism are believed to occur at times in mongolism. Hypothyroidism secondary to hypopituitarism (pituitary myxedema) is often difficult to distinguish from the primary variety, because both are characterized by retardation of growth and other endocrinal disturbances. When pituitary secretion is at fault, replacement therapy with thyroidal principles rectifies only those disturbances related directly to the hypothyroidism.

Laboratory Findings

Just as with symptoms and signs, the extent of the laboratory abnormalities in hypothyroidism depend upon severity and age of onset. In classical cases not receiving replacement therapy the basal metabolic rate and the serum levels of protein-bound iodine and radioactive iodine are all depressed. The uptake of radioactive iodine over the gland is almost negligible when there is absence or atrophy of the thyroid but may be unusually high if the hypothyroidism is associated with goitrous enlargement of the gland. The red cell count and hemoglobin level tend to be normocytically low, and the bone marrow is hypoplastic. The total leukocyte count is usually not reduced, because a moderate absolute lymphocytosis tends to overshadow any mild depression in the absolute granulocyte count. Platelets may be abundant or diminished. The red cell sedimentation rate may be accelerated. The output of urinary creatine is reduced, as is the creatine-creatinine ratio. The serum phosphatase activity is usually subnormal, and the serum carotene elevated. The serum cholesterol tends to be increased; a rise 6 to 10 weeks after a trial period of thyroid extract therapy is of diagnostic significance (p. 521).

HYPERTHYROIDISM

The syndrome usually seen in children is the diffuse toxic goiter of Graves' disease. A multinodular or discrete adenoma in a child is suggestive of carcinoma.

Laboratory Findings

In a pronounced case of hyperthyroidism the basal metabolic rate, serum protein-bound iodine level, and uptake of radioactive iodine are all well above the normal range, indicating an accelerated rate of thyroid activity. Care must be taken in interpreting results when only one of these tests gives elevated readings, since there are many sources of error. In clinically questionable cases a battery of normal results excludes the diagnosis of hyperthyroidism. The various components of the serum lipids, including cholesterol, may be in the low-normal or moderately subnormal range, but these estimations are of little assistance in differential diagnosis. Mild anemia or lymphocytosis may be present. Alterations in the blood sugar curves are not diagnostic. The urine creatine and the creatine-creatinine ratio go up.

BIBLIOGRAPHY

BASAL METABOLISM

Alexander, J. G., Evaluation of a Method of Estimating the Basal Metabolic Rate, J. Clin. Path. 4:381, 1951.

740

Endocrine System

Benedict, F. G., and F. B. Talbot, Metabolism and Growth from Birth to Puberty, Carnegie Inst. Wash. Publ. 302, 1921.

Benjamin, H., and A. A. Weech, Basal Heat Production in Relation to Growth: A Longitudinal Study on Normal Infants Six to Twenty Months of Age, Am. J. Dis. Child. 65:1, 1943.

Bierring, E., "Standard Metabolism of Boys," Levin & Munksgaard, Copenhagen, 1931.

Boothby, W. M., and I. Sandiford, Normal Values of Basal or Standard Metabolism: A Modification of the DuBois Standards, Am. J. Physiol. 90:290, 1929.

Clagett, D. D., and M. L. Hathaway, Basal Metabolism of Normal Infants from Three to Fifteen Months of Age, Am. J. Dis. Child. 62:967, 1941.

Dreyer, G., The Normal Basal Metabolism in Man, and Its Relation to the Size of the Body and Age, Expressed in Simple Formulae, Lancet 2:289, 1920.

Iliff, A., V. A. Lee, and R. C. Lewis, Interpretation of Basal Metabolic Rate of Children of Unusual Body Build, Pediatrics 8:616, 1951.

Karlberg, P., Determination of Standard Energy Metabolism (Basal Metabolism) in Normal Infants, Acta paediat. vol. 41, suppl. 89, 1952.

Lamb, M. W., Basal Metabolism of 8 Nursery School Children Determined at 3 Month Intervals, Am. J. Dis. Child. 70:220, 1945.

Levine, S. Z., T. H. McEachern, M. A. Wheatley, E. Marples, and M. D. Kelly, Respiratory Metabolism in Infancy and in Childhood. XV. Daily Energy Requirements of Normal Infants, Am. J. Dis. Child. 50:596, 1935.

—— and E. Marples, The Respiratory Metabolism in Infancy and Childhood. XII. A Biometric Study of Basal Metabolism in Normal Infants, Am. J. Dis. Child. 41:1332, 1931.

—— and J. R. Wilson, The Respiratory Metabolism in Infancy and in Childhood. I. Basal Metabolism of Children, Am. J. Dis. Child. 31:323, 1926.

Lewis, R. C., A. M. Duval, and A. Iliff, (a) Basal Metabolism of Normal Boys and Girls from 2 to 12 Years Old Inclusive: Report of a Further Study, Am. J. Dis. Child. 65:834, 1943. (b) Standards for Basal Metabolism of Children from 2 to 15 Years of Age, Inclusive, J. Pediat. 23:1, 1943.

——, ——, and ——, Effect of Repeated Determinations on Basal Metabolism of Children, Am. J. Physiol. 140:461, 1944.

——, A. Iliff, and A. M. Duval, Comparative Accuracy of Closed Circuit Bedside Method and Open Circuit Chamber Procedure for Determination of Basal Metabolism, J. Lab. & Clin. Med. 28:1238, 1943.

——, G. M. Kinsman, and A. Iliff, Basal Metabolism of Normal Boys and Girls from 2 to 12 Years Old, Inclusive, Am. J. Dis. Child. 53:348, 1937.

Stevenson, S. S., P. Wirth, R. Bastiani, and T. S. Danowski, Some Effects of Exogenous Thyroid or Thyroxin upon Premature Infants, Pediatrics 12:263, 1953.

Talbot, F. B., Basal Metabolism Standards for Children, Am. J. Dis. Child. 55:455, 1938.

Vogelius, H., Basal Metabolism of Girls and the Use of Metabolic Standards, Acta med. scandinav. suppl. 165, 1945.

Wolman, I. J., Basal Metabolism in Childhood: Current Progress, Am. J. M. Sc. 211:733, 1946.

PROTEIN-BOUND IODINE DETERMINATIONS

Danowski, T. S., S. J. Huff, L. H. Erhard, M. Price, M. Brown, P. Wirth, and S. S. Stevenson, Protein-bound Iodine Levels in Normal and in Diabetic Children, A.M.A. Am. J. Dis. Child. 84:5, 1952.

——, S. Y. Johnston, W. C. Price, M. McKelvy, S. S. Stevenson, and E. R.

McCluskey, Protein-bound Iodine in Infants from Birth to One Year of Age, *Pediatrics* 7:240, 1951.

Hallman, B. L., P. K. Bondy, and *M. A. Hagewood,* Determination of Serum Protein-bound Iodine as a Routine Clinical Procedure, *A.M.A. Arch. Int. Med.* 87:817, 1951.

Means, J. H., Comparison of Tests of Thyroid Function, *Bull. New York Acad. Med.* 26:583, 1950.

RADIOIODINE

Jaffe, H. L., and *R. E. Ottoman,* Evaluation of Radioiodine Test for Thyroid Function, *J.A.M.A.* 143:515, 1950.

Lowrey, G. H., W. H. Beierwalters, I. Lampe, and *H. J. Gomberg,* Radioiodine Uptake Curve in Humans. II. Studies in Children, *Pediatrics* 4:627, 1949.

McConahey, W. M., C. A. Owen, and *F. R. Keating, Jr.,* A Clinical Appraisal of Radioiodine Tests of Thyroid Function, *J. Clin. Endrocrinol.* 16:724, 1956.

Oliner, L., R. M. Kohlenbrener, T. Fields, and *R. H. Kunstadter,* Thyroid Function Studies in Children: Normal Values for Thyroidal I[131] Uptake and PBI[131] Levels up to the Age of 18, *J. Clin. Endocrinol.* 17:61, 1957.

Rall, J. E., The Role of Radioactive Iodine in the Diagnosis of Thyroid Disease, *Am. J. Med.* 20:719, 1956.

Silverman, S. H., and *L. Wilkins,* Radioiodine Uptake in the Study of Different Types of Hypothyroidism in Childhood, *Pediatrics* 12:288, 1953.

Van Middlesworth, L., Radioactive Iodine Uptake of Normal Newborn Infants, *A.M.A. Am. J. Dis. Child.* 88:439, 1954.

HYPOTHYROIDISM

Akerrén, Y., Early Diagnosis and Early Therapy in Congenital Cretinism, *Arch. Dis. Childhood* 30:254, 1955.

Cooke, R. E., and *E. B. Man,* Management of Hypothyroidism in Infancy and Childhood, *Pediatrics* 17:617, 1956.

Fisher, D. A., G. D. Hammond, and *D. E. Pickering,* The Hypothyroid Infant and Child, *A.M.A. Am. J. Dis. Child.* 90:6, 1955.

Herlitz, G., Iodine and Sporadic Goiter in Childhood, *Acta paediat.* 41:556, 1952.

Hutchison, J. H., and *E. M. McGirr,* Hypothyroidism as an Inborn Error of Metabolism, *J. Clin. Endocrinol.* 14:869, 1954.

Lawson, D., On the Prognosis of Cretinism, *Arch. Dis. Childhood* 30:75, 1955.

McGirr, E. M., and *J. H. Hutchison,* Dysgenesis of the Thyroid Gland as a Cause of Cretinism and Juvenile Myxedema, *J. Clin. Endocrinol.* 15:668, 1955.

Reilly, W. A., Thyroid Disorders in Childhood, *Advances Pediat.* 9:137, 1957.

Talbot, N. B., E. H. Sobel, J. W. McArthur, and *J. D. Crawford,* "Functional Endocrinology From Birth Through Adolescence," Harvard University Press, Cambridge, 1952.

Van Wyk, J. J., The Use of Thyroid in Pediatric Practice, *Quart. Rev. Pediat.* 10:212, 1955.

Wilkins, L., G. W. Clayton, and *M. Bethrong,* Development of Goiters in Cretins without Iodine Deficiency: Hypothyroidism due to Apparent Inability of the Thyroid Gland to Synthesize Hormone, *Pediatrics* 13:235, 1954.

—— and *W. Fleischmann,* The Dianosis of Hypothyroidism in Children, *J.A.M.A.* 116:2459, 1941.

——, ——, and *W. Block,* Hypothyroidism in Childhood: Sensitivity to Thyroid Medication as Measured by Serum Cholesterol and Creatine Excretion, *J. Clin. Endocrinol.* 1:14, 1941.

HYPERTHYROIDISM

Allen, R. E., E. Rose, and *E. K. Rose,* Juvenile Thyrotoxicosis: Results of Treatment in 30 Cases, *Pediatrics* **14**:38, 1954.

Hardy, J. D., and *C. Riegel,* The Laboratory Diagnosis of Hyperthyroidism: A Practical Analysis of Current Methods, with Presentation of Illustrative Cases, *Am. J. M. Sc.* **221**:359, 1951.

Kunstadter, R. H., and *A. F. Stein,* Treatment of Thyrotoxicosis in Children with Thiourea Derivatives, *Pediatrics* **6**:244, 1950.

CHAPTER 65

Adrenal Cortex

ANATOMY

The adrenal cortex is separable morphologically into three fairly distinct concentric zones. There is the outermost narrow *zona glomerulosa* consisting of clumps and loops of pyramidal cells, the middle wider *zona fasciculata* made up of large polygonal cells in columnar arrangement, and the innermost narrow *zona reticularis* which is a plexus of small more deeply staining cells.

Prominent during the neonatal period only is the transitory *zona fetalis,* or so-called "fetal cortex," a broad band of palely staining cells situated between the cortex and medulla. Of as yet unelucidated physiologic significance, this zone begins to atrophy in the first few days after birth, regardless of whether the infant has been born at full term or prematurely. During the second week it undergoes most marked involution. Some shrunken epithelial cells may remain until 3 to 6 months, and fibrous tissue remnants may persist until the first or second birthday.

During the first 2 weeks of age the adrenals are relatively large. In full-term newborn infants each adrenal has an average weight of about 3.5 gm, with a range of 1.5 to 6 gm. There are no recognizable sex differences. In premature infants the weight is less, in proportion to body weight. After involution of the fetal zone the mean weight is slightly under 2 gm at 3 months of age. Cortex and medulla then grow very slowly, reaching about 2.5 gm by the second year and 7 or 8 gm at puberty.

Newer cytologic, histochemical, and extraction studies have brought out some suggestive correlations between physiologic activities and histologic appearances. The fasciculata and reticular layers atrophy when the pituitary is damaged or extirpated, whereas the glomerulosa layer does not. The glomerulosa zone perhaps secretes the hormones which are related to renal control of water and electrolytes. The fasciculata appears to secrete many of the oxysteroids, including corticosterone and cortisone, which affect the metabolism of sugar, fat, and proteins and are related to antibody production and reactions in disease states. The reticularis seems the major source of the androgenic hormones which accelerate protein metabolism and evoke masculinization.

REGULATION OF ELECTROLYTES

The internal distribution and renal excretion of potassium, sodium, and chloride seems to be affected significantly by all the known biologically active corticosteroids. Aldosterone seems to exert the most potent sodium-retaining effect.

When elaboration of these "salt-and-water," "electrolyte-regulating," or "aldosterone-like" hormones is inadequate, as in Addison's disease, potassium is reabsorbed from the glomerular filtrate in excess of normal and sodium is excreted in unusual amounts. The sodium lost in the urine carries chloride and water along with it and tends to dehydrate the blood stream and tissues. The retained potassium may depress the myocardium and skeletal muscles if in abundance (p. 582). Normal electrolyte levels do not exclude the diagnosis of Addison's disease when a patient shows the classical clinical picture, since in the absence of a crisis the serum sodium and chloride levels may not be reduced and a rise in serum potassium may be minimal or even absent. The finding of a serum sodium level of less than 135 mEq per liter in a suspected case, however, practically establishes the diagnosis. Early laboratory signs of a crisis are low serum sodium and chloride levels, a rise in packed cell volume denoting dehydration and hemoconcentration, a rise in the blood urea nitrogen, and a fall in blood pressure.

An abundance of sodium in the urine in a patient with a subnormal blood sodium level and receiving a low sodium diet is a sign of adrenocortical hypofunction. In a normal subject with a low sodium intake the urine will be free or nearly free of this element. A normal individual can continue almost indefinitely with a salt-free diet, whereas a patient with Addison's disease will become very ill within a few days. Adrenalectomized animals may live indefinitely when given sodium chloride freely. Human beings with Addison's disease need hormonal support as well.

Study of the urine for the presence of sodium after its withdrawal from the diet ("salt-deprivation test") is of fairly good reliability for detection of adrenocortical deficiency. This test is safe only with hospitalized patients under careful observation, while intravenous saline solution and adrenal cortical extracts are kept on hand for an emergency. This approach should not be employed unless other tests have given unrevealing results.

An excess of salt-and-water hormones within the body is followed typically by retention of sodium and water, enhanced excretion of urinary potassium, and decline in both plasma and intracellular potassium. Laboratory studies sometimes show a slight increase in the plasma levels of sodium and bicarbonate and a diminution in potassium and chloride. If pronounced, this combination is known as hypopotassemic hypochloremic alkalosis.

BLOOD RESPONSES

The responses of the eosinophils, in the absence of allergic or parasitic or other disorders which affect the eosinophil level (Chap. 15), are presumptive but far from reliable indicators of adrenal cortical status. The usual normal range is from 100 to 400 eosinophils per cu mm. A persistently high count may be a sign of diminished adrenal activity. A count below 100 and usually below 50, provided the bone marrow is not hypoplastic, may coincide with increased cortical activity.

In the 4-hour corticotropin test a dose of 25 mg (or proportionately less if the subject is an infant) is injected intramuscularly and the level of circulating eosinophils followed. In the 48-hour corticotropin test an initial 25-mg dose is given, followed by 10 mg every 6 hours for a total of 48 hours. Eosinophil counts are taken at intervals until 4 hours after the final injection. In general, a failure of the eosinophils to fall more than 50 per cent is taken as a sign of reduced adrenal cortical function.

Corticotropin, cortisone, and some of the other adrenal hormones in effective therapeutic dosages act in the direction of correcting hematologic disturbances referable to functional depression of the bone marrow. In normal subjects the absolute number of neutrophils typically rises within a few hours, to become 25 to 100 per cent higher than the pretreatment level. Lymphocytes may fall transitorily in the first few days of therapy, but exhibit no consistent change thereafter. Eosinophils are usually depressed. With corticotropin the red cell readings sometimes drop transiently in the first few days, due to hemodilution.

The intermediary mechanisms by which these hormones exert their remedial action in marrow aplastic states, thrombocytopenic purpura, and childhood leukemia as yet remain unknown.

Influence on Inflammatory States

Experimental observations indicate that in bacterial infections an antagonistic effect is exerted by cortisone-like hormones on inflammatory vascular dilatation, increased permeability of blood vessels, and diapedesis of leukocytes. This permits the bacteria to multiply more freely within the tissues of the host and facilitates inflow of organisms into the blood stream. At the same time the toxemic and febrile responses of the body may be depressed, giving rise to a false impression of clinical improvement.

In inflammatory and other diseases unrelated to microbial spread, such as rheumatoid arthritis and bronchial asthma, the reduction in the vascular and mesenchymal responses may result in marked benefit to the patient.

These hormones seem to inhibit some interactions between antibodies and antigens. In serum sickness, rheumatic fever, and allergic states, the clinical disturbances are ameliorated. In bacterial infections, this repression of immune processes may deprive the host of a major resistance mechanism. Organisms such as *Aspergillus niger, Monilia albicans,* or the slowly growing tubercle bacillus may find the internal environment more favorable for multiplication.

PLASMA GLUCOSE RESPONSES

Some adrenocortical hormones favor the production of glucose from protein and fat and retard its utilization by the tissues. When a single therapeutic dose of corticotropin is injected into an individual with normal adrenal function, the plasma glucose level will usually rise to 100 or even 120 mg per 100 ml. This is effected also by other physiologic influences in addition to the adrenal steroids. Disturbances due to all other mechanisms must therefore be excluded before plasma glucose responses related to the adrenal can be evaluated.

With the intravenous glucose tolerance test, a patient with hypoadrenocorticism tends to experience an unusual degree of hypoglycemia after the initial hyperglycemia, as a consequence of unusual sensitivity to the endogenous insulin evoked by a test dose of sugar (p. 505). Conversely, a patient with hyperadrenocorticism tends to have an unusual persistence of the hyperglycemia because of the antiinsulin behavior of the adrenal steroids. With the insulin tolerance test, a small injection of insulin given to a patient with hypoadrenocorticism will usually depress the blood sugar level to an abnormal degree and for a prolonged time. Symptoms of hypoglycemia may result and may not be relieved until carbohydrate is administered.

OTHER TESTS OF ADRENAL CORTICAL FUNCTION

Methods are being developed and standardized for isolation and quantitative measurement of the individual corticosteroids which are found in the human circulation. Exploratory studies have indicated that 17-hydroxycorticosterone (compound F) and corticosterone (compound B) are present nearly always; also aldosterone and other compounds which seem conjugated. The plasma corticosteroid level varies normally between 5 and 20 μgm per 100 ml within a 12-hour period. Significant rises follow the intravenous injection of ACTH.

In congenital virilizing adrenocortical hyperplasia (the adrenogenital syndrome), Bongiovanni and Eberlein found that the adrenal cortex secretes excessive quantities of androgens as reflected in the high secretion of 17-ketosteroids in the urine. On the other hand, the level of compound F in the blood is exceptionally low and fails to rise after administration of ACTH. Interestingly, the urine of most patients contains large quantities of pregnanetriol, a reduction product of 17-hydroxyprogesterone. This finding suggests an inability of the adrenal cortex to convert 17-hydroxyprogesterone into compound F. It is in accord with the hypothesis that the anterior pituitary secretes an excessive amount of ACTH in an attempt to stimulate the production of compound F; the adrenal cortex responds by liberating an abundance of androgenic steroids which produce the clinical disturbance. The high urinary output of 17-ketosteroids in this disease (p. 363) is suppressed by cortisone therapy, whereas the high urinary output in virilizing adrenal tumor remains unaffected by the therapy.

BIBLIOGRAPHY

ADRENAL MORPHOLOGY

Greep, R. O., and *H. W. Deane,* The Cytology and Cytochemistry of the Adrenal Cortex, *Ann. New York Acad. Sc.* **50:**596, 1949.

Hasner, E., The Size of the Adrenals in Children (Grandeur des surrénales chez les enfants), *Acta chir. scandinav.* **99:**51, 1949.

O'Donnell, W. M., S. Fajans, and *J. G. Weinbaum,* Human Adrenal Cortex after Administration of ACTH and Cortisone: Morphologic Changes, *A.M.A. Arch. Int. Med.* **88:**28, 1951.

Tahka, H., On the Weight and Structure of the Adrenal Glands and the Factors Affecting Them, in Children of 0–2 Years, *Acta paediat.* vol. 40, suppl. 81, 1951.

ADRENAL PHYSIOLOGY AND DISTURBANCES

Bongiovanni. A. M., Evaluation of Adrenal Cortical Function in Pediatrics: Methods, *Am. J. M. Sc.* **220:**697, 1950.

———, Physiology of the Adrenal Cortex in Infancy and Childhood, *Am. J. M. Sci.* **222:**710, 1951.

——— and *W. R. Eberlein,* Clinical and Metabolic Variations in the Adrenogenital Syndrome, *Pediatrics* **16:**628, 1955.

Burdick, W. F., R. O. Warthen, J. E. Cassidy, and *W. W. Welsh,* Addison's Disease in a Five and One-half Year Old Boy, *Am. J. Dis. Child.* **80:**975, 1950.

Daeschner, C. W., J. H. Moyer, and *L. W. Able,* Pheochromocytoma in a Four-year-old Child: Renal Hemodynamic, Pharmacologic, and Radiographic Studies, *J. Pediat.* **45:**141, 1954.

Gardner, L. I. (ed.), "Adrenal Function in Infants and Children: A Symposium," Grune & Stratton, Inc., New York, 1956.

———, Adrenocortical Metabolism of the Fetus, Infant, and Child, *Pediatrics* **17:**897, 1956.

Geppert, L. J., W. A. Spencer, and *A. M. Richmond,* Adrenal Insufficiency in Infancy: A Clinical Classification, Review and Report of a Case, *J. Pediat.* **37:**1, 1950.

Gold, J. J., Blood Corticoids: Their Measurement and Significance—A Review, *J. Clin. Endocrinol.* **17:**296, 1957.

Hain, A. M., The Excretion of 17-Ketosteroids and Gonadotrophin in Children: Normal and Abnormal Cases, *Arch. Dis. Childhood* **22:**152, 1947.

Lanman, J. T., Adrenal Function in Premature Infants. I. Infants without Recognized Disease, *Pediatrics* **11:**120, 1953. II. ACTH-treated Infants and Infants Born of Toxemic Mothers, *ibid.* **12:**62, 1953.

Rose, E. K., H. T. Enterline, J. E. Rhoads, and *E. Rose,* Adrenal Cortical Hyperfunction in Childhood, *Pediatrics* **9:**475, 1952.

Simpson, S. L., Adrenal Hyperfunction and Function, *Bull. New York Acad. Med.* 27:723, 1951.

Wilkins, L., The Diagnosis of the Adrenogenital Syndrome and Its Treatment with Cortisone, *J. Pediat.* 41:860, 1952.

Williams, A., and *M. J. Robinson,* Addison's Disease in Infancy, *Arch. Dis. Childhood* 31:265, 1956.

CHAPTER 66

Ovaries and Vagina

OVARIES

The mature ovary of the infant weighs 0.5 to 1 gm; of the adult woman, about 5 gm. Primitive follicles, each composed of a primitive ovum encircled by a single layer of epithelial cells, are present at birth or begin to develop immediately afterward. These originate just beneath the surface layer of cuboidal germinal epithelium. When puberty is reached, individual follicles begin to run through their full cycle of oogenesis, one for each intermenstrual period. Each cycle commences with swelling and proliferation of the granulosa cells which surround the ovum. Clear serous fluid, the liquor folliculi, forms on one side as the granulosa cells disintegrate locally. The ovum then begins to enlarge and divide and soon extrudes the first polar body. The follicle enlarges, reaches the surface of the ovary, and when 1 to 1.5 cm in diameter, ruptures to discharge the ovum. Follicles often start to mature simultaneously in groups, but all but one regress before the cycle is very far along.

Clotted blood fills the ruptured follicle to form the corpus hemorrhagicum. The granulosa cells, epithelioid in character, then proliferate rapidly to form the corpus luteum. If the ovum is not fertilized the corpus luteum begins to shrink about the eighth to tenth day after follicular rupture and soon becomes a white scarred area of hyalinization, the corpus albicans. If conception occurs the corpus luteum persists until the fourth month of gestation.

Simple Cysts

During infancy the ovaries often exhibit minor degrees of follicular maturation, to be followed by recession, cyst formation, and scarring. The enlarging follicles may measure 1 to 2 mm in diameter, and the cysts up to 7 mm in diameter. Some of the cysts may have an outer granulosa cell layer, others may not. Hemorrhages into the cysts are rare.

This follicle and cyst development is most marked in early infancy and attains its peak at about the fourth month. The phenomenon is probably related to the maternal chorionic hormones. Spontaneous regression is the almost invariable rule, but the large ovarian cysts which arise occasionally in later girlhood may have their origin as such small follicular cysts which continue to grow.

749

Estrogens and Progesterone

The naturally occurring estrogens in women—estradiol, estrone, and estriol—are derived principally from the ovary. When administered to castrated female animals or immature women they stimulate growth of the vagina, uterus, and mammary glands. A number of pharmaceutically synthesized compounds have a parallel action.

Estrogens from the mother are transmitted to the infant throughout the fetal period. Their action produces the mild hypertrophy of the labia and uterus and the glycogen in the vaginal epithelium of the newborn female infant. The breast enlargement with secretion of "witch's milk" at the end of the first weeks is referable either to these estrogens or to a hypothesized hormonal prolactin of autogenous or maternal origin.

Progesterone, produced both by the corpus luteum and the placenta, brings about those changes throughout the matured female genital tract which are important for reception and support of the embryo. The adrenal cortex is able to produce progesterone in some endocrinopathies but probably does not do so under normal circumstances. Imbalance between the rhythm of secretion of ovarian estrogens and progesterone is a principal cause of the irregularities of menstruation and other endometrial disorders which may become manifest during and after puberty.

MENSTRUAL CYCLE. During the first 2 weeks of the cycle the content of FSH (follicle-stimulating hormone) in the blood increases rapidly. This leads the ripening follicle in the ovary to pour forth estrogens; and these in turn stimulate the uterine endometrium.

At about the fourteenth day of the cycle the circulating FSH begins to decline. At this time the follicle ruptures and ovulation occurs. Other pituitary gonadotropins then appear—LH (luteinizing hormone) and LTH (luteotropin). These stimulate the conversion of the ruptured follicle into a corpus luteum, which in turn releases estrogens and progesterone. After 10 days the luteinizing pituitary hormones decline and the corpus luteum regresses into a corpus albicans. The uterine mucosa coincidentally begins to desquamate.

When the endometrial desquamation is over the mucosa is only about 1 mm in thickness and consists essentially of a flat or basal layer. As regenerative proliferation occurs, the newly forming glands are narrow and straight or spiral and the stromal cells become numerous. By the time of ovulation the endometrium is about 3 mm in thickness.

The secretory phase begins with ovulation and is the direct response to the combined estrogen-progesterone stimulation from the corpus luteum. The mucosa becomes thicker (about 6 mm) and differentiates into basalis, spongiosa, and compacta layers. Premenstrually the mucosal glands become even more tortuous and distended, the stroma cells are swollen and thin-walled, and infiltration with phagocytic leukocytes takes place. Menstruation begins with hemorrhagic necrosis of the spongiosa and compacta.

Laboratory Aids in the Study of Ovarian Function

Recognition of disease of the ovary is made chiefly from clinical phenomena. Laboratory tests are used for specific problems.

VAGINAL SMEARS. The cells of the vaginal epithelium are small and rounded when circulating estrogens are inadequate; larger, flatter, cornified, and richer in glycogen when estrogens are circulating. By weekly vaginal smear examinations one can follow the course of the ovarian cycle and often detect poor or irregular estrogenic stimulation when present. In adolescent hypomenorrhea due to slow sexual underdevelopment the cells undergo cyclic changes even though of minor degree, whereas in true sexual infantilism no such response can be seen. Serial studies can assist in following the response of a patient to hormonal therapy, if the earlier cellular responses were those of estrogenic deficiency. In precocious puberty induced by ovarian tumors which secrete estrogens the vaginal epithelium will show the characteristic response.

TECHNIQUE OF VAGINAL SMEAR. Clean the vulva with wet cotton. Spread the vulvar lips and introduce a cotton applicator or aspirator tube through the hymenal orifice, being careful to avoid brushing against the external structures. Transfer the removed material to glass slides.

To study cell morphology one may immerse the slide in a mixture of equal parts of ether and ethyl alcohol and stain later by the method of Shorr. To search for glycogen, place an unfixed dried slide face down over a vessel containing Lugol's iodine solution. Many cells will be stained by the iodine vapor if estrogen activity has stimulated glycogen formation.

URINARY SEDIMENT. The epithelial cells in the urinary sediment of older girls, derived from the urethra, are said to undergo the same cyclic changes as the vaginal epithelium. In the absence of circulating estrogens the urinary cells tend to be small and rounded, whereas when these are circulating the cells are larger and cornified.

VAGINAL pH. At birth the vaginal hydrogen-ion concentration is acid, near 5.5. This acidity subsides during the neonatal period, as the glycogen fades from the epithelial cells. Throughout childhood the vaginal secretion remains neutral or moderately alkaline (pH 6.8 to 8.2). At puberty the vaginal acidity returns as the ovarian hormones stimulate the synthesis of glycogen within the vaginal epithelium. Breakdown of this glycogen in desquamated cells by the local bacteria liberates lactic and related acids. In problems of sexual precocity in young girls, the finding of an acid intravaginal pH is suggestive that ovarian estrogens are being produced.

ENDOMETRIAL CURETTAGE. The functional status of the ovaries is reflected in the appearance of the endometrial fragments obtained by curettage or biopsy. A normal secretory picture is indicative of normal ovulation. Persistent hyperplasia of the mucosa in repeated examinations denotes unusual secretion of estrogens. Persistent atrophy is indicative of ovarian deficiency, though one cannot tell from the histology whether the deficiency is primarily ovarian or secondary to pituitary insufficiency.

Curettage of the uterus is more important in the management of excessive bleeding than in amenorrhea. It is usually not done under 35 years of age unless tuberculosis or some other local disease of the endometrium is suspected. Adequate information as to whether the genital tract is being exposed to estrogen stimulation can ordinarily be obtained from study of vaginal smears.

BASAL BODY TEMPERATURE. Beyond puberty, daily readings of the body temperature taken at 7:00 A.M., before arising in the morning, may show a sudden increase of 1°F within a few days of normal ovulation. In anovulatory menstrual cycles this rise does not take place.

URINE ESTROGENS. Since chemical methods are cumbersome and difficult, estrogens in the urine for clinical purposes are ordinarily evaluated by bioassay. Estrogenic activity is estimated by noting the changes induced in spayed adult female rats by 24-hour urine specimens. Trace amounts are barely detectable in the urine of younger boys and girls. By approximately 2 years before the onset of menstruation the average girl begins to exhibit increasing urinary estrogenic activity. Excretion fluctuates rhythmically with the menstrual cycle, being higher in the latter half. Unusual amounts may be excreted in premature adolescence induced by granulosa-cell tumors or choriocarcinomatous teratomas.

PREGNANEDIOL. Progesterone itself does not appear in the urine, but some steroid derivatives do, and notably pregnanediol. Its absence during the latter part of a menstrual cycle indicates absence of a functionally active corpus luteum, and hence failure of ovulation.

PITUITARY GONADOTROPINS. See page 764.

Ovarian Hypofunction

MENARCHE. Menstrual bleeding ordinarily commences between 10 and 14 years of age. The first episodes are usually anovulatory, i.e., not associated with a full cycle of follicular changes within the ovary. The onset of menstruation antedates by one or more years the onset of reproductive fertility.

AMENORRHEA. Defective secretory activity by the ovaries seems to be the basis for amenorrhea, hypomenorrhea, oligomenorrhea, and related disturbances, except when the uterus itself is malformed or otherwise diseased. Hypoplasia or atrophy of the genital structures may be present if the ovarian failure is severe or of long duration.

In primary amenorrhea, early womanhood is reached without menstruation ever taking place. In secondary amenorrhea the menses cease entirely or almost entirely after having once been established.

GONADAL DYSGENESIS (TURNER'S SYNDROME). Typical features, usually first recognized at puberty, are primary amenorrhea, infantilism of the sexual organs, sparse axillary and pubic hair, and short stature. Urinary excretion of 17-ketosteroids and estrogens is low. Bone age is slightly retarded before puberty, more marked thereafter. Other severe anomalies are often associated, especially webbed neck, coarctation of the aorta, cubitus valgus, or syndactylism.

These patients have the external configuration and cultural and psychologic expressions of females, but studies of the tissue cells have indicated that the majority, if not all, are histologically males.

STUDY FOR SEX CHROMOSOMES. Study of cells from most organs of the body has shown that most cell nuclei of females exhibit a stainable chromatin mass that is not present in the nuclei of males. This mass, about 1 μ in diameter, in skin and mucosal cells occurs just inside the nuclear membrane. Tissue for study may accordingly be taken from a skin biopsy or scrapings of the mucosa of the mouth. Neutrophils in the peripheral blood may also be examined: 2 to 8 per cent of cells of females have a small club-shaped protrusion from one of the nuclear lobes. These protrusions are ordinarily less numerous in males.

Ovarian Dysfunction

FUNCTIONAL UTERINE BLEEDING. This is the name given to prolonged or excessive or irregular discharge of uterine blood which cannot be traced to obvious lesions of the cervix, uterus, or adnexae. The endometrium as obtained by curettage may appear atrophic, hyperplastic, normally proliferative (preovulatory or estrogenic), normally secretory (postovulatory or progestational), or show a "mixed" pattern of different stages.

Many girls during and just beyond adolescence experience episodes of prolonged and profuse bleeding during the years that menstruation is being established. This variety of abnormal bleeding tends to be self-limited and rarely has serious significance, though secondary anemia of the iron-deficiency type may result. The mother is usually in more need of reassurance than the adolescent herself. The possibility of a blood dyscrasia should always be considered.

Ovarian Hyperfunction

Tracking down the cause of premature sexual development in a female child requires a thorough analysis of the family background, case history, physical concomitants, and laboratory results. Interpretation of studies of the circulating and excreted hormones usually requires consultation with an endocrinologist familiar with the vagaries of the tests themselves and their results in systemic endocrinal disturbances. In general, gonadotropins appear in the urine when the anterior pituitary is being stimulated or when pregnancy is present and chorionic epithelium is active. An excess of estrogens in the urine may be derived from premature follicular development, an epithelializing cyst, a granulosa cell tumor, or a teratomatous chorionepithelioma. Urinary pregnanediol in detectable amounts signifies luteinized tissue in the ovaries. The 17-ketosteroid excretion may be somewhat elevated, especially with some adrenal tumors. The serum alkaline phosphatase may be moderately elevated in the presence of bone changes related to polyostotic fibrous dysplasia. Tests for thyroid function may point in the direction of hyperthyroidism.

VAGINA

Bacterial Flora

At birth the vagina is sterile, but assorted and diverse bacteria become demonstrable within 12 hours. Doederlein's Gram-positive lactobacillus becomes predominant by the third day, remains in the ascendancy for the first 2 weeks, and then fades from prominence. It does not reappear in significant numbers until the prepubertal return of glycogen to the vaginal cells.

When treating chronic vaginitis in a child the beneficial action of sulfonamides and antibiotics can be enhanced, if need be, by the coincidental administration of estrogenic hormone for a week to a month to stimulate local glycogen formation and growth of Doederlein's bacillus. Most vaginal pathogens are inhibited by an acid environment.

Vulvovaginitis

BACTERIAL INFECTIONS. Infection with inflammation of the vulvovaginal tract of infants and children is caused nearly always by the hemolytic streptococcus, the gonococcus, or the pneumococcus. Other bacteria such as staphylococci, colon bacilli, diphtheroids, Shigella, or Monilia are sometimes recovered, often in mixed cultures, but are rarely responsible for irritative phenomena. Diphtheritic and herpetic vaginitis have been described. Foreign bodies and vesicovaginal fistulas should always be thought of. Masturbation can excite vaginitis and interfere with recovery. Vulvovaginitis caused by streptococci and pneumococci is often associated with and secondary to infections elsewhere in the body caused by these organisms.

With modern chemotherapy, nearly all children with bacterial vulvovaginitis can be treated successfully by the oral route. Bacterial measures for identifying the causative organism consist of smear and culture.

In the direct smear one searches primarily for intracellular Gram-negative diplococci which morphologically resemble gonococci. Possibilities for error in either direction are numerous, so that one should be cautious in recognizing or excluding this organism solely from the findings in a smear. Therefore, and also because of the medicolegal and social implications attached to the diagnosis of gonorrheal vaginitis, one should also prepare a culture from the depths of the vagina on a medium and in an atmosphere favorable to the growth of gonococci. Suspicious colonies should be fully identified.

TRICHOMONIASIS. *Trichomonas vaginalis* is a pear-shaped protozoan about the size of a white blood cell. It has four anterior flagellae and an undulating membrane extending along its side for one-half to two-thirds of its length. The oval nucleus is situated near the front end, and the pointed axostyle protrudes posteriorly. When caught in debris the organism exhibits rapid changes in shape.

Chronic vaginal trichomoniasis ordinarily does not begin to appear until puberty. There is no conclusive evidence that *Tr. vaginalis* represents an adaptation of *Tr. hominis* to the vagina.

The vaginal discharge may be thin and watery, or thick and yellowish. The diagnosis is made by recovery of the parasite from the inflamed area.

The patient reports for examination without taking a douche or medication in the previous 24 hours. Samples of vaginal secretion are collected from the vagina with an aspirating tube. These are examined microscopically in a fresh wet preparation, mixed when thick with a little Ringer's solution or normal saline. Covering the slide with a cover slip is not essential. Incubating a portion of the material for 4 to 6 hours at 37°C will often reveal motile trichomonads when the immediate examination has failed.

The parasites are best detected with the low power of the microscope, and their identity confirmed with the high power. Any motile flagellated protozoan found in the vagina can be assumed to be *Tr. vaginalis.*

If infection in urethra or bladder is suspected, a hanging drop preparation may be made of a centrifuged specimen of the residual urine, obtained by catheterization. Purulent material from Bartholin's or Skene's glands may be examined directly.

HERPES SIMPLEX VULVOVAGINITIS. When primary infection with herpes simplex virus takes the form of an acute vulvovaginitis, the area becomes reddened and edematous and exhibits vesicles or superficial shallow ulcers. The diagnosis is established by demonstration of the herpes simplex virus in the lesion or of the development of neutralizing serum antibodies during convalescence. Diphtheria, impetigo, ammoniacal dermatitis, and accidental vaccination with vaccine virus also come into the differential diagnosis.

Foreign Body

The presence of an introduced foreign object should always be suspected with every stubborn vaginal discharge which is resistant to therapy. Rectal palpation and lower abdominal x-rays are two methods of diagnosis. If these approaches are negative, the vaginal tract can be inspected directly through a small nasal or otologic speculum.

BIBLIOGRAPHY

OVARY

Costin, M. E., Jr., and R. L. J. Kennedy, Ovarian Tumors in Infants and in Children, Am. J. Dis. Child. 76:127, 1948.

Polhemus, D. W., Ovarian Maturation and Cyst Formation in Children, Pediatrics 11:588, 1953.

Schwartz, O. H., C. C. Young, Jr., and J. C. Crouse, Ovogenesis in the Adult Human Ovary, Tr. Am. A. Obstet. Gynec. & Abdom. Surgeons 59:263, 1948.

Soffer, L. J., Diagnosis of Endocrine Disease: Clinical and Laboratory Considerations, Bull. New York Acad. Med. 29:101, 1953.

Wharton, L. R., "Gynecology," 2d ed., W. B. Saunders Company, Philadelphia, 1947.

MENSTRUATION

Bicker, W., Amenorrhea and Oligomenorrhea, Etiology and Treatment, Am. J. Obst. & Gynec. 56:893, 1948.

Fluhmann, C. F., Menometrorrhagia during Adolescence, J.A.M.A. 135:557, 1947.

Novak, E., Uterine Bleeding with Special Reference to the Functional Type, J. Internat. Coll. Surgeons 11:9, 1948.

Simell, G., On the Menarche Age of Finnish Women, Acta paediat. vol. 41, suppl. 84, 1952.

HYPOOVARIANISM

Silver, H. K., and C. H. Kempe, Ovarian Agenesis (Congenital Aplastic Ovaries) in Children, A.M.A. Am. J. Dis. Child. 85:523, 1953.

Wilkins, L., and W. Fleischmann, Ovarian Agenesis: Pathology, Associated Clinical Symptoms and the Bearing on the Theories of Sex Differentiation, J. Clin. Endocrinol. 4:357, 1944.

HYPEROVARIANISM

Mason, L. W., Precocious Puberty, J. Pediat. 34:730, 1949.

Pray, L. G., Sexual Precocity in Females: Report of Two Cases, Pediatrics 8:684, 1951.

Seckel, H. P. G., W. W. Scott, and E. P. Benditt, Six Examples of Precocious Sexual Development. I. Studies in Diagnosis and Pathogenesis, Am. J. Dis. Child. 78:484, 1949.

VAGINA

Boisvert, L., and *D. N. Walcher*, Hemolytic Streptococcal Vaginitis in Children, *Pediatrics* 2:24, 1948.

Hardy, G. C., Vaginal Flora in Children, *Am. J. Dis. Child.* 62:939, 1941.

Krugman, S., Primary Herpetic Vulvovaginitis, *Pediatrics* 9:585, 1952.

MacDonald, E. M., and *A. L. Tatum*, The Differentiation of Species of Trichomonads by Immunological Methods, *J. Immunol.* 59:309, 1948.

McGuiness, W. J., and *R. C. Telling*, Vulvovaginitis in a Child Due to *Shigella flexneri, Brit. M. J.* 2:1424, 1950.

Mukherjee, C., Gonococcal Vulvovaginitis in Infants and Children: A Study of 240 Cases, *Arch. Dis. Childhood* 25:262, 1950.

Schauffler, G. C., "Pediatric Gynecology," Year Book Publishers, Chicago, Ill., 1953.

Trussell, R. E., "*Trichomonas vaginalis* and Trichomoniasis," Charles C Thomas, Springfield, Ill., 1947.

Weinstein, L., Bacterial Flora of Human Vagina, *Yale J. Biol. & Med.* 10:247, 1938.

HISTOLOGIC DIFFERENTIATION OF SEX

Davidson, W. M., and *D. R. Smith*, A Morphological Sex Difference in the Polymorphonuclear Leucocytes, *Brit. M. J.* 2:6, 1954.

Greenblatt, R. B., O. M. de Acosta, E. Vázquez, and *D. F. Mullins, Jr.*, Oral Mucosal Smears in Detection of Genetic Sex, *J.A.M.A.* 161:683, 1956.

Grumbach, M. M., J. J. Van Wyk, and *L. Wilkins*, Chromosomal Sex in Gonadal Dysgenesis (Ovarian Agenesis): Relationship to Male Pseudohermaphrodism and Theories of Human Sex Differentiation, *J. Clin. Endocrinol.* 15:1161, 1955.

Moore, K. L., and *M. L. Barr*, Nuclear Morphology, According to Sex, in Human Tissues, *Acta anat.* 21:197, 1954.

CHAPTER 67

Testes

ANATOMY

The testis consists essentially of two functional parts. The long and convoluted seminiferous tubules provide and nourish the germ cells through their complex evolution into spermatozoa. The interstitial polyhedral cells of Leydig have as their principal activity the furnishing of androgenic hormones to support spermatogenesis and control the secondary sex characteristics.

The diagnostic advances in testicular biopsy have made it important for the physician to be familiar with the histologic changes during normal growth and in pertinent endocrinal disturbances.

Fetal and Newborn Periods

In the latter third of gestation the tubules appear as small solid cords 50 to 75 μ in diameter. The tubular cells are of two varieties. The majority (ultimately destined to become Sertoli cells) form undifferentiated syncytial-like structures, with small nuclei which stain intensely. Distributed among them in small numbers are large clear-cut cells that appear to be primary germ cells (spermatogonia).

At the time of birth the tubules are separated from one another by broad masses of Leydig cells which fill the interstitium. These Leydig cells differ from those of the adult in having less lipid and being free from cytoplasmic crystalloids or pigment. Within a few hours after birth they begin to shrink and involute, but are usually recognizable for a few months. The fetal hyperplasia of the Leydig cells appears to be a response to the maternal chorionic gonadotropin transferred across the placenta.

Childhood

Until the onset of puberty the histologic appearance of the testis remains essentially unchanged with the interstitial cells of Leydig not recognizable. The tubules are narrow, lined with compact ovoid or cuboidal cells in a double layer, and have suggestive rather than definite central lumens. A few mitoses may be seen. The fibrous tissue stroma is loose and myxomatous.

Puberty

Starting at 9 to 11 years of age the pattern changes more and more in the direction of sperm formation. The tubules become broader (average diameter, 72 to 85 μ) and are more coiled and contorted. The lining epithelium proliferates into multiple layers, with many of the cells having swollen cytoplasm and rounded nuclei. Mitoses are more numerous, and Sertoli cells appear. One can recognize spermatogonia, primary spermatocytes, secondary spermatocytes, and even some spermatids. Clumps of interstitial cells can be recognized after about age 9, cytologically resembling those of the fetus. These changes coincide with the appearance in the urine of gonadotropins and 17-ketosteroids in appreciable quantity.

Adulthood

The adult pattern of fully active spermatogenesis and well-defined interstitial cells is usually achieved between 11 and 15 years of age, or sometimes later. The tubules are broad and uniform and actively producing spermatozoa. The Leydig cells form small islands among the tubules and contain pigment and other inclusions. The supporting tissue is fibrous and rich in collagen.

Spermatogenesis begins with the spermatogonia. These are relatively large primary germinal cells resembling in size and structure the primitive sex cells of young embryos. They go through several successive mitotic divisions and metamorphoses. The majority of the daughter cells are converted first into small type B spermatogonia, and later into the resting or primary spermatocytes. A few, however, revert back to original size and appearance, and after a resting period divide again to start another cycle of proliferation. The primary spermatocytes proliferate by meiosis or reduction-division, a process in which the chromosomes divide once but the cell body divides twice, with the result that the nuclei of the resultant cells contain but half of the original number of chromosomes. The secondary spermatocytes thus produced are soon converted into spermatids, or immature true spermatozoa. The spermatids in turn undergo a complex series of progressive changes termed spermiogenesis as they mature into free spermatozoa. The Sertoli elements are large cells holding and nourishing the outer cells of the seminiferous epithelium. Their large light nuclei are spaced along the basement membrane, while their cytoplasm is believed to fuse into a syncytium.

PITUITARY CONTROL

The physiologic maturation and functioning of the Leydig or interstitial cells appears to be governed by the pituitary luteinizing hormone or LH (also known as the interstitial cell-stimulating hormone or ICSH). Growth of the tubules and maturation of the spermatogonia and spermatids appear to be governed by the follicle-stimulating hormone or FSH. Both these gonadotropic hormones commence their activity in normal boys a year or more before puberty. The interstitial cells of the testes began to elaborate testosterone and testosterone-like androgens shortly before puberty.

HYPOGONADISM

Hypogonadism is a loose term, applied when either the production of sperm cells or the activity of the interstitial cells is impaired. When both are affected one sometimes speaks of "panhypogonadism." The clinical manifestations are conditioned by the character and degree of the testicular defect, the age at which the deficiency begins, and the presence or lack of pituitary stimulation. Study of the microscopic development of the testis in biopsy specimens, and semen examination in males past puberty, are useful approaches to the appraisal of the development of the component parts.

All children are hypogonadal up to the onset of puberty. Even when both testes have been removed by surgery or destroyed by trauma or infection or other lesions in early childhood, growth and maturation proceed normally through the childhood years. Since occasional normal boys do not spontaneously exhibit the beginning of pubertal androgenic activity until age 15 or 16, or even rarely until age 20, the diagnosis of hypogonadism is difficult to establish during the early teen years. It may be suspected earlier when there has been known injury to the testes.

From clinical studies alone it is usually not possible to determine whether an observed deficiency in the masculinization of an adolescent boy or young man is due primarily to testicular failure or to pituitary failure. Differentiation can be facilitated by a trial with chorionic gonadotropin therapy. The secondary sexual characteristics will be stimulated to development if the pituitary is inactive, whereas failure of improvement is a sign of absence or defect of the interstitial cells.

When pubertal growth of the testicular tubules does not take place, the testes will fail to undergo the increase in size characteristic of that age. In primary pituitary lesions the output of urinary gonadotropins is either below normal or absent, whereas in primary testicular failure it is often increased.

Testicular biopsy in pituitary gonadotropin deficiency reveals small undeveloped seminiferous tubules and few or absent interstitial cells—the appearance resembling that shown by prepuberal boys. Chorionic gonadotropic hormone therapy stimulates the interstitial cells and tubular size, but not the germinal epithelium. If this therapy is discontinued the interstitial cells and tubules return to the immature state in a few months. Testosterone initiates the maturation of the tubules, but not of the interstitial cells.

There is considerable evidence that infertility in some adult males has its incipiency in the childhood years. Body configuration and external genitalia attain normal proportions, presumably because of adequate interstitial cell activity, but spermatogenesis and tubular architecture remain that of a younger age period.

Undescended Testis

The cryptorchid testis before puberty resembles histologically its descended normal mate. Once puberty has begun, however, the undescended testis shows poor development of the seminiferous epithelium, and this may not be resumed fully after surgical correction. Interstitial cell growth appears to be unimpaired both before and after operation unless surgical trauma has been severe.

It is problematic whether an undescended testis in an abnormal position will ever achieve full spermatogenesis even when surgical correction is performed in the first few years of life.

Hyalinization of the Seminiferous Tubules

This condition is part of a syndrome of unknown cause which is characterized consistently by abnormally small testes, azoospermia, and a high urinary gonadotropin output. With less uniformity there is gynecomastia ("Klinefelter's syndrome"), eunuchoidal habitus, and underdevelopment of some of the secondary sexual characteristics. Puberty starts in a normal fashion but may not continue to completion. Excretion of urinary 17-ketosteroids may vary from normal to very low. Urinary estrogens are not increased. Testicular biopsy reveals progressive sclerosis of the lamina propria and basement membrane of the seminiferous tubules and retardation of spermatogenesis. The end result is progressive and complete disappearance of all germinal and Sertoli cells and complete hyalinization of the tubules. The interstitial cells which remain tend to be clumped.

Systemic Disease

Minor illnesses such as colds and streptococcic throat infections may transitorily depress spermatogenesis, resulting in a decrease in the sperm count. More severe acute illness may lead to a more profound depression, lasting at times as long as 3 months. Chronic illnesses such as congenital heart disease or tuberculosis may retard the onset of puberty and cause apparently irreversible sclerosis in some of the tubules.

Myotonic Dystrophy

This is a disease with a pronounced familial tendency that may become apparent before, during, or some time after puberty. In males, the muscular dystrophy is usually associated with polyglandular deficiency and testicular atrophy. In the few cases studied there was a normal urinary excretion of estrogens, a low excretion of 17-ketosteroids, and a variable excretion of gonadotropins. The testicular atrophy is due to progressive tubular sclerosis usually with an increased prominence of interstitial cells.

HYPERGONADISM

True Precocious Puberty

In this disturbance the initiating cause seems to lie in the hypothalamus. This activates the pituitary, which in turn releases one or both of the gonadotropic hormones. Secondary sex characteristics develop, and growth of the skeleton and musculature is accelerated, but the output of urinary gonadotropins and 17-ketosteroids is increased only moderately if at all. In the so-called complete precocious puberty the testes are large, the semen contains well-formed spermatoza, and a testicular biopsy reveals the adult type of seminiferous tubules along with an abundance of large interstitial cells. In the so-called incomplete form, on testicular biopsy the tubules are immature but the interstitial cells are exceptionally abundant and form large confluent masses.

Pseudoprecocious Puberty

Premature masculinization in a young boy without pituitary disease can be caused by an interstitial cell tumor or chorionepithelioma, adrenocortical hyperplasia or tumor, or excessive therapeutic use of chorionic gonadotropin or testosterone. With any of these conditions the urinary output of 17-ketosteroids tends to be excessive. In adrenal cortical hyperplasia (adrenogenital syndrome), testicular biopsy shows the gonads immature in all respects. In the other conditions there may be some tubular dilatation and lumen formation, incomplete differentiation of the lining cells, and perhaps suggestive spermatogenic activity. The interstitial cells of Leydig are not large or prominent, as they are in true precocious puberty.

BIBLIOGRAPHY

ANATOMY; PHYSIOLOGY

Albert, A., L. O. Underdahl, L. F. Greene, and *N. Lorenz,* Male Hypogonadism. I. The Normal Testis, *Proc. Staff Meet. Mayo Clin.* 28:409, 1953.

Goldzieher, J. W., and *E. C. Hamblen,* Andrologic Endocrinology; Correlation of Clinical Symptoms, Urinary Hormone Excretion and Testicular Cytology, *Surg., Gynec. & Obst.* 85:583, 1947.

Greulich, W. W., R. I. Dorfman, H. R. Catchpole, C. I. Solomon, and *S. S. Culotta,* Somatic and Endocrine Studies of Puberal and Adolescent Boys, *Monogr. Soc. Res. in Child Develop.* vol. 7, no. 33, 1942.

Nelson, W. O., et al., Biology of the Testes, *Ann. New York Acad. Sc.* 55:543, 1952.

Schonfeld, W. A., Primary and Secondary Sexual Characteristics: Study of Their Development in Males from Birth through Maturity with Biometric Study of Penis and Testes, *Am. J. Dis. Child.* **65**:535, 1943.

Talbot, N. B., and *E. H. Sobel,* Endocrine and Other Factors Determining the Growth of Children, *Advances Pediat.* **2**:238, 1947.

———, ———, *J. W. McArthur,* and *J. D. Crawford,* The Testes, chap. 6 in "Functional Endocrinology from Birth through Adolescence," Harvard University Press, Cambridge, Mass., 1952.

HYPOGONADISM

del Castillo, E. B., A. Trabucco, and *F. A. de la Balze,* Syndrome Produced by Absence of the Germinal Epithelium without Impairment of the Sertoli or Leydig Cell, *J. Clin. Endocrinol.* **7**:493, 1947.

Heller, C. G., and *W. O. Nelson,* Hyalinization of the Seminiferous Tubules Associated with Normal or Failing Leydig-cell Function: Discussion of Relationship to Eunuchoidism, Gynecomastia, Elevated Gonadotrophins, Depressed 17-ketosteroids and Estrogens, *J. Clin. Endocrinol.* **5**:1, 1945.

——— and ———, Classification of Male Hypogonadism and a Discussion of the Pathologic Physiology, Diagnosis and Treatment, *J. Clin. Endocrinol.* **8**:345, 1948.

Hotchkiss, R. S., Diagnosis of Testicular Deficiencies, *Bull. New York Acad. Med.* **27**:510, 1951.

Klinefelter, H. F., Jr., E. C. Reifenstein, Jr., and *F. Albright,* Syndrome Characterized by Gynecomastia, Aspermatogenesis without A-leydigism and Increased Excretion of Follicle-stimulating Hormone, *J. Clin. Endocrinol.* **2**:615, 1942.

Nelson, W. O., and *C. G. Heller,* The Testis in Human Hypogonadism, *Recent Prog. Hormone Res.* **3**:197, 1948.

HYPERGONADISM

Jacobsen, A. W., and *M. T. Macklin,* Hereditary Sexual Precocity: Report of a Family with 27 Affected Members, *Pediatrics* **9**:682, 1952.

Jungck, E. C., A. M. Thrash, A. P. Ohlmacher, A. M. Knight, Jr., and *L. Y. Dyrenforth,* Sexual Precocity Due to Interstitial-cell Tumor of the Testis: Report of 2 Cases, *J. Clin. Endocrinol.* **17**:291, 1957.

Rusche, C., Twelve Cases of Testicular Tumors Occurring during Infancy and Childhood, *J. Pediat.* **40**:192, 1952.

Seckel, H. P. G., W. W. Scott, and *E. P. Benditt,* Six Examples of Precocious Sexual Development: Studies in Diagnosis and Pathogenesis, *Am. J. Dis. Child.* **78**:484, 1949.

Sobel, E. H., R. C. Sniffen, and *N. B. Talbot,* The Testis: V. Use of Testicular Biopsies in the Differential Diagnosis of Precocious Puberty, *Pediatrics* **8**:701, 1951.

Walker, S. H., Constitutional True Sexual Precocity, *J. Pediat.* **41**:251, 1952.

Weinberger, L. M., and *F. C. Grant,* Precocious Puberty and Tumors of the Hypothalamus: Report of a Case and Review of Literature, with Pathophysiologic Explanation of Precocious Sexual Syndrome, *Arch. Int. Med.* **67**:762, 1941.

CHAPTER 68

Pituitary

ANTERIOR LOBE

The pituitary gland weighs about 0.5 mg in the adult, and proportionately less in growing children. Its anterior segment displays three types of glandular cells—acidophilic (eosinophilic), basophilic, and chromophobic. The growth hormone appears to come from the eosinophilic cells, and the gonadotropic hormones from the basophilic cells. The precise origins of the other hormones—thyrotropic, corticotropic, and lactogenic—are as yet undetermined. The chromophobic cells appear to be endocrinally inert.

Because of the multiplicity of elaborated principles, disorders of the anterior pituitary give rise to complex patterns of disturbances which usually are difficult to classify precisely. There may be an excess or deficiency in the production of one or more hormones without parallel involvement of the remainder. Disorders in pituitary function can be recognized and interpreted more readily from the clinical and endocrinal phenomena exhibited by the patient than from the results of specific laboratory tests.

Growth Hormone

Excessive activity of the growth hormone (somatotropin) can produce gigantism in various forms, and the level of blood phosphorus may be elevated a little. Deficiency in growth hormone leads to dwarfism or infantilism. As yet, there is no simple laboratory test for direct evaluation of this hormone, but bioassay methods are being developed.

Gonadotropins

Several pituitary gonadotropins are recognized: (1) the follicle-stimulating principle (FSH) which controls spermatogenesis in the male or maturation of the ovarian follicles in the female, and (2) the luteinizing or interstitial-cell-stimulating principle (LH) which controls Leydig (interstitial) cell development and activity or corpus luteum formation.

764

The presence of FSH is demonstrated and assayed by study of changes induced in the sex organs of immature rats or mice. The assay methods most widely used are based on increases in uterine weight induced by extracts of 24-hour urine specimens. A so-called "mouse unit" is the amount of hormone which will double the weight of the uterus of a 21-day-old mouse; this is equivalent to approximately 0.2 rat unit (RU).

Demonstrable quantities of gonadotropins are not excreted until about the eighth year by individuals of either sex. Boys then begin to exhibit small amounts, which reach the adult male level of approximately 6 RU per day at about 15 years of age. Girls display a more pronounced increase, rising to about 15 RU at 16 years of age and subsiding to about 9 RU at age 20. This urine level is usually maintained until a later rise begins at about age 40. There is wide variation from individual to individual and often rhythmic fluctuations in women during the menstrual cycle.

In children with precocious sex development the urine often shows undue gonadotropic activity when the condition is induced by hypothalamic or pituitary stimulation, but none when induced by primary ovarian tumors.

Overproduction of the pituitary gonadotropic hormones leads to sexual precocity along with exaggerated height and increased bone age. Diagnostic studies for such disturbances include roentgenographic study of the pituitary fossa as well as study of the urine. Gonadotropin production is excessive also in the syndromes of ovarian agenesis (p. 753) and sometimes in primary testicular hypoplasia (p. 760) after the age of 10 or 11 years. Deficiency of gonadotropic hormones results in hypoplasia of the genital organs.

Thyrotropin

Difficulty attends the differentiation between primary hypothyroidism and that secondary to absence of pituitary stimulation. In both situations the serum concentrations of cholesterol and carotene are elevated and that of protein-bound iodine is low. In primary thyroid gland failure the production of pituitary thyrotropic hormone has been found enhanced, but measuring the output of this hormone is technically difficult.

Corticotropin (Adrenocorticotropin, ACTH)

Quantitative methods for assay of circulating corticotropic hormone are not yet widely available. In general, when hyperactivity of the adrenal cortex is due to pituitary stimulation the urinary excretion of 17-ketosteroids and 11-oxycorticosteroids is elevated (p. 363). When cortisone therapy which inhibits pituitary activity is given to such patients the abnormal output subsides, whereas with autonomous adrenal tumors it remains unaltered.

With hypoadrenalism due to pituitary failure the urinary content of these steroids remains abnormally low.

Hypopituitarism

When many functions are involved, this may show itself as Simmonds' disease, Frohlich's syndrome, idiopathic pituitary dwarfism, or hypopituitarism secondary to primary athyrosis. When hypopituitarism is severe, and especially if an organic lesion of the gland is present, the typical patient may show a very low level of basal metabolism, a low blood pressure, hypogonadic phenomena, reduced blood level of fasting glucose, and a slow blood glucose recovery rate after a test dose of insulin. Prolonged undernutrition, whether from semistarvation, intestinal disease, renal insufficiency, or chronic illness, will sometimes induce a reversible or so-called functional hypopituitarism.

POSTERIOR LOBE

Histologically this segment of the gland is made up of a loose meshwork of neurocytes, covered by a thin epithelial layer. Of the secreted principles the antidiuretic hormone is the one of most importance in pediatrics. The oxytocic principle, oxytocin, brings about contraction of the pregnant uterus in the mature woman. The vasoconstrictor principle, vasopressin, induces constriction of the muscularis of the peripheral arterioles, resulting in hypertension, and has some antidiuretic action.

The posterior pituitary also appears to bear some relation to emptying of the lactating mammary gland. Suckling at the nipple seems to reflexly liberate a posterior pituitary hormone, which in turn causes other elements of the breast to contract; this facilitates the flow of milk.

Antidiuretic Hormone

This stimulates water reabsorption by the kidney at the level of the lower tubules. Liberation of this hormone seems to be evoked by a minimal rise in the osmotic pressure of the blood. The *osmoreceptors* which are activated by hypertonicity seem to lie in the distribution of the carotid arterial system, but their exact nature and location are not known. It is presumed that they lie in the hypothalamus and are responsive to the osmotic status of the blood in the carotid artery. The hypothalamus in turn appears to govern the posterior pituitary through nerve pathways, since transection of the pituitary stalk and its contained neurons is followed by a deficiency in posterior pituitary activity similar to that which occurs when this part of the gland is destroyed.

Primary diabetes insipidus is believed to be a manifestation of inadequate production of this hormone. In the rare patients with so-called nephrogenic diabetes insipidus the production of hormone is apparently adequate but the tubules of the kidney seem refractory to its action.

Laboratory Studies for Diabetes Insipidus

The subcutaneous or intravenous administration of 2 units of aqueous posterior pituitary extract per square meter of body surface to an older child with diabetes insipidus will reduce urine volume and raise the urinary specific gravity above 1.015 for several hours, if the disturbance is of pituitary origin, but will be of no benefit if it is a primary renal tubular defect (p. 424).

In the "water-loading" test, as outlined by Weil, an intravenous infusion of 5 per cent glucose solution equivalent to 20 ml per kg body weight is given at a constant rate for 1 hour, after a moderate period of fluid restriction. The rate is then changed to 15 ml per kg per hour for 45 minutes. Urine collections are made at 15-minute intervals during and for 60 minutes after the infusions. A peak of diuresis occurs normally 60 to 90 minutes after the start of the infusion. In diabetes insipidus states, provided the patient is not dehydrated beforehand, there is no diuretic peak and the excretion of water is prolonged.

As a supplementary test, after a high rate of urine flow has been established by the infusion of 5 per cent glucose solution for 60 minutes as described above, one may give a 2.5 per cent solution of sodium chloride at a rate of 15 ml per kg per hour for 45 minutes. In normal subjects these maneuvers will bring about a sharply reduced output of urine having a high specific gravity. In diabetes insipidus whether of pituitary or renal origin, and also in chronic renal insufficiency, this antidiuretic response will be diminished or absent.

The antidiuretic hormone of the posterior pituitary may be released in normals by violent emotions, acetylcholine, nicotine, morphine, anesthesia, surgical operations, or injections of hypertonic saline. It has been suggested that if unresponsiveness lies in the osmoreceptor mechanisms rather than in the pituitary itself, an antidiuretic response after a 5 per cent glucose infusion will be induced by nicotine but not by hypertonic saline.

BIBLIOGRAPHY

PITUITARY

Klinefelter, H. F., Jr., F. Albright, and *G. C. Griswold,* Experience with a Quantitative Test for Normal or Decreased Amounts of Follicle-stimulating Hormone in the Urine in Endocrinological Diagnosis, *J. Clin. Endocrinol.* 3:529, 1943.

Pickering, D. E., and *E. R. Miller,* Thyrotropic Hormone in Infants and Children: Differentiation between Primary and Hypopituitary Hypothyroidism, *A.M.A. Am. J. Dis. Child.* 85:135, 1953.

Silver, H. K., W. Kiyasu, J. George, and *W. C. Deamer,* Syndrome of Congenital Hemihypertrophy, Shortness of Stature, and Elevated Urinary Gonadotropins, *Pediatrics* 12:368, 1953.

Talbot, N. B., E. H. Sobel, J. W. McArthur, and *J. D. Crawford,* The Anterior

Pituitary, chap. 7, The Posterior Pituitary, chap. 8, in "Functional Endocrinology from Birth through Adolescence," Harvard University Press, Cambridge, Mass., 1952.

van Dyke, H. B., The Regulation of Water Excretion by the Neurohypophysis, *Bull. New York Acad. Med.* 29:24, 1953.

Weil, W. B., Jr., The Evaluation of Renal Function in Infancy and Childhood, *Am. J. M. Sc.* 229:678, 1955.

West, J. R., and *J. G. Kramer,* Nephrogenic Diabetes Insipidus, *Pediatrics* 15:424, 1955.

White, A., Hormones of the Adenohypophysis, *Bull. New York Acad. Med.* 29:11, 1953.

Wilkins, L., "The Diagnosis and Treatment of Endocrine Disorders in Childhood and Adolescence," Charles C Thomas, Springfield, Ill., 1950.

CHAPTER 69

Bacterial Infections: General Considerations

IMPORTANCE OF THE BACTERIOLOGY LABORATORY

The experienced practitioner is able to diagnose and treat most of the acute bacterial infections of childhood (e.g., tonsillitis, bronchitis, otitis media, furunculosis) without recovery or identification of the etiologic organisms. Bacteriologic studies are called for (1) when an infection is protracted or progressive despite treatment, (2) when an infection is severe or of uncertain origin, so that exact knowledge of the invading organism and its antibiotic sensitivities is needed (e.g., septicemia, pyogenic meningitis, chronic pyuria), (3) when an infection is being thoroughly studed for epidemiologic or investigative reasons, (4) when the possible presence of a bacterial infection in a patient must be excluded or confirmed, or (5) when it is important to know whether a convalescent patient or a clinically well contact is harboring a pathogenic organism.

Every specimen for bacteriology must be collected properly and delivered immediately. It should be submitted with adequate information, so that the smears and cultures will be prepared according to the requirements of the problem at hand. Conferences between clinician and bacteriologist always contribute to the best management of the patient and optimal interpretation of results.

Tests to determine whether specific immune reactions have developed or are developing in the skin or serum can be invaluable adjuncts to the study of some bacterial infections. These responses are of little immediate assistance in the earliest stages, however, since they usually do not become positive until a week or more has passed. Furthermore, one cannot always be certain that a particular illness being studied is necessarily the cause of a positive immune reaction; the responsivity may have antedated the illness or be anamnestic in character.

Determination of the antibiotic sensitivities of a pathogen is usually more important for therapeutics than knowledge of the exact genus and species. Indeed, the antibiotic susceptibilities of many pathogenic bacteria can be ascertained within 12 to 24 hours (p. 933), even though several days or weeks may be required for precise identification.

APPROPRIATE CULTURE MEDIA

The pathogenic bacteria differ widely in their cultural responses to nutrients, moisture, pH, oxygen, and environmental temperature. There is no single or "universal" cultural environment which will favor the growth of all organisms. For primary culture the best media are those made with either meat infusions or beef extract, though simple enzymatic protein hydrolysates in the form of "peptone" mixtures with added salts and vitamins are being substituted more and more. Dyes, buffer salts, agar, carbohydrates, and other growth-promoting substances are introduced as indicated.

The average well-equipped hospital bacteriologic laboratory has available in its refrigerator some 50 or more different media. The more complex of these are for primary isolation of possible pathogens and are utilized with individual problems according to the probabilities of success. The rest contain selected sugars or simpler nutrients for subcultural exploration of single or multiple biochemical properties. Every manual of medical bacteriology contains extended lists of culture media which are grouped according to the class of organisms being sought for in specimens from patients and subgrouped for differentiation and identification within specific families of organisms. Establishing the subspecies of a strain often requires specific serums for quelling tests, agglutination, and related properties.

Many of the bacteria responsible for human infections will grow on media containing serum, blood, or ascitic fluid, under atmospheric conditions of oxygen tension at 37°C. Others, such as the meningococci, Bacteroides and Clostridia, cannot be cultivated unless anaerobic or microaerobic (reduced oxygen tension) conditions are provided.

Enterococci thrive at 25 or 45°C, environmental extremes which inhibit most other pathogens. They will grow also under other adverse conditions, such as in media having a pH of 9.6 or containing 6.5 per cent sodium chloride or 0.1 per cent methylene blue.

PHARYNGEAL FLORA

The throats of American children without obvious respiratory tract infections, if cultured during the summer months, will as a rule reveal the presence of *Neisseria catarrhalis, Staphylococcus albus,* or viridans streptococci. In the colder seasons of the year there usually will be, in addition, beta hemolytic streptococci, pneumococci, or influenza bacilli. Meningococci are rarely recovered from routine throat cultures unless specifically searched for. Infants who are vomiting or ill with diarrhea not infrequently show enteric bacteria such as *Escherichia coli,* Proteus, Pseudomonas, or enterococci.

The giving of penicillin or erythromycin as therapy for any infection tends to depress the pharyngeal growth of the usual Gram-positive organisms, since most of these are susceptible. With occasional infants, the giving of an antibiotic is followed by proliferation of resistant Gram-negative enterobacteria; this in turn may cause a "superinfection" in the form of pharyngitis, otitis media, or bronchopneumonia.

Pharyngeal specimens for bacteriologic examination are procured by rubbing a pair of cotton-tipped swabs over the tonsillar areas and wall of the pharynx. One swab is used for making a direct smear if desired; the other for inoculation of culture media.

The varieties of bacterial species which will be recovered on culture will depend as much on the processes of culture as on the flora of the area. To search for diphtheria organisms one inoculates Loeffler's or a similar culture medium; for the relatively slow growing influenza bacilli, a special selective medium such as Levinthal's; for any intestinal tract bacilli which may have ascended to the throat, EMB or Endo agar plates or similar media favorable for growth of Enterobacteriaceae. The comparative numbers and size of the different colonies which grow out do not necessarily represent the comparative numerical distribution of these species on the pharyngeal mucous membrane.

Microscopic examination of a direct smear is usually omitted when searching for pneumococci, staphylococci, hemolytic streptococci, and similar pathogenic cocci. Controlled cultures have shown that the full gamut of bacteria in the flora is much more likely to be revealed if the material on the swab, instead of being spread immediately over blood agar or other plates, is first inoculated into a test tube containing blood broth. The surfaces of the plates are then smeared with a loopful of the broth and incubated at 37°C until examination next day. If the swab does not reach the laboratory within an hour or two, the more vigorous species will proliferate and may inhibit the growth of other bacteria which may be more pathogenic. Should the original swab be permitted to dry, any contained meningococci or intestinal pathogens will lose their viability within a few hours and most of the other pathogens will not survive more than a half day.

Throat smears stained with Loeffler's methylene blue will demonstrate the organisms of diphtheria, thrush, and Borrelia (Vincent's) stomatitis. Direct smear examinations are of little help in recognizing other forms of stomatitis and pharyngitis. Direct typing of cocci or bacilli in "rusty" sputum with antipneumococcic and antiinfluenzal serums is no longer used for facilitating the recognition of pneumonia caused by these bacteria. A preponderance of Gram-negative bacilli suggests an influenzal or Klebsiella infection. Ziehl-Neelsen stains are applied to the slide when searching for tubercle bacilli.

NASAL AND UPPER NASOPHARYNGEAL FLORA

If a cotton-tipped moist sterile bacteriologic swab is applied to the mucous membrane of the anterior nares of a healthy child and then cultured, a few colonies of nonpathogenic staphylococci, Neisseria, or diphtheroids will usually be recovered. Cultures of the middle meatus will be sterile unless an upper respiratory tract infection has developed.

Swabs for culturing the upper nasopharynx are prepared by dipping a 7-in. length of flexible wire in collodion and then covering one end with a small bit of cotton. The distal end of the wire should be bent into a large loop as protection against the swab being accidently swallowed. Swabs are sterilized in pairs within plugged test tubes. With the head held immobile, cultures are taken by gently passing swabs through both nares with a revolving motion until the posterior nasopharyngeal wall is reached. These are left in place for a full minute before being withdrawn.

During the months when respiratory tract infections are numerous, or at any season when an individual has an acute illness of this sort, a diversity of respiratory tract pathogens may be found—pneumococci, hemolytic staphylococci, hemolytic or viridans streptococci, influenza bacilli, Klebsiella, Proteus, or Pseudomonas. When such infections remain persistent despite empirical antibacterial therapy, bacteriologic studies comprising antibiotic sensitivity studies as well as local measures become indispensable for intelligent management. The pathogens encountered most frequently in this situation will be strains of staphylococci, Proteus, or Pseudomonas which are resistant to the antimicrobial drugs being given.

With rhinitis of vasomotor or allergic origin the mucoid watery discharge is sterile or shows only saprophytes on culture.

In the presence of a lower respiratory tract infection the organisms revealed by nasopharyngeal swabbing reflect the flora of the tract more accurately than does material collected from the throat through the oral cavity. With bacterial bronchitis or pneumonia one may encounter pneumococci, streptococci, influenza bacilli, or other respiratory tract pathogens. With whooping cough during the early catarrhal stage, *Hemophilus pertussis* can often be grown from secretions obtained in the postnasal space (p. 809).

A special situation of epidemiologic interest relates to the staphylococcic carrier state of hospitalized individuals. Numerous studies have shown that pathogenic strains of staphylococci become much more prevalent in the nasopharynx and feces of patients within a few days after their admission to a hospital. Employees in these institutions also exhibit a high carrier rate. The endemic persistence and transference of these strains is believed to bear an etiologic relationship to the well-known phenomenon of secondary infection in hospitalized patients caused by staphylococci which are resistant to the antibiotics used in those hospitals (p. 817).

EAR CULTURES

Secretion cultured from the external auditory canal in otitis media while the eardrum remains unruptured may yield staphylococci, diphtheroids, and miscellaneous other organisms, but these are not the causative agents. When found in association with a purulent aural discharge they should be viewed as external contaminants.

Cultures obtained from inflamed middle ears by needle aspiration through the eardrum usually uncover the presence of pneumococci, influenza bacilli, beta hemolytic streptococci, or (infrequently) Gram-negative bacilli. One cannot predict the causative agent of an otitis media from a nasopharyngeal culture. The latter typically yields multiple potential pathogens. However, an organism not in the nose or throat is not likely to be recovered from the middle ear.

Because of the not infrequent relationship of the influenza bacillus to otitis media, antibiotics such as penicillin and Novobiocin which are effective against most Gram-positive pathogens but not all Gram-negative ones may fail to eradicate completely a middle-ear infection.

BACTEREMIA

The patterns of disease reflect the interactions between (1) the biologic characteristics of the invading bacterial strain and (2) the character and efficiency of the physiologic defenses of the host. Understanding of the interplay of mechanisms which govern pathogenicity and resistance in different diseases and of the causes of variations among individual cases of any one disease is still in the early descriptive phase.

In most clinically mild infections the local proliferation of the organisms calls forth, within a day or less, an equally rapid mobilization of defensive mechanisms on the part of host. In more severe infections the pathogenic bacteria usually gain access to the blood stream and may be demonstrated there during the so-called early or invasive stage. Except when the plasma or certain organs prove exceptionally susceptible to the invader, the septicemia usually clears promptly and blood cultures become negative. The bacteria may persist, however, in a local area such as lung, peritoneum, joint, or meninges. Should the patient later become debilitated or the bacteria gain local ground and proliferate, the blood stream may be entered once more. A positive blood culture then becomes a much more unfavorable prognostic sign, since it heralds the possibility of metastatic spread. In salmonellosis and a few other infections the initial septicemia may continue for several weeks.

A customarily nonpathogenic organism recovered in a blood culture should never be interpreted summarily as a "contaminant." Almost any "nonvirulent" inhabitant of the stools, skin, or respiratory tract may acquire a foothold in some tissue and produce disease when the resistance mechanisms are diminished. Every large clinic has seen incontestable instances of local or general infections caused by coliform bacilli, *Staphylococcus albus,* enterococci, Neisseria, *Bacillus subtilis,* diphtheroids, and atypical strains of streptococci, pneumococci, and influenza bacilli. Invasion by such comparatively nonpathogenic strains occurs not infrequently in newborn, premature, and severely malformed infants and in children of all ages with an advanced illness such as nephritis, leukemia, hydrocephalus, or generalized tuberculosis.

Surface surgical procedures such as tonsillectomy or dental extraction, and especially incision of abscesses, open up channels by which bacteria can invade the circulation. Postoperative blood cultures have been positive in nearly half the cases in some series. Many of the organisms thus recovered are of varieties deemed "nonpathogenic." Their presence is nearly always transient. When some part of the body is diseased, however, such as an obstructed urinary tract, a hydrocephalus, or a valvular endocarditis, this form of septicemia may result in a serious metastatic lesion.

Possession of capsules by strains of such pyogenic organisms as pneumococci, hemolytic streptococci, influenza bacilli, and Klebsiella appears to favor resistance to local phagocytosis and enhances pathogenicity. Once an encapsulated organism is engulfed by a leukocyte, however, whether locally or in the blood stream, it is as a rule destroyed rapidly. Nonencapsulated bacteria which can survive parasitically in the interior of cells, such as typhoid bacilli, tubercle bacilli, and Brucella, typically give rise to stubborn or chronic infections.

Septicemia in Early Infancy

Premature infants and infants of neonatal age are peculiarly likely to develop septicemia when ill with a bacterial infection anywhere in the body. The most frequent bacterial invaders during infancy are streptococci, staphylococci, and colon or coliform bacilli. Almost any known pathogen, however, including those which almost never produce serious disease in older children, may be implicated. The portal of entry is usually related to the customary habitat of the organism. Pneumococci, streptococci, and influenza bacilli enter from the respiratory tract or conjunctiva; staphylococci from skin pustules, umbilical granuloma, or surface wounds; colon and coliform organisms, Proteus, Pseudomonas, and enterococci from the gastrointestinal or genitourinary tract. Sometimes no local area of infection is discoverable. While bacteria are in an infant's blood stream, a culture of catheterized urine will nearly always yield the same organism.

Bacteremia with or without metastatic lesions in the internal organs can give rise to shock, hypotension, respiratory distress, vascular collapse, bleeding phenomena, electrolyte disturbances, gastrointestinal symptoms, jaundice, or other indications of systemic prostration and intoxication. The intermediate incitants are thought to be the endotoxins liberated by the bacteria. Fever may not appear. Waddell, Balsley, and Grossmann found positive blood cultures in 23 (65 per cent) of 34 infants 7 to 16 days of age who were exhibiting anorexia and weight loss. Prior to the advent of the sulfonamides and antibiotics the outcome of such bacteremia at this early age was often fatal.

Subacute Bacterial Endocarditis

This disease may be caused by almost any bacterium. Fever, cardiac murmurs, anemia, and splenomegaly are among the prominent symptoms. The total leukocyte count may or may not be elevated. The neutrophils show an abundance of toxic granulations and immature forms. There is prominent rouleaux formation of the red cells and an elevated sedimentation rate. Large reticuloendothelial cells may appear in numbers in the blood stream as the illness progresses.

To destroy the invading organisms which lie deep in fibrin or necrotic avascular tissue, an antibiotic with both fibrin-penetrating and bacteria-killing properties must be given in high dosage for a prolonged period. Relapses are frequent with antibiotics which are essentially bacteriostatic (Chap. 76).

The great majority of childhood cases are caused by *Streptococcus viridans* or enterococci. *Streptococcus viridans* can nearly always be eradicated by penicillin, which is bactericidal. Most strains of enterococci are resistant to penicillin alone, but a combination with streptomycin or bacitracin has often proved synergistically successful. With cases caused by other organisms, such as Brucella, diphtheroids, influenza bacillus, Pseudomonas, Proteus, or fungi, the drugs to be used must be selected from the results of antibiotic sensitivity tests.

BLOOD CULTURE PROCEDURES

When requesting a culture one should inform the laboratory which organism is suspected and what antimicrobial medication the patient has been receiving. If a chronic infection such as brucellosis or salmonellosis is suspected it is advisable to discontinue all medications and wait 2 or 3 days before taking the culture. It is always advisable, whenever possible, to take the culture before treatment is instituted.

In most infections the results are most likely to be positive in the first day or days of the illness. With brucellosis and subacute bacterial endocarditis the chances of success are best when the specimen is taken during a febrile period.

A single isolation of a saprophyte or questionable pathogen is always difficult to interpret. When this occurs a subsequent culture should be taken in the effort to obtain the same organism. In our laboratory it is the practice to inoculate routinely two bottles of culture medium at the time the blood is withdrawn and to place much more emphasis on a positive result when the same organism grows in both bottles.

Sterile bottles already filled with satisfactory culture media are available commercially. These are especially applicable for use in offices where requests for blood cultures are relatively infrequent and have the advantage of reducing external contamination because manipulation is minimized.

Prior administration of an antibiotic or other chemotherapeutic agent to a patient who may have septicemia tends to suppress the recovery of organisms from the blood stream.

Several modifications of technique are available to overcome this difficulty in part. The enzyme penicillinase specifically inactivates any penicillin contained in a blood sample and enables the pathogenic organisms, if still viable, to grow. Para-aminobenzoic acid, which has a molecular structure similar to that of the sulfonamides and is an essential metabolite for most bacteria, will counteract many of the effects of sulfonamides when added to culture media. Cysteine hydrochloride and some other reducing compounds may help to neutralize streptomycin. Cultures with inactivators added should be incubated for at least 10 days before being read as negative, because a lag of a few days often occurs before the organisms resume their growth.

Another approach toward overcoming the possible inhibitory activity of any antibiotic is by diluting its concentration in the blood sample. This is done by adding very small amounts of blood to comparatively large amounts of culture medium—for example, 0.5 ml of blood to 200 ml of broth.

A more complicated maneuver is to pass an oxalated or heparinized blood specimen through a small Seitz filter with aseptic precautions. The pad will trap any microorganisms which may be present. This is then dropped in the culture medium after being washed with sterile water to remove any residue of absorbed antibiotic.

BIBLIOGRAPHY

THROAT AND NASOPHARYNGEAL FLORA

Bloomfield, A. L., The Significance of Bacteria Found in the Throats of Healthy People, Bull. Johns Hopkins Hosp. 32:33, 1921.

Commission on Acute Respiratory Diseases, Bacteriological Findings in Undifferentiated and Other Acute Respiratory Diseases, Medicine 26:465, 1947.

————, Problems in Determining the Bacterial Flora of the Pharynx, Proc. Soc. Exper. Biol. & Med. 69:45, 1948.

————, The Single Throat Culture as an Index of the Bacterial Flora of the Respiratory Tract, Am. J. Hyg. 50:168, 1949.

Cunliffe, A. C., Incidence of Staph. aureus in the Anterior Nares of Healthy Children, Lancet 2:411, 1949.

Goldman, J. L., S. M. Bloom, and C. Herschberger, Bacteriologic and Clinical Interpretation of the Flora of the Nose and Nasopharynx in Children, J. Pediat. 44:299, 1954.

Haffner, F. D., E. Neter, and *M. I. Rubin,* Penicillin and Its Effect in Producing a Predominant Gram-negative Bacillary Flora in Upper Respiratory Tract of Children, *Pediatrics* 6:262, 1950.

Kneeland, Y., Jr., The Upper Respiratory Flora of Infants, *J. Exper. Med.* 51:617, 1930.

Lipman, M. O., J. A. Coss, Jr., and *R. H. Boots,* Changes in the Bacterial Flora of the Throat and Intestinal Tract during Prolonged Oral Administration of Penicillin, *Am. J. Med.* 4:702, 1948.

McCurdy, R. S., and *E. Neter,* Effects of Penicillin and Broad-spectrum Antibiotics on Emergence of a Gram-negative Bacillary Flora in Upper Respiratory Tract of Infants, *Pediatrics* 9:572, 1952.

Mortimer, E. A., Jr., and *R. L. Watterson, Jr.,* A Bacteriologic Investigation of Otitis Media in Infancy, *Pediatrics* 17:359, 1956.

Sanders, S. H., Persistent Nasal Symptoms in Children, *J.A.M.A.* 157:1205, 1955.

Tompkins, V., and *J. C. Macauley,* A Characteristic Cell in Nasal Secretions during Prodromal Measles, *J.A.M.A.* 157:711, 1955.

Warthin, A. S., Occurrence of Numerous Large Giant Cells in Tonsils and Pharyngeal Mucosa in the Prodromal Stage of Measles: Report of Four Cases, *Arch. Path.* 11:864, 1931.

SEPTICEMIA

Cates, J. E., and *R. V. Christie,* Subacute Bacterial Endocarditis: A Review of 442 Patients Treated in 14 Centres Appointed by the Penicillin Trials Committee of the Medical Research Council, *Quart. J. Med.* 20:93, 1951.

Coventry, K. J., and *C. Isbister,* A Bacteriological and Clinical Study of Infection in Newborn Babies in a Maternity Hospital Nursery, *M. J. Australia* 2:394, 1951.

Gulotta, G. A., and *S. E. Pascucci,* Subacute Bacterial Endocarditis in a Rheumatic Colony, *Bull. St. Francis Sanatorium (Roslyn, N.Y.)* 9:43, 1952.

King, E. S., Routine Blood Cultures in Pediatrics, *North Carolina M. J.* 9:30, 1948.

Kotin, P., Techniques and Interpretation of Routine Blood Cultures: Observations in Five Thousand Consecutive Patients, *J.A.M.A.* 149:1273, 1952.

Rhoads, P. S., J. R. Sibley, and *C. E. Billings,* Bacteremia Following Tonsillectomy: Effect of Preoperative Treatment with Antibiotics in Postoperative Bacteremia and in Bacterial Content of Tonsils, *J.A.M.A.* 157:877, 1955.

Lopage, C. P., and *F. A. Langley,* Acute Bacterial Endocarditis with a Positive Blood Culture in a Child Aged One Year, *Arch. Dis. Childhood* 22:253, 1947.

Silverman, W. A., and *W. E. Homan,* Sepsis of Obscure Origin in the Newborn, *Pediatrics* 3:157, 1949.

Todd, R. M., Septicemia of the Newborn, *Arch. Dis. Childhood* 23:102, 1948.

Waddell, W. W., Jr., R. E. Balsley, and *W. Grossman,* The Significance of Positive Blood Cultures in Newborn Infants, *J. Pediat.* 33:426, 1948.

CONTROL OF INFECTIONS IN CHILDREN

Cruickshank, R., Prevention and Control of Infection, *Brit. M. J.* 1:25, 1950.

Edsall, E., Active and Passive Immunity of the Infant, *Ann. New York Acad. Sc.* 66:32, 1956.

Frazer, M. J. L., A Study of Neonatal Infections in the Nurseries of a Maternity Hospital, *Arch. Dis. Childhood* 23:107, 1948.

MacLeod, C. M., Interactions of Host, Microbe and Chemotherapeutic Agent, *Bull. New York Acad. Med.* 31:427, 1955.

Moncrieff, A., Infection in the Newborn Baby, *Brit. M. J.* 1:1, 1953.

Rubbo, S. D., Infection: A Hospital Problem, *M. J. Australia* 35:627, 1948.

Saslaw, S., Practical Applications of Bacteriologic Studies in the Diagnosis of Infectious Diseases, *Postgrad. Med.* 8:184, 1950.

Shwartzman, G., Advances in the Diagnosis of Bacterial Infections, *Bull. New York Acad. Med.* 26:617, 1950.

Smith, M. H. D., The Transmission of Infections, *Pediatrics* 14:1, 1954.

Spaulding, E. H., The Role of the Bacteriologist in the Diagnosis and Control of Acute Infectious Diseases, *M. Clin. North America* 34:1589, 1950.

CHAPTER 70

Bacterial Infections: Specific Diseases

BACTEROIDES INFECTIONS

The Bacteroides genus is made up of a number of biologically related species of nonsporulating Gram-negative bacilli which are anaerobic, highly pleomorphic, and usually nonmotile. In humans they are intestinal saprophytes, though at times recoverable from the pharynx or outer genital tract. Growth in culture media is so slow that it may take 4 to 8 days for colonies to become apparent.

Human infections due to Bacteroides are rare. The species most commonly recovered have been *Bact. fragilis, Bact. funduliformis,* and *Bact. necrophorus.* These are sometimes encountered in mixed infections caused by intestinal bacteria; they then occur in association with *Escherichia coli, Clostridium welchii,* and anaerobic streptococci. Some of the fusiform bacilli seen in association with oral spirochetes in stomatitis appear to be Bacteroides.

Organisms of this group have been recorded as having caused septicemia, tonsillitis, otitis media, lung abscess, empyema, appendicitis, and peritonitis. Septicemia may be followed by metastatic lesions anywhere in the body, the most frequent sites being the lungs, joints, and liver. The prognosis is then exceedingly grave. It is probable that Bacteroides would be isolated more frequently if slowly growing anaerobic bacteria were looked for specifically in such disorders.

Success in treatment of Bacteroides infections seems to depend upon eradication of purulent foci and application of suitable antimicrobial therapy. Most strains are resistant to penicillin, sulfonamides, and streptomycin, but may be moderately sensitive to one or more of the broad-spectrum antibiotics. Combined therapy with several antibiotics is recommended.

BRUCELLOSIS

Epidemiology

Brucellosis (undulant fever) can be caused by any of three species of Brucella: *Br. abortus* (which infects cows chiefly), *Br. melitensis* (goats and swine chiefly), and *Br. suis* (swine chiefly). It is feasible to distin-

779

guish these three species from each other by biochemical reactions and less satisfactorily by immunologic differences. *Br. abortus* and *Br. suis* are the frequent sources of brucellosis in adults. *Br. suis* tends to cause the most severe form of illness.

An estimated 40,000 to 100,000 human cases occur annually in the United States. Chronic infections, usually not diagnosed, are believed to outnumber the acute by a ratio of at least 10:1. Most of the patients are farmers or employees of packing plants, who acquire the disease through direct or indirect contact with infected animals or animal products.

Brucella organisms pass readily through the unbroken skin. Spread from human to human is rare if it occurs at all. The best approach to control is to eradicate the disease from the animal population by immunizing young uninfected animals with specific vaccine and by destroying all infected animals when detected clinically or by serologic testing.

The low prevalence of cases among users of contaminated unpasteurized milk is ascribed to (1) the inhibitive effect of human digestive fluids, (2) the dilution of infected milk with clean milk, and (3) the probability that many strains of Brucella isolated from dairy cows are relatively avirulent for man.

Clinical Manifestations

In human beings the organisms localize in the reticuloendothelial cells, whence they migrate at intervals into the blood and other tissues. The resulting clinical picture is protean. There may be a single acute febrile illness, a long-continued chronic disease, or latent disease without recognizable signs.

Correct diagnosis is contingent upon laboratory confirmation of clinical suspicion. Unfortunately the results of laboratory approaches, except during acute febrile episodes, are often negative and disappointing.

Bacteriology

Recovery of Brucella organisms from the patient is the only unequivocal method for establishing the existence of the disease. Cultures should be taken from the blood, bone marrow, or other obviously involved sites whenever the diagnosis is suspected. Special nutrient media are utilized. In addition to inoculating the patient's blood directly into suitable media, one may first permit the collected blood to coagulate in a sterile dry tube and then prepare cultures from the clot after removal of the serum. This latter maneuver is recommended for chronically ill patients whose serum may contain neutralizing substances.

Incubation should be in a carbon dioxide–containing atmosphere for 4 to 6 weeks before cultures are read as negative. Morphologically the organisms are small Gram-negative coccobacilli which do not clump.

Properly carried out blood cultures taken during the initial stage or during exacerbations of the illness yield the organisms in a high proportion of cases. It is advisable to take several such cultures, preferably daily for 7 to 10 days, since the number of organisms per unit of circulating blood are usually few and their appearance sporadic. They are sometimes recoverable from the arterial blood after the administration of epinephrine. Blood cultures are usually negative when there are no agglutinins against Brucella in the serum.

Cultures of bone marrow aspirates are more likely to be positive. About 2 to 3 ml of bloody marrow should be withdrawn for this purpose.

Positive cultures are occasionally secured with aspirates of cervical or other lymph nodes which enlarge during febrile exacerbations. Other sites which are clearly infected may give successful cultures, such as the cerebrospinal fluid when symptoms of meningoencephalitis are present or lymph nodes excised from patients with protracted disease. Guinea pig inoculation of blood, urine, or material from infected tissues is often successful and is advisable when there is contamination with other organisms.

Whether a Brucella strain recovered from a patient is *melitensis, suis,* or *abortus* can be ascertained with fair certainty by macroscopic tube agglutination tests using specific antisera and a freshly isolated culture. Knowledge of the animal source of the infection is of aid in recognizing the species.

In vitro a recovered strain of Brucella organisms may be susceptible to penicillin, streptomycin, the sulfonamides, or a broad-spectrum antibiotic in moderate concentrations. Therapy with any of these substances is not consistently successful, since relapses are frequent afterward. The best therapeutic results are obtained with a combination of an antibiotic or antibiotics and a sulfonamide.

Serologic Tests

The blood agglutination reaction is a valuable aid in diagnosis when done carefully with standardized antigens. Antigens and test procedures differ widely. A "standard" antigen has been proposed by Spink, McCullough, Hutchings and Mingle. In general, the higher the level of serum agglutinins, the more likely is it to represent a true infection. Most culturally proven cases have a titer of at least 1:80. Lower readings have questionable diagnostic value. Agglutinins are sometimes demonstrable by diluting the serum. The rapid slide test is helpful for immediate presumptive results, but its use should be restricted to this purpose. The definitive titer should be ascertained by the test tube dilution method.

A level of 1:320 or higher in a properly performed test is a strong indication that the patient has active brucellosis. A rise during an illness also has considerable significance.

The agglutinin response remains elevated for about a year after recovery from brucellosis and then begins to fall. It may persist below 1:100 for some years. A sign of successful treatment of the infection with antibiotics is a gradual diminution in titer over the ensuing weeks or months.

Therapeutic injections of Brucella antigen, as have been given at times, usually evoke the appearance of agglutinins. This may confuse the interpretations for months or years thereafter. A small amount of antigen injected for skin testing is enough to induce the appearance of agglutinins when previously absent, even when the injection site shows no reaction. Any rise in titer soon after a skin test must be interpreted with caution, though such an occurrence may be a sign of previous infection or latent illness.

One source of possible error when positive agglutination is obtained is cross agglutination with related antigens from some other infection. Agglutinins for Brucella, often in high titer, sometimes appear after a recent attack of tularemia, salmonellosis, or shigellosis. Immunization against cholera may likewise evoke these antibodies. Conversely, occasional brucellosis patients with a high titer of specific antibodies may exhibit serum agglutinins for *Pasteurella tularense* or *Vibrio comma*. Such antibodies can be differentiated from Brucella-induced agglutinins by reciprocal absorption tests. Febrile illnesses due to other organisms are not known to produce a positive Brucella response except perhaps as an anamnestic phenomenon.

Results with the complement-fixation and opsonocytophagic tests agree in general with those obtained with the agglutination test. Being more complicated, they may readily give false results from minor variations in the technical procedure.

Skin Testing

Several antigens are available for determining the dermal sensitivity of man for Brucella. Performance and significance are essentially the same as with the tuberculin reaction. An erythematous area 1 cm or more in diameter in 48 hours represents a positive reading. It is presumed that individuals with reactive skin tests have at some time in the past been exposed to Brucella sufficiently to become sensitized, with or without ever having clinically recognizable brucellosis. In the United States, 10 to 25 per cent of healthy adults give positive skin reactions. The prevalence in children is much less. With most positive reactors no history of a disease resembling brucellosis in the past can be elicited. A positive reaction cannot be used to distinguish an active infection from an inactive or healed one with persisting skin allergy.

The responsiveness of the skin test develops late in an attack and may persist for years thereafter. Conversely, it is sometimes negative even in a severe infection. Hence skin testing is of little service as a diagnostic procedure. In fact, a skin test should not be performed early in an obscure febrile illness, or at least not before other diagnostic tests have been performed, since the injection calls out immune bodies and thenceforth renders unreliable all other serologic diagnostic procedures.

The chief usefulness of skin testing is in large-scale surveys of population groups. It occasionally helps to rule out brucellosis in a patient with an obscure disease in whom this possibility is deemed highly unlikely for other reasons.

Other Laboratory Findings

Most patients have a normal total leukocyte count or even a mild leukocytopenia. A mild to moderate absolute lymphocytosis is not unusual, with many of the cells being the so-called "atypical" forms resembling those of infectious mononucleosis. The erythrocyte sedimentation rate may or may not be elevated. A mild anemia is often seen.

DIPHTHERIA

An infection with the diphtheria bacillus *Corynebacterium diphtheriae* typically consists of the formation of an inflammatory membrane in the pharynx or nose. Tracheobronchitis, wound infections, conjunctivitis, vaginitis, otitis media, subacute bacterial endocarditis, and omphalitis of the newborn may also be caused by this organism. The infective site is usually on some surface of the body, readily accessible to cultural investigation. Bacilli may be found in blood or urine in the first few days, terminally, or in the rare patients with endocarditis. The constitutional disturbances result from absorption of an exotoxin produced in the local lesion. The route of spread is from human to human, usually by airborne droplets or dust particles. Some milk-borne epidemics have been described.

Laboratory abnormalities which may appear in patients include proteinuria, elevated blood urea, diminished serum phospholipids, and increased serum globulin. The leukocyte count as a rule is between 10,000 and 20,000 per cubic millimeter, owing to a neutrophil increase. A count over 25,000 suggests a very severe illness or a superimposed complication. With postdiphtheritic neuritis the spinal fluid cell count remains normal, but the protein content is usually elevated for some months.

Bacteriology

C. diphtheriae organisms are Gram-positive rodlike nonmotile nonsporulating bacilli which tend to group themselves side by side or at angles with each other. They may be slender or stubby, straight or curved, inconstant in length and width, and frequently swollen at the ends. They stain deeply and may take a reddish-purple color in methylene blue preparations. They frequently contain two or three irregular metachromatic aggregations of protoplasm known as *granules*, though these may vary from one to six.

Similar but nontoxicogenic and nonpathogenic bacilli are often recoverable from the body surfaces. Not even the most experienced observer can always distinguish on morphologic grounds alone the "diphtheroid" organisms from true *C. diphtheriae*.

C. diphtheriae thrives on simple media which contain peptones. Loeffler's coagulated blood serum medium is widely employed because it is deficient in nutrients which are essential for the growth of streptococci, pneumococci, and most of the other inhabitants of the nasopharyngeal area. On Loeffler's medium the colonies lack a distinctive appearance. On blood agar they are small, gray, smooth, and convex types. The colony appearances on solid agar media containing potassium tellurite, which is bactericidal for many other organisms, form the primary basis for dividing the virulent strains into three types. Since other bacterial genera sometimes give identical colony formation on tellurite media, it is important to carry out microscopic identification using two typical colonies.

The *gravis* colonies are the largest. Typically these have a dull surface with a dark-gray center and a higher or "daisy-headed" periphery, or sometimes a smoother slightly crenated surface with an "escarpment" edge. *Gravis* strains will almost always ferment starch with the liberation of acid and prove toxicogenic when tested with guinea pigs. Strains with typical colony characteristics but which fail to ferment starch or agglutinate with antisera to *gravis* types I to V have been designated *gravoid* by some workers.

The *intermedius* colonies are pin-point and low, with uneven surfaces and edges. They are gray or black or gray with black centers. They ferment glucose but not starch or sucrose and do not hemolyze red cells. A group of closely related strains, termed *minimus*, has unusually small colonies, tends to ferment sucrose or glucose slowly, and may or may not elaborate an exotoxin. Members of the other groups do not ferment sucrose (saccharose).

The *mitis* colonies are also small and usually smooth, black, and domelike. They ferment glucose, but not starch or sucrose, and usually produce a small zone of beta hemolysis on blood agar.

Each cultural variety of *C. diphtheriae* can be subdivided into a number of immunologic serotypes when tested with serums from injected rabbits or human convalescents. Within each of the three groups these types, labeled numerically, are highly specific with little serologic overlapping, but cross agglutination can be marked between individual members of different groups. Qualitatively the exotoxin appears to be the same, regardless of the exact serotype.

The diphtheroid bacilli, such as *C. pseudodiphtheriae*, tend to grow much more luxuriantly than *C. diphtheriae* on plain agar, have dull flat hard nonhemolytic colonies on blood agar, usually do not ferment starch or glucose, and do not react with anti-*diphtheriae* sera. To be certain of the differentiation, one must carry out toxigenic or virulence tests with guinea pigs.

Epidemiology

Tracing of the spread of diphtheria through populations is much facilitated when the strain or strains recoverable from patients and carriers are typed. Interestingly, the distribution and number of the different types of *C. diphtheriae* endemic in any geographic area alter with the passage of time. These changes in type sometimes can be correlated with variations in the severity of the cases in that area. Diphtheria due to *gravis* stains tends to be the most severe, and some outbreaks of "bull-neck" diphtheria have been associated with *gravis* type II. Numerous outbreaks of diphtheria in immunized populations have been traced to variant or new strains to which there had been no exposure in recent years.

In the United States the severity of clinical diphtheria shows little correlation with the groups and types of the causative strains. Mild, severe, or fatal cases may be caused by any type.

Once the character of an epidemic strain has been identified and its toxicogenicity established by guinea pig tests, the serotyping of diphtheria organisms recovered from carriers may be an inferential approach for determining whether such organisms are virulent or nonvirulent.

The increasing number of outbreaks of clinical diphtheria in immunized populations can be ascribed not only to the introduction of new and highly virulent strains, but paradoxically also to the vigorous programs of antidiphtheria immunization. By depressing the prevalence of carriers of virulent organisms, the repeated contact with the organisms which appears to be essential for the sustaining of resistance in those previously immunized is diminished. Numerous surveys of American populations with Schick tests indicate that 20 to 40 per cent of individuals immunized as infants lose their immunity by the time of entering junior high school.

Diphtheria carriers and patients with diphtheria remain constant threats to populations that are not wholly immune. The true carrier state may be transient, recurrent, or highly persistent. Organisms may be harbored in the tonsils, adenoids, nasal mucosa, postnasal space, gingival groves, or middle ear. Atypical attacks with little or no toxemia may occur in subjects with waning immunity. Bacteriologic culture is necessary for diagnosis.

Procuring of Specimens

Cultures from tonsils, throat, nasopharynx, wounds, skin lesions, ear discharges, and other sites are taken by rubbing and rotating the cotton-tipped ends of sterile applicators over all suspected areas. The applicator should not come in contact with the saliva, tongue, or other surfaces of the mouth. Smears on glass slides should be made also. The entire surface of a slant of fresh moist Loeffler's blood serum medium is then inoculated as soon as possible and the swabs left in the tubes with the projecting ends broken off. In surveys for carriers the applicators from nose and throat may be used to inoculate the same slant, but when clinical diphtheria is suspected these two sites should be cultured separately. The culture tubes containing the broken ends of the swabs should be forwarded to the laboratory immediately, along with information regarding the hour of collection, source of the culture, and clinical problem presented.

Additional cultures may be prepared in the laboratory from the swabs or the surface of the Loeffler's slant. Plates of tellurite medium can be inoculated in order to ascertain the *gravis, mitis,* or *intermedius* type, if desired. It is often advisable to inoculate a blood agar plate for incubation at 37°C for 24 hours, in order to ascertain the possible presence of streptococci and other pathogens. Colony typing and tests for toxin production are ordinarily not made unless specially arranged for.

Loeffler cultures may be examined microscopically after 8 or 10 hours incubation at 37°C. If diphtheria-like organisms are not apparent another examination is made after 18 to 24 hours. At that time it is better to make subcultures than to hold the original cultures for 48 hours.

Direct smears of exudate from a mucosal or skin surface may be reported after microscopic study as "organisms resembling diphtheria bacilli in smear" or "no organisms resembling diphtheria bacilli in smear." Typical diphtheria organisms in cultures from clinically suspected cases need no further identification, except perhaps to determine the type for epidemiologic purposes, and the report should be forwarded at once. Diphtheria-like organisms in cultures from presumed carriers or from sites other than the nasopharynx should be identified further by tests for fermentation and toxin production. The report should state also whether fusospirochetal organisms or hemolytic streptococci were seen in the smears or cultures.

Tests for Toxin Production

Demonstration of toxin production by the intradermal virulence test is the only dependable way for differentiating pathogenic diphtheria bacilli from nonpathogenic diphtheroids. A favorite method is to inject suspensions from a pure 1-day subculture intradermally into several areas on the shaved back or flank of a guinea pig or rabbit. After 4 hours the animal is given an intra-abdominal injection of diphtheria antitoxin. After 30 minutes the skin injections are repeated. If the organism produces toxin, only those sites injected before the antitoxin will become erythematous or necrotic in 2 or 3 days.

While the soluble exotoxin is the principal factor in producing the myocardial, adrenal, neural, and other injuries of diphtheria, unmistakable nasopharyngeal and systemic disease has been caused by strains which have not elaborated any toxin demonstrable by the intracutaneous animal test.

Antibiotic Sensitivities

Most strains of diphtheria bacilli are highly sensitive in vitro to penicillin. The minimum complete inhibiting range for penicillin in the studies of Jackson et al. was 0.2 to 0.8 μgm per ml. Somewhat less effective were the broad-spectrum antibiotics and neomycin and streptomycin. Several antibiotics may be given in a severe illness to arrest the inflammation as quickly as possible. Since antibiotics do not neutralize circulating diphtheria toxin, specific antitoxin is necessary also. The therapy should be begun as soon as the disease is suspected. Cultures should be taken first. It is important to remember that diphtheria may complicate streptococcic pharyngitis or rhinitis.

Detection of Immunity

The Schick test measures the skin response to exactly 0.1 ml of dilute toxin on the flexor surface of one forearm. A *negative* reaction is one in which no inflammatory changes are noted when the test is read 5 to 7 days later. This signifies the presence of immunity and corresponds usually to a concentration of 0.01 to 0.03 unit of circulating antitoxin per ml of blood serum. A *positive* reaction, reflecting absence of immunity, is an area of erythema at the site of toxin injection which develops at 24 hours and reaches a maximum on the fourth to seventh day. A *pseudo* reaction—a tuberculin-like allergic response to the proteins in the toxin—is local erythema which begins at 18 hours, attains a maximum at 24 to 48 hours, and then fades away gradually or abruptly. To avoid being confused by this response, many physicians at the time of the Schick test inject the other forearm with similar material which has been heat-inactivated or diluted 1:100 with a physiologic solution of sodium chloride.

To detect antitoxin in a subject's blood one can incubate some of his serum with diphtheria toxin for 30 minutes under standard conditions, and then perform an intradermal test in a shaved guinea pig with the mixture. Unneutralized toxin produces marked redness and some necrosis, whereas neutralized toxin gives only slight redness.

BACTERIAL ENTERIC INFECTIONS

Enterobacteriaceae

This taxonomic name is applied to the great family of Gram-negative nonsporulating bacilli whose members reside principally in the intestinal tract of mammals, birds, and man. Nearly all grow readily on standard media, ferment glucose with or without gas formation, and reduce nitrates to nitrites.

Hundreds of species are contained in Enterobacteriaceae. Differentiation is not always easy because of the many which are intermediate or "transitional." The major groups and genera are Salmonella, Shigella, Escherichia, Proteus, Klebsiella-Aerobacter, Alkalescens-Dispar, and Paracolobactrum or "coliform," which includes Arizona, Ballerup-Bethesda, and Providence groups.

Precise classification of any recovered strain of Gram-negative bacilli is based upon its motility, cultural and biochemical responses, and immunologic and antigenic reactions. Most hospital laboratories are able to recognize the principal human pathogens and to place an unusual organism in the broad group to which it belongs. For full identification or corroboration a culture may have to be forwarded to a reference laboratory which specializes in serologic typing of enteric bacteria.

Infections caused by Enterobacteriaceae spread as a rule from person to person. The organisms are disseminated through direct contact or contamination of food, milk, or water.

Escherichia coli

BIOCHEMICAL REACTIONS. The members of the genus Escherichia are Gram-negative nonsporulating lactose-fermenting bacilli, usually motile, which with many confusing exceptions exhibit characteristic biochemical reactions in culture media. The principal organism is *Esch. coli*. Usually classified under the term "coliform" are several other bacteriologically related families of bacilli which also ferment lactose; these include the paracolon bacilli and the Klebsiella group.

Typical strains of *Esch. coli* grow readily. On agar media they form circular convex colonies which usually have smooth edges. They usually ferment lactose, dextrose, maltose, mannitol, and xylose. They rarely attack citrate, urea, adenitol, or inositol; do not form mucus; and usually give negative Voges-Proskauer and positive methyl red and indole reactions. A capsule may be present. Growth is inhibited somewhat on desoxycholate-citrate and other selective Salmonella-Shigella agar media in the first 18 to 24 hours. Encapsulated strains with the capacity to hemolyze red cells seem to be the most likely to induce morbid processes in humans.

CLASSIFICATION BY SEROTYPING. Antigenically the members of the *Esch. coli* group have a diverse and complex structure. The strains have been divided into numerous subgroups and subtypes on the basis of three classes of contained antigens: O, K, and H (the Kauffmann-Knipschildt-Vahlne schema). The O or somatic antigens are thermostable and usually carbohydrates. The K or coating antigens consist of the A thermostable and the L and B thermolabile capsular and envelope antigens. If present, H flagellar antigens are also thermolabile; when cultures are feebly motile these are poorly developed and difficult to identify. The K antigens may prevent agglutination of the whole organisms by O antisera and must first be selectively destroyed by boiling or autoclaving. As a general rule these antigens do not serologically overlap those of the Salmonella group and the H antigens do not undergo phasic variation. The serologic properties are much less labile than the cultural and biochemical reactions.

At least 137 different O antigens, 78 K antigens, and 40 H antigens have thus far been differentiated serologically. Because of the large number of reagent materials which are required and complicated refinements of technique, the complete serologic description of strains is performed only by special laboratories. The state laboratories in this country either carry out such identification themselves or transfer the cultures to the Communicable Disease Center of the U.S. Public Health Service in Atlanta, Ga., for that purpose.

Most normal individuals possess serum agglutinating antibodies against the K component of the coliform organisms present in their stools. Serum titers may be as high as approximately 1:3,000, though most readings fall between 1:40 and 1:640. Interestingly, fecal extracts may also contain agglutinins for homologous coliform organisms during the acute stages of infantile diarrhea or in early convalescence, though fluctuations of titer are not well correlated with the clinical course of diarrhea. These fecal agglutinins are believed to come from extracellular fluid transuded across the intestinal wall.

Esch. coli strains inhabit the human intestinal tract as saprophytes, but occasionally give rise to infections. In older children the infections are usually local, occurring in the urogenital tract, appendix, peritoneum, or elsewhere. In young infants, and especially during the neonatal and prematurity periods, the infections may be more severe or generalized, e.g., septicemia, meningitis, or osteomyelitis.

Table 70-1. *Eschericia coli* Strains Associated with Diarrhea

O antigen	K antigen	H antigen
26	B₆	NM,* 11
55	B₅	NM, 2, 4, 6, 7, 8, 10, 21
86	B₇	NM, 8, 9, 10, 11, 34
86	L	2
111	B₄	NM, 2, 4, 11, 12, 16, 21
112†	B₁₁	NM
119	B₁₄	NM, 6, 9, 18, 27
124	B₁₇	NM, 19, 30, 32
125 †	B₁₅	19, 21
126	B₁₆	NM, 2, 27
127a	B₈	NM
128 †	B₁₂	2, 8, 9, 10, 12

SOURCE: Condensed from Ewing, W. H., *Ann. New York Acad. Sc.* 66:64, 1956.
* Nonmotile.
† Several subtypes are recognized, for example, 112*a* and 112*c*.

ANTIBIOTIC SENSITIVITIES. Strains of *Esch. coli* and other Enterobacteriaceae differ markedly in their sensitivity to antibiotics in the serum concentrations given by the customary therapeutic dosages. With in vitro tests most strains prove highly susceptible to polymyxin B, neomycin, and the sulfonamides. They are often moderately susceptible to the broad-spectrum antibiotics, and irregularly to streptomycin. Sensitivity to penicillin is extremely variable, perhaps because many strains have the property of elaborating a penicillinase. Few strains are inhibited by bacitracin or erythromycin.

RELATION TO EPIDEMIC GASTROENTERITIS. It is now accepted that certain strains of *Esch. coli* can cause infantile gastroenteritis. One strain belongs to O group 55 and contains the B_5 and H_6 antigens, for example, and accordingly is termed *Esch. coli* $O55:B_5:6$. The pathogenic serotypes which thus far have been found associated with diarrheal disease are listed in Table 70-1.

Attacks of gastroenteritis in outbreaks associated with these organisms have had somewhat distinctive features—toxemia, diarrhea, vomiting, anorexia, severe dehydration, pronounced loss of weight, and a tendency to relapse. The incubation period in contact cases appears to be 3 to 20 days, usually 8 to 12 days. The stools are sometimes described as having a "seminal" odor. During the height of the symptoms the same strain of *Esch. coli* organisms may be recovered from the nasopharynx as from the stools. Diarrheal symptoms have been induced in healthy infants and adults by the feeding of these strains under experimental conditions.

One or more of the broad-spectrum antibotics usually prove more effective than penicillin, streptomycin, or bacitracin in arresting or preventing these illnesses and reducing the death rate. Neomycin has been highly effective in many epidemics.

PROCEDURE FOR DEMONSTRATION OF PATHOGENIC *Esch. coli* STRAINS. When searching for a causative organism in infantile gastroenteritis, a fresh rectal swab, or less preferably a fecal specimen, is planted on the selective media employed for recovery of the enteric pathogens—eosin-methylene blue (EMB) agar, Salmonella-Shigella (SS) agar, and tetrathionate broth. A blood agar plate is also inoculated, since Escherichia do not grow well on these other media which are preferential for Salmonella and Shigella. *Esch. coli* and coliform strains, if present, usually grow out in abundance on blood agar. So will streptococci, staphylococci, yeasts, and most other aerobes. These latter are identified separately by standard bacteriologic procedures. Experienced bacteriologists look for small, compact, flat, nonhemolytic colonies with regular margins, as contrasted with the larger, more irregular, and often hemolytic colonies of other strains of *Esch. coli*. When growth of the pathogenic strain is profuse, as often happens during the period of active symptoms, the cultures may emit the odor suggestive of semen.

If no suspicious Salmonella or Shigella strains are detectable on the selective media, 5 to 10 colonies which appear to be *Esch. coli* are removed and subcultured individually in nutrient broth and other media which corroborate their species identity. After 18 to 24 hours the organisms are tested with polyvalent serum containing antibodies against a pool of O antigens representing those strains which are believed to be pathogenic for humans. If agglutination occurs the organisms are then serotyped once more with individual grouping serums. Such cultures may be sent to a reference laboratory for full serologic identification, including subtyping.

The antiserums needed for the identification of pathogenic *Esch. coli* cultures are prepared from living organisms and therefore contain agglutinins for the B or surface antigens as well as for the deeper-lying O antigens. Young 24-hour cultures of the organisms are first tested with diluted typing serums. Other batches of the same suspensions are heated at 100°C to inactivate the B antigens, cooled, and then retested similarly with the same serums to determine the O antigens. Experience has shown that strong, instant agglutinations in this procedure may be accepted as positive identification of the strains being studied.

Specific antibodies develop in a fair proportion of cases during the recovery period. Laurell and associates found specific anti-O agglutinins in the titer range of 1:40 to 1:160 in serum specimens from 20 of 45 affected infants. Only 3 of 71 controls had titers as high as 1:40. The agglutinins disappeared gradually after convalescence.

Paracolon Bacilli

Many strains of Gram-negative bacilli are similar in their cultural and morphologic behavior to the Escherichia, but ferment lactose very slowly if at all. The so-called "anaerogenic" varieties produce acid from lactose without gas. The collective terms "coliform," "paracolon bacilli," and "Paracolobactrum" are often applied to the members of this group. Paracolon bacilli have been isolated at times from normal stools, from the stools of patients with gastroenteritis, and from the urine of patients with chronic pyelonephritis. Their clinical significance in the latter situations is still uncertain. Cultures may be sent to reference laboratories for precise study if desired.

ARIZONA GROUP. These Gram-negative gelatin-liquefying series of coliform organisms are separated from the paracolon bacteria because as a rule they ferment lactose within 2 weeks of incubation. Many of the O and H antigens are similar to those of Salmonella. At least 29 O groups and 96 serotypes were identified by Edwards, McWhorter, and Fife in 1956.

The Arizona organisms are common causes of infections in reptiles, fowls, lower mammals, and very occasionally in humans. Several outbreaks of severe gastroenteritis in man have been reported as due to their presence. Serum agglutinins against the homologous strain tend to develop in patients with a protracted illness.

BETHESDA-BALLERUP GROUP. These bacilli behave biochemically somewhat like the salmonellae, except that they often ferment lactose and sometimes sucrose. Serologically, at least 32 distinctive O and 88 H antigens were recognized by West and Edwards in 1954, permitting subclassification into 167 serotypes.

The members of the Bethesda-Ballerup group, like other paracolon bacilli, may be found in human stools. Whether they can cause enteric or other infections is questionable. Their clinical importance lies in their superficial resemblance to the salmonellae, with which they can be readily confused in the early steps of the bacteriologic search for pathogens in stools.

PROVIDENCE GROUP. These paracolon bacilli seem to be intermediate biologically between the Shigella and the Proteus groups. They are recovered occasionally from normal and from diarrheal stools; their pathogenicity is questionable.

Alkalescens-Dispar Group

This group comprises those strains of Gram-negative bacilli previously known as *Shigella alkalescens* (*Alcaligenes faecalis, Bacillus faecalis* or *alcaligenes*) and *S. dispar*. They are unlike Shigella in many biochemical and immunologic characteristics and resemble more closely the Escherichia with whom they share many somatic antigens. A scheme of serologic identification has been developed which permits differentiation into at least eight bacterial subtypes.

Ordinarily harmless, these sometimes invade human tissues, especially in patients already ill with other infections or illnesses. Bacteremia, meningitis, arthritis, enteritis, conjunctivitis, and infections of the lymph nodes, appendix, kidney, or biliary tract may arise, or sometimes a syndrome resembling rheumatic or typhoid fever.

Later, during convalescence, agglutinin titers from 1:32 up to 1:512 may appear in the patient's serum against the causative strain, and lower titers against the other members of the group. Of diagnostic significance is a low agglutinin level at the beginning of the illness, followed by a rise after several weeks.

Salmonella Infections (Salmonellosis)

The salmonellae are Gram-negative nonsporulating bacilli which do not ferment lactose, sucrose, or adonitol. They break down glucose usually with gas production, are motile as a rule, and possess other characteristic biochemical reactions which are of importance in their recognition. Over 200 distinct but serologically related antigenic types have been recovered to date from man, animals, and animal products served as human foods. Some salmonellae (*S. typhosa, S. paratyphi* A and *B*) are primarily human strains which are rarely recovered from animals. Others are much more prevalent in animals but are potentially pathogenic for man (*S. pullorum; S. abortus equi*).

BACTERIOLOGY. The Kauffmann-White schema by which the various strains are identified according to antigenic structure is the one used most generally for classification. The individual combinations of the O or somatic antigens (referred to by Roman numerals) and H or flagellar antigens (referred to by small letters of the alphabet) establish the identity. At least 30 major O antigens and 57 H antigens—the latter often exhibiting phasic variability—can be separately agglutinated. Strains are often named in accordance with the geographic location where first recovered.

About 98 per cent of the Salmonella strains from human patients fall into the first five somatic groups of the Kauffmann-White classification. The preliminary diagnostic differentiation is accordingly made with these group-specific serums.

Group A (somatic antigens I, II, XII) has one major component, S. *paratyphi A.*

Group B (IV, V, XII) includes S. *paratyphi B₁* and *B₂*, S. *typhi-murium,* and many others.

Group C (VI, VII, VIII) includes, among others, S. *choleraesuis,* S. *montevideo,* S. *oranienburg,* and S. *paratyphi C.* Those in subgroup C_1 contain antigens VI and VII. Those in subgroup C_2 contain antigen VIII.

Group D (IX, XII) includes S. *gallinarum* and S. *miami,* among others.

Group E (III, X, XV) includes S. *anatum* and S. *newington.*

To establish the identity of a Salmonella organism one first tests it with a polyvalent serum containing all these major somatic antigens. If agglutination is obtained, the organism is then tested further with the separate grouping serums to place it in one of the various groups listed above. From the behavior exhibited and the reactions with Vi and other special H serums and bacteriophages, the precise nature of the strain can usually be elucidated. The cultural behavior of the organism must be considered as well as its serologic responses, since many paracolon bacilli contain antigens similar to or identical with the O antigens of Salmonella. The fact that only a minority of the strains produce most of the human infections expedites the serotyping in clinical laboratories. Stool cultures are usually more successful than blood or urine cultures for recovering the organisms from patients.

SYMPTOMATOLOGY. In general, Salmonella infections occur in three overlapping clinical patterns: an acute gastroenteritis, a septicemia-like syndrome, and localized extraintestinal infections. These may be produced by any of the Salmonella strains, although there is a statistical tendency for certain symptom patterns to be closely correlated with certain strains. Septicemia is more often due to S. *choleraesuis* ("*suipestifer*"), S. *typhosa,* S. *montevideo,* S. *newport,* S. *oranienburg,* S. *panama,* and S. *paratyphi A, B₁, B₂, and C.* Gastroenteritis is more often due to S. *typhi-murium,* S. *montevideo,* S. *oranienburg,* S. *newport,* S. *enteritidis,* S. *panama,* and S. *give.* Localized extraintestinal infections such as otitis, pneumonia, pyuria, meningitis, arthritis, and osteomyelitis can be caused by any strain.

The gastroenteritis resembles bacillary dysentery but is more likely to have a watery than a bloody diarrhea. The younger the patient the more severe tend to be the symptoms and the longer the course. Affected infants, especially if malnourished to begin with, are likely to suffer from constitutional toxicity with fever, dehydration, and electrolytic imbalances. Other agents which can also produce diarrhea, such as Shigella and intestinal protozoa, are not infrequently found in association. The usual sources of infection are human carriers, especially food handlers; insufficiently cooked food; domestic pets; and infected farm animals and their products. The portal of entry is nearly always the gastrointestinal tract. Young children and especially infants are more likely to have recognizable disturbances and to be seriously ill than are older children and adults. Sometimes the salmonellosis develops as a complication or sequel of an infection caused by some other organism. Patients should always be handled with hygienic precautions.

Expectant mothers when hospitalized for delivery should be asked whether they have had an intestinal infection in the preceding week or two. If so, they should be admitted under isolation precautions and their stools should be cultured.

Like the other Gram-negative bacilli the salmonellae tend to be more susceptible in laboratory tests to streptomycin and the broad-spectrum antibiotics than to penicillin, erythromycin, or the sulfonamides. It is well known clinically that chloramphenicol is usually more effective in therapy of acute symptoms than are the other antibiotics.

PUBLIC HEALTH REPORTING. In most American communities the reporting of infections caused by Salmonella organisms is still limited to cases of typhoid and paratyphoid fever and outbreaks of food poisoning. It would be a step forward to expand the reporting of every kind of salmonellosis, since any Salmonella organism can produce typhoid-like disease and epidemics of gastroenteritis.

S. typhi-murium INFECTIONS. S. typhi-murium was formerly known as Bacterium aertrycke, Bacillus pestis caviae, the "Breslau" bacillus, and the "mouse-typhoid" bacillus. It is a natural pathogen of rodents, and especially of mice, in which it gives rise to a septicemic and often fatal illness. A common cause of bacterial food poisoning, it is frequently recovered from outbreaks in institutional and other groups after ingestion of contaminated food. Gastrointestinal symptoms are most prominent, though typhoid-like infective states and pyogenic localizations are far from rare. Extreme toxemia or even fatal prostration is occasionally seen. The case fatality rate is about 6 per cent. Many outbreaks of diarrhea and septicemia in newborn nurseries have been caused by this type.

TYPHOID FEVER. In the Kauffmann-White system the Salmonella strain which is the cause of typhoid fever contains the O or somatic antigens IX and XII, and the H or flagellar antigen d. The Vi or "virulence" component often also present is believed to offer resistance to phagocytosis. Strains rich in Vi antigen will be agglutinated by serums rich in Vi antibodies but may not react with serums containing the specific anti-O agglutinins alone.

Bacteriology. In untreated typhoid fever one finds bacteriologic as well as clinical indications of generalized septicemia. Blood cultures are positive for S. *typhosa* in about 90 per cent of untreated patients during the first week of illness, 75 per cent during the second week, and 30 per cent during the third week. With stool cultures, only about 10 per cent are positive in the first week, about 20 per cent in the second week, 50 per cent in the third week, and 80 per cent during convalescence. Bile cultures, more difficult to obtain, often continue to remain positive for weeks or months after convalescence. The urine contains viable typhoid bacilli in about 30 per cent of patients during the second week of illness.

Serologic Responses. The agglutinin or Widal reaction is less dependable than the bacteriologic approach for making the diagnosis of typhoid fever but has to be relied on when cultural attempts to isolate the organisms have been unsuccessful.

Patients with typhoid fever begin to show agglutinins against both the O and the H antigens after the first week, and these attain a peak at about the fifth or sixth week. The readings vary from 1:80 to 1:280 or higher. The titers against O and H antigens do not necessarily run parallel, and some patients fail to develop antibodies against H. The O antigen also appears in the urine and may be tested for there. After the sixth week the serum levels begin to fall, and in about half the cases are down to normal levels by the eighth week. A positive O titer in an individual who had not been recently vaccinated is of greater diagnostic significance than a positive H titer.

Agglutinins to the Vi antigen may also appear, but not as consistently, and rarely in the absence of the O or H agglutinins. For these reasons the Vi antigen is usually not included in routine serologic studies of patients with suspected typhoid fever.

The agglutinin responses may fail to rise until late in the illness, in exceptional patients. Because of this a single negative report does not exclude the possibility of this disorder. In such doubtful situations the test should be made again after a time interval. Titers above 1:40 for both H and O are usually exhibited by carriers and by normal subjects who have received prophylactic typhoid vaccination within the preceding year or so.

A rise in serum titer during the course of a febrile illness is presumptive evidence afforded by the Widal reaction. Serum from patients recovering from S. *typhosa* infections will usually show cross agglutination with the other Salmonella strains which possess the same somatic antigens, such as S. *enteriditis* and S. *paratyphi* A and B. The reverse is also true. A reaction which is persistently negative throughout a febrile illness lasting several weeks is valuable negative evidence against typhoid fever, but does not rule out other varieties of salmonellosis caused by organisms which are lacking in the antigens contained in S. *typhosa* itself.

One diagnostic limitation of the Widal test is that patients who have had a Salmonella infection or received typhoid vaccine inoculations in the past may exhibit a transitorily positive response during other bacterial and viral infections—the so-called anamnestic reaction. There is no arbitrary titer above which the agglutination reaction may be adjudged significant or diagnostic. Normal individuals who have never had typhoid fever or received typhoid vaccine rarely have agglutinin titers greater than 1:20 or 1:40.

A new development is the subtyping of serologically homogeneous Vi-type strains of S. *typhosa* (and of S. *paratyphi B*) by study of differential susceptibility to specifically adapted bacteriophages. This highly specialized procedure is carried out in central laboratories. Specific phage typing has become an invaluable aid in epidemiologic investigations of typhoid fever, since strains recovered from persons infected from a common source invariably belong to the same type.

The widely used heat-killed phenol-preserved typhoid vaccine calls forth antibodies which are predominantly of the anti-O type. These tend to fade away in about 6 months, but the anti-H agglutinins may persist in low titer for a longer period. The alcohol-killed and preserved vaccine results in a greater production of Vi antibodies, but whether such a vaccine actually has an augmented immunizing value remains to be demonstrated. The use of vaccines simultaneously containing dead paratyphoid bacilli does not reduce the immunizing efficiency against typhoid fever itself and may even enhance it.

Other laboratory abnormalities in typhoid fever patients are a progressive normochromic anemia which may need supportive transfusions in a severe case. The absolute granulocyte count is usually in the low normal range, but rises for a time if septic complications develop.

Antibiotic Therapy. Most of the chemotherapeutic and antibiotic agents will inhibit the growth of S. *typhosa* in vitro. Chloramphenicol, however, seems the most effective in treatment. Its action in vivo appears to be bacteristatic rather than bactericidal, suppressive rather than curative. Relapses or recurrences are not uncommon while it is being given.

SALMONELLA CARRIER STATE. Many persons who have had a Salmonella infection continue to excrete the pathogenic organism in the stool for weeks or months after all clinical manifestations have subsided. Since excretion is intermittent rather than continuous, the customary practice of adjudging an individual as a noncarrier when three successive stool specimens have failed to yield the bacilli is not entirely reliable. After typhoid fever, even when stool cultures have been negative over a period of 6 months, culture of bile collected by duodenal tube may reveal the typhoid organism still present.

Eradication of Salmonella from asymptomatic carriers is sometimes very difficult. It is doubtful that current antimicrobial drugs can selectively destroy small numbers of pathogenic bacteria which may be living symbiotically within the bacteria-crowded environment of the large intestine.

Shigellosis (Bacillary Dysentery)

CLINICAL ASPECTS. Acute gastroenteritis with tenesmus, fever, and diarrhea is caused typically by the Shigella genus of bacteria. The onset is usually sudden. The cecum, colon, and rectum are the principal sites of inflammation, and sometimes the lower ileum as well. In infants and young children the diapers soak up the watery contents, leaving a characterisitic coating of yellow-green mucus and pus, admixed frequently with flecks or streaks of blood. Microscopy of the feces reveals a rich content of single and clumped leukocytes, with red cells frequently not present. Isolation of the organisms by fecal culture is as successful with mild as with severe cases and bears no relation to the number of bowel evacuations per day. Other syndromes occasionally produced are obscure fevers, septicemia, localized abscesses, and invasion of the urinary tract.

The infection is spread most commonly by direct contact with carriers or indirectly through toilet facilities used by infected persons. Spread may also be through the medium of water supplies or uncooked foods which are contaminated with infected fecal matter. Flies may spread the organism from unsanitary privies.

After an attack of dysentery, many patients continue to excrete the organisms erratically in the feces for many months. Prolonged administration of a sulfonamide or antibiotic to which the strain is sensitive is recommended for such chronic symptomless carriers but does not always prove successful.

BACTERIOLOGY. The numerous members of the Shigella genus are aerobic, nonencapsulated, nonmotile Gram-negative bacilli. They grow well on the usual media and display distinctive cultural reactions. Antigenically they exhibit considerable overlapping of their somatic or O antigens and envelope or K antigens. Some of these antigens coincide with those of other species of Gram-negative bacilli.

Classification of the Shigella genus begins with arrangement into four main classes, A, B, C, and D. These in turn are subdivided into at least 30 serotypes.

Group A, known also as S. *dysenteriae,* comprises those strains which do ferment mannitol. The best-known subtypes are the *shiga, ambigua, shiga-kruse, schmitzii,* and Large-Sachs group. Current policy is to refer to these by type numerals rather than by eponyms. S. *dysenteriae* is believed to be the only class which produces an exotoxin.

Group B, S. *flexneri,* contains those organisms formerly called S.

paradysenteriae Flexner. At least six subgroups, referred to by number, have been identified.

Group C, S. *boydii,* has at least seven subtypes.

Group D, S. *sonnei,* is made up of strains which break down lactose after prolonged incubation. Some authorities include S. *dispar* in this group.

SEROLOGY. Serum agglutinins against the bacilli recoverable from the stools develop in some patients, but as a rule these do not reach an appreciable titer until the second week or later. Study of the serologic response is of value primarily for establishing the correctness of the diagnosis when earlier bacteriologic studies have failed to yield the organisms. Serums from normal subjects only infrequently give readings higher than 1:50, whereas after the active disease the titer may rise transitorily to 1:100, 1:500, or higher.

The mechanism which leads to recovery appears to be largely a tissue immunity localized in the intestinal mucosa. Except in S. *flexneri* infections this immunity seems to last but a few months, since reinfection with the same or a similar strain may take place after that interval. This perhaps explains why anti-Shigella bacterial vaccines have not proved satisfactory.

LABORATORY RECOGNITION. The diagnosis is accomplished primarily by the successful isolation of Shigella organisms from a rectal swab or less preferably from a stool itself. Specimens must be cultured as soon as possible after collection and protected from chilling while en route to the bacteriologist. Flecks of purulent mucus when present should be teased out and utilized for the culture. The technique to be followed is the same as for Salmonella. From the same specimen two different serotypes of Shigella, or even a concurrent Salmonella strain, may be recovered.

Bacilli which on morphologic and cultural grounds appear to be shigellae should be tested with group-specific serums. The precise subtype identification is generally done in reference laboratories to which the strains are sent.

ANTIBIOTIC SENSITIVITIES. As a general rule the sulfonamide drugs are not highly effective in rendering stools Shigella-free. Zimmerman, Cooper, and Graber found that 30 per cent of adults with proved shigellosis and treated with sulfadiazine were still excreting viable organisms after eight days of treatment. The broad-spectrum antibiotics eradicated Shigella from the stools within 2 days, though this clearance may have been impermanent. Clinical benefit has been described after therapy with neomycin, polymyxin B, or bacitracin.

OTHER LABORATORY FINDINGS. Leukocytosis is a usual concomitant. The fever, anorexia, and excessive loss of water in the stools may lead to dehydration and ketosis. Sigmoidoscopic examination reveals the sigmoidal mucosa to be intensely hyperemic, friable, edematous, and coated with mucopurulent exudate; erosions with hemorrhagic bases may be seen. Material wiped from the surface of such inflamed areas is an excellent source of material for culture and for microscopic search for pus cells and erythrocytes.

GONOCOCCIC INFECTIONS

The gonococcus *Neisseria gonorrhoeae* is not a common pathogen in the childhood age period. The usual sites of infections are the urethral tract, the vaginal area (p. 754), and the conjunctiva of the eye. To establish the diagnosis both smears and cultures are needed. A serologic complement-fixation test is available but rarely used.

Laboratory Diagnosis

The purulent exudates from an acutely inflamed area, when smeared and stained, will usually show an abundance of Gram-negative bean-shaped pairs of cocci situated intracellularly. In more chronic lesions only an occasional pus cell will contain these typical diplococci. Other Gram-negative cocci will usually be present in the smear, leading to difficulties in recognition.

Cultures are more reliable and are best made immediately. If a delay is unavoidable, the swab (or urine) may be stored in a refrigerator for a few hours only. The exudate is smeared on sugar medium reinforced with sterile serum or ascitic fluid and incubated at 37°C in about 10 per cent carbon dioxide. Suspicious small opalescent colonies which turn black in the test for oxidase are assumed to be Neisseria. These should be subcultured and inoculated both in standard media and the reinforced medium. Other Neisseria species such as *N. catarrhalis, N. pharyngis, N. sicca, N. flavescens,* and even the meningococcal *N. meningitidis* will grow in both media, whereas gonococci will grow only in the special medium.

The sediment from urine cultures of male patients will sometimes yield gonococci on culture when these are present in the urogenital tract. The urine should be collected by voiding and should preferably be a morning specimen.

Therapy

Gonococci display considerable strain variation in susceptibility to the various antibiotics. Every recovered strain should be tested in vitro with a battery of antimicrobial agents, and appropriate therapy based on the results.

An acute infection should not be considered cured until at least three negative smears and cultures have been obtained over a 3-week period. Chronic cases require intensive therapy and longer posttreatment observation.

Ophthalmia Neonatorum

This may be associated with the presence of gonococci, staphylococci, diphtheroids, or other organisms. Inclusion bodies are not infrequently found in swabs of the conjunctiva, regardless of whether or not organisms can be cultured. Ocular prophylaxis of gonococcic infection in the newborn infant can be attained by instilling 1 per cent silver nitrate solution. Local and systemic therapy with different antibiotics and sulfonamides is currently being explored as replacement for silver nitrate solution, since the latter often induces a transient chemical conjunctivitis.

Gonococcic Vaginitis. See page 754.

INFLUENZA BACILLUS INFECTIONS

Hemophilus influenzae (Pfeiffer's bacillus) is a common cause of pyogenic infections in infancy. It can give rise to nasopharyngitis, otitis media, sinusitis, tracheobronchitis, croup, bronchopneumonia, empyema, meningitis, pyarthosis, conjunctivitis, vaginitis, and assorted other diseases. The organism is usually a direct primary invader, especially during infancy. The portal of entry is usually the nasopharynx, with later dissemination through the blood stream. Hence the nasopharyngeal or throat culture will prove positive for *H. influenzae* nearly always, even when the infection is predominant elsewhere in the body. The pathogenic effects are often produced conjointly with the influenza virus, the streptococcus, the pneumococcus, or other organisms which cause respiratory tract disease. Epidemiologic and serologic surveys have shown that most normal children possess marked resistance to *H. influenzae* infections after 2 to 3 years of age.

Bacteriology

H. influenzae is an encapsulated pleomorphic Gram-negative bacillus. In smears of infected cerebrospinal fluid, pleural aspirates, and other infective exudates the predominant forms are coccobacillary, often poorly staining and occurring in pairs. Careful scrutiny, however, will usually reveal a few rodlike organisms among the rounded forms. The latter may be mistaken for pneumococci or even pleuropneumonia-like organisms if the Gram staining is imperfect. They are sometimes arranged in short chains, simulating streptococci. Nonlethal exposures to antibiotic solutions may accentuate these changes. Elongated forms predominate in young cultures; these may be irregular or bent and sometimes contain polar bodies.

H. influenzae thrives best on culture media which contain hemolyzed blood. In synthetic media the nutrient factors x (hemin) and v (yeast) are essential for growth. Colonies less than 24 hours old display iridescence when viewed by transmitted light.

CLASSIFICATION. The pathogenic varieties of *H. influenzae* can be sub-classified serologically as types *a, b, c, d, e,* and *f,* on the basis of specific polysaccharide antigens within their capsules. Most childhood infections due to *H. influenzae* prove to be type *b.* This type tends to persist in the nasopharynx for long periods after recovery.

The precise nature of a recovered strain can be identified serologically by agglutination tests, capsular swelling reactions (quelling), and precipitin tests for the specific soluble polysaccharide of the capsule. The capsular polysaccharides of types *a, b,* and *c* are immunologically similar to and exhibit cross reactions with polysaccharides from a few of the pneumococcic types. The nonencapsulated or R strains of *H. influenzae,* which form rough colonies, are not pathogenic and do not react with any of the typing sera. These may be transformed into any desired encapsulated type-specific strain by exposure to the desoxyribonucleic acid extractable from that type.

ANTIBIOTIC SENSITIVITIES. Most strains are sensitive to streptomycin, sulfonamides, polymyxin B, and the broad-spectrum antibiotics, especially when first isolated. Susceptibility to penicillin is unusual, except with mutant forms resistant to streptomycin. Severe *H. influenzae* infections, such as purulent meningitis, are best treated by combinations of suitable antimicrobial drugs.

Koch-Weeks Bacillus

Acute conjunctivitis is not infrequently attended by the presence of this species of Gram-negative bacilli, which morphologically and culturally is similar to *H. influenzae.*

Morax-Axenfeld Bacillus

This organism, more correctly termed *Moraxella lacunata* or *Hemophilus duplex,* is another biologically related nonencapsulated Gram-negative short bacillus occurring in pairs or short chains, found in some conjunctival and corneal infections. This organism or the Koch-Weeks bacillus may be encountered in epidemics of conjunctivitis of presumed viral origin and is thought to be a secondary invader in that circumstance.

KLEBSIELLA-AEROBACTER INFECTIONS

Bacteriology

Klebsiella-Aerobacter constitutes a large group of Gram-negative bacilli which are encapsulated, nonsporulating, nonmotile, and which form large mucoid colonies on agar media. They ferment most carbohydrates including adonitol and inositol with the liberation of acid and gas, may or may not liquefy gelatin, usually metabolize citrate, usually do not produce indole, and give a negative methyl red reaction. In stained smears they appear as pleomorphic rods, often paired, with capsules which are usually recognizable even by this technique. Serologically it is possible to distinguish different types on the basis of capsular or K antigens, somatic smooth or O antigens, and somatic rough or R antigens. At least 72 K antigens and 3 distinct O antigens have been recognized thus far. Identification if desired is ordinarily restricted to the K antigen, since acapsular forms are required for recognition of the O antigen. The K antigens are referred to by numbers rather than name; recovered strains are diagnosed as type 1, type 2, etc. The capsules swell enormously when specific antiserum is added to hanging drop preparations.

The members of this group show so much overlapping in their biochemical reactions that no single cultural test or group of tests can be used to differentiate among them. In the past, the term *Aerobacter aerogenes* has been applied to strains recovered from the respiratory tract, and Friedländer bacillus (*Bacillus mucosus capsulatus*) to those from the intestine and urinary tracts. But morphologically and culturally these are so similar that any distinction based on site of isolation is artificial and invalid.

Most of the strains in this group can be distinguished from colon bacilli on the basis of their differences in culture with four critical tests—the I M Vi C reaction—as follows:

Organism	Indole production	Methyl red reaction	Voges-Proskauer reaction	Citrate utilization
Escherichia coli	+	+	−	−
Klebsiella-Aerobacter	−	±	+	+
	(usually)			(usually)

Pathogenicity

Klebsiella are found occasionally in normal stools and respiratory passages and in soil, water, and room dust. They are frequent secondary invaders in the sputum of patients with bronchiectasis, tuberculosis, and other respiratory tract infections. They often cause a destructive cavitating form of pneumonia which tends to have delayed resolution; in these instances they are generally demonstrable in the sputum. Infection may localize anywhere, in the form of appendicitis, meningitis, stomatitis, osteomyelitis, cystitis, pyelonephritis, deep abscesses, or infected wounds. Bacteremia appears to be transient, since blood cultures are as a rule negative. Diarrhea and vomiting are common accompaniments of Klebsiella infections in infancy. Some epidemics of diarrhea and respiratory disease have been attributed to dissemination of these organisms through air droplets or fomites. There is no practical procedure for the study of antibodies in the serum of patients suspected of having such infections.

No direct relationships have been found between serologic type, clinical character of the infection, and antibiotic sensitivities. A decided tendency to local abscess formation seems to prevent adequate access of antimicrobial agents. In pneumonia, for example, the organism may reappear in the sputum and be still sensitive in vitro after bacteriologically guided therapy has been discontinued.

LACTOBACILLUS RELATIONSHIPS

The lactobacilli are nonmotile nonsporulating Gram-positive pleomorphic rods which are found normally in the mouth, vagina, and gastrointestinal tract. Their differentiation into distinct species is still under study. They are essentially nonpathogens, but may bear some relation to softening of the teeth during childhood.

Dental Caries

A current explanation of dental caries is that tooth decay results from acids derived from lactobacilli and related microorganisms acting upon carbohydrates within the mouth. Decalcification of the inorganic portion is thought to be accompanied or followed by disintegration of the organic substance of the tooth. This theory calls for the action of numerous concurrent factors: (1) Fermentable carbohydrate-containing foods must be frequently ingested, and fragments left adherent to the teeth after the food is swallowed. (2) Certain specialized enzymes must be present in the patient's saliva in order to react with the teeth; a tough adherent bacterial plaque appears essential for this. (3) The teeth must be soluble in weak organic acids and not otherwise resistant to the destructive action of acids. (4) Bacteria which are both acid-forming and acid-tolerating must occur in abundance about the teeth. The theory states further that in caries-resistant individuals the lactobacilli are absent from the mouth and digestive tract and the blood agglutinin titer to lactobacilli is high; that saliva from caries-resistant mouths will not support the growth of lactobacilli and will not permit the formation of acid as rapidly as will saliva from susceptible mouths in the presence of sugar. Among the oral organisms deemed capable of producing sufficient local acidity to decalcify teeth are leptothrix, some strains of streptococci, and above all the lactobacilli—especially *Lactobacillus acidophilus*.

Penicillin, dibasic ammonium phosphate, amino acid products, and some other agents are being tried experimentally to rid children's mouths of these so-called aciduric organisms. It is also advised that the consumption of fermentable sugars be reduced and that the teeth be brushed and the mouth rinsed with water immediately after every meal which includes carbohydrates. Since at least 12 or 13 enzymes and coenzymes are essential for the breakdown of sucrose into lactic acid, it has been seriously suggested that oral acid formation could be inhibited by incorporating some nontoxic chemical inhibitor of enzyme activity in all sugar-containing foods. The lactobacilli produce a low pH, can live in a highly acid environment, and are consistently present in the saliva of children with active caries.

PERFORMANCE OF LACTOBACILLUS COUNTS. The child is given paraffin to chew, and the saliva expectorated into a test tube. The tube is placed on a shaking machine to break up the clumps of bacteria. A sample of 1 ml of saliva is then transferred to a tube containing 4 ml of broth adjusted to pH 5 and mixed thoroughly; 0.1 ml of this saliva-broth mixture is then spread over the surface of a tomato-agar Petri dish with a sterile glass rod or spreader. The plates are incubated at 37.5°C for 4 days. The number of recognized lactobacillus colonies times 50 equals the count per milliliter of saliva.

CLINICAL ASPECTS. The majority of individuals with active dental caries have lactobacillus counts ranging between 1,000 and 1 million per ml of saliva, whereas only occasional caries-free individuals have counts this high. When individuals with high counts are placed on diets low in refined carbohydrates, reexamination after several months as a rule will show virtual disappearance of the organisms. For these reasons the lactobacillus count is frequently taken as an indicator of the activity of tooth decay in a given mouth and as a guide for prognosis as to what will happen in the near future. A number of interested laboratories will perform lactobacillus counts on samples of saliva sent to them by dentists.

Another concept for dental decay postulates the existence of some as yet unidentified substance or substances, possibly a vitamin or trace element, which can make the teeth able to resist acids or other destructive factors.

MENINGOCOCCIC INFECTIONS

Bacteremia and meningitis and other infections caused by *Neisseria meningitidis* are encountered sporadically in all seasons, though least often in the summer months. Epidemics break out at approximately 8- to 12-year intervals in the United States as a whole. Patients often have an upper respiratory infection for a few days, followed by meningococcemia for about a day and then an extension to the leptomeninges.

The number of frank infections is only a small fraction of the total number of persons who become subclinically attacked during an epidemic, to judge from the great number of so-called "carriers" who can be detected by nasopharyngeal cultures at those times. In fact, survey of a population by throat cultures in any season will nearly always uncover a few individuals who are harboring some strain of these organisms.

Clinical Aspects

Meningococcic bacteremia can be so fulminant as to cause death before meningeal localization has taken place. Most of the fatal cases in current years are of this acute character. Illnesses which progress more slowly give the physician time to institute antimicrobial therapy, which is usually lifesaving when vigorously pursued. In rapidly fatal cases the prominent manifestations are those of fever, shock, prostration, circulatory collapse, and widespread hemorrhages. An endotoxin liberated from the meningococcus into the circulation is believed to explain this constitutional response. The adrenals often, but not invariably, show gross or microscopic hemorrhages at autopsy; the condition may then be termed the Waterhouse-Friderichsen syndrome.

If meningitis is suspected, the cerebrospinal fluid should be cultured and a microscopic study made of the Gram-stained smear of the centrifuged sediment. Organisms are sometimes demonstrable in the cerebrospinal fluid in the first day of illness, while the fluid itself still appears uninvolved in the routine cytologic and chemical tests (p. 450).

When a physician encounters a sick infant with suspected meningococcemia in a home and concludes that hospitalization is imperative, he may first take a nasopharyngeal swab for culture and collect a few milliliters of the patient's blood in a sterile tube for later bacteriologic study. He should then administer immediately a large dose of penicillin or some other antibiotic or sulfonamide, in order to check the advance of the illness. The intravenous route is preferable whenever feasible. A lag of a few hours may mean the difference between simple septicemia and meningeal involvement, or even between recovery and death.

Bacteriologic Grouping

Meningococci are small Gram-negative diplococci, usually occurring in pairs with flattened adjacent sides. The strains isolated from patients and carriers fall into specific serologic groups. These are determined by the immunologic reactions of their carbohydrate capsules, shown by agglutination and quelling tests. Most epidemics prove to be due to group I, whereas sporadic cases are more apt to be caused by group II or group IIA. Group ("type") IV is rare now, but appears to have caused epidemics in years past. Strains in groups II and IIA are more prone to cause low-grade chronic septicemia without meningeal involvement.

Group I organisms when recovered from a carrier are usually encapsulated and prove virulent for mice. This type of carrier is adjudged as a menace to others. The finding of group I strains in increasing numbers among carriers is an omen that an outbreak of meningococcic infections may be near.

Occasional individuals carry meningococci in their nasopharynx for years. Those strains usually prove to be of group II, though they may contain so little carbohydrate that their colony formation is "rough" and their mouse virulence negligible.

Before the advent of modern antimicrobial agents, when the only good therapy was specific antimeningococcic serum, it was important to identify all meningococci by group in order to administer the proper monovalent therapeutic serum. For epidemiologic reasons this immunologic identification is still advisable.

Cultural Study

When a child is ill with what may be a meningococcic infection, cultures should be taken from both the nasopharynx and blood stream, and of course from the cerebrospinal fluid when meningitis is suspected.

These materials should be planted in prewarmed culture media as quickly as possible. The organism grows best in media which contain blood or serum or certain other important nutrients and when the incubation is done in a moist atmosphere containing 5 to 10 per cent carbon dioxide. It is killed by heat, cold, and drying. Typical colonies are smooth and translucent. Yellow pigment is not produced, which helps in differentiation from *Neisseria flava* and other members of the Neisseria genus which rarely may also cause a septicemic or meningeal infection. Recognition of *N. meningitidis* is accomplished by colony appearance, positive reaction to the oxidase test, sugar fermentation reactions, and agglutinability or capsular swelling with the proper typing serums.

Cultures from fresh skin lesions or early arthritic effusions often prove positive. Organisms are demonstrated in skin lesions by scraping fresh hemorrhages and pressing a clean glass slide over the oozing point, after which the slide is stained with the Gram stain and examined microscopically.

The best method for detecting carriers and subclinical infections is by recovery of meningococci from the posterior nasopharyngeal wall. This area may be approached through the nostrils or the oral cavity. When it is not feasible to inoculate the swab immediately on culture medium, its tip may be left in 1 ml of sterile defibrinated horse blood at room temperature for as long as 5 hours without adversely affecting the likelihood of colony growth.

The nasopharyngeal culture is less likely to be successful than cultures prepared from the blood stream or cerebrospinal fluid. Blood cultures are most often positive early, while the rash is appearing and before the meninges have been invaded. All bacteriologic studies should be done before antimicrobial therapy is begun.

Antibiotic Sensitivities

The present-day approach to the therapy of meningococcic infections consists in administering one or more antibiotics parenterally and orally, usually in combination with a sulfonamide, in large and frequent doses. Most meningococci are highly susceptible to penicillin, the broad-spectrum antibiotics, and the soluble sulfonamides.

MIMEAE INFECTIONS

The Mimeae constitute a loosely defined group of pleomorphic Gram-negative cocci, diplococci, and rods which have many biochemical and serologic properties in common. The pertinent variety, with numerous serotypes, is *Mima polymorpha*. Isolated instances of meningitis, endocarditis, conjunctivitis, and other infections produced by one or another of these have been reported. They are found not infrequently in urine cultures from patients with genitourinary infections and may be mistaken for *Neisseria gonorrhoeae*.

The majority of strains when tested in vitro seem to be sensitive to the tetracyclines and resistant to streptomycin, chloramphenicol, and penicillin.

INFECTIONS CAUSED BY PASTEURELLA

The Pasteurella species of human pathogenicity are *Pasteurella multocida*, *P. pestis*, *P. pseudotuberculosis*, *P. tularensis*, and possibly *P. pneumotropica*. The pasteurellae in general are small, easily grown, aerobic, Gram-negative coccoid or ovoid rods which may be motile or show bipolar staining by special methods. *P. multocida* is a common cause of hemorrhagic septicemia in animals and birds.

Pasteurellosis

Human infections due to *P. multocida* are probably not as rare as published reports would indicate. About half the infections follow an animal bite (usually that of a cat); they tend to remain localized but sometimes produce generalized symptoms. Other cases have followed contact with infected cattle, pigs, rats, or rabbits and have resulted in enteritis, conjunctivitis, meningitis, pyelonephritis, sinusitis, and similar lesions. There is evidence that *P. multocida* may be carried in the respiratory passages for months, to produce local disease after a superimposed local injury, e.g., a brain abscess after a skull fracture. The organisms may be mistaken for *Hemophilus influenzae* in routine bacteriologic studies. Some strains have been sensitive to therapy with chlortetracycline. Meyer states that the serums of patients tested during subacute Pasteurella infections have yielded agglutination or complement-fixation titers in dilutions as high as 1:3,200 when tested with the strain isolated from the lesions.

Plague

P. pestis organisms are Gram-negative pleomorphic rods which show prominent bipolar staining when first recovered from infected rodents or man. Even though epidemic plague has disappeared from North America, isolated cases are occasionally seen, usually following contact with infected squirrels, chipmunks, prairie dogs, rats, or mice. Insects spread the disease to man. Either the bubonic or the pneumonic symptom complex may be produced. Patients often have a positive blood culture in the first few days of acute symptoms. The organisms may also be recovered from the sputum or from the fluid recovered by puncture of an inflamed bubo. They are susceptible to the sulfonamides, streptomycin, and some of the broad-spectrum antibiotics.

Tularemia

P. tularensis occurs as short single nonmotile Gram-negative rods which are pleomorphic and frequently coccoid. Growth is best on special media containing hen's egg yolk or blood and cystine. Since the organism is highly infective for man, the antigens used in serologic studies are prepared from an attenuated strain. The disease is spread by contact with infected animals or water and by the bites of deer flies and ticks. Many laboratory workers have become infected while investigating dead animals or studying live cultures.

Blood cultures occasionally show the organisms up to the twelfth day of illness. To recover the organisms from sputum, cerebrospinal fluid, pleural fluid, or macerated tissue, it is best to inject the material into chick embryos or guinea pigs or other animals. Direct bacteriologic cultures are less likely to be positive.

SERUM AGGLUTININS. Specific agglutinins begin to appear in the sera of patients in the second week, reach their peak in the third and fourth weeks, and persist at moderate levels for at least a year thereafter. The titer of agglutinins may be 1:10 or 1:20 by the end of the first week of illness and rise a week or two later. Failure of specific agglutinins to appear after symptoms have persisted for 2 weeks or more is presumptive evidence that the illness is some disease other than tularemia.

With the exception of antigens from *Brucella abortus* and *Br. melitensis*, a patient's serum will show no cross agglutination with antigens from other bacteria. Serums from suspected cases of tularemia or undulant fever should be tested with both sets of antigens. Marked serologic differences in speed of reactivity and final titer aid in differentiating between these diseases.

Vaccination of individuals with tularemic antigens brings about an elevation in serum titer to 1:320 or 1:640 at first, followed by subsidence to 1:40 or 1:80 after a few months, which then persists. It has been noted that the onset of tularemia in previously vaccinated individuals is accompanied by a transitory fall in serum titer in the early phases, followed by a steady rise to a much higher level than that originally evoked by the vaccination itself.

PERTUSSIS (WHOOPING COUGH)

Advanced cases with the characteristic coughing paroxysms present a picture which is so typical that the astute clinician rarely has need for laboratory tests. In mild, early, or atypical cases, on the other hand, positive laboratory results can be most helpful in establishing the existence of this disease.

Laboratory abnormalities are often undemonstrable when pertussis develops in previously immunized children.

Bacteriology

Hemophilus pertussis is a small ovoid nonmotile Gram-negative encapsulated bacillus which attacks the tracheobronchial tree of susceptible children. It grows best on complex media such as the potato-blood-agar-glycerol mixture of Bordet-Gengou. A weak concentration of penicillin is often incorporated in this medium to reduce the growth of susceptible bacteria. Freshly isolated strains from children with whooping cough are in the form known as phase 1. Important antigenic constituents are an agglutinogen and a toxin. Most immunologic studies have been done with the agglutinogen, because of the indications that immunity in pertussis is largely antibacterial rather than antitoxic.

CULTURES. The most reliable guide to diagnosis in suspected cases is the actual recovery of *H. pertussis* from the respiratory tract. Prompt recognition is desirable in order to isolate the patient and institute treatment early. Proper cultural studies yield *H. pertussis* in a high percentage of specimens taken in the first week of onset of symptoms, when catarrhal symptoms are prominent. Thereafter, bacteriologic success declines rapidly. It is unusual to recover the organisms once the paroxysmal stage has been reached.

There are several approaches for obtaining specimens of infected secretions for culture. In our hands the nasopharyngeal swab seems to yield the highest percentage of positive cultures. Cough plates are feasible with older children, especially when used in duplicate or triplicate, though the number of bacterial colonies which grow out and have to be differentiated is much greater. Expectorated sputum containing tracheal secretions may also be used for culture but is almost impossible to obtain in patients under 5 or 6 years of age. Laryngeal suction is cumbersome, and its success is no higher than with the other methods.

All cultures should be kept in the incubator at 37°C for at least 7 days. *H. pertussis* colonies are tiny, rounded, and pearly gray, surrounded by a faint zone of hemolysis. Organisms in suspicious colonies are identified by their morphology, staining reaction, and agglutination in specific antiserum available for testing purposes.

Direct microscopic study of the sputum or nasopharyngeal mucus is of no value in diagnosis, since *H. influenzae* and other Gram-negative bacilli are indistinguishable morphologically from *H. pertussis* and may be present in the flora.

NASOPHARYNGEAL SWAB. The technique of culturing the upper pharynx through the nose is described on page 772. The swabs with their coating of mucus and pus are rubbed in a drop of penicillin solution previously placed upon the culture plate if the culture medium itself does not have penicillin in it. The material is then streaked over the plate surface with a platinum loop.

COUGH PLATE. Two Petri dishes containing freshly prepared solid culture medium are placed in succession about 5 in. from the mouth, while the child coughs repeatedly upon them. The plates may be rotated slowly to obtain uniform distribution of the droplets. If the child is not old enough to cough voluntarily, a paroxysm of coughing may be induced by compressing the trachea from the anterior surface of the neck or by irritating the posterior pharyngeal wall with an applicator or tongue depressor. Passage of a nasopharyngeal swab may induce coughing when all other methods fail.

LARYNGEAL SUCTION. A slender rubber catheter is inserted orally to the larynx while the patient coughs and gags. A rubber bulb at the free end is alternately compressed and released until sputum becomes visible in the glass irrigating tip which connects the catheter and bulb. The catheter is then withdrawn. The irrigating tip containing the sputum is detached from its rubber connection and placed in a Petri dish for immediate transport to the laboratory. The sputum is cultured in the same manner as described for nasopharyngeal swabs.

ANTIBIOTIC SENSITIVITIES. Most freshly isolated strains of *H. pertussis* prove to be highly sensitive in vitro to polymyxin B, moderately sensitive to the broad-spectrum antibiotics and penicillin, and weakly sensitive to streptomycin.

The partial symptomatic improvement which follows therapy with most antibiotics seems to be due to depression of other pathogenic bacteria acting symbiotically with *H. pertussis*. It is much more difficult to recover *H. pertussis* from the nasopharynx after antibiotic therapy has been given.

Serum Antibodies

Antibacterial antibodies—agglutinins, opsonins, and complement-fixing and mouse-protection antibodies—appear during the third week of illness and subside after convalescence. Tests for these antibodies have not proved of much assistance in the diagnostic study of questionable or borderline cases. Positive agglutinations in dilutions 1:200 or higher do not appear until late in the disease. The sera of many normal children give positive agglutinations in dilutions up to 1:100.

A rapid test for serum antibodies has been devised in which a small amount of finely granular pertussis antigen, stained with methylene blue, is mixed with a drop of serum on a glazed surface. The drop is rocked back and forth for a minute. The blue-colored antigen becomes clumped if the serum contains appreciable antipertussis agglutinating antibodies. This test when properly performed shows a good correlation with the more precise tube dilution methods when specific antibodies are present in more than borderline concentrations.

About 90 per cent of children who have received prophylactic injections of dead bacilli within the preceding few months will show a positive serum complement-fixation test with a killed suspension of whole organisms. About 25 per cent of nonimmunized children also have positive titers, possibly as a manifestation of a previous subclinical infection. Most children with a high titer of circulating antibodies are resistant to whooping cough. However, many with no circulating antibodies demonstrable are also resistant; it has been suggested that these may have a "tissue" immunity.

Skin Tests

A positive skin reaction to the agglutinogen injected intradermally is believed to be an indication of immunity, whereas positive reaction to the toxin is thought, like the Schick test, to indicate susceptibility. Neither of these approaches has received wide acceptance.

Blood Leukocyte Picture

An attack of pertussis occasionally calls forth a rise in the absolute lymphocyte count, often to above 10,000 per cu mm and sometimes above 50,000 per cu mm. This lymphocytic response begins in the early catarrhal stage and reaches its maximum in the paroxysmal stage. The lymphocytes are of small size and show no morphologic abnormalities. They evidently come from the lymph nodes, since the bone marrow shows no increase in these cells. A neutrophilic leukocytosis may occur simultaneously, especially when secondary infection is present. A neutrophilic leukocytopenia is not unusual.

Parapertussis Infections

A respiratory tract infection resembling whooping cough, but less severe and of shorter duration, can be produced by *Hemophilus parapertussis*. This is also a short ovoid nonmotile Gram-negative bacillus. Colonies are similar to but larger than those of *H. pertussis* on Bordet-Gengou medium and grow readily on plain agar.

Bronchiseptica Infections

The motile Gram-negative bacillus known as *Brucella bronchiseptica*, which produces a respiratory tract disease in dogs, will in rare instances cause pertussis-like symptoms in children. Sneezing may be more prominent than coughing. *Br. bronchiseptica, H. parapertussis,* and *H. pertussis,* though related closely in biologic and infective characteristics, are culturally and serologically distinguishable.

INFECTIONS WITH PLEUROPNEUMONIA-LIKE ORGANISMS

Minute pleomorphic organisms similar to those which cause pleuropneumonia in cattle have been recovered from many species of animals, with some of whom they are clearly pathogenic. They occur also in the female genital tract and in the throat and saliva of a high percentage of normal human beings.

Bacteriology

The following criteria define the group, according to Sabin: (1) They grow and develop in cell-free culture media, producing large protoplasmic masses with "chromatin" bodies, globules, filaments, "rings," and filterable bodies 125 to 250 mμ in size which are the minimal reproductive units. (2) They give rise on suitable solid media to minute deeply imbedded colonies with a central dark nipplelike structure or vacuolar meshwork. They appear to be distinct from ordinary bacteria, filterable viruses, and rickettsiae. Strains from human cases seem biologically different from those recovered from infected animals.

When searching for the presence of pleuropneumonia-like organisms (PPLO), one spreads the fluid to be cultured over the surface of a special agar-containing medium which contains ascitic fluid or serum. This is then incubated aerobically for 2 to 7 days at 37°C. The agar plate is inspected for growth by inverting it (without removing the cover) and examining under the low power of the microscope. Typical colonies are minute and round, with a dense center and thinner periphery. Since they grow into the agar, the medium must not be too solid and clear enough to permit the passage of light. When rubbed with a loop or needle the colonies remain undisturbed, unlike bacterial growths which are easily moved. They can be cut out and stained with Dienes stain, which they take deeply and characteristically. Organisms are not recognizable in stained preparations of lesions.

Recovered strains vary considerably in their in vitro resistance to the antibiotics and sulfonamides. Streptomycin and the broad-spectrum antibiotics are perhaps the most effective.

Pathogenicity

The importance of these organisms in human infections is still controversial. There is some evidence that they may cause so-called "nonspecific" infections in the eye, joints, meninges, and the male urogenital tract. They have been recovered from the urine in some cases of pyuria of unknown cause, from the cerebrospinal fluid of a few children with meningitis, and from the blood in sundry other affections including chronic arthritis, urethritis, and anaphylactoid purpura. They may be searched for in inflammatory material from the joints, eyes, or urogenital tract when ordinary bacteria are not demonstrable and a virus etiology appears improbable. We have succeeded in recovering these organisms only twice in over 200 consecutive catheterized urine cultures of children with chronic pyuria, and the pathogenetic importance in those two cases was highly doubtful.

Colonies of some bacteria, when cultivated on solid media containing high concentrations of penicillin, may at times assume gross and microscopic appearances identical with those of the pleuropneumonia-like organisms—the so-called L type of growth. Subcultures on penicillin-free media will be followed by a reversion to the original bacterial forms or no growth at all.

These organisms are best viewed as being of special interest to the bacteriologist rather than the clinician.

PNEUMOCOCCIC INFECTIONS

Epidemiology

The infections produced most frequently by pneumococci occur in the respiratory passages and contiguous areas. These infections include sinusitis, otitis media, laryngitis, mastoiditis, conjunctivitis, and the lobar, lobular, and interstitial varieties of pneumonia. Septicemia, empyema, peritonitis, meningitis, and other more remote diseases develop from spread through hematogenous or lymphatic channels. Pneumococcic infections of the respiratory passages are often preceded or accompanied by influenza, measles, or the common cold.

As many as 50 per cent of healthy children may carry pneumococci of one or several types in their upper respiratory passages during the winter season. Hence, when a strain of pneumococcus is recovered from the secretions in this area during a respiratory tract infection, one cannot always be certain that this is the primary cause of the infection.

Otitis media, sinusitis, and bronchopneumonia often seem to be "mixed" infections induced by several organisms. Such multiple combinations often include pneumococci of two or more types, or a pneumococcus with a staphylococcus or streptococcus or the influenza bacillus. In prematurely born or otherwise debilitated infants, less pathogenic organisms such as *Pseudomonas aeruginosa* or even *Micrococcus catarrhalis* may be associated with the pneumococcus.

Bacteriology

More than 75 serologic types of pneumococci have been recognized, the differentiation being based on the antigenic capsular polysaccharides. Unlike what obtains with adults and older children in whom types I, II, and III have caused at least half of all cases of lobar pneumonia, pneumonia in younger children and infants is usually due to XIV, VI, XIX, and V and other higher-numbered types. Lobular and interstitial bronchopneumonia are the most frequent in infants under 2 years of age, whereas lobar pneumonia is most common above that age. In general, the nonpathogenic strains of pneumococci belong to the highest-numbered types.

In pneumonia, otitis media, empyema, meningitis, and other pneumococcic infections the same type of organism is more likely to be recovered from the nasopharyngeal mucus than from the throat. Bacteriologic procedures such as these outlined below will succeed in detecting the offending microorganism in nearly every untreated child with bacterial pneumonia.

PROCEDURES FOR CULTURES. As described on page 772, a sterilized fine-wire swab is moistened with sterile saline, advanced through the nostril to the posterior pharyngeal wall, and left in position for a full minute to collect mucus before being withdrawn. The swab is then inserted into a small quantity of sterile broth in a test tube and forwarded immediately to the laboratory. Here the wire swab is withdrawn and used to inoculate plates of blood agar, influenza bacillus medium, and selective media for Gram-negative colon organisms.

If a direct smear examination is also desired, two swabs are prepared. The direct smear when stained with methylene blue will often show numerous leukocytes and large lancet-shaped encapsulated diplococci if the patient has pneumococcic pneumonia.

On the culture plates the colonies of most of the pathogens will become evident by 24 hours. Any colonies of pneumococci or influenza bacilli which develop are used for typing if desired.

Cultures of the blood taken in the early phases of pneumonia and other severe pneumococcic infections are more likely to be positive than those obtained later and should be procured before chemotherapy is given. In general, especially with patients not receiving such treatment, the persistence of circulating organisms indicates that immune bodies are not being developed at an appreciable rate and bespeaks a poor prognosis. Cultures of the clear fluid which may appear transitorily in greater or lesser quantities within the pleural cavities of patients with pneumonia are usually sterile; bacteria when present herald an impending empyema.

ANTIBIOTIC SENSITIVITIES. Pneumococci are highly susceptible to penicillin, the broad-spectrum antibiotics, and erythromycin. Sensitivity is greatest to penicillin, complete inhibition being obtained in vitro by concentrations of less than 0.05 μgm per ml. The serologic type is unimportant. There is as yet no evidence that the strains of pneumococci now being isolated from the human population are any less sensitive to penicillin than those prevalent 10 years ago.

TYPING. Typing of pneumococci is no longer necessary for the treatment of pneumonia, since antipneumococcic serum therapy is no longer given except in rare situations. (In fact, specific antipneumococcic serums even for typing purposes are now almost unavailable for purchase.) The therapeutic effectiveness of sulfonamides and antibiotics is independent of the precise numerical type. For epidemiologic reasons it may be advisable when possible to secure a sample of nasopharyngeal mucus for typing and culture when a child with pneumonia is first seen, prior to the initial dose of antimicrobial therapy. If sulfonamides were administered prior to this, adding para-aminobenzoic acid to the culture medium may aid in recovery of the organism.

PROTEUS INFECTIONS

The Proteus organisms are pleomorphic Gram-negative bacilli which are highly motile, do not ferment lactose, and spread rapidly over solid media. They are normal inhabitants of sewage, manure, and human feces. They show overlapping antigenically with some of the rickettsiae. On the basis of biochemical reactions the members of this group have been subdivided by Rustigian and Stuart into four subgroups—*Pr. vulgaris, Pr. mirabilis, Pr. morganii,* and *Pr. rettgeri.* Kauffmann has suggested that *Pr. vulgaris* and *Pr. mirabilis* be considered together under the designation of *Pr. hauseri* because of the close serologic similarity.

Any Proteus strain may produce gastroenteritis, meningitis, arthritis, peritonitis, pyelonephritis, bacteremia, or wound or other infections. They frequently are secondary invaders at sites of tissue injury and are especially likely to attack premature or debilitated infants. Their growth and pathogenicity in a patient appears to be favored by the giving of antibiotics to suppress other more pathogenic bacteria.

Proteus strains recovered from patients exhibit wide differences in susceptibility to the different antibiotics. They usually show partial rather than total inhibition when exposed to antibiotics in the concentrations usually attained with standard therapeutic dosages. They are able to become refractory quickly to those agents. Streptomycin is perhaps the most potent effective agent, but polymyxin B, penicillin, sulfonamides, or the broad-spectrum agents may be effective with certain strains.

Combinations of several antimicrobial drugs in high dosage, selected by in vitro sensitivity tests, is important in the therapy of Proteus infections.

PSEUDOMONAS AERUGINOSA INFECTIONS

The 30-odd members of the Pseudomonas family are Gram-negative nonencapsulated motile bacilli which occur widely in soil, water, and sewage. They have distinctive chemical reactions and tend to produce water-soluble pigments. *Ps. aeruginosa,* the only important species pathogenic for men, elaborates two pigments—pyocyanin which is bluish green and fluorescin which is greenish yellow. This organism is a common inhabitant of the stools and skin of normal individuals. In children it will occasionally give rise to infections in the meninges, joints, conjunctiva, skin, middle or outer ear, gastrointestinal tract, respiratory tract, skin wounds, or other areas. These infections are sometimes primary, but more often the organism seems to take over as a secondary invader. There is epidemiologic evidence that it can sometimes play a causative role in infantile diarrhea, both in sporadic cases and institutional outbreaks.

With primary infections of the skin or intestine the initial lesions are small ecchymotic areas which rapidly necrose and ulcerate and expand peripherally. Blood cultures in the early stages of these infections are usually positive despite absence of fever. Metastatic abscesses are not uncommon. The development of pathogenicity seems to be favored by prematurity, infancy, debility, tissue injury, or antibiotic inhibition of normal bacterial flora.

Antibiotic sensitivities are inconstant. Most strains, if not already resistant to the currently available antibiotics, develop resistance rapidly on exposure to these. It ordinarily requires only a few culture transfers in vitro to render a strain insensitive to very high concentrations of any of the antibiotics, except perhaps polymyxin B. Strains have been encountered which are not only resistant to high concentrations of streptomycin, but actually need these concentrations of streptomycin in the environment in order to proliferate. Obviously the therapeutic administration of streptomycin to patients infected with such strains will only aggravate their illness.

. Laboratory and clinical experiences have demonstrated the value of following the chemotherapy of Pseudomonas infections by repeated in vitro sensitivity studies. Combined therapy with three antimicrobial agents is said to be sometimes more effective when the organism thrives in the presence of any one or two in combination.

Because of their high adaptability, *Ps. aeruginosa* and other occasional Pseudomonas strains proliferate in stools or injured tissues whenever antibacterial agents have repressed other organisms and may assume enhanced virulence under these conditions. This is often seen when children with cystic fibrosis of the pancreas or congenital urinary tract malformations are given prophylactic antibiotic therapy. For this reason, prophylaxis against bacterial infections in circumstances where secondary growth of Pseudomonas may occur should consist either of administering one antibiotic intermittently or changing frequently from one antibiotic to another.

Serologic tests are not needed for diagnosis, since the organisms grow so readily on all standard media. After recovery from a severe *Ps. aeruginosa* infection some patients will exhibit agglutination titers as high as 1:1,000 against the responsible strain. Typing antisera can be prepared for epidemiologic studies by injection of rabbits with organisms recovered from epidemic situations.

RAT-BITE FEVERS

These may follow the bite of a rat or of some other animal rarely. Local inflammation at the site of the bite is followed by lymphangitis, fever, arthritis, macular skin eruptions, and symptoms referable to the central nervous system or respiratory or intestinal tracts. The constitutional phenomena may recur sporadically for months after the local wound has healed. Either of two biologically unrelated pathogenic organisms, *Streptobacillus moniliformis* or *Spirillum minus,* may be the causative agent. The streptobacillus is more prone to give rise to a shorter illness with arthritis and rashes, whereas the spirillum tends to have a longer incubation period, a relapsing course, regional lymphadenitis, and an indurated lesion at the bite. Penicillin and the broad-spectrum antibiotics are helpful in therapy.

Haverhill Fever

This name is sometimes applied to the form of rat-bite fever caused by *Streptobacillus moniliformis* (*Streptothrix muris ratti, Asterococcus muris, Actinomyces muris*), which is a pleomorphic Gram-negative chainlike bacillus. A milk-borne epidemic caused by this bacillus has been described. The organism is often recoverable by direct culture of suspected material or its injection into mice or embryonated eggs.

A specific streptobacillary antigen is available for serum tests. Agglutinins in titer of 1:80 or higher, which may be adjusted as diagnostic, become demonstrable in 1 to 3 months after onset of the illness, and persist for months or years. A positive intradermal reaction will be found during convalescence when the skin is injected with an antigen prepared from the organism.

Spirillum Fever (Sodoku)

This very similar infection is caused by the spiral Gram-negative flagellated *Spirillum minus* (*Spirillum morsus muris, Spirocheta morsus muris*). Its presence may be demonstrated by inoculation of hamsters, guinea pigs, or white mice with the patient's blood or extracts of biopsied lesions. Darkfield study of the plasma of patients or inoculated animals after they become ill may show the spirilla in the blood and local lesions. They may also be demonstrated by this method within the exudate from the primary lesion or secondary exanthematous patches.

The flocculation tests for syphilis, but not the complement-fixation test, are often positive with *Spirillum minus* infections, but only exceptionally with *Streptobacillus moniliformis* infections.

STAPHYLOCOCCIC INFECTIONS

Classification of Staphylococci

The staphylococci are now classified as a group within the genus Micrococcus, with the following recognized species: *Micrococcus pyogenes* var. *aureus* (*Staphylococcus aureus*), *M. pyogenes* var. *albus* (*S. albus*), *M. citreus, M. aurantiacus* (*S. aurantiacus*), and *M. epidermidis* (*S. epidermidis*). All grow well at 37°C on most bacteriologic media, and nearly all strains are aerobic. Most of the staphylococci recovered from human lesions belong to the *S. aureus* species, though *S. albus* and rarely *S. citreus* and other species have at times been recovered from mild infections. Subclassification of *M. pyogenes* by serologic and related methods is as yet clinically impractical, though several avenues of progress in this direction are opening up.

Most strains elaborate one or another of two intracellular polysaccharides distinguishable by precipitin tests. Those which fall into the so-called group A of Julianelle and Weighard are usually pathogenic, those in group B are usually benign and saprophytic. The pathogenic strains on the whole produce pigment more abundantly, liquefy gelatin more quickly, and are more likely to ferment mannitol. Studies with immune sera indicate that the pathogenic strains are agglutinated by such sera, whereas the nonpathogenic strains are not. More refined analysis with technics of agglutinin absorption have established the occurrence of at least nine serologic subgroups among the pathogenic varieties.

Pathogenic strains will often produce a plasma-clotting enzyme known as coagulase, a necrotizing soluble exotoxin, four separate hemolysins, a leukocyte-destroying enzyme known as leukocidin, a fibrinolysin, a "spreading" factor similar to hyaluronidase, or a heat-stable enterotoxin. These toxins and enzymes may be elaborated in individually varying amounts by different strains of pathogenic staphylococci and contribute to the tissue-invading properties.

Since coagulase, with occasional exceptions, is produced only by disease-producing strains of human or animal origin, testing for this substance is included routinely in the standard bacteriologic study of staphylococci in clinical laboratories. The test consists of incubating a small amount of fresh citrated or oxalated plasma from rabbits or humans with a small amount of the culture at 37°C. Clotting is usually evident in 3 hours with pathogenic strains, though it may not occur until 24 hours. The rapidity and intensity of the reaction have no direct relation to the severity of symptoms in the patient.

Phage Typing

By studies with specific staphylococcic bacteriophages it is feasible to identify the majority of strains of coagulase-positive staphylococci by their lytic susceptibility to specific staphylococcic bacteriophages. The Staphylococcus Reference Laboratory of the British Public Health Laboratory Service currently employs a basic set of about 21 of these phages, which are segregated in three groups—groups I, II, and III. Staphylococcic strains which are lysed by other known phages may be placed in group IV. The phages have been divided also into the serologic groups A, B, F, and L according to their responses in serum neutralization tests.

Individual strains of staphylococci are denoted by the "patterns" of phages which lyse them strongly. For example, one may be known as 6/53/77; another as 6/7/47/53/54/75+ (the appending of the + sign indicates that the strain was lysed weakly by additional phages).

The bacteriophage approach is the best for tracing the origin of staphylococcic infections. For example, in an outbreak of food poisoning, a suspected foodstuff may be incriminated by showing that the staphylococci isolated from it are identical in phage type with those obtained from the feces or vomitus of patients. Most staphylococci which produce outbreaks of enterotoxin food poisoning or acute enterocolitis following antibiotic therapy seem to belong to the broad group III. Phage typing has also been of assistance in the detecting of carriers and in the tracing of routes of spread during epidemics. Most strains of staphylococci from acute cases of impetigo contagiosa seem to be lysed solely by phage 71.

Antibiotic Sensitivities

Most strains of *M. pyogenes* when first recovered from nonhospitalized patients prove to be sensitive to therapeutic concentrations of many of the common antibiotics or sulfonamides, at least to a moderate extent. Once therapy has been begun, however, specifically resistant organisms tend to emerge within a few days. One biochemical property possessed by most penicillin-resistant strains is the capacity to elaborate penicillinase in comparative abundance.

Because resistant strains appear so frequently, it is wise to administer whatever chemotherapeutic agent is being employed in high dosages from the beginning, in order quickly to attain high serum concentrations.

The antibiotic susceptibility pattern should be ascertained by vitro studies with all serious staphylococcic illnesses. A combination of two or more antibiotics will occasionally be more potent in preventing bacterial growth than will a single agent.

Within institutions which consistently use one antibiotic in therapy, the staphylococci recovered from patients usually prove insusceptible to that antibiotic. This is true even with patients not receiving such therapy. The majority of such strains which prove resistant to penicillin and the broad-spectrum antibiotics are usually found to belong in phage group III. However, strains resistant to one or more antibiotics may be found in all phage groups.

This phenomenon of the high incidence of similar phage patterns among "hospital staphylococci" suggests that one or a few related strains are progenitors and are responsible for cross-infectional spread from patient to patient or from carriers of antibiotic-resistant staphylococci among the hospital personnel. Resistant strains are maintained not only in the purulent discharges of patients, but also in the nasal passages, throats, feces, and skin of carriers. In the populace at large, a similar but lesser increase in the prevalence of antibiotic-resistant staphylococci is believed by some to be taking place, though this has been disputed.

Patients who are receiving an antimicrobial agent orally for some other clinical reason often excrete staphylococci resistant to that agent in their stools. Should any of these strains be producers of staphylococcic enterotoxin, a diarrhea may ensue which in part at least may be a response to this toxin. The development of such a staphylococcic or micrococcic "enteritis" can be minimized if the antimicrobial substance is prescribed in the lowest effective dose. When such a staphylococcic diarrhea occurs, it can usually be eliminated by a change in the therapeutic agent.

Human Infections

Staphylococci can cause disease in any part of the body. Pneumonia, empyema, pericarditis, osteomyelitis, arthritis, otitis media, meningitis, impetigo, focal abscesses, or wound suppuration may all result from staphylococcic invasion. Fever, malaise, leukocytosis, gastroenteritis, and anemia may all be produced, of intensity which depends to some extent on the enzyme- and toxin-producing properties of the infective strain. Underlying debilitating conditions favor the progress of such infections.

Septicemia is a frequent concomitant of most severe inflammatory lesions. This may be perpetuated by a local thrombophlebitis of veins in the area. The therapeutic administration of staphylococcic antitoxin may alleviate some of the constitutional signs of intoxication but will not hamper the invasive spread of the organisms.

In nurseries for newborns a virulent strain can give rise to epidemics of pustular skin eruptions. These in turn may lead to subcutaneous abscesses, conjunctivitis, pneumonia, lung or breast abscesses, or other troublesome or even fatal complications.

There are indications that injections of vaccines made from autogenous cultures of chemically killed pathogenic staphylococci may be of assistance in treating stubborn chronic staphylococcic infections.

Laboratory Diagnosis

There can be little doubt of the diagnosis if staphylococci are recovered from the blood stream or local lesions or from internal suppurative foci at necropsy. When the area is inaccessible during life a heavy growth of staphylococci from the nasopharynx or sputum is presumptive evidence. Otherwise the diagnosis must depend on clinical criteria. Positive skin reactions to staphylococcic filtrates are given by a majority of all individuals over 1 year of age. Serum antibody levels may or may not be elevated during or after an active infection.

Staphylococcic pigment is best demonstrable if the organisms recovered from blood, pus, or body discharges are grown under aerobic conditions on solid media which contain a carbohydrate such as glucose, lactose, or mannitol. The exhibition of hemolysis is of interest, but its absence does not rule out pathogenicity. The coagulase test is of much more significance in this respect. Penicillinase should be incorporated in the culture medium if the patient is receiving penicillin, or para-aminobenzoic acid if a sulfonamide is being given. When staphylococcic food poisoning is suspected the enterotoxin can be demonstrated by injecting filtrates of cultures into kittens or monkeys.

Staphylococci exposed to sublethal doses of antibiotics can undergo misleading alterations in appearance. In cultures taken from a patient soon after the beginning of treatment the cell bodies may show distortions, swellings, and unevenness or loss of Gram-staining quality.

Pseudomembranous Enterocolitis

This a shocklike syndrome associated with diarrhea, which may suddenly complicate acute gastroenteritis or follow major surgery of the gastrointestinal tract. Its development seems to follow the giving of oral antimicrobial agents which inhibit the normal intestinal flora and permit an overgrowth of antibiotic-resistant staphylococci. Direct staining of the fecal discharges in suspected cases often reveals great numbers of Gram-positive cocci, and confirmation of their proliferation is given by stool cultures made on blood agar or other media which favor their growth. If the condition is recognized, therapy should be in the form of some other antimicrobial agent to which the staphylococci are found susceptible.

Antibiotic-resistant strains of Pseudomonas and other intestinal organisms have been suspected at times of being responsible for this syndrome.

STREPTOCOCCIC INFECTIONS

Classification

Streptococci are widely distributed in nature. Homer Swift has classified the species which are of clinical importance under four chief divisions on the basis of their metabolic behavior and biologic and cultural characteristics.

The so-called *hemolytic* division contains the human strains which are mainly hemolytic on blood agar and tend to produce soluble hemolysins in serum broth; this production of clear zones about colonies is known as *beta hemolysis*. The organisms in this division also elaborate group-specific polysaccharides or *C antigens*. They are subdividable into 11 main serologic groups: A, B, C, E, F, G, H, K, L, M, and O. The majority of pathogenic strains belong to group A.

The members of the *viridans* division can convert hemoglobin to a brown or green derivative (*alpha hemolysis*) and resemble pneumococci in many ways.

The members of the *enterococcus* division are typically found in the gastrointestinal tract and can grow at temperatures and salt concentrations lethal for most other streptococci (p. 770). They elaborate the group-specific D carbohydrate and are nonhemolytic.

The members of the *Streptococcus lactis* or milk-souring division can coagulate milk, are nonhemolytic, and elaborate the group-specific N carbohydrate. Though highly important to dairy bacteriology these are only rarely found in man.

Group A Streptococci

Group A streptococci are frequent inhabitants of the respiratory tract of man and can produce septicemia or inflammatory invasion in any part of the body. They are known also as *Str. hemolyticus, Str. pyogenes,* and *Str. epidemicus.* The variant forms which produce scarlet fever are sometimes called *Str. scarlatinae.* They have their optimal growth at 37°C, exhibit a clear zone of beta hemolysis on blood agar plates, and are nonsoluble in bile. Capsules can usually be demonstrated by special techniques. They contain, or produce during growth, a considerable variety of antigens, toxins, and enzymes. Important constituents are the type-specific M proteins and the related T substances, also proteins. Some strains elaborate both the M and the T components, others only one. Often produced also are nucleoproteins or P substances, erythrogenic toxins, streptokinase (fibrinolysin), streptococcic desoxyribonuclease (streptodornase), hemolysins (streptolysins O and S), proteinase, hyaluronic acid, and hyaluronidase. Infected individuals tend to develop specific antibodies against most of these substances. Immunologic methods have been devised for the quantitative estimation of antibodies against the C substances, M and T proteins, nucleoproteins, fibrinolysin, hemolysin, and hyaluronidase. Most pathogenic strains are susceptible to penicillin in minimal concentrations of 0.03 units per ml and do not acquire resistance on continued exposure to sublethal concentrations.

SUBTYPING. Griffith's serologic method has differentiated over 40 component types within group A, designated by number. Recognition of these group A types is based essentially on the behavior with type-specific anti-M serums as studied by agglutination, precipitation, bacteriostatic, or mouse protection tests.

Clinical experience usually fails to show any relation between the Griffith types of the group A hemolytic streptococci and their disease-producing capacities. Outbreaks of scarlet fever or other streptococcic infections can be due to almost any type. Infections with types 12 or 4 are unusually likely to be followed by acute glomerulonephritis.

Type identification can be useful in tracking down the source and manner of spread of institutional epidemics. In such epidemics most of the patients will be found to be infected with the same strain of streptococci, which also will be recoverable from the throats of a high percentage of apparently uninfected carrier contact. During interepidemic and endemic periods the types prevalent in the population are diverse and unrelated.

ERYTHROGENIC TOXINS. These are soluble products which when injected intracutaneously in at least 100-fold dilution will give rise to an area of erythema in nonimmune individuals. If the red area has a diameter of more than 10 mm in 6 to 24 hours after injection, the individual is said to have a positive Dick reaction. Cross-neutralization tests with specific antitoxic serums indicate the existence of at least five of these erythrogenic toxins. The production of such toxins by different strains of group A streptococci is inconstant and highly variable.

Individuals susceptible to any of these toxins, when infected with a streptococcic strain which is a rich producer, exhibit the clinical phenomena which collectively comprise what is known as scarlet fever. Repeated attacks of scarlet fever are ascribed to infections with other streptococcic strains which produce erythrogenic toxins different from the one or ones in the antecedent attacks. Following illnesses of this sort, or a series of injections with a pool of erythrogenic toxins, the immunized individual will no longer exhibit the peculiar constitutional responses of scarlet fever when infected with organisms which produce the same toxins. This immunity is essentially antitoxic only; no protection is conferred against further infections with group A streptococci.

STREPTOKINASE (FIBRINOLYSIN). This is an extracellular activator enzyme produced by the growth of various groups of hemolytic streptococci and especially those of group C. Streptokinase activates the fibrinolytic proenzyme in the euglobulin fraction of human plasma designated as plasminogen. The capacity of a pathogenic streptococcic strain to form streptokinase in vitro seems to bear no direct relation to any clinical feature of the illness or its complications.

Antistreptokinase (Antifibrinolysin). Infection with a streptokinase-producing streptococcus is typically accompanied by the development in the serum of the patient of a specific antagonistic substance, antistreptokinase, able to inhibit the activation of the conversion of plasma fibrinolysin. Laboratory measurement of antistreptokinase (antifibrinolysin) activity is based upon the time required for a plasma clot from the individual under study to resist lysis by a broth culture of a standard strain of streptococci.

Inasmuch as many pathogenic strains of group A streptococci do not produce much streptokinase, the absence of a rise in this antibody does not exclude the possibility of a recent streptococcic infection. Since the techniques of measurement have not been universally agreed upon, each laboratory which performs this and related streptococcic tests usually includes in the report a statement as to the normal limits of variation with the method employed.

The other important antistreptococcic antibody, antihyaluronidase, gives more consistent results in laboratory approaches to recognition of rheumatic fever (p. 828).

Streptococcic Desoxyribonuclease (Streptodornase)

One or more pus-liquefying enzymes, known collectively as streptococcic desoxyribonuclease or streptodornase, are produced by nearly all group A strains and most of those in group B. A similar desoxyribonuclease may also be produced by pneumococci and some other bacteria. These enzymes act directly on extracellular desoxyribonucleoprotein and desoxyribonucleic acid, which are important constituents of cell nuclei and make up 30 to 70 per cent of the sediment in thick purulent exudates.

Streptodornase is antigenic. A specific antistreptodornase develops in significant amounts in 50 per cent of patients with streptococcic infections, with titers which rarely rise above 300 units per ml by the standard methods of measurement. Injections of commercial preparations of streptodornase are nearly always followed by rises in titer to between 1,000 and 32,000 units.

A mixture of streptokinase and streptodornase has been accepted for therapeutic purposes by the Council on Pharmacy and Chemistry of the American Medical Association. This mixture, in addition to proteolytic and fibrinolytic activity, stimulates a local outpouring of both fluid and phagocytes at the site of application.

Hyaluronidase and Antihyaluronidase

A hyaluronic acid-splitting enzyme is produced by many group A streptococci, as indicated by the eventual finding of antihyaluronidase in the blood stream of most infected individuals. It has not been possible to correlate the intensity of hyaluronidase production in cultures with the pathogenicity of infecting strains in disease states.

After acute streptococcic infections the capacity to neutralize streptococcic hyaluronidase rises to a peak in the third week or sometimes later. Antihyaluronidase antibodies can be found in most infants in the first few months of life, presumably as the result of passive transfer from their mothers. These fade away in later infancy. They begin to reappear at about 3 to 5 years of age, but are not widely prevalent in the population until adulthood is reached. Exceptionally high readings are encountered in acute rheumatic fever, whereas in quiescent rheumatic fever the findings are comparable to those of normal children.

The range of titers for antihyaluronidase antibodies overlaps that of rises in nonrheumatic children after acute streptococcic infections (p. 828).

A so-called nonspecific hyaluronidase inhibitor has also been demonstrated. The concentration of this inhibitor can be estimated by observing the inhibitory effect of a subject's serum upon a lytic system consisting of hyaluronidase from bovine testicles and a hyaluronic acid substrate prepared from human umbilical cords. Good and Glick reported that serums from patients with convalescent or inactive rheumatic fever have a subnormal content of this inhibitor.

Hemolysins

Most group A streptococci liberate one or another or both of two separable red cell–disrupting enzymes known respectively as streptolysins S and O. Streptolysin O is elaborated also by other hemolytic streptococci, whereas S has been found only in those of group A. Still other unrelated hemolysins may be produced by organisms from any of the other fundamental divisions of streptococci.

Since blood from horses often contains considerable antistreptolysin O, whereas that from rabbits does not, the latter is preferred for blood agar studies of hemolytic streptococci, particularly when deeply planted colonies are being cultured.

Streptolysin S does not act as an antigen. The antistreptolysin S titer in convalescent patients rarely goes above 30 units and is usually less than 20 units.

Antistreptolysin O Titers

Streptolysin O acts as a specific antigen which can lead to the production of an antistreptolysin O antibody in man or animals following infection with streptolysin O–producing strains of streptococci. This antibody is stable and quantitatively measurable. Satisfactory tests can be carried out with sera which have been stored aseptically at 3°C for several years. Of patients convalescent from streptococcic infections, 75 to 90 per cent display a demonstrable rise in antistreptolysin O in their serum. This appears in gradually increasing titer to reach a peak at about 4 weeks and may persist for many months. In infants and young children the response may be feeble or pronounced but of short duration.

The antistreptolysin titers of normal subjects vary with their ages and the geographic areas of residence. Population surveys have shown that mean antibody levels are lowest in the Southwest and Southeast and highest in the Middle West and Far West regions of the United States. The normal range of variation is so wide, however, that single determinations must be interpreted with caution in studies of the etiology of human disease.

Newborn infants usually possess this antibody in titers reasonably close to those of their mothers. The levels practically disappear in the first few months, remain negligible during infancy, and rise gradually after the second year of life. The average titer in Northern children 10 to 15 years of age is about 1:200 units, with 15 to 25 per cent giving negative readings. After adolescence the levels tend to decline, so that the titers for young adults average about 1:100 units. These measurable quantities reflect the ubiquitous prevalence of streptococcic infections within the population.

It is probably of importance that the antistreptolysin responses tend to be proportional to the severity and duration of the streptococcic infections. Titers are much higher when there are late nonsuppurative complications of streptococcic disease than when recovery has been prompt and uneventful.

Children in whom group A streptococcic infection is followed by rheumatic fever tend to produce exceptional amounts of various antistreptococcic antibodies and to maintain these levels for prolonged periods of time. Their antistreptolysin readings tend to be as high as 1:2,500 at the peak and to maintain levels of 1:200 or higher for as long as a half year thereafter, in 85 to 90 per cent of the patients.

Streptococcic Diseases (Streptococcosis)

The reaction patterns of the human being to streptococcic infections change characteristically with increasing age. In infants under 6 months of age the typical group A streptococcic infection may either be asymptomatic or appear as a brief mild illness with mild pharyngeal injection, irregular fever, and thin nasal discharge. In older infants and children up to about 4 years of age the illness is more likely to be prolonged and to last several weeks. Suppurative lesions such as otitis media, cervical adenitis, and infections of the skin occur in untreated cases with fair frequency.

In older children and young adults the typical streptococcic infection tends to consist of an acute inflammatory reaction in the throat and upper respiratory passages. In fact, more than half the instances of acute tonsillitis, pharyngitis, or laryngitis in later childhood are caused by group A streptococci. The illness typically has an abrupt febrile onset and a short stormy course. Suppurative complications which may occur include sinusitis, otitis media, lymphadenitis, appendicitis, pneumonia, peritonitis, osteomyelitis, vaginitis, or meningitis. A short-lived immunity, lasting a few weeks or months, usually follows an acute streptococcic illness which has been permitted to run its course without early chemotherapy.

In all streptococcic infections the peripheral leukocyte count tends to rise to between 12,000 to 20,000, because of an increase in neutrophils. This is helpful in making the differentiation from the common cold and other respiratory tract infections due to viruses, since in the latter the leukocyte count tends to remain within normal limits and the neutrophils may be depressed.

Throat and nose cultures from patients with streptococcic infections generally show an abundance of these organisms, whereas cultures from normal children show only small numbers if any. As a general rule, the organisms recovered from the nasopharynx and from other infected sites will all be of the same subtype.

Streptococci are expelled in large numbers in droplets and droplet nuclei when a carrier or patient with an infection in the throat or especially in the nasal passages coughs, sneezes, talks, or exhales rapidly. Infected handerchiefs and bedding are other routes of transmission. Infants and children with infected skin lesions can be the source of widespread secondary illnesses in hospital wards. All patients with acute streptococcic infections should be kept in isolation, and their disease treated with vigor as quickly as possible.

With patients receiving cortisone or corticotropin, acute infections due to streptococci or other bacteria may advance with unusual rapidity at the same time that the constitutional signs of intoxication in the patient may be depressed. Evidence from experimental pathology indicates that these hormones depress the cellular and other inflammatory reactions of the body but do not enhance bacterial growth per se.

As mentioned, some of the streptococcic antibodies—antistreptolysin O, antihyaluronidase, antistreptokinase, antidornase—will usually rise in the serum following a streptococcic infection. These responses are not of much diagnostic assistance at the time of onset or at the height of the illness, and the performance of the tests is too complicated for use in routine laboratories. Formation of these antibodies may be suppressed partially or even completely if adequate chemotherapy has been given.

Antibiotic Therapy

Penicillin has proved highly effective as therapy. Erythromycin and the broad-spectrum antibiotics are also satisfactory for preventing or treating suppurative complications though they are perhaps slower in overcoming the initial symptoms. Full therapeutic dosages of these substances are best continued for 7 to 10 days, else the infection may recur or sequelae such as rheumatic fever develop. The sulfonamides on the whole are less effective against streptococci; their use is advised only when allergic sensitivity or some other difficulty interferes with the use of penicillin or other antibiotic. One difficulty which attends the institution of prompt therapy of this sort is that the individual may be left with little or no natural immunity, so that a fresh streptococcic infection may begin immediately after recovery.

Streptococci and Scarlet Fever

Scarlet fever is no longer viewed as a specific infection, but rather as a disease syndrome that can be caused by any strain of group A streptococci which produces a potent erythrogenic toxin. The attack may be interpreted analytically as a double reaction—an acute local infection with a tendency toward septic complications by a highly invasive streptococcus, along with an acute constitutional toxemia induced by the erythrogenic toxin of the invader. The rash is an indicator of the individual's susceptibility to this toxin. During every epidemic of scarlet fever one will find many individuals in the population with a streptococcic throat infection caused by the same erythrogenic strain, but with no associated rash. Individual insusceptibility or immunity to the toxin appears to be the deciding factor.

In untreated scarlet fever, the phenomena caused by the toxin, even when extremely severe, are usually over within a few days. These phenomena are not inhibited by chemotherapy, but can be abruptly terminated as a rule by specific antitoxic therapeutic serum, whether of human or animal origin. Penicillin or related antibiotics are needed for prompt control of the infection itself.

The majority of untreated patients with scarlet fever and other streptococcic infections will continue to exhibit positive throat or nose cultures for group A streptococci for at least 1 month after the onset of the illness, and often for several months. The therapeutic administration of penicillin for 10 days to 2 weeks will as a rule eradicate these organisms.

Streptococci and Rheumatic Fever

An infection with group A streptococci typically precedes by a few weeks the first attack or active recurrence of rheumatic fever. A flare-up of the disease in a patient subacutely ill may be induced by streptococci of a different serologic type.

During acute flare-ups most patients exhibit unusually high serum levels of one or more of the antistreptococcic antibodies, especially antistreptolysin and antihyaluronidase. In interpreting such serologic data one must always bear in mind that positive reactions mean fundamentally that the individual had a streptococcic infection within the preceding half year. They are not pathognomonic or specific for rheumatic fever. According to Harris, when the antistreptolysin titer is within normal limits there is only one chance in seven that a patient under study has rheumatic fever. In nearly half the patients with rheumatic fever the antihyaluronidase titers exceed those seen after streptococcic infections without this sequel. The level or changes in titers are not proportional to the activity of the rheumatic fever.

Rises in antistreptolysin and antihyaluronidase are seen occasionally in patients with rheumatoid arthritis and even more often in acute glomerulonephritis, but the frequency and the maxima of the titers are less than in acute rheumatic fever. After scarlet fever the changes are the same as after other uncomplicated streptococcic infections.

Since individuals in apparent good health may have high titers for any of these various antibodies, especially if they have had a streptococcic infection in the preceding half year, and since not all patients with rheumatic fever have titers above the wide normal range, the results of the determinations are of diagnostic value only when negligibly low or excessively high. Even then they must be viewed as presumptive rather than as specific adjuncts to diagnosis.

OTHER LABORATORY FINDINGS. In chronically affected cases the changes in red cell sedimentation rate usually run parallel with the activity of the rheumatic fever symptoms. An exception to this rule occurs in the presence of cardiac failure resulting from rheumatic myocarditis, in which the rate may transitorily appear as normal. This may lead the uninformed to believe that a patient's condition is improving rather than actively growing worse. In chorea uncomplicated by carditis the sedimentation rate is usually normal. In early acute rheumatic carditis the sedimentation rate is more often normal than rapid.

In addition to elevations in specific antistreptococcic antibodies, the gamma globulin content of the plasma often goes up. This may be an expression of a general increase in antibody formation. The plasma mucoproteins also tend to be elevated (p. 542).

The red cell and hemoglobin levels typically undergo a normochromic depression in chronic cases; they are within normal limits in more than half the acute cases. The leukocyte and differential white cell count tend to remain unaltered except perhaps for the appearance of some leukocytes with toxic granules and of relatively more band forms. The urine in a minority of patients exhibits mild proteinuria or microscopic hematuria. The vital capacity falls only when cardiac decompensation develops; a rise in this measurement may be the first sign of improvement when a patient has severe heart failure. Other laboratory studies such as blood cultures are of value chiefly for the exclusion of complications or other diseases. Histologic study of excised subcutaneous nodules can be of value in confirming the existence of rheumatic fever.

PREVENTION OF RHEUMATIC FEVER. Prompt recognition of streptococcic respiratory infections and their adequate treatment with penicillin or other antistreptococcic antibiotics is a major approach to the prevention of rheumatic fever. In such suspected infections it is best to procure a throat culture before starting the antibiotic program. If the throat culture indicates that streptococci are absent, the therapy may be discontinued after 48 hours; otherwise, or if no culture is made, it should be maintained for 10 days.

Sulfonamides given continuously to population groups have been demonstrated to prevent streptococcic infections and rheumatic fever. However, treatment of an established streptococcic infection with a sulfonamide may not prevent a complicating attack of rheumatic fever, whereas penicillin will. The reason for this difference seems to be that sulfonamides are bacteriostatic for group A hemolytic streptococci, whereas penicillin is bactericidal. Furthermore, sulfonamides may influence adversely the activity of rheumatic fever when already established.

All patients hospitalized for rheumatic fever must be guarded against contact with other patients having illnesses which may be associated with streptococci, such as scarlet fever, erysipelas, acute glomerulonephritis, acute tonsillitis, or even mild upper respiratory infections. They must also not be exposed to employees or visitors or other patients who may be carriers of group A streptococci. Dust or lint from bedding, hand-kerchiefs, and clothing in the immediate environment of a person who is expelling streptococci from his mouth or nose are potential sources of in-fection, as are also uncleaned dishes, glassware, cutlery, and related utensils.

It is advisable that prophylactic treatment with penicillin or other anti-biotic be continued after the initial program of therapy, or initiated whenever a patient is first seen without active symptoms. The prophy-laxis should be continued through all seasons of the year until at least to the age of 18 years, and in older subjects for at least 5 years from the last attack.

Hemolytic Streptococci Other Than Group A

It has already been mentioned that nearly all streptococcic infections are caused by hemolytic streptococci belonging to some serotype of group A. Streptococci of groups B, C, F, E, G, H, K, L, M, or O are re-covered occasionally from the nose and throat of presumedly healthy in-dividuals and less frequently from patients with infections. Of these, members of groups C, G, and O are the most common producers of human disease. Streptococci of bovine mastitis (*Str. agalactiae,* group B), though widely distributed and found often in raw milk, are probably of little public-health importance to man. They are sometimes encountered as saprophytes in the human throat and vagina. Anaerobic streptococci (e.g., *Str. foetidus, Str. anaerobius, Str. putridus*) appear to play a role in the production of putrefactive wounds and other infections associated with gangrene.

Viridans Streptococci

The members of this division are so designated because a green or brown pigment is formed about colonies on blood agar and in the depths of blood broth cultures (alpha hemolysis). Low-power magnification re-veals intact red cells within a zone of partial hemolysis and discoloration about each colony, especially those deep in the agar. The green or brown discoloration sometimes does not develop in the first 24 hours of incuba-tion. There are wide differences in the degree and amount of the color change produced.

Attempts to subdivide these streptococci into serologic subgroups have not been wholly successful. Nine different varieties have been recognized by Swift. The variety known as *Streptococcus MG,* sometimes found in human mouths, is believed to have a symbiotic role in patients with primary atypical penumonia. *Str. SBE* (*sanguis*) appears to be one of the more common causes of subacute bacterial endocarditis. *Str. salivarius,* a frequent inhabitant of the mouth, nose, and intestine, has also been associated with subacute bacterial endocarditis. The other named varieties are known as *mitis, bovis, equinus, thermophilus, acidominimis,* and *uberis.*

The viridans streptococci differ widely among themselves in their susceptibility to the individual antibiotics and sulfonamides. In vitro cultural studies for sensitivity are therefore essential for adequate therapy. For subacute bacterial endocarditis the dosages of the indicated agent or combination of agents should be as high as can be tolerated, since these organisms tend to be enveloped by a fibrinous layer difficult to penetrate.

Enterococci (Group D Streptococci)

These are widely distributed in the intestinal tract and vagina of humans and are not infrequent in cow's milk. They elaborate the group-specific D carbohydrate and possess distinctive cultural hardiness such as the ability to grow in the presence of 40 per cent bile or milk containing 0.1 per cent methylene blue. They are also able to grow at extremes of temperature (60°C for 30 minutes) and in salt concentrations of 6.5 per cent sodium chloride which inhibit or kill most other streptococci. Their hardiness is shown also in their relative or complete insensitivity to therapeutic dosages of sulfonamides and the antibiotics. Combined therapy with several agents is advisable in these infections.

The majority of recovered strains fall into a few well-defined groups named numerically on the basis of antigenic and serologic relationships. Individual species which have received names are *Str. fecalis, Str. higue-faciens, Str. zymogenes,* and *Str. durans.*

Enterococci are sometimes recovered from the urinary tract, the blood stream, or inflammatory exudates of man. They may cause subacute bacterial endocarditis. Some strains are believed to aggravate the intestinal lesions of chronic ulcerative colitis. Outbreaks of so-called food poisoning have been traced to contamination of cheese, meat, bologna, pie filling, canned evaporated milk, and other foods by nonhemolytic streptococci of the enterococcus group.

Streptococcus lactis (Group N Streptococci)

This division comprises *Str. lactis* and *Str. cremoris.* These strains occur in plants and in milk and cream; they are almost never pathogenic. Culturally they resemble the enterococci, but can be readily differentiated by their serologic agglutinability with group N antiserum.

TETANUS

The spores of the tetanus bacillus are ubiquitously distributed. They occur not only in soil and excreta of horses and other grazing animals but have been recovered from human feces in as many as 40 per cent of one series of reported cases. The risk of wound contamination is therefore much greater than the prevalence of cases in the nonimmunized population would indicate. Evidently the environment in most wounds is unfavorable to the multiplication of tetanus bacilli, or else many individuals have an acquired immunity from frequent exposure and subclinical infections. It is significant, nevertheless, that almost as many cases of tetanus occur as a sequel to trivial skin injuries, which may be so superficial as to escape notice, as follow severe burns or deep wounds containing imbedded soil or other foreign material.

Bacteriology

Clostridium tetani is a long slender nonmotile Gram-positive rod which tends to show round terminal spores in culture preparations. It grows anaerobically, forming spreading hemolytic colonies with irregular edges. Penicillin is the most effective of the currently available antimicrobial agents.

It is not possible to distinguish toxicogenic from nontoxicogenic and nonpathogenic species by morphology alone. This can be accomplished only by animal injections. A small inoculum of recovered culture or a bit of infected tissue is injected subcutaneously into the legs of mice or guinea pigs. In half of the animals the infected matter is first mixed with 1,000 units of tetanus antitoxin. If tetanus toxin is present, the animals not receiving the antitoxin will exhibit either local spasm of the extremity or generalized intoxication with rapidly developing prostration, convulsions, and death.

Wounds are usually investigated for tetanus organisms by direct culture of purulent exudate or of excised tissue macerated in sterile salt solution. These approaches succeed in yielding positive cultures in only a minority of patients with the actual disease. Conversely, recovery of tetanus-like organisms from a wound does not necessarily mean that the patient has tetanus, since these may be nontoxicogenic contaminating strains. A negative bacteriologic report in the presence of suspicious clinical findings should be ignored, and vigorous treatment instituted nevertheless.

True *Cl. tetani* will not grow within a wound unless oxygen is absent. The latter circumstance can be brought about by the coincident presence of necrotic tissue, foreign materials, or tetanus toxin itself. Once the organisms begin to proliferate they produce exotoxin, and this permits growth to continue. Spores will sometimes remain locally for months in a viable but dormant state, to be activated by a later superadded injury, perhaps only a blow.

Pathogenesis of Tetanus

Tetanus bacilli have little invasiveness. They produce disease by the elaboration and diffusion of their soluble exotoxin, known as tetanospasmin. Tetanospasmin is a neurotoxin which stimulates the neuromuscular end organs to sustained muscle spasm and the motor nerve cells of the spinal cord, medulla, and pons to convulsive seizures. The mode of spread along nerve trunks is still unsettled. Once united with tissue cells the toxin is no longer neutralizable by antitoxin in any amount.

In tetanus neonatorum the portal of entry is usually an infected umbilical stump, although contaminated circumcisions have also been incriminated. Umbilical infections are still unnecessarily prevalent, however, in rural areas or where the unhygienic custom of placing dung or soot on the umbilical stump are still practiced. The prognosis is more grave when the umbilicus is purulent grossly than when its appearance is normal.

Clinical Aspects

Tetanus in human beings is usually characterized by constitutional intoxication with recurrent generalized tonic spasms. Local spasm of the area around the primary site of infection is unusual, with the possible exception of involvement of the muscles about the lower face (*lockjaw*) in wounds of the head or neck. The incubation period is highly variable, and may be prolonged for many weeks. In general the shorter the incubation period the more grave the illness and the prognosis.

Therapy

Useful symptomatic measures include cleansing or even excision of the wound when practicable, complete rest with anticonvulsive sedation in a dark room, oxygen inhalation, gavage feedings, and parenteral fluids. Tracheotomy is sometimes necessary in the presence of laryngeal spasm or inability to swallow. The most important single factor is the constant attendance of a highly skilled nurse.

Penicillin is advisable in large and frequent dosage for probable in vivo effect on the *Cl. tetani* and to counteract secondary infection. Other antimicrobial agents are administered as indicated to control other associated microorganisms. Large quantities of antitoxin are also needed, even though the symptoms progress once the tetanus toxin has entered the nerve cells. It has been advised that patients be given tetanus toxoid injections during or subsequent to recovery in order to establish a full active immunity.

Laboratory Measurement of Immunity

Most individuals after a course of prophylactic injections of tetanus toxoid will maintain for several years an antitoxin level at or above 0.1 unit of antitoxin per ml of serum, as measured by the standard neutralization test using mice. With previously immunized individuals whose titer has fallen below the protective level, a "booster" injection of tetanus toxoid will usually evoke a satisfactory rise in titer within a matter of days. This serum concentration is thought to be the minimum for maintenance of immunity.

TUBERCULOSIS

Bacteriology

Mycobacterium tuberculosis is a hardy acid-fast aerobic bacillus 1 to 4 μ in length which grows slowly on proper media. Human, bovine, and avian varieties are recognized. The only other species of Mycobacterium pathogenic for man is *M. leprae,* the leprosy bacillus. Patients are sometimes encountered with active pulmonary lesions clinically indistinguishable from tuberculosis who persistently exhibit in the sputum a chromogenic acid-fast bacillus which differs culturally from *M. tuberculosis* and may or may not be pathogenic for guinea pigs. A murine type of tubercle bacillus, pathogenic for voles and mice, is *M. muris.* Many of the filamentous nocardiae are also acid-fast.

Among the nonpathogenic species which are sometimes found in situations where *M. tuberculosis* is being looked for are *M. smegma,* the smegma bacillus, *M. butyricum,* the butter bacillus, and *M. phlei,* the timothy bacillus. These and related saprophytic mycobacteria grow more rapidly on artificial media, usually produce more yellow-orange pigment, and tend to be less acid-fast. One cannot always, however, rely on cultural reactions for differentiating these various species from each other. Tubercle bacilli are the only ones which will produce disease in laboratory animals, except that *M. leprae* is pathogenic for the rat. Differences in pathogenicity for animals may be used for recognizing the three main varieties of tubercle bacilli.

	Human	Bovine	Avian
Guinea pig	+++	++++	+
Rabbit	+	+++	++
Susceptible mice	++	++	+
Chicken	0	0	+++

Nonvirulent strains of any of these give atypical responses with animal tests.

Human strains grow well on solid egg media or in the presence of glycerin and are called eugonic. Most bovine strains grow poorly on media containing egg or glycerin, and hence are called dysgonic. Avian organisms grow more readily on artificial media than either of the mammalian types. All varieties are killed by proper pasteurization when present in milk.

Nearly all human cases of tuberculosis in the United States are caused by the human type of organism, with the respiratory system being involved primarily. Tuberculosis caused by the bovine bacillus comes from the ingestion of unpasteurized milk from infected cows and is likely to be most prominent in the intestinal tract, bones, or joints. Human disease due to avian strains is rare if it occurs at all.

Tubercle bacilli contain lipids, which in some way are related to the property of acid fastness and the tendency of invaded tissues to form tubercles. They contain proteins which are responsible for the positive "tuberculin" skin reaction and constitutional symptoms in individuals who have or have had an infection caused by this organism. Polysaccharide fractions can also be isolated.

Most strains are susceptible both in vitro and in vivo to streptomycin, dihydrostreptomycin, aminosalicylic acid (PAS), and isoniazid and various derivatives. Neomycin inhibits growth of some strains, but its high toxicity and the pronounced tendency for the emergence of resistance have restricted its use in therapy.

Continued administration of any of these therapeutic agents for more than 3 months may result in disappearance of the organism from the local discharges or in emergence of a strain which is no longer susceptible. Administration of two of these in combination tends to delay the emergence of drug-resistant strains for a longer period and thereby appears to prolong the period in which therapy may be effective. There is not full agreement among clinicians, however, as to the significance to be attached to recovery of a drug-resistant strain of tubercle bacilli from a patient during treatment with that drug. Resistant strains are recovered occasionally from patients who never received a therapeutic agent previously.

Drug therapy alone is not sufficient for adequate treatment of tuberculosis. The administration must be coordinated with a broad program of medical and surgical treatment, preferably in a special hospital division. In cutaneous tuberculosis (lupus vulgaris) the addition of high dosage of vitamin D such as calciferol (vitamin D_2) has been found helpful.

BCG

Bacillus Calmette-Guérin is an attenuated strain of human tubercle bacilli which, when given to uninfected tuberculin-negative children, confers some degree of resistance against the naturally acquired disease. It is recommended chiefly for infants who are likely to be exposed to infection or who live in conditions which favor the spread of the disease. It should not be given to individuals who already have a tuberculous infection as indicated by a positive tuberculin reaction.

The BCG cultures used in the preparation of vaccines are propagated in laboratories which conduct no other bacteriologic procedures and where the personnel are checked periodically to be sure they remain free from tuberculosis. The vaccine should be given within 14 days of the last preceding negative tuberculin test. Preliminary tuberculin testing may be omitted with newborn infants being vaccinated in the first few days of life. If the skin tuberculin reaction is still negative 2 months or more after a BCG injection, or if the reaction becomes positive and then disappears subsequently, revaccination is advised for those who need the protection.

Tuberculin Testing

The application of a test with tuberculin is a most important diagnostic procedure whenever even a remote possibility of tuberculosis exists. A positive skin reaction to old tuberculin (OT) or to its purified protein derivative (PPD) indicates that tubercle bacilli have been harbored in the body and that the tissues have become sensitized. During infancy all positive skin reactions must be construed as indicating an active infection. Above the infancy period, a positive reaction does not necessarily denote the presence of disease activity at the time of the test. Patients who are moribund or starved or who are ill with measles, influenza, or perhaps other febrile diseases may lose temporarily a previously present skin reactivity.

Most pediatric clinics prefer to use OT for routine testing. The standard Mantoux intradermal test is done with 0.1 ml of a 1:10,000 dilution (0.01 mg), after 48 hours. If this is negative the test may be repeated with 0.1 ml of a 1:1,000 dilution (0.1 mg) and occasionally with a 1:100 dilution (1.0 mg) in special diagnostic situations. With PPD, when the initial intradermal dose is 0.00002 mg with no reaction, this may be followed after 2 days by a second test with 0.005 or 0.0025 mg. The Vollmer patch test, which employs filter paper impregnated with OT and fastened by adhesive tape to the skin of the back, is very convenient for office practice. Results are believed to be comparable with those from the first testing strengths of either intradermal OT or PPD.

Practically all cases of childhood tuberculosis can be detected by the proper application of tuberculin testing, apart from the exceptions mentioned. About 90 per cent of children who are sensitive to tuberculin will exhibit a positive skin reaction with the first testing strengths of OT or PPD and with the patch test. No child should be adjudged a negative tuberculin reactor, however, until after being tested with the second strength of PPD or OT. Skin testing should be employed whenever tuberculosis is being looked for, except that with tuberculosis of the eye and with some forms of bone or joint tuberculosis the testing may be followed by a flare-up of the lesions. The skin response following BCG vaccination is usually slight or moderate and appears within 3 to 8 weeks following successful vaccination. Should a greater sensitivity to tuberculin develop subsequently, this may reflect a superimposed infection with virulent bacilli.

Recovery of Organisms

The most convincing confirmation of the tuberculous character of a lesion is the finding of tubercle bacilli in its contents or discharges. Acid-fast bacilli found by direct microscopy are not always true tubercle bacilli. It is always best to verify the morphologic diagnosis in the initial specimen by recovery of the organisms in culture and by the further demonstration of their virulence by guinea pig inoculation. Smears alone are adequate for following the response to therapy after the existence of tuberculosis in a patient has been shown.

The specimen, whether sputum, urine, cerebrospinal fluid, or pus from a wound, may be looked at directly in a stained smear or if watery can be subjected to centrifugation and a smear made of the deposit at the bottom of the centrifuge tube. Thick purulent matter may have to be liquefied beforehand by mixing with some weak digestant such as 3 per cent sodium hydroxide solution.

Search for acid-fast bacilli under the microscope should be continued for at least 5 minutes. The longer the time spent in searching the smear, the more likely the probability of success if the patient has tuberculosis. *M. tuberculosis* may be present in very small numbers and often occurs in small clumps. The observation is more reliable when multiple clumps of *M. tuberculosis* are found.

About half of the specimens of urine and cerebrospinal fluid which give positive results by culture or guinea pig inoculation do not reveal detectable bacillin in the direct staining of the sediment. Further pursuit of the organisms by these methods in suspected cases is obviously advisable when the direct smear is negative.

Sputum

Older children are usually able to produce sputum for bacteriologic studies. This is best collected in the early morning. The child should be instructed to brush his teeth, take a drink of water, and then cough up sputum into a wide container held before the mouth. When the volume is scanty the collection may be continued for 24 hours, meanwhile keeping contamination by saliva to a minimum.

With infants and children under 6 years who are too young to expectorate, sputum frequently can be secured by placing a square of dry sterile gauze over the end of the finger and introducing this into the throat near the base of the tongue. The gagging which ensues promptly may bring up material for examination and culture.

Gastric Washings

With younger children, who normally swallow rather than expectorate their sputum, the fasting gastric contents may be aspirated and the contents cultured. Gastric lavage of patients with roentgen lung changes and a positive skin reaction to tuberculin frequently yields tubercle bacilli (p. 672). Tubercle bacilli seem able to survive contact with childhood gastric secretions for at least 12 to 24 hours. This holds particularly when the content of pepsin and hydrochloric acid is weak, as after an overnight interval. For best success the cultures should be planted as soon as possible after the specimen is collected. The results of direct study of the gastric washings by smear examination can be misleading, because normal individuals frequently exhibit nonpathogenic acid-fast bacteria in their gastric contents.

Culture

The development in recent years of excellent media for the growth of tubercle bacilli has resulted in the widespread adoption of this approach for recovery of the organisms. Cultures usually display recognizable growth in less than a month, and often within $2\frac{1}{2}$ to 3 weeks. Cultures should be kept under observation for at least 2 months, however, since occasional strains require that much time to show themselves.

Nonpathogenic mycobacteria which may appear on culture media usually grow more rapidly and form softer, smoother, and more deeply pigmented colonies than true tubercle bacilli. When colony appearances do not permit clear differentiation the culture may be injected into guinea pigs to test for virulence.

Guinea Pig Inoculation

Young guinea pigs (300 to 350 gm), when injected intraperitoneally or subcutaneously with material containing viable tubercle bacilli, will succumb to tuberculosis as a rule within 2 months. The reading can sometimes be accelerated by testing the animal's skin with tuberculin every few weeks and carrying out a pathologic examination as soon as the skin reaction becomes positive. All injected animals who survive for 2 months should be killed and examined for necropsy evidence of tuberculosis. Gross lesions which contain acid-fast bacilli on microscopy are evaluated as a positive result.

A variant procedure is to inject previously inoculated animals subcutaneously with a large dose of OT at about 4 weeks after the first injection. Animals which have become sensitized by the development of tuberculosis will usually die within 2 days.

With large series of specimens a few will prove positive by guinea pig inoculation when negative by culture, but an equal number will prove positive by culture when negative by guinea pig inoculation. Guinea pig inoculation establishes the pathogenicity of any acid-fast organism which may have been recovered and thereby has an advantage over the cultural method. Unfortunately, the much greater expense, work, and time required and the propensity of these animals to succumb to intercurrent infections have led most laboratories to abandon such animal studies. Cultural studies are deemed adequate except (1) with urine and gastric specimens in which other acid-fast mycobacteria may be present and have to be differentiated from *M. tuberculosis* and (2) with the suspected presence of bovine tubercle bacilli which are difficult to cultivate but highly virulent for the guinea pig. The latter possibility is very exceptional in this country and does not come into consideration with routine cases.

It should be emphasized that the percentage of positive results with all bacteriologic examinations for tuberculosis depends on the number of specimens which are examined. One or two negative reports do not rule out the disease.

Histopathologic Examination

Excised lymph nodes or portions of organs suspected of tuberculous involvement should always be studied histologically for so-called tuberculous granulation tissue. Characteristically this is made up of epithelioid cells, giant cells, fibroblasts, and lymphocytes, with or without caseation. Experience with tissue examinations has made it clear, however, that such formations may appear in other granulomatous lesions. Brucellosis, histoplasmosis, coccidioidomycosis, Hodgkin's disease, syphilis, cat-scratch disease, lymphopathia venereum, sarcoidosis, fungal infections, and other diseases will sometimes give rise to tissue reactions which can simulate tuberculosis closely or even be indistinguishable from it. Occasionally, also, the histologic formations in tuberculosis may differ markedly from the typical pattern. It is advisable, therefore, that all suspected surgically removed tissue be divided into two portions. One portion is prepared for histologic examination. The other is macerated and utilized for bacteriologic smear, culture, and guinea pig inoculation as indicated.

Hemagglutination Test

In this serologic procedure an antigen is employed which consists of sheep red cells coated with water-soluble polysaccharide fractions derived from old tuberculin. Such "activated" red cells will often exhibit specific agglutination when mixed with serum from a tuberculous patient. The serum is heated first to inactivate the complement, and then freed from antibodies unrelated to the tuberculous infection by undergoing a preliminary mixing with sheep red cells.

The serologic approach as yet has not proved sufficiently dependable to be used as an indicator of the presence of active tuberculosis in the absence of other accepted diagnostic criteria. Most, though not all, children with negative tuberculin skin tests and no clinical evidence of tuberculosis have a negligible hemagglutinin titer. Conversely, many children with active tuberculosis have levels of circulating hemagglutinins within the normal range, especially those under 6 years of age. Hence an elevated titer may be suggestive of tuberculosis in a suspected case, but its absence does not rule out the active disease.

The prior performance of a tuberculin skin test in older children will occasionally bring about a mild rise in hemagglutinin titer regardless of whether the skin response to the tuberculin proves positive or negative. It is important, therefore, to secure the blood specimen for serologic testing at the same time or before the tuberculin test is studied when studying a child for suspected tuberculosis.

Hematologic Phenomena

In childhood tuberculosis the occurrence of fever and other clinical symptoms are signs that the infection is active. In addition to such overt manifestations, serial blood studies at biweekly or monthly intervals furnish helpful information as to the trend of changes. The red cell count and hemoglobin level tend to be normochromically depressed while the infectious process is active and to revert to normal as improvement occurs, especially when supplemental iron and other nutrients are furnished in abundance during the recovery period. The red cell sedimentation rate is often but not necessarily elevated in tuberculosis of moderate severity. The total leukocyte count usually remains within the normal range throughout the illness. Monocytes are often increased in the early stages, followed by a rise in the absolute number of lymphocytes as improvement begins. The serum gamma globulin level rises early in the illness; it subsides during convalescence or shortly before death in refractory cases.

BIBLIOGRAPHY

BACTEROIDES INFECTIONS

Biegelman, P. M., and L. A. Rantz, Clinical Significance of Bacteroides, Arch. Int. Med. 84:605, 1949.

Fisher, A. M., and V. A. McKusick, Bacteroides Infections: Clinical, Bacteriological and Therapeutic Features of Fourteen Cases, Am. J. M. Sc. 225:253, 1953.

BRUCELLOSIS

Castaneda, M. R., and C. Carrillo-Cardenas, A New Approach to Treatment of Brucellosis, Am. J. M. Sc. 226:504, 1953.

Harris, H. J., Chronic Brucellosis: The Unsatisfactory Status of Current Diagnostic Methods, Am. J. Pub. Health 39:870, 1949.

———, Antibiotic and Antigenic Therapy of Brucellosis with Special Reference to the Chronic Disease: A Report of 421 Cases, Antibiotics & Chemother. 3:982, 1953.

Magoffin, R. L., P. Kabler, W. W. Spink, and D. S. Fleming, An Epidemiologic Study of Brucellosis in Minnesota, Pub. Health Rep. 64:1021, 1949.

Spink, W. W., The Laboratory in the Diagnosis of Brucellosis, Am. J. Clin. Path. 22:201, 1952.

———, Epidemiologic and Clinical Studies on Brucellosis, 1937–52, Tr. & Stud. Coll. Physicians Philadelphia 21:51, 1953.

———, N. B. McCullough, L. M. Hutchings, and C. K. Mingle, Diagnostic Criteria for Human Brucellosis, J.A.M.A. 149:805, 1952.

———, ———, ———, and ———, A Standardized Antigen and Agglutination Technic for Human Brucellosis, *Am. J. Clin. Path.* 24:496, 1954.

Stanfield, C. A., P. W. Taylor, and *H. R. Morgan,* Some Important Antigenic Relationships in the Serologic Diagnosis of Brucellosis, *Am. J. Clin. Path.* 22:211, 1952.

Valdes, J. M., C. Piantoni, and *A. S. Segura,* Neurobrucelosis en el niño, *Arch. argent. pediat.* 24:165, 1953.

DIPHTHERIA

Amies, C. R., The Pathogenesis of Diphtheria, *J. Path. & Bact.* 67:25, 1954.

Bruyn, H. B., H. Brainerd, and *B. W. Leppla,* Penicillin in the Treatment of Diphtheria, *Am. J. M. Sc.* 219:408, 1950.

Cohen, P., H. Schneck, E. Dubow, and *S. Q. Cohlan,* The Changed Status of Diphtheria Immunity, *Pediatrics* 3:630, 1949.

Fanning, J., An Outbreak of Diphtheria in a Highly Immunized Community, *Brit. M. J.* 1:371, 1947.

Ferris, A. A., Serological Types of *Corynebacterium diphtheriae* in Australia, *J. Path. & Bact.* 62:165, 1950.

———, Type-specific Agglutinins in *Corynebacterium diphtheriae* Infections, *J. Path. & Bact.* 62:157, 1950.

Fisher, A. M., and *S. Cobb,* Clinical Manifestations of the Severe Form of Diphtheria, *Bull. Johns Hopkins Hosp.* 83:297, 1948.

Frobisher, M., Jr., E. I. Parsons, and *E. Updyke,* The Correlation of Laboratory and Clinical Evidence of Virulence of *C. diphtheriae, Am. J. Pub. Health* 37:543, 1947.

Greenberg, I., and *D. S. Fleming,* The Effect of Inherited Antibodies on the Active Immunization of Infants, *J. Pediat.* 36:143, 1950.

Hartley, P., W. J. Tulloch, M. Anderson, W. A. Davidson, J. Grant, W. M. Jamieson, C. Neubauer, R. Norton, and *G. H. Robertson,* A Study of Diphtheria in Two Areas of Great Britain, *Med. Res. Council (Great Britain), Spec. Rep.* 272, 1950.

Hewitt, L. F., Serological Typing of *C. diphtheriae, Brit. J. Exper. Path.* 28:338, 1947.

Jackson, G. G., S. Chang, E. H. Place, and *M. Finland,* Sensitivity of Diphtheria Bacilli and Related Organisms to Nine Antibiotics, *J. Pediat.* 37:718, 1950.

Karelitz, S., H. King, and *I. S. Rubinstein,* Aureomycin Treatment of Diphtheria and Diphtheria Carriers, *J. Pediat.* 39:544, 1951.

——— and *V. A. Spinelli,* Penicillin Treatment of Diphtheria Carriers, *Pediatrics* 3:639, 1950.

Naiditch, M. J., and *A. O. Bower,* Diphtheria: A Study of 1,433 Cases Observed during a Ten-year Period at the Los Angeles County Hospital, *Am. J. Med.* 17:229, 1954.

ESCHERICHIA AND COLIFORM ORGANISMS

Bruner, D. W., P. R. Edwards, and *A. S. Hopson,* The Serological Classification of the Ballerup Group of Paracolon Bacilli, *J. Infect. Dis.* 85:290, 1949.

Edwards, P. R., and *W. H. Ewing,* "Identification of Enterobacteriaceae," Burgess Publishing Co., Minneapolis, 1955.

———, *A. C. McWhorter,* and *M. A. Fife,* The Arizona Group of Enterobacteriaceae in Animals and Man: Occurrence and Distribution, *Bull. World Health Organ.* 14:511, 1956.

——— and *M. G. West,* Unusual Types of Enteric Bacteria, *J. Infect. Dis.* 87:184, 1950.

Ewing, W. H., M. W. Taylor, and M. C. Hucks, The Alkalescens-Dispar Group, Pub. Health Rep. 65:1474, 1950.

———, K. E. Tanner, and D. A. Dennard, The Providence Group: An Intermediate Group of Enteric Bacteria, J. Infect. Dis. 94:134, 1954.

Felsenfeld, O., and V. M. Young, Studies in Salmonellosis in North and South America, Am. J. Trop. Med. 29:483, 1949.

Frank, V. F., C. Wilcox, and M. Finland, In Vitro Sensitivity of Coliform Bacilli to Seven Antibiotics (Penicillin, Streptomycin, Bacitracin, Polymyxin, Aerosporin, Aureomycin and Chloromycetin), J. Lab. & Clin. Med. 35:188, 1950.

Frantzen, E., Biochemical and Serological Studies on Alkalescens and Dispar Strains, Acta path. et microbiol. scandinav. 27:236, 1950.

———, "Biochemical and Serological Studies of the Alkalescens-Dispar Group," Munksgaard, Copenhagen, 1952.

Herweg, J. C., J. N. Middelkamp, and H. K. Thornton, Escherichia coli Diarrhea: The Relationship of Certain Serotypes of Escherichia coli to Sporadic and Epidemic Cases of Infantile Diarrhea, J. Pediat. 49:629, 1956.

Kauffmann, F., "The Differentiation of Escherichia and Klebsiella Types," American Lecture Series 84, Charles C Thomas, Springfield, Ill., 1950.

———, "Enterobacteriaceae," 2d ed., Munksgaard, Copenhagen, 1954.

Murphy, W. J., and J. F. Morris, Two Outbreaks of Gastroenteritis Apparently Caused by a Paracolon of the Arizona Group, J. Infect. Dis. 86:255, 1950.

Schaub, I. G., The Cultural Differentiation of Paracolon Bacilli, Bull. Johns Hopkins Hosp. 83:367, 1948.

Seligmann, E., I. Saphra, and M. Wassermann, Salmonella Infections in the U.S.A., J. Immunol. 54:69, 1946.

Stuart, C. A., et al., Biochemical and Antigenic Relationships of the Paracolon Bacteria, J. Bact. 45:101, 1943.

———, M. M. Galton, and V. McGann, Antigenic Studies of 765 Paracolobactrum intermedium Cultures, J. Bact. 56:411, 1948.

Weinstein, L., and E. Wasserman, Bacterium alcaligenes (Alcaligenes faecalis) Infections in Man, New England J. Med. 244:662, 1951.

West, M. G., and P. R. Edwards, The Bethesda-Ballerup Group of Paracolon Bacteria, Pub. Health Serv. Publ. 362, 1954.

GASTROENTERITIS AND ESCH. COLI STRAINS

Dupont, A., On the Occurrence of Escherichia coli 55: B₅6 and E. coli 111: B 4 in Fecal Samples from Infants with Diarrhea Disease and in a Control Material, Acta paediat. 40:95, suppl. 83, 1951.

Epidemic and Endemic Diarrheal Diseases of the Infant (Conference), Ann. New York Acad. Sc. 66:3, 1956.

Ferguson, W. W., and R. C. June, Experiments on Feeding Adult Volunteers with Escherichia coli 111, B 4, A Coliform Organism Associated with Infant Diarrhea, Am. J. Hyg. 55:155, 1952.

Gorzynski, E. H., and E. Neter, Study on the in Vitro Efficacy of Neomycin and Streptomycin on Subgroups of Escherichia coli Associated with Diarrheal Disease of Infants, Antibiotics & Chemother. 3:798, 1953.

Laurell, G., J. H. Magnusson, E. Frisell, and B. Werner, Epidemic Infantile Diarrhea and Vomiting, Acta paediat. 40:302, 1951.

Modica, R. I., W. W. Ferguson, and E. F. Ducey, Epidemic Infantile Diarrhea Associated with Escherichia coli 111, B 4, J. Lab. & Clin. Med. 39:122, 1952.

Neter, E., R. F. Korns, and R. E. Trussell, Association of Escherichia coli Serogroup O111 with Two Hospital Outbreaks of Epidemic Diarrhea of the Newborn Infant in New York State during 1947, Pediatrics 12:377, 1953.

———, *C. R. Webb, C. N. Shumway,* and *M. R. Murdock,* Study of Etiology, Epidemiology and Antibiotic Therapy of Infantile Diarrhea, with Particular Reference to Certain Serotypes of *Escherichia coli, Am. J. Pub. Health* **41**:1490, 1951.

Rabe, E. F., and *D. L. Dunphy,* Agglutinating Substances for Homologous Coliform Organisms: Observations on Their Occurrence in the Serum and Feces of Infants, *Am. J. Dis. Child.* **78**:717, 1949.

Smith, J., and *W. H. Galloway,* The Sensitivity to Antibiotics of Strains of Bacteria Coli Associated with Infantile Gastro-enteritis, *Arch. Dis. Childhood* **28**:30, 1953.

Vahlne, G., Serological Typing of the Colon Bacteria, with Special Reference to the Occurrence of *B. coli* in Man under Normal and Pathological Conditions, Particularly in Appendicitis, *Acta path. et microbiol. scand.* suppl. 62, 1945.

Wolfish, M. G., Acute Gastroenteritis: A Review of 518 Cases Treated at the Hospital for Sick Children during 1951 and 1952, *J. Pediat.* **43**:675, 1953.

SALMONELLOSIS

Abramson, H., Infection with *Salmonella typhimurium* in the Newborn: Epidemiologic and Clinical Considerations, *Am. J. Dis. Child.* **74**:576, 1947.

Batson, H. C., Typhoid Fever Prophylaxis by Active Immunization, *Pub. Health Rep.* suppl. 212, 1949.

Bauer, F. K., and *A. G. Bower,* Typhoid Fever of Short Duration, *Am. J. M. Sc.* **222**:174, 1951.

Clyde, W. A., Jr., Salmonellosis in Infants and Children: A Study of 100 Cases, *Pediatrics* **19**:175, 1957.

Edwards, P. R., Salmonella and Salmonellosis, *Ann. New York Acad. Sc.* **66**:44, 1956.

Epstein, H. C., A. Hochwald, and *R. Ashe,* Salmonella Infections of the Newborn Infant, *J. Pediat.* **38**:723, 1951.

Henderson, L. L., Salmonella Meningitis: Report of Three Cases and Review of One Hundred and Forty-four Cases from the Literature, *Am. J. Dis. Child.* **75**:351, 1948.

Jones, J., and *H. F. Lee, Salmonella suipestifer* Infection in Children: A Report of Eighteen Cases, *Am. J. M. Sc.* **211**:723, 1946.

Kauffmann, F., "The Diagnosis of Salmonella Types," American Lecture Series No. 62, Charles C Thomas, Springfield, Ill., 1950.

Ling, C., J. Liu, and *T. Chen,* A Comparative Study of Bile, Marrow, Blood, Stool, Urine Cultures and Widal Reaction in Typhoid and Paratyphoid Fevers: An Analysis of 31 Cases, *Chinese Med. J.* **66**:66, 1948.

Lundgoot, L., Typhoid Fever: A Review of 68 Cases at Children's Hospital from 1937 to 1947, *Clin. Proc. Children's Hosp. Washington, D.C.* **3**:289, 1947.

Neter, E., Microbiologic Aspects of Salmonellosis in Children, *New York J. Med.* **48**:412, 1948.

Savage, W., Problems of Salmonella Food-poisoning, *Brit. M. J.* **2**:317, 1956.

Scroggie, A., H. Garces, and *A. C. y J. Agliati,* Salmonellosis intestinal en el lactante, *Rev. chil. pediat.* **24**:46, 1953.

Shaughnessy, H. J., F. Friewer, and *A. Snyder,* Comparative Efficiency of Rectal Swabs and Fecal Specimens in Detecting Typhoid and Salmonella Cases and Carriers, *Am. J. Pub. Health* **38**:670, 1948.

Stock, A. H., F. B. Warner, A. F. Catto, and *A. Ashute,* Rectal Swab Method for Isolating *Eberthella typhosa*: Its Use in a Typhoid Epidemic, *Am. J. Clin. Path.* **17**:759, 1947.

SHIGELLOSIS

Cooper, M. L., J. Tepper, and *H. M. Keller,* Studies in Dysentery Vaccination. IV. Primary Vaccination of Children with Monovalent Vaccines of Shigella, *J. Immunol.* 60:189, 1948.

Feig, M., Epidemic Shigella Gastroenteritis (Bacillary Dysentery) in an Endemic Area. II. Age-specific Clinical Aspects, *Pediatrics* 11:145, 1953.

Felsen, J., and *W. Wolarsky,* Acute and Chronic Bacillary Dysentery and Chronic Ulcerative Colitis, *J.A.M.A.* 153:1069, 1953.

Hutchinson, R. I., Some Observations on the Method of Spread of Sonne Dysentery, *Month. Bull. Min. Health,* 15:110, 1956.

Neter, E., The Genus Shigella and Shigellosis, *Am. J. Digest. Dis.* 15:213, 1948.

Zimmerman, L. E., M. Cooper, and *C. D. Graber,* Bacteriologic Studies in an Epidemic of Bacillary Dysentery in Korea: Serotypes of Shigella and Salmonella Recovered and Bacteriologic Response to Sulfadiazine, Chloramphenicol, Terramycin, Aureomycin and Streptomycin, *Am. J. Clin. Path.* 22:549, 1952.

GONOCOCCIC INFECTIONS

Gocke, T. M., C. Wilcox, and *M. Finland,* Antibiotic Spectrum of the Gonococcus, *Am. J. Syph.* 34:265, 1950.

Hajek, J. P., M. J. Pelczar, and *J. E. Faber,* Variations in the Fermentative Capacity of Neisseriae, *Am. J. Clin. Path.* 20:630, 1950.

OPHTHALMIA NEONATORUM

Allen, S. H., and *L. E. Barrere,* Prophylaxis of Gonorrheal Ophthalmia of the Newborn, *J.A.M.A.* 141:522, 1949.

Bickel, J. E., Sodium Sulfacetimide for the Prophylaxis of Gonorrheal Ophthalmia Neonatorum, *J. Pediat.* 37:854, 1950.

Elliott, R. A., Ophthalmia Neonatorum: A Review of the Prophylactic Methods at Present in Use, *Month. Bull. Min. Health* 11:135, 1952.

Franklin, H. C. and *L. N. Loeb,* Bacterial Flora in Eyes of Newborn Infants during First Forty Hours of Life, *J. Pediat.* 32:251, 1948.

Sorsby, A., The Incubation Period of Ophthalmia Neonatorum, *J. Obst. & Gynaec. Brit. Emp.* 54:842, 1947.

Stuart, R. D., and *D. McWalter,* Primary Meningococcal Conjunctivitis in Children, *Lancet* 1:246, 1948.

INFLUENZA BACILLUS INFECTIONS

Alexander, H. E., Transformation Reaction in *Hemophilus influenzae, Bull. New York Acad. Med.* 28:350, 1952.

———— and *G. Leidy,* Determination of Inherited Traits of *H. influenzae* by Desoxyribonucleic Acid Fractions Isolated from Type-specific Cells, *J. Exper. Med.* 93:345, 1951.

Applebaum, E., and *J. Nelson,* Streptomycin in the Treatment of Influenzal Meningitis: A Study of Ninety Cases, with 96.6 per cent Recovery, *J.A.M.A.* 143:715, 1950.

Finland, M., and *C. Wilcox, In Vitro* Susceptibility of *Hemophilus influenzae* to Seven Antibiotics (Penicillin, Streptomycin, Bacitracin, Polymyxin, Aerosporin, Aureomycin and Chloromycetin), *Am. J. Clin. Path.* 20:335, 1950.

Foley, G. E., H. Schwachman, M. McGarry, and *W. D. Winter, Jr.,* Morphologic Characteristics and Antibiotic Resistance of *Hemophilus influenzae, Am. J. Dis. Child.* 78:659, 1949.

Fothergill, L. D., and *J. Wright,* Influenzal Meningitis: The Relation of Age Incidence to the Bactericidal Power of Blood against Causal Organism, *J. Immunol.* 24:273, 1933.

Koch, R., and *M. J. Carson,* Management of *Hemophilus influenzae,* Type B, Meningitis: Analysis of 128 Cases, *J. Pediat.* 46:18, 1955.

McCrumb, F. R., Jr., H. E. Hall, J. Imburg, A. Merideth, R. Helmhold, J. Defillo, and *T. E. Woodward,* Treatment of *Hemophilus influenzae* Meningitis with Chloramphenicol and Other Antibiotics, *J.A.M.A.* 145:469, 1951.

McMorrow, K. J., and *F. H. Top,* Treatment of *Hemophilus influenzae* b Meningitis: Report of 67 Cases, *Pediatrics* 5:452, 1950.

Rabe, E. F., Infectious Croup. III. *Hemophilus influenzae* Type B Croup, *Pediatrics* 2:559, 1948.

Wilkins, R. B., F. J. Jarvis, and *R. L. King,* Purulent Pericarditis Due to *Hemophilus influenzae,* Type B, *Am. Heart J.* 42:749, 1951.

Wood, S. H., F. J. Buddingh, and *B. F. Abberger, Jr.,* An Inquiry into the Etiology of Acute Bronchiolitis of Infants, *Pediatrics* 13:363, 1954.

KLEBSIELLA-AEROBACTER INFECTIONS

Edwards, P. R., and *M. A. Fife,* Studies on the Klebsiella-Aerobacter Group of Bacteria, *J. Bact.* 70:382, 1955.

Eisenberg, G. M., J. M. O'Loughlin, and *H. F. Flippin,* Distribution and In Vitro Antibiotic Susceptibility of Klebsiella (Kauffmann), *J. Lab. & Clin. Med.* 43:707, 1954.

Faucett, R. L., and *H. Miller,* Stomatitis in Infants Caused by *B. mucosus capsulatus, Pediatrics* 1:458, 1948.

Holowach, J. S., L. Thurston, and *H. J. Wohltmann,* Chronic Friedländer Pneumonia in Infancy, *J. Pediat.* 41:430, 1952.

Kauffmann, F., "The Differentiation of Escherichia and Klebsiella Types," Charles C Thomas, Springfield, Ill., 1951.

Lemke, C. E., and *L. E. Gates,* Distribution and Antibiotic Sensitivity in Fifty-five Strains of *Klebsiella pneumoniae, J. Lab. & Clin. Med.* 38:889, 1951.

Nataro, M., D. Shapiro, and *A. T. Gordon,* Acute Primary Klebsiella Pneumonia, *J.A.M.A.* 144:12, 1950.

Obrinsky, W., R. E. Dormont, R. E. L. Fowler, and *F. Ruhstaller,* Friedländer-Aerogenes Infections in Infancy, *Am. J. Dis. Child.* 80:621, 1950.

Sternberg, S. D., C. Hoffman, and *B. M. Zweifler,* Stomatitis and Diarrhea in Infants Caused by *Bacillus mucosus capsulatus, J. Pediat.* 38:509, 1951.

LACTOBACILLUS RELATIONSHIPS

Boyd, J. D., V. D. Cheyne, and *K. E. Wessels,* Is the Salivary Lactobacillus Count a Valid Index of Activity of Dental Caries? *Proc. Soc. Exper. Biol. & Med.* 71:535, 1949.

Schlesinger, E. R., and *D. B. Ast,* Use of Fluoride Compounds in Prevention of Dental Caries, *Advances Pediat.* 9:191, 1957.

Sugar and Dental Caries: A Symposium, *J. California State Dent. A.,* vol. 26, no. 3, May–June, 1950.

MENINGOCOCCEMIA

Aycock, W. L., and *J. H. Mueller,* Meningococcus Carrier Rates and Meningitis Incidence, *Bact. Rev.* 14:115, 1950.

Branham, S. E., Value of Typing Meningococci, *Am. J. Pub. Health* 35:233, 1945.

Banks, H. S., Meningococcosis, a Protean Disease, *Lancet* 2:635, 677, 1948.

Daniels, W. B., Meningococcic Bacteremia, *Arch. Int. Med.* **81**:145, 1948.

Hedrich, A. W., Recent Trends in Meningococcal Disease, *Pub. Health Rep.* **67**:411, 1952.

Love, B. D., Jr., and *M. Finland,* In Vitro Susceptibility of Meningococci to Eleven Antibiotics and Sulfadiazine, *Am. J. M. Sc.* **228**:534, 1954.

Thomas, L., and *J. H. Dingle,* Investigations of Meningococcal Infection. I. Bacteriological Aspects, *J. Clin. Invest.* **22**:353, 1943.

PASTEURELLA INFECTIONS

Cavanaugh, D. C., and *S. F. Quan,* Rapid Identification of *Pasteurella pestis, Am. J. Clin. Path.* **23**:619, 1953.

Eskey, C. R., and *V. H. Haas,* Plague in the Western Part of the United States, *Pub. Health Bull.* 254, 1940.

Foshay, L., Tularemia, *Ann. Rev. Microbiol.* **4**:313, 1950.

Hausmann, G. H., and *M. Tully,* Cat-bite and Scratch Wounds with Consequent Pasteurella Infection of Man, *Am. J. Clin. Path.* **15**:312, 1945.

Lewis, M. L., Fatal Meningitis with Septicemia Caused by *Pasteurella multocida, Am. J. Clin. Path.* **23**:241, 1953.

Meyer, K. F., Pasteurella, chap. 19 in "Bacterial and Mycotic Infections of Man," R. J. Dubos (ed.), 2d ed., J. B. Lippincott Company, Philadelphia, 1952.

————, Pasteurella Infections, *M. Clin. North America* February, 1955, p. 3.

Neter, E., E. H. De Kleine, and *R. W. Egan,* Treatment with Aureomycin of Localized *Pasteurella multocida* Infection, *J. Pediat.* **38**:242, 1951.

Ransmeier, J. C., and *C. L. Ewing,* The Agglutination Reaction in Tularemia, *J. Infect. Dis.* **69**:193, 1941.

Snyder, G. A. C., and *N. J. Vogel,* Human Infection by *Pasteurella pseudotuberculosis:* Report of a Case with Recovery, *Northwest Med.* **42**:14, 1943.

PERTUSSIS

Alexander, H. E., C. MacPherson, and *W. Redman,* Quantitative Method for Measuring *H. pertussis* Antibody, *Pediatrics* **5**:443, 1950.

Barysh, N., Use of the Pertussis Agglutinogen Skin Test in a Well Baby Clinic, *Pediatrics* **7**:48, 1951.

Cockburn, W. C., and *H. D. Holt,* A Comparison of the Results Obtained with Prenasal and Postnasal Swabs in the Diagnosis of Pertussis, *Month. Bull. Min. Health* **7**:156, 1948.

Day, E., and *W. L. Bradford,* Susceptibility of *Hemophilus parapertussis* to Certain Antibiotics, *Pediatrics* **9**:320, 1952.

Felton, H. M., Pertussis: Current Status of Prevention and Treatment, *Pediat. Clinics North America* February, 1957, p. 271.

Hazen, L. N., G. G. Jackson, C. Shih-Man, E. H. Place, and *M. Finland,* Antibiotic Treatment of Pertussis: Comparison of Penicillin, Aureomycin, Chloramphenicol and Terramycin in 150 Cases, *J. Pediat.* **39**:1, 1951.

Kohn, J. L., L. W. Wannamaker, S. R. Kaplan, and *K. S. Shepard,* The Use of Pertussis Agglutinogen Skin Test during Active Infection with Whooping Cough, *J. Pediat.* **36**:614, 1950.

McGovern, J. P., Passive Intraperitoneal Mouse Protection Test in a Study of Immune Response to *H. pertussis* Vaccination, *Pediatrics* **5**:38, 1950.

Shih-Man, C., Pertussis Due to *Brucella bronchiseptica:* Case Report, *Pediatrics* **6**:227, 1950.

Wells, E. B., C. Shih-Man, G. G. Jackson, and *M. Finland,* Antibiotic Spectrum of *Hemophilus pertussis, J. Pediat.* **36**:752, 1950.

Zuelzer, W. W., and W. E. Wheeler, Parapertussis Pneumonia: Report of Two Fatal Cases, J. Pediat. 29:493, 1946.

PLEUROPNEUMONIA-LIKE ORGANISMS

Carlson, H. J., S. Spector, and H. G. Douglas, Possible Role of Pleuropneumonia-like Organisms in Etiology of Disease in Childhood, A.M.A. Am. J. Dis. Child. 81:193, 1951.

Davis, J. H., and L. H. Arnstein, Pleuropneumonia Organism Meningitis Complicating Ruptured Meningocele: Report of Case with Recovery, Pediatrics 11:381, 1953.

Morton, H. E., P. F. Smith, and R. Keller, Prevalence of Pleuropneumonia-like Organisms and the Evaluation of Media and Methods for Their Isolation from Clinical Material, Am. J. Pub. Health 42:913, 1952.

Paine, T. F., Jr., R. Murray, I. Pearlmutter, and M. Finland, Brain Abscess and Meningitis Associated with Pleuropneumonia-like Organism: Clinical and Bacteriological Observations in Case with Recovery, Ann. Int. Med. 32:554, 1950.

Sabin, A. B., The Pleuropneumonia Group, chap. 30 in R. J. Dubos (ed.), "Bacterial and Mycotic Infections of Man," 2d ed., J. B. Lippincott Company, Philadelphia, 1952.

PNEUMOCOCCIC INFECTIONS

Alexander, J. D., Jr., H. F. Flippin, and G. M. Eisenberg, Pneumococcic Meningitis: Study of One Hundred Two Cases, A.M.A. Arch. Int. Med. 91:440, 1953.

Austrian, R., R. Rosenblum, and the Pneumonia Study Group, The Relative Efficacy of Erythromycin (Ilotycin) and of Penicillin in the Treatment of Pneumococcal Lobar Pneumonia, Am. J. M. Sc. 226:487, 1953.

Dowling, H. F., and M. H. Lepper, The Effect of Antibiotics (Penicillin, Aureomycin, and Terramycin) on the Fatality Rate and Incidence of Complications in Pneumococcic Pneumonia, Am. J. M. Sc. 222:396, 1951.

Heffron, R., "Pneumonia, with Special Reference to Pneumococcus Lobar Pneumonia," The Commonwealth Fund, New York, 1939.

Hendry, E., A Clinical and Bacteriological Survey of Pneumonia in Childhood, Arch. Dis. Childhood 17:111, 1942.

Holzel, A., and B. Wolman, The Prognosis of Pneumonia in Infancy and Childhood, Arch. Dis. Childhood 25:282, 1950.

Jackson, G. G., T. M. Gocke, C. Wilcox, and M. Finland, In Vitro Susceptibility of Pneumococci to Seven Antibiotics (Penicillin, Streptomycin, Bacitracin, Polymyxin, Aerosporin, Aureomycin and Chloromycetin), Am. J. Clin. Path. 20:218, 1950.

Smillie, W. G., and O. F. Jewitt, The Relationship of Immediate Family Contact to the Transmission of Type Specific Pneumococci, Am. J. Hyg. 32:79, 1940.

White, G. B., E. S. Robinson, and L. A. Barnes, "The Biology of Pneumococcus: The Bacteriological, Biochemical and Immunological Characters and Activities of Diplococcus pneumoniae," The Commonwealth Fund, New York, 1938.

PROTEUS BACILLUS INFECTIONS

Bogdanovitch, A., Neonatal Arthritis Due to Proteus vulgaris, Arch. Dis. Childhood 23:65, 1948.

Frank, P. F., In Vitro Sensitivity of Bacillus proteus and Pseudomonas aeruginosa to Seven Antibiotics (Penicillin, Streptomycin, Bacitracin, Polymyxin, Aerosporin, Aureomycin and Chloromycetin), J. Lab. & Clin. Med. 35:205, 1950.

Labrinacos, P., Mélissalsis and vassardanis: sur une épidémie d'affection gastrointestinale à Proteus vulgaris, Arch. franç. pédiat. 10:714, 1953.

Neter, E. R., and *R. H. Farrar, Proteus vulgaris* and *Proteus morganii* in Diarrheal Disease of Infants, *Am. J. Digest. Dis. & Nutrition* 10:344, 1943.

Rustigian, R., and *C. A. Stuart,* The Biochemical and Serological Relationships of the Genus Proteus, *J. Bact.* 49:419, 1945.

Walker, S. H., Polymyxin B in Pseudomonas and Proteus Enteritis, *J. Pediat.* 41:176, 1952.

Yow, E. M., Development of Proteus and Pseudomonas Infections during Antibiotic Therapy, *J.A.M.A.* 149:1184, 1952.

PSEUDOMONAS INFECTIONS

Coleman, J. M., and *F. C. Lowry,* Acute Purulent Arthritis (*B. pyocyaneus*) in a Premature Infant, *Pediatrics* 7:347, 1951.

Erwin, C. P., B. A. Waisbren, and *R. Kruse,* Clinical and Laboratory Studies of Infections Due to *Pseudomonas aeruginosa* and Pseudomonas Species, *Am. J. M. Sc.* 226:525, 1953.

Florman, A. L., and *N. Schifrin,* Observations on a Small Outbreak of Infantile Diarrhea Associated with *Pseudomonas aeruginosa, J. Pediat.* 36:758, 1950.

Garrard, S. D., J. B. Richmond, and *M. M. Hirsch, Pseudomonas aeruginosa* Infection as a Complication of Therapy in Pancreatic Fibrosis (Mucoviscidosis), *Pediatrics* 8:482, 1951.

Geppert, L. J., H. J. Baker, B. I. Copple, and *E. J. Pulaski,* Pseudomonas Infections in Infants and Children, *J. Pediat.* 41:555, 1952.

Hoffman, M. A., and *L. Finberg,* Pseudomonas Infections in Infants Associated with High-humidity Environments, *J. Pediat.* 46:626, 1955.

Hunter, C. A., and *P. R. Ensign,* An Epidemic of Diarrhea in a New-born Nursery Caused by *Pseudomonas aeruginosa, Am. J. Pub. Health* 37:1166, 1947.

Hayes, E. R., and *E. Yow,* Meningitis Due to *Pseudomonas aeruginosa* Treated with Polymyxin B, *Am. J. M. Sc.* 220:633, 1950.

Walker, S. H., Polymyxin B in Pseudomonas and Proteus Enteritis, *J. Pediat.* 41:176, 1952.

Yow, E. M., and *E. S. Townsend,* A Comparison of the Sensitivity of *Pseudomonas aeruginosa* to Various Antibiotics, *Antibiotics & Chemother.* 3:709, 1953.

RAT-BITE FEVERS

Adams, J. M., and *C. M. Carpenter,* Rat-bite Fevers, *Med. Clin. North America* February, 1955, p. 101.

Humphreys, F. A., A. G. Campbell, M. W. Driver, and *G. N. Hatton,* Rat Bite Fever, *Canad. J. Pub. Health* 41:66, 1950.

Place, E. H., and *L. E. Sutton, Jr.,* Erythema Arthriticum Epidemicum (Haverhill Fever), *Arch. Int. Med.* 54:659, 1934.

Steen, E., Rat Bite Fever: Report of a Case with Examination of *Haverhillia moniliformis, Acta path. et. microbiol. scandinav.* 28:17, 1951.

Watkins, C. G., Ratbite Fever, *J. Pediat.* 28:429, 1946.

Wooley, P. V., Jr., and *M. Dowell,* Ratbite Fever Due to *Streptobacillus moniliformis, J. Pediat.* 33:507, 1948.

STAPHYLOCOCCIC INFECTIONS

Anderson, E. S., and *R. E. O. Williams,* Bacteriophage Typing of Enteric Pathogens and Staphylococci and Its Use in Epidemiology, *J. Clin. Path.* 9:94, 1956.

Barber, M., and *J. E. M. Whitehead,* Bacteriophage Types in Penicillin-resistant Staphylococcal Infection, *Brit. M. J.* 2:565, 1949.

Blair, J. E., The Staphylococci, chap. 13 in R. J. Dubos (ed.), "Bacterial and Mycotic Infections of Man," 2d ed., J. B. Lippincott Company, Philadelphia, 1952.

———— and *M. Carr*, The Bacteriophage Typing of Staphylococci, *J. Infect. Dis.* 93:1, 1953.

Brodie, J., M. R. Kerr, and *T. Sommerville,* The Hospital Staphylococcus: A Comparison of Nasal and Faecal Carrier States, *Lancet* 1:19, 1956.

Christie, R., and *E. V. Keogh,* Physiological and Serological Characteristics of Staphylococci of Human Origin, *J. Path. & Bact.* 51:189, 1940.

Crichton, J. U., Chronic Staphylococcal Enteritis in Infants, *J. Pediat.* 49:553, 1956.

Draper, F., and *G. W. Brown,* Staphylococcal Enteritis in Children, *M. J. Australia* 1:469, 1946.

Fairlie, C. W., and *R. E. Kendall,* Fatal Staphylococcus Enteritis Following Penicillin and Streptomycin Therapy, *J.A.M.A.* 153:90, 1953.

Felsen, J., J. Lapin, W. Wolarsky, A. J. Weil, and *I. Fox,* Staphylococcic Infections in Hospital Nurseries and Pediatrics Wards, *A.M.A. Am. J. Dis. Child.* 81:534, 1951.

Finland, M., and *T. H. Haight,* Antibiotic Resistance of Pathogenic Staphylococci: Study of Five Hundred Strains Isolated at Boston City Hospital from October 1951, to February 1952, *A.M.A. Arch. Int. Med.* 91:143, 1953.

Fusillo, M. H., R. N. Roerig, and *K. F. Ernst,* Phage Typing the Antibiotic-resistant Staphylococci. IV. Incidence and Phage Type Relationship of Antibiotic-resistant Staphylococci among Hospital and Nonhospital Groups, *Antibiotics & Chemother.* 4:1202, 1954.

Jackson, G. G., H. F. Dowling, and *M. Lepper,* Bacteriophage Typing of Staphylococci. II. Epidemiologic Studies among Patients, Household Contacts, and Hospital Personnel, *J. Lab. & Clin. Med.* 44:29, 1954.

Julianelle, L. A., and *C. W. Weighard,* The Immunological Specificity of Staphylococci, *J. Exper. Med.* 62:11, 23, 31, 1935.

Kanof, A., B. Epstein, B. Kramer, and *I. Mauss,* Staphylococcal Pneumonia and Empyema, *Pediatrics* 11:385, 1953.

Kirby, W. M. M., and *J. J. Ahern,* Changing Pattern of Resistance of Staphylococci to Antibiotics, *Antibiotics & Chemother.* 3:831, 1953.

Lee, H. F., and *R. B. Wilson, C. E. Brown,* and *T. P. Reed,* Impetigo and Acute Infectious Exfoliative Dermatitis of the Newborn Infant (Ritter's Disease), *J. Pediat.* 41:159, 1952.

Martyn, G., Staphylococci in the Newborn: Their Coagulase Production and Resistance to Penicillin and Streptomycin, *Brit. M. J.* 1:710, 1949.

Prissick, F. H., Antibiotic-resistant Staphylococci and Related Infections, *Am. J. M. Sc.* 225:299, 1953.

Rogers, D. E., The Current Problem of Staphylococcal Infections, *Ann. Int. Med.* 45:748, 1956.

Scott, T. J., R. M. Young, and *H. Fanger,* Incidence of Staphylococci Associated with Enteritis and Their Sensitivity to Antibiotics, *Am. J. Clin. Path.* 25:1315, 1955.

Smith, W., J. H. Hale, and *M. M. Smith,* The Role of Coagulase in Staphylococcal Infections, *Brit. J. Exper. Path.* 28:57, 1947.

Staphylococcal Infections (Conference), *Ann. New York Acad. Sc.* 65:57, 1956.

Surgalla, M. J., and *G. M. Dack,* Enterotoxin Produced by Micrococci from Cases of Enteritis after Antibiotic Therapy, *J.A.M.A.* 158:649, 1955.

Tager, M., and *H. B. Hales,* Quantitative Coagulase and Toxin Production by Staphylococci in Relation to the Clinical Source of the Organisms, *Yale J. Biol. & Med.* 20:41, 1947.

STREPTOCOCCIC INFECTIONS

Bernardin, R. M., M. A. Fyala, and *A. C. LaBoccetta,* Scarlet Fever: Diagnostic Value of the Dick Test, White Blood Cell Counts, Throat Cultures and Desquamation, *Am. J. Dis. Child.* 78:314, 1949.

Breese, B. B., Treatment of Beta Hemolytic Streptococcic Infections in the Home: Relative Value of Available Methods, *J.A.M.A.* **152**:10, 1953.

—— and *F. A. Disney*, The Accuracy of Diagnosis of Beta Streptococcal Infections on Clinical Grounds, *J. Pediat.* **44**:670, 1954.

Cook, G. T., W. H. H. Jebb, and *R. Knox*, Serological Grouping of 2662 Consecutive Strains of Beta-haemolytic Streptococci, *Month. Bull. Min. Health* **8**:214, 1949.

Denny, F. W., L. W. Wannamaker, and *E. O. Hahn*, Comparative Effects of Penicillin, Aureomycin and Terramycin on Streptococcal Tonsillitis and Pharyngitis, *Pediatrics* **11**:7, 1953.

Dick, G. F., and *G. H. Dick*, A Skin Test for Susceptibility to Scarlet Fever, *J.A.M.A.* **82**:265, 1924.

Evans, A. C., and *A. L. Chinn*, The Enterococci: With Special Reference to Their Association with Human Disease, *J. Bact.* **54**:495, 1947.

Finland, M., C. Wilcox, and *P. F. Frank*, In Vitro Sensitivity of Human Pathogenic Strains of Streptococci to Seven Antibiotics, *Am. J. Clin. Path.* **20**:208, 1950.

Gordon, J. E., and *J. H. Janney*, Antistreptolysin Content of the Sera of Normal Infants and Children, *J. Pediat.* **18**:587, 1941.

Griffith, F., The Serological Classification of *Streptococcus pyogenes*, *J. Hyg.* **34**:542, 1934.

Kwantes, W., and *J. R. E. James*, Hemolytic Streptococci on the Neonatal Umbilicus, *Brit. M. J.* **2**:576, 1956.

Lancefield, R. C., A Serological Differentiation of Human and Other Groups of Hemolytic Streptococci, *J. Exper. Med.* **57**:571, 1933.

Laurell, G., Airborne Infections. IV. The Control of Dustborne Streptococcal Infections in Children's Wards, *Acta paediat.* **37**:237, 1949.

Loosli, C. G., M. H. D. Smith, J. Cline, and *L. Nelson*, The Transmission of Hemolytic Streptococcal Infections in Infant Wards with Special Reference to "Skin Dispersers," *J. Lab. & Clin. Med.* **36**:342, 1950.

McCarty, M. (ed.), "Streptococcal Infections," Columbia University Press, New York, 1954.

Rantz, L. A., J. M. Di Caprio, and *E. Randall*, Antistreptolysin O and Antihyaluronidase Titers in Health and in Various Diseases, *Am. J. M. Sc.* **224**:194, 1952.

——, *M. Maroney*, and *J. M. Di Caprio*, Antistreptolysin O Response Following Hemolytic Streptococcus Infection in Early Childhood, *A.M.A. Arch. Int. Med.* **87**:360, 1951.

——, ——, and ——, Hemolytic Streptococcal Infection in Childhood, *Pediatrics* **12**:498, 1953.

Rhoads, P. S., G. Y. Youmans, and *R. Rosi*, Duration of the Infection in Scarlet Fever, *Ann. Int. Med.* **32**:30, 1950.

Stoppelman, M. R., Antihyaluronidase Content of Serum in Children Suffering from Hemolytic Streptococcal Infections, Rheumatic Fever and Other Diseases, *Acta paediat.* **39**:510, 1950.

Streptokinase—Streptodornase, *J.A.M.A.* **151**:1290, 1953.

Ström, J., Penicillin Treatment and Immunity to Scarlatina, *Acta paediat.* **43**:267, 1954.

Swift, H., The Streptococci, chap. 12 in R. J. Dubos (ed.), "Bacterial and Mycotic Infections of Man," 2d ed., J. B. Lippincott Company, Philadelphia, 1952.

Tunevall, G., Antistreptolysin Titre in School Children, *Acta paediat.* **35**:218, 1948.

Wehrle, P. F., H. A. Feldman, and *K. Kuroda*, Effect of Penicillins V and G on Carriers of Various Groups of Streptococci in a Children's Home, *Pediatrics* **19**:208, 1957.

Wheeler, S. M., and *G. E. Foley*, Serologic Types of Hemolytic Streptococci Isolated from Scarlet Fever in Massachusetts, 1942–1943, *New England J. Med.* **231**:287, 1944.

RHEUMATIC FEVER

Blount, R., J. A. Orbison, A. P. Long, and *G. N. Schumann,* An Epidemic of Rheumatic Fever in Japan and South Korea, *U.S. Armed Forces Med. J.* 3:43, 1952.

Diehl, A. M., T. R. Hamilton, I. C. Keeling, and *J. S. May,* Long-acting Repository Penicillin in Prophylaxis of Recurrent Rheumatic Fever, *J.A.M.A.* 155:1466, 1954.

Good, R. A., and *D. Glick,* Mucolytic Enzyme Systems. IX. Nonspecific Hyaluronidase Inhibitor in Rheumatic Fever, *J. Infect. Dis.* 86:38, 1950.

Harris, S., and *T. N. Harris,* Serologic Response to Streptococcal Hemolysin and Hyaluronidase in Streptococcal and Rheumatic Infection, *J. Clin. Invest.* 29:351, 1950.

Harris, T. N., Studies on the Relation of the Hemolytic Streptococcus to Rheumatic Fever. I. Review of Serologic Literature, *Am. J. Dis. Child.* 76:411, 1949.

—— and *S. Harris,* Studies in the Relation of the Hemolytic Streptococcus Infection to Rheumatic Fever. V. Streptococcal Anti-hyaluronidase (Mucin-clot-prevention) Titers in the Sera of Patients with Rheumatic Fever, Streptococcal Infection and Others, *Am. J. M. Sc.* 217:174, 1949.

——, ——, and *R. L. Nagle,* Studies in the Relation of the Hemolytic Streptococcus to Rheumatic Fever. VI. Comparison of Streptococcal Antihyaluronidase with Antibodies to Other Streptococcal Antigens in the Serum of Patients with Rheumatic Fever and Acute Streptococcal Infection: Mucin Clot Prevention Test, *Pediatrics* 3:482, 1949.

Kelley, V. C., Acute Phase Reactants. I. Serum Nonglucosamine Polysaccharides in Patients with Rheumatic Fever and Related Conditions, *J. Pediat.* 40:405, 1952.

——, *R. A. Good,* and *I. McQuarrie,* Serum Mucoproteins in Children in Health and Disease with Special Reference to Rheumatic Fever, *Pediatrics* 5:824, 1950.

McCarty, M., Present State of Knowledge Concerning Pathogenesis and Treatment of Rheumatic Fever, *Bull. New York Acad. Med.* 28:307, 1952.

Quinn, R. W., S. J. Liao, and *J. P. Quinn,* Antistreptolysin "O," Antihyaluronidase and Streptococcal Agglutinin Titers in Seventh and Eighth Grade School Children from Two Connecticut Cities: A Serological and Environmental Study, *Am. J. Hyg.* 54:331, 1951.

Rammelkamp, C. H., L. W. Wannamaker, and *F. W. Denny,* The Epidemiology and Prevention of Rheumatic Fever, *Bull. New York Acad. Med.* 28:321, 1952.

Roberts, E., Use of Sulfonamides and Penicillin to Prevent Recurrence of Rheumatic Fever, *A.M.A. Am. J. Dis. Child.* 85:643, 1953.

Statements of American Heart Association Council on Rheumatic Fever and Congenital Heart Disease, *J.A.M.A.* 151:141, 1953.

Stollerman, G. H., The Prevention of Rheumatic Fever by the Use of Antibiotics, *Bull. New York Acad. Med.* 31:165, 1955.

Taran, L. M., and *J. M. Jablon,* Eight Years Experience with the Hemolytic Streptococcus Group A, in a Rheumatic Colony of Children, *Bull. St. Francis Sanatorium* 8:1, 1951.

Waksman, B. H., The Etiology of Rheumatic Fever: A Review of Theories and Evidence, *Medicine* 28:143, 1949.

Ziegra, S. R., and *A. G. Kuttner,* Reappearance of Abnormal Laboratory Findings in Rheumatic Patients Following Withdrawal of ACTH or Cortisone, *Am. J. M. Sc.* 222:516, 1951.

TETANUS

Press, E., Desirability of the Routine Use of Tetanus Toxoid, *New England J. Med.* 239:50, 1948.

Spivey, O. S., C. G. Grulee, Jr., and *B. T. Hickman,* Tetanus Neonatorum, *J. Pediat.* 42:345, 1953.

Stafford, E. S., T. B. Turner, and L. Goldman, On the Permanence of Anti-tetanus Immunization, Ann. Surg. 140:563, 1954.

Turner, T. B., E. S. Stafford, and L. Goldman, Studies on the Duration of Protection Afforded by Active Immunization against Tetanus, Bull. Johns Hopkins Hosp. 94:204, 1954.

Wohltmann, H. J., Clinical Conference, St. Louis Children's Hospital: A Case of Tetanus, J. Pediat. 43:220, 1953.

TUBERCULOSIS

Anderson, H. W., R. V. Platou, and S. Spatafora, Middlebrook-Dubos Hemagglutination Reaction: Study of the Test in Children, Pediatrics 8:498, 1951.

Bailey, W. H., Resistance of Mycobacterium tuberculosis to Chemotherapeutic Agents, Am. J. Clin. Path. 21:241, 1951.

Buhler, V. B., and A. Pollak, Human Infection with Atypical Acid-fast Organisms: Report of Two Cases with Pathologic Findings, Am. J. Clin. Path. 23:363, 1953.

Cohen, A. C., and G. C. Glinsky, Virulence of Isoniazid-resistant Tubercle Bacilli in Man, Am. J. M. Sc. 230:70, 1955.

Feldman, W. H., D. W. Hutchison, V. M. Schwarting, and A. G. Karlson, Juvenile Tuberculosis Infection, Possibly of Avian Type, Am. J. Path. 25:1183, 1949.

Ferebee, S. H., and F. W. Appel, Resistance to Streptomycin of Tubercle Bacilli Isolated from Patients Treated with Streptomycin, Pub. Health Rep. 66:277, 1951.

Josiukas, A., T. E. Roy, and G. Boyd, The Middlebrook-Dubos Hemagglutination Test for Tuberculosis in Children and Adults, J. Clin. Invest. 33:1415, 1954.

Levin, B. M., H. Kaufman, and J. De La Huerga, Gamma Globulin Studies in Tuberculosis in Children, A.M.A. Am. J. Dis. Child. 83:26, 1952.

Middlebrook G., Antigens of Tubercle Bacillus Involved in Hemagglutination and Hemolysis Reactions, Bull. New York Acad. Med. 28:474, 1952.

Mullahy, M. E., Detection of Acid-fast Bacilli, Am. J. Clin. Path. 20:672, 1950.

Peden, V. H., K. E. Vincent, and E. Rich, The Use of Serial Hemagglutination Tests in Following the Course of Tuberculosis in Children, Pediatrics 14:340, 1954.

Riley, E. A., Chemotherapy of Tuberculosis, Am. J. M. Sc. 226:552, 1953.

Segard, E. C., G. E. Thompson, Acid-fast Bacilli as Contaminants, Am. J. Clin. Path. 22:294, 1952.

Shane, S. J., J. H. Laurie, C. Riley, and M. Boutilier, Effect of Combined Therapy (Dihydrostreptomycin and PAS) on the Emergence of Streptomycin-resistant Strains of Tubercle Bacilli, New England J. Med. 246:132, 1952.

Soltys, M. A., C. A. St. Hill, and I. Ansell, "Tubercle Bacillus and Laboratory Methods in Tuberculosis," E. & S. Livingstone, Ltd., London, 1952.

Symposium on Tuberculosis in Infancy and Childhood, Am. Rev. Tuberc. vol. 74, no. 2, pt. 2, 1956.

Timpe, A., and E. H. Runyon, The Relationship of "Atypical" Acid-fast Bacteria to Human Disease: A Preliminary Report, J. Lab. & Clin. Med. 44:202, 1954.

Weed, L. A., Introduction: Symposium on Laboratory Diagnostic Methods in Tuberculosis, Am. J. Clin. Path. 21:673, 1951.

CHAPTER 71

The Spirochetal Infections

SYPHILIS

Darkfield Microscopy

In severe cases of congenital syphilis, before treatment is instituted, it is sometimes feasible to find *Treponema pallidum* in darkfield preparations of skin lesions or of scrapings from the wall of the umbilical vein. The procedure is the same as with the study of chancres in adults. Material from mucous membrane ulcerations are often contaminated by the nonpathogenic spirochetes *T. microdentium, T. macrodentium, T. vincenti,* or *T. buccale,* which are similar in appearance to *T. pallidum* and may be confused with it. As a general rule, spirochetes are not discoverable in lesions of congenital syphilis except when serologic responses and roentgenologic osseous changes are well marked and unmistakable. It is useless to search for spirochetes in any lesion once therapy with an antibiotic has been begun.

Exudate from the surface of a chancre-like lesion is preferably collected in the laboratory and examined immediately for spirochetes by the darkfield method. If the patient is seen elsewhere, the exudate may be aspirated into a capillary glass tube. After the ends are sealed with drug-free petroleum jelly, the tube may be sent unhurriedly to the laboratory, even through the mails. *T. pallidum* is demonstrable on the surface of a primary lesion in abundance during the first 2 weeks and with diminishing frequency thereafter as the serologic reactivity begins to rise. Gloves should be worn when collecting specimens from acute skin or mucous membrane lesions for darkfield microscopy in order to protect the examiner from accidental infection.

T. pallidum is recognizable morphologically by the tightly wound regular coils, the rotation on its long axis like a corkscrew, the slow forward and backward movements, and the tendency to bend its body most often near the middle. All *T. pallidum* in a single preparation are more or less uniform in size, shape, and motility, whereas nonpathogenic spirochetes exhibit wide variations in these characteristics.

853

Serologic Testing

Serodiagnostic tests for syphilis depend upon the occurrence in serum or cerebrospinal fluid of *reagin*—a nonspecific globulin component which is capable of flocculating alcohol-soluble *lipid antigens* from beef heart and other mammalian tissues under suitable test conditions. With the precipitation or flocculation techniques the floccules become grossly visible; with the complement-fixation techniques, the floccules, too small to be seen, evidence their presence by absorbing or fixing complement. Cholesterol and lecithin are usually added to the test mixtures in order to facilitate the reactions.

By adjusting the technical conditions, serum from practically every normal person can be made to react with these lipid antigens. The difference in reactivity between nonsyphilitic and syphilitic serums appears to be of degree rather than of kind—quantitative rather than qualitative. In diseases other than spyhilis the circulating reactive substance is sometimes augmented also—probably in association with excess production of globulins. The so-called standard tests have their components so balanced as to give a minimum of positive reactions with serums from nonsyphilitic individuals and a maximum with serums from those who are syphilitic. An important recent advance has been the extraction from alcoholic extracts of beef heart of the complex of phosphatidic acids known as cardiolipin. The advantages of the cardiolipin-containing antigens are stability, reproducibility, and fewer nonsyphilitic-postive reactions.

All of the serologic methods for testing for syphilis are based upon interactions of biologic substances—reagin, beef heart lipid extracts, cardiolipin, complement. All require meticulous efforts to achieve standardization, "ripening," and exact titration. Every good serologic laboratory continually (1) verifies positive and doubtful readings by rechecks with a second technique (usually a complement-fixation test when the first reading is with a flocculation test, and vice versa), (2) exchanges specimens with reference laboratories or other laboratories of excellent reputation, (3) correlates the results of tests with clinical observations in a well-run clinic for syphilis.

Apart from a number of individualized techniques performed chiefly in the laboratories of their originators, the accepted methods for qualitative serologic testing in the United States include the following flocculation procedures: APHA (American Public Health Association) reference test, Eagle tests, Hinton tests, Kahn tests, Kline tests, Mazzini tests, Rein-Bossak tests, the VDRL (Venereal Disease Research Laboratory) tests, and also the Kolmer-Wassermann complement-fixation tests. Each method has its merits and disadvantages from the viewpoints of sensitivity, specificity, and technical conduct. Since all are based upon the same physicochemical phenomenon the dissimilarities among them are essentially minor.

Results are often reported under the generic term *serologic test for syphilis,* abbreviated STS, without the name of the exact procedure employed being given. The flocculation tests are easier to carry out and more widely utilized. When two different tests are deemed necessary to authenticate any results obtained, it is customary to carry out both a flocculation and a complement-fixation test. For screening of large population groups, quick tests of excessively high sensitivity—"presumptive" or "exclusion" tests—are often employed to rule out the completely negative reactors. All serums with weak or positive reactivity with these methods must be retested by a less sensitive but more dependable method.

REACTIVITY. Except when the attending syphilologist explicitly requests otherwise, reports from most laboratories are phrased as "reactive," "weakly reactive," or "nonreactive." Reactive (positive) means that a complete reaction was given by a standard test, and nonreactive (negative) means the opposite. Weakly reactive (doubtful) signifies that an incomplete reaction was given by the serum specimen or that several techniques coincidentally employed gave conflicting results. Since weakly reactive readings correspond to the lowest unitage in the quantitative procedures, it is pointless to seek verification of such a report by requesting titrations from the same individual. The responses with weakly reactive serums may be inconstant even in the same laboratory on consecutive days, as the result of slight variations in the patient's status or the potency of the reagents.

Quantitative methods of assay measure either (1) the least amount of complement, (2) the smallest amount of antigen, or (3) the least amount of serum needed to give a positive reaction. The standard quantitative Kahn technique, for example, employs serial serum dilutions of 1:2, 1:4, 1:8, 1:16, 1:32, 1:64, and higher, if necessary. In reporting results of quantitative titrations it has been recommended that the endpoint titer be reported in terms of the greatest dilution in which the tested specimen produces a reactive (positive) result and that the term *dils,* a contraction of the word dilution, be used to identify these dilution reactivity end points. Differences in positivity of no more than one or two dilutions in successive tests with any of these methods cannot be deemed significant.

NONSYPHILITIC POSITIVE REACTIVITY. Erroneous apparent reactivity may result from inadequately cleaned glassware, careless collection of blood resulting in foaming, contamination, or hemolysis, or errors in technical performance of the test.

Nonsyphilitic individuals occasionally show some reactive substance in the serum as an aftereffect of a recent infection or other ailment. The occurrence of such positive reactivity among normal individuals in routine surveys has ranged from 1 in 700 to 1 in several thousand, depending in part upon the character and state of health of the population and the specificity of the test employed. Of special importance to pediatrics are the newborn infants in whom reagin is transferred across the placenta to a nonsyphilitic child from a treated (or perhaps untreated) syphilitic mother (see below).

Positive reactions to the tests for syphilis are found in 50 per cent or more of patients with the other treponemal diseases—pinta, bejel, yaws. Positive or doubtful reactions may be encountered in leprosy (40 to 60 per cent of patients); malaria (20 to 100 per cent); vaccinia (4 to 40 per cent); rat-bite fevers, relapsing fever, leptospirosis, infectious hepatitis, primary atypical pneumonia, and infectious mononucleosis (up to 30 per cent). Positive responses are found occasionally (2 to 5 per cent) in pulmonary tuberculosis; the exanthemata; acute bacterial infections including pneumonia, scarlet fever, and the common cold; malignant tumors; after injections of vaccines; and in other infections and intoxications. Positive reactivity caused by these illnesses usually lasts 3 weeks to 3 months and rarely more than 6 months. The reactivity with cardiolipin-containing antigens is more likely to be negative or of lower titer than with other antigens.

The childhood population of many Central American countries exhibits an approximately 15 per cent incidence of nonsyphilitic positive reactions with the Kahn and Mazzini flocculation tests which use lipid antigens. With the VDRL, Kline, and Rein-Bossak flocculation tests which utilize cardiolipin antigens, and the Kolmer complement-fixation test with either lipid or cardiolipin antigens, the incidence of such nonspecific positive reactions is only 2 to 5 per cent.

Polyarteritis nodosa, rheumatoid arthritis, rheumatic fever, and disseminated lupus erythematosus occasionally give rise to persistent serologic reactivity—"biologic false positive" (BFP). In fact, nonsyphilitic patients with disseminated lupus erythematosus may exhibit positive serologic reactivity for one or more years before the lupus erythematosus becomes recognizable clinically.

Another approach to differentiating nonsyphilitic reactivity from that due to syphilis is by repeated quantitative tests. Nonsyphilitic positive reactions tend to exhibit a well-defined curve of rise and fall in titer in specimens taken week after week, whereas the syphilis curve is more stable or fluctuates erratically.

A "weak" reaction in a child having no known history of syphilis is usually of nonsyphilitic origin. This should be confirmed by negative results of tests on the parents, normal physical and x-ray findings, and a negative reading when the test is repeated several weeks or months later.

Acquired Syphilis

Acquired syphilis in early childhood may result from asexual contact with some adult ill with secondary syphilis. Extragenital chancres arising under these conditions are usually small and may escape detection. Whenever such a case is encountered the source of the contagion must be tracked down. All other children in the household should be studied by repeated examinations and serologic tests for 3 months from the last known exposure.

The incubation period of a chancre is usually about 3 weeks after contact. In untreated cases, serum reactivity becomes detectable about 1 week after the chancre begins. It rises during the ensuing month, to reach and remain at an approximate plateau for the next 2 years or longer while the secondary stage runs its course with recurrent lesions of skin and mucous membranes. The level then subsides slowly and eventually disappears in an estimated 25 per cent of patients with untreated late syphilis.

The contour and height of the reactivity curve during the secondary and later phases of syphilis differ widely from patient to patient. A single quantitative estimation is of no value as a measure of the severity of the illness, the degree of immunity, or the prognosis.

Every child who has been treated for acquired syphilis should be examined regularly thereafter, and a quantitative serologic test made at each visit. It often takes many months for the readings to return to a nonreactive level. Should the titer fail to drop or clinical evidences of relapse appear, another course of therapy may be administered according to the judgment of the attending physician. One must remember that in latent or treated syphilis an intercurrent infection can bring about a transitory rise in titer.

Congenital Syphilis

This disease varies greatly in clinical severity. Sometimes the symptoms are prominent at birth, suggesting that the fetus was infected early and heavily and that opposing immune influences were scanty or absent. More often, however, the neonatal infant appears superficially normal and syphilis is not detectable until a positive serology report or later signs and symptoms disclose its existence. In 85 per cent of infants with congenital syphilis the serologic tests are reactive at birth, and in nearly all the remainder the serum will become reactive or signs of disease will become apparent before the age of 4 months.

The earlier the diagnosis of congenital syphilis can be established and treatment begun, the better the prospects for complete cure and achievement of seronegativity. Penicillin is deemed the most satisfactory therapeutic agent for congenital syphilis at this writing, though some other antibiotics seem effective also.

Even though clinical evidences of healing become apparent within a few days after penicillin treatment is begun, serum reactivity does not begin to decline until after a few months, more rapidly with infants than with older children. Serologic reversals are lowest in patients with clinical neurosyphilis. About half of the treated children who become seronegative after penicillin do so during the first posttreatment year, about 75 per cent during the second year, and about 90 per cent by 2½ years. The remainder may remain seropositive indefinitely.

Seronegativity is attained ultimately by about 85 per cent of children who are under 2 years of age at the beginning of treatment, by about 40 per cent of those between 2 and 4 years, but by less than 10 per cent of those over 4 years. Once serologic nonreactivity is attained there is almost no likelihood of relapse.

Children who retain serum reactivity after all clinical evidences of active syphilis have been eradicated by energetic treatment are known as seroresistant. Those who were under 2 years of age at the beginning of treatment usually have weak quantitative titers, such as 4 units or less. Titers up to 15 units or more are not infrequent in seroresistant children who were between 2 and 4 years of age at the beginning of treatment, and up to 128 units in those above 4 years of age.

Newborn Infants Born to Syphilitic Mothers

Treatment during pregnancy in order to protect the infant is not thought necessary for syphilitic women who have had adequate treatment prior to pregnancy and who have lost their seroreactivity. Treatment is also not recommended for adequately treated mothers with seroresistance, particularly when the syphilis is late and the titer remains low in repeated tests. Additional treatment is advised for pregnant women whose serologic responses to previous therapy have been unsatisfactory or when there is doubt as to their remaining under close observation during this pregnancy. Women whose syphilis is congenital or acquired in early childhood almost never transmit the disease to their offspring.

When an infant's serologic reactivity is due to passive transfer of maternal reagin, his titer will be approximately the same as that of his mother. Approximately 70 per cent of such infants become seronegative in the first month, and the remainder before the fourth or fifth month. On the other hand, when the infection was contracted in utero and eradicated by penicillin given during the last months of pregnancy, the infant titer may be considerably higher than that of the mother.

Every infant born to a treated or untreated syphilitic mother should receive a serologic test at least once monthly for 4 months. These should be quantitative whenever reactivity is present. A spontaneously decreasing titer and absent physical findings should lead one to withhold treatment and trust that complete disappearance of the seroreactivity will establish the absence of the disease. Contrariwise, a rapid appearance of reagin in the first few months after the cord blood has been negative, or a sudden rise in titer in blood already reactive, is suggestive of active infection. Roentgenography in such circumstances may reveal bone changes of congenital syphilis. As a rule, however, seroreactivity usually precedes the appearance of clinical symptoms. Therapy should be begun as soon as the diagnosis is clear, even if there are no confirmatory skin eruptions or x-ray bone changes.

Nonsyphilitic seroreactivity sometimes arises in early infancy after injections of immunizing vaccines or after vaccinia, chickenpox, or other acute infections. This reactivity deviates from that of true syphilis in being of comparatively low titer and fades away spontaneously after a few weeks or months.

Serologic Problems

The final decision as to whether or not serologic reactivity means the existence of syphilis rests on evaluation of the total evidence. Seroreactivity in a child who seems clinically well and has no history indicative of syphilis, or who has had a recent acute illness, should be studied further. Beyond infancy, the few weeks required for verification procedures will not alter the prognosis materially. If the serologic reading is of very low titer, the probability is much against syphilis being present. If the reactivity subsides spontaneously in tests repeated at weekly or biweekly intervals and physical examinations are negative, syphilis can be safely ruled out. If the reactivity persists, serial quantitative tests should be made to determine the trend of change in titer, if any. The development of seroreactivity in an infant with an initially negative test is much more suggestive of congenital syphilis than is seroreactivity demonstrable at birth. The treponemal immunization test (see below) should always be applied to the study of questionable cases, provided arrangements can be made for its performance. The tests for syphilis should be repeated with other methods and in other laboratories. Inquiry should be made as to whether antibiotic therapy has been given briefly in the past for some acute infection, since that may temporarily depress syphilis and its serologic titer. Roentgenograms of the long bones in infants can provide helpful diagnostic information.

In every study for syphilis, at least one serologic examination of the cerebrospinal fluid should be made to determine the presence or absence of asymptomatic neurosyphilis, except when one is reasonably sure that the patient's serum reactivity is nonsyphilitic.

Treponemal Immobilization Test (TPI Test)

This procedure, developed by Nelson and Mayer in 1949, is based on the finding that serums from syphilitic animals or humans contains a truly specific antibody which in the presence of complement will immobilize suspensions of live *Treponema pallidum* organisms. The immobilizing antibody has been shown by absorption techniques to be different and distinct from that which gives reagin activity in syphilitic serums.

In acquired syphilis the immobilizing antibody appears in the serum in 5 to 15 days after the beginning of a chancre, coinciding with the development of the reagin antibody. The titer rises rapidly, reaches a plateau in 2 to 3 months, and then persists indefinitely, as a rule, unless treatment is begun in the primary or early secondary phases of the infection. It disappears from the blood more slowly than the reagin antibody. In congenital syphilis a positive reaction is present at birth. Positive findings in a treated patient do not necessarily signify a need for further therapy.

Positive reactions are found very infrequently in normal subjects or those with nontreponemal diseases. Cross reactions may be given with the other treponematoses such as pinta, bejel, and yaws. The cerebrospinal fluid may show the antibody in neurosyphilis.

The immobilization test is utilized mainly for differentiating serologic reactivity due to syphilis itself from the so-called biologic false positive reactivity encountered occasionally with the more usual techniques in nonsyphilitic patients ill with other diseases. The test is useful also in detecting the presence of acquired syphilis in the minority of patients who have the disease in a late stage but whose blood is nonreactive to tests for reagin.

In performing the procedure, all steps including the collection of the initial specimen require perfect asepsis. A fresh treponemal suspension prepared from syphilomas of rabbits infected with the Nichols strain, 1.7 ml in volume, is mixed in a test tube with 0.2 ml of serum to be tested and 0.1 ml of complement obtained from guinea pigs. Controls are tested simultaneously. The tubes are incubated at 35°C in Brewer anaerobic jars with 5 per cent carbon dioxide and 95 per cent nitrogen. The percentage of motile organisms is determined by examining 50 successive treponemes for microscopic motility at the end of 16 hours. If specific antibodies are present in the serum the majority of the spirochetes will be immobilized and killed as well. At the termination of each test failing to produce immobilization, the contents are tested to establish the presence of active complement and eliminate the possibility of false negative results. Serum for testing should be obtained before antibiotics are administered, since trace amounts of these can also inactivate spirochetes.

The procedure is complicated and subject to numerous technical pitfalls and requires infected rabbits to supply the living treponemes. The test has therefore been limited thus far to a handful of experimental laboratories, to which specimens should be submitted. If it can be simplified satisfactorily, however, it may ultimately replace the "standard" serologic tests which utilize lipid antigens to detect nonspecific reagin.

Newer procedures related to *T. pallidum* immobilization (TPI) are *T. pallidum* immune adherence (TPIA) and *T. pallidum* agglutination (TPA). As antigens the two latter procedures utilize killed treponemes, which can be stored under refrigeration for months.

Endemic Syphilis

Spread through unclean childhood populations by nonvenereal routes, this form of the disease occurs almost exclusively in tropical and Eastern Mediterranean areas. Secondary and tertiary (gummatous) lesions are frequent, whereas primary lesions are usually not seen. Activity appears to die out before adult life.

Table 71-1. Pathogenic Spirochetes and Resultant Diseases

Parasite	Vector	Disease
Treponema		
pallidum	Human beings	Syphilis
pertenue	Human beings	Yaws
carateum	Human beings	Pinta
Leptospira		
icterohemorrhagiae	Rodents	Weil's disease
canicola	Dogs	Canicola fever
pomona	Pigs, calves	Swineherd's disease
grippotyphosa	Rodents	Water fever; mud fever
hebdomadis	Mice, voles	Seven-day fever
autumnalis		Pretibial fever
mitis	Pigs	
suis	Pigs	
bovis	Cattle	
ballum	Mice	
bataviae	Rats, mice, mongooses	
alexi	Rats	
Borrelia		
recurrentis	Ticks, lice	Relapsing fever
vincenti		Stomatitis
muris (*Spirillum*		
minus)	Rodents	Rat-bite fever

LEPTOSPIROSIS

Numerous distinct strains of species of Leptospira have been identified as etiologic causes of acute human illnesses (Table 71-1). Weil's disease, caused by *Lept. icterohemorrhagiae,* is transmitted to man through contact with water such as sewer water which has been contaminated with the urine of infected rats, mice, dogs, or voles. Canicola fever, spread by dogs infected with *Lept. canicola,* is uncommon, but may be contracted by contact with the dog's saliva or urine. A serious form of leptospirosis may spread through dairy herds, though human infection from contaminated milk apparently does not occur.

Clinical Manifestations

Fever and malaise are the usual symptoms and typically last 1 to 2 weeks. These symptoms are often mistaken for influenza or may be so mild as to be ignored. Hepatomegaly with or without jaundice is often noted. A tendency to spontaneous hemorrhages is almost as common; this appears to be due primarily to capillary injury since the known blood-coagulation factors show little or no change.

Many patients exhibit a mild aseptic meningitis with headache, stiff neck, and minor cerebrospinal fluid changes. These begin early. The protein content of the cerebrospinal fluid tends to be slightly elevated and the sugar content normal. The cell count is between 10 and 300 per cu mm, with lymphocytes predominant. Live leptospirae are sometimes demonstrable. Distinctive is an icteric tint if the patient is jaundiced, since in most jaundiced patients with meningeal disturbances the bile pigments do not penetrate the cerebrospinal fluid.

Iritis, iridocyclitis, or chorioretinitis develops not infrequently in 1 to 8 months after the systemic infection has run its course. The eye lesions are ophthalmologically indistinguishable from those encountered in tuberculosis, syphilis, and nonspecific uveitis. The leptospiral origin may be suspected from the clinical history, but laboratory confirmation in the form of abnormally high antibody titers in the serologic tests should be sought for. One case has been reported in which puncture of the anterior chamber of the eye and aspiration and culture of the aqueous humor succeeded in recovering Leptospira organisms, later identfied as *Lept. alexi.*

Demonstration of Organisms

Leptospirae usually circulate in the patient's blood stream during the acute febrile phase of the illness.

When the infestation is severe a direct smear or darkfield preparation of the blood will sometimes show the organisms. As a rule, however, one has to resort to cultural or animal inoculation techniques for their demonstration.

In the hands of trained workers, direct cultures on proper media will be positive in the majority of cases, more often than will be animal inoculations. Cultures should be held for a full 28 days before being read as negative. All recovered strains are subcultured and identified by serologic tests.

For animal studies one may use young guinea pigs, hamsters, mice, or chick embryos. Darkfield examination of cultures of the heart blood of these animals, beginning 4 days after the inoculation, will frequently succeed in demonstrating the spirochetes if present. Most animals succumb within 2 weeks with generalized hemorrhages and jaundice. If not, they are killed.

Suspensions of livers and kidneys are then examined with the darkfield micro-scope or inoculated into culture media. Guinea pigs are relatively resistant to *Lept. canicola,* but young hamsters are susceptible.

Leptospirae are excreted in the urine of patients after the first week, and this may continue for a month or more. They can be seen by darkfield ex-amination if in abundance; otherwise cultures or animal inoculations are needed. The urine also tends to contain pus cells, hyaline casts, and protein. Oliguria or anuria with azotemia may be seen in severe cases. Permanent renal damage is rare. A sudden diuresis is an early sign of recovery.

Serum Antibodies

Specific antibodies against the causative leptospirae usually appear in the patient's serum in the second or third weeks of illness.

In the so-called agglutinin-lysin test, living or freshly formalinized leptospirae are mixed with the serum and the reaction followed microscopically. Agglutina-tion takes place first, followed by lysis. Titers of 1:100 or higher are deemed significant. Since cross agglutination among the various species is common, absorption procedures may be needed to determine the precise species. The agglutinin lysins reach their maximum in 3 to 8 weeks, remain at a high level between 1:400 and 1:100,000 for some months, and then subside to ap-proximately 1:300 where they may persist for many years. Therefore, when utilizing the serologic approach for establishing the diagnosis, one should test at least two serum specimens collected several weeks apart in order to detect any rise in titer. The agglutinin-lysin test is most useful in serologic surveys of human populations to detect the prevalence of past infections.

The complement-fixation reaction, which uses mechanically disintegrated leptospirae as the antigen, is a simpler procedure. Complement-fixing anti-bodies appear during the second or third weeks, earlier than the agglutinin lysin antibodies, but do not remain long after convalescence. A rise in titer to 1:32 or 1:256 from an initial 1:4 or 1:8 may be interpreted as positive. The com-plement-fixation test responds to a wide variety of leptospiral antigens. It is useful in the clinical recognition of active cases even though it may fail to identify the precise causative species.

Serial serum tests for leptospiral antibodies are indicated in all otherwise unexplained cases of meningeal inflammation with a lymphocytic pleocytosis, with the first test early in the illness. Some patients may show a rise in agglutinin-lysin antibodies but not in complement-fixing antibodies, and vice versa. Proven cases have been seen in which significant amounts of either anti-body have failed to develop.

Precise identification of leptospiral strains requires the employment of antibody absorption procedures, performed at a reference laboratory.

INFECTIONS CAUSED BY BORRELIA

Relapsing Fever

This acute infection characteristically gives rise to short bouts of fever and malaise recurring every 2 to 9 days. The causative organism may be *Borrelia (Treponema) recurrentis* or a biologically related spirochete. In the United States the disease is transmitted by infected ticks; in other parts of the world it may be spread either by ticks or the body louse *Pediculus humanus.*

Laboratory identification is accomplished by (1) direct demonstration of the parasites in the circulating blood during febrile periods in darkfield examination of stained thin or thick smears, or (2) injecting white mice with the patient's blood and later finding the spirochetes in the blood of the animals.

Vincent's Stomatitis

In this poorly defined disorder one frequently finds in the oral exudate both a large spirochete *Borrelia vincenti* and a Gram-negative fusiform bacillus *Bacillus fusiformis (Fusobacterium plaut-vincenti)*. The spirochetes are best demonstrated by darkfield illumination or by staining with dilute crystal violet. With the latter the coils are difficult to detect and the appearance is that of bent hairs. The fusiform bacilli, best brought out by Gram-staining or smears, have tapering pointed ends and usually occur in pairs.

Rat-bite Fevers. See page 816.

PINTA AND YAWS

The spirochetes which cause pinta (*Treponema carateum*) and yaws (*T. pertenue*) have the same morphologic appearances as the spirochete of syphilis (*T. pallidum*), even with the phase contrast or electron microscope approaches. Immunologically, also, the serologic responses which are induced—flocculation, complement fixation, and treponemal immobilization and agglutination—are not sufficiently unlike to be specifically diagnostic (Willcox). Differentiation rests upon clinical manifestations.

BIBLIOGRAPHY

SYPHILIS

Beerman, H., The Treponemal Immobilization Test, Am. J. M. Sc. **226**:425, 1953.
Bundesen, H. N., and *H. C. S. Aron,* How to Evaluate Positive Kahn Tests in Infants, J. Ven. Dis. Inform. **31**:185, 1950.
Chacko, C. W., The Clinical Value of the Treponema Immobilization Test in the Diagnosis and Control of Syphilis, J. Clin. Path. **6**:227, 1953.
Curtis, A. C., K. Kitchen, A. O'Leary, H. Rattner, C. R. Rein, G. Schoch, W. Shaffer, and *U. J. Wile,* Penicillin Treatment of Syphilis, J.A.M.A. **145**:1223, 1951.

Henchett, L. J., and *M. E. Perry,* Results of Penicillin Treatment in Congenital Syphilis, *J. Ven. Dis. Inform.* 31:277, 1950.

Ingraham, N. R., Jr., and *H. Beerman,* The Present Status of Penicillin in the Treatment of Syphilis in Pregnancy and Infantile Congenital Syphilis, *Am. J. M. Sc.* 219:433, 1950.

Ledbetter, R. K., Jr., The Treponema Immobilization Test: A Diagnostic Aid to the Clinician, *J.A.M.A.* 160:1392, 1956.

MacPherson, D. J., R. K. Ledbetter, Jr., and *V. E. Martens,* Test for Immobilization of *Treponema pallidum:* Correlation with Some of the Standard Serologic Tests for Syphilis, *Am. J. Clin. Path.* 25:89, 1955.

Manual of Serologic Tests for Syphilis, *Pub. Health Serv. Publ.* 411, 1955.

Moore, J. E., and *W. B. Lutz,* The Natural History of Systemic Lupus Erythematosus: An Approach to Its Study through Chronic Biologic False Positive Reactors, *J. Chron. Dis.* 1:297, 1955.

Moore, J. W., and *C. F. Mohr,* Biologically False Positive Serologic Tests for Syphilis: Type, Incidence and Cause, *J.A.M.A.* 150:467, 1952.

Nelson, N. A., and *V. R. Struve,* Prevention of Congenital Syphilis by Treatment of Syphilis in Pregnancy, *J.A.M.A.* 161:869, 1956.

Nelson, R. S., Jr., and *M. M. Mayer,* Immobilization of *Treponema pallidum* in Vitro by Antibody Produced in Syphilitic Infection, *J. Exper. Med.* 89:369, 1949.

Shaffer, L., and *C. Courville,* Effectiveness of Penicillin in the Prevention of Congenital Syphilis, *A.M.A. Arch. Dermat. & Syph.* 63:91, 1951.

Stout, G. W., and *J. C. Cutler,* Serology Problems (Syphilis) in Central America, *J. Ven. Dis. Inform.* 32:237, 1951.

Willcox, R. R., Treponemal Diseases of Children in the Tropics, *J. Trop. Pediatrics* 1:191, 1956.

Wolman, I. J., Positive Reactions to the Kahn Test for Syphilis; Their Incidence and Meaning in Healthy American Men: A Survey of 82,070 U.S. Maritime Service Enrollees, *Am. J. M. Sc.* 212:280, 1946.

LEPTOSPIROSIS

Beamer, P. R., Treatment of Leptospirosis with Antibiotics, *Ann. New York Acad. Sc.* 55:1195, 1952.

Chesney, G., Leptospira canicola in a Girl and Her Puppy, *Month. Bull. Min. Health* 10:78, 1951.

Coffey, J. H., I. Dravin, and *W. C. Dine,* Swineherd's Disease (Aseptic Meningitis) Due to *Leptospira pomona, J.A.M.A.* 147:949, 1951.

Gochenour, W. S., Jr., R. H. Yager, P. W. Wetmore, and *J. A. Hightower,* Laboratory Diagnosis of Leptospirosis, *Am. J. Pub. Health* 43:405, 1953.

Leroy, E. P., A. Goldman, M. Goldin, and *S. J. Bolonik,* Fatal Canicola Fever with Autopsy Findings, *Pediatrics* 9:20, 1952.

Schubert, J. H., and *D. S. Martin,* Evaluation of Serologic Tests for Leptospirosis, *J. Lab. & Clin. Med.* 48:155, 1956.

Wolff, J. W., "Laboratory Diagnosis of Leptospirosis," Charles C Thomas, Publisher, Springfield, Ill., 1954.

Woodward, T. E., R. S. Diaz Rivera, and *J. A. Hightower,* The Various Clinical Manifestations of Leptospirosis, *Bull. New York Acad. Med.* 29:642, 1953.

Yager, R. H., and *W. S. Gochenour, Jr.,* Current Problems in the Field of Leptospirosis, *Am. J. Pub. Health* 43:411, 1953.

CHAPTER 72

Infections Caused by Fungi

Superficial invasions of the skin or hair, commonly known as ringworm, are the most frequent fungal infections. Generalized invasions are referred to in terms of the respective organisms, such as histoplasmosis, coccidioidomycosis, and so on (Table 72-1).

Fungi may be sought for by direct microscopic examination of material from lesions, by mycologic cultures, by inspection of affected hairs for fluorescence under ultraviolet light, or by histologic study of biopsied tissue fragments. Sensitization of the host is demonstrable in a few of the diseases by acquired skin reactivity or by positive serologic responses to antigenic extracts of the fungi.

Table 72-1. Fungus Infections of Pediatric Importance in the United States

Disease	Usual site of involvement	Usual causative organism
Actinomycosis	Lung	*Actinomyces israeli*
Aspergillosis	Lung, ear	*Aspergillus fumigatus*
Blastomycosis	Skin, lung	*Blastomyces dermatitidis*
Coccidioidomycosis	Lung	*Coccidioides immitis*
Cryptococcosis	Meninges	*Cryptococcus neoformans*
Dermatomycosis (ringworm)	Scalp, skin	Microsporum (3 species)
		Trichophyton (11 species)
		Epidermophyton floccosum
Geotrichosis	Lung	Geotrichum, several species
Histoplasmosis	Generalized	*Histoplasma capsulatum*
Moniliasis	Mouth, nail bed	*Candida (Monilia) albicans*
Mucormycosis	Nose, viscera	Mucor
Nocardiosis	Lung, brain	*Nocardia asteroides*
Sporotrichosis	Skin, viscera	*Sporotrichum schenckii*
Tinea versicolor	Skin	*Malassezia (Microsporon) furfur*

Nonpathogenic fungi frequently contaminate the oral cavity and open skin lesions and may be found in the air of offices and hospital wards. Among them are species of Penicillium, Aspergillus, Monilia, Cephalosporium, Fusarium, Streptomyces, Cryptococcus, Ustilago, Alternaria, Nigrospora, Pullularia, Mucor, Rhizopus, etc. These often grow out on

866

media inoculated with material from lesions and may be mistaken for the cause of disease.

Serologic tests are unsatisfactory for the evaluation of most cases of fungus infection. Complement-fixing antibodies have been described in blastomycosis, coccidioidomycosis, histoplasmosis, moniliasis, and some others.

GENERAL PRINCIPLES OF LABORATORY EXAMINATION

Direct Microscopic Study

Material for examination may be taken from the mouth by a loop or swab; from the centers of affected patches in the hair or scalp by a forceps; or from infected skin or nails by scraping the edges of the lesions with a scalpel or edge of a glass slide after preliminary cleansing with 70 per cent alcohol. The suspected material is placed on a glass slide, and a drop of 10 per cent sodium or potassium hydroxide solution added. The slide is passed through a flame several times to destroy the epidermal structures (avoid overheating). A cover glass is then superimposed and pressed down. An inserted drop of methylene blue stain is sometimes helpful. The heat and alkali clear away much of the tissue and debris, giving to the fungus a refractile appearance which is readily seen in dim illumination. These unstained wet preparations are preferable for study for all fungi, except that *H. capsulatum* is best seen in Giemsa's stain, and *N. asteroides* with the standard Ziehl-Neelsen method. Whenever feasible, cultures and tissue biopsies for staining should be taken as well as slide preparations.

Robinson and associates recommend the use of an ink-potassium hydroxide solution for microscopic identification of fungi which cause superficial mycotic infections. Scrapings from lesions on the feet, crural areas, nails, or elsewhere are added to a few drops of a mixture of equal parts of 20 per cent potassium hydroxide solution and Parker Superchrome blue-black ink. After some minutes any spores or hyphae which are present will be stained and will stand out clearly.

Culture

Cultures may be planted on a variety of special media, depending on the requirements of the precise fungus being looked for. They are usually held at 25°C or room temperature. The usual media are Sabouraud's agar, thiamine-dextrose agar, cornmeal agar, Littman oxgall agar, gelatin, blood agar containing antibiotics, brain-heart infusion agar, and thioglycollate broth. Material for culture should be obtained sterilely whenever practical and planted promptly after collection. It is often helpful to first expose material being cultured for fungi to a solution containing bactericidal concentrations of both penicillin and streptomycin for several hours, in order to destroy coexisting bacteria. Since most fungi grow better at room temperature, whereas pathogenic bacteria require elevated temperatures, contamination of mycologic cultures by bacteria from human sources is not common. Most fungi grow aerobically, but Actinomyces thrives best in an anaerobic environment. Colonies are usually ready for examination after 10 to 20 days. Cultures should be held for a month before being discarded as negative because some fungi grow slowly.

Fungi differ in colony pattern, pigment production, and microscopic structure and arrangement of hyphae, spores, and related structures. Most well-equipped laboratories can recover a pathogenic fungus and recognize the general botanical class to which it belongs. For more precise identification the culture is forwarded to a mycologic department. Experience is needed to attach proper significance to rate, texture, and luxuriance of colony growth, sharpness of colony border, and relationship of the components under the low power of the microscope. Taxonomic recognition is based on gross appearances of the colonies (yeast, yeastlike, or filamentous), architecture of the filaments, types of spore produced (sexual or asexual), and locations, modes of formation, and appearances of these spores.

Handling of Specimens

When immediate examination is not feasible, suspected hairs and skin scales may be placed in a dry Petri dish or folded paper and sent to a reference laboratory for direct examination and culture. Tissue biopsies, pus from abscesses, scrapings from the edges of ulcers, and samples of peripheral blood, bone marrow, or cerebrospinal fluid may be sent in sterile vials or test tubes. If the laboratory is more than a few hours away, some of the infected matter should be planted on suitable media immediately and the cultures forwarded along with the specimen. Otherwise an overgrowth of saprophytes may invalidate the results. Pertinent information including the character of the disease suspected always should accompany the specimen. Pure cultures forwarded for identification should be sent in sturdy test tubes of standard size, plugged with cotton.

SPECIFIC MYCOSES

Most fungi enter the body through inhalation, or sometimes through the intestinal wall. Person-to-person spread is almost unknown. The usual pathogenic species are *Actinomyces bovis* or *israeli, Aspergillus fumigatus, Blastomyces dermatitidis* and *brasiliensis, Coccidioides immitis, Cryptococcus neoformans, Geotrichum candidum, Histoplasma capsulatum, Nocardia asteroides,* and *Sporotrichum Schenkii.*

Pulmonary lesions may be acute, subacute, or chronic and debilitating or asymptomatic. Differentiation must always be made from tuberculosis, bronchiectasis, bacterial pneumonitis, sarcoidosis, and related disturbances. Correct recognition rests upon (1) the exclusion of tuberculosis and other conditions by proper diagnostic procedures, (2) the repeated recovery of pathogenic fungi in smears or cultures of the bronchial secretions, and (3) when applicable, demonstration of positive serum or skin reactions (e.g., histoplasmin) with antigens from the presumptive organism.

Invasion of other viscera can take place by direct extension from the lungs and pleura or through hematogenous or lymphatic routes. Such systemic extensions tend to be chronic and progressive. Healing, when it occurs, tends to leave fibrous scars which may become partly calcified.

The widespread utilization of the broad-spectrum antibiotics for bacterial diseases has been followed by a significant increase in generalized and fatal infections caused by fungi, and especially *Candida albicans*. All patients with debilitating illnesses who are receiving these antibiotics should be watched carefully for early signs of fungal invasion.

Actinomycosis

This rare disease is usually caused by the human strain *Actinomyces israeli* and not infrequently by the bovine strain *Actinomyces bovis*. The latter has been recovered occasionally from the gums of apparently healthy individuals.

Lesions begin as stubborn progressive infections of the jaw, neck, lungs, chest wall, cecum, or appendiceal area. Since tuberculosis, nocardiosis, and actinomycosis may be similar clinically, all specimens studied for actinomyces should be studied simultaneously for tubercle bacilli and nocardia.

In infected material the colonies appear as gray or pale-yellow flecks known as *sulfur granules*. These are small bodies less than a millimeter in diameter.

Pus is spread over the bottom of a sterile Petri dish, diluted with salt solution if too thick, and inspected for granules with a hand lens. Suspicious granules or pus droplets are picked with a platinum loop and transferred to a glass slide, a few drops of 10 per cent sodium or potassium hydroxide solution added, and a cover slip superimposed and pressed down firmly. If the granules are hard, a drop of concentrated acetic acid may be introduced first for decalcifying.

The preparation is inspected microscopically under dim light for the presence of interlacing radiating mycelia which often have club-shaped hyaline-like formations at their periphery. The cover glass may then be removed, and the granules dried, rinsed, and stained with Gram stain to bring out the Gram-positive mycelia. Spores are not evident. In old granules the mycelia may be coated with pink-staining hyaline matter and be more clearly demonstrable with carbol fuchsin stain. Sulfur granules having this microscopic pattern are essentially pathognomonic for actinomycosis.

Cultures are made by inoculating emulsified granules or suspected exudate onto infusion broth, blood agar plates, Sabouraud's medium, and thioglycollate medium. These should be prepared in duplicate, placing one set anaerobically and the other aerobically at 37°C, except that the Sabouraud's cultures are kept at room temperature. *Actinomyces israeli* is anaerobic whereas Nocardia is aerobic. Israeli strains give rise to rough colonies on solid media, and bovis to smooth colonies. Animal inoculations to prove pathogenicity are usually unsuccessful.

Histologic studies of the wall of a chronic suppurative area will show chronic inflammation. Granules consisting of Gram-positive branching mycelia are present not uncommonly.

Aspergillosis

Aspergilli are saprophytic molds which are found everywhere, along with Penicillium and Mucor. Their spores contaminate food, exposed culture media, and open wounds. One species, *Aspergillus fumigatus*, can occasionally give rise to stubborn chronic granulomas in the skin, external ear, nasal sinuses, bronchi, or lungs.

The mycologic diagnosis is established by the finding of spores and mycelial fragments in the sputum or other discharges and by recovering the characteristic conidiophores and long spore chains in culture media. One must make sure that this rapidly growing fungus is not a contaminant concealing another truly pathogenic but slower growing fungus in the same specimen.

Blastomycosis

This infection, known also as North American blastomycosis, is uncommon in children. The causative fungus is *Blastomyces dermatitidis*, a rounded double-walled budding yeastlike organism. Its diameter is usually 8 to 10 μ, but small forms measuring only 2 to 4 μ which superficially resemble histoplasma are sometimes found in sputum or in human tissue at autopsy. On Sabouraud's medium at room temperature the fungus produces white filaments or hyphae which project above the surface.

Systemic blastomycosis usually begins in the respiratory tract. Granulomatous, suppurative, or necrotic lesions with foreign-body giant cells may appear subsequently in any part of the body, but are most frequent in the skin, lungs, and bones. The sputum ultimately becomes purulent and blood-streaked and shows the specific organism either extracellularly or inside giant cells or macrophages. The causative organism is often not demonstrable in tissue sections. The cutaneous blastomycosis which results from direct penetration of the organisms into the skin is found usually on an exposed part of the body and rarely spreads beyond the underlying subcutaneous tissue. Skin testing and complement-fixation reactions aid in establishing the diagnosis.

A fungal extract known as blastomycin is used for skin testing. Since a common antigen seems to be present, skin tests with blastomycin, coccidioidin, and histoplasmin should be performed simultaneously when a systemic mycosis is suspected. The extract related to the patient's disease will evoke the most pronounced reaction. The skin response to blasto-mycin usually remains positive after clinical cure.

COMPLEMENT FIXATION. Responses with an antigen prepared from *Bl. dermatitidis* are positive only while there is generalized tissue invasion. Reversal of a positive complement fixation to negative indicates inactivity of the disease. A positive skin response combined with a negative comple-ment fixation is a prognostically favorable sign.

Coccidioidomycosis

Coccidioides immitis grows in branching hyphae which break up into rounded thick-walled arthrospores which are dustlike, durable, and highly infectious. This fungus is prevalent in the arid regions of the Southwest-ern United States. Its particles are widely air-borne; when inhaled in quantity they can cause a primary infection of the lungs. Rarely, a break in the skin can give rise to a local infection. Malaise, fever, cough, chest pains, and aches in various parts of the body are common symptoms of the early or invasion stage. The sputum may be blood-tinged. Very often the entire illness terminates at this stage, after a few days.

In a minority of patients the pulmonary infection becomes prolonged and may simulate pulmonary tuberculosis. Roentgenography of the chest then shows diffuse infiltrations. Cavitations sometimes ensue. The red cell sedimentation rate is elevated, and mild leukocytosis is often present. Erythema nodosum or eosinophilia complicate about 20 per cent of the cases. As the lung lesions heal they leave calcifications which may be in-distinguishable roentgenologically from those caused by histoplasmosis, blastomycosis, or tuberculosis. Exceptionally coccidioidomycosis becomes progressive, spreading through the body and eventually leading to death, with specific meningitis as a frequent terminal development.

SKIN TEST. A positive skin response to the fungus extract coccidioidin typically develops within 2 to 7 weeks after the infection begins. This ma-terial is injected intradermally as 0.1 ml of a 1:1,000 or 1:10,000 solution. In sensitized individuals it gives a tuberculin-like reaction in 48 hours.

Skin reactivity, once acquired, may persist for years. Many residents in endemic areas exhibit a skin reaction in the absence of demonstrable signs of the disease, except perhaps for a residual pulmonary calcification. Newborn infants show a negative skin reaction, even when their mothers' tests are positive. Positive reactions in endemic areas have been noted with infants as young as 1 month of age. Repeated skin testing does not sensitize the skin of the patient or evoke the appearance of antibodies. Patients with a pronounced skin sensitivity to coccidioidin may also give a weakly positive skin reaction with histoplasmin or blastomycin.

COMPLEMENT FIXATION. A low complement-fixation titer, in general, means a minimal or past infection and may continue for years after all signs of activity of the disease have gone. A high or rising titer in successive examinations indicates a serious or progressive infection. A falling titer is a good prognostic sign. In newborn infants one may find such antibodies, derived from the mother by passive transfer. In most cases of coccidioidal meningitis the cerebrospinal fluid also contains specific complement-fixing antibodies.

RECOVERY OF ORGANISMS. *C. immitis* is sometimes culturable from the sputum, gastric contents, pus, biopsy tissue, or other body materials, using mycologic media. The procedure is hazardous, since air-borne spores may form.

Mice may be injected intraperitoneally or guinea pigs intratesticularly with questionable colonies or other infected materials. *C. immitis* when present leads to local lesions in a week or 10 days, followed by death. The exudates or tissues are then examined for typical spherules. Blastomyces also will infect these animals.

BIOPSY. Tissue studies can be carried out with unstained slide and cover-slip preparations containing a few drops of 10 per cent potassium or sodium hydroxide solution. The parasites, sometimes intracellular, appear as nonbudding thick-walled doubly refractile spherules 10 to 80 μ in diameter and filled with small rounded endospores.

According to Smith, the diagnosis of coccidioidomycosis cannot be established beyond doubt without laboratory evidence. The skin test with coccidioidin should be made first, since skin reactivity develops before serologic antibodies, except sometimes with disseminated lesions. Complement-fixing antibodies need not be looked for if the skin test is negative. The bacteriologic or histologic demonstration of *C. immitis* is difficult and requires considerable time.

Cryptococcosis (Torulosis)

Cryptococcus neoformans is a budding thick-walled yeastlike fungus, 3 to 10 μ in diameter, exclusive of its thick refractile gelatinous capsule. The capsule can be demonstrated readily in india ink preparations of strains freshly isolated from human or animal tissue, but becomes attenuated on subculture in artificial media.

C. neoformans differs from other related species in being pathogenic for mice. It enters the human through the lungs or skin, or perhaps through the gastrointestinal tract, to produce local cysts which are filled with organisms. Other organs may be invaded secondarily, including the central nervous system. There are no generally accepted procedures for demonstrating antibodies in the blood serum of patients or for performing skin tests. Occasionally the organisms in tissues become calcified.

Material from infected sites is often mucilaginous in character. Purulent discharges or infected spinal fluid should be centrifuged and the sediment examined in a fresh wet microscopic preparation containing added india ink. Care should be taken to avoid mistaking the rounded organisms for red cells or lymphocytes. On blood agar and Sabouraud's medium the slowly growing colonies may be mucoid or dry, smooth or irregular, tan or brown. Mycologic methods are available for differentiating *C. neoformans* from the nonpathogenic yeasts.

The presence of these organisms in human material can be demonstrated by injecting the material intraperitoneally into white mice. After several weeks normal saline is introduced into the cavity, aspirated, and examined for cryptococci.

Dermatomycoses

Tinea capitis or annular ringworm of the scalp is limited almost entirely to childhood. The typical lesions are rounded scaly patches of baldness 1 to 4 cm across, which on close inspection reveal hair shafts broken off close to the scalp. Local inflammation, sometimes associated, can vary from a mild low-grade folliculitis, usually with a few serous crusts, up to marked erythema with tissue edema and pustular follicles (kerion). The regional lymph nodes may be enlarged.

The patches are most frequent on or above the occiput but can begin anywhere where hair is found. Spontaneous cures are sometimes seen, but the lesions usually persist until puberty if left untreated. Boys are affected more often than girls. Energetic public-health measures become essential whenever cases begin to appear in a community.

Hair shafts attacked by Microsporum will exhibit a green fluorescence when examined under a Wood's light, which is an ultraviolet lamp with a selective filter that screens out all except the ultraviolet rays. The fluorescence is extremely easy to detect in a dark room and often reveals small or mild patches undetectable in daylight. Hairs infected with Trichophyton fluoresce very little if at all. Complete epilation of diseased hairs, which is an integral part of treatment, can be done more easily under the ultraviolet light.

It is important to identify the responsible fungus. Mixed infections are rare. *M. audouini,* which gives rise to epidemics, is sometimes called the "human type." It is pathogenic chiefly for children and is disseminated directly from child to child. The next most common strain is *M. lanosum,* known as the "animal type" because spread to the human occurs ordinarily from cats and dogs. Lesions exhibit more local inflammation and are more susceptible to therapy than those caused by *M. audouini.* In Mexico and Puerto Rico a large percentage of cases are due to the endothrix-like fungus *Trichophyton tonsurans,* and such cases are becoming less rare in the United States. This variety is practically always derived from human sources, is more difficult to detect, and is usually more refractory to treatment. It does not disappear at puberty as do the other forms, but may persist into adult life. Infected areas have a speckled or "black dot" appearance.

MYCOLOGIC DIAGNOSIS. Suspected hairs can be placed on a glass slide in a drop of warmed (not hot) saline or 5 to 10 per cent sodium or potassium hydroxide solution and examined microscopically under a cover glass. Hairs which are invaded with either variety of Microsporum (the two cannot be differentiated microscopically) will be covered with a mass or "mosaic" of circular spores smaller in size than a red cell. These surround the hair shaft, occasionally penetrate its center, and have new filaments. If a trichophyton is responsible, there will be larger spores often arranged in chains, the filaments will be more numerous, and the hair shaft will be heavily invaded. The rare pathogen known as *Achorion schoenleini* gives rise to small air bubbles within the shaft.

Skin scrapings may yield a species belonging to one of three genera of dermatophytes: *Microsporum* (3 species: *canis, gypseum, audouini*), *Trichophyton* (about 10 species: *mentagrophytes, rubrum, megnini, gallinae, tonsurans, sulphureum, schoenleini, verrucosum, ferrugineum,* and *violaceum*), or *Epidermophyton* (one species: *floccosum*). In the skin and nails any of these appear as filaments (mycelia), or in the hair as spores produced by fragmentation of mycelia (arthrospores).

On solid media the dermatophytes produce filamentous colonies containing distinctive asexual spores. Their microscopic structure on Sabouraud's glucose agar at room temperature is a chief approach to the exact identification of genus and species.

Slants of Sabouraud's medium can be kept in sealed tubes or bottles on the office shelf and inoculated with suspected hairs as patients present themselves. Cultures are made by placing or rubbing the hair on Sabouraud's agar (4 per cent glucose, 2 per cent agar, 1 per cent peptone) and incubating at room temperature. Growths should be passed on to a trained mycologist for subculture and identification.

Geotrichosis

Geotrichum can produce a systemic mycosis similar to coccidioidomycosis and blastomycosis. The genus is large and consists chiefly of saprophytic species. In rare individuals the skin or mucous membranes may be attacked. Lung lesions can resemble chronic pulmonary tuberculosis. Cough, low-grade fever, and anorexia are usually present. When there is no complicating bacterial infection, the sputum tends to be white and mucoid and to contain grayish flakes.

Geotrichum can be cultured from the sputum on Sabouraud's medium. It can be identified by the rectangular arthrospores formed by the segmentation of the hyphae.

Histoplasmosis

In its severe form this disease is a generalized infection with *Histoplasma capsulatum*. There is usually hepatosplenomegaly, anemia, granulocytopenia, and sometimes thrombocytopenia. At necropsy, disseminated granulomas are found.

A much milder form of histoplasmosis is distributed widely through the Eastern Central region of the United States. Some of these cases begin with an acute episode of pneumonitis, with lung lesions which may calcify instead of resolving.

MYCOLOGIC DIAGNOSIS. This often can be established in the disseminated disease by recovery of the invading fungus. Material for cultures is taken from the blood, sputum, bone marrow aspirate, excised lymph nodes, or surface of a mucous membrane ulcer. This is spread over Sabouraud's or blood agar plates, which are then sealed to conserve moisture and incubated both at 37°C and at room temperature. Growth is usually evident in 8 to 10 days but may not appear until as late as 4 weeks. A penicillin-streptomycin mixture may be added to the medium if bacteria are present also in the inoculum. Sputum which may be contaminated with other fungus spores such as Candida should be injected intraperitoneally into mice. After 4 weeks these animals are killed and their livers and spleens cultured for Histoplasma. Attempted bacteriologic confirmation of the diagnosis of histoplasmosis in the acute benign form is usually unsuccessful.

H. capsulatum grows as a mold at room temperatures and as a yeast at 37°C. In the moldlike phase, cultures form slow-growing colonies, usually with mycelia which are white at first but gradually become light brown. Distinctive characteristics are two types of spores on the terminal branches: spherical spiny microconidia 3 to 4 μ in diameter and spherical or clavate macroconidia 8 to 12 μ in diameter with fingerlike appendages on the surface. In the yeast phase, which is the form found in the tissues, the cells are egg-shaped, 3 to 4 μ in length, and reproduce by budding at the smaller end.

BIOPSY IDENTIFICATION. Surgically removed infected tissues typically show central necrosis with spindle-shaped connective tissue cells palisaded along the margins. Epithelioid granulomas, often with Langhans giant cells, may appear in the lungs. Masses of histoplasma organisms, best demonstrated by the periodic acid-Schiff stain, appear as rounded basophilic bodies surrounded by clear zones, within swollen and sometimes multinucleated reticuloendothelial cells. Unlike most other pathogenic fungi, these invaders are rarely found outside reticuloendothelial cells in human lesions.

HISTOPLASMIN SENSITIVITY. A skin test is performed with 0.1 ml of a 1:100 dilution of the antigen extract histoplasmin, injected intradermally. A positive cutaneous reaction consists of an erythematous indurated area with a surrounding zone of edema measuring at least 0.5 cm in diameter. This becomes maximum in 2 to 3 days. Erythema alone is not interpreted as a positive response.

Skin sensitivity to histoplasmin is a sign of present or past infection. Patients with rapidly progressing lesions may give a negative response. In some endemic areas, so great a percentage of the population exhibits skin sensitivity from early childhood that its occurrence is of little diagnostic aid in suspected active cases. Most of these asymptomatic reactors have no demonstrable serum antibodies.

Histoplasmin often induces a positive skin response in blastomycosis, and occasionally in coccidioidomycosis; when necessary one may use the corresponding skin-test antigens simultaneously, noting the comparative size of the skin reactions.

SEROLOGIC TESTS. Complement fixation, precipitin, and other immunologic reactions, utilizing histoplasmin or the yeast phase of *H. capsulatum* as antigen, are often positive in generalized infections of minimal and moderate severity. These antibodies appear early in the illness. They subside after a few weeks or months in minimal infections, but persist in acute and progressive infections. In the terminal stages they often disappear.

Serums from patients with blastomycosis typically show minimal or negative reactivity to histoplasmin, but serums from patients with active histoplasmosis sometimes react almost as strongly with blastomyces antigen. It has been advised, therefore, that suspected cases of either disease be tested with both antigens.

Moniliasis

Candida is an oval budding yeastlike fungus 2 to 5 μ in diameter. In infancy it will sometimes produce a superficial stomatitis characterized by whitish patches on the oral membranes (thrush), but may also give rise to paronychiae, omphalitis, vulvovaginitis, esophagitis, and perianal or bronchopulmonary infections. Many stubborn forms of intertrigo in the corners of the mouth (perlèche), or on the folds of the neck or groin or buttocks, or behind the ears are due to invasion by Candida. Occasional instances of spread to the lungs, liver, spleen, lymph nodes, or meninges have been reported. Thrush infections of the mouth in infants are not to be regarded lightly, since spread into the esophagus may be followed by anorexia, dehydration, and other secondary complications, and even a fatal outcome. Disseminated lesions are occasionally seen in patients of all ages who have been ill with other systemic diseases.

Candidae are normal inhabitants of room dust and the intestinal tract and may be found in the mouth, skin, or vagina of normal individuals. They appear in the sputum of children with bronchiectasis or tuberculosis. They may become prominent in the stools of patients receiving oral antibiotics or sulfonamides which inhibit the growth of the normal fecal flora, and in such circumstances may be associated with troublesome irritation of the perianal mucutaneous area.

The species most often recovered from infants and children is *Candida albicans*. Other species which may be encountered are *C. albicans* var. *stellatoidea, C. tropicalis, C. krusei,* and *C. parapsilosis.*

MYCOLOGIC DIAGNOSIS. Sputum or other material from the skin or mucous membranes may be smeared and studied in a wet slide and cover-slip preparation, or fixed on a slide and then stained with the Gram stain. Scrapings from the skin or nails may be mounted in a 10 per cent solution of sodium or potassium hydroxide and warmed gently for microscopic examination. The typical yeastlike cells, with occasional hyphal filaments, will be seen.

All strains of suspected *C. albicans* should be studied mycologically to make certain of their identity and to rule out nonpathogenic yeastlike fungi which may be accidental contaminants. The presence of Candida in sputum should not be deemed diagnostic of pulmonary moniliasis unless these are found regularly in successive examinations.

Growth occurs readily in aerobic conditions on corn meal agar, blood agar plates, and Sabouraud's medium, at both 37°C and at room temperature. Surface colonies are rounded, cream-colored, and give off a pronounced yeastlike odor. In corn meal agar or other nutritionally deficient media one finds pseudomycelia chains of elongated cells with attached clusters of large, rounded chlamydospores. The other species of Candida do not form chlamydospores in this circumstance.

Serologic tests are of little aid, since a high percentage of normal individuals have agglutinins for *C. albicans* in their serum.

Mucormycosis

This infection is caused by members of the fungus family Mucoraceae, which have nonseptate hyphae. The Mucoraceae occur in abundance as dark saprophytic molds in soil and manure and on fruits and starchy substances such as bread. The two genera which have been pathogenic to man in rare instances have been Mucor and Rhizopus. These do not produce disease in humans except when there is some serious metabolic or wasting disease such as diabetes mellitus or uremia.

The portal of entry is usually the nasal passages, but may be the lung or gastrointestinal tract. Suppuration develops and spreads locally or to remote viscera. The organisms can be cultured readily from the lesions with mycologic procedures. Patients may exhibit a positive tuberculin-like reaction to intradermal injections of dead organisms.

Nocardiosis

Nocardia is a genus of aerobic fragmenting nonsporulating fungi resembling Actinomyces. Nine species have been identified thus far. Those which have caused the reported cases of human disease are *N. asteroides, N. madurae,* and *N. brasiliensis,* as a rule.

Most human illnesses caused by *N. asteroides* have been chronic pulmonary or foot infections. Nocardiosis should be considered a diagnostic possibility in chronic lung infections when efforts to demonstrate tuberculosis are consistently unsuccessful.

Pus or sputum may contain colonies resembling the sulfur granules of actinomycosis, but softer and often colored. Microscopically they consist of interlacing Gram-positive mycelia without peripheral club formation. Most non-acid-fast strains appear to be saprophytes.

Colored colonies grow on enriched nutrients media and Sabouraud's glucose agar, at both incubator and room temperatures. Pathogenicity can be demonstrated by animal inoculation. Since these organisms are susceptible to the chemicals used in concentrating sputum or gastric washings for tubercle bacilli, cultures should be prepared before the concentrating procedure.

Sporotrichosis

Sporotrichum schenckii gives rise to subacute or chronic granulomatous infections which begin in the skin and progress as an ascending lymphadenitis. Entry is through a break in the skin, induced by trauma. Children are infected only rarely. The single-celled fusiform organisms are demonstrated by culture of tissue lesions on Sabouraud's glucose agar or similar media.

Tinea Versicolor

Tinea versicolor with its disseminated fawn-colored macules is caused by the fungus *Malassezia* (*Microsporon*) *furfur*. Scrapings from scaly skin areas, when mounted on a slide and warmed gently in a few drops of 10 per cent solution of potassium or sodium hydroxide, show clusters of round thick-walled cells 3 to 8 μ in diameter, associated with short, straight fragments of mycelium. Cultural studies are usually not carried out, since the organism does not grow on the standard media for fungi.

BIBLIOGRAPHY

FUNGI

Ajello, L., Collecting Specimens for the Laboratory Demonstration and Isolation of Fungi, *J.A.M.A.* **146**:1581, 1951.

Beamer, P. R., Immunology of Mycotic Infections, *Am. J. Clin. Path.* **25**:66, 1955.

Conant, N. F., D. T. Smith, R. D. Baker, J. L. Callaway, and *D. S. Martin,* "Manual of Clinical Mycology," 2d ed., W. B. Saunders Company, Philadelphia, 1954.

Delamater, E. D., Technic and Identification of Fungi of Medical Interest, *Am. J. Clin. Path.* **18**:235, 1948.

Dubos, R. J., "Bacterial and Mycotic Infections of Man," chaps. 31 and 32, J. B. Lippincott Company, Philadelphia, 1952.

Haley, L. D., Mycotic Diseases in Pediatric Practice, *J. Pediat.* **41**:104, 1952.

Kligman, A. M., D. M. Pillsbury, and *H. Mescon,* Improved Technic for Diagnosing Ringworm Infections and Moniliasis, *J.A.M.A.* **146**:1563, 1951.

Lewis, G. M., W. Sachs, and *M. E. Hopper,* Mycologic and Histologic Technics in the Study of Superficial Fungous Infections, *A.M.A. Arch. Dermat. & Syph.* **63**:622, 1951.

Nickerson, W. J., "Biology of the Pathogenic Fungi," Chronica Botanica, Waltham, Mass., 1947.

Raptery, A., and *F. W. Hartman,* Adjuncts to Mycologic Diagnosis, *Am. J. Clin. Path.* **21**:133, 1951.

Robinson, H. M., Jr., M. M. Cohen, R. C. V. Robinson, and *E. S. Bereston,* Simplified Office Procedures for Mycological Diagnosis, *J.A.M.A.* **160**:537, 1956.

Schwarz, J., and *M. L. Furcolow,* Some Epidemiologic Factors and Diagnostic Tests in Blastomycosis, Coccidioidomycosis and Histoplasmosis, *Am. J. Clin. Path.* **25**:261, 1955.

Wilson, J. W., and *O. A. Plunkett,* Practical Medical Mycology: The Culture of Fungi as an Office Procedure, *Arch. Dermat. & Syph.* **59**:414, 1949.

Zimmerman, L. E., Fatal Fungus Infections Complicating Other Diseases, *Am. J. Clin. Path.* **25**:46, 1955.

BLASTOMYCOSIS

Potenza, L., C. Lares Campos, and *M. Feo,* Paracoccidioidosis infantil en Venezuela: Aspecto del parasito a la luz polarizada, *Arch. venez. puericult. y pediat.* **16**:7, 1953.

Smith, J. G., Jr., J. S. Harris, N. F. Conant, and *D. T. Smith,* An Epidemic of North American Blastomycosis, *J.A.M.A.* **158**:641, 1955.

Weed, L. A., North American Blastomycosis, *Am. J. Clin. Path.* **25**:37, 1955.

COCCIDIOIDOMYCOSIS

Baum, G. L., and *J. Schwarz,* Coccidioidomycosis: A Review, *Am. J. M. Sc.* **230**:82, 1955.

Campbell, C. C., and *G. E. Binkley,* Serologic Diagnosis with Respect to Histoplasmosis, Coccidioidomycosis, and Blastomycosis and the Problem of Cross Reactions, *J. Lab. & Clin. Med.* **42**:896, 1953.

Cohen, R., and *R. Burnip,* Coccidioidin Skin Testing during Pregnancy and in Infants and Children, *California Med.* **72**:31, 1950.

Faber, H. K., Coccidioidomycosis, in Brennemann-McQuarrie, "Practice of Pediatrics," vol. II, chap. 14, sec. II, W. F. Prior Co, Hagerstown, Md., 1957.

Friedman, L., D. Pappagianis, R. J. Berman, and *C. E. Smith,* Studies on *Coccidiodes immitis:* Morphology and Sporulation Capacity of Forty-seven Strains, *J. Lab. & Clin. Med.* **42**:438, 1953.

Mead, I., Coccidioidomycosis in Children, *J.A.M.A.* **146**:85, 1951.

Smith, C. E., Coccidioidomycosis, *Pediat. Clin. North America,* February, 1953, p. 127.

————, *M. T. Saito,* and *S. A. Simons,* Pattern of 39,500 Serological Tests in Coccidioidomycosis, *J.A.M.A.* **160**:546, 1956.

Townsend, T. E., and *R. W. McKey,* Coccidioidomycosis in Infants, *A.M.A. Am. J. Dis. Child.* 86:51, 1953.

CRYPTOCOCCOSIS

Baker, R. D., and *R. K. Haugen,* Tissue Changes and Tissue Diagnosis in Cryptococcosis: A Study of 26 Cases, *Am. J. Clin. Path.* 25:14, 1955.

Benham, R. W., The Genus Cryptococcus, *Bact. Rev.* 20:189, 1956.

Cox, L. B., and *J. C. Tolhurst,* "Human Torulosis: A Clinical Pathological and Microbiological Study with a Report of Thirteen Cases," Melbourne University Press, Melbourne, 1946.

Littman, M. L., and *L. E. Zimmerman,* "Cryptococcosis," Grune & Stratton, Inc., New York, 1956.

O'Neill, F. J., A. Necomb, and *C. S. Nielsen,* Cryptococcus Meningitis, *U.S. Nav. M. Bull.* 49:300, 1949.

DERMATOMYCOSIS

Beare, J. M., and *E. A. Cheeseman,* A Localized Outbreak of Tinea Capitis (*M. audouini*) in Northern Ireland, *Arch. Dis. Childhood* 26:149, 1951.

Georg, L. K., Trichophyton tonsurans Ringworm: A New Public Health Problem, *Pub. Health Rep.* 67:53, 1952.

Schwartz, L., S. M. Peck, I. Botvinick, A. L. Leibovitz, and *E. S. Frazier,* Control of Ringworm of the Scalp among School Children in Hagerstown, Maryland, *Pub. Health Bull.* 294, 1944–1945.

Scully, J. P., C. S. Livingood, and *D. M. Pillsbury,* The Local Treatment of Tinea Capitis Due to *M. audouini:* The Importance of Inflammatory Reaction as an Index of Curability, *J. Invest. Dermat.* 10:111, 1948.

Warner, M. P., and *F. E. Grove,* A Study of Forty Cases of Ringworm of the Scalp in Hagerstown Schools, 1950 and 1951, Washington County, Maryland, *J. Pediat.* 43:267, 1953.

HISTOPLASMOSIS

Beadenkopt, W. G., and *G. G. Loosli,* Histoplasmosis, Tuberculosis, and Coccidioidomycosis, *J.A.M.A.* 146:621, 1951.

Binford, C. H., Histoplasmosis: Tissue Reactions and Morphologic Variations of the Fungus, *Am. J. Clin. Path.* 25:25, 1955.

Emmons, C. W., Histoplasmosis, *Bull. New York Acad. Med.* 31:627, 1955.

Furcolow, M. L., Further Observations on Histoplasmosis: Mycology and Bacteriology, *Pub. Health Rep.* 65:965, 1950.

Grayston, J. T., and *M. L. Furcolow,* The Occurrence of Histoplasmosis in Epidemics: Epidemiological Studies, *Am. J. Pub. Health* 43:665, 1953.

Klingberg, W. G., Generalized Histoplasmosis in Infants and Children, *J. Pediat.* 36:728, 1950.

Lynch, J. F., and *E. B. Alpern,* Results of Histoplasmin Skin Testing in Children from the St. Louis, Mo., Area, *J. Pediat.* 38:51, 1951.

Peterson, J. C., and *A. Christie,* Histoplasmosis and Pulmonary Calcifications, *Am. Rev. Tuberculosis* 57:361, 1948.

——— and ———, Histoplasmosis, *Pediat. Clin. North America* February, 1955, p. 127.

Rohn, R. J., and *W. H. Bond,* The Value of Routine Bone Marrow Culture for *Histoplasma capsulatum* in Pediatric Hematology, *Blood* 8:329, 1953.

Silverman, F. N., J. Schwarz, and *M. E. Lahey,* Histoplasmosis, *Am. J. Med.* 19:410, 1955.

MONILIASIS

Baird, K. H., Unusual Syndrome Associated with *Candida albicans* Infection, *Pediatrics* 4:730, 1949.

Carpenter, A., Studies on Candida. I. Identification of 100 Yeastlike Fungi Isolated from Children, *Am. J. Clin. Path.* 25:98, 1955.

Cohen, A. C., Pulmonary Moniliasis, *Am. J. M. Sc.* 226:16, 1953.

Gausewitz, P. L., F. S. Jones, and *G. Worley, Jr.,* Fatal Generalized Moniliasis, *Am. J. Clin. Path.* 21:41, 1951.

Hamil, B. M., Bronchopulmonary Mycosis: Simultaneous Primary Occurrence in Four Children and Their Mother with Subsequent Healing by Diffuse Miliary Calcification: A Twelve Year Observation, *Am. J. Dis. Child.* 79:233, 1950.

Holzel, A., Skin Thrush in Early Infancy, *Arch. Dis. Childhood* 28:412, 1953.

Lederer, H., and *R. M. Todd,* Thrush in Infancy, *Arch. Dis. Childhood* 24:200, 1949.

Martin, D. S., C. P. Jones, K. F. Yao, and *L. E. Lee, Jr.,* A Practical Classification of the Monilias, *J. Bact.* 34:99, 1937.

McGovern, J. J., R. H. Parrott, C. W. Emmons, S. Ross, F. G. Burke, and *E. C. Rice,* The Effect of Aureomycin and Chloramphenicol on the Fungal and Bacterial Flora of Children, *New England J. Med.* 248:397, 1953.

Nilsby, I., and *A. Norden,* Studies of the Occurrence of *Candida albicans, Acta. med. scandinav.* 133:340, 1949.

Winter, W. D., Jr., and *G. E. Foley,* Candida Infections in Children with Neoplastic Disease: Influence of Therapy with Antibiotics and Steroid Hormones, *Pediatrics* 18:595, 1956.

Wright, E. T., J. H. Graham, and *T. H. Sternberg,* Treatment of Moniliasis with Nystatin, *J.A.M.A.* 163:92, 1957.

MISCELLANEOUS FUNGUS INFECTIONS

Ballenger, C. N., Jr., and *D. Goldring,* Nocardiosis in Childhood, *J. Pediat.* 50:145, 1957.

Harris, J. S., Mucormycosis: Report of a Case, *Pediatrics* 16:857, 1955.

Hertzog, A. J., T. S. Smith, and *M. Goblin,* Acute Pulmonary Aspergillosis: Report of a Case, *Pediatrics* 4:331, 1949.

Kaliski, S. R., M. L. Beene, and *L. Mattman,* Geotrichum in Blood Stream of an Infant, *J.A.M.A.* 148:1207, 1952.

Kunstadter, R. H., A. Milzer, and *F. Whitcomb,* Bronchopulmonary Geotrichosis in Children, *Am. J. Dis. Child.* 79:82, 1950.

McQuown, A. L., Actinomycosis and Nocardiosis, *Am. J. Clin. Path.* 25:2, 1955.

Weil, M. L., J. T. Cuttino, and *A. M. McCabe,* Pure Granulomatous Nocardiosis, *Pediatrics* 3:345, 1949.

CHAPTER 73

Viral and Rickettsial Infections

Many of the virus infections may be subgrouped according to the kind of tissue which they chiefly attack—skin, respiratory tract, central nervous system, or other organ systems. This form of approach is somewhat arbitrary, since not all viruses are monotropic. For example, lymphocytic choriomeningitis may occasionally involve the respiratory tract without any noticeable central nervous system phenomena. Mumps may localize itself exclusively in the meninges, pancreas, or epididymotesticular area. Yellow fever is predominantly hepatotropic, but neurotropic and viscerotropic strains are known also. Some of these diseases such as parotid mumps, smallpox, or varicella are usually identifiable without any special tests. Epidemiologic information that a suspected viral disease is prevalent in the environment is of presumptive aid in a diagnostic problem.

Whether the animal viruses are living organisms or nonliving chemical substances remains in the realm of hypothesis. Their complex molecular structure is known to consist of nucleic acids, carbohydrates, lipids, biotin, riboflavin, metals, and other components of protoplasm. Duplication and proliferation take place only inside living cells, through perverted routes of intracellular metabolism. The strain differences responsible for alterations in pathogenicity are believed to originate in genetic mutations similar to those of bacteria. Ultrafiltration, high-speed centrifugation, and electron microscopy make it feasible to determine the approximate size and even the shape of viruses, but diameter in millimicrons seems to have little relation to selective tissue affinities.

Laboratory approaches fill a practical need when symptoms of presumably viral origin are somewhat nonspecific and capable of being caused by different agents. Examples are the pulmonary lesions caused by influenza, psittacosis, and Q fever; the conjunctival inflammation caused by trachoma, epidemic keratoconjunctivitis, inclusion blennorrhea, adenoviruses, and Newcastle disease virus; the skin lesions caused by typhus, Rocky Mountain spotted fever, and rickettsialpox; the stomatitis induced by herpes simplex and herpangina; and the meningeal and cerebral irritation evoked by mumps, herpes simplex, poliomyelitis, and other varieties of meningoencephalitis.

882

The great growth of virology in the past two decades has made it clear that some viruses can induce antibody responses and other expressions of immunity without inducing any signs or symptoms. With poliomyelitis and mumps the subclinical infection is more frequent than the overt illness. Furthermore, latent carrier states may occur with many viral and rickettsial agents such as those of serum hepatitis, herpes simplex, psittacosis, and the numerous dormant viruses recoverable from the gastrointestinal tract.

VIRUS DIAGNOSTIC LABORATORIES

Comparatively simple procedures are now available which permit of rapid recognition of the diseases caused by many known viruses and rickettsiae. The two major approaches are (1) direct isolation of the infectious agent, and (2) study of the human host for immune responses. For such investigations it is usually necessary to consult a reference virus laboratory. These give instructions as to the nature and care of the specimens to be collected, perform the tests indicated by the particular case, and advise in the interpretation of the results obtained. Every physician should be familiar with the location and scope of the diagnostic center closest to his community (Table 73-1).

Table 73-1. Virus Diagnostic Laboratories in the United States

Communicable Disease Center, Montgomery, Ala.
Viral and Rickettsial Disease Laboratory, 1392 University Avenue, Berkeley 2, Calif.
Los Angeles City Department of Health, 10975 Wilshire Boulevard, Los Angeles 24
Affiliated Hospitals of Northwestern University Medical School, Chicago
Illinois Department of Health, Division of Laboratories, Chicago
Michael Reese Hospital, Department of Microbiology, Chicago
Massachusetts State Department of Public Health, Diagnostic Laboratory, 281 South
    Street, Jamaica Plain, Mass.
University of Minnesota, State Health Laboratories, Minneapolis
Rocky Mountain Laboratory, Hamilton, Mont.
New York State Department of Health, Division of Laboratories and Research,
    Laboratories for Virology, Albany 1
University of Rochester, School of Medicine, Rochester Health Bureau Laboratories,
    Rochester, N.Y.
State University of New York, College of Medicine, Department of Bacteriology and
    Parasitology, Syracuse, N.Y.
Children's Hospital, Virus Diagnostic Laboratory, 1740 Bainbridge Street, Philadelphia 46
Medical College of South Carolina, Virus Diagnostic Laboratory, 16 Lucas Street,
    Charleston 16, S.C.
Texas State Health Department, Bureau of Laboratories, Austin, Tex.

Embryonated hens' eggs, tissue cultures, adult mice, suckling mice, hamsters, rabbits, and guinea pigs are utilized as indicated for the direct recovery of viruses, and complement fixation, virus neutralization, and hemagglutination-inhibition procedures for the demonstration of serum antibodies.

With every specimen it is essential to attach pertinent information. This should report the clinical picture or suspected diagnosis, the date of onset of the illness, the date the specimen was obtained, dates of any previous specific prophylactic inoculations, and pertinent epidemiologic facts. For special problems, prior consultation with the laboratory director is advisable with respect to choice of proper specimens and probability of success in the particular instance.

RECOVERY OF VIRUS

For actual isolation of a virus or rickettsia one must collect, as early in the illness as possible, specimens from the part of the body most likely to harbor the agent—throat washings, saliva, sputum, feces, blood, spinal fluid, or tissue. The specimens should be placed in test tubes with rubber stoppers or tightly stoppered bottles or jars, and sealed with tape. They are then sent to the laboratory as quickly as feasible, in a manner which will maintain the viability of any infective agent present. This usually means freezing and shipping in an insulated container packed with solid carbon dioxide. Several specimens, taken at 1- or 2-day intervals during the stage of acute illness, enhance the likelihood of successful isolation of an infective agent.

Recovery of an infective agent by inoculation of experimental hosts or tissue cultures, and later exact identification, often takes too long to have much immediate therapeutic utility. Furthermore, many of the viruses and especially those of the neurotropic group are in the blood and other body fluids only during the incubation period and the first few days of illness.

Isolation of a virus from a patient does not necessarily establish the true nature of the illness. Stools of a child recovering from a clinically obscure febrile infection with mild meningeal irritation may contain the virus of Coxsackie or of poliomyelitis, and yet some other infective agent may have been the cause of the actual illness. Demonstration of the influenza virus in the lung of an infant dying of bronchopneumonia is not proof that this virus was related to the lethal illness.

Procedures which may be applied to the problem of recovery and recognition of a suspected viral agent depend upon its known capacity to survive and multiply in living hosts or organ cells derived therefrom. Embryos of developing chicks, experimental animals (white mice usually), and especially tissue cultures are utilized most frequently.

Tissue Cultures

In appropriate living cultures of various tissue cells, many viruses after an appropriate incubation exposure can induce distinctive reactions ranging from syncytium formations (measles) to destructive necrosis (poliomyelitis). These changes may be made evident by simple means such as direct microscopy or alterations in the chemical characteristics of the growth medium. Portions of the infected tissue culture are then mixed with standardized antibodies against different possible viruses, and these mixtures inoculated into fresh tissue cultures. The virus-antibody inoculum which can not induce growth serves to identify the virus which is present. This technique can be used with poliomyelitis, measles, varicella, herpes simplex, equine encephalitis, mumps, and influenza.

So-called HeLa cells are used widely for tissue culture of viruses. These cells, derived originally from an epithelial carcinoma of the cervix from a patient designated as He——— La———, thrive and multiply profusely in ordinary test tubes when supplied with a relatively simple nutrient medium. They support the growth of the poliomyelitis viruses, the adenoviruses, and a few others.

ANTIBODY RESPONSES

With practically all virus diseases which have systemic spread, specific antibodies appear in the circulation in detectable amounts during or soon after illness. Since serum specimens for immunologic testing can be procured easily and the procedures performed efficiently and economically, this approach to diagnosis is the most widely used.

Since a single positive reading may be the consequence of an earlier illness or a vaccination, establishing a diagnosis by serologic means rests on *at least a fourfold increase* in titer of specific antibodies between the acute and the convalescent phase of the illness. Hence two serum samples are required. One is taken as early as possible in the acute phase of the suspected viral illness, and the second several weeks later. The different varieties of antibodies in any disease may develop at different rates, but nearly always at least one will be demonstrable relatively early, and it or another will persist for a year or longer.

A sample of 10 to 20 ml of blood or 5 to 10 ml of serum is usually required. This should be collected in a dry clean sterile tube, preferably after a few hours of fasting. The larger amounts are helpful in the event that tests have to be made with many antigens, or repeated because of equivocal results. When facilities for centrifugation are not available, the clotted blood should be forwarded immediately, provided it will reach the laboratory within 24 to 48 hours. Otherwise the serum should be separated and kept refrigerated in a corked sterile tube until sent to the laboratory.

If shipping is to be delayed for several weeks, the serum should be stored frozen in a sealed ampoule or in a thick-walled test tube with a cork or rubber stopper which is sealed with paraffin or adhesive tape. Hemolysis results when whole clotted blood is frozen. Glass containers should not be filled beyond one-third of their volume, to prevent bursting during freezing.

Blood and serum may be sent in the usual mailing containers, packed to avoid breakage; they do not have to be mailed in the frozen condition. If a cold agglutinin test is to be made, the whole blood should not be refrigerated before the clot is removed from the serum.

Complement-fixation Tests

Complement-fixation tests are now available for many of the viral and rickettsial diseases. Patterned after the familiar complement-fixation test for syphilis, these employ viral or rickettsial antigens which are obtained usually from commercial sources. "Positive" and "negative" serums are used as controls.

Most complement-fixation tests are specific for individual viruses. When cross reactions indicate common antigenic components, the highest titer indicates the infective agent. A positive result in a single test conveys no exact information concerning the severity of the infection or the interval since its occurrence.

Neutralization Tests

When an unknown serum is incubated with a suspension of living virus or rickettsia in suitable proportions and the mixture inoculated into susceptible hosts, protection will be given if the serum contains specific antibodies in sufficient amount. This approach may be used in reverse by mixing an unknown agent which needs identification with separate serums containing known specific antibodies. For quantitation of antibodies the inoculum is kept constant with some agents and the serum is diluted serially; with others the volumes of serum are kept unaltered and the infective preparation is diluted.

Hemagglutination-inhibition Test

The viruses of influenza, mumps, Newcastle disease, smallpox, and vaccinia can be absorbed on to the surfaces of the red cells of many animal species and will thereafter agglutinate those cells. Chicken red cells are customarily used. This hemagglutination phenomenon is inhibited specifically and quantitatively by antibody-containing serum. Inhibition titers are read in serum dilutions set up as in bacterial agglutination tests. Here also a rise in titer during convalescence must be at least fourfold before it is deemed diagnostic of a recent illness.

NONSPECIFIC APPROACHES

Skin

In herpes simplex, varicella, and herpes zoster one can usually demonstrate multinucleated giant cells in scrapings from the surface of the base of a vesicle. Tissue taken with a sharp knife edge is spread on a glass slide, permitted to dry, and then stained with Giemsa, methylene blue, or Wright's stain. Typical cells show two to six large vesicular nuclei crowded together in an abnormally large basal epithelial cell. These cytologic changes are not found in vaccinia, rickettsialpox, dermatitis herpetiformis, and other vesicular or vesiculopustular eruptions. In urticaria pigmentosa a similarly made preparation will reveal mast cells filled with basophilic granules.

In smallpox one may be able to demonstrate the Guarnieri inclusion bodies. Proven to be aggregates of the true virus particles or elementary bodies, these cytoplasmic inclusions are found in the papular and vesicular lesions and disappear when pustular changes develop, at about the tenth day of illness.

They are acidophilic or basophilic and occupy most of the cytoplasm. Vaccinia and varicella do not produce these formations to any extent. Failure to find inclusion bodies in skin scrapings, however, does not exclude the diagnosis of smallpox. It is of interest that live smallpox virus can be recovered from skin lesions at all stages, even the dry crusts, and that smears or extracts of pustules are satisfactory antigens for specific immunologic tests.

In molluscum contagiosum the characteristic cytoplasmic inclusion bodies are demonstrated by spreading the cheesy exudate from the nodules on a glass slide and adding a drop of Lugol's iodine solution or 1:2,000 brilliant cresyl blue in saline. The smear is then examined under the dry high-power objective of the microscope. Large oval molluscum bodies if present will take a deep-brown color with Lugol's solution and are blue with brilliant cresyl blue.

Eye

Trachoma and inclusion conjunctivitis are two viral conjunctival diseases with many features in common. Their causative agents are large and seem taxonomically related to the psittacosis-lymphogranuloma family of viruses, since group antibodies appear in the serum of patients. Within the conjunctival and corneal exudate of acute cases the infective rounded elementary bodies, about 0.25 μ in diameter, form masses which appear as cytoplasmic inclusion bodies. The latter are demonstrable by examination of scrapings from the conjunctival epithelium or of material expressed from inflamed follicles. Smears are fixed for 5 minutes in methyl alcohol and then stained for 1 hour at 37°C in diluted neutral Giemsa stain. In trachoma, in addition, one finds necrotic debris and macrophages full of cellular fragments.

Epidemic keratoconjunctivitis is a viral disease characterized by nonpurulent inflammation of the conjunctiva, preauricular lymphadenitis, and superficial punctate corneal opacities. The diagnosis can be substantiated by direct recovery of an adenovirus from conjunctival secretions or by demonstration of specific neutralizing antibodies against the virus appearing during convalescence.

Nonspecific Serologic Tests

In the repertory of diagnostic viral and rickettsial procedures are several serologic procedures which are performed with nonviral antigens. The heterophil antibody test with selective absorption reactions is useful with suspected infectious mononucleosis (p. 204). The cold agglutinin and the streptococcus MG agglutination tests tend to be positive in "primary atypical pneumonia" (p. 830). Variations of the Weil-Felix test with Proteus OX antigens aid in the recognition and differentiation of some of the rickettsial diseases (p. 900).

NOTES ON LABORATORY ASPECTS OF SOME VIRAL INFECTIONS

Poliomyelitis

Laboratory tests are essential for accurate diagnosis of nonparalytic poliomyelitis, and, at times, even for the paralytic form. Widespread use of vaccination can be expected to reduce the incidence of cases to a level where true poliomyelitis will be more sporadic and diagnosis more difficult. Attacks in previously vaccinated children may often be mild and atypical. Illnesses which simulate nonparalytic poliomyelitis can be produced by the viruses of mumps, herpes simplex, and lymphocytic choriomeningitis, and possibly also by the Coxsackie or ECHO viruses (see below).

Typical severe poliomyelitis can be recognized with reasonable assurance from the clinical phenomena and the cerebrospinal fluid findings (p. 458). Fatal cases exhibit more or less characteristic histopathologic lesions in brain and spinal cord.

RECOVERY OF VIRUS. Demonstrable virus in the blood in this disease is limited to the first day or two of symptoms. Throughout the acute stages virus may be recovered from the nasopharyngeal secretions, and for some weeks afterwards from the fecal discharge. In fresh autopsy material it is recoverable occasionally from central nervous tissue and rarely from the mesenteric lymph nodes.

Man himself appears to be the chief vector in transmission. All attempts to find an animal reservoir have been unsuccessful. Fecally contaminated material from patients or healthy carriers is the probable source of epidemic spread. Many ambulatory and asymptomatic individuals in epidemic areas have the virus in their stools. House flies and sewage in such areas may also carry the virus, presumably from contamination with human feces. Milk has been implicated as the vehicle of spread in one epidemic.

Most of the strains of poliomyelitis virus which have been isolated from patients can be grouped immunologically into three types, designated 1, 2, and 3. The majority of cases in most epidemics are caused by one single type. No correlation has been demonstrated between individual virus types, severity of clinical manifestations, and serologic reactivity.

One of the three types of poliomyelitis can usually be recovered from the stools of most paralyzed individuals, but from only half of those diagnosed as having nonparalytic poliomyelitis. This latter observation suggests that some of these illnesses may have been caused by other agents. Interestingly, the virus is usually demonstrable in the stools of about one-third of all persons having household contact with a clinically diagnosed case of poliomyelitis, even though they have had no recent symptoms of illness. Among these, the virus carrier rate is much higher with persons who have recently seemed ill or have been exposed to a paralytic patient or are under 10 years of age. The percentage of positive fecal samples among asymptomatic household contacts usually reaches its peak at 3 weeks after the first appearance of symptoms in the household.

ANTIBODY RESPONSES IN ACUTE POLIOMYELITIS. Complement-fixing antibodies and those which neutralize the virus in protection tests begin to appear in the blood within a few days after the onset of the illness. The titers rise rapidly in the next few weeks, and then persist indefinitely or decline gradually over many years. An illness caused by a virus of one type will sometimes evoke antibodies in low titer against the other types.

Mixed pools of gamma globulin prepared from human whole blood usually contain antibodies against all three types of virus. Controlled epidemiologic studies have indicated that injections of such gamma globulin into children can result in a passive transfer of protective immunity which lasts for at least 4 weeks if an adequate amount is given (0.14 ml per lb body weight).

ANTIBODY RESPONSES FOLLOWING VACCINATION. It is believed that an individual to be fully protected against poliomyelitis must acquire immunity against all three types, and that a paralytic or nonparalytic attack or a series of injections of a vaccine from one type will fail to protect fully against the other two. Formalin-killed Salk vaccines containing the three types of viruses propagated in tissue culture will call forth the corresponding serum antibodies when injected into subjects who do not have these antibodies, and will elicit rises in titer when antibodies are already present.

Salk has reported that the total amount of virus antigen injected appears to be the chief determinant of the intensity of the immune response. The first two primary injections, spaced 2 to 6 weeks apart, usually bring about moderate increases in titer against all three virus types; the third, or booster, injection, given 7 months or more later, enhances markedly the levels of antibody induced by the primary series. It also affords a third chance for primary sensitization in the event that an impotent preparation had been given in the primary series or the recipient had been unresponsive at that time.

Rabies

Complement-fixation and mouse protection tests are available for the study of rabies in experimental animals and have been used to appraise immunity in man. Positive tests will appear 3 weeks after vaccination. The fact that immune bodies develop in patients and animals has led to a recent revival of interest in the use of hyperimmune antirabies rabbit and horse serum to supplement protective vaccination. The diagnosis in human cases depends almost entirely on the history of exposure and the manifestations shown clinically by the biting animal and the bitten man.

STUDY OF THE ANIMAL. It is most important to know whether a dog or other animal who has bitten a human being is ill with the disease. Approximately 50 per cent of rabid animals excrete virus in the saliva. Those whose saliva does not contain virus are presumed to be noninfective for humans.

Every effort should be made to catch the animal and keep him in isolation for at least 2 weeks. If he is infected he will almost always show signs of the illness within a few days, and expire before this isolation period is over. Since injections of immunizing vaccine are expensive, time-consuming, and not without risk, and since most biting dogs are not infected, this procedure of observation has many advantages over the routine administration of vaccine to all bitten humans.

When the animal dies or is destroyed, the head should be packed in a water-tight container with cracked ice. Solid carbon dioxide should not be used since this renders the tissue unfit for microscopy. The specimen is then rushed to the nearest laboratory which is equipped for diagnosis. There the brain is examined for Negri bodies by study of impressions on a glass slide from un-fixed tissue and of routine histologic studies of cerebral cortex, cerebellum, and Ammon's horn. Negri bodies are oval or round eosinophilic formations 2 to 10 μ in diameter, occurring singly or in small numbers within the cytoplasm of large neurons. They must not be confused with the irregular lighter-staining inclusion bodies produced by the distemper virus. They are found in the majority of animals dying of rabies. When they are not found, or if it is desired to confirm the diagnosis, a portion of the brain tissue is injected intracerebrally into white mice, which are highly susceptible and succumb within 21 days, exhibiting neurologic symptoms and the formation of Negri bodies.

The Meningoencephalitides

Most of the viruses which produce meningoencephalitis do so by direct invasion of the central nervous system. The more common in North America (excluding poliomyelitis) are rabies, St. Louis encephalitis, western equine encephalitis, eastern equine encephalitis, and lymphocytic choriomeningitis. These, with the probable exception of lymphocytic cho-riomeningitis, appear to be arthropod-borne, as shown by epidemiologic studies and direct recovery of the viruses from mosquitoes and assorted ticks and mites. Exceptionally, the viruses of mumps, Coxsackie infection, herpes simplex, or Newcastle disease may attack the central nervous system; in several such instances the viruses have been isolated from cerebral specimens. Identification of the causative agent is based on specific virology studies utilizing serum, cerebrospinal fluid, throat swabs, nasopharyngeal washings, or stool extracts as indicated; and also on the results of histopathologic examinations and inoculations with postmortem material.

NEUROPATHOLOGY. The neuropathologic changes are much the same in all these diseases. Hence the etiology is usually not determinable either from clinical observation, cerebrospinal fluid changes (Chap. 39), or the character of the microscopic central nervous system lesions of fatal cases. When the changes are advanced the cerebral tissue shows focal lesions consisting of neuronal necrosis with or without neuronophagia, aggregations of glial cells, and perivascular accumulations of lymphocytes. Infiltrations with phagocytes of various types are sometimes evident. The meninges may show infiltrations with lymphocytes, monocytes, or even neutrophils. Occasional blood vessels may have inflammation of the walls or thrombi in their lumens. In lymphocytic choriomeningitis there occurs usually, in addition, a pronounced lymphocytic infiltration of the chorioid plexuses, ependyma, and meninges.

RECOVERY OF VIRUS. Patients with any of the viral encephalitides presum-ably experience a fleeting viremia in the initial phase of the infection. Only in lymphocytic choriomeningitis is it worthwhile to try to isolate the causative virus from the blood stream at the time the patient comes under medical observation. With the same exception the active agents have only rarely been recovered from human cerebrospinal fluid.

Recovery of virus from central nervous tissue of fatal cases is often successful. Fragments from the brain and spinal cord should be taken aseptically as soon as feasible after death. These are preserved frozen or in glycerol until after the histopathologic examination has established that a viral encephalitis was the cause of death.

ANTIBODY TESTS. Specific complement-fixing and virus-neutralizing antibodies make their appearance in the serum of most encephalitic patients during convalescence. The complement-fixing antigens for the tests are derived from mice brain, tissue culture, or chick embryo material, depending on circumstances. Antigens are now available for testing for eastern and western equine encephalomyelitis, St. Louis encephalitis, lymphocytic choriomeningitis, and mumps. Serologic cross reactions between eastern and western equine encephalitis and between St. Louis and Japanese B encephalitis are usual, but the antibodies are in higher titer with the homologous virus.

POSTINFECTIOUS ENCEPHALITIS. The encephalitic complications which follow measles, chickenpox, German measles, vaccinia, smallpox, and lymphogranuloma venereum are of uncertain pathogenesis. The typical pathologic lesion is one of patchy demyelination, very different from the neuronal disintegration and lymphocytic infiltration of the encephalitides of unequivocal viral invasion. It has been suggested that this lesion is the product of some sort of local antigen-antibody union within the brain tissue.

Coxsackie Virus Infections

The Coxsackie viruses are found not infrequently in the feces of human beings and occasionally in throat washings. The significance of their occurrence in individuals who are not ill, and in patients with poliomyelitis, is still subject to investigation. Over 20 immunologic types have been recognized.

When injected into infant mice these viruses induce fatal destructive lesions. Two distinct groups of these viruses known as A and B have been differentiated: Those in group A produce degenerative changes in mouse muscles only, whereas those in group B produce changes in the central nervous system as well.

Some members of group A can give rise to the disease entity known as herpangina. Seen chiefly in young children, this is a short-lived febrile epidemic infection with ulcerating vesicles in the throat and posterior regions of the mouth, often associated with vomiting and gastroenteritis.

Some members of group B can produce Bornholm disease (epidemic pleurodynia, myalgia), characterized by fever, severe pain in the chest or abdomen, and pharyngitis. The illness is of short duration and is probably more frequent in children than in adults. Members of group B have at times seemed responsible for minor febrile illnesses and also for some instances of aseptic meningitis.

Infection with a Coxsackie virus may be suspected from the clinical manifestations, but laboratory confirmation is required for positive establishment of the diagnosis. In general, this consists either of the demonstration of the virus in material procured from fecal discharges or swabs of the throat or anus or the finding of a rise in serum antibodies between the early and convalescent phases of the illness. The ubiquity of the Coxsackie viruses in human feces makes it unsafe to establish an atypical attack of illness as being caused by Coxsackie virus when a strain of this virus is recovered solely from the stool, or even when antibodies to such a strain are found in the patient's serum.

Mumps

The diagnosis of mumps parotitis can usually be made with confidence from the manifestations exhibited by the patient, especially when an epidemic prevails in the community. Sporadic and unusual cases, however, or instances of isolated orchitis or aseptic lymphocytic meningitis may be puzzling clinically and require laboratory confirmation. Isolation of the virus by inoculation of chick embryos or tissue cultures is of practical usefulness for diagnosis.

The virus of mumps will agglutinate the red cells of chickens, humans, and some other animal species. This hemagglutination will be inhibited when an individual's serum contains mumps antibodies, if the serum is mixed with mumps antigen before the latter is added to the red cells. Rises in agglutination-inhibition titer are dependable for the recognition of an acute or recent infection with mumps but are less reliable for the diagnosis of a past attack. Fourfold increases or greater are usually demonstrable between blood specimens collected early in the disease and later in the convalescent phase.

Many patients also develop antibodies against the virus of Newcastle disease of fowls during or after an attack of mumps. This is ascribed to an antigenic component common to the two species of viruses.

Yellow Fever

This disease has been divided epidemiologically into two main varieties —the classic urban yellow fever transmitted from man to man by the *Aedes aegypti* mosquito and the jungle variety in which man becomes only accidentally infected from strains of virus endemic for monkeys and other animals. During epidemics the diagnosis usually can be made from the clinical story, but laboratory confirmation is needed for sporadic and atypical cases.

The injection of a patient's serum intracerebrally into mice, up to the fifth day of illness, will usually produce encephalitis. Further studies are then needed to identify this infective agent as the yellow fever virus.

In a typical attack the content of antibodies rises markedly. Accordingly a sample of serum may be taken as soon as the disease is suspected, and a second sample 2 or 3 weeks later, during convalescence. A rise in titer, or the presence of antibodies in the second but not the first sample, is of diagnostic importance.

Pathologic changes in the liver may be studied in a biopsy specimen if deemed advisable or in postmortem material from fatal cases. The usual findings are midzonal parenchymal necroses with masses of eosinophilic hyaline-like cytoplasm (Councilman bodies) scattered lightly through the lobule. Fatty degeneration is also prominent. Nuclear inclusion bodies are seen in experimental animals but almost never in man.

ACUTE RESPIRATORY TRACT INFECTIONS

The catarrhal inflammatory illnesses of the upper respiratory tract may be produced by viruses, by bacteria, or by both kinds of agents acting in conjunction or sequentially. Antibiotics and sulfonamides are of little or no value for therapy of the viral components apart from the psittacosis group, but tend to counteract or inhibit the bacteria.

So many resemblances and so much overlapping exist in the patterns of the catarrhal respiratory tract infections among children that differentiation into distinct entities on symptomatic grounds alone is often difficult. A practical classification from the *clinical* point of view is the following: (1) common cold, (2) influenza, (3) acute respiratory tract disease, (4) acute bacterial pharyngitis, and (5) viral respiratory tract infection complicated by bacterial invasion. Inflammation of the respiratory tract may occur also in diphtheria, pneumonia, measles, rickettsialpox, poliomyelitis, infectious mononucleosis, psittacosis, herpangina, Q fever, lymphocytic choriomeningitis, herpes simplex, and other diseases; or may be caused by pneumococci, streptococci, meningococci, staphylococci, influenza bacilli, or other bacteria, viruses, or fungi.

Common Cold (Rhinitis, Coryza)

This is characterized by catarrhal nasal inflammation, a short incubation period of 1 to 3 days, a mild fever in some patients, and a total duration when uncomplicated of from 2 to 5 days. The lymphoid tissue in the nasopharyngeal area may swell. Similar illnesses can be transmitted to well human volunteers or chimpanzees by nasal instillation of bacteria-free filtrates of the nasal washings of patients, collected during the period of active symptoms. Prior mixing of these secretions with serum from convalescent patients will inactivate the infective agent. Simple specific laboratory tests are not available. In the early stages the abundant nasal secretion may be comparatively cell-free and show no specific bacteria on culture. Later it may contain large numbers of neutrophils and viable bacteria, and often some eosinophils. The inflammatory changes tend to be especially pronounced if there already exists an allergic rhinopathy; eosinophils are then more abundant. The peripheral and differential leukocyte counts show no significant changes. The red cell sedimentation rate and the serum titers of antistreptolysin, cold hemagglutinins, and heterophil and other antibodies remain unaltered.

Influenza

By symptoms alone it is often difficult to differentiate influenza from other acute respiratory tract illnesses. The true influenza viruses are more likely to give rise to a sudden onset, high fever, severe constitutional symptoms, and inflammation of the nasal mucosa, whereas the undifferentiated diseases tend to have a prominent pharyngitis, laryngitis, or bronchitis. These differences are of statistical importance chiefly, not very useful in the study of individual patients. Frequent simultaneous or secondary complications are otitis media, sinusitis, or bronchopneumonia, caused usually by streptococci, staphylococci, pneumococci, or influenza bacilli, often in combination.

The influenza viruses can be isolated by inoculation of nasal or pharyngeal washings from patients in the early stages. Recovered strains are then identified by immunologic procedures.

The main antigenic groups which thus far have been recognized are A, B, and C. Variant strains of influenza viruses A and B have been the most frequent causes of epidemics in the past few years; influenza C virus has been encountered only a few times in sporadic cases. Those which are similar to but not identical with A are known collectively as A-prime. For most purposes only the group need be identified, using hemagglutination inhibition or complement fixation.

EPIDEMIOLOGY. An international program to study influenza and aid physicians and health officials in the control of the disease has been set up by the World Health Organization. As soon as a significant outbreak of suspected influenza is encountered, regional laboratories embark on serologic testing of patients for the presence of influenza antibodies. Efforts are also made to recover the virus from some of the patients. Every strain thus isolated is then subjected to a complete antigenic analysis by a central reference laboratory. All new strains are considered for possible inclusion in protective vaccines. In the United States this program is under the direction of the Public Health Service.

Influenza spreads rapidly. A strain causing epidemics in the Southern Hemisphere during the winter may give rise to epidemics in the Northern Hemisphere a few months later. For example, a strain of A-prime virus isolated in South Africa and Australia during June, 1950, was found to be identical with that causing a severe outbreak in Liverpool, England, in January, 1951. Closely similar and probably identical strains gave rise to epidemics in western Europe, Japan, and the United States during 1952. Successful vaccination against influenza requires inclusion in the vaccine of the precise strain which threatens to cause a regional epidemic. Hence it is essential to isolate and identify the potentially prevalent strain before an epidemic becomes widespread.

Acute Respiratory Tract Disease

An abundance of epidemiologic and bacteriologic evidence indicates that nonbacterial and presumably viral agents can be responsible primarily for many of the acute infections which afflict the nose, pharynx, larynx, trachea, and bronchi during the colder months of the year. The same epidemic infective agent apparently can produce a variety of clinical responses in different individuals. Conversely, clinically similar illnesses may be produced by different agents. Some of these causative viral agents have already been identified and differentiated.

Routine laboratory findings in these illnesses are much the same as with the common cold. Throat cultures reveal no abnormal bacterial flora. Blood cultures are sterile. The nasal discharge or sputum may contain pus cells. During convalescence the peripheral blood may contain occasional atypical lymphocytes, resembling somewhat those of infectious mononucleosis.

ADENOVIRUS INFECTIONS. Research in respiratory tract viruses has been stimulated greatly by the discovery in 1953 of hitherto unknown cytopathogenic viruses which could be grown in tissue culture from apparently healthy adenoids removed surgically. This group of so-called "adenoviruses" in 1956 numbered at least fourteen serologically distinct types pathogenic for human beings. Previously termed the APC (adenoidal-pharyngeal-conjunctival) viruses, they are nonpathogenic for laboratory animals, heat-labile, filtrable, and resistant to antibiotics. Group-specific and type-specific contained antigens can be demonstrated. Types 1, 2, 4, 5, and 6 have been found in tonsil and adenoid tissues and nasopharyngeal secretions. Type 3 has been found in anal swabbings and conjunctival and nasopharyngeal secretions. Type 7 has been found in throat washings, and type 8 in conjunctival and corneal scrapings. One or another of these viruses have been associated with outbreaks of acute respiratory tract illnesses, often attended by conjunctivitis. It seems probable that they may be one cause of acute bronchiolitis and acute laryngotracheobronchitis in infants and small children.

EXUDATIVE NONBACTERIAL PHARYNGITIS. This poorly defined disorder, of as yet unestablished etiology, is a constitutionally prostrating illness with a distinctive yellow-white or gray exudate on the tonsils and oropharyngeal membranes. The exudate is thin and usually patchy; it originates within the follicles of the tonsils, and may involve only the crypts.

INFECTIOUS CROUP. In this syndrome the typical course is that of an upper respiratory tract infection which involves the larynx early and may spread downward to the tracheobronchial passages. The symptom-complex is most prevalent during the winter months, in children between 1 and 7 years of age. Among 347 cases studied by Rabe at New Haven, Conn., 22 seemed due to diphtheria, 28 to the type B influenza bacillus, and the remainder to unknown agents assumed to be viruses perhaps accompanied by bacteria.

PRIMARY ATYPICAL PNEUMONIA (VIRUS PNEUMONIA, ACUTE INTERSTITIAL PNEUMONITIS). This is a poorly defined lower respiratory tract syndrome. Some outbreaks seem to be due to viral agents, inasmuch as careful bacteriologic investigations are noncontributory. Many authorities believe that this form of illness may result from virus invasion, acting synergistically with bacteria which normally are merely nasopharyngeal saprophytes. Symptoms are usually not prostrating, but fever, cough, and weakness may continue for a month or more. Roentgenograms may show mottlings or scattered opacities which are out of proportion to the scanty physical signs over the chest. The pathologic lesions in the lung are those of acute focal bronchiolitis, patch interstitial and alveolar exudate, and some atelectasis and emphysema. Sputum when present may be blood-streaked, but not rust-colored as in bacterial pneumonia.

Laboratory Findings. The leukocyte count typically remains in the normal range, with no neutrophil increase to suggest a primary or secondary bacterial invasion. A mild lymphocytosis may be demonstrable. The red cell sedimentation rate is usually elevated and does not return to normal until after the symptoms and the lung x-ray changes have subsided. "Atypical lymphocytes" may appear in the blood stream during convalesence.

Nonspecific Serum Antibodies. In some epidemics, nonspecific cold hemagglutinins and agglutinins for Streptococcus MG can be found in about one-third of untreated older children and adults, not necessarily coincidentally, and less frequently in infants and young children. In general, the more severe the illness the more likely are these nonspecific antibodies to appear, and the higher the serum concentrations. The changes in titer between early in the disease and convalescence should be at least fourfold to be adjudged diagnostic.

The cold hemagglutinin test is based on the capacity of serum from a patient to agglutinate a diluted suspension of human group O red cells at a temperature of 0 to 5°C in a dilution of 1:32 or higher. Hemagglutination at 37°C does not take place except when the titer in the cold is extremely high. These agglutinins appear usually in the second week of the illness, attain a peak in the third or fourth week, and then decline gradually. Serum to be tested should be kept warm until the clot is separated or rewarmed to 37°C before this is done. If the specimen has been placed in the refrigerator by mistake, a convalescent titer of 1:20 or more may be deemed abnormal. The serum from healthy subjects without respiratory tract infections will rarely give a reaction with this test in dilutions above 1:16.

Streptococcus MG is a nonhemolytic streptococcus which appears to be distinct serologically from other species of streptococci. The organism is not the cause of this form of pneumonia, but a suspension may be agglutinated by a patient's serum in a dilution titer of 1:20 or higher, during or immediately after an attack.

VIRAL BRONCHIOLITIS OF INFANCY (BRONCHIOLITIS, CAPILLARY BRONCHIO-LITIS). This is a symptomatic entity restricted chiefly to the first 2 years of life. Characteristic features are coryza, cough, low fever, and progressive dyspnea with cyanosis, produced by inflammatory changes in the bronchi and bronchioles. Bacteria sometimes seem to play a role as secondary invaders and may cause superimposed bacterial pneumonia which may be fatal.

Evidence for the viral origin of these attacks lies in (1) coexistence of a viral-like catarrhal reaction in the upper respiratory passages, (2) normal bacterial flora usually present in the nasopharynx, (3) occurrence of a mononuclear cell exudate in the peribronchial and peribronchiolar tissues, and (4) the finding in a few outbreaks of acidophilic cytoplasmic inclusion bodies within the cells of the tracheobronchial epithelium and pulmonary alveoli and to a lesser extent in other organs.

Acute Bacterial Pharyngitis ("Strep Throat")

Hemolytic streptococci frequently cause a primary pharyngitis, tonsillitis, or laryngitis in children over 4 years of age (see p. 826). Most of these cases can be traced to contact with other cases or carriers, but some outbreaks have been food- or milk-borne. It is questionable whether pneumococci or influenza bacilli can cause respiratory tract infections in the absence of a concomitant virus.

Combined Viral and Bacterial Infections

Many of the respiratory tract infections seen in children, especially during the winter and spring, seem to be expressions of the symbiotic action of pathogenic bacteria with a respiratory tract virus. In most instances the virus appears to be the initiating offender, though both forms of agents may attack simultaneously. The bacteria most prevalent in this symbiotic association are pneumococci, hemolytic streptococci, viridans streptococci, influenza bacilli, and staphylococci. Meningococci, Klebsiella, or other Gram-negative bacilli are sometimes implicated. Several contiguous segments of the respiratory tract are usually affected. The diagnosis applied is based on the anatomic area in which the inflammation is most prominent—sinusitis, otitis media, laryngitis, bronchitis, bronchopneumonia, laryngotracheobronchitis, and so on. Migration of the bacteria may lead to septicemia, meningitis, osteomyelitis, or other remote infections. An example of this mode of spread for such infections is the frequent association of purulent meningitis due to meningococci, pneumococci, influenza, bacilli, streptococci, or staphylococci with an otitis media, sinusitis, or upper respiratory tract infection caused by the same organism.

The pneumonia which follows measles or influenza, as in the great influenza pandemic of 1917–1918, is typically an acute interstitial bacterial bronchopneumonia, though there may be wide deviations from this pattern. The sputum and postmortem lung cultures often yield a mixture of bacterial species— staphylococci, influenza bacilli, hemolytic streptococci, viridans streptococci, pneumococci of various types, and even *Escherichia coli* or coliform organisms in rare instances. When the lung lesions are those of purulent bronchitis or bronchiolitis the predominant organism is likely to be the influenza bacillus. Lobar and lobular pneumonia are usually associated with pneumococci or streptococci; and pulmonary necroses or abscesses with staphylococci.

Even though the antibiotics are ineffective in respiratory tract infections of purely viral origin, except perhaps for primary atypical pneumonia, many physicians nevertheless treat such illness with antibiotics or sulfonamide drugs, as prophylaxis against the development of complications caused by bacteria.

Sudden Death in Infancy

Microscopic studies of tissues of apparently well infants who expire suddenly after a few minor constitutional symptoms are making it increasingly clear that the precipitating cause of death in most of these cases is a fulminating respiratory tract infection. For example, in 31 such well-nourished New York City infants found dead while in apparent good health, in whom the gross necropsy findings were insufficient to explain death, Werne and Garrow found acute inflammatory lesions in the upper or lower respiratory passages and related structures in every instance. Bacteriologic studies in 24 of the infants yielded cultures of hemolytic staphylococci in 11 and hemolytic streptococci in 3. These authors concluded also that the "mononuclear pneumonia" and "giant cell pneumonia" proposed by others are not true entities. Mononuclear cells proliferate readily in response to many stimuli, including a protracted death agony. Mononuclear infiltrations were noted frequently in another series of well infants whose lives were terminated by known violence.

Enteric Viruses

The alimentary tract of children will sometimes contain viruses which can cause hepatitis, poliomyelitis, Coxsackie, influenza, mumps, herpes simplex, or adenovirus infections. A group of other enteric viruses with no evident pathogenic attributes has been found in the past few years by the newer tissue culture approaches. For convenience, these latter are termed "enteric cytopathogenic human orphan" (ECHO) viruses. Cross-neutralization tests have made it possible thus far to differentiate at least nineteen numbered antigenic types. The clinical significance of some of these is as yet unknown. A few have been found only in children in the first 10 years of life. It has been suggested that some may prove to be saprophytic variants of poliomyelitis or respiratory tract viruses. Ramos-Alvarez and Sabin, who studied rectal swabs of children in several cities, recovered these viruses from 5 per cent of children in Cincinnati, 15 per cent in Mexico City, and 10 per cent in Veracruz.

RICKETTSIAL DISEASES

The rickettsiae are Gram-negative coccobacillary microorganisms which are classified biologically as intermediate between bacteria and viruses. Though visible under the microscope, they appear unable to grow outside living cells. With the exception of the large causative agent of Q fever, most rickettsiae are just large enough to be caught by fine bacteriologic filters. The diseases they produce in man have been divided into five classes on the basis of immunologic cross reactions:

1. Spotted fever group
   a. Rocky Mountain spotted fever
   b. Rickettsialpox
   c. Related tick-borne rickettsioses in Europe, Africa, Mexico, South America, and elsewhere
2. Typhus group
   a. Epidemic typhus fever
   b. Brill's disease
   c. Murine typhus fever
3. Q fever
4. Scrub typhus (tsutsugamushi disease)
5. Miscellaneous trench fever
   a. Trench fever
   b. Colorado tick fever

Complement-fixing, Weil-Felix, or other antibodies arise early in most rickettsial infections unless a vigorous program of chemotherapy is begun early in the illness. In the latter event, diagnostically high titers may not appear until well along in convalescence or sometimes not at all.

Spotted Fever Group

ROCKY MOUNTAIN SPOTTED FEVER. This acute febrile disease is produced by widespread dissemination of *Rickettsia rickettsii* throughout the body. It is acquired from the bite of the wood tick *Dermacentor andersoni,* the dog tick *D. variabilis,* and perhaps other related insects. Wild rodents (squirrels, rabbits, wood rats, chipmunks, etc.) are the animal reservoir of the infectious agent.

After an incubation period of 2 to 12 days the child who is bitten by an infected tick experiences an initial period of prostration and fever, followed in a few days by a spreading generalized rash. In the pre-eruptive stage one may find a positive tourniquet test and a low or normal leukocyte count with an increase in the polymorphonuclear cells. A subsequent leukocytosis is usually a manifestation of a secondary bacterial infection. Adults frequently have a moderate monocytosis, but this is unusual in children.

As the illness progresses the red cell and hemoglobin levels fall. Hypoproteinemia, hypoelectrolytemia, and nitrogen retention can be found, ascribable in part to a shift of body fluids from the vascular to the extravascular spaces. Since this fluid shift may contribute to a later peripheral vascular collapse, supportive fluid and electrolyte therapy are needed. Abnormalities of the urine and cerebrospinal fluid are frequent. The liver function tests may also show abnormalities. Secondary bronchopneumonia and related bacterial infection develop in about half the cases unless chemotherapy is given.

Isolation and identification of the infectious agent by laboratory approaches requires trained personnel, a special laboratory, guinea pigs or other animals, and the maintenance of known rickettsial strains with which cross-immunity tests can be carried out. The Weil-Felix and complement-fixation reactions are more practical aids in diagnosis.

Weil-Felix Reaction. This phenomenon is based on the evoking by most pathogenic rickettsiae of agglutinins against the strains of Proteus X bacillus known as OX19, OX2, and OXK. The antigenic overlapping between these bacteria and the rickettsial organisms appears to be accidental. The OX19 agglutination usually becomes high in endemic or murine typhus, in Rocky Mountain spotted fever, and in epidemic or louse-borne typhus. The OXK agglutination tends to rise only in tsutsugamushi fever. None of the Proteus X strains become agglutinated in rickettsial and Q fever. The OX2 titer is most likely to rise as high as or even higher than the OX19 titer in Rocky Mountain spotted fever, but such rise is not invariable or absolutely specific.

In rickettsial diseases the Weil-Felix response is usually elevated to a peak level of between 1:160 and 1:5,120 dilutions. Two successive serum specimens should be examined. The first should be obtained as soon as a rickettsial disease is suspected, to serve as a base line for repeat tests. This is particularly important with children who may have once received antityphus inoculations. The titer tends to rise significantly during the second week of the illness and early convalescence and fades away in late convalescence. The Weil-Felix agglutination therefore cannot be used to demonstrate a past infection with a rickettsial disease.

One difficulty with the Weil-Felix reaction is that occasional children free from rickettsial or obvious Proteus bacillus infections may exhibit a titer up to 1:160 or rarely even up to 1:640.

Complement Fixation. Specific soluble antigens are available for complement-fixation tests. These have the superiority over the Weil-Felix approach in being more specific, though some overlapping of reactivity takes place among the rickettsial diseases. Results of the tests in Rocky Mountain spotted fever are usually interpreted as positive if these antibodies become demonstrable in serum dilutions of 1:10 or higher at about the second week of illness. Once these antibodies appear they persist for at least 6 to 8 years, in contrast to the Weil-Felix antibodies which usually fade away in a few weeks.

RICKETTSIALPOX. This is a newly recognized acute febrile illness caused by *Rickettsia akari*. The vector is the rodent mite (*Allodermanyssus sanguineus*) which is an ectoparasite of the house mouse (*Mus musculus*).

The initial focal lesion at the site of the insect bite is followed within a week by fever and other systemic symptoms. A papulovesicular eruption develops 1 to 10 days later. Routine laboratory studies reveal no characteristic changes other than a granulocytopenia and lymphocytosis, or sometimes a transitory monocytosis up to 5 per cent of all the leukocytes. The monocytes are often vacuolated and may resemble the altered cells of infectious mononucleosis. The heterophil antibodies do not rise, and the Weil-Felix tests are negative.

The diagnosis is based clinically on the overt features during the acute illness. From the laboratory standpoint, it is often possible to transmit the rickettsiae to mice, chick embryos, and guinea pigs by direct injection of patient's blood taken during the early period of symptoms. If animals are not immediately available, the blood may be stored in the frozen state for later recovery of the organisms.

Complement-fixing antibodies begin to appear in the blood about a week after the onset of fever and reach their peak 3 or 4 weeks later. The antigen is prepared from rickettsiae grown in chick embryos. For diagnosis a blood specimen is taken early in the illness and again 2 to 7 weeks later. A significant rise in titer will be demonstrated. Readings usually fall in the range 1:32 to 1:128. Most convalescent serum specimens also react with the antigen for Rocky Mountain spotted fever.

Typhus Group

CLASSICAL (EPIDEMIC, LOUSE-BORNE) TYPHUS FEVER. This is an acute febrile disease with chills, fever, headache, hypotension, and gastrointestinal disturbances as early symptoms, followed often by a macular rash lasting 2 or 3 days. The liver and spleen may be enlarged. The leukocyte count varies from 3,000 to 20,000 with a neutrophilia when there is secondary infection, but no eosinophilia. The red cell and hemoglobin levels fall. The urine shows proteinuria and signs of renal irritation. Dehydration, hypochlorhydria, and nitrogen retention may appear, more marked in the severe cases. The cerebrospinal fluid often shows a mild pleocytosis. The rickettsiae in all types of typhus fever are susceptible to the broad-spectrum antibiotics.

The cause of the disease is *Rickettsia prowazeki*. This is spread from man to man by the human body louse, *Pediculus humanus corporis*, and to a lesser extent by the human head louse, *P. humanus capitis*.

The laboratory approaches to diagnosis are the same as for Rocky Mountain spotted fever. Guinea pigs injected with patient's blood in the early stages of the illness will become ill with the disease. The Weil-Felix reaction becomes positive on the fifth to eighth day and continues for some weeks. The complement-fixation titer rises rapidly after the first week and may persist for years. Little or no cross reactions are given with the specific antigens for the other rickettsial diseases, with the exception of positive but lower titers for the antigen of murine typhus.

BRILL'S DISEASE (RECRUDESCENT OR SPORADIC TYPHUS). This is a typhus-like infection which is seen most often in foreign-born subjects who have come to this country from areas where typhus fever is endemic. Routine laboratory tests show no significant abnormalities. The Weil-Felix titer is usually at 1:40 or lower. The complement-fixation titer after the first week is usually 1:320 to 1:5,120 with the antigen from epidemic typhus, and 1:20 to 1:2,560 with the antigen from murine typhus. Rickettsiae recovered from early cases by louse-feeding experiments have seemed identical with *R. prowazeki* of classic epidemic typhus.

MURINE (ENDEMIC, FLEA-BORNE) TYPHUS FEVER. This less severe form of typhus is seen in all parts of the world. It is a naturally occurring disease of rats and mice. The causative agent is *Rickettsia mooseri*, which is transferred sporadically and as it were accidentally to man by the bite of the rat or shrew louse, *Polyplax spinulosus*, of the rat flea, *Xenopsylla cheopis*, or of the squirrel flea, *Xenopsylla astia*. Serologic procedures are the methods of choice in diagnosis. To establish that *R. mooseri* is responsible, the serum complement-fixation titer should be higher against antigen from this organism than from *R. prowazeki*.

Q Fever

This infection, caused by *Rickettsia (Coxiella) burnetii*, is characterized by a sudden onset, fever, headache, and malaise, followed often by an attack of interstitial pneumonitis. The course may vary from a subclinical infection to a severe illness lasting weeks or months, or even become chronic. Most patients have been stockyard workers, laboratory workers, dairy workers, and residents of dairy areas. The most likely mode of infection seems to be the inhalation of or contact with contaminated dust or other material from infected animals. Very few childhood cases have been recognized. Potential sources are infected cows, sheep, goats, milk from these animals, wild animals, and a wide variety of ticks.

Rickettsiae can be demonstrated in the patient's blood during the acute stages of the illness. Because of the great danger of infecting laboratory workers this approach is to be avoided except with special problems. The broad-spectrum antibiotics seem of some value in therapy, but rickettsiemia is still demonstrable by animal inoculation after their administration is begun. Specific antibodies may develop more slowly, however.

The serologic approach is used widely for establishing the diagnosis. One specimen of patient's blood is taken early in the illness, and another at 14 to 21 days later. Both sera are tested simultaneously for complement-fixing antibodies or agglutinins, employing an antigen prepared from the parasite. When only one serum specimen is obtainable from a suspected patient, a titer of 1:128 or higher has been deemed diagnostic. Readings of 1:32 or 1:64 are suggestive of an infection in the recent past. Cross reactions with the typhus fever and spotted fever antigens are rare.

PSITTACOSIS–LYMPHOGRANULOMA VENEREUM DISEASES

The two most important pathogens for man in this biologic group, which is intermediate between the rickettsiae and viruses, are those which induce psittacosis and those which induce lymphogranuloma venereum. The causative agents are coccoid elementary bodies 300 to 500 $\mu\mu$ in diameter. They stain tinctorially and can be seen with the oil-immersion microscopic lens. They can infect mice and other laboratory animals and may be propagated in chick embryos or tissue cultures. The serum reactions of patients convalescent from either illness show considerable antigenic overlapping.

Psittacosis (Ornithosis)

This is an avian infection which can be transmitted to man through contact with infected parrots, parakeets, pigeons, doves, canaries, finches, ducks, turkeys, and other birds. Symptoms are predominately constitutional and pulmonary; the illness resembles stubborn influenza, atypical pneumonia, or typhoid fever. A large spleen is sometimes found.

LABORATORY DIAGNOSIS. During the first 2 weeks of illness, the causative virus, *Miyagawanella psittaci*, can usually be recovered from patients by injection of blood, throat washings, vomitus, or sputum into white mice. Complement-fixing antibodies to the specific antigen begin to appear in the blood by the end of the first week after onset of symptoms and rise during the following weeks. However, when antibiotics are being taken the appearance of antibodies may be delayed until 4 to 6 weeks. Once present they persist for months or even years. Many dealers and breeders of birds regularly have serum complement-fixing titers of 1:8 to 1:32. A serum titer of 1:16 or higher may be deemed presumptive evidence for the diagnosis of psittacosis in a patient who displays suggestive symptoms even when a history of contact with birds cannot be obtained. One must exclude lymphogranuloma venereum on clinical grounds, since patients with this disease also exhibit a positive antibody response with the psittacosis antigen during the period of acute illness. The reverse is also true. It has been feasible also to elicit specific skin reactions in patients with psittacosis by the intradermal injections of extracts of the psittacosis agent.

Lymphogranuloma Venereum

Though essentially a disease of adults spread by venereal contact, lymphogranuloma venereum may appear occasionally in children in the form of inguinal adenitis, rectal stricture, or arthritic effusions; cervical node involvement has also been described. Infection in the child can usually be attributed to contact with an infected parent. The nature of the illness may be suspected from the physical findings and epidemiologic history.

In both psittacosis and lymphogranuloma venereum there is a tendency for leukopenia and a mild normochromic anemia to appear early in the disease, with a leukocytosis in the later stages. The red cell sedimentation rate is usually increased. Mild proteinuria is not uncommon.

SURGICAL BIOPSY. Affected tissue removed for biopsy shows acute or chronic inflammatory tuberculous-like reactions, often with central abscesslike necroses. The inflammatory tissue contains epithelioid cells which are sometimes multinucleated, along with plasma cells, lymphocytes, and neutrophilic leukocytes. Staining with the Machievello, Castenada, or Noble techniques reveals large basophilic intracytoplasmic inclusion bodies within large macrophages. These formations in a purulent discharge are sometimes demonstrable by suitable stains.

RECOVERY OF AGENT. Intracerebral injection of mice with suspected material usually infects the animals and permits identification of the causative agent. The yolk sacs of embryonated hen's eggs may also be employed.

FREI TEST. Skin tests with a sterilized extract of pus from buboes of known cases (the Frei antigen) are usually positive. A similar antigen prepared from the yolk sacs of infected eggs is commercially available (Lygranum). A positive reaction consists of an area of induration measuring 6 by 6 mm or more which appears in 2 to 4 days. The skin reaction usually becomes positive in 1 to 6 weeks after the onset of the secondary adenitis which follows the usually unrecognized small primary lesion.

ANTIBODY TESTS. Complement-fixation tests almost always become positive in about a month and remain positive as long as the causative agent persists in the host. Obtained titers may range from 1:6 up to 1:1,000. Rises in titer in successive tests are of great significance. Single titers of 1:32 usually indicate the existence of the infection, though individuals with early syphilis or with recent or recovered psittacosis often given positive reactions with the lymphogranuloma antigen.

BIBLIOGRAPHY

DIAGNOSIS OF VIRAL DISEASES

Ayres, J. C., and *R. F. Feemster,* Serologic Tests in the Diagnosis of Infectious Diseases, *New England J. Med.* 243:996, 1043, 1950.

Blank, H., C. F. Burgoon, G. D. Baldridge, P. L. McCarthy, and *F. Urbach,* Cytologic Smears in Diagnosis of Herpes Zoster and Varicella, *J.A.M.A.* 146:1410, 1951.

——— and *G. Rake,* "Viral and Rickettsial Diseases of the Skin, Eye and Mucous Membranes of Man," Little, Brown & Co., Boston, 1955.

Cohen, S., The Enzymes of the Host Cell as a Requirement for Virus Synthesis, *Ann. New York Acad. Sc.* 54:902, 1952.

Cox, H. R., Specific Complement-fixing Diagnostic Antigens for Viral and Rickettsial Disease, *Am. J. Pub. Health* 38:351, 1948.

Harding, B. H., N. J. Schmidt, and O. E. Hepler, Some Pitfalls in the Performance and the Interpretation of Results of Serologic Tests for Virus and Rickettsial Diseases, *A.M.A. Arch. Path.* 57:447, 1954.

Milzer, A., Routine Laboratory Diagnosis of Virus and Rickettsial Diseases: Results of an Eighteen Months Study, *J.A.M.A.* 143:219, 1950.

Rivers, T. M., "Viral and Rickettsial Infections of Man," 2d ed., J. B. Lippincott Company, Philadelphia, 1952.

Robbins, F. C., and T. H. Weller, Application of Tissue Culture Methods to the Study of Viral Infections, *Pediatrics* 13:283, 1954.

Sigel, M. M., The Role of the Virologist in the Diagnosis of Acute Infectious Diseases, *M. Clin. North America* 34:1605, 1950.

Utz, J. P., R. H. Parrott, and J. A. Kasel, Diagnostic Virus Laboratory for Clinical Service, *J.A.M.A.* 163:350, 1957.

HERPES SIMPLEX

Buddingh, G. J., D. I. Schrum, J. C. Lanier, and D. J. Guidry, Studies of the Natural History of Herpes Simplex Infections, *Pediatrics* 11:595, 1953.

Crouse, H. V., L. L. Coriell, H. Blank, and T. F. McN. Scott, Cytochemical Studies on the Intranuclear Inclusion of Herpes Simplex, *J. Immunol.* 65:119, 1950.

Florman, A. L., and R. L. Mindlin, Generalized Herpes Simplex in an Eleven-day-old Premature Infant, *A.M.A. Am. J. Dis. Child.* 83:481, 1952.

Quilligan, J. J., Jr., and J. L. Wilson, Fatal Herpes Simplex Infection in a Newborn Infant, *J. Lab. & Clin. Med.* 38:742, 1951.

Scott, T. F. McN., L. Coriell, H. Blank, and C. F. Burgoon, Some Comments on Herpetic Infection in Children with Special Emphasis on Unusual Clinical Manifestations, *J. Pediat.* 41:835, 1952.

Zuelzer, W. W., and C. S. Stulberg, Herpes Simplex Virus as the Cause of Fulminating Visceral Disease and Hepatitis in Infancy, *A.M.A. Am. J. Dis. Child.* 83:421, 1952.

SMALLPOX AND VACCINIA

Bigler, J. A., and E. L. Slotkowski, Smallpox Vaccination with Prolonged Vaccinia, *Pediatrics* 7:24, 1951.

Bohls, S. W., and J. V. Irons, Chorio-allantoic Membrane Infection as a Diagnostic Test for Smallpox, *Am. J. Pub. Health* 32:300, 1942.

Downie, A. W., The Laboratory Diagnosis of Smallpox, *Month. Bull. Min. Health* 5:114, 1946.

———, K. McCarthy, and A. Macdonald, Laboratory Methods in the Diagnosis of Alastrim, *Month. Bull. Min. Health* 11:227, 1952.

Gray, F. G., A Familial Spread of Vaccinia with One Death: Isolation and Identification of the Virus, *Bull. Johns Hopkins Hosp.* 82:538, 1948.

Kempe, C. H., Passive Immunity to Vaccinia in Newborns: Placental Transmission by Antibodies, *Yale J. Biol. & Med.* 24:328, 1952.

———, T. O. Berge, and B. England, Hyperimmune Vaccinal Gamma Globulin: Source, Evaluation, and Use in Prophylaxis and Therapy, *Pediatrics* 18:177, 1956.

Marsden, J. P., Variola Minor, *Month. Bull. Min. Health* 11:74, 1952.

Parker, R. F., "Variola and Vaccinia: Diagnostic Procedures for Virus and Rickettsial Diseases," p. 83, American Public Health Association, New York, 1948.

van Rooyen, C. E., and *G. D. Scott,* Smallpox Diagnosis with Special Reference to Electron Microscopy, *Canad. J. Pub. Health* **39**:467, 1948.

Wolman, M., Application of the Feulgen Reaction to the Laboratory Diagnosis of Smallpox, *Proc. Soc. Exper. Biol. & Med.* **74**:85, 1950.

POLIOMYELITIS

Bhatt, P. N., M. Brooks, and *J. P. Fox,* Extent of Infection with Poliomyelitis Virus in Household Associates of Clinical Cases as Determined Serologically and by Virus Isolation Using Tissue Culture Methods, *Am. J. Hyg.* **61**:287, 1955.

Bodian, D., and *S. Paffenbarger, Jr.,* Poliomyelitis Infection in Households. Frequency of Viremia and Specific Antibody Response, *Am. J. Hyg.* **60**:83, 1954.

Brown, G. C., and *D. C. Smith,* Serologic Response of Infants and Preschool Children to Poliomyelitis Vaccine, *J.A.M.A.* **161**:399, 1956.

Francis, T., Jr., Approach to Control of Poliomyelitis by Immunological Methods, *Bull. New York Acad. Med.* **31**:259, 1955.

Hammon, W. McD., L. L. Coriell, P. F. Wehrle, C. R. Klimt, and *J. Stokes, Jr.,* Evaluation of Red Cross Gamma Globulin as a Prophylactic Agent for Poliomyelitis, *J.A.M.A.* **150**:757, 1952.

Melnick, J. L., M. Ramos-Alvarez, F. L. Black, A. J. Girardi, and *D. Nagaki,* Poliomyelitis Viruses in Tissue Culture. VII. Experiences With Viral and Serological Diagnostic Procedures, *Yale J. Biol. & Med.* **26**:465, 1954.

Miller, C. A., and *P. Kamitsuka,* The Recovery of Poliomyelitis Viruses from Fecal Samples of Poliomyelitis Patients and Household Contacts, *Am. J. M. Sc.* **231**:607, 1956.

National Foundation for Infantile Paralysis Committee on Typing, Immunologic Classification of Poliomyelitis Viruses. VII. Discussion of Results and Comparative Program for the Typing of Two Hundred and Thirty Strains, *Am. J. Hyg.* **58**:74, 1953.

"Poliomyelitis: Papers and Discussions Presented at the Third International Poliomyelitis Conference," J. B. Lippincott Company, Philadelphia, 1955.

Sabin, A. B., Immunity in Poliomyelitis, With Special Reference to Vaccination, World Health Organization: *Monograph Series No. 26,* p. 297, Geneva, 1955.

Salk, J. E., Antigenic Potency of Poliomyelitis Vaccine: Influence on Degree and Duration of Vaccine Effect, *J.A.M.A.* **162**:1451, 1956.

Svedmyr, A., J. F. Enders, and *A. Holloway,* Complement-fixation with the Three Types of Poliomyelitis Viruses Propagated in Tissue Culture, *Am. J. Hyg.* **57**:50, 1953.

Weller, T. H., Advances in the Laboratory Diagnosis of Poliomyelitis, *J.A.M.A.* **156**:16, 1954.

———, *J. F. Enders, F. C. Robbins,* and *M. B. Stoddard,* Studies on the Cultivation of Poliomyelitis Viruses in Tissue Culture. I. The Propagation of Poliomyelitis Viruses in Suspended Cell Cultures of Various Human Tissues, *J. Immunol.* **69**:645, 1952.

RABIES

Damon, S. R., and *T. F. Sellers,* A Note on the Probability of Error in the Diagnosis of Rabies by Microscopic Search for Negri Bodies, *J. Lab. & Clin. Med.* **27**:71, 1941.

Hodes, H. L., Present-day Problems in Rabies, *Bull. New York Acad. Med.* **31**:569, 1955.

Hosty, T. S., and *F. R. Hunter,* Incidence of Reactions to Antirabies Horse Serum, *Pub. Health Rep.* **68**:789, 1953.

Johnson, H. N., Significance of the Negri Body in the Diagnosis and Epidemiology of Rabies, *Illinois M. J.* 81:382, 1942.

Leach, C. N., Comparative Methods of Diagnosis of Rabies in Animals, *Am. J. Pub. Health* 28:162, 1938.

Steele, J. H., and *E. S. Tierkel,* Rabies Problem and Control: A Nation-wide Program, *Pub. Health Rep.* 64:785, 1949.

Webster, L. T., and *J. R. Dawson,* Early Diagnosis of Rabies by Mouse Inoculation, *Proc. Soc. Exper. Biol. & Med.* 32:570, 1935.

VIRAL MENINGOENCEPHALITIS

Apley, J., Lymphocytic Meningitis with Lung Involvement Occurring in Childhood, *Arch. Dis. Childhood* 22:18, 1947.

Ayres, J. C., and *R. F. Feemster,* Public-health Aspects of the Virus Encephalitides, *New England J. Med.* 240:966, 1949.

———— and ————, Serologic Tests in the Diagnosis of Infectious Diseases, *New England J. Med.* 243:996, 1034, 1950.

Blattner, R. J., and *F. M. Heys,* Encephalitis: Isolation and Identification of Virus from Body Fluids of Human Subjects, *Pediatrics* 3:303, 1949.

Chanock, R. M., and *A. B. Sabin,* The Hemagglutinin of St. Louis Encephalitis Virus. III. Properties of Normal Inhibitors and Specific Antibody: Use of Hemagglutination-inhibition for Diagnosis of Infection, *J. Immunol.* 70:302, 1953.

Eberlein, W. R., and *C. P. Lynxwiler,* The Clinical Picture of Mumps Meningoencephalitis and Report of a Case without Parotitis, *J. Pediat.* 31:513, 1947.

Greenberg, M., and *E. Appelbaum,* Postvaccinal Encephalitis: A Report of 45 Cases in New York City, *Am. J. M. Sc.* 216:565, 1948.

Hammon, W. McD., Encephalitis in "Diagnostic Procedures for Virus and Rickettsial Diseases," pp. 187–217, American Public Health Association, New York, 1948.

MacCallum, F. O., The Laboratory Diagnosis of Virus Infections of the Central Nervous System, *Month. Bull. Min. Health* 10:267, 1951.

Meyer, E., and *R. K. Byers,* Measles Encephalitis: A Follow-up Study of Sixteen Patients, *A.M.A. Am. J. Dis. Child.* 84:543, 1952.

Olitsky, P. K., and *J. Casals,* Viral Encephalitides, chap. 2 in T. M. Rivers (ed.), "Viral and Rickettsial Infections of Man," 2d ed., J. P. Lippincott Company, Philadelphia, 1952.

Scott, T. F. McN., Encephalitis Associated with the Exanthems, Mumps and Vaccination Procedures, *M. Clin. North America* 36:1627, 1952.

Van Hagen, K. O., and *R. N. Baker,* Infectious Neuronitis, Present Concepts of Etiology and Treatment, *J.A.M.A.* 151:1465, 1952.

COXSACKIE VIRUS INFECTIONS

Clark, E. M., D. S. Knowles, F. T. Shimada, A. J. Rhodes, R. C. Ritchie, and *W. L. Donohue,* Coxsackie Virus in Urban Sewage, *Canad. J. Pub. Health* 42:103, 1951.

David, J. K., Jr., D. Leavitt, and *B. F. Howitt,* Vesicular Pharyngitis: Its Relationship to the Coxsackie Group of Viruses, *Pediatrics* 8:672, 1951.

Kravis, L. P., K. Hummeler, M. Sigel, and *H. I. Lecks,* Herpangina: Clinical and Laboratory Aspects of an Outbreak Caused by Group A Coxsackie Viruses, *Pediatrics* 11:113, 1953.

Lazarus, A. S., E. A. Johnston, and *J. E. Galbraith,* An Outbreak of Epidemic Pleurodynia with Special Reference to the Laboratory Diagnosis of Coxsackie Virus Infections, *Am. J. Pub. Health* 42:20, 1952.

McLeod, D. L., A. J. Beale, G. A. McNaughton, and *A J. Rhodes,* Clinical Features of Aseptic Meningitis Caused by Coxsackie-B Virus, *Lancet* 2:701, 1956.

Melnick, J. L., The Coxsackie Group of Viruses, *Ann. New York Acad. Sc.* 56:587, 1953.

Parrott, R. H., S. Ross, F. G. Burke, and *E. C. Rice,* Herpangina: Clinical Studies of a Specific Infectious Disease, *New England J. Med.* 245:275, 1951.

Silverthorne, N., C. Anglin, J. B. J. McKendry, D. S. Knowles, E. M. Clark, F. T. Shimada, A. J. Rhodes, T. E. Roy, R. C. Ritchie, and *W. L. Donohue,* Studies on Poliomyelitis in Ontario. V. Further Observations on the Recovery of Coxsackie Viruses from Cases of Clinical Poliomyelitis, *Canad. M. A. J.* 65:536, 1951.

van Creveld, S., La Maladie de Bornholm, *Arch. franç. pediat.* 9:689, 1952.

MUMPS

Aikawa, J. K., and *G. Meiklejohn,* The Serologic Diagnosis of Mumps: A Comparative Study of Three Methods, *J. Immunol.* 62:261, 1949.

Cabasso, V. J., and *R. J. Hoagland,* Mumps Skin Test during a Mumps Epidemic, *J.A.M.A.* 152:1527, 1953.

Enders, J. F., S. Cohen, and *L. W. Kane,* Immunity in Mumps. II. The Development of Complement-fixing Antibody and Dermal Hypersensitivity in Human Beings Following Mumps, *J. Exper. Med.* 81:119, 1945.

Feller, A. E., and *W. S. Jordan, Jr.,* Serologic Studies of Mumps Employing Complement-fixation and Agglutination-inhibition, *J. Lab. & Clin. Med.* 36:360, 1950.

Henle, G., S. Harris, and *W. Henle,* The Reactivity of Various Human Sera with Mumps Complement-fixation Antigens, *J. Exper. Med.* 88:133, 1948.

Maris, E. P., J. F. Enders, J. Stokes, Jr., and *L. W. Kane,* Immunity in Mumps. IV. The Correlation of the Presence of Complement-fixing Antibody and Resistance to Mumps in Human Beings, *J. Exper. Med.* 84:323, 1946.

COMMON COLD

Andrewes, C. H., Adventures among Viruses: Some Properties of Viruses, *New England J. Med.* 242:161, 1950. Adventures among Viruses: Epidemic Influenza, *ibid.* 242:197, 1950. Adventures among Viruses: The Puzzle of Common Cold, *ibid.* 242:235, 1950.

Paul, J. H., and *H. L. Freese,* An Epidemiological and Bacteriological Study of the "Common Cold" in an Isolated Arctic Community (Spitsbergen), *Am. J. Hyg.* 17:517, 1933.

Topping, N. H., Research on the Common Cold, *Bull. New York Acad. Med.* 25:530, 1950.

Ward, T. G., and *D. F. Proctor,* Isolation of a Common Cold Virus in Chick Embryos and the Clinical Manifestations It Produces in Human Volunteers, *Am. J. Hyg.* 52:91, 1950.

INFLUENZA

Chu, C. M., C. H. Andrewes, and *A. W. Gledhill,* Influenza in 1948–1949, *Bull. World Health Org.* 3:187, 1950.

Expert Committee on Influenza, Report, *World Health Organ. Techn. Rep.* 64, 1953.

Finland, M., M. W. Barnes, and *E. B. Wells,* Influenza Viral Infections in Boston, Sept. 1947 to Aug. 1949: A Study of the Serologic Response of Patients and of the Antigenic Differences among the Influenza Viruses That Were Isolated, *J. Lab. & Clin. Med.* 37:88, 1951.

Hennessen, W. A., Antigenic Analysis of Influenza: B Strains Isolated in 1952, *Bull. World Health Organ.* 6:481, 1952.

Hilleman, M. R., R. P. Mason, and *N. G. Rogers,* Laboratory Studies on the 1950 Outbreak of Influenza, *Pub. Health Rep.* 65:771, 1950.

Hummeler, K., L. P. Kravis, and *M. M. Sigel,* A Rapid Method for Identification of Newly Isolated Influenza Viruses, *J. Bact.* 64:253, 1952.

Isaacs, A., A. W. Gledhill, and *C. H. Andrewes,* Influenza A Viruses, *Bull. World Health Organ.* 3:187; 5:149; 6:287, 481, 1950.

Kirber, M. W., and *W. Henle,* A Comparison of Influenza Complement-fixation Antigens Derived from Allantoic Fluids and Membranes, *J. Immunol.* 65:229, 1950.

Maxwell, E. S., T. G. Ward, and *T. E. Van Metre, Jr.,* The Relation of Influenza Virus and Bacteria in the Etiology of Pneumonia, *J. Clin. Invest.* 28:307, 1949.

Stokes, J., Jr., and *I. J. Wolman,* The Probable Synergism of Human Influenza Virus and *Staphylococcus aureus* in a Rapidly Fatal Respiratory Infection, *Internat. Clin.* (n.s. 3), 1:115, 1940.

Taylor, R. M., Studies on Survival of Influenza Virus between Epidemics and Antigenic Variants of the Virus, *Am. J. Pub. Health* 39:171, 1949.

ACUTE RESPIRATORY TRACT DISEASE

Adams, J. M., Acute Respiratory Diseases: Etiologic, Diagnostic and Therapeutic Considerations, *Pediatrics* 19:129, 1957.

Bell, J. A., W. P. Rowe, J. I. Engler, R. H. Parrott, and *R. J. Huebner,* Pharyngoconjunctival Fever: Epidemiological Studies of a Recently Recognized Disease Entity, *J.A.M.A.* 157:1083, 1955.

Conference on Viruses in Search of Disease, New York Academy of Science, *Section on Biology,* May 24–25, 1956.

Dingle, J. H., Atypical Pneumonia, *Advances Pediat.* 2:194, 1947.

————— and *A. E. Feller,* Noninfluenzal Viral Infections of the Respiratory Tract, *New England J. Med.* 254:465, 1956.

Enders, J. F., J. A. Bell, J. H. Dingle, T. Francis, Jr., M. R. Hilleman, R. J. Huebner, and *A. M. M. Payne,* "Adenoviruses": Group Name Proposed for New Respiratory Tract Viruses, *Science* 124:119, 1956.

James, D. G., Primary Atypical Pneumonia, *J.A.M.A.* 151:810, 1953.

Manson, G., Acute Respiratory Disease with Special Reference to Pathogenesis, Classification and Diagnosis, *J. Pediat.* 43:599, 1953.

Morgan, H. R., and *M. Finland,* Serologic Findings in Patients with Primary Atypical Pneumonia, *Am. J. Clin. Path.* 18:593, 1948.

Rabe, E. F., Infectious Croup, *Pediatrics* 2:255, 1948; 2:415, 1948; 2:559, 1949.

Ward, R., Recent Discoveries in the Etiology of Acute Respiratory Infections: The Adenoviruses, *J. Pediat.* 49:480, 1956.

Woolridge, R. L., J. T. Grayston, J. E. Whiteside, and *M. Friedman,* Etiologic Studies of Febrile Respiratory Disease in Navy Recruits with Emphasis on APC Viruses, *Fed. Proc.* 15:540, 1956.

VIRAL BRONCHIOLITIS OF INFANCY

Adams, J. M., Primary Pneumonitis in Infancy, *J.A.M.A.* 138:1142, 1948.

—————, Primary Virus Pneumonitis with Cytoplasmic Inclusion Bodies: Study of an Epidemic Involving Thirty-two Infants, with Nine Deaths, *J.A.M.A.* 116:925, 1941.

Morgan, E. A., J. A. Turner, A. J. Rhodes, A. M. Peach, E. Zaiman, and *D. Duncan,* Observations on the Etiology of Acute Laryngotracheobronchitis, Toronto, 1953–1954, *Canad. M.A.J.* 75:638, 1956.

Wood, S. H., G. J. Buddingh, and *B. F. Abberger, Jr.,* An Inquiry into the Etiology of Acute Bronchiolitis of Infants, *Pediatrics* 13:363, 1954.

SUDDEN DEATH DURING INFANCY

Adelson, L., and *E. R. Kinney,* Sudden and Unexpected Death in Infancy and Childhood, *Pediatrics* 17:663, 1956.

Arey, J. B., and *J. Sotos,* Unexpected Death in Early Life, *J. Pediat.* 49:523, 1956.

Deamer, W. C., and *H. U. Zollinger,* Interstitial "Plasma Cell" Pneumonia of Premature and Young Infants, *Pediatrics* 12:11, 1953.

Gormsen, H., On Interstitial Plasma Cell Pneumonia in Infants, *Acta paediat.* 39:291, 1950.

Gruenwald, P., and *M. Jacobi,* Mononuclear Pneumonia in Sudden Death or Rapidly Fatal Illness in Infants, *J. Pediat.* 39:650, 1951.

Werne, J., and *I. Garrow,* Sudden Apparently Unexplained Death during Infancy. I. Pathologic Findings in Infants Found Dead, *Am. J. Path.* 29:633, 1953. II. Pathologic Findings in Infants Observed to Die Suddenly, *ibid.,* 29:817, 1953.

ENTERIC VIRUSES

Committee on ECHO Viruses, Enteric Cytopathogenic Human Orphan (ECHO) Viruses, *Science* 122:1187, 1955.

Karzon, D. T., A. L. Barron, W. Winkelstein, Jr., and *S. Cohen,* Isolation of Echo Virus Type 6 during Outbreak of Seasonal Aseptic Meningitis, *J.A.M.A.* 162:1298, 1956.

Ramos-Alvarez, M., and *A. B. Sabin,* Characteristics of Poliomyelitis and Other Enteric Viruses Recovered in Tissue Culture from Healthy American Children, *Proc. Soc. Exp. Biol. & Med.* 87:655, 1954.

―――― and ――――, Intestinal Viral Flora of Healthy Children Demonstrable by Monkey Kidney Tissue Culture, *Am. J. Pub. Health* 46:295, 1956.

RICKETTSIAL DISEASES

Schubert, J. H., S. M. Stanford, and *E. J. Tiffany,* Comparative Evaluation of Several Complement Fixation Techniques for Laboratory Diagnosis of the Rickettsioses, *J. Lab. & Clin. Med.* 37:388, 1951.

van der Scheer, J., E. Bohnel, and *H. R. Cox,* Diagnostic Antigens for Epidemic Typhus, Murine Typhus, and Rocky Mountain Spotted Fever, *J. Immunol.* 56:365, 1947.

Wilder, R. M., The Rickettsial Diseases: Discovery and Conquest, *Arch. Path.* 49:479, 1950.

Wolbach, S. B., Rickettsiae and Rickettsial Diseases of Man: A Survey, *Arch. Path.* 50:612, 1950.

RICKETTSIALPOX

Barker, L. P., Rickettsialpox, Clinical and Laboratory Study of Twelve Hospitalized Cases, *J.A.M.A.* 141:1119, 1949.

LaBoccetta, A. C., H. L. Israel, A. M. Perri, and *M. M. Sigel,* Rickettsialpox: Report of Four Apparent Cases in Pennsylvania, *Am. J. Med.* 13:413, 1952.

Rose, H. M., Rickettsialpox, *New York J. Med.* 48:2266, 1948.

――――, *Y. Kneeland, Jr.,* and *C. D. Gibson,* Treatment of Rickettsialpox with Aureomycin, *Am. J. Med.* 9:300, 1950.

TYPHUS FEVER

Harrell, G. T., Treatment of Rocky Mountain Spotted Fever with Antibiotics, *Ann. New York Acad. Sc.* 55:1027, 1952.

Knight, V., and *F. Ruiz-Sanchez,* Treatment of Endemic and Epidemic Typhus with Antibiotics, *Ann. New York Acad. Sc.* 55:992, 1952.

Murray, E. S., G. Baehr, G. Shwartzman, R. A. Mandelbaum, N. Rosenthal, J. C. Doane, L. B. Weiss, S. Cohen, and *J. C. Snyder,* Brill's Disease. I. Clinical and Laboratory Diagnosis, *J.A.M.A.* 142:1059, 1950.

National Research Council, Division of Medical Sciences, Committee on Pathology, with Collaboration of Armed Forces Institute of Pathology, Pathology of Epidemic Typhus: Report of Fatal Cases Studied by United States of America Typhus Commission in Cairo, Egypt, during 1943–1945, *A.M.A. Arch. Path.* 56:397, 512, 1953.

Plotz, H., The Interpretation of the Weil-Felix Agglutination Test in Rocky Mountain Spotted Fever, *J. Lab. & Clin. Med.* 31:982, 1946.

—— and *K. Wertman,* The Use of the Complement-fixation Test in Rocky Mountain Spotted Fever, *Science* 95:441, 1942.

——, ——, and *R. L. Reagan,* Laboratory Aids in the Diagnosis of Rocky Mountain Spotted Fever, *Bull. U.S. Army M. Dept.* 79:40, 1944.

Q FEVER

Berge, T. O., and *E. H. Lennette,* World Distribution of Q Fever: Human, Animal and Arthropod Infection, *Am. J. Hyg.* 57:125, 1953.

Irons, J. V., J. N. Murphy, Jr., and *D. M. Wolfe,* Q Fever in the United States. III. Serologic Observations in an Outbreak among Stock Handlers and Slaughterhouse Workers, *J.A.M.A.* 133:819, 1947.

Lennette, E. H., W. H. Clark, F. W. Jensen, and *C. J. Toomb,* Q Fever Studies. XV. Development and Persistence in Man of Complement-fixing and Agglutinating Antibodies to *Coxiella burnetii, J. Immunol.* 68:591, 1952.

PSITTACOSIS—LYMPHOGRANULOMA VENEREUM DISEASES

Bedson, S. P., C. F. Barwell, E. J. King, and *L. W. J. Bishop,* The Laboratory Diagnosis of Lymphogranuloma Venereum, *J. Clin. Path.* 2:241, 1949.

Fitz, R. H., G. Meiklejohn, and *M. D. Baum,* Psittacosis in Colorado, *Am. J. M. Sc.* 229:252, 1955.

Maclachlan, W. W. G., G. E. Crum, R. F. Kleinschmidt, and *P. F. Wehrle,* Psittacosis, *Am. J. M. Sc.* 226:157, 1953.

Meyer, K. F., The Psittacosis-Lymphogranuloma Group, chap. 20 in T. M. Rivers (ed.), "Viral and Rickettsial Infections of Man," 2d ed., J. P. Lippincott Company, Philadelphia, 1952.

—— and *B. Eddie,* The Value of the Complement Fixation Test in the Diagnosis of Psittacosis, *J. Infect. Dis.* 65:225, 1939.

Nyberg, L. O., and *C. E. Sonck,* Lymphogranuloma Inguinale in Children: Report of 2 Cases, *Acta paediat.* 39:433, 1950.

Packer, H., and *A. D. Dulaney,* Diagnostic Tests in Granuloma Inguinale, *Am. J. Syph.* 33:68, 1949.

Roth, D., and *R. Schulick,* Isolated Cervical Lymphogranuloma Venereum in a Child, *Pediatrics* 8:489, 1951.

Sigel, M. M., L. S. Cole, and *O. Hunter,* Mounting Incidence of Psittacosis, *Am. J. Pub. Health* 43:1418, 1953.

St. John, E., and *F. B. Gordon,* Studies on the Immunological Relationships of the Psittacosis-Lymphogranuloma Venereum Group of Viruses, *J. Infect. Dis.* 80:297, 1947.

Wolins, W., Ornithosis (Psittacosis): A Review, with a Report of Eight Cases Resulting from Contact with the Domestic Pekin Duck, *Am. J. M. Sc.* 216:551, 1948.

TRACHOMA AND EPIDEMIC KERATOCONJUNCTIVITIS

Braley, A. E., Intracellular Bodies of the Conjunctival Epithelial Cells, *Arch. Ophth.* 24:681, 1940.

Jawetz, E., L. Hanna, S. J. Kimura, and *P. Thygeson,* A New Type of APC Virus from Follicular Conjunctivitis, *Am. J. Ophthalmol.* 41:231, 1956.

Rake, G., M. F. Shaffer, and *P. Thygeson,* Relationship of Agents of Trachoma and Inclusion Conjunctivitis to Those of Lymphogranulomapsittacosis Group, *Proc. Soc. Exper. Biol. & Med.* 49:545, 1942.

Thygeson, P., Trachoma and Inclusion Conjunctivitis, chap. 21 in "Viral and Rickettsial Infections of Man," 2d ed., J. P. Lippincott Company, Philadelphia, 1952.

CHAPTER 74

Systemic Protozoan Infections

LEISHMANIASIS

The Leishmania are parasitic protozoa which multiply by simple fission in human beings. Morphologically the species responsible for the different Leishmania infection are indistinguishable from one another. Identification depends upon clinical and biologic phenomena. *Leishmania donovani* causes the kala-azar which occurs in parts of Africa, India, and China. *L. infantum* is responsible for the kala-azar which occurs in children in countries bordering on the Mediterranean. *L. tropica* causes Oriental sore (Aleppo, Bagdad, or Delhi boil). *L. brasiliensis* causes the cutaneous and mucocutaneous leishmaniasis (espundia, uta, chiclero's ulcer) found in Mexico and most of Central and South America.

Kala-azar

Children with this chronic infection exhibit recurrent fever, enlargement of the liver and spleen and lymph nodes, malnutrition, anemia, weakness, leukocytopenia in the absence of complicating infection, and a tendency to bleed. The source of contagion is presumedly the bite of infected sandflies of the genus Phlebotomus. The fly acquires the parasite by sucking the peripheral blood or biting a skin lesion of an infected human or perhaps of an infected dog. The disease has occasionally been transmitted through transfusion from an infected donor.

LABORATORY DIAGNOSIS. The organisms may be recovered from the blood or organ aspirates by culture in special media or by inoculation of hamsters or other animals with such material. In cultures the organisms are elongated and flagellated, 14 to 20 μ in length, "leptomonad" forms. In the peripheral blood and in organ aspirates they tend to be oval or rounded, nonflagellated, and 2 to 4 μ in length. These so-called "Leishman-Donovan bodies" occur chiefly in the reticuloendothelial cells and monocytes, where they display a large semilunar nucleus opposite to a deeper-staining red-shaped parabasal body. The cytoplasm appears pale blue in Wright's or Giemsa's stain. They are easily seen in aspirates of the bone marrow, spleen, liver, or lymph nodes. The marrow approach is preferable.

913

In chronic cases the circulating neutrophils may be reduced and the monocytes increased, often to as much as 25 per cent of all the leukocytes. The thrombocytes are usually diminished in numbers. Both the bleeding and the coagulation times are prolonged in advanced cases. Evidence that a hypersplenic mechanism underlies most of these blood changes is found in the hyperplasia of the bone marrow and in the leukocytosis, thrombocytosis, and rises in red cell and hemoglobin levels which follow splenectomy.

The serum albumin level is nearly always below normal (1 to 4 gm per 100 ml) whereas the serum globulin level is elevated (3 to 9 gm per 100 ml). These serum protein alterations underlie the use of the presumptive or formol gel test. When one drop of commercial formalin (36 per cent formaldehyde) is added to one drop of patient's serum in a small test tube at room temperature, the serum becomes opaque immediately and within 30 minutes is white and jellylike. Such a positive reaction is exhibited by most patients after the infection has been active for several months. This response is not pathognomonic; it may be obtained in advanced cases of tuberculosis, nephrosis, leprosy, liver cirrhosis, uremia, malignancy, and parasitic tropical diseases. Several other related tests based on altered serum proteins have also been proposed, such as Chopra's antimony test, Napier's aldehyde test, and Sia's precipitative reaction. Most children exhibit a positive serologic test for syphilis with the lipid antigens.

MALARIA

Malaria in North America may be due to any of three species: *Plasmodium vivax*, the cause of tertian (benign tertian) malaria, *P. malariae*, the cause of quartan malaria, and *P. falciparum*, the cause of aestivo-autumnal (malignant tertian or subtertian) malaria. Infections due to *P. ovale* occur in Africa, South America, and the Philippines.

Some childhood patients experience the classical cycle of recurrences of chills and fever. More often, however, and especially in infancy, the disturbance manifests itself in the form of infrequent rises in temperature, or splenomegaly, or anemia of obscure origin, or chills during intercurrent infections only. Many of the cases have their origin in a blood transfusion, the donor being an unwitting carrier of vivax malaria. Associated findings of laboratory interest which are sometimes seen are proteinuria, icterus, splenomegaly, and leukocytopenia. *Blackwater fever*, that poorly understood hemoglobinuric complication of falciparum infection, is a rarity in childhood.

Laboratory Diagnosis

When malaria is suspected the only reliable laboratory approach is the blood smear. Satisfactory serologic or skin tests have not been perfected. Fresh blood may be studied as a cover-slip preparation under the darkfield microscope, with which procedure any intracellular parasite will call attention to itself as a dancing or ameboid point of light. With fixed preparations, which are preferred because they permit better scrutiny and identification, Giemsa's or Wright's stain or some other modification of the Romanowsky technique may be employed. Fluorescent microscopy can be used if the equipment is available. Recommended for staining malarial parasites is certified American-made Giemsa stain.

LIFE CYCLES OF THE PARASITES. The best care of a patient with malaria calls for an understanding of at least the rudiments of the life cycle of the malarial parasites on the part of the physician. The parasites pass their sexual phase in the anopheline mosquito, with the important consequence that live sporozoites remain lodged in the salivary glands. When the mosquito bites a human, these are injected into the subcutaneous tissues. The sporozoite forms circulate only for some minutes, until they are picked up by the tissue cells, including those of the liver parenchyma. Within the liver an exoerythrocytic rhythm of asexual multiplication begins. About every 8 or 10 days infected parenchymal cells rupture and discharge hundreds of new merozoites or schizonts. Some of these are phagocytized, some enter other liver cells to continue the repetitive pattern, and the majority enter red blood cells and proliferate as trophozoites.

In all forms of malaria the youngest forms within the red cells appear as a circle of cytoplasm with a small dot of chromatin and a central vacuole. This arrangement gives rise to a "signet ring" appearance. The chromatin and cytoplasm divide progressively until numerous merozoites are produced. In vivax and quartan infections the brown granules of metabolized hemoglobin become visible as one or two intracellular aggregates, whereas in falciparum malaria the pigment clumps early, often before the chomatin has broken up. The growing merozoites ultimately rupture the red cell membrane, to liberate cytoplasmic residues and other toxic substances which if abundant enough give rise to a paroxysm or chill.

Along with the merozoites a few gametocytes or sexual forms are produced. These are recognizable within the red cells as small compact blue-staining bodies with a red granule of chromatin. When such red cells are not ingested by a biting mosquito these gametocytes die within a few days. The small male forms are known as microgametocytes; the large female forms, macrogametocytes. These undergo further development and unite only if they reach the gastric cavity of the mosquito.

THIN VS. THICK FILMS. Either thin or thick blood films can be used in the search for malarial parasites. The thin film has the advantage of permitting more ready identification of the exact plasmodial species and is therefore preferred by the beginner. The thick film takes in much more blood in the same unit area and is therefore more likely to detect light infestations such as occur in new or chronic cases. Various staining methods are available.

The thin film permits study of the red cells and leukocytes, the thick film does not. In the stained thin film of an active case the granulocytes are usually reduced below normal, though they may increase during paroxyms, with many immature forms. The lymphocytes and monocytes tend to increase. Granules of malaria pigment are often seen in the blood leukocytes in heavy infestations. The red cells, in addition to contained parasites, often have central pallor and show anisocytosis, polychromatophilia, and basophilic stippling. In acute cases the anemia is usually normocytic in character; micro- or macrocytosis is indicative of a superimposed nutritional or hepatic disturbance or of a long-standing chronic infection. Direct destruction of the red cells by the parasites is the predominant cause of the anemia. In tertian malaria the parasitized red cells often appear swollen.

The novice is wise to prepare and stain thick and thin films on opposite ends of the same slide. The thin portion is smeared first. Better fixation is secured if the slides are left to stand a few hours before being stained. If they must be kept unstained for a few days they should be stored in a cool or cold place and protected from condensation of moisture.

For therapy and prognosis it is important to distinguish between vivax or quartan malaria on the one hand and falciparum on the other. Modern drugs can suppress malarial attacks very quickly. Mosquito-borne vivax or quartan infections relapse eventually in about half of the cases, whereas those transmitted by injected blood are not likely to recur. Most falciparum infections remain cured permanently.

If falciparum infection is recognized, therapy should be begun at once because of the potentially severe character of the symptoms which develop with each paroxysm. With the other forms of malaria, immediacy of treatment is not so urgent.

For satisfactory microscopy a good blue-white light and eyepieces of moderate magnification (6 to 8X) are best. The smears are examined under oil immersion. With thick films one starts at the edge and moves toward the thicker central portion. Focusing up and down is necessary to scrutinize all layers. The hemoglobin is usually lysed by the Giemsa stain, but the parasites lie in pink areas suggesting the size and shape of the cells which contained them. Where the red cells are heaped and crowded the parasites may seem shrunken and dense but are still identifiable.

When a patient is having symptoms the peripheral blood will almost invariably contain enough parasites to permit their detection with a fixed smear. Hence if two such smears collected morning and evening for three successive days are negative for parasites when searched for by a trained worker, the symptoms displayed by the patient are almost certainly not due to malaria. At least 100 oil-immersion fields, however, should be examined before a negative diagnosis is made, or even more if the findings are doubtful. An experienced worker can scrutinize 100 fields of a good thick film in 3 to 5 minutes. The first parasite is found, as a rule, within the first 20 to 30 fields. Several parasites should be recognized before a film is read as positive. With a thin smear it is important to spend up to a half hour on inspection of the slide. A dot or particle should not be interpreted as a parasite if there is any possibility of its being a platelet or other artifact. The rings may appear incomplete in the thick smear, but the red dots of the chromatin remain readily identifiable.

Asymptomatic carriers usually have negative blood smears, except when the parasites have escaped from their reservoir in the liver or elsewhere and are multiplying in the blood stream to the point where there will soon be a recurrence of paroxysms. If the carrier state is suspected and repeated thick-film examinations are negative, an injection of epinephrine may drive the parasites from the tissue capillaries into the circulating blood stream. Another approach is to aspirate the bone marrow and prepare films in the same manner as thick blood films. This may help to uncover falciparum carriers.

With individuals infected with vivax or quartan malaria the plasmodia are detectable at any time within the circulating red cells. It is not necessary to wait for a bout of fever before collecting the blood specimen. With falciparum infections, on the other hand, one examination may show no parasites whereas another made 12, 24 or 36 hours later may uncover a shower of young forms.

In tertian and quartan infections, older trophozoites or presegmenting or segmenting schizonts may be seen in the films, depending on the stage of the maturation cycle and whether one or more "broods" are in the patient. The gametocytes circulate coincidentally with the asexual forms and disappear with them when immunity develops or treatment begins.

In falciparum malaria the red cells containing the more mature parasites are held in the peripheral capillaries where they produce symptoms by impeding the oxygen supply of various vital organs. Hence only cells containing young parasites, or gametocytes at times, are free in the circulating blood except in very severe infestations. When only young forms are seen in the film, one can be reasonably positive that the patient has falciparum malaria. The mature falciparum gametocytes are not detectable until 7 to 10 days after the initial parasitemia. They may persist for an indefinite period after the asexual forms have been eradicated by antimalarial therapy.

REPORTING. The report of the blood film examination for malaria should recount (1) all species found, (2) their stages of maturation, and (3) the approximate numbers of each. If a leukocyte count is done simultaneously with the preparation of the thick smear, the number of parasites per cubic millimeter of blood can be estimated from the numerical ratio of the parasites to the leukocytes.

TOXOPLASMOSIS

Toxoplasma gondii are curved or crescentic protozoa with pointed extremities. They are 4 to 7 μ long and 2 to 4 μ wide. In smears stained with Wright's or Giemsa's stain the eccentric nuclei appear red and the cytoplasm blue. A small reddish paranuclear body lies in the cell opposite to the nucleus. The organisms often occur in pairs or clusters (pseudocysts), especially when in reticuloendothelial cells.

Obvious human disease due to invasions by *T. gondii* is rare, but latent asymptomatic infections are not uncommon. Most of the active infantile cases are believed to have their beginning before birth, through transplacental transfer from the mother. Premature birth or death in utero are frequent. The principal lesions occur in the central nervous system and eyes, where they take the form of meningoencephalitis, cerebral degeneration with calcification, uveitis, and chorioretinitis. The liver and spleen may be enlarged. Physical and psychomotor growth are retarded. The source of contagion in older children and adults is unknown, but entry is perhaps by insect vectors or inhalation of contaminated droplets through the lungs.

Nearly all childhood infections are of congenital origin. The severity of the clinical manifestations during the neonatal period seems to depend on the gestational age at which the infection was contracted from the mother. In late infections the chorioretinopathy, cerebral calcification, hydrocephalus, or microcephaly may be absent. No instances have been recorded of more than one sibling having the congenital disease.

Siim has described in children and adults discrete lymph node enlargement, often generalized, which lasted many months. From the excised large nodes *T. gondii* was isolated. Seroreactions became positive after about a month. Microscopy of lymph node sections revealed reticulum cell hyperplasia and scattered islands of large eosinophilic cells.

Laboratory Diagnosis

ISOLATION OF VIABLE TOXOPLASMA. Sometimes the parasites can be recognized microscopically in smears of centrifuged cerebrospinal fluid, but direct visualization of the organisms from other sites is almost never successful. However, they may be isolated by injection of the concentrated sediment from blood, bone marrow, splenic aspirate, cerebrospinal fluid, or possibly sputum into the peritoneum and brains of mice, hamsters, and guinea pigs. Several transfers of brains and viscera from animal to animal may be necessary before the parasite adapts itself and is able to produce overt infection.

BIOPSY EXAMINATION. Fragments of skin, lymph nodes, bone marrow, liver, or spleen may be imbedded and stained with standard procedures and examined microscopically. Zenker-formalin fixation gives better preparations than formalin alone. The toxoplasma appear as intracellular clumps of deep-staining spherical bodies. Suspected structures must be differentiated from other protozoa and fungi such as *Histoplasma capsulatum,* Cryptococcus (Torula), Encephalitozoon, Sarcosporidia, and Leishmania.

DEMONSTRATION OF ANTIGEN IN VENTRICULAR FLUID. A rapid and fairly reliable test, if proper animals are available, is to centrifuge the ventricular fluid from infants with subacute toxoplasmosis, and then introduce 0.1 ml of the supernatant fluid intracutaneously into normal guinea pigs and guinea pigs already infected with latent chronic toxoplasmosis. If toxoplasma are present in the fluid, a large area of erythema and induration will appear in 24 hours at the injection sites in the infected animals, but not in controls.

SEROLOGIC APPROACHES. Two quantitative antibody tests have proved trustworthy with infants and small children: the dye or cytoplasm-modifying test and the complement-fixation test. These have been simplified and standardized and can be performed in special diagnostic laboratories, such as that of the Parasitology and Mycology Section of the Communicable Disease Center, United States Public Health Service. Specimens from probable cases are forwarded through the State Departments of Health.

Each submitted specimen should consist of at least 5 ml of sterile clear serum, or 10 ml of sterile whole blood. Preservatives should not be added, since these can interfere with the test. Serums from both mother and infant should be sent in whenever the congenital form of the disease is suspected. Interpretation of the serologic tests in adults still constitutes a research problem.

Dye (Cytoplasm-modifying) Test. In this procedure, devised by Sabin and Feldman, a suspension of organisms mixed with a complement-like accessory factor from human serum is added to a series of dilutions of the patient's serum in the presence of methylene blue solution buffered to pH 11. If the patient's serum contains specific antibodies the cytoplasm will not take the blue stain. The highest dilution of serum in which at least half the organisms have unstained cytoplasm is taken as the antibody titer. A titer of less than 1:16 is of doubtful significance if the prozone phenomenon can be excluded. Most normal individuals do not have titers exceeding 1:64. For screening purposes each serum may be tested in 1:16, 1:64, and 1:256 dilutions. If staining is still inhibited in the 1:256 dilution, the test should be repeated with higher dilutions in order to ascertain the actual titer.

Complement-fixation Test. In this test a soluble extract of infected chorioallantoic membranes of chick embryos is used as the complement-fixing antigen. This antigen, unlike that for the dye test, is stable in the frozen or lyophilized states. The complement-fixing antibody appears later and disappears earlier than the dye-modifying antibody. Serums with titers as low as 1:2 will always contain significant amounts of dye-modifying antibody. Newborn infants with active congenital toxoplasmosis may have no complement-fixing antibody despite a high dye test titer. Since a negative complement-fixation does not rule out toxoplasmosis, this test should not be used by itself for diagnostic purposes.

SKIN TESTING. In this test the intracutaneous injection of a toxoplasma complement-fixing antigen known as "toxoplasmin" results in a tuberculin-like reaction in some of the individuals who have specific antibodies in their serum. The skin sensitivity develops late in the infection. Many children with proved congenital toxoplasmosis give negative skin reactions. Conversely, a positive reaction may be exhibited when the dye test titer is below the pathognomonic titer of 1:8. The skin test is therefore deemed of little practical diagnostic value except in old or chronic infections and in population surveys.

CLINICAL CORRELATIONS. When a human being becomes infected with toxoplasma, the dye (cytoplasm-modifying) antibody usually makes its appearance within 10 to 20 days, rises quickly to levels of 1:256 to 1:4,000 or higher, and may persist at these high levels for 5 years or more. Sabin, Eichenwald, Feldman, and Jacobs attribute the presence of this antibody in most individuals to inapparent or unrecognized infection. The complement-fixing antibody arises later and fades away earlier than the dye test antibody.

Because toxoplasma antibodies are so prevalent in the normal population, the presence of such antibodies, in any titer, does not prove that associated clinical manifestations are due to toxoplasma. A sharply rising titer with the dye test antibody, or a dye test titer of 1:256 or more which remains constant for several weeks while the complement-fixing antibody changes from negative to 1:8 or more or increases sharply in titer, signifies a recent infection.

The diagnosis of congenital toxoplasmosis should not be made if the dye test antibody cannot be demonstrated in the child, no matter how high the titer may be in the mother's serum. The diagnosis can be made with assurance when the titer in the dye test is 1:256 or more in both mother and child, provided the latter is older than 4 months. When a younger infant has a high dye test titer, the test should be repeated after 4 months of age. The titer will still be elevated in the second test if the first reading was due to infection. If negative, or if much lower, however, the high initial reading is attributed to passive transfer of maternal antibody to the infant.

When an infant in the first weeks of life has a high dye test titer, complement-fixation tests are indicated with both mother and child. The finding of high titers of both antibodies in the mother, in the absence of complement-fixing antibody in the infant, indicates a current active infection.

With children over the age of 6 years, a dye test titer less than 1:256 in mother or child or both does not exclude the diagnosis if the child exhibits clinical manifestations compatible with congenital toxoplasmosis. A negative or low titer in maternal serum within 3 years after delivery ordinarily rules out toxoplasmosis in the child. If the dye test is positive, a toxoplasmin skin test is usually followed by an anamnestic rise in titer.

Serologic diagnostic testing seems warranted with infants in the neonatal period who display unexplained encephalitis, jaundice, hepatomegaly, or splenomegaly, especially when hydrocephalus, microcephaly, cerebral calcifications, or chorioretinitis are also present. Serologic tests for toxoplasmosis are positive in about 80 per cent of infants with these disturbances. The tests are indicated also in later infancy and childhood when convulsions, hydrocephalus, microcephaly, or psychomotor retardation occur together with chorioretinopathy; cerebral calcification is often but not necessarily apparent in these older ages. Positive serologic results in suspected older children are uncommon except when chorioretinopathy is marked. The tests are almost never positive in other forms of cerebral or ocular damage of neonatal or congenital origin or the chorioretinitis of unknown cause acquired after birth.

BIBLIOGRAPHY

LEISHMANIASIS

Ginandes, G. H., Kala-azar in Children, *Am. J. Dis. Child.* 48:1336, 1934.

Kirk, R., The Differentiation and Nomenclature of Leishmania, *Parasitology* 39:263, 1943.

Leahy, H. F., Kala-azar, *Am. J. Dis. Child.* 57:1085, 1939.

Ramos, R., W. Oppenheimer, and *J. Prats*, Diagnosi, decorso e prognosi del kala-azar infantile, *Il Lattante* 24:1, 1955.

Scott, A. V., and *P. L. Fan*, Kala-Azar in Children: Clinical Analysis of 314 Cases, *Chinese M. J.* 61A:145, 1943.

MALARIA

Eckstein, A., Weitere Beobachtungen zur Frage der angeborenen Malaria, *Ann. paediat.* 169:381, 1947.

Einhorn, N. H., and *W. J. Tomlinson*, Estivoautumnal (*Plasmodium falciparum*) Malaria: A Survey of 493 Cases of Infection with *Plasmodium falciparum* in Children, *Am. J. Dis. Child.* 72:137, 1946.

Russell, P. F., L. S. West, and *R. D. Manwell*, "Practical Malariology," W. B. Saunders Company, Philadelphia, 1946.

Simmons, J. S., and *C. J. Gentzkow*, "Medical and Public Health Laboratory Methods," Lea & Febiger, Philadelphia, 1955.

Walker, A. J., Laboratory Diagnosis of Malaria, *Am. J. Clin. Path.* 22:495, 1952.

Wilcox, A., Manual for the Microscopic Diagnosis of Malaria in Man, *Nat. Inst. Health Bull.* 180, rev. 1950.

Williams, C. D., Clinical Malaria in Children, *Lancet* 1:441, 1940.

Wright, F. H., Accidental Transmission of Malaria through the Injection of Whole Blood, *J. Pediat.* 12:327, 1938.

TOXOPLASMOSIS

Cathie, I. A. B., and *J. A. Dudgeon*, The Laboratory Diagnosis of Toxoplasmosis, *J. Clin. Path.* 2:259, 1949.

Feldman, H. A., and *A. B. Sabin*, Skin Reactions to Toxoplasmic Antigen in People of Different Ages without Known History of Infection, *Pediatrics* 4:798, 1949.

Frankel, J. K., and *S. Friedlander,* Toxoplasmosis: Pathology of Neonatal Disease, Pathogenesis, Diagnosis, and Treatment, *Pub. Health Publ.* 141, 1951.

Humphries, J. M., and *C. G. Grulee, Jr.,* Toxoplasmosis: Methylene-blue Dye Tests and Mouse-antigen Skin Test in One Hundred Two Hospitalized Children, *A.M.A. Am. J. Dis. Child.* 84:580, 1953.

Report of Conference on "Some Protozoan Diseases of Man and Animals: Anaplasmosis, Babesiosis and Toxoplasmosis" Part III. Toxoplasmosis, *Ann. New York Acad. Sc.* vol. 64, art. 2, p. 152, 1956.

Ruchman, I., Occurrence of Toxoplasma Neutralizing Antibodies in Various Disease Conditions, *J. Lab. & Clin. Med.* 33:87, 1948.

Sabin, A. B., Complement Fixation Test in Toxoplasmosis and Persistence of the Antibody in Human Beings, *Pediatrics* 4:443, 1949.

———, *H. Eichenwald, H. A. Feldman,* and *L. Jacobs,* Present Status of Clinical Manifestations of Toxoplasmosis in Man, Indications and Provisions for Routine Serologic Diagnosis, *J.A.M.A.* 150:1063, 1952.

——— and *H. A. Feldman,* Persistence of Placentally Transmitted Toxoplasmic Antibodies in Normal Children in Relation to Diagnosis of Congential Toxoplasmosis, *Pediatrics* 4:660, 1949.

Siim, J. C., Acquired Toxoplasmosis: Report of Seven Cases with Strongly Positive Serologic Reactions, *J.A.M.A.* 147:1641, 1951.

———, Toxoplasmosis Acquisita Lymphonodosa: Clinical and Pathological Aspects, *Ann. New York Acad. Sc.* 64:185, 1956.

CHAPTER 75

Arthropod Infestations

SPIDER BITE

The black widow spider, *Latrodectus mactans*, has been found in nearly all parts of the United States and seems to be increasing in numbers.

The body of the female averages 1.3 cm in length. The legs and body are a glossy black and covered with short black hairs. The ventral abdominal surface shows a red marking resembling an hourglass. The designation "black widow" arises from its habit of devouring the much smaller male after mating. The full-grown female appears to be the more poisonous, particularly when distended with eggs. It does not bite except when cornered or compressed, as between skin and clothing. The male almost never bites a human. The venom is more potent than that of a rattlesnake and has its most damaging activity on the nerve endings.

A bite is followed by a distinctive syndrome which may be confused with acute surgical disease of the abdomen. Immediately following the bite a transient excruciating local pain begins. This is usually followed by local edema and redness of the skin. Within 15 minutes a "burning sensation" spreads centrifugally from the site of the bite to involve the whole body. About a half hour later come sudden cramplike pains in the abdomen, extremities, and back; weakness, restlessness, fear, headache, nausea, and vomiting; and burning of the soles of the feet. Paralysis, cyanosis, dyspnea, and urinary retention may follow. Children often have convulsions. On examination, in addition to local erythema, there may be a boardlike nontender abdomen, hypersensitivity of the skin, tenderness in the muscles, muscle spasm with flexion of extremities, shock, slow pulse, moderate leukocytosis, and proteinuria. Intravenous calcium gluconate in 10 per cent solution gives immediate relief of muscle spasm and pain.

SCABIES

The mite which causes scabies, *Sarcoptes scabiei*, should be searched for in all suspected cases. Microscopically the female is an oval 8-legged mite 400 μ in length, with head fused with the thorax. The male is similar in appearance but smaller. They produce itching macules and pustules and skin burrows 1 to 10 mm in length.

To find the parasites the papular skin lesions, whether on wrists, fingers, fingerwebs, abdomen, genitalia, buttocks, or other parts, are scraped or sliced with a sterile sharp knife blade. The material obtained is transferred to a glass slide, dissolved in 10 to 20 per cent sodium or potassium hydroxide, covered with a glass slip, and examined with both low- and high-power microscopy. If the parasite is present one may find the adult forms, skeletal parts, eggs, larvae, or scybalae.

The size of individual lesions is to some extent determined by the allergic sensitivity of the skin. In children, especially infants, the scalp and face may be involved. One should find and treat all infested contacts and give prophylactic treatment to those who have been in intimate contact with the patient. The object of treatment is the killing of all mites, including their larvae and ova. Itching after treatment may indicate failure in cure but is more likely to result from allergic reactions to the dead parasites. Children, particularly infants, often exhibit dermatitis as the result of the medications. Scabies should be suspected in all children with furunculosis, ecthyma, pyoderma, or impetigo.

PEDICULOSIS

Pediculus humanus corporis, *P. humanus capitis*, and *Phthirius pubis*, the three human body lice, infest the respective regions of the body that their names indicate. They are six-legged insects measuring 0.5 to 4 mm in length. The diagnosis is made from the appearance and distribution of the lesions and the finding of the lice or eggs ("nits"), the latter attached by their blunt end.

The body louse is a vector for epidemic typhus, relapsing fever, and trench fever. It inhabits the clothing preferentially and uses the skin mainly for feeding purposes. With suspected infestations it is necessary to examine the underclothing most thoroughly for both active parasites and nits, since absence of these forms on the body surface does not exclude the diagnosis.

Infestation with the head louse is best recognized by finding the nits on the hairs. This insect can be infected experimentally with rickettsiae, but its role in the transmission of diseases is very minor.

The pubic or crab louse is broad, whereas the head and body lice are slender. The nits of all three are superficially identical. The crab louse may attack any hairy surface, but especially the pubic area, axillae, eyelashes, and eyebrows. It has not been demonstrated to be the vector of any major disease.

TICK BITES

The principal ticks which attack man in the United States are *Dermacentor andersonii*, the Western or wood tick, and *D. variabilis*, the Eastern or dog tick. These can transmit the rickettsiae of Rocky Mountain spotted fever and of related diseases in the spotted fever groups (p. 899).

Tick Paralysis

This appears to be caused by a neurotropic toxin found in the saliva of pregnant females of both *D. andersonii* and *D. variabilis*. The first symptoms are irritability followed by ataxia. Flaccid paralysis typically begins in the legs and progressively ascends the trunk up to the neck in approximately 48 hours. Reflexes become diminished or absent. All laboratory examinations including that of the spinal fluid are within normal limits. Unless the tick is removed, cerebral symptoms in the form of ocular palsy, impaired speech and swallowing, and finally respiratory paralysis and death may occur. Treatment consists of immediate removal of the tick and supportive measures as indicated. Recovery is complete in about 4 days.

Before removing the tick, which frequently remains on the patient after biting, the physician should first kill it with ether or ethyl chloride spray and then remove it with a forceps which is later sterilized. Otherwise his own fingers may become contaminated.

PAPULAR URTICARIA

This not uncommon disease of infancy and childhood is characterized by pruritic lichenified papules which are distributed characteristically in greatest abundance on the extensor and exposed surfaces of the arms and legs and on the face and neck, but only exceptionally on the trunk. The lesions appear in the warm seasons and tend to break out in crops. Secondary infection is a not unusual sequel to the bloody crusts elicited by scratching.

The usual cause has been found to be contact with the dog flea *Ctenocephalides canis*, the cat flea *Ct. felis*, or the human flea *Pulex irritans*. Exposure may be through infested dogs or cats, cellar debris, sand boxes, upholstered furniture, or heavy pile rugs. Bites of head lice (*Pediculus humanus capitis*) or bed bugs (*Cimex lectularius*) occasionally produce similar lesions. Most of the childhood cases will show positive skin reactions with antigens prepared from one or another of these insects.

RAT MITE DERMATITIS

A diffuse pruritic skin eruption can be caused by bites of the rat mite, *Lyponyssus bacoti*. The lesions appear as macules, papules, vesicles, wheals, pustules, or excoriations, often in combination. Areas most frequently attacked are the face, hands, ankles, and other parts of the body where clothing fits tightly.

The diagnosis is established by identification of the parasite. As described by Haggard, unfed mites are lively and so small as to be barely visible. Engorged females are about 1 mm in diameter, yellow-gray in color, and easier to catch. In infested rooms they are on the walls, ceilings, and crevices near stoves and hot-water pipes. They can be dislodged with a soft camel's-hair brush and placed in a test tube or white paper cup and may be preserved for entomologic study with 70 or 95 per cent alcohol.

BIBLIOGRAPHY

ARTHROPOD INFESTATIONS

Blank, H., B. Shaffer, M. C. Spencer, and *W. C. Marsh,* Papular Urticaria: Study of the Role of Insects in Its Etiology and the Use of DDT in Its Treatment, *Pediatrics* **5**:408, 1950.

Costa, J. A., Tick Paralysis on the Atlantic Seaboard: Study of Incidence during Poliomyelitis Season with Report of a Case and Review of Published Cases, *A.M.A. Am. J. Dis. Child.* **83**:336, 1952.

Greer, W. E. R., Arachnidism: Effect of Calcium Gluconate in Six Cases, *New England J. Med.* **240**:5, 1949.

Haggard, C. N., Rat Mite Dermatitis in Children, *Pediatrics* **15**:322, 1955.

Howell, J. B., Office Diagnosis of Scabies, *Arch. Dermat. & Syph.* **62**:144, 1950.

Huss, C. B., Head Louse Infestation in School Children: A Comparative Trial of Insecticides, *Month. Bull. Min. Health* **8**:112, 1949.

Kittrell, A. M., Tick Paralysis, *J.A.M.A.* **147**:1561, 1951.

Mellanby, K., C. G. Johnson, and *W. C. Bartley,* The Treatment of Scabies, *Brit. M. J.* **2**:1, 1942.

Stock, P. G., Scabies and Pediculosis, *Month. Bull. Min. Health* **6**:214, 1947.

CHAPTER 76

Chemotherapy: General Considerations

The number of safe antibiotic substances which exert a direct depressive or lethal activity upon pathogenic bacteria and some rickettsiae is increasing year by year. The ones most widely available in the United States at this writing are penicillin in various forms, streptomycin (and dihydrostreptomycin), erythromycin, chlortetracycline (Aureomycin), oxytetracycline (Terramycin), chloramphenicol (Chloromycetin), tetracycline (Achromycin, Panmycin, Polycycline, Tetracyn), polymyxin B, bacitracin, novobiocin (Albamycin, Cardelmycin, Cathomycin), oleandomycin (Matromycin), nystatin (Mycostatin), and vancomycin (Vancocin). All do not act against the same organisms, nor necessarily in the same way. Intelligent administration of these, often in combination with each other or sulfonamides or other drugs, has made many of the bacterial diseases which presented grave problems to the clinician only two decades ago readily curable or at least ameliorable.

A few antibiotics such as penicillin and streptomycin are bactericidal in some circumstances, bacteriostatic in others. The majority, however, and especially those in the so-called "broad-spectrum" group (chlortetracycline, oxytetracycline, tetracycline, and chloramphenicol) are purely bacteriostatic in the usual therapeutic situations.

Many bacterial strains which in vitro seem readily susceptible to an antibiotic may not be eliminated when this agent is applied in recommended dosage to an infection caused by them. In the laboratory, the procedures for measuring the minimal concentration of an antibiotic necessary to inhibit bacterial growth tend to be performed at conditions optimal for growth. Within the body, bacteria often proliferate slowly or are otherwise quiescent metabolically and are much less susceptible to antibiotic action.

Local circumstances at the infected site are contributory also. Organisms trapped in clotted blood or fibrin or in the meningeal spaces may be shielded from the threshold concentration of antibiotic to which they are highly susceptible and which may be present in the environmental blood stream and tissue fluids. Diffusion may be hampered, or the anti-

927

biotic may even be absorbed by the inflammatory exudate. Such difficulties can sometimes be overcome by prescribing extremely high doses or by injecting streptolysin and streptodornase locally as adjuvants (p. 824).

Organisms which have penetrated intracellularly but are still viable may be protected similarly from contact with the antibiotic. It has been suggested that the favorable effects of added corticotropin or cortisone in the therapy of typhoid fever and some rickettsial diseases is through the mechanism of lysing the membranes of the cells which contain ingested organisms and thereby making their surfaces more permeable.

Repeated subculturing of pathogenic strains which have been suppressed by an antibiotic will often reveal the persistence of resting viable forms which can multiply once more after successive dilutions remove the inhibitory substance. This bacteriostatic phenomenon is demonstrable typically with the broad-spectrum antibiotics. Penicillin, especially when combined with streptomycin or a sulfonamide, will often prove to have been completely bactericidal.

BACTERIAL RESISTANCE

In bacteriologic cultures, many bacterial strains will show a significant decrease in numbers for 1 or 2 days as those individuals which are sensitive are killed off by an added antibiotic, and then increase once more as the resistant ones proliferate. This phenomenon appears to occur also in vivo and explains some of the exacerbations which occur after the giving of an antibiotic has induced some transitory clinical improvement.

Another mechanism by which bacterial progeny can become more resistant is that of mutational adaptation. Mutations become manifest as alterations in structure, metabolic behavior, nutritional requirements, specific virulence, or drug resistance. Most of the mutations which favor bacterial resistance during antibiotic therapy are believed to take place independently of its administration. The antibiotic functions as a selecting agent, permitting only those mutants which are adaptable to its presence to survive and proliferate. Mutations may be induced also by such artifices as irradiation with x-rays or radioactive materials or by exposure to other physical or chemical agents such as ultraviolet light or the nitrogen mustards. Mutant forms which are as adaptable to the environment as their prototypes will maintain themselves side by side with their parent strains.

Strains of bacteria have been isolated which after exposure to sublethal concentrations of an antibiotic have developed mutational forms which require the presence of the antibiotic for further growth and proliferation. Should such a dependent strain develop during the therapy of a human infection, its virulence would be enhanced as the antibiotic continues to be given.

The capacity of bacteria to develop variant resistant forms when exposed to antibiotics relates directly to clinical problems. Acquiring of resistance can often be discouraged by administering simultaneously a combination of two or even three agents possessing differing modes of action. The chances of emergence of doubly or triply resistant mutants become almost negligible in that circumstance, even though singly resistant mutants might evolve readily were the exposures to the antibiotics separately spaced. This approach is highly advisable when treating infections caused by staphylococci, Pseudomonas, Proteus, or other Gram-negative bacilli, since these can often exhibit resistance to most antibiotics within a few days after therapy is begun. The same principle holds for the chemotherapy of tuberculosis. It is best to administer two of the effective agents simultaneously, such as aminosalicylic acid, isoniazid, and streptomycin or dihydrostreptomycin.

ANTIBIOTICS IN THERAPY

Pediatric Considerations

The general principles which underlie the application of antibiotics in the therapy of bacterial diseases are broadly the same for infants and children as for adults.

The offending organism must be isolated and identified at least presumptively; the antibiotic administered must be one to which it is susceptible; the dosage and route of administration must provide an effective concentration of the antibiotic throughout the area of infection; and the therapeutic program must be continued sufficiently long to protect against a resurgence of bacterial growth after the antibiotic is stopped.

Organ site as a rule is less important than the character of the bacterium, but local features also affect the therapy. Thus meningeal infection must be treated with an antibiotic which will penetrate the cerebrospinal fluid spaces in adequate concentration.

The antibiotics in common use are either sufficiently water-soluble to yield therapeutically adequate levels in the body fluids or are converted into soluble active derivatives after being absorbed. With most infections one proceeds on the assumption that diffusion is free and that the concentrations of antibiotic in the plasma, extracellular fluid, lymph spaces, and infected areas are all about the same. Major exceptions to this generalization exist in those situations in which a body membrane, abscess wall, or necrobiotic barrier may hinder the penetration of the antibiotic —for example, osteomyelitis, empyema, bronchiectasis, meningitis, purulent arthritis, or walled-off abscesses. The bacteriostatic activity of the antibiotic may aid the natural defense mechanisms in preventing the spread of the infection but may fail to eradicate the bacterium, even after many weeks of treatment.

Susceptibility to an antibiotic is not always predictable from identi-fication of the species. This is particularly true with respect to infections caused by staphylococci, Proteus, and Pseudomonas organisms and Gram-negative bacilli generally. Thus staphylococci which are insensitive to penicillin are being recovered with great frequency in recent years, and strains resistant to other antibiotics hitherto deemed effective are also on the increase. With potentially stubborn infections such as pyelo-nephritis, osteomyelitis, and subacute bacterial endocarditis it is most important to establish the identity and antibiotic sensitivity of the offend-ing organism as soon as possible and to administer sufficiently high dosages of antibiotics to discourage the emergence of adaptative resistant forms. Cultures and sensitivity determinations should be repeated at periodic intervals if the infection persists or returns.

It is sometimes said that a given dosage of an antibiotic is "adequate" for mild or moderately severe infections but "inadequate" for severe infections. Evaluation of an infectious process in these terms describes only the clinical phenomena exhibited by the patient, including his ca-pacity to overcome by physiologic mechanisms the danger of septicemia and metastatic spread. Of perhaps equal importance in judgment regard-ing dosage, however, are (1) the susceptibility of the invading organisms to the antibiotic and (2) its accessibility within the tissues to the concen-tration of the antibiotic which will be attained in the blood stream. Many a small localized abscess, with no signs or symptoms deemed "severe," has failed to subside until massive doses or even local injections of the anti-biotic have been given.

Antibiotic therapy of most acute infections, if the causative organism is susceptible, should lead to satisfactory clinical improvement in 24 to 48 hours. The successful therapeutic agent should nevertheless be continued for at least several days after the infection has overtly sub-sided, and for a week longer with streptococcic infections (p. 829).

All antibiotics should be prescribed at a dosage level which is high enough to elicit the desired therapeutic effect rapidly. Overdosage pro-duces no greater therapeutic benefit and magnifies the risk of allergic sensitization and other toxic complications. Underdosage favors the de-velopment of bacterial resistance. When a choice of antibiotics is avail-able, the one to be preferred with children is that which can be given orally, provided that absorption is compatible with the need.

Superinfections

An occasional sequel of therapy with an antibiotic agent is the pro-liferation of insensitive organisms. Within the nasopharynx, for example, therapy with penicillin, streptomycin, erythromycin, or a broad-spectrum antibiotic tends to bring about a practically complete disappearance of hemolytic streptococci, pneumococci, and sensitive staphylococci, along with a diminution in the saprophytic Neisseria. Suppression of these cocci may be followed by the proliferation of insusceptible staphylococci, organisms of the coli and coliform groups, and Proteus or Pseudomonas. Emergence of this resistant flora in children under 3 years of age is sometimes associated with fever and other clinical manifestations.

Similarly, within the colon, the giving of streptomycin, polymyxin, a nonabsorbable sulfonamide, or a broad-spectrum antibiotic by mouth tends to suppress susceptible organisms. The customary profusion of *Escherichia coli* within the intestinal tract becomes replaced by a proliferation of Proteus, Pseudomonas, coliform organisms, staphylococci, and enterococci. The change in flora becomes evident within 4 days of treatment or earlier and may continue for as long as a week after the antibiotic is discontinued. Yeasts and *Candida albicans* also become more abundant. Other fungi such as *C. tropicalis* and *C. parakrusei*, previously undetectable, may become culturable. Irritative moniliasis of the mouth or perianal skin sometimes develops. In debilitated patients a generalized invasion by *C. albicans* may follow.

With resistant bacterial infections one should repeat the cultural studies as often as feasible, in order to discover emergence of any secondary pathogenic bacteria. The therapeutic addition of another antibiotic agent, to which the newly predominant organism is sensitive, then becomes advisable.

Sometimes the use of antibiotics is accompanied by fever, which persists as long as these are being given. The mechanism is believed to be absorption of toxins produced by the staphylococci and other organisms which proliferate in the intestines while the more usual saprophytes are suppressed.

Combinations of Antibiotics

As mentioned, it is a common practice to administer two or more antimicrobial agents concomitantly when treating infections which are constitutionally severe or whose bacterial cause has as yet been unascertained. This is done with the hope that at least one of the drugs will be effective or that the combination may exert an additive or synergistic antibacterial action. Furthermore, exposing the bacterial population to several agents reduces the likelihood of resistant variants.

The possible combinations of antibiotics with each other and the effective sulfonamides are almost innumerable. A few have special therapeutic merit. Penicillin together with streptomycin can be of great benefit in peritonitis and other infections caused by multiple organisms. As a rule this is more effective than a combination of penicillin or streptomycin with any broad-spectrum antibiotic. A tetracycline with streptomycin or a sulfonamide or both is much more effective against brucellosis than any of these alone. Penicillin with sulfonamides is usually successful in severe infections caused by pneumococci, streptococci, or influenza bacilli—for example, pyogenic meningitis. Aminosalicylic acid, isoniazid, and similar drugs are important adjuvants to the streptomycin therapy of tuberculosis. Streptomycin and sulfones are given for the therapy of leprosy, and penicillin combined with specific antitoxin is the best for diphtheria. Mixed therapy is advisable for subacute bacterial endocarditis, for deep infections caused by coagulase-positive staphylococci or fecal streptococci (enterococci), and for stubborn urinary tract infections due to Proteus, Pseudomonas, or some strains of coliform bacilli.

Contrariwise, in certain situations the use of multiple therapeutic agents may result in antagonistic interference. Organisms susceptible to penicillin are usually rendered less sensitive when a bacteriostatic antibiotic is given simultaneously, since the lethal activity of penicillin is maximal when bacteria are in the phase of logarithmic multiplication and minimal when growth is quiescent.

It is wisest, therefore, to reserve the use of chemotherapeutic combinations to situations where past experience has established such benefit. Problem cases are best treated with the help of information regarding the antibiotic sensitivities of the bacterial strain recovered from the individual patient. When the use of more than a single agent seems necessary, it is advisable to give effective dosages of each agent and thereby obtain an additive effect. Antagonism appears to be elicited only when the tissue fluid concentrations are inadequate or marginal.

LABORATORY ASSAY OF ANTIBIOTIC CONCENTRATIONS

Serial Dilution Methods

These expose freshly inoculated broth cultures to progressive dilutions of an antibiotic in order to estimate the minimal antibiotic concentration necessary to inhibit bacterial growth. After proper incubation the first tube in which bacteria cease to grow is read as the end point. Minimal growth is generally recognizable by the formation of sediment or visible turbidity.

A somewhat similar procedure is to use agar culture plates which contain serial dilutions of antibiotics. These may be prepared in quantity and stored for 3 to 4 weeks without loss of potency. By sectoring the surface several organisms can be studied on the same plate. A group of small standard cylinders, usually of porcelain, may be placed on plates which have been freshly spread or seeded with suspensions of the organism. Dilutions of the unknown solution of the antibiotic are then introduced into the cylinders, and also a set of control dilutions of known potency. After incubation for some hours, growth of the organism will be apparent on the plates, with circular zones of inhibition about those cylinders which contain concentrations above which the organism is sensitive. The so-called cup-plate method is very similar except that the test and control solutions are deposited in cuplike cavities cut into the agar.

These approaches measure bacteristasis primarily. To ascertain whether the bacteria are still viable, subcultures or plate counts must be made from areas where the bacterial populations have been inhibited by the antibiotic.

Disk Method

This consists of placing sterile antibiotic-impregnated disks of filter paper on agar culture plates which have been inoculated with a fresh subculture or with material from a patient. A circular macroscopic zone of inhibition of microbial growth indicates bacteriostatic or bactericidal activity of the antibiotic. The size of the zone is contingent upon the pH and other nutrient properties of the medium, the concentration of the antibiotic and its physical capacity to diffuse outward, the circumstances of incubation, and the suitability of the culture medium for the bacterial strain. The number of organisms in the inoculum is not relevant. For clinical purposes it is important that the inhibitory activity of the disks correspond with that of plasma levels attained in patients receiving adequate dosage schedules.

The degree of sensitivity of any bacterium is indicated chiefly by its response to the concentration of antibiotic on the disk, though the width of the zone of inhibition is not entirely without meaning. A 2-mm zone of inhibition at a low concentration is of much more significance than a 15-mm zone at a high concentration. One should not draw comparative inferences from the widths of the inhibition zones to different antibiotics or with different bacteria.

The advantages of the disk method are simplicity and economy, the lack of need for a uniform inoculum, and the speed with which results are secured (rarely over 1 or 2 days) from the time the specimen is received. Comparative studies have indicated a close parallel between the readings from disks impregnated with increasing strengths of antibiotics and a corresponding series of tubes or cylinders.

Reporting of Readings

In studies with the disk procedure the usual report will state that a given organism recovered from a patient is "resistant" or "susceptible" to the antibiotics to which it has been exposed on a culture plate. These, of course, are relative terms. The comparative standards for such a report should be the minimal aqueous dilutions which experience has shown will kill or inhibit this organism in patients receiving the antibiotics, provided of course that the organism is not harbored in sites where these concentrations cannot be attained.

Antibiotic-impregnated disks are so calibrated that the thresholds for macroscopic inhibition of bacterial colony growth correspond approximately to plasma levels attainable by therapeutic dosages. These disks are often prepared with two or even three increasing concentrations of an antibiotic (Table 76-1).

The sensitivity of an organism to an antibiotic is described as follows:

Susceptible, when all the disks containing the various concentrations of the antibiotic are surrounded by zones of inhibition of growth

Moderately susceptible, when growth occurs around the disk of lowest concentration but is inhibited around those of higher concentration

Slightly susceptible, when there is no inhibition around the two disks of lower concentration, and only around the disk of highest concentration

Resistant, when growth occurs around all disks

Degrees of susceptibility are sometimes deduced from the size of the zone of macroscopic inhibition. This is a far from reliable criterion.

Table 76-1. Concentrations of Antibiotics Utilized in Testing for Inhibition of Bacterial Growth with Filter-paper Disks on Agar Plates

| Antibiotic | Concentration in disk | | |
	Lowest	Intermediate	Highest
Bacitracin	2 units	10 units	20 units
Carbomycin	2 μgm	5 μgm	15 μgm
Chloramphenicol	5 μgm	10 μgm	30 μgm
Chlortetracycline	5 μgm	10 μgm	30 μgm
Erythromycin	2 μgm	5 μgm	15 μgm
Neomycin	5 μgm	10 μgm	30 μgm
Novobiocin	5 μgm	50 μgm	100 μgm
Nystatin	10 units		100 units
Oleandomycin	2 μgm		15 μgm
Oxytetracycline	5 μgm	10 μgm	30 μgm
Penicillin	2 units	5 units	10 units
	(1.2 μgm)	(3 μgm)	(6 μgm)
Polymyxin B *	5 units	10 units	30 units
Streptomycin and dihydrostreptomycin	2 μgm	10 μgm	30 μgm
Tetracycline	5 μgm	10 μgm	30 μgm

* 1 μgm is equivalent to 10 units.

Clinical Applications

All the serial dilution methods require considerable time and experience for their performance. They are used primarily for pharmaceutic assays, for research, and for exceptional clinical problems relating to resistant organisms such as may be encountered with subacute bacterial endocarditis or infections which relapse during therapy. The disk method is much more suitable for routine studies by medical technologists whose formal training in academic bacteriology has been limited.

Laboratory studies of bacterial sensitivity to antibiotics are useful clinically for (1) all infections which are severe or puzzling enough to require bacteriologic cultures, (2) those in which antibiotic therapy on an empirical or presumptive basis has not proved rapidly effective, (3) those in which insufficient therapy may result in the acquiring of resistance to the antibiotic by a bacterial strain originally sensitive to it, (4) those which are caused by a mixture of bacteria, in order to select an antibiotic or group of antibiotics which will be active therapeutically against every strain present.

Nearly always, therapy with a given antibiotic will be unsuccessful if the highest concentration used in the disk test fails to depress growth of the pathogen in vitro.

In stubborn infections it is sometimes necessary to titrate the concentration of antibiotic attained in the patient's body fluids by the dosage being given. This is done by applying one of the tube dilution methods to fresh cultures of the organism responsible for the infection. Such sensitivity tests have their special usefulness in infections caused by bacteria whose strains can exhibit great variability in susceptibility— for example, staphylococci, enterococci, or Proteus organisms. Recourse to these tests is not necessary when the pathogenic organism is of a species which is known to be always highly susceptible to an antibiotic. Thus pneumococci and hemolytic streptococci are sensitive almost invariably to penicillin.

Paper disks have been impregnated for sensitivity tests with combinations of antibiotics. This approach is of limited value with cultures from sources, such as sputum, which contain assorted organisms. The occurrence of a zone of inhibition will not indicate whether the bacterial growth has been suppressed by only one of the constituents or whether the presence of both is necessary. It has not been shown as yet that such disks will uncover any significant synergistic or antagonistic antibacterial properties inherent in specific combinations.

Antibiotics in Market Milk

Traces of antibiotics are demonstrable occasionally in the milk distributed by dairy plants. These traces have their origin in treatments given to cows which are being treated for evident or suspected mastitis. Since most instances of mastitis are due to bovine streptococci, and particularly to *Streptococcus agalactiae,* penicillin is the antibiotic administered most frequently. However, inasmuch as this disease may be caused by other organisms such as the Corynebacteria or members of the coli-aerogenes group, other antibiotics such as dihydrostreptomycin, streptomycin, the tetracyclines, neomycin, bacitracin, or sulfonamides are often given also.

The treatments consist usually of local injections of an antibiotic preparation into an infected udder or "quarter." A severely infected animal may receive four infusions within 48 hours. The extent of this practice in the country is shown by the fact that more than 75 tons of antibiotics is sold annually for treatment of bovine mastitis.

Experience has shown that substantially the entire amount of infused antibiotic is eliminated in 3 days by regular milking. Hence all such preparations sold for mastitis therapy must carry a warning on the label: "Milk from treated quarters should be discarded or used for purposes other than human consumption for at least 72 hours after the last treatment." Disregard of this warning appears to be responsible for the antibiotic residues found in most of the milk on the American market.

A nationwide survey of market milk for contamination with antibiotics was conducted by the Food and Drug Administration in 1955–1956. Tested were 1,640 samples of pasteurized and 66 samples of market raw milk, collected from the 48 states and the District of Columbia. Of the total of 1,706 samples, 101 (5.9 per cent) contained residues of penicillin as confirmed by the penicillinase identity test. One sample contained both penicillin and streptomycin. The concentrations of penicillin found ranged from 0.003 to 0.55 units per ml. Seventeen others (approximately 1 per cent) appeared to contain one of the tetracyclines, bacitracin, or a combination of these antibiotics.

These minute amounts appear to be of no clinical significance. They cannot be detected in the blood stream of an individual who drinks such milk and almost certainly will not affect the bacterial flora normally existing in the colon or respiratory tract. It is highly improbable that enough would be absorbed to evoke symptoms of hypersensitivity in an allergic individual already sensitized.

BIBLIOGRAPHY

BIOLOGY OF ANTIBIOTICS

Council of the Pharmaceutical Society of Great Britain, "Antibiotics: A Survey of Their Properties and Uses," 2d ed., The Pharmaceutical Press, London, 1952.

Davis, B. D., Bacterial Genetics and Drug Resistance, Pub. Health Rep. 67:376, 1952.

Dowling, H. F., M. H. Lepper, and G. G. Jackson, Clinical Significance of Antibiotic-resistant Bacteria, J.A.M.A. 157:327, 1955.

Eagle, H., R. Fleischman, and M. Levy, Development of Increased Bacterial Resistance to Antibiotics. I. Continuous Spectrum of Resistance to Penicillin, Chloramphenicol and Streptomycin, J. Bacteriol. 63:623, 1952.

——— and A. K. Saz, Antibiotics, Ann. Rev. Microbiol. 9:173, 1955.

Finland, M., Some Observations on Changing Patterns of Resistance of Certain Common Pathogenic Bacteria to Antimicrobial Agents, "Antibiotics Annual 1954–1955," Medical Encyclopedia, Inc., New York, 1955.

Florey, H. W., E. Chain, N. G. Heatley, M. A. Jennings, A. G. Saunders, E. P. Abraham, and M. E. Florey, "Antibiotics: A Survey of Penicillin, Streptomycin, and Other Antimicrobial Substances from Fungi, Actinomycetes, Bacteria and Plants," Oxford University Press, New York, 1949.

Garrod, L. P., The Reactions of Bacteria to Chemotherapeutic Drugs, Brit. M. J. 1:206, 1951.

Hobby, G. L., The Current Status of the Development of Antimicrobial Agents, Bull. New York Acad. Med. 31:181, 1955.

Jawetz, E., J. B. Gunnison, and *R. S. Speck,* Studies on Antibiotic Synergism and Antagonism: The Interference of Aureomycin, Chloramphenicol and Terramycin with the Action of Streptomycin, *Am. J. M. Sc.* 222:404, 1951.

McCurdy, R. S., and *E. Neter,* Effects of Penicillin and Broad-spectrum Antibiotics on the Emergence of a Gram-negative Bacillary Flora in the Upper Respiratory Tract of Infants, *Pediatrics* 9:572, 1952.

Romansky, M. J., M. H. Fusillo, E. Caldwell, and *E. D. Robin,* The Synergistic Action and Potential Applications of Antibiotic Combinations, *M. Clin. North America* 35:535, 1951.

Weinstein, L., M. Goldfield, and *T. W. Chang,* Infections during Chemotherapy: A Study of Their Frequency, Type and Predisposing Factors, *New England J. Med.* 251:247, 1954.

Welch, H., W. R. Jester, and *J. M. Burton,* Antibiotics in Fluid Market Milk: Third Nationwide Survey, *Antibiotics & Chemother.* 6:369, 1956.

——, *W. A. Randall, R. J. Reedy,* and *J. Kramer,* Bacterial Spectrum of Erythromycin, Carbomycin, Chloramphenicol, Aureomycin and Terramycin, *Antibiotics & Chemother.* 2:693, 1952.

LABORATORY CONTROL

Bondi, A., Jr., E. H. Spaulding, D. Smith, and *C. C. Dietz,* A Routine Method for the Rapid Determination of Susceptibility to Penicillin and Other Antibiotics, *Am. J. M. Sc.* 213:221, 1947.

Eisenberg, G. M., Bacterial Susceptibility to Antibiotics, *Am. J. M. Sc.* 223:600, 1952.

—— and *J. M. O'Loughlin,* Bacterial Susceptibility to Antibiotics. III. Study of Activity in Vitro of Combinations of Antibiotics, *Am. J. Clin. Path.* 23:1040, 1953.

Fairbrother, R. W., and *G. Martyn,* The Disc Technique for Determining Sensitivity to the Antibiotics, *J. Clin. Path.* 4:374, 1951.

Gunnison, J. B., and *E. Jawetz,* Sensitivity Tests with Combinations of Antibiotics: Unsuitability of Disc Method, *J. Lab. & Clin. Med.* 42:163, 1953.

Jackson, G. G., E. E. Vicher, and *J. W. Soska,* Clinical Observation of Changes in Sensitivity of Bacteria to Antibiotics, *Am. J. Clin. Path.* 23:297, 1953.

Lind, H. E., The Rationale of Routine Antibiotic Sensitivity Determinations, *Antibiotics & Chemother.* 3:672, 1953.

—— and *E. Swanton,* Routine Bacteriologic Sensitivity Determinations in Antibiotic Treatment, *Antibiotics & Chemother.* 2:30, 1952.

Neter, E., M. R. Murdock, and *E. H. Kunz,* The Influence of the Composition of Culture Media on Growth Inhibition by Various Microorganisms by Antibiotic Discs, *Antibiotics & Chemother.* 2:35, 1952.

Spaulding, E. H., Laboratory Aspects of Antibiotic Therapy, *Pediatrics* 8:406, 1951.

Waisbren, B. A., C. Carr, and *J. Dunnette,* The Tube Dilution Method of Determining Bacterial Sensitivity to Antibiotics, *Am. J. Clin. Path.* 21:884, 1951.

Welch, H., Antibiotic Sensitivity Testing, *Antibiotic Med.* 2:309, 1956.

THERAPEUTIC APPLICATIONS

Alexander, H. E., Guides to Optimal Therapy in Bacterial Meningitis, *J.A.M.A.* 152:662, 1953.

Brown, H. W. (ed.), Use of Antibiotics in Tropical Disease: Symposium, *Ann. New York Acad. Sc.* 55, art. 6:967, 1952.

Dowling, H. F., M. H. Lepper, and *G. G. Jackson,* When Should Antibiotics Be Used in Combination?, *J.A.M.A.* 151:813, 1953.

Eisenberg, G. M., J. D. Alexander, Jr., and *H. F. Flippin,* Combined Antibiotic Therapy in Refractory Urinary Tract Infections, *J.A.M.A.* **152**:1302, 1953.

Hunt, A. D., Jr., Antibiotics in Pediatric Practice, *M. Clin. North America* **36**:1607, 1952.

Karelitz, S., Choice of an Antibiotic: An Interpretative Review, *J. Pediat.* **42**:478, 1953.

—— and *N. Schifrin,* Antibiotic and Sulfonamide Therapy in Communicable Diseases, *Postgrad. Med.* **11**:17, 1952.

Rossi, E., Die Antibiotica im Kindesalter, *Helvet. paediat. acta* **7**:397, 1952.

Spink, W. W., Clinical Problems Relating to the Management of Infections with Antibiotics, *J.A.M.A.* **152**:585, 1953.

Welch, H., "Principles and Practice of Antibiotic Therapy," Medical Encyclopedia, Inc., New York, 1954.

CHAPTER 77

Individual Antibiotics

PENICILLIN

Pharmacology

Penicillin is an organic compound elaborated by certain strains of *Penicillium notatum* and possessing the empirical formula $C_5H_{11}O_2NS$. It is available in over 30 different pharmaceutic variants, which are marketed commercially under innumerable trade names. These differ from one another chemically in the radicals and side chains which are attached to the therapeutically active penilloaldehyde portion of the molecule, and clinically with respect to best routes of administration, speeds of absorption and excretion, and concentrations attained in the various tissues and body fluids.

In human infections penicillin is active against the streptococci, pneumococci, meningococci, gonococci, lactobacilli, diphtheria bacilli, Clostridia, many of the treponema and leptospira, and the psittacosis group of agents to a lesser extent. The effect is either bacteriostatic or bactericidal, depending principally upon the phase of growth of the organism. In threshold dosages the rate at which penicillin kills susceptible bacteria is proportional to its concentration. Penicillin is most active during rapid bacterial growth or so-called logarithmic multiplication and may be ineffective when the organisms are in a resting state.

Some organisms undergo morphologic distortions when exposed to sublethal concentrations of penicillin. Gram-positive cocci, for example, may enlarge but not divide, so that their cell bodies become enormously swollen. *Salmonella typhosa* and *Clostridium welchii* may form long continuous chains. Staphylococci undergo lysis. Pneumococci exhibit no recognizable changes and continue to react with type-specific serum though permanently unable to reproduce.

DEFINITION OF UNIT. The original Oxford unit of penicillin was "that amount of penicillin contained in one milliliter of a certain buffer solution containing ether" (Heatley, 1944). This arbitrary measure is still used as the unit when referring to potency, but more permanent crystalline standards have been prepared for general use. The international unit, agreed on by a conference held under the auspices of the Permanent Commission of Biological Standardization of the League of Nations Health Organisation, has been defined as "the specific penicillin activity contained in 0.6 micrograms of the International Penicillin Standard." The latter is a pure crystalline sodium salt of benzyl-penicillin and is approximately equivalent to the original Oxford unit.

Penicillinase

This is a bacterial enzyme, or family of enzymes, which hydrolyzes and inactivates penicillin. Some resistant strains (e.g., staphylococci) produce it liberally, whereas others (e.g., *Salmonella typhosa*) do not. All the penicillin-resistant strains of staphylococci recovered from human cases have been producers of penicillinase, and this contributes to their resistance. A sterile preparation of penicillinase may be introduced into cultures of blood or body fluids from patients receiving penicillin therapeutically, for the purpose of counteracting any inhibition of bacterial growth by traces of penicillin in the specimen.

Plasma Levels in Relation to Therapy

The clinical effectivness of penicillin is contingent upon several variables. Those compounds which are absorbed rapidly give rise to plasma levels which are high but only transitorily sustained, as exemplified to extreme degree by aerosol inhalations. Other preparations, such as "repository" procaine penicillin in oil with added 2 per cent aluminum monostearate, release penicillin into the body fluids for a longer time but in lower concentrations.

In vitro studies have shown that the bactericidal activity of penicillin against most susceptible strains of bacteria is maximal at concentrations of 0.1 to 0.5 unit per ml. With 0.03 to 0.1 unit per ml the effect is bacteriostatic only—the organisms do not multiply but still remain viable. Raising the concentration above the lethal level does not accelerate the bactericidal action.

In clinical evaluations, the minimal "therapeutically desirable level" in the plasma seems to be at least 0.03 unit per ml. Even though not bactericidal, this induces sufficient bacteriostasis to support significantly the normal intrinsic body defenses. The recommended schedules of therapy for the diverse available forms of penicillin tend to yield plasma levels in excess of 0.03 unit per ml during most of the treatment period.

If a child is given a single intramuscular injection of crystalline sodium or potassium penicillin in dosage of approximately 11,000 units per kg (5,000 units per lb), the plasma level will be about 16 units per ml at 30 minutes, 6 units at 1 hour, 0.3 unit at 3 hours, and 0.03 unit at 5 hours. An intramuscular injection of penicillin A in dosage of 14,000 units per kg (6,000 units per lb) will give levels which average about 3 units per ml at 30 minutes, 2 units at 3 hours, and 0.45 unit at 24 hours. Intramuscular injections of 1,100 units per kg (500 units per lb) when repeated at 3-hour intervals will maintain the plasma level at or near 0.1 unit per ml.

When procaine penicillin is given intramuscularly in dosage of 13,000 units per kg (6,000 units per lb), the plasma level reaches a peak of 1.75 to 2 units per ml in 30 minutes, and then falls slowly so that at 24 hours it is still about 0.1 unit per ml in most individuals.

Benzathine penicillin is absorbed more slowly than are other forms of crystalline penicillin. A single intramuscular dose of 1.2 million units produces blood levels up to 0.2 μgm ($\frac{1}{5}$ unit) per ml in an hour, and 0.02 to 0.04 μgm for from 1 to 2 weeks thereafter. To eliminate the streptococcic carrier state in preventive programs for recurrence of rheumatic fever, a monthly injection of 1.2 million units seems to have a place with patients who are irregular or careless in taking daily oral doses of sulfonamides or simple penicillin. When taken at 8-hour intervals oral benzathine maintains plasma levels above 0.1 unit of penicillin per ml.

From 5 to 30 per cent (average 15 per cent) of penicillin taken orally is absorbed from the gastrointestinal tract. Accordingly, for a desired plasma level, an oral dose should be five to ten times as great as that of an intramuscular injection. The oral route with proportionally enhanced doses has been found to be as dependable as the intramuscular route with the majority of infections amenable to penicillin therapy. Intramuscular injection of an aqueous preparation which is absorbed quickly is preferable for gastrointestinal disturbances (diarrhea, vomiting), for fulminating infections (septicemia, meningitis), and when continuously high penicillinemia is needed to overcome a resistant organism or to penetrate a sequestered site (osteomyelitis, meningitis, subacute bacterial endocarditis).

When potassium penicillin is administered orally to children in the form of 200,000 units as an initial dose, followed by 100,000 units at 4-hour intervals, plasma levels above 0.03 unit per ml are maintained for at least 2 hours. When 300,000 units of the same preparation is given at 12-hour intervals, this plasma level is maintained for 2 to 4 hours.

The giving of a renal blocking agent such as probenecid in adequate amount retards the excretion of penicillin, resulting in plasma levels which are five- to ten-fold higher and more sustained. The optimal dosage of probenecid with smaller children was found by Coriell and associates to be an initial dose of 25 mg per kg, followed by 10 mg per kg every 6 hours. With children weighing over 50 kg, the initial dose was 1 to 2 gm followed by 500 mg every 6 hours. Coincident administration of a dose of 6,000 to 11,000 units of potassium penicillin G per kg every 6 to 8 hours gave average penicillin serum levels of 0.5 unit per ml at 1 hour, 0.46 unit at 2 hours, and 0.32 unit at 3 hours.

Blood penicillin concentrations are higher and last longer after an oral dose of phenoxymethyl penicillin (penicillin V) than after a comparable oral dose of penicillin G. The renal blocking agent probenecid will elevate further the blood penicillin V levels; combined treatment with penicillin V is one means of achieving a sustained high plasma level in the oral therapy of serious infections.

Penicillin does not enter normal cerebrospinal fluid in measurable amounts with the standard dosage schedules. With extremely large intramuscular injections of water-soluble preparations, such as 1 million to 2 million units of crystalline penicillin G, levels of above 1 unit per ml may be sustained for several hours. The cerebrospinal fluid is penetrated much more readily when the meninges are diseased.

More than half the penicillin which is absorbed or injected is excreted by the kidneys, with most being lost in a few hours. Urine concentrations of 40 to 100 units per ml are not unusual. The level depends upon the size of the dose, route of administration, and rate of urine formation. Penicillin is an excellent urinary tract antiseptic for infections caused by organisms possessing any degree of sensitivity. The pH of the urine appears to be of minor significance.

Infections sometimes fail to subside with dosages and routes of administration of penicillin which would be expected to kill off the organisms as indicated by in vitro testing. This may be the result of temporary inhibition of the growth of the organisms by local factors. Bacteria when dormant can be refractory to penicillin in superlethal concentrations. In this contingency the desired therapeutic result is facilitated by administering the penicillin for a prolonged period or by adding a second antimicrobial agent such as streptomycin whose action against organisms is less dependent upon their growth status. There is also the possibility that the bacterial species has developed resistant forms through mutation or other selective mechanisms.

The infections in ambulatory children for which penicillin therapy is usually given without preliminary laboratory studies include impetigo, acute lymphadenitis, furuncles, scarlet fever, and especially nasopharyngitis and its complications of sinusitis, otitis media, tonsillitis, laryngitis, and bronchitis. The majority of these infections are associated with pneumococci, streptococci, staphylococci, or influenza bacilli, often in combination. When the strains of staphylococci or influenza bacilli are penicillin-resistant, which is not unusual, defervescence and clinical improvement may not ensue within a day or two after the penicillin treatment is begun. Other antimicrobial agents should then be employed.

With more severe infections which require hospitalization, such as septicemia, meningitis, or peritonitis, the management should be less empirical. The proper antimicrobial agent or combination of agents should be selected according to clinical judgment and the results of in vitro laboratory tests.

STREPTOMYCIN

Pharmacology

Streptomycin is elaborated by a species of actinomycetes known as *Streptomyces griseus*. It has the empirical formula $C_{21}H_{39}O_{12}N_7$, and its chemical structure has been identified as N-methyl-l-glucosamido-strepto-sidostreptidine. The pharmaceutic preparations generally procurable are the crystalline form, streptomycin sulfate and streptomycin trihydro-chloride calcium chloride.

When two atoms of hydrogen are added catalytically the resulting product is dihydrostreptomycin, which possesses essentially the same therapeutic and antimicrobial activities as streptomycin itself.

Streptomycin has nearly as wide an antibacterial spectrum as does penicillin. It is not used as extensively for infections with Gram-positive organisms because of its weaker potency, need for parenteral admin-istration, higher rate of toxic reactions, and greater tendency to evoke resistant strains. The most important of the susceptible pathogenic bac-teria against which streptomycin is used are various members of the Salmonella, Shigella, Klebsiella, Hemophilus, Pasteurella, Brucella, and Mycobacteria groups. Some strains of Proteus and Pseudomonas are also susceptible, particularly when the drug is first given. Spore forms of bacteria are much more resistant than vegetative forms. It is of inter-est that some of the bacteria which are highly sensitive to low concen-trations in vitro, such as the Brucella varieties which are killed by con-centrations of less than 10 μgm per ml, prove to be relatively refractory when streptomycin is administered as therapy. The viruses, treponemas, fungi, spirochetes, rickettsiae, and protozoa are not affected by strepto-mycin, as a rule.

Streptomycin can be either bacteriostatic or bactericidal, depending on the concentration achieved. With some organisms it appears to affect adversely the enzyme systems concerned with cell division. With others, in sublethal concentrations, it actually seems to stimulate growth.

Because many susceptible bacteria tend to develop resistant strains within a few generations after exposure to streptomycin, it is important to commence the therapy with large dosages so as to eradicate all patho-gens completely before such refractory strains can appear.

Resistant strains are less likely to be produced when streptomycin is combined with some other antimicrobial agent. In the therapy of tuber-culosis, for example, aminosalicylic acid or isoniazid may be added for this purpose. Penicillin together with streptomycin seems to exert a syner-gistic action against many bacteria; this combination is one of the best for therapy of unelucidated infections giving rise to severe or prostrating symptoms. Sulfonamides will often show synergism when given with streptomycin.

Streptomycin does not pass readily through the wall of the gastro-intestinal tract. Hence the oral route is used only to inhibit Gram-negative organisms within the intestine, such as those which produce diarrhea. Following intramuscular injections it is rapidly absorbed and excreted. It passes the placenta readily; the concentrations in the cord blood and amniotic fluid soon after an injection is given to a parturient mother will approximate about one-half the maternal level for an hour or so after delivery. Significant amounts do not enter the cerebrospinal fluid except when meningitis or some other meningeal inflammatory process is active.

Definition of Unit

One international unit (IU) of streptomycin is equivalent to 1 microgram (μgm) of crystalline streptomycin base. Hence 1 mg contains 1,000 IU. Of the two salts commonly employed in therapy, pure streptomycin sulfate has a potency of 788 IU per mg, and the calcium chloride complex 779 IU. Crystalline dihydrostreptomycin sulfate has a potency of 725 IU per mg, and the amorphous form about 650 IU per mg in terms of standard dihydromycin units.

The assay methods are in general the same as for penicillin assay, though more careful attention must be given to hydrogen-ion concentration. Most assays are carried out at a pH between 7.8 and 8.0.

Plasma Levels in Relation to Therapy

Following an intramuscular injection the concentration in the plasma is maximal within 30 minutes, the extent of the peak being proportional to the amount received. The serum concentration 1 hour after an intramuscular injection is the same as after an intravenous injection of the identical amount; hence the latter route of administration has been largely discontinued. Streptomycin taken orally is excreted in abundance in the stools, and its appearance in the blood is almost undetectable.

In infants and children an intramuscular injection of 11 mg per kg (5 mg per lb) every 6 hours gives plasma levels which fluctuate from 5 to 45 μgm per ml. This appears to be a desirable therapeutic range for most infections. High peaks with intervening low levels seem to give as much benefit as continuously sustained high levels. Care should be exerted to avoid plasma levels in excess of 50 μgm per ml for more than a week, since this regimen is conducive to the production of the neurotoxic signs of vestibular dysfunction or deafness.

About 50 per cent or more of the quantity injected appears in the urine within 24 hours, with the greater part in the first 12 hours. A much smaller percentage is excreted in the bile. If the kidneys are damaged, the renal excretion becomes much diminished and the blood levels may be sustained at exceptional levels for a protracted period. With poor kidney function, therefore, the quantities given should be much reduced and the plasma concentrations followed by laboratory assay in so far as feasible. In newborn infants the rate of excretion is unusually low also, presumably because of renal immaturity, and the same consideration holds.

ERYTHROMYCIN (ERYTHROCIN, ILOTYCIN)

Pharmacology

This antibiotic is produced by *Streptomyces erythreus* and has the approximate formula $C_{39}H_{73}NO_{13}$. Like penicillin it is more active against Gram-positive than against Gram-negative organisms. *Hemophilus pertussis, Neisseria gonorrheae, Corynebacterium diphtheriae,* and certain strains of Brucella and Clostridia, however, are also sensitive to some degree. Since it is comparatively inactive against coliform and enteric bacilli, moniliasis and other gastrointestinal symptoms are unlikely to follow its use. It may be of value against rickettsiae and certain larger viruses and against *Endamoeba histolytica.* Its action is not only bacteriostatic, but slowly bactericidal as well.

Most erythromycin-sensitive strains of *Micrococcus pyogenes* (*Staphylococcus aureus*) will acquire resistance gradually when subcultured repeatedly in increasing concentrations of this antibiotic. Such resistant strains of staphylococci are being encountered with increasing frequency in hospital populations, presumably as a result of spread from old patients to new arrivals (p. 819).

Since erythromycin is destroyed by a pH below 2.0, tablets have been prepared for oral use which are coated to resist the action of gastric acid but which disintegrate in the alkaline medium of the intestine. Flavored suspensions of erythromycin stearate are available for pediatric use. These may be given without relation to food intake. From 0.3 to 0.6 mg of erythromycin per gm of feces is excreted by adults taking 300 mg every 6 hours.

With six children given approximately 1.5 mg of erythromycin per lb of body weight at 4-hour intervals for three doses by Sylvester and Josselyn, the blood concentrations 2 hours after the third dose ranged from 0.64 to 2.5 μgm per ml. Since most susceptible staphylococci and other organisms are inhibited in vitro by concentrations of 0.7 μgm per ml or less, this dosage would seem adequate for such infections. Higher dosages may produce mild intestinal symptoms, apparently as a direct action on gastrointestinal motility. *H. influenzae* and *H. pertussis* are not usually inhibited until concentration of 2.5 μgm per ml or more are attained. A dosage schedule for children of 6 to 8 mg of erythromycin per kg of body weight every 6 hours can be expected to give average serum concentrations of 1.3 μgm per ml at 2 hours, 0.6 μgm at 4 hours, and 0.1 to 0.4 μgm at 6 hours. Passage into the cerebrospinal fluid in the absence of infection is poor, but levels of 1 μgm per ml or higher have been detected in the presence of pyogenic meningitis.

An estimated 15 per cent of administered erythromycin is excreted into the urine in biologically active form following a single intravenous dose. Concentrations in the urine vary from 8 to 32 μgm per ml following the usual program of oral therapy. The more concentrated the urine, as judged by specific gravity, the higher the content of the antibiotic.

Since the renal excretion of erythromycin appears to be filtrative rather than secretory, and since a major portion is eliminated into the bile rather than through the kidneys, it is unlikely that the simultaneous administration of probenecid would raise significantly its plasma concentration.

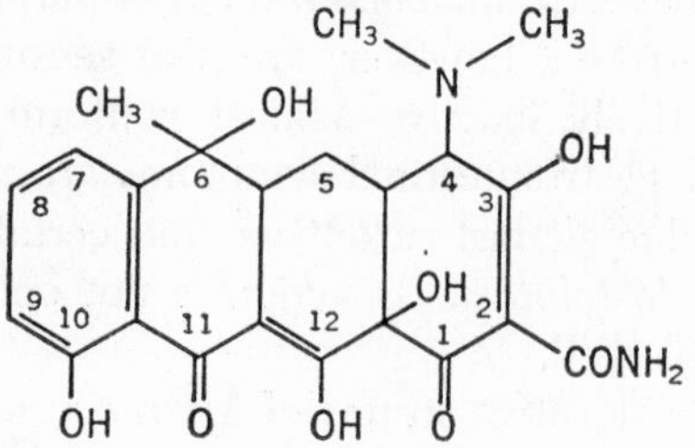

Tetracycline

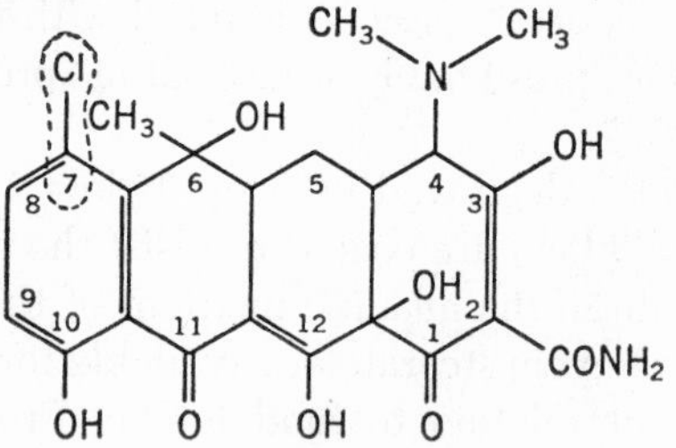

Chlortetracycline

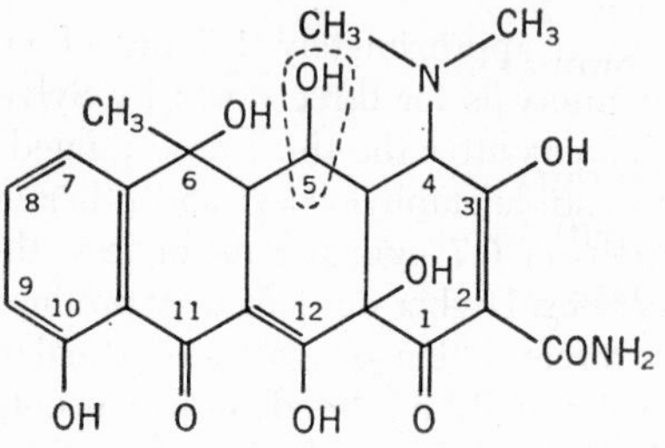

Oxytetracycline

Structural Relationships of the Tetracyclines

THE BROAD-SPECTRUM ANTIBIOTICS

This term is applied collectively to a group of antibiotics which have an exceptionally wide range of bacteriostatic effectiveness. The best known are chlortetracycline (Aureomycin), oxytetracycline (Terramycin), tetracycline (various trade names), and chloramphenicol (Chloromycetin) (see diagram above). The mechanisms of their action are obscure and not necessarily the same with each. They are sometimes bactericidal in extremely high concentrations.

Pharmacology

In therapeutic concentrations these antibiotics inhibit many strains of Salmonella, Neisseria, Proteus, Pseudomonas, Corynebacteria, Brucella, colon and coliform bacilli, and other Gram-positive and Gram-negative pathogens. They are therapeutically helpful in some diseases caused by the larger viruses (psittacosis, lymphogranuloma venereum), in some rickettsial infections (typhus, scrub typhus, Q fever, rickettsialpox), and to a lesser extent with some protozoan diseases including amebic dysentery. Their value in spirochetosis (Treponema, Borrelia, and Leptospira infections) and other tropical diseases is still under exploration.

Individual strains of susceptible species often exhibit differences in their susceptibility to one or another of these three substances. Chloramphenicol has proved the most effective in infections due to *Salmonella typhosa* and the rickettsiae which cause typhus fever, scrub typhus, and Rocky Mountain spotted fever.

All are effective when given orally. They can be administered intravenously when patients are vomiting, comatose, or otherwise very ill or when exceptionally high plasma levels are desired. Direct diffusion into normal cerebrospinal fluid after oral or intravenous administration is erratic and often negligible, with chloramphenicol and tetracycline the most soluble and penetrating. In pyogenic meningitis of various kinds the results are nevertheless favorable.

The plasma levels attained and the therapeutic results with oral administration are usually satisfactory with doses every 6 or 8 hours. All are excreted in large amounts in the urine following oral and parenteral administration. Probenecid and similar agents do not significantly enhance the peak levels or the duration of retention within the body.

Most susceptible pathogens do not develop resistant forms under therapy, except perhaps after prolonged exposure. Proteus and Pseudomonas and staphylococci are prominent exceptions.

Chlortetracycline (Aureomycin)

This yellow antibiotic is produced by selected strains of *Streptomyces aureofaciens* and is marketed as crystalline Aureomycin hydrochloride. It contains a chloride radical attached to carbon atom 7 on the tetracycline ring. The solution which will inhibit the growth in vitro of most clinically susceptible bacteria is ordinarily 1 to 3 μgm per ml and often weaker. Chlortetracycline is usually active against *Salmonella typhosa* in vitro but of relatively little worth in the therapy of typhoid fever in man.

This antibiotic when given at the recommended dosage schedules is absorbed from the gastrointestinal tract quickly and almost completely.

With larger dosages the excess in the lower segments of the bowel may cause irritation in some patients. Surgeons sometimes give large amounts for the purpose of reducing the bacteria in the intestine before bowel surgery.

When chlortetracycline is given orally on a 4-hour schedule of 11 mg per kg (5 mg per lb), the serum levels are usually maintained between 1 and 3 μgm per ml. Higher dosage schedules give only slightly higher levels. Six-hour schedules of 2.5 mg per kg maintain the plasma levels at approximately 1.0 μgm per ml, and of 5 mg per kg at approximately 1.5 μgm per ml. The latter is deemed adequate for mild or moderate infections with susceptible organisms, and a 10- to 11-mg dosage for more severe infections such as septicemia or pyogenic meningitis. Dosages of 50 mg daily have been advised for prophylaxis against cross infections in hospitals caring for premature infants. With an intravenous dosage of 7 mg per kg (3 mg per lb), a plasma level of 8 to 10 μgm per ml may be transitorily attained. The concentration in normal cerebrospinal fluid with the usual dosage schedules is only 0.1 to 0.2 μgm per ml.

The concentration of biologically active chlortetracycline attained in the urine is approximately 50 to 150 times that in the blood. For this reason systemic administration is helpful in many infections of the urinary tract. With patients who are excreting large amounts of dilute urine the concentration of the antibiotic is decreased along with that of the other urinary constiutents.

Oxytetracycline (Terramycin)

This is produced by the soil actinomycete *Streptomyces rimosa,* so named because on solid media its colony surfaces are fissured and cracked. It is sold commercially in the form of the crystalline hydrochloride. The molecular architecture is closely similar to that of chlortetracycline, but with a hydroxyl group attached to carbon 5 and no chloride attached to carbon 7.

According to in vitro sensitivity tests the minimal concentration of tetracycline necessary to inhibit sensitive strains of microorganisms is usually considerably below 4 μgm per ml. Satisfactory therapeutic recovery in illnesses such as childhood pneumonia due to staphylococci, pneumococci, or streptococci can be obtained with the customary oral dosage schedule of 10 mg per kg every 6 hours, which maintains plasma levels of 1 to 2 μgm per ml. A 6-hour schedule of 20 to 30 mg per kg orally or 7 mg per kg intravenously may, after 24 hours, maintain a serum level as high as 8 μgm per ml.

The usual therapeutic schedule maintains the urinary content at 50 to 200 μgm per ml. Larger dosages produce higher urinary concentrations. The concentration in cerebrospinal fluid of normals with any treatment regime is negligible, though occasionally it may reach 1.2 μgm per ml. During purulent meningitis, however, levels in the fluid are often of the magnitude of 2.5 μgm per ml after large intravenous or intramuscular injections.

Tetracycline (Tetracyn, Polycycline, Achromycin)

This broad-spectrum antibiotic has a molecular structure very similar to that of oxytetracycline (Terramycin) and chlortetracycline (Aureomycin), but lacks the attached oxy- or chloride radical (see diagram on p. 946). In general it is more soluble, more stable chemically, and its untoward effects fewer and less severe. It is absorbed readily and rapidly from the gastrointestinal tract, where local reactions are unusual.

Despite the closely related chemical structures of these three analogues, laboratory and clinical studies indicate that some strains of staphylococci, enterococci, Klebsiella, Proteus, and coliform and other organisms show disparity in their sensitivities to these agents.

Serum and urine concentrations are approximately the same as with similar doses of chlortetracycline or oxytetracycline, whether given orally or intravenously. Effective concentrations can be maintained with adequate doses given orally every 6 hours. A total oral dosage of 25 mg per kg per day with children brings about a level of 0.6 μgm in 4 hours and a sustained level of 1.2 μgm after 24 hours. Entry into normal cerebrospinal fluid spaces is more prompt and higher concentrations are attained than with either oxytetracycline or chlortetracycline. After several adequate oral doses the concentrations of tetracycline in the cerebrospinal fluid of meningitis may range from 1.25 to 5 μgm per ml.

Chloramphenicol (Chloromycetin)

This was first recovered from a Venezuelan streptomycete related to the streptothricin-forming *Streptomyces lavendulae* and known from its origin as *S. venezuelae*. It has the empirical formula $C_{16}H_{12}O_5N_2Cl_2$ and the organic configuration of D-(-)threo-2-dichloracetamino-1-p-nitrophenyl-1, 3-propanediol. The pharmaceutic products come either from fermentative or synthetic manufacture and appear to have identical antibacterial properties. Microbiologic and chemical assay methods are available. The latter often gives higher readings, since it fails to distinguish between active forms of the drug and inactive degradation products. Growth of most susceptible organisms in vitro is inhibited by concentrations of 12 μgm per ml or less.

Blood concentrations are related directly to the amounts administered. With the crystalline preparation, almost complete absorption in the upper gastrointestinal tract and high diffusibility explain rapid attainment of high blood serum concentrations and low residues in the feces. Because excretion into the urine is likewise rapid, administration at intervals of not more than 6 hours, and preferably not more than 4 hours, is advisable for effective blood concentrations. When a single oral dose is taken the plasma concentration usually reaches a peak in approximately 2 hours but sometimes not until 6 hours or more. This is followed by a gradual disappearance over the ensuing 24 hours. The height of the peak and the mean level are proportional to the amount given.

The palmitic ester must be hydrolyzed in the intestine before the chloramphenicol base is available for absorption. The blood level rises more slowly and does not attain as high a level as with the crystalline form, but is sustained for a longer period. Plasma levels above 10 μgm per ml in newborn infants can be maintained by a 6-hourly dose of 25 mg per kg.

The usual recommendation for infants and children is 50 to 100 mg per kg per day, in divided dosage every 6 to 8 hours until the fever is abated, followed by half of this or 25 to 50 mg per kg for at least several days of afebrile convalescence. With severe infections due to insensitive microorganisms, dosages even above 100 mg per kg, divided at intervals of 4 to 6 hours, may be utilized. Total daily amounts of 100 mg per kg or higher give plasma levels from 20 to 50 μgm per 100 ml. Therapeutic levels are attained more rapidly by a double dosage given initially.

In children without meningitis the cerebrospinal fluid concentration is from 6 to 62 per cent of that of the plasma, with a mean of approximately 25 per cent. Plasma levels of 25 to 40 μgm per ml are advisable to be sure of cerebrospinal fluid levels of at least 5 μgm per ml. Diffusion is negligible with plasma levels below 10 μgm per ml.

Even though more than 90 per cent is excreted into the urine as an inactive nitro derivative, chloramphenicol exerts excellent chemotherapeutic activity in urinary tract infections caused by susceptible organisms.

Because of the possibility of permanent bone marrow depression (p. 329), this important antibiotic should be used only for illnesses for which no other antibiotic will serve equally well. The majority of such cases have occurred after a prolonged high dosage, though some have followed only a few doses.

NOVOBIOCIN

This antibiotic, produced biosynthetically in special nutrient media by *Streptomyces spheroides* and *S. niveus,* is marketed commercially under the trade names Albamycin (Upjohn), Cathomycin (Merck), and Cardelmycin (Pfizer).

Like penicillin, novobiocin is acid in character, and its monosodium salt is readily soluble in water. In vitro studies have indicated that it is highly effective against staphylococci and many other Gram-positive pathogens and also against a few Gram-negative ones. Its action appears to be bacteriostatic in weak solutions, bactericidal in higher concentrations. Antagonism or cross resistance between novobiocin and the other familiar antibiotics has not been noted to any extent.

Studies with children by Lin and Coriell have shown that a dosage regimen of 5 mg per kg body weight every 6 to 8 hours maintains serum levels between 20 and 30 μgm per ml more or less continuously. This range is much higher than the minimal inhibitory concentration in vitro, which for many susceptible pathogens appears to be less than 1 μgm per ml. Individual variations are pronounced.

Diffusion into the cerebrospinal fluid is poor. The concentration attained is less than 1 per cent of that of blood serum even in the presence of bacterial meningitis. The poor penetration may be related to the observation that much of the drug in the circulation seems combined loosely with the serum proteins.

The principal excretory route for novobiocin appears to be the gastrointestinal tract. Much of the orally ingested drug is absorbed through the intestinal mucosa, to be later concentrated in the liver and discharged into the bile. Urinary concentrations with the usual oral dosages as a rule are higher than the corresponding plasma levels and the minimal inhibitory concentrations for most susceptible bacteria. Inconstant amounts may appear in ascitic and pleural effusions.

Novobiocin can be helpful therapeutically in infections caused by staphylococci, streptococci, pneumococci, corynebacteria, pasteurellae, and some resistant strains of *Proteus vulgaris.* Since novobiocin was made widely available only in 1956, most staphylococcic strains which have been resistant to other antibiotics are still susceptible, but contact with novobiocin is followed by the rapid acquiring of specific resistance.

BACITRACIN

Bacitracin consists of the antibiotic substance or substances produced by growth of *Bacillus subtilis,* strain Tracy 1. One unit is equivalent to 26 μgm of the Federal Food and Drug Administration working standard. It is effective in vitro against many Gram-positive organisms, such as the streptococci, pneumococci, staphylococci, micrococci, and corynebacteria in the aerobic group and clostridia, streptococci, and micrococci in the anaerobic group. It is ineffective against the Gram-negative organisms, except for the gonococci and the meningococci. Spirochetes are highly susceptible. *Endamoeba histolytica* is also susceptible.

The use of bacitracin is restricted largely to local application for the reason that, when given systemically, it produces nephrotoxic manifestations in about two-thirds of the patients. Bacitracin may be applied topically to superficial skin or eye lesions in the forms of ointments or wet dressings or as irrigations in chronic sinus or nasal infections. When given orally it is destroyed in the gastrointestinal tract, so that even large oral dosages do not produce detectable blood levels.

Should it be deemed advisable to give bacitracin intramuscularly because of the susceptibility of an invading organism to it in a stubborn infection, the precautions outlined by the manufacturer should be followed. The nephro-toxic effects become manifest first in the form of proteinuria, so that urine analy-sis should be performed daily. The proteinuria usually becomes moderate on the third to fifth day of treatment and then subsides. Parallel to the pro-teinuria, leukocytes and granular casts usually appear in the urine; erythrocytes are rare. The urine should be kept at a pH of 6 or over by the administration of sodium bicarbonate or some other alkali by mouth at the time of each in-tramuscular dose of bacitracin. In about 3 per cent of the patients the urinary output may fall and the nonprotein nitrogen level of the blood will rise. Hence it is advisable during the therapy to give liberal amounts of fluids, measure the 24-hour intake and output of fluids, and determine the plasma nonprotein nitrogen before and twice weekly during therapy. The therapeutic program should be discontinued if the proteinuria and the appearance of formed ele-ments in the urine become pronounced or if a significant decrease in urinary output or a progressive rise in nitrogen retention should occur. A preexisting renal lesion is not necessarily a contraindication for the use of bacitracin; such cases often fail to experience further renal injury during its administration. Nevertheless, such patients should be followed with particular care.

When given intravenously or intramuscularly, bacitracin does not pass readily through the normal blood-brain barrier and reaches the cerebro-spinal fluid only in an insignificant concentration. When the meninges are severely inflamed, however, the cerebrospinal fluid has a considerably higher level. In stubborn meningeal infections caused by staphylococci or other organisms against which other antibiotics are ineffective, bacitracin has been injected intrathecally at times with good therapeutic results.

Bacitracin and some of the other antibiotics, especially penicillin, often have a synergistic action against some strains of organisms. This may be ascertained in vitro. Combinations may be more effective than either alone. Antagonism between bacitracin and other antibiotics has thus far not been reported.

POLYMYXIN B

Polymyxin is the generic name given to a group of related basic poly-peptide antibiotics produced by strains of the spore-forming soil bac-terium *Bacillus polymyxa* (*B. aerosporus* Greer). Letters of the alphabet are used to differentiate these related substances. All are rapidly bacteri-cidal when given in adequate amounts. This may explain the infrequent development of resistant strains during therapy.

Polymyxin B is the least toxic of the polymyxins adequately studied. Marketed as the sulfate (Aerosporin), it is given by intramuscular in-jection for the treatment of infections caused by Gram-negative bacilli, especially those which are more susceptible to this than to other anti-microbial therapeutic agents. Numerous strains of Klebsiella, *Hemophilus influenzae,* and Shigella are sensitive to polymyxin B sulfate concentrations of 0.005 to 2 μgm per ml. Most strains of *Escherichia coli* are highly sensitive. Proteus and Pseudomonas are sometimes susceptible.

The usual intramuscular daily dosage of 2.5 mg per kg body weight, given at 4- to 8-hour intervals to children, provides therapeutic blood serum levels of 1 to 8 μgm per ml. The peak concentration is reached in 30 minutes to 2 hours, one-half the peak level is still present after 6 hours, and detectable amounts persist up to 12 hours.

Since polymyxin B does not diffuse readily into the cerebrospinal fluid it should also be administered intrathecally for meningitis caused by susceptible organisms. Solutions for intrathecal injection are prepared by adding 10 ml of sterile isotonic sodium chloride solution to 50 mg of the powdered drug. Solutions containing procaine, as available for intramuscular use, must not be given intrathecally. Polymyxin B may be of some value in the treatment of cryptococcosis.

Its toxicity in doses below 3 mg per kg body weight is low when given parenterally. Neurotoxic disturbances such as dizziness, mild weakness, and parethesias are usually subjective and do not contraindicate the therapy. The kidney tubules are sometimes injured, giving rise to proteinuria or nitrogen retention. The possibility of this complication makes it important to keep the patients under close laboratory observation. The drug may be given in the presence of a preexisting renal lesion provided watch is kept for aggravation of the renal disease. With impaired renal function the serum levels can be maintained at 2.5 μgm per ml by dosage of 20 mg every 8 hours.

Much of the polymyxin which is given intramuscularly is excreted into the urine, giving rise to high concentrations there. This makes it useful in the therapy of urinary tract infections due to Gram-negative organisms such as susceptible strains of *E. coli, A. aerogenes* and *Pseudomonas aeruginosa.* The urinary excretion of polymyxin B is progressive for the first 12 hours after an injection and subsides during the next 12 hours. Kagan and associates reported that after intramuscular injection of 0.8 mg per kg, six normal children showed levels of 0.2 to 48 μgm (average 28.2 μgm) at 2 hours and 0.2 μgm at 4 hours.

Since approximately 98 per cent of orally given polymyxin is not absorbed from the intestinal tract, toxic systemic manifestations do not attend this route of administration. Good results have been reported in the treatment of childhood enteritis caused by Shigella and Pseudomonas. Results in Salmonella and nonspecific gastroenteritis and in typhoid fever have been equivocal.

Polymyxin B may be applied topically for the treatment of skin and surface infection caused by susceptible Gram-negative bacilli, especially *Ps. aeruginosa,* and to prevent contamination of wounds or burns by these organisms. Sterile dry powder is dissolved in distilled water or isotonic sodium chloride solution to prepare concentrations of 0.1 to 0.25 per cent.

NEOMYCIN

Neomycin, obtained from *Streptomyces fradiae,* is bactericidal against most Gram-positive and Gram-negative pathogenic organisms. It is water-soluble and can withstand the digestive secretions and products of bacterial growth. Absorption from the gastrointestinal tract is minimal. Only about 3 per cent of what is taken orally is excreted into the urine. Emergence of resistant strains among originally susceptible pathogens occurs rarely if at all.

A single dose taken by mouth will suppress the usual bacterial inhabitants of the large bowel within 24 hours; hence neomycin is often employed for this purpose in abdominal surgery. When it is given orally at high dosage levels or for some days there often occurs the local proliferation of Monilia, but usually without symptoms of monilial infection.

Neomycin is not recommended for general use internally because of ototoxic and nephrotoxic effects which have been observed at times following intramuscular injections. It is sometimes given intramuscularly for stubborn systemic or urinary tract infections caused by staphylococci, Proteus, Pseudomonas, and other susceptible organisms which cannot be eradicated by other forms of therapy. Granular casts frequently appear in the urine in this circumstance, indicative of nephrotoxicity. Surface wounds and infections are treated by neomycin applied locally, often in combination with another antibiotic such as bacitracin or polymyxin.

NITROFURANTOIN (FURADANTIN)

This is an antimicrobial nitrofuran recommended for oral administration in the treatment of bacterial infections of the urinary tract. Many strains of both Gram-negative and Gram-positive bacteria are found to be sensitive on in vitro testing. From 40 to 50 per cent of what is ingested orally is excreted into the urine. A single 50-mg dose given to a child with an average 200-ml urine secretion in a 6-hour period yields an average urinary concentration of 12.5 mg per 100 ml. The urinary content is entirely active from an antibacterial standpoint. Plasma levels with the standard dosages are low, in the range of 0.1 to 0.2 mg per 100 ml. Cerebrospinal fluid levels are under the border of measurability.

Practically all the ingested drug is absorbed, less than 5 per cent being found in the stools.

NYSTATIN (MYCOSTATIN)

This powdery product of *Streptomyces noursei* is fungistatic and fungicidal in media and animals. It may be of value in prophylaxis and therapy of candidiasis and some of the other mycoses.

BIBLIOGRAPHY

PENICILLIN

Barnett, H. L., H. McNamara, S. Shultz, and *R. Tompsett,* Renal Clearances of Sodium Penicillin G, Procaine Penicillin G, and Inulin in Infants and Children, *Pediatrics* 3:418, 1949.

Bayne, G. M., J. Gylfe, S. Carfagno, and *W. P. Boger,* Benzethacil (Bicillin): A Report of the Penicillemia Following Its Oral Administration in Man, *Am. J. M. Sc.* 225:190, 1953.

Beyer, K. H., "Pharmacological Bases of Penicillin Therapy," Charles C Thomas, Springfield, Ill., 1950.

Clarke, H. T., J. R. Johnson, and *R. Robinson* (eds.), "The Chemistry of Penicillin," Princeton University Press, Princeton, N.J., 1949.

Cohlan, S. Q., J. M. Lewis, and *E. Seligmann,* Blood Levels of Penicillin with Oral Use of Buffered and Unbuffered Solutions: Studies on a Series of Infants and Children, *Am. J. Dis. Child.* 75:15, 1948.

Coriell, L. L., C. Labra, E. Saltzman, and *T. F. McN. Scott,* An Evaluation of Benemid (P-(Di-N-Propylsulfamyl)-Benzoic Acid) Dosage Schedule in Children, *J. Pediat.* 42:292, 1953.

Doxiadis, S. A., J. L. Emery, and *S. M. Stewart,* Oral Penicillin in Children, *Brit. M. J.* 1:16, 1951.

Eagle, H., Experimental Approach to the Problem of Treatment Failure with Penicillin. I. Group A Streptococcal Infection in Mice, *Am. J. Med.* 13:389, 1952.

——, *R. Fleischman,* and *A. D. Musselman,* Effect of Schedule of Administration on the Therapeutic Efficacy of Penicillin: Importance of the Aggregate Time Penicillin Remains at Effectively Bactericidal Levels, *Am. J. Med.* 9:280, 1950.

Hildick-Smith, G., T. F. McN. Scott, and *C. M. Whitlock,* Penicillin Regimens in Pediatric Practice: Study of Blood Levels, *Pediatrics* 5:97, 1950.

Huang, N. N., and *R. H. High,* Comparison of Serum Levels Following Administration of Oral and Parenteral Preparations of Penicillin to Infants and Children of Various Age Groups, *J. Pediat.* 42:657, 1953.

International Standard and Unit for Penicillin, *League of Nations Bull. Health Organ.* vol. 12, no. 2, 1945–1946.

Karlberg, P., G. Sterner, and *G. Wallmark,* Aerosol-penicillin Therapy for Infants and Children, *Ann. paediat.* 175:263, 1950.

Kern, R. A., and *N. A. Wimberley,* Penicillin Reactions: Their Nature, Growing Importance, Recognition, Management and Prevention, *Am. J. M. Sc.* 226:357, 1953.

Lipman, M. O., J. A. Coss, Jr., and *R. H. Boots,* Changes in the Bacterial Flora of the Throat and Intestinal Tract during Prolonged Oral Administration of Penicillin, *Am. J. Med.* 4:702, 1948.

Martin, W. J., D. R. Nichols, and *F. R. Heilman,* Observations on Clinical Use of Phenoxymethyl Penicillin (Penicillin V), *J.A.M.A.* 160:928, 1956.

Murray, J., and *E. M. Crawford,* Penicillin Blood Levels in Babies, *Lancet* 2:147, 1951.

Weinstein, L., G. K. Daikos, and *T. S. Perrin,* Studies on the Relationship of Tissue Fluid and Blood Levels of Penicillin, *J. Lab. & Clin. Med.* 38:712, 1951.

Welch, H., W. A. Randall, and *F. D. Hendricks,* Serum Concentrations of Penicillin

Following Administration of Various Preparations of Dibenzylethylenediamine Dipenicillin G (DBED Penicillin), *Antibiotics & Chemother.* 3:1053, 1953.

STREPTOMYCIN

Alexander, H. E., G. Leidy, W. Redman, and *E. Simakow,* Experimental Basis for Prediction of Therapeutic Efficacy of Streptomycin in Infections Caused by Gram Negative Bacilli, *Pediatrics* 5:78, 1950.

Applebaum, E., and *J. Nelson,* Streptomycin in the Treatment of Influenzal Meningitis: A Study of Ninety Cases, with 96.6 Per Cent Recovery, *J.A.M.A.* 143:715, 1950.

Bogen, E., Laboratory Aspects of Streptomycin, *J.A.M.A.* 140:469, 1949.

Holzel, A., G. Martyn, and *L. Apter,* Streptomycin Treatment of Infantile Diarrhoea and Vomiting, *Brit. M. J.* 2:454, 1949.

Hunt, A. D., Jr., and *M. B. Fell,* Streptomycin Intramuscular Dosage per Unit Body Weight Correlated with Serum Levels in Infants and Children, *Pediatrics* 4:163, 1949.

Welch, H., Streptomycin and Dihydrostreptomycin, chap. 4 in "Principles and Practice of Antibiotic Therapy," Medical Encyclopedia, Inc., New York, 1954.

ERYTHROMYCIN

Freeman, L. C., and *R. B. Scott,* Erythromycin in Treatment of Pyoderma in Children, *J. Pediat.* 42:669, 1953.

Haight, T. H., and *M. Finland,* Laboratory and Clinical Studies on Erythromycin, *New England J. Med.* 247:227, 1952.

Herrell, W. E., "Erythromycin," Medical Encyclopedia, Inc., New York, 1955.

Josselyn, L. E., and *J. C. Sylvester,* Absorption of Erythromycin, *Antibiotics & Chemother.* 3:63, 1952.

Kirby, W., M. M. Maple, M. Francis, and *B. O'Leary,* Erythromycin Serum Concentrations Following Administration in Acid-resistant Tablets, *Antibiotics & Chemother.* 3:473, 1953.

Martin, W. J., D. R. Nichols, and *J. E. Geraci,* The Present Status of Erythromycin, *Proc. Staff Meet. Mayo Clin.* 22:609, 1953.

Smith, J. W., R. W. Dyke, and *R. S. Griffith,* Absorption Following Oral Administration of Erythromycin, *J.A.M.A.* 151:805, 1953.

Sylvester, J. C., and *L. E. Josselyn,* Absorption of Erythromycin. II. Erythromycin Stearate, *Antibiotics & Chemother.* 3:930, 1953.

CHLORTETRACYCLINE

Dowling, H. F., M. H. Lepper, E. R. Caldwell, Jr., R. L. Whelton, and *R. L. Brickhouse,* The Concentration of Aureomycin in Urine and Cerebrospinal, Pleural and Ascitic Fluids after Oral and Intravenous Administration, *J. Clin. Invest.* 28:983, 1949.

Hines, L. R., An Appraisal of the Effects of Long-term Chlortetracycline Administration, *Antibiotics & Chemother.* 6:623, 1956.

Lepper, M. H., "Aureomycin (Chlortetracycline)," Medical Encyclopedia, Inc., New York, 1957.

Olshaker, B., S. Ross, A. Recinos, Jr., and *E. Twible,* Aureomycin in the Treatment of Pneumonia in Infants and Children, *New England J. Med.* 241:289, 1949.

Schwachman, H., G. E. Foley, and *C. D. Cook,* Aureomycin in Pediatrics: A Review, *J. Pediat.* 38:91, 1951.

Snelling, M. B., and *R. Johnson,* The Value of Aureomycin in Prevention of Cross Infection in the Hospital for Sick Children, *Canad. M. A. J.* 66:6, 1952.

Whitlock, C. M., Jr., A. D. Hunt, Jr., and *S. G. Tashman,* Studies on the Administration, Absorption, Distribution and Excretion of Aureomycin in Children, *Pediatrics* 6:827, 1950.

OXYTETRACYCLINE

Baker, H. J., and *E. J. Pulaski,* Effects of Terramycin on Fecal Flora, *Ann. New York Acad. Sc.* 53:324, 1950.

Coodin, F. J., Studies of Terramycin in Premature Infants, *Pediatrics* 12:652, 1953.

Hunt, A. D., Jr., R. S. Kelley, L. L. Coriell, M. L. Murphy, S. G. Tashman, and *C. Stevens,* Studies on Absorption and Distribution of Terramycin in Children, *Pediatrics* 9:607, 1952.

Koch, R., Blood and Cerebrospinal Fluid Levels of Intramuscular Oxytetracycline, *J. Pediat.* 46:44, 1955.

Musselman, M. M., "Terramycin (Oxytetracycline)," Medical Encyclopedia, Inc., New York, 1956.

O'Regan, C., and *S. Schwarzer,* Intramuscular Terramycin: Laboratory and Clinical Studies in Children, *J. Pediat.* 44:172, 1954.

Rivers, J. A., and *V. M. Sborov,* The Effect of Terramycin on the Intestinal Flora, *Gastroenterology* 17:546, 1951.

Sayer, R. J., J. C. Michel, F. C. Moll, and *W. M. M. Kirby,* Terramycin: Clinical, Pharmacologic, and Bacteriologic Studies, *Am. J. M. Sc.* 221:256, 1951.

Wooding, C. H., Jr., and *R. B. Scott,* Terramycin in Treatment of Pneumonias of Childhood: A Report of Ten Cases, *J. Pediat.* 38:423, 1951.

TETRACYCLINE

Dowling, H. F., "Tetracycline," Medical Encyclopedia, Inc., New York, 1955.

Eisenberg, G. M., E. L. Foltz, A. J. Palazollo, and *H. F. Flippin,* Laboratory and Clinical Observations on Tetracycline, in "Antibiotics Annual 1954–1955," Medical Encyclopedia, Inc., New York, 1955.

Finland, M., E. M. Purcell, S. S. Wright, and *E. H. Kass,* Clinical and Laboratory Observations of a New Antibiotic Tetracycline, *J.A.M.A.* 154:561, 1954.

Minsky, A. A., S. Schwarzer, and *M. B. Milberg,* Tetracycline in Pediatric Practice: Pharmacology and Therapeutic Efficacy, in "Antibiotics Annual 1954–1955," Medical Encyclopedia, Inc., New York, 1955.

Putnam, L. E., F. D. Hendricks, and *H. Welch,* Tetracycline: A New Antibiotic, *Antibiotics & Chemother.* 3:1183, 1953.

Waddington, W. S., G. G. Bergy, R. L. Nielsen, and *W. M. M. Kirby,* Tetracycline: Clinical and Pharmocologic Studies, *Am. J. Med. Sc.* 228:164, 1954.

Welch, H., W. A. Randall, R. J. Reedy, and *E. J. Oswald,* Variations in Antimicrobial Activity of the Tetracyclines, *Antibiotics & Chemother.* 4:741, 1954.

CHLORAMPHENICOL

Burnell, J. M., and *W. M. M. Kirby,* Serum Concentrations of Chloramphenicol Following Intravenous and Intramuscular Administration, *J. Lab. & Clin. Med.* 38:234, 1951.

Deane, G. E., J. E. Furman, A. R. Bentz, and *T. E. Woodward,* Treatment of Meningitis with Chloromycetin Palmitate, *Pediatrics* 11:368, 1953.

Hodgkinson, R., Blood Dyscrasias Associated with Chloramphenicol: An Investigation into the Cases in the British Isles, *Lancet* 1:285, 1954.

Kelly, R. S., A. D. Hunt, Jr., and *S. G. Tashman,* Studies on the Absorption and Distribution of Chloramphenicol, *Pediatrics* 8:362, 1951.

Lewis, C. N., L. E. Putnam, F. D. Hendricks, I. Kerlan, and *H. Welch,* Chloramphenicol (Chloromycetin) in Relation to Blood Dyscrasias with Observations on Other Drugs: A Special Survey, *Antibiotics & Chemother.* 2:601, 1952.

O'Brien, D., The Absorption of Chloramphenicol in the Newborn, *Arch. Dis. Childhood* 28:66, 1953.

Roy, T. E., E. Kroeger, G. Craig, D. Cohen, G. A. McNaughton, and *N. Silverthorne,* Studies on the Absorption of Chloramphenicol in Normal Children in Relation to the Treatment of Meningitis, *Antibiotics & Chemother.* 2:505, 1952.

Smadel, J. E., Chloramphenicol (Chloromycetin) in Treatment of Infectious Diseases, *Am. J. Med.* 7:671, 1949.

Woodward, T. E., and *C. Wisseman,* "Chloromycetin (Chloramphenicol)," Medical Encyclopedia, Inc., New York, 1957.

Yow, E. M., F. M. Taylor, J. Hirsch, R. A. Frankel, and *H. E. Carnes,* Chloromycetin Palmitate, *J. Pediat.* 42:151, 1953.

NOVOBIOCIN

Carroll, G., The Changing Flora in Urinary Infections in This Antibiotic Age, *J. Urol.* 73:609, 1955.

Frost, B. M., M. E. Valiant, L. McClelland, M. Solotorovsky, and *A. C. Cuckler,* The Antimicrobial Activity of Cathomycin, a New Antibiotic, "Antibiotics Annual," p. 918, Medical Encyclopedia, Inc., New York, 1955–1956.

Lin, F. K., and *L. L. Coriell,* Novobiocin: A Laboratory and Clinical Evaluation, *Antibiot. Med.* 2:268, 1956.

Symposium on Novobiocin, *Antibiot. Med.* 2:201, 1956.

Wright, W. W., L. E. Putman, and *H. Welch,* Novobiocin: Serum Concentrations and Urinary Excretion Following Oral Administration in Man, *Antibiot. Med.* 2:311, 1956.

BACITRACIN

Bacitracin: Accepted by the Council on Pharmacy and Chemistry of the American Medical Association, *J.A.M.A.* 145:822, 1951.

Finnerty, E. F., Bacitracin in Dermatology: Its Effectiveness in Topical Therapy, *New England J. Med.* 245:14, 1951.

Friedberg, C. K., and *M. E. Bader,* Acute Staphylococcic Endocarditis Cured with the Aid of Bacitracin, *J.A.M.A.* 147:46, 1951.

Longacre, A. B., and *R. Waters,* Parenteral Bacitracin in Surgical Infections, *Am. J. Surg.* 81:599, 1951.

Teng, P., Further Experiences in Treatment of Septic Meningitis with Bacitracin, *Arch. Neurol. & Psychiat.* 64:861, 1950.

POLYMYXIN B

Florman, A. L., and *N. Shifrin,* Observations on a Small Outbreak of Infantile Diarrhea Associated with *Pseudomonas aeruginosa, J. Pediat.* 36:758, 1950.

Hopper, J., Jr., E. Jawetz, and *F. Hinman, Jr.,* Polymyxin B in Chronic Pyelonephritis: Observations on the Safety of the Drug and on Its Influence on the Renal Infection, *Am. J. M. Sc.* 225:402, 1953.

Kagan, B. M., D. Krevsky, A. Milzer, and *M. Locke,* Polymyxin B and Polymyxin E, *J. Lab. & Clin. Med.* 37:402, 1951.

Newton, B. A., The Properties and Mode of Action of the Polymyxins, *Bact. Rev.* 20:14, 1956.

Polymyxin: Report of the Council on Pharmacy of the American Medical Association, *J.A.M.A.* 150:1219, 1952.

NEOMYCIN

Duncan, G. G., C. F. Clancy, J. R. Wolgamot, and *B. Beidleman,* Neomycin: Results of Clinical Use in Ten Cases, *J.A.M.A.* **145:**75, 1951.

Jawetz, E., "Polymyxin, Neomycin, Bacitracin," Medical Encyclopedia, Inc., New York, 1956.

NITROFURANTOIN

MacLeod, P. F., G. S. Rogers, and *B. R. Anzlowar,* The Nitrofurans in Clinical Medicine, *Internat. Rec. Med.* **169:**561, 1956.

NYSTATIN

Candidiasis (Moniliasis) and its Management with Mycostatin, *Monogr. Therapy* (*Squibb*), **2:**1, 1957.

Sternberg, T. H., and *V. D. Newcomer* (eds.), "Therapy of Fungus Diseases: An International Symposium," Little, Brown & Company, Boston, 1955.

CHAPTER 78

Sulfonamides

The fundamental constituent of the therapeutically active sulfonamides is a benzene ring having a sulfonamido group ($-SO_2NH$) attached to one carbon atom and an amino group ($-NH_2$) at the para or opposite position. Radicles which are added to the sulfonamido group are called N^1 substituents, and to the amino group, N^4 substituents. Altering the relative positions of the sulfonamido and amino groups, or attaching another radicle to the benzene ring itself, usually destroys the antibacterial activity.

Thousands of sulfonamide compounds have been synthesized and investigated. Only those which have minimal toxicity and potent antibacterial activity in vivo are made available pharmaceutically.

Estimation of the concentration of sulfonamides in the blood (and other body fluids) can be carried out by two standard approaches: (1) the method of Marshall and Bratton, which diazotizes the sulfonamide and completes it with naphthylethylenediamine or some similar reagent to produce a red color, or (2) the method of Werner, which treats the body fluid with Ehrlich's reagent to produce a yellow color. The intensity of either color is proportional to the amount of sulfonamide present. Phenacetin and local anesthetics of the procaine group will react with these reagents, so that care must be taken to avoid contamination of specimens from patients with these substances when carrying out any determinations.

Sulfonamides may kill organisms which are multiplying rapidly but will merely inhibit them in other phases of growth. Within the body, where natural suppressive mechanisms are operative, their action is mainly that of bacteriostasis.

In general the bacteriostatic capacity of any sulfonamide is related to its ability to counteract para-aminobenzoic acid, which is an essential nutrient for most bacteria. Sulfonamides interfere with its metabolic utilization, and vice versa. Some amino acids, especially methionine, and some of the peptones and other products produced by necrotic tissue and pus may also interfere with the action of the sulfonamides.

Metabolic resistance to sulfonamides is often acquired by bacteria after therapeutic exposures which continue for some days or weeks. This phenomenon, when resistance is not initially present, makes it advisable to commence any therapeutic program with large dosages and to change to some other form of therapy should clinical improvement not appear within a few days. The possibility of the development of resistant strains also casts some theoretical doubt on the efficacy of prolonged administration of a sulfonamide in small dosage as prophylaxis against recurrent bacterial infections.

PLASMA LEVELS

The many therapeutically satisfactory sulfonamides differ in their solubility, absorbability, concentrations obtained in the blood and body fluid, rate of excretion, and antimicrobial effects. Sulfanilamide, sulfadiazine, sulfamerazine, and sulfisoxazole (Gantrisin), for example, are readily soluble and rapidly absorbed when taken by mouth. Other compounds such as sulfaguanidine and succinylsulfathiazole tend to be poorly absorbed; they remain in the lumen of the bowel and exert their action upon the bacteria locally present.

When a patient is given a customary oral dose of soluble sulfonamide the blood concentration rises to a peak in 4 to 8 hours and then subsides slowly over the next 48 hours. With sulfadiazine, the height of this peak, subject to individual variation, may fall between 1 and 7 mg per 100 ml. Larger oral doses give higher blood levels, but the augmentation is not directly proportional. With a large initial dose followed by smaller doses every 4 to 6 hours, the blood level is usually maintained between 3 and 10 mg per 100 ml after the first 24 hours. Food exerts a negligible effect on absorption. A subcutaneous injection of a soluble sulfonamide raises the blood level more rapidly. This route is sometimes preferred at the onset of therapy of a severe infection such as pyogenic meningitis or when a patient is vomiting and cannot take medication by mouth. The chemical methods in routine use measure the blood levels of free sulfonamide, which is the biologically active form; they do not react with the acetylated or other derivatives which are inactive.

When a sulfonamide reaches the blood stream some of it combines with and is "bound" to the plasma proteins. The balance diffuses rapidly through the body fluids and tissues with the exception of bone and fat. The level attained in the cerebrospinal fluid varies from 20 to 100 per cent of the level in the blood, depending on the character of the sulfonamide employed and the state of permeability of the blood-brain barrier.

The major route for excretion of most absorbed sulfonamides is into the urine. From 10 to 50 per cent may be as acetylated and therapeutically inactive derivatives (p. 402).

As with the antibiotics, a clear relation exists in vitro between the concentration of a sulfonamide in the culture medium and the threshold capacity of a bacterial strain to grow in its presence. The presumption is that the same relation occurs in vivo and that the levels in plasma and other body fluids should be sufficiently high to suppress the growth of the pathogenic bacteria within the body. Blood concentrations which may be deemed adequate to suppress susceptible organisms have been shown by experience to be approximately 10 to 15 mg per 100 ml for sulfadiazine and sulfamerazine in severe infections; 6 to 10 mg in moderate infections; and 2 to 3 mg for prophylaxis. Since toxic reactions are frequent at the higher blood levels, the dosage should be kept to the minimum necessary for the desired therapeutic result.

THERAPY

Mixtures of two, three, or more sulfonamides are often administered concurrently, in total amounts approximating what would be given as a single drug. Such combinations are more soluble in the blood and urine, are much less nephrotoxic, give rise to fewer sensitivity reactions, and sometimes seem therapeutically more effective than any of the individual members in comparable total dosage. Sulfadiazine and sulfamerazine are usually included, with sulfamethazine, sulfacetamide, or sulfathiazole as a third or fourth ingredient. With such combinations it is more feasible to give very large doses and obtain unusually high blood and cerebrospinal fluid concentrations when necessary.

Sulfonamides in reasonable dosages have been found efficacious to at least some extent in the therapy of infections caused by staphylococci, hemolytic streptococci, bacilli, Clostridia, Brucella, plague bacilli, and some varieties of Shigella, including the Flexner and Schmitz strains. Sulfonamides exhibit also considerable potency against the virus of lymphogranuloma inguinale and possibly against the trachoma virus. Only occasional strains of viridans streptococci, enterococci, Proteus, Pseudomonas, and Klebsiella are susceptible. Acquired resistance may develop with almost every organism after repeated exposures.

At least one of the antibiotics is effective also against nearly every one of the above-mentioned pathogens and often is more effective. The use of sulfonamides is ordinarily reserved in this country to situations (1) where a proper antibiotic is for some reason unavailable, (2) where a patient has an idiosyncracy to the antibiotic which contraindicates its use, (3) where an auxiliary agent is needed to serve as an adjuvant to the antibiotic in severe or resistant infections or to depress the development of resistant strains of bacteria, (4) where the lower cost of sulfonamides as compared to that of antibiotics is an important consideration, or (5) where the pathogenic organisms have been found resistant to all antibiotics employed, as occurs at times in chronic pyelonephritis or bronchopulmonary infections.

The degree of sensitivity or resistance of a bacterial strain to a sulfonamide can be assayed for clinical purposes by planting the organism in a series of suitably prepared plates or tubes containing graded amounts of sulfonamide within the range attainable in a patient's blood. Readings are interpreted as with the antibiotics. A cruder method is to plant a diluted culture on the surface of a standard blood agar plate and then place upon it a drop of thick watery paste made from the sulfonamide to be tested. Control plates are prepared with organisms already known to be susceptible and resistant. The degree of inhibition of growth around the sulfonamide drop is an indicator of the presence or absence of susceptibility.

BIBLIOGRAPHY

SULFONAMIDES

Hawking, F., and *J. S. Lawrence,* "The Sulphonamides," Grune & Stratton, Inc., New York, 1951.

Nortley, E. H., "The Sulfonamides and Allied Compounds," Reinhold Publishing Corporation, New York, 1948.

Rhoads, P. S., C. E. Billings, and *V. J. O'Conor,* Antibacterial Management of Urinary Tract Infections, *J.A.M.A.* 148:165, 1952.

Ross, S., C. Rite, F. G. Burke, J. J. McGovern, R. H. Parrott, and *J. P. McGovern,* Treatment of Meningitis Due to *Hemophilus influenzae, New England J. Med.* 247:541, 1952.

Schweinburg, F. B., and *A. M. Rutenberg, In vitro* Sensitivity of Bacteria to Sulfonamide Combinations as Compared to Single Sulfonamides, *Proc. Soc. Exper. Biol. & Med.* 74:480, 1950.

Wieder, S., and *W. Elias,* Triple Sulfonamides in Urinary Tract Infections, *Internat. Rec. Med.* 169:572, 1956.

Yow, E. M., Observations on the Use of Sulfisoxazole (Gantrisin) in 1000 Consecutive Patients, with Particular Reference to the Frequency of Undesirable Side Effects, *Am. Pract. & Digest Treat.* 4:521, 1953.

———, A Re-evaluation of Sulfonamide Therapy, *Ann. Int. Med.* 43:323, 1955.

CHAPTER 79

Obscure Generalized Diseases

CAT-SCRATCH DISEASE (CAT-SCRATCH FEVER, BENIGN INOCULATION LYMPHORETICULOSIS)

This is an apparently infectious disorder which usually follows the scratch of a cat, but has been seen after skin injuries caused by splinters, thorns, and porcupine quills. Three to five days later, in approximately half the cases, a primary lesion develops at the site of the scratch in the form of a red or purple inflammatory lesion which may become crusted or pustular. Two to three weeks later one or more regional lymph nodes becomes enlarged. These may be tender and sometimes go on to suppuration. The overlying skin is usually inflamed. Fever, malaise, and leukocytosis are not uncommon during this stage. A minority of the patients have an evanescent rash. Several instances of complicating acute meningoencephalitis, which may end fatally, have been described. The nodes remain enlarged for several weeks or months, and then subside spontaneously. A low-grade conjunctivitis may follow a scratch of the eyelid region.

The etiologic agent is unknown. The epidemiology and natural history of the infection suggest an infectious process, but bacteriologic cultures prove consistently sterile. Cats which spread the disease are not sick themselves. It is believed that the infective agent is derived from some sources in the environment and carried passively on the surface of the claws and other sources of scratch. Efforts to transmit the disease to chick embryos and laboratory animals by virologic techniques have been unsuccessful to date.

Skin Testing

An antigen for intradermal testing can be prepared from pus aspirated from a suppurating node. The material is diluted 1:5 with isotonic salt solution, heated to 57°C for 1 hour on 2 successive days, and then preserved with added 0.5 per cent phenol or similar drug. Infected patients show a tuberculin-like skin reaction in 48 hours after an intradermal injection of 0.1 ml of this antigen. Because local discoloration persists oc-

964

casionally for several days without other evidences of reactivity, it has been recommended that the reading be taken as positive when there is a local area of induration at least 4 mm in diameter, with a surrounding zone of erythema 1 cm or more in diameter.

Lymph Node Biopsy

Surgical excision of lymph nodes is ordinarily not recommended except when the diagnosis is in doubt or when large abscesses have formed.

In the early stages the nodes are swollen and soft. On microscopy they show proliferation of the reticulum cells and zonelike infiltrations of neutrophils and plasma cells about small central foci of necrosis; the reticulum cells may assume an epithelioid appearance in these areas. Multinucleated cells similar to the Sternberg cells of Hodgkin's disease or the foreign-body giant cells of the Langhans type are inconstantly present. In the more advanced stages the nodes may be firmer and show gross foci of yellow purulent softening. These foci are large necrotic areas containing debris, fibrin, and neutrophils, encircled by a zone of epithelioid cells and fibroblasts infiltrated with lymphocytes, monocytes, neutrophils, and giant cells.

This cellular reaction pattern is nonspecific. Similar formations may develop in tularemia, lymphogranuloma venereum, sporotrichosis, and even glandular tuberculosis. Stains and cultures for bacteria, fungi, and tubercle bacilli are negative. Large intracytoplasmic inclusion bodies, such as occur in lymphogranuloma venereum, are uncommon in cat-scratch disease.

Other Laboratory Findings

The red cell sedimentation rate is often elevated. Complement-fixation tests with the lymphogranuloma venereum antigen have been positive in a minority of cases. Other serologic tests, such as agglutination for *Pasteurella tularensis,* are regularly negative.

CYTOMEGALIC INCLUSION DISEASE

This is a rare disturbance in which inclusion bodies are found within the nuclei or cytoplasm of enlarged tissue cells. It is presumed that the cause is the same as yet unidentified virus which forms the inclusion bodies which are not infrequently encountered as an incidental finding in the salivary glands of older children and adults at autopsy.

The reported childhood cases tend to fall into two major groups. Most often the illness is found at birth or in the neonatal period. It may stimulate erythroblastosis fetalis or give rise to microcephaly or other disturbances. Most affected infants, usually prematurely born, will exhibit jaundice, hepatosplenomegaly, hemolytic anemia and reticulocytosis on the first or second day of life. They may have thrombocytopenia with bleeding manifestations. The Coombs test is negative. Microscopy of the urine may reveal large desquamated renal epithelial cells containing the inclusion bodies (p. 388). All such severely affected infants survive only a few weeks or months. Inclusion cells may be found in any organ of the body. The most frequent sites have been the liver, kidney, and pancreas.

Less commonly the disease becomes evident after the neonatal period but usually before the fifth year. A few instances have been recorded in adults. These patients succumb to a progressively debilitating disturbance. Cytomegalic inclusion cells in small numbers are found at autopsy in a few organs.

GARGOYLISM

This is a familial disturbance which manifests itself clinically in bony deformities, clouded corneae, mental deficiency, and enlarged liver and spleen. Not all these features need be present in every case. The disorder is not sex-linked.

Histologically one finds an abnormal intracellular substance within the connective tissues, various organs, and the neurons of the central and autonomic nervous system. This infiltrating substance, as yet unidentified, is thought to be a lipoidal or lipid-carbohydrate complex.

There are no distinctive laboratory findings which are pathognomonic. The neutrophils or other cells in the circulation often contain abnormal basophilic granular formations (p. 227).

HODGKIN'S DISEASE

This disease, of unknown cause, exhibits a variable but progressive course in childhood. Discrete enlargement of the cervical lymph nodes is the most frequent initial symptom. This is usually unilateral and may be on either side. Enlargement of other nodes, hepatomegaly, and splenomegaly often develop later.

Laboratory studies in the earlier stages typically show only a slight anemia and a normal leukocyte count. The sedimentation rate is nearly always elevated. No test is even presumptively diagnostic, other than biopsy of affected tissue. Even this examination is not always satisfactory, because of similarity of the histologic lesions at times to neoplasms or to inflammatory granulomas such as those of tuberculosis.

GAUCHER'S DISEASE

There are two clearly defined constitutional disorders, Gaucher's disease and Niemann-Pick disease, in which the reticuloendothelial system accumulates lipid substances. It is still unsettled whether the intracellular accumulations in these disorders are of normal or abnormal metabolic substances or whether these substances originate within the cells themselves or are filtered from the blood stream or lymph where they may be circulating in trace concentrations.

Gaucher's disease is characterized by abnormal storage of large amounts of galactosidocerebroside (kerasin) and glucosidocerebroside in inconstant proportions within the cells of the reticuloendothelial system. The disease is usually found in whites, chiefly Jewish, and is not sex-linked. When it becomes apparent in early infancy it runs a comparatively rapid course and carries a grave prognosis. In older children and adults the course is slow and protracted.

There are no distinctive biochemical blood changes. The plasma lipids, including cholesterol and lecithin, are within normal limits, except in terminal cachexia when they may be low. The cerebroside content of the blood serum is not demonstrably elevated. The subclinical jaundice shown by some individuals has been thought to be due to increased blood destruction. Despite the heavy infiltration of the liver with Gaucher cells the results of routine liver function tests are usually normal.

Gaucher cells are distinctively large, 20 to 40 or more μ in diameter, and pale, round, or polyhedral. Their nuclei are small, eccentrically placed, and often multiple. The cytoplasm is finely mottled, with pale-staining deposits supported by wavy fibrils. The cytoplasmic deposits do not react with any of the usual staining reagents for lipids; vacuoles when they occur are artifacts resulting from fixation. There are no cellular reactive changes in the contiguous tissues.

The peripheral blood shows depressive changes in advanced cases. There may be leukopenia, neutropenia, anemia, or thrombocytopenia. The anemia is usually normocytic and of moderate degree, but may be macrocytic. The depression of the cellular elements is attributable to Gaucher cell infiltration of the bone marrow, or inanition of the patient, or occasionally also to hypersplenism secondary to the enormous splenic enlargement. The reduced platelets may be responsible for the prolonged epistaxis, bleeding spongy gums, and scattered petechiae and ecchymoses so frequently seen in the late stages.

The bone marrow is usually infiltrated with the characteristic cells, discoverable by aspiration or biopsy (p. 335). The typical cells are also demonstrable by splenic puncture, but this procedure carries some danger. They will also be revealed by diagnostic biopsy of the liver or large internal lymph nodes. The subcutaneous lymph nodes may not contain the characteristic cells in any quantity; aspiration of these structures does not always give positive results.

NIEMANN-PICK DISEASE

In this disorder the reticuloendothelial system and many organs such as the brain and liver undergo an extreme degree of intracellular glycerophosphatide accumulation, particularly of sphingomyelin. Lecithin is present also in enhanced amounts. The cephalin content is not increased.

The disease is equally common in boys and girls, who are usually of Jewish origin. It nearly always ends fatally within the first 2 years. A very few cases have been seen in older children.

The most prominent clinical features are retarded growth and mental development, enlargement of the liver and spleen, and a red fovea centralis in the macular region of the eye. The blood may show moderate normochromic anemia. About one-third of the cases exhibit a neutrophilic leukocytosis, usually moderate but sometimes pronounced. There may also be a mild monocytosis (up to 5 per cent); in a minority of cases the cytoplasm and even the nuclei of the monocytes may contain prominent vacuoles. Occasional immature red cells, plasma cells, or reticulum cells may also be found. The platelet level is as a rule normal, though thrombocytopenia with hemorrhagic diathesis has been reported a few times. Leukopenia is not seen.

The reticuloendothelium contains the so-called Niemann-Pick foam cells, not necessarily in abundance. These are about the same size and shape as Gaucher cells, up to 40 μ in diameter. They differ in having the cytoplasm packed with equal-sized rounded droplets and some additional ones inside the nucleus. These droplets are stainable with Sudan III and Nile blue sulfate and other fat stains but do not reduce osmic acid. At autopsy droplets of lipid, in small numbers, are found also within the cells of vascular endothelium, nervous and connective tissues, and parenchyma of most other organs, enlarging these cells and changing their normal appearance.

Biopsy of the spleen, liver, or internal lymph nodes will establish the diagnosis, but bone marrow aspiration is simple and equally reliable (p. 335). The superficial lymph nodes may have a meager content of these cells.

The total serum lipids may be normal or enhanced. Readings as high as 1,610 and 1,430 mg per 100 ml have been described. The total serum cholesterol is only occasionally elevated. The ratio of free to total cholesterol may be disturbed, with free cholesterol constituting 35 to 95 per cent of the total. The phospholipid level of the serum is not increased. Serum phosphorus and alkaline phosphatase may be high, or the calcium low. The cerebrospinal fluid may have a moderate increase in protein (50 to 250 mg per 100 ml), with no pleocytosis or other changes.

Genetic Transmission

Both Gaucher's disease and Niemann-Pick disease follow the recessive pattern of mendelian inheritance. Since neither gene has any appreciable prevalence within the population, the diseases occur but rarely. When several cases are encountered in a family they are almost always siblings of the same generation.

Attempts have been made to identify genetic carriers by search of the bone marrow aspirate for the characteristic cells. Occasional individuals with subclinical Gaucher's disease have been detected, but none to our knowledge with Niemann-Pick disease.

LETTERER-SIWE DISEASE
(NONLIPID RETICULOENDOTHELIOSIS)

Occurring in infancy or the first few years of life, this disease is characterized by progressive hyperplasia of the reticuloendothelial system, enlargement of the spleen and lymph nodes and often of the liver, a maculopapular rash, seborrhea, destructive lesions in the bones, a tendency to anemia, thrombocytopenia, and hemorrhage, susceptibility to infections, and an outcome which is often but not invariably fatal.

The diagnosis in suspected cases is best confirmed by biopsy of a lymph node and demonstration of overgrowth of reticulum cells with finely granular cytoplasm and no excess fat deposits. The bone marrow aspirate may show an increased number of these cells (p. 336). The peripheral blood smear may show a granulocytic leukocytosis, sometimes with mild eosinophilia. Leukocytopenia is often seen, with the lymphocyte as the predominant cell. There are no abnormal leukocytes in the blood smear. The erythrocytopenia which is often present tends to be normochromic in character. The blood chemistry findings are not typically abnormal. At necropsy one finds focal accumulations of reticulum cells, often with eosinophils in the lymph nodes, lungs, skin, spleen, liver, bone marrow, and other locations.

HAND-SCHÜLLER-CHRISTIAN DISEASE AND
EOSINOPHILIC GRANULOMA OF BONE

These diseases, closely related to each other, tend to be restricted in distribution of lesions to one or more focal areas in the bones and contiguous structures (p. 335). Large lipid-containing "foam" cells accompany the proliferating histiocytic cells, eosinophils, and scattered multinucleated giant cells at the sites of infiltration but are not associated with consistent systemic changes. Diabetes insipidus may occur in Hand-Schüller-Christian disease as a result of infiltration about the pituitary stalk.

There are no specific changes of a laboratory nature apart from the histologic lesions demonstrable by biopsy.

Because of the absence of any alteration in cholesterol or other fractions of the serum lipids, these two disorders, together with xanthoma disseminata of the skin, are sometimes referred to as the normocholesteremic xanthomatoses. The fat-containing cell formations in inflammatory tissue and in true tumors, such as the lipomas and nevoxanthoendothelioma, are also not associated with any increase in any of the serum lipid fractions.

Other Xanthomatoses

In idiopathic hyperlipemia, the nephrotic syndrome, glycogen storage disease, and a few other conditions (p. 522), the enormously enhanced levels of serum neutral fat along with moderate increases in cholesterol and phospholipids may lead to xanthomatous lesions in the skin and elsewhere. These recede as the hyperlipemia subsides. The serum in these cases appears creamy or milky.

SARCOIDOSIS

Of unknown cause, this chronic disease becomes manifest in the form of granulomatous noncaseating infiltrations which may appear in any of the organs. The clinical course varies from spontaneous subsidence within a few months or years to stagnant persistence or slow progress. Overt symptoms are usually minimal or absent, though episodes of malaise and fever may develop acutely. Secondary bacterial infections may be superimposed. Pulmonary lesions are often discovered in routine roentgenograms of the chest.

Histopathology

The diagnosis is best established by microscopic study of tissue from an involved area—bone marrow aspirates, needle biopsy of the liver, or fragments of the skin, tonsils, or excised deeper structures. Superficial lymph nodes are usually affected and lend themselves readily to biopsy. Preference should be given to a cervical node, which is the least likely to show confusing nonspecific inflammation from other causes. Even a tiny node may exhibit the typical lesion.

The cellular reactions are the same regardless of site. These consist of proliferation and agglomeration of epithelioid cells into circumscribed masses resembling somewhat those of miliary tuberculosis. Langhans giant cells may be seen about deeply staining structures which appear to be calcium granules. The infiltrations may or may not be encapsulated. Attendant lymphocytes and central foci of necrosis are uncommon. Efforts to demonstrate fungi or acid-fast bacteria in the involved areas are unsuccessful, though special stains and culture for these should always be carried out to exclude the possibility of an error in diagnosis.

Other Laboratory Findings

The skin tuberculin reaction is negative unless this disease is present also. Active cases often have a marked increase in serum globulins; this produces an elevation in total serum protein level, often above 8 gm per 100 ml, and a reversal of the albumin-globulin ratio. The serum levels of calcium, phosphorus, phosphatase, bilirubin, or nonprotein nitrogen are elevated occasionally, though the degree of changes cannot be correlated with the site of the infiltrations or severity or duration of the disease. The red cell sedimentation rate tends to be rapid while the process is active and to recede to normal as the lesions heal.

A minority of the patients exhibit a mild normochromic anemia. About one-fourth have an eosinophilia amounting to 5 to 25 per cent of all the leukocytes. The monocytes are usually increased a little. Infiltration of the bone marrow spaces by sarcoid tubercles may cause hemopoietic depression of extramedullary hemopoiesis. Splenomegalic involvement may evoke a hypersplenic syndrome or thrombocytopenia or acquired hemolytic anemia.

STILL'S DISEASE

A leukocytosis of 15,000 per cu ml is nearly always present in the early stages of this disorder, with a neutrophilic outpouring amounting to 80 to 90 per cent of all leukocytes. This leukocytosis does not subside under antibiotic therapy. The bone marrow exhibits a hyperplasia of cells of the granulocyte series; sometimes the myelocytes escape into the blood stream in small numbers. In the late stages of the disease there is not infrequently a terminal bone marrow hypoplasia, reflected peripherally as a thrombocytopenia, granulocytopenia, and erythrocytopenia.

BIBLIOGRAPHY

CAT-SCRATCH DISEASE

Daeschner, C. W., G. W. Salmon, and F. M. Heys, Cat-scratch Fever, J. Pediat. 43:371, 1953.

Daniels, W. B., and F. G. MacMurray, Cat Scratch Disease; Nonbacterial Regional Lymphadenitis: A Report of 60 Cases, Ann. Int. Med. 37:697, 1952.

Debré, R., Accidents nerveux de la maladie des griffes du chat, Bull. Acad. nat. méd. 454:24, 1952.

Greer, W. E. R., and C. S. Keefer, Cat-scratch Fever: A Disease Entity, New England J. Med. 244:545, 1951.

McGovern, J. J., L. J. Kunz, and F. M. Blodgett, Nonbacterial Regional Lymphadenitis ("Cat-scratch Fever"), New England J. Med. 252:166, 1955.

Stevens, H., Cat Scratch Fever Encephalitis, A.M.A. Am. J. Dis. Child. 84:218, 1952.

Winship, T., Pathologic Changes in So-called Cat-scratch Fever: Review of Findings in Lymph Nodes of 29 Patients and Cutaneous Lesions of 2 Patients, Am. J. Clin. Path. 23:1012, 1953.

CYTOMEGALIC INCLUSION DISEASE

Bacala, J. C., and R. J. Burke, Generalized Cytomegalic Inclusion Disease: Report of a Case and Review of Literature, J. Pediat. 43:712, 1953.

Bellamy, J., Cytomegalic Inclusion-body Disease Occurring in Twins, *Am. J. Clin. Path.* 24:1040, 1954.

Cappell, D. F., and *M. N. McFarlane,* Inclusion Bodies (Protozoan-like Cells) in the Organs of Infants, *J. Path. & Bact.* 59:385, 1947.

Dyckman, J., and *J. Bellamy,* Histochemical Studies in Cytomegalic Inclusion Disease, *A.M.A. Arch. Path.* 56:360, 1953.

Fetterman, G. H., A New Laboratory Aid in the Clinical Diagnosis of Inclusion Disease of Infancy, *Am. J. Clin. Path.* 22:424, 1952.

Margileth, A. M., The Diagnosis and Treatment of Generalized Cytomegalic Inclusion Disease of the Newborn, *Pediatrics* 15:270, 1955.

Mercer, R. D., S. Luse, and *D. H. Guyton,* Cytomegalic Inclusion Disease, *Pediatrics* 11:502, 1953.

Wyatt, J. P., J. Saxton, R. S. Lee, and *H. Pinkerton,* Generalized Cytomegalic Inclusion Disease, *J. Pediat.* 36:271, 1950.

GARGOYLISM

Dawson, I. M. P., The Histology and Histochemistry of Gargoylism, *J. Path. & Bact.* 67:587, 1954.

Henderson, J. L., A. R. MacGregor, S. J. Thannhauser, and *R. Holden,* The Pathology and Biochemistry of Gargoylism, *Arch. Dis. Childhood* 27:230, 1952.

Lindsay, S., W. A. Reilly, T. J. Gotham, and *R. Skahen,* Gargoylism. II. Study of Pathological Lesions and Clinical Review of 12 Cases, *Am. J. Dis. Child.* 76:239, 1948.

Strauss, L., The Pathology of Gargoylism and Review of the Literature, *Am. J. Path.* 24:855, 1948.

HODGKIN'S DISEASE

Howard, J. E., and *S. J. Yanez,* Hodgkin's Disease in Childhood (Enfermedad de Hodgkin en el niño), *Rev. chil. de pediat.* 25:205, 1954.

LIPID STORAGE DISEASES AND RETICULOENDOTHELIOSES

Batson, R., J. Shapiro, A. Christie, and *C. M. Riley,* Acute Nonlipid Disseminated Reticuloendotheliosis, *A.M.A. Am. J. Dis. Child.* 90:323, 1955.

Beerman, H., Lipid Diseases as Manifested in the Skin, *Med. Clin. North America* 35:433, 1951.

MacKelvie, A. A., and *W. W. Park,* Letterer-Siwe Disease, *Arch. Dis. Childhood* 25:93, 1950.

Orchard, N. P., Letterer-Siwe's Syndrome: Report of a Case with Unusual Peripheral Blood Changes, *Arch. Dis. Childhood* 25:151, 1950.

Uzman, L. L., The Lipoprotein of Gaucher's Disease, *A.M.A. Arch. Path.* 51:329, 1951.

van Creveld, S., The Lipoidoses, *Advances Pediat.* 6:190, 1953.

Videbaek, A., Niemann-Pick's Disease: Acute and Chronic Type, *Acta paediat.* 37:95, 1949.

SARCOIDOSIS

Bruschi, M., and *J. S. Howe,* Classification of the Hematologic Variations and Abnormalities Associated with Boeck's Sarcoid: Review of the Literature, *Blood* 5:478, 1950.

Curtis, A. C., and *R. H. Grekin,* Sarcoidosis III: A Review, *M. Clin. North America* 33:31, 1949.

McCort, J. J., R. H. Wood, J. B. Hamilton, and *D. E. Ehrlich,* Sarcoidosis: A

Clinical and Roentgenologic Study of Twenty-eight Proved Cases, *Arch. Int. Med.* 80:293, 1947.

Naumann, O., Kasuistischer Beitrag zur Kenntnis der Schaumauschen "benignen Granulomatose" (Morbus Besnier-Boeck-Schaumann), *Ztschr. Kinderh.* 60:1, 1938.

Posner, I., Sarcoidosis: Case Report, *J. Pediat.* 20:486, 1942.

CHAPTER 80

Poisonings

A survey of fatal accidents from poisoning in young children, conducted by Dr. Katherine Bain of the Children's Bureau, revealed that over 400 deaths from this cause are recorded annually in the United States in children under 5 years of age. Salicylates, especially aspirin, barbiturates, and other drugs kept in homes accounted for about one-third of the deaths. Among the other toxic agents were petroleum products (kerosene, lighter fluid, carbon tetrachloride, etc.) lead, lye, arsenic, bleaching agents, antifreeze solutions, naphthalene moth balls, furniture polish, insecticides, and noxious foodstuffs such as toadstools and wild berries.

The possibility of accidental poisoning must always be considered whenever a child exhibits symptoms which are otherwise unexplainable. Overt signs which may give a clue are usually lacking, though one should look at the mucous membranes for the cyanosis secondary to methemoglobinemia and smell the breath for the odor of garlic which attends phosphorus ingestion or of oil of bitter almond in poisoning with cyanides or nitrobenzene.

Interrogation of the family and neighbors will often bring out statements regarding contact with or ingestion of known poisonous substances.

For laboratory identification of a possible poison, the effort should be made to obtain for analysis specimens of the urine, of the stomach contents by collecting vomitus or by gastric lavage, and of blood for abnormal hemoglobins and toxic substances.

Roentgen studies of the bones will show abnormal densities at the growing ends when there has been chronic absorption of lead, bismuth, or phosphorus.

Convulsions may be a manifestation of hypoxia, hypocalcemia, or central nervous stimulation (e.g., camphor, strychnine). Hypocalcemic convulsions or tetany may be due to poisoning by fluorides, oxalates or organic insecticides, and may be controllable with calcium therapy.

Suppression of urine formation can be a manifestation of generalized collapse or of a more specific necrotoxic action by mercury, bismuth, or

974

carbon tetrachloride. Severe acidosis can result from phenol derivatives, formaldehyde, methanol, or salicylates.

When the exact composition of a suspected toxic mixture is not known, a direct inquiry to the manufacturer or processor, if necessary by telephone, will usually secure the information regarding the ingredients.

The following pages deal only with those poisons which can be identified quickly by a clinical laboratory not specializing in toxicologic analyses and not discussed in preceding chapters (for salicylates see p. 644).

ANILINE AND DERIVATIVES

Aniline-containing inks, dyes, and wax crayons have been responsible at times for the production of cyanosis and anoxia. Methemoglobinemia and Heinz bodies within the red cells may be produced. A discussion of the pathogenesis and control of the methemoglobinemia is given on page 112).

BORON

Boron may enter the body from boric acid or borax. Talcum powders which contain about 5 per cent of boric acid appear to be safe. Most of the reported cases of boric acid poisoning caused by toxic absorption have been associated with the repeated application of the full-strength powder to large areas of denuded or inflamed skin of young infants. Studies by Fisher and associates have indicated that blood boric acid levels up to several milligrams per 100 ml do not produce ill effects and that these levels are not exceeded when talcum powders containing 5 per cent boric acid are used daily for several months.

Trace amounts of boric acid being excreted into the urine will produce a color change in paper impregnated with turmeric. A positive color reaction will not indicate whether the child has toxic concentrations of boron in the blood or tissues.

KEROSENE

Toxic manifestations may result from the ingestion of only a few milliliters of kerosene or similar petroleum derivatives. Upper respiratory tract symptoms are the rule, usually with demonstrable roentgenologic signs of lung consolidations. The central nervous and gastrointestinal systems may show clinical signs of irritation. Positive findings in the urine are not unusual, consisting of the presence of protein, reducing substances, or acetone. Leukocytosis occurs frequently.

LEAD

Once lead has been absorbed into the body, whether from gastrointestinal or respiratory tract or skin, it is transported by the blood stream to many parts of the body. Any lead which may be taken up first by the soft structures does not remain there long but reenters the circulation to be excreted in the feces or urine, or stored in the bones. The circulating and recirculating lead gives rise to untoward symptoms when physiologic circumstances are favorable for this effect.

The concentration of lead in the blood does not always run parallel to clinical manifestations; a patient may exhibit symptoms of lead poisoning when the blood level is low, and vice versa. Readings above 0.06 mg per 100 ml of whole blood in children are usually of significance, provided the analyses are accurately done. In the series of 54 children with lead poisoning reported by Deane, Heldrich, and Bradley the content of lead in whole blood ranged from 0.080 mg to 0.730 mg per 100 ml, and averaged 0.250 mg per 100 ml. Most of the children with lead poisoning in our experience have had blood levels between 0.050 and 0.200 mg per 100 ml.

When lead poisoning is treated with calcium disodium ethylene-diaminetetraacetate (CaEDTA), this compound releases its calcium and replaces it with lead. The lead-containing complex passes freely through the body membranes, enters the plasma, and is excreted by the kidney. In children the lead content of blood may rise significantly during the first few days of the therapy period without producing ill effects.

One frequent manifestation of lead poisoning is an excess of protoporphyrin III in the blood and the urine (p. 354). The source appears to be the erythropoietic cells of the marrow. Normal red cells contain approximately 13 μgm per 100 ml protoporphyrin III. In lead poisoning this intracellular constituent becomes much increased, often to 500 μgm per 100 ml or higher.

Anemia of hypochromic character is present almost invariably when the intoxication is subacute or chronic. There may be stippling and related changes in the blood and bone marrow (p. 82). The cerebrospinal fluid may show abnormalities when the central nervous system is affected (p. 468). The 24-hour urinary lead output may be increased at times. Roentgenograms of the long bones usually show increased density at the ends of the shafts except in very acute or minimal intoxications.

MERCURY

Acute poisoning is most often produced by accidental ingestion of mercuric chloride (corrosive sublimate), though other mercuric salts are sometimes implicated. Metallic mercury itself is not poisonous until converted into some derivative. The mercurous salts such as mercurous chloride (calomel) are insoluble and nontoxic unless changed within the body to mercuric compounds. Once absorbed, the mercuric salts act principally on the liver and kidneys; in the latter organ they destroy the renal tubular epithelium and give rise to anuria followed by uremia. The patient may recover if given proper supportive therapy for the anuria for a week or more.

Of special interest to pediatrics is the growing belief that acrodynia (acrocyanosis) is a reaction to trace amounts of ingested mercury. Infants and young children are affected chiefly. Ammoniated mercury ointment, calomel in "teething powders" or worm cures, mercury bichloride used for rinsing diapers, and mercury amalgam in dental fillings are potential sources of the poisoning. Occasional patients excreting mercury have no detectable source of exposure. The fact that thousands of children are treated with drugs containing mercury and excrete it in their urine whereas only a few acquire acrodynia-like symptoms suggests that individual idiosyncracy plays a major role.

Metabolic studies in infants with acrodynia have shown an excessive loss of electrolytes from the body, mainly through the kidney. Urinary excretion of chloride tends to be abnormally high. Plasma bicarbonate tends to be elevated, plasma chloride low, and plasma sodium normal or low. The blood levels of hemoglobin, hematocrit, leukocytes, and plasma protein usually exceed those for normal children of the same age. These disturbances, the generalized dehydration, and many other symptoms can be explained theoretically as the result of a persistent renal tubular injury induced by mercury. The mercury, when ingested, is believed to be deposited in the bones and then steadily liberated. Some affected infants have been said to improve strikingly when given oral sodium chloride, 6 to 8 gm a day, with or without adrenal cortical salt-retaining hormones.

Overactivity of the sympathetic nervous system as an intermediate mechanism is suggested by the manifestations of hypertension, tachycardia, sweating, and occasional hyperglycemia.

BAL unites with heavy metals in the tissue fluids, including mercury, and thereby prevents their combining with the SH groups of the intracellular enzymes. The BAL-metal combinations then find their way to the urine. BAL has accordingly been advised for therapy of acrodynia. An unusual urinary elimination of mercury in suspected acrodynia following BAL administration can be of assistance in diagnosis.

PHOSPHORUS

Yellow Phosphorus

Toxic symptoms may be produced by as little as 15 mg of this substance. The most common route of childhood poisoning is by ingestion of proprietary rat poisons and roach and vermin mixtures (pastes, powders, or seeds), which contain 1 to 4 per cent of yellow phosphorus. It may also be absorbed by inhalation or through the skin. Matches and fireworks no longer contain this substance. Red phosphorus, the other physical form of elementary phosphorus, is unabsorbable and nontoxic unless contaminated by traces of yellow phosphorus.

Acute phosphorus poisoning is classically divided into three stages. The first stage, which begins promptly after the ingestion of the poison and lasts 6 to 8 hours, is that of severe gastroenteritis, with abdominal pain, nausea, vomiting, and shock. The breath, vomitus, and feces give off a pathognomonic odor of garlic. The second stage is a symptom-free period of 1 to 3 days which sometimes lasts as long as 10 days. The third stage is characterized by systemic toxemia and signs of liver damage. The gastroenteritis returns, the liver enlarges rapidly, icterus develops, and spontaneous hemorrhages appear. Leukopenia with monocytosis may be present. The urine shows characteristic changes—oliguria, hematuria, lipuria, and cast formation, with crystals of leucine, tyrosine, cystine, or peptone-like substances in the sediment. The urine, feces, or vomitus may be luminescent. The electrocardiogram shows changes in the T wave and ST segments in leads 1, 2, and 4.

Laboratory studies show interference with bilirubin excretion; disturbed liver function; abnormal dextrose tolerance curves; and other signs of liver damage. The decreased fibrinogen level, together with toxic changes in the capillaries and possible other blood changes, leads to hemorrhage. The nitrogenous metabolites of the urine rise, and especially the ammonia. The nonprotein nitrogen content of the blood is increased, with amino acid fraction ranging from 10 to 30 mg per 100 ml. The blood cholesterol may be low, with a diminished proportion of cholesterol esters. Death is usually precipitated by shock, liver failure, massive hemorrhage, or nervous system degeneration. The phosphate level of the serum tends to fall to levels around 3 to 2 mg per 100 ml. Several weeks later, in patients who survive, dense transverse lines become evident at the epiphyseal ends of the long bones.

BIBLIOGRAPHY

MISCELLANEOUS POISONINGS

Alway, R. H., "Accidental" Ingestion of Poisons in Childhood, *Postgrad. Med.* 11:239, 1952.

Bain, K., Death Due to Accidental Poisoning in Young Children, *J. Pediat.* 44:616, 1954.

Jacobziner, H., and **H. W. Raybin**, Accidental Poisonings in Childhood and Their Prevention, *J. Pediat.* 49:592, 1956.

McNally, W. D., Kerosene Poisoning in Children: A Study of 204 Cases, *J. Pediat.* 48:296, 1956.

Ryan, D. C., Acute Accidental Poisoning in Children, Its Incidence, Diagnosis and Treatment, *M. J. Australia* 2:702, 1951.

Selwyn, J. G., and *F. A. Dark,* The Identification of Barbiturate Drugs in Gastric Contents and Urine, *J. Clin. Path.* 3:152, 1950.

BORON POISONING

Boggs, T. R., Jr., and *H. G. Anrode,* Boric Acid Poisoning Treated by Exchange Transfusion: Report of a Case, *Pediatrics* 16:109, 1955.

Ducey, J., and *W. D. Brooke,* Transcutaneous Absorption of Boric Acid, *J. Pediat.* 43:644, 1953.

Fisher, R. S., H. C. Freimuth, K. A. O'Connor, and *V. Johns,* Boron Absorption from Borated Talc, *J.A.M.A.* 157:503, 1955.

Goldbloom, R. B., and *A. Goldbloom,* Boric Acid Poisoning: Report of Four Cases and a Review of 109 Cases from the World Literature, *J. Pediat.* 43:631, 1953.

MacGillivray, P. C., and *M. S. Fraser,* Boric Acid Poisoning in Infancy Arising from the Treatment of Napkin Rash, *Arch. Dis. Childhood* 28:484, 1953.

LEAD

Bessman, S. P., and *E. C. Layne, Jr.,* Distribution of Lead in Blood as Affected by Edathamil Calcium-Disodium, *A.M.A. Am. J. Dis. Child.* 89:292, 1955.

————, *M. Rubin,* and *S. Leikin,* The Treatment of Lead Encephalopathy: A Method for the Removal of Lead during the Acute Stage, *Pediatrics* 14:201, 1954.

Bradley, J. E., A. E. Powell, W. Niermann, K. R. McGrady, and *E. Kaplan,* The Incidence of Abnormal Blood Levels of Lead in a Metropolitan Pediatric Clinic, *J. Pediat.* 49:1, 1956.

Burrows, N. F. E., J. Rendle-Short, and *D. Hanna,* Lead-poisoning in Children: Report of Five Cases, with Special Reference to Pica, *Brit. Med. J.* 1:329, 1951.

Cantarow, A., and *M. Trumper,* "Lead Poisoning," The Williams & Wilkins Company, Baltimore, 1944.

Deane, G. E., F. J. Heldrich, Jr., and *J. E. Bradley,* The Use of BAL in the Treatment of Acute Lead Encephalopathy, *J. Pediat.* 42:409, 1953.

Giannattasio, R. C., A. V. Bedo, and *M. J. Pirozzi,* Lead Poisoning, Observations in Fourteen Cases, *A.M.A. Am. J. Dis. Child.* 84:316, 1952.

Karpinski, F. E., Jr., F. Rieders, and *L. S. Girsh,* Calcium Disodium Versenate in the Therapy of Lead Encephalopathy, *J. Pediat.* 42:687, 1953.

McFadzean, A. J. S., and *L. J. Davis,* On the Nature and Significance of Stippling in Lead Poisoning, with Reference to the Effect of Splenectomy, *Quart. J. Med.* 18:57, 1949.

Sidbury, J. B., Jr., Lead Poisoning: Treatment with Disodium Ethylenediamine-tetra-acetate, *Am. J. Med.* 18:932, 1955.

Tanis, A. L., Lead Poisoning in Children Including Nine Cases Treated with Edathamil Calcium-Disodium, *A.M.A. Am. J. Dis. Child.* 89:325, 1955.

Wolman, I. J., Hematology of Lead Poisoning in Childhood, *Am. J. Med. Sc.* 232:688, 1956.

MERCURY AND ACRODYNIA

Drukker, J., Mercury Poisoning as Cause of Acrodynia, *Nederl. tijdschr. geneesk.* 96:884, 1952.

Fanconi, G., and *A. Botsztejn,* Die Feersche Krankheit (Akrodynie) und Queck-silvermedikation, *Helvet. paediat. acta* 3:264, 1948.

Fischer, A. E., and *H. L. Hodes,* Subacute Mercury Poisoning (Acrodynia) Caused by Protiodide of Mercury, *J. Pediat.* 40:143, 1952.

Holzel, A., and *T. James,* Mercury and Pink Disease, *Lancet* 1:441, 1952.

McCoy, G. E., Acrodynia Following the Use of Bichloride of Mercury Diaper Rinse: Report of 2 Cases, *J. Indiana M. A.* 43:1095, 1950.

Warkany, J., and *D. M. Hubbard,* Acrodynia and Mercury, *J. Pediat.* 42:365, 1953.

——— and ———, Adverse Mercurial Reactions in the Form of Acrodynia and Related Conditions, *A.M.A. Am. J. Dis. Child.* 81:335, 1951.

Wilson, V. K., M. L. Thomson, and *A. Holzel,* Mercury Nephrosis in Young Children, with Special Reference to Teething Powders Containing Mercury, *Brit. M. J.* 1:358, 1952.

PHOSPHORUS

Johnston, J. M., Parathion Poisoning in Children, *J. Pediat.* 42:286, 1953.

Rubitsky, H. J., and *R. M. Myerson,* Acute Phosphorus Poisoning, *Arch. Int. Med.* 83:164, 1949.

Index

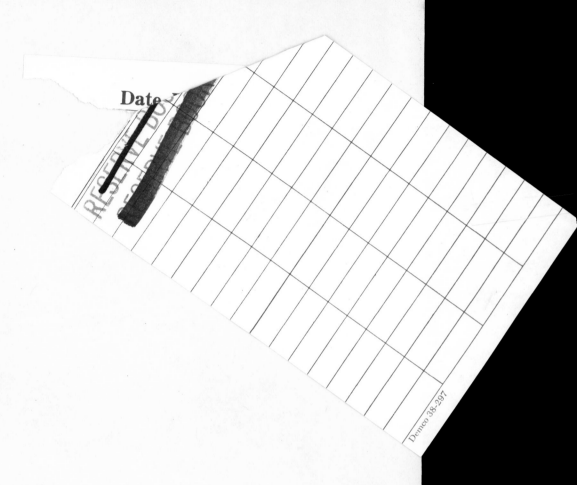